Health Informatics

(formerly Computers in Health Care)

Kathryn J. Hannah   Marion J. Ball
Series Editors

Health Informatics Series
(formerly Computers in Health Care)

Series Editors
Kathryn J. Hannah Marion J. Ball

Dental Informatics
Integrating Technology into the Dental Environment
L.M. Abbey and J. Zimmerman

Ethics and Information Technology
A Case-Based Approach to a Health Care System in Transition
J.G. Anderson and K.W. Goodman

Aspects of the Computer-Based Patient Record
M.J. Ball and M.F. Collen

Performance Improvement Through Information Management
Health Care's Bridge to Success
M.J. Ball and J.V. Douglas

Strategies and Technologies for Healthcare Information
Theory into Practice
M.J. Ball, J.V. Douglas, and D.E. Garets

Nursing Informatics
Where Caring and Technology Meet, Third Edition
M.J. Ball, K.J. Hannah, S.K. Newbold, and J.V. Douglas

Healthcare Information Management Systems
A Practical Guide, Second Edition
M.J. Ball, D.W. Simborg, J.W. Albright, and J.V. Douglas

Healthcare Information Management Systems
Cases, Strategies, and Solutions, Third Edition
M.J. Ball, C.A. Weaver, and J.M. Kiel

Clinical Decision Support Systems
Theory and Practice
E.S. Berner

Strategy and Architecture of Health Care Information Systems
M.K. Bourke

Information Networks for Community Health
P.F. Brennan, S.J. Schneider, and E. Tornquist

Informatics for the Clinical Laboratory
A Practical Guide
D.F. Cowan

(Continued after index)

Edward H. Shortliffe

Editor

James J. Cimino

Associate Editor

Biomedical Informatics

Computer Applications in Health Care and Biomedicine

Third Edition

With 229 Illustrations,
Including 4 Color Plates

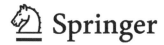 Springer

Edward H. Shortliffe, MD, PhD, MACP
Department of Biomedical Informatics
Columbia University Medical Center
New York, NY 10032-3720
USA

James J. Cimino, MD, FACP
Department of Biomedical Informatics
Columbia University Medical Center
New York, NY 10032-3720
USA

Series Editors:
Kathryn J. Hannah, PhD, RN
Adjunct Professor
Department of Community Health Science
Faculty of Medicine
The University of Calgary
Calgary, Alberta T2N 4N1
Canada

Marion J. Ball, EdD
Fellow, IBM Center for Healthcare
   Management
Business Consulting Services
Baltimore, MD 21205
and
Professor
Johns Hopkins University
School of Nursing
Baltimore, MD 21205

Library of Congress Control Number: 2006921549

ISBN 978-0-387-28986-1   e-ISBN 978-0-387-36278-6   Printed on acid-free paper.

Printed in the United States of America

9 8 7 6 (Corrected at 6th printing 2010)

springer.com

Dedicated to Donald A. B. Lindberg, whose innovative research and visionary leadership of the National Library of Medicine have transformed both the field of biomedical informatics and the institution to which he has dedicated much of his professional life.

Series Preface

This series is directed to healthcare professionals who are leading the transformation of health care by using information and knowledge. Launched in 1988 as Computers in Health Care, the series offers a broad range of titles: some addressed to specific professions such as nursing, medicine, and health administration; others to special areas of practice such as trauma and radiology. Still other books in the series focus on interdisciplinary issues, such as the computer-based patient record, electronic health records, and networked healthcare systems.

Renamed Health Informatics in 1998 to reflect the rapid evolution in the discipline, the series will continue to add titles that contribute to the evolution of the field. In the series, eminent experts, serving as editors or authors, offer their accounts of innovations in health informatics. Increasingly, these accounts go beyond hardware and software to address the role of information in influencing the transformation of healthcare delivery systems around the world. The series also will increasingly focus on "peopleware" and organizational, behavioral, and societal changes that accompany the diffusion of information technology in health services environments.

These changes will shape health services in the new millennium. By making full and creative use of the technology to tame data and to transform information, health informatics will foster the development of the knowledge age in health care. As coeditors, we pledge to support our professional colleagues and the series readers as they share advances in the emerging and exciting field of health informatics.

Kathryn J. Hannah
Marion J. Ball

Preface to the Third Edition

Just as banks cannot practice modern banking without financial software, and airlines cannot manage modern travel planning without shared databanks of flight schedules and reservations, it has become impossible to practice modern medicine, or to conduct modern biological research, without information technologies. Life scientists are generating data at a rate that defies traditional paper-and-pencil methods for information management and data analysis. Health professionals also recognize that a large percentage of their activities relates to information management—for example, obtaining and recording information about patients, consulting colleagues, reading the scientific literature, planning diagnostic procedures, devising strategies for patient care, interpreting results of laboratory and radiologic studies, or conducting case-based and population-based research. It is complexity and uncertainty, plus society's overriding concern for patient well-being, and the resulting need for optimal decision making, that set medicine apart from many other information-intensive fields. Our desire to provide the best possible health and health care for our society gives a special significance to the effective organization and management of the huge bodies of data with which health professionals and biomedical researchers must deal. It also suggests the need for specialized approaches and for skilled scientists who are knowledgeable about biology, clinical medicine, and information technologies.

Information Management in Biomedicine

Although the application of computers to biomedicine is recent, the clinical and research influence of biomedical-computing systems is already remarkably broad. Clinical information systems, which provide communication and information-management functions, are now installed in essentially all healthcare institutions. Physicians can search entire drug indexes in a few seconds, using the information provided by a computer program to anticipate harmful side effects or drug interactions. Electrocardiograms (ECGs) are typically analyzed initially by computer programs, and similar techniques are being applied for interpretation of pulmonary-function tests and a variety of laboratory and radiologic abnormalities. Devices with embedded microprocessors routinely monitor patients and provide warnings in critical-care settings, such as the intensive-care unit (ICU) or the operating room. Both biomedical researchers and clinicians regularly use computer programs to search the medical literature, and modern clinical research would be severely hampered without computer-based data-storage techniques and statistical analysis systems. Advanced decision-support tools also are emerging from research laboratories, are being integrated with patient-care systems, and are beginning to have a profound effect on the way medicine is practiced.

Despite this growing use of computers in healthcare settings and biomedical research, and a resulting expansion of interest in learning more about biomedical computing, many life scientists, health-science students, and professionals have found it difficult to obtain a comprehensive and rigorous, but nontechnical, overview of the field. Both practitioners and basic scientists are recognizing that thorough preparation for their professional futures requires that they gain an understanding of the state of the art in biomedical computing, of the current and future capabilities *and* limitations of the technology, and of the way in which such developments fit within the scientific, social, and financial context of biomedicine. In turn, the future of the biomedical computing field will be largely determined by how well health professionals and biomedical scientists are prepared to guide the discipline's development. This book is intended to meet this growing need for well-equipped professionals. The first edition appeared in 1990 (published by Addison-Wesley) and was used extensively in courses on medical informatics throughout the world. It was updated with a second edition (published by Springer) in 2000, responding to the remarkable changes that occurred during the 1990s, most notably the introduction of the World Wide Web and its impact on adoption and acceptance of the Internet. Like the first two editions, this new version provides a conceptual framework for learning about computer applications in medical care and biology, for critiquing existing systems, and for anticipating future directions that the field may take. In many respects, this new edition is very different from its predecessors, however. Most important, it reflects the remarkable changes in computing and communications that continue to occur, most notably in communications, networking, and health information technology policy and the exploding interest in the role that information technology must play in systems integration and the melding of genomics with innovations in clinical practice and treatment. In fact, the name of the book has been changed from *Medical Informatics* to *Biomedical Informatics,* reflecting (as is discussed in Chapter 1) both the increasing breadth of the basic discipline and the evolving new name for academic units, societies, research programs, and publications in the field. In addition, new chapters have been introduced, while others have been revamped. We have introduced new chapters on cognitive science, natural language processing, imaging informatics, consumer health informatics, and public health informatics. The previous chapters on bioinformatics and imaging systems have also undergone major revisions. All other chapters have been significantly rewritten and updated as well. Those readers who are familiar with the first two editions will find that the organization and philosophy are unchanged, but the content is either new or extensively updated.*

This book differs from other introductions to the field in its broad coverage and in its emphasis on the field's conceptual underpinnings. Our book presumes no health- or computer-science background, but it does assume that readers are interested in a comprehensive summary of the field that stresses the underlying concepts, and it introduces technical details only to the extent that they are necessary to meet the principal goal. It thus differs from an impressive early text in the field (Ledley, 1965) that emphasized

---

* As with the first two editions, this book has tended to draw both its examples and its contributors from North America. There is excellent work in other parts of the world as well, although variations in healthcare systems, and especially financing, do tend to change the way in which systems evolve from one country to the next. The basic concepts are identical, however, so the book is intended to be useful in educational programs worldwide.

technical details but did not dwell on the broader social and clinical context in which biomedical computing systems are developed and implemented.

Overview and Guide to Use of This Book

This book is written as a text so that it can be used in formal courses, but we have adopted a broad view of the population for whom it is intended. Thus, it may be used not only by students of medicine and of the other health professions, but also as an introductory text by future biomedical computing professionals, as well as for self-study and for reference by practitioners. The book is probably too detailed for use in a 2- or 3-day continuing-education course, although it could be introduced as a reference for further independent study.

Our principal goal in writing this text is to teach *concepts* in biomedical informatics—the study of biomedical information and its use in decision making—and to illustrate them in the context of descriptions of representative systems that are in use today or that taught us lessons in the past. As you will see, biomedical informatics is more than the study of computers in biomedicine, and we have organized the book to emphasize that point. Chapter 1 first sets the stage for the rest of the book by providing a glimpse of the future, defining important terms and concepts, describing the content of the field, explaining the connections between biomedical informatics and related disciplines, and discussing the forces that have influenced research in biomedical informatics and its integration into medical practice and biological research.

Broad issues regarding the nature of data, information, and knowledge pervade all areas of application, as do concepts related to optimal decision making. Chapters 2 and 3 focus on these topics but mention computers only in passing. They serve as the foundation for all that follows. A new Chapter 4 on cognitive science issues enhances the discussions in Chapters 2 and 3, pointing out that decision making and behavior are deeply rooted in the ways in which information is processed by the human mind. Key concepts underlying system design, human–computer interaction, educational technology, and decision making are introduced in this chapter.

Chapters 5 and 6 introduce the central notions of computer hardware and software that are important for understanding the applications described later. Also included is a discussion of computer-system design, with explanations of important issues to consider when reading about specific applications and systems throughout the remainder of the book.

Chapter 7 summarizes the issues of standards development, focusing in particular on data exchange and issues related to sharing of clinical data. This important and rapidly evolving topic warrants inclusion given the evolution of the national health information infrastructure and the increasingly central role of standards in enabling clinical systems to have their desired influence on healthcare practices.

Chapter 8 is a new chapter that addresses a topic of increasing practical relevance in both the clinical and biological worlds: natural language understanding and the processing of biomedical texts. The importance of these methods is clear when one considers the amount of information contained in free-text dictated notes or in the published biomedical literature. Even with efforts to encourage structured data entry in clinical systems, there will likely always be an important role for techniques that allow computer systems to extract meaning from natural language documents.

Chapter 9 is another new chapter, this one developed in response to the growing complexity and size of the radiology systems chapters that had appeared in the first two editions. In this volume, we divide the former material into two chapters, one on Imaging and Structural Informatics (Chapter 9 in the *Methods* section of the book) and the other on Imaging Systems in Radiology (Chapter 18). This division has allowed us to separate the conceptual underpinnings, as represented in methods and imaging techniques, from the applications issues, highlighted in the world of radiological imaging and image management (e.g., in picture archiving and communication systems).

Chapter 10 addresses the key legal and ethical issues that have arisen when health information systems are considered. Then, in Chapter 11, the challenges associated with technology assessment and the evaluation of clinical information systems are introduced.

Chapters 12 through 22 survey many of the key biomedical areas in which computers are being used. Each chapter explains the conceptual and organizational issues in building that type of system, reviews the pertinent history, and examines the barriers to successful implementations.

Chapter 23 provides a historical perspective on changes in the way society pays for health care. It discusses alternative methods for evaluating the costs and the benefits of health care, and suggests ways in which financial considerations affect medical computing. The book concludes in Chapter 24 with a look to the future—a vision of how informatics concepts, computers, and advanced communication devices one day may pervade every aspect of biomedical research and clinical practice.

The Study of Computers in Biomedicine

The actual and potential uses of computers in health care and biomedicine form a remarkably broad and complex topic. However, just as you do not need to understand how a telephone or an ATM machine works to make good use of it and to tell when it is functioning poorly, we believe that technical biomedical-computing skills are not needed by health workers and life scientists who simply wish to become effective computer users. On the other hand, such technical skills are of course necessary for individuals with a career commitment to developing computer systems for biomedical environments. Thus, this book will neither teach you to be a programmer, nor show you how to fix a broken computer (although it might motivate you to learn how to do both). It also will not tell you about every important biomedical-computing system or application; we shall use an extensive bibliography to direct you to a wealth of literature where review articles and individual project reports can be found. We describe specific systems only as examples that can provide you with an understanding of the conceptual and organizational issues to be addressed in building systems for such uses. Examples also help to reveal the remaining barriers to successful implementations. Some of the application systems described in the book are well established, even in the commercial marketplace. Others are just beginning to be used broadly in biomedical settings. Several are still largely confined to the research laboratory.

Because we wish to emphasize the concepts underlying this field, we generally limit the discussion of technical implementation details. The computer-science issues can be learned from other courses and other textbooks. One exception, however, is our emphasis on the details of decision science as they relate to biomedical problem solving (Chapters 3 and 20). These topics generally are not presented in computer-science courses, yet they play a central role in the intelligent use of biomedical data and knowledge. Sections on medical decision making and computer-assisted decision support accordingly include more technical detail than you will find in other chapters.

All chapters include an annotated list of Suggested Readings to which you can turn if you have a particular interest in a topic, and there is a comprehensive listing of References at the end of the book. We use **boldface** print to indicate the key terms of each chapter; the definitions of these terms are included in the Glossary at the end of the book. Because many of the issues in biomedical informatics are conceptual, we have included Questions for Discussion at the end of each chapter. You will quickly discover that most of these questions do not have "right" answers. They are intended to illuminate key issues in the field and to motivate you to examine additional readings and new areas of research.

It is inherently limiting to learn about computer applications solely by reading about them. We accordingly encourage you to complement your studies by seeing real systems in use—ideally by using them yourself. Your understanding of system limitations and of what you would do to improve a biomedical-computing system will be greatly enhanced if you have had personal experience with representative applications. Be aggressive in seeking opportunities to observe and use working systems.

In a field that is changing as rapidly as computer science is, it is difficult ever to feel that you have knowledge that is completely current. However, the conceptual basis for study changes much more slowly than do the detailed technological issues. Thus, the lessons you learn from this volume will provide you with a foundation on which you can continue to build in the years ahead.

The Need for a Course in Biomedical-Computing Applications

A suggestion that new courses are needed in the curricula for students of the health professions is generally not met with enthusiasm. If anything, educators and students have been clamoring for *reduced* lecture time, for more emphasis on small group sessions, and for more free time for problem solving and reflection. A 1984 national survey by the Association of American Medical Colleges found that both medical students and their educators severely criticized the traditional emphasis on lectures and memorization. Yet the analysis of a panel on the General Professional Education of the Physician (GPEP) (Association of American Medical Colleges, 1984) and several subsequent studies and reports have specifically identified biomedical informatics, including computer applications, as an area in which new educational opportunities need to be developed so that physicians and other health professionals will be better prepared for clinical practice. The AAMC has recommended the formation of new academic units in biomedical informatics in our medical schools, and subsequent studies and reports have continued to stress the importance of the field and the need for its inclusion in the educational environments of health processionals.

The reason for this strong recommendation is clear: *The practice of medicine is inextricably entwined with the management of information.* In the past, practitioners handled medical information through resources such as the nearest hospital or medical-school library; personal collections of books, journals, and reprints; files of patient records; consultation with colleagues; manual office bookkeeping; and (all-too-often flawed) memorization. Although all these techniques continue to be valuable, the computer is offering new methods for finding, filing, and sorting information: online bibliographic-retrieval systems, including full-text publication; personal computers or PDAs, with database software to maintain personal information and reprint files; office-practice and clinical information systems to capture, communicate, and preserve key elements of the medical record; consultation systems to provide assistance when colleagues are inaccessible or unavailable; practice-management systems to integrate billing and receivable functions with other aspects of office or clinic organization; and other online information resources that help to reduce the pressure to memorize in a field that defies total mastery of all but its narrowest aspects. With such a pervasive and inevitable role for computers in clinical practice, and with a growing failure of traditional techniques to deal with the rapidly increasing information-management needs of practitioners, it has become obvious to many people that a new and essential topic has emerged for study in schools that train medical and other health professionals.

What is less clear is how the subject should be taught, and to what extent it should be left for postgraduate education. We believe that topics in biomedical computing are best taught and learned in the context of health-science training, which allows concepts from both the health sciences and computer science to be integrated. Biomedical-computing novices are likely to have only limited opportunities for intensive study of the material once their health-professional training has been completed.

The format of biomedical-informatics education is certain to evolve as faculty members are hired to develop it at more health-science schools, and as the emphasis on lectures as the primary teaching method diminishes. Computers will be used increasingly as teaching tools and as devices for communication, problem solving, and data sharing among students and faculty. In the meantime, biomedical informatics will be taught largely in the classroom setting. This book is designed to be used in that kind of traditional course, although the Questions for Discussion also could be used to focus conversation in small seminars and working groups. As resources improve in schools, integration of biomedical-computing topics into clinical experiences also will become more common. The eventual goal should be to provide instruction in biomedical informatics whenever this field is most relevant to the topic the student is studying. This aim requires educational opportunities throughout the years of formal training, supplemented by continuing-education programs after graduation.

The goal of integrating biomedicine and computer science is to provide a mechanism for increasing the sophistication of health professionals, so that they know and understand the available resources. They also should be familiar with biomedical computing's successes and failures and its research frontiers and its limitations, so that they can avoid repeating the mistakes of the past. Study of biomedical computing also should improve their skills in information management and problem solving. With a suitable integration of hands-on computer experience, computer-based learning, courses in clinical problem solving, and study of the material in this volume, health-science students will be well prepared to make effective use of computer-based tools and information management in healthcare delivery.

The Need for Specialists in Biomedical Informatics

As mentioned, this book also is intended to be used as an introductory text in programs of study for people who intend to make their professional careers in biomedical informatics. If we have persuaded you that a course in biomedical informatics is needed, then the requirement for trained faculty to teach the courses will be obvious. Some people might argue, however, that a course on this subject could be taught by a computer scientist who had an interest in biomedical computing or by a physician or biologist who had taken a few computing courses. Indeed, in the past, most teaching—and research—has been undertaken by faculty trained primarily in one of the fields and later drawn to the other. Today, however, schools are beginning to realize the need for professionals trained specifically at the interfaces among biomedicine, computer science, and related disciplines such as statistics, cognitive science, health economics, and medical ethics. This book outlines a first course for students training for careers in the biomedical informatics field. We specifically address the need for an educational experience in which computing and information-science concepts are synthesized with biomedical issues regarding research, training, and clinical practice. It is the *integration* of the related disciplines that traditionally has been lacking in the educational opportunities available to students with career interests in biomedical informatics. If schools are to establish such courses and training programs (and there are growing numbers of examples of each), they clearly need educators who have a broad familiarity with the field and who can develop curricula for students of the health professions as well as of engineering and computer science.

The increasing introduction of computing techniques into biomedical environments will require that well-trained individuals be available not only to teach students, but also to design, develop, select, and manage the biomedical-computing systems of tomorrow. There is a wide range of context-dependent computing issues that people can appreciate only by working on problems defined by the healthcare setting and its constraints. The field's development has been hampered because there are relatively few trained personnel to design research programs, to carry out the experimental and developmental activities, and to provide academic leadership in biomedical computing. A frequently cited problem is the difficulty a health professional (or a biologist) and a technically trained computer scientist experience when they try to communicate with one another. The vocabularies of the two fields are complex and have little overlap, and there is a process of acculturation to biomedicine that is difficult for computer scientists to appreciate through distant observation. Thus, interdisciplinary research and development projects are more likely to be successful when they are led by people who can effectively bridge the biomedical and computing fields. Such professionals often can facilitate sensitive communication among program personnel whose backgrounds and training differ substantially.

It is exciting to be working in a field that is maturing and having a beneficial effect on society. There is ample opportunity remaining for innovation as new technologies evolve and fundamental computing problems succumb to the creativity and hard work of our colleagues. In light of the increasing sophistication and specialization required in computer science in general, it is hardly surprising that a new discipline should arise at that field's interface with biomedicine. This book is dedicated to clarifying the definition and to nurturing the effectiveness of that discipline: biomedical informatics.

Edward H. Shortliffe
New York, N.Y.

James J. Cimino
New York, N.Y.
February 2006

Acknowledgments

In the 1980s, when Larry Fagan, Gio Wiederhold, and I decided to compile the first comprehensive textbook on what was then called medical informatics, none of us predicted the enormity of the task we were about to undertake. Our challenge was to create a multi-authored textbook that captured the collective expertise of leaders in the field yet was cohesive in content and style. The concept for the book first developed in 1982. We had begun to teach a course on computer applications in health care at Stanford University School of Medicine and had quickly determined that there was no comprehensive introductory text on the subject. Despite several collections of research descriptions and subject reviews, none had been developed with the needs of a rigorous introductory course in mind.

The thought of writing a textbook was daunting due to the diversity of topics. None of us felt he was sufficiently expert in the full range of important subjects for us to write the book ourselves. Yet we wanted to avoid putting together a collection of disconnected chapters containing assorted subject reviews. Thus, we decided to solicit contributions from leaders in the respective fields to be represented but to provide organizational guidelines in advance for each chapter. We also urged contributors to avoid writing subject reviews but, instead, to focus on the key conceptual topics in their field and to pick a handful of examples to illustrate their didactic points.

As the draft chapters began to come in, we realized that major editing would be required if we were to achieve our goals of cohesiveness and a uniform orientation across all the chapters. We were thus delighted when, in 1987, Leslie Perreault, a graduate of our training program, assumed responsibility for reworking the individual chapters to make an integral whole and for bringing the project to completion. The final product, published in 1990, was the result of many compromises, heavy editing, detailed rewriting, and numerous iterations. We were gratified by the positive response to the book when it finally appeared, and especially that of students of biomedical informatics who have often come to us at scientific meetings and told us about their appreciation of the book.

As the 1990s progressed, however, we began to realize that, despite our emphasis on basic concepts in the field (rather than a survey of existing systems), the volume was beginning to show its age. A great deal had changed since the initial chapters were written, and it became clear that a new edition would be required. The original editors discussed the project and decided that we should redesign the book, solicit updated chapters, and publish a new edition. Leslie Perreault by this time was a busy Director at First Consulting Group in New York City and would not have as much time to devote to the project as she had when we did the first edition. With trepidation, in light of our knowledge of the work that would be involved, we embarked on the new project.

As before, the chapter authors did a marvelous job, trying their best to meet our deadlines, putting up with editing changes that were designed to bring a uniform style to the book, and contributing excellent chapters that nicely reflected the changes in the field in the preceding decade.

No sooner had the second edition appeared in print than we started to get inquiries about when the next update would appear. We began to realize that the maintenance of a textbook in a field such as biomedical informatics was nearly a constant, ongoing process. By this time I had moved to Columbia University and the initial group of editors had largely disbanded to take on other responsibilities, with Leslie Perreault no longer in New York City. Accordingly, as plans for a third edition began to take shape, my Columbia colleague Jim Cimino joined me as the new associate editor, whereas Drs. Fagan, Wiederhold, and Perreault continued to be involved as chapter authors. Once again the authors did their best to try to meet our deadlines as the third edition took shape. This time we added several chapters, attempting to cover additional key topics that readers and authors had identified as being necessary enhancements to the earlier editions. We are once again extremely appreciative of all the authors' commitment and for the excellence of their work on behalf of the book and the field.

The completed third edition reflects the work and support of many people in addition to the editors and chapter authors. Particular gratitude is owed to Andi Cimino, our developmental editor whose rigorous attention to detail was crucial given the size and the complexity of the undertaking. At Springer we have been delighted to work on this edition with the responsible editors, first with Laura Gillan and, subsequently, with Michelle Schmitt-deBonis. Katharine Cacace has also played a key coordinating role at our interface with Springer and the production processes for the volume.

The unsung hero of the effort has been my assistant, Eloise Wender, who has shouldered the burden for creating the Name Index and for updating the Glossary in the third edition. These are arduous tasks that needed to be undertaken with great care, and I am grateful to Eloise for the attention to detail that she provided in helping with these important elements of the final product.

Edward H. Shortliffe
New York, N.Y.
February 2006

Contents

UNIT I RECURRENT THEMES IN BIOMEDICAL INFORMATICS

UNIT II BIOMEDICAL INFORMATICS APPLICATIONS

UNIT III BIOMEDICAL INFORMATICS IN THE YEARS AHEAD

Contributors

Russ B. Altman, MD, PhD, FACP, FACMI
Professor, Department of Genetics, Stanford University, Stanford, CA 94305, USA

Suzanne Bakken, RN, DNSc, FACMI, FAAN
Alumni Professor, School of Nursing; Professor, Department of Biomedical Informatics, Columbia University, New York, NY 10032, USA

Octo Barnett, MD, FACP, FACMI
Senior Scientific Director, Laboratory of Computer Science, Massachusetts General Hospital; Professor of Medicine, Harvard Medical School, Boston, MA 02114, USA

Patricia Flatley Brennan, RN, PhD, FAAN, FACMI
Moehlman Bascom Professor, School of Nursing and College of Engineering, University of Wisconsin, Madison, WI 53792, USA

James F. Brinkley, MD, PhD, FACMI
Research Professor, Structural Informatics Group, Departments of Biological Structure, Medical Education and Biomedical Informatics, and Computer Science and Engineering, University of Washington, Seattle, WA 98195, USA

James J. Cimino, MD, FACMI, FACP
Professor, Departments of Biomedical Informatics and Medicine, Columbia University, New York, NY, 10032 USA

William M. Detmer, MD, MSc
President, Unbound Medicine, Inc.; Clinical Assistant Professor, Department of Health Evaluation Sciences, University of Virginia School of Medicine, Charlottesville, VA 22908, USA

Parvati Dev, PhD, FACMI
Director, SUMMIT Research Laboratory; Senior Scientist, School of Medicine, Stanford University, Stanford, CA 94305, USA

Alain C. Enthoven, BA, MPhil, PhD
Professor Emeritus, Graduate School of Business, Stanford University, Stanford, CA 94305, USA

Lawrence M. Fagan, MD, PhD, FACMI
Associate Director, Biomedical Informatics Training Program, Stanford University, Stanford, CA 94305, USA

Andrew Friede, MD, MPH, FACMI
Vice President for Health Affairs, Constella Health Sciences, Constella Group, LLC, Atlanta, GA 30329, USA

Carol Friedman, PhD, FACMI
Professor, Department of Biomedical Informatics, Columbia University, New York, NY 10032, USA

Charles P. Friedman, PhD, FACMI
Professor, Center for Biomedical Informatics, University of Pittsburgh, Pittsburgh, PA 15213, USA

Alan M. Garber, MD, PhD, FACP
Staff Physician, Department of Veterans Affairs Palo Alto Health Care System, Palo Alto, CA 94304, USA; Henry J. Kaiser Professor and Director, Center for Primary Care and Outcomes Research/Center for Health Policy, Stanford University, Stanford, CA 94305, USA

Reed M. Gardner, PhD, FACMI
Professor, Department of Medical Informatics, University of Utah, Salt Lake City, UT 84132, USA

Kenneth W. Goodman, PhD
Associate Professor, Departments of Medicine and Philosophy; Director, Bioethics Program, University of Miami, Miami, FL 33136, USA

Robert A. Greenes, MD, PhD, FACMI, FACR, FSCAR
Professor, Department of Radiology, Harvard Medical School; Harvard-MIT Division of Health Sciences and Technology; Distinguished Chair in Biomedical Informatics and Director, Decision Systems Group, Department of Health Policy & Management, Harvard School of Public Health; Decision Systems Group, Brigham and Women's Hospital, Boston, MA 02115, USA

W. Edward Hammond, PhD, FACMI
Professor, Fuqua School of Business, Department of Community and Family Medicine, Department of Biomedical Engineering, Duke University, Durham, NC 27715, USA

William R. Hersh, MD, FACMI, FACP
Professor and Chair, Department of Medical Informatics and Clinical Epidemiology, Oregon Health and Science University, Portland, OR 97239, USA

Edward P. Hoffer, MD, FACP, FACC, FRCP(C), FACMI
Associate Professor of Medicine, Harvard Medical School, Senior Scientist and Assistant Director, Laboratory of Computer Science, Massachusetts General Hospital, Boston, MA 02114, USA

Stephen B. Johnson, PhD, FACMI
Associate Professor, Department of Biomedical Informatics, Columbia University, New York, NY 10032, USA

David R. Kaufman, PhD
Associate Research Scientist, Departments of Biomedical Informatics and Psychiatry, Columbia University, New York, NY 10032, USA

Clement J. McDonald, MD, FACP, FACMI
Director, Regenstrief Institute, Regenstrief Professor of Medical Informatics; Distinguished Professor of Medicine, Indiana University School of Medicine, Indianapolis, IN 46202, USA

Randolph A. Miller, MD, FACP, FACMI
Donald A.B. and Mary M. Lindberg, University Professor, Department of Biomedical Informatics, Vanderbilt University Medical Center, Vanderbilt University, Nashville, TN 37232, USA

Sean D. Mooney, PhD
Assistant Professor of Medical and Molecular Genetics, Indiana University School of Medicine, Indianapolis, IN 46202, USA

Mark A. Musen, MD, PhD, FACMI, FACP
Professor, Stanford Medical Informatics, Department of Medicine, Stanford University, Stanford, CA 94305, USA

Patrick W. O'Carroll, MD, MPH, FACPM, FACMI
Regional Health Administrator, U.S. Public Health Service Region X, U.S. Department of Health and Human Services, Seattle, WA 98121, USA

Douglas K. Owens, MD, MS
Senior Investigator, Department of Veterans Affairs Palo Alto Health Care System, Palo Alto, CA 94304, USA; Professor of Medicine, Center for Primary Care and Outcomes Research, Stanford University, Stanford, CA 94305, USA

Judy Ozbolt, PhD, RN, FAAN, FACMI
Professor and Director, Graduate Program in Nursing Informatics, The University of Maryland School of Nursing, Baltimore, MD 21201, USA

Vimla L. Patel, PhD, DSc, FACMI
Departments of Biomedical Informatics and Psychiatry, Columbia University, New York, NY 10032, USA

Leslie E. Perreault, MS
Consultant, San Diego, CA, USA

Thomas C. Rindfleisch, MS, FACMI
Director Emeritus, Lane Medical Library, School of Medicine, Stanford University, Palo Alto, CA 94305, USA

M. Michael Shabot, MD, FACS, FCCM, FACMI
Director, Surgical Intensive Care and Medical Director, Enterprise Information Services, Cedars-Sinai Medical Center, Los Angeles, CA 90048, USA; Professor, Department of Surgery, David Geffen School of Medicine, University of California, Los Angeles

Yuval Shahar, MD, PhD
Head, Medical Informatics Research Center, Head, Graduate Program Information Systems Engineering, Deputy Dean for Research, Faculty of Engineering, Ben-Gurion University of the Negev, Beer-Sheva 84105, Israel; Consulting Associate Professor, Stanford Medical Informatics, Stanford University, Stanford, CA 94305, USA

Edward H. Shortliffe, MD, PhD, FACMI, MACP
Rolf H. Scholdager Professor and Chair, Department of Biomedical Informatics, Professor of Medicine and Computer Science, Columbia University, New York, NY 10032, USA

Sara J. Singer, MBA
Senior Research Scholar, Center for Health Policy, Stanford University, Stanford, CA 94305, USA; Doctoral Candidate, Department of Health Policy, Harvard University, Boston, MA 02613, USA

Harold C. Sox, MD, MACP
Editor, Annals of Internal Medicine, American College of Physicians, Philadelphia, PA 19106, USA

Justin B. Starren, MD, PhD, FACMI
Associate Professor, Departments of Biomedical Informatics and Radiology, Columbia University, New York, NY 10032, USA

P. Zoë Stavri, MLS, PhD
Consultant, Chambersburg, PA 17201, USA

Paul C. Tang, MD, MS, FACMI, FACP
Vice President and Chief Information Officer, Palo Alto Medical Foundation, Palo Alto, CA 94301, USA; Associate Clinical Professor of Medicine, University of California, San Francisco, CA 94143, USA

Lynn Harold Vogel, PhD
Vice President and Chief Information Officer, University of Texas MD Anderson Cancer Center, Houston, TX 77030, USA; Adjunct Assistant Professor, Department of Biomedical Informatics, Columbia University, New York, NY 10032, USA

Gio Wiederhold, PhD, FACMI, FACM, FIEEE
Professor Emeritus, Departments of Computer Science, Electrical Engineering, and Medicine, Stanford University, Stanford CA 94305

Jeremy C. Wyatt, MBBS, DM, FRCP, FACMI
Professor of Health Informatics, Centre for Health Informatics, University of Dundee, Dundee, Scotland

William A. Yasnoff, MD, PhD, FACMI
Managing Partner, NHII Advisors, Arlington, VA 22201

Unit I
Recurrent Themes in Biomedical Informatics

1
The Computer Meets Medicine and Biology: Emergence of a Discipline

EDWARD H. SHORTLIFFE AND MARSDEN S. BLOIS†

After reading this chapter, you should know the answers to these questions:

- Why is information management a central issue in biomedical research and clinical practice?
- What are integrated information management environments, and how might we expect them to affect the practice of medicine, the promotion of health, and biomedical research in coming years?
- What do we mean by the terms *medical computer science*, *medical computing*, *biomedical informatics*, *clinical informatics*, *nursing informatics*, *bioinformatics*, and *health informatics*?
- Why should health professionals, life scientists, and students of the health professions learn about biomedical informatics concepts and informatics applications?
- How has the development of modern computing technologies and the Internet changed the nature of biomedical computing?
- How is biomedical informatics related to clinical practice, biomedical engineering, molecular biology, decision science, information science, and computer science?
- How does information in clinical medicine and health differ from information in the basic sciences?
- How can changes in computer technology and the way medical care is financed influence the integration of medical computing into clinical practice?

1.1 Integrated Information Management: Technology's Promise[1]

After scientists had developed the first digital computers in the 1940s, society was told that these new machines would soon be serving routinely as memory devices, assisting with calculations and with information retrieval. Within the next decade, physicians and other health workers had begun to hear about the dramatic effects that such technology would have on medical practice. More than five decades of remarkable progress in computing have followed those early predictions, and many of the original prophesies have

---

[1] Portions of this section are adapted from a paper presented at Medinfo98 in Seoul, Korea (Shortliffe, 1998a).
† Deceased

come to pass. Stories regarding the "information revolution" fill our newspapers and popular magazines, and today's children show an uncanny ability to make use of computers as routine tools for study and entertainment. Similarly, clinical workstations are now available on hospital wards and in outpatient offices. Yet many observers cite the health care system as being slow to understand information technology, to exploit it for its unique practical and strategic functionalities, and to incorporate it effectively into the work environment. Nonetheless, the enormous technological advances of the last two decades—personal computers and graphical workstations, new methods for human–computer interactions, innovations in mass storage of data, personal digital assistants, the Internet and the World Wide Web, wireless communications—have all combined to make routine use of computers by all health workers and biomedical scientists inevitable. A new world is already with us, but its greatest influence is yet to come. This book will teach you both about our present resources and accomplishments *and* about what we can expect in the years ahead.

It is remarkable that the first personal computers did not appear until the late 1970s, and the World Wide Web dates only to the early 1990s. This dizzying rate of change, combined with equally pervasive and revolutionary changes in almost all international health care systems during the past decade, makes it difficult for health care planners and institutional managers to try to deal with both issues at once. Yet many observers now believe that the two topics are inextricably related and that planning for the new health care environments of the twenty-first century requires a deep understanding of the role that information technology is likely to play in those environments.

What might that future hold for the typical practicing clinician? As we shall discuss in detail in Chapter 12, no clinical computing topic is gaining more attention currently than is the issue of electronic health records (EHRs). Health care organizations are finding that they do not have systems in place that allow them to answer questions that are crucially important for strategic planning and for their better understanding of how they compare with other provider groups in their local or regional competitive environment. In the past, administrative and financial data were the major elements required for such planning, but comprehensive clinical data are now also important for institutional self-analysis and strategic planning. Furthermore, the inefficiencies and frustrations associated with the use of paper-based medical records have become increasingly clear (Dick and Steen, 1991 [revised 1997]), especially when inadequate access to clinical information is one of the principal barriers that clinicians encounter when trying to increase their efficiency in order to meet productivity goals for their practices.

1.1.1 *Electronic Health Records: Anticipating the Future*

Many health care institutions are seeking to develop integrated clinical workstations. These are single-entry points into a medical world in which computational tools assist not only clinical matters (reporting results of tests, allowing direct entry of orders by clinicians, facilitating access to transcribed reports, and in some cases supporting telemedicine applications or decision-support functions) but also administrative and financial topics (e.g., tracking of patients within the hospital, managing materials and inventory, supporting personnel functions, and managing the payroll), research (e.g., analyzing the outcomes associated with treatments and procedures, performing quality assurance, supporting clinical trials, and implementing various treatment protocols), scholarly information (e.g., accessing digital libraries, supporting bibliographic search, and providing access to drug information databases), and even office automation (e.g., providing access to spreadsheets, word processors). The key idea, however, is that at the heart of the evolving clinical workstation lies the medical record in a new incarnation: electronic, accessible, confidential, secure, acceptable to clinicians and patients, and integrated with other types of nonpatient-specific information.

Inadequacy of the Traditional Paper Record

The paper-based medical record is woefully inadequate for meeting the needs of modern medicine. It arose in the nineteenth century as a highly personalized "lab notebook" that clinicians could use to record their observations and plans so that they could be reminded of pertinent details when they next saw the same patient. There were no bureaucratic requirements, no assumptions that the record would be used to support communication among varied providers of care, and few data or test results to fill up the record's pages. The record that met the needs of clinicians a century ago has struggled mightily to adjust over the decades and to accommodate to new requirements as health care and medicine have changed.

Difficulty in obtaining information, either about a specific patient or about a general issue related to patient management, is a frustrating but common occurrence for practitioners. With increasing pressures to enhance clinical productivity, practitioners have begun to clamor for more reliable systems that provide facile, intuitive access to the information they need at the time they are seeing their patients. The EHR offers the hope for such improved access to patient-specific information and should provide a major benefit both for the quality of care and for the quality of life for clinicians in practice.

Despite the obvious need for a new record-keeping paradigm, most organizations have found it challenging to try to move to a paperless, computer-based clinical record (see Chapters 12 and 13). This observation forces us to ask the following questions: "What is a health record in the modern world? Are the available products and systems well matched with the modern notions of a comprehensive health record?" Companies offer medical record products, yet the packages are limited in their capabilities and seldom seem to meet the full range of needs defined within our complex health care organizations.

The complexity associated with automating medical records is best appreciated if one analyzes the *processes* associated with the creation and use of such records rather than thinking of the record as an object that can be moved around as needed within the institution. For example, on the input side (Figure 1.1), the medical record requires the integration of processes for data capture and for merging information from diverse sources. The contents of the paper record have traditionally been organized chronologically—often a severe limitation when a clinician seeks to find a specific piece of information that could occur almost anywhere within the chart. To be useful,

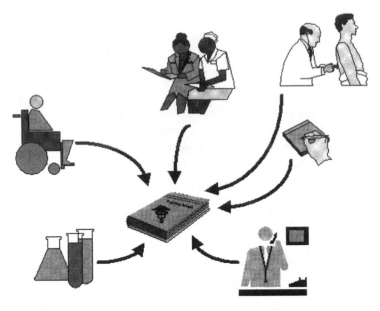

Figure 1.1. Inputs to the medical record. The traditional paper medical record is created by a variety of organizational processes that capture varying types of information (notes regarding direct encounters between health professionals and patients, laboratory or radiologic results, reports of telephone calls or prescriptions, and data obtained directly from patients). The record thus becomes a merged collection of such data, generally organized in chronological order.

the record system must make it easy to access and display needed data, to analyze them, and to share them among colleagues and with secondary users of the record who are not involved in direct patient care (Figure 1.2). Thus, the computer-based medical record is best viewed not as an object, or a product, but rather as a set of processes that an organization must put into place, supported by technology (Figure 1.3). Implementing electronic records is inherently a systems-integration task; it is not possible to buy a medical record system for a complex organization as an off-the-shelf product. Joint development is crucial.

The Medical Record and Clinical Trials

The arguments for automating medical records are summarized in Chapters 2 and 12 and in the Institute of Medicine's report on computer-based patient records (CPRs; Dick and Steen, 1991 [revised 1997]). One argument that warrants emphasis is the importance of the electronic record in supporting **clinical trials**—experiments in which data from specific patient interactions are pooled and analyzed in order to learn about the safety and efficacy of new treatments or tests and to gain insight into disease processes that are not otherwise well understood. Medical researchers are constrained today by clumsy methods for acquiring the data needed for clinical trials, generally relying on manual capture of information onto datasheets that are later transcribed into

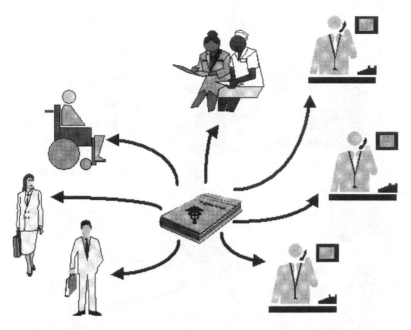

Figure 1.2. Outputs from the medical record. Once information is collected in the traditional paper medical record, it may be provided to a wide variety of potential users of the chart. These users include health professionals and the patients themselves but also a wide variety of "secondary users" (represented here by the individuals in business suits) who have valid reasons for accessing the record but who are not involved with direct patient care. Numerous providers are typically involved in a patient's care, so the chart also serves as a means for communicating among them. The mechanisms for displaying, analyzing, and sharing information from such records results from a set of processes that often vary substantially across several patient care settings and institutions.

computer databases for statistical analysis (Figure 1.4). The approach is labor-intensive, fraught with opportunities for error, and adds to the high costs associated with randomized prospective research protocols.

The use of EHRs offers many advantages to those carrying out clinical research. Most obviously, it helps to eliminate the manual task of extracting data from charts or filling out specialized datasheets. The data needed for a study can be derived directly from the EHR, thus making research data collection a by-product of routine clinical record keeping (Figure 1.5). Other advantages accrue as well. For example, the record environment can help to ensure compliance with a research protocol, pointing out to a clinician when a patient is eligible for a study or when the protocol for a study calls for a specific management plan given the currently available data about that patient. We are also seeing the development of novel authoring environments for clinical trial protocols that can help to ensure that the data elements needed for the trial are compatible with the local EHR's conventions for representing patient descriptors.

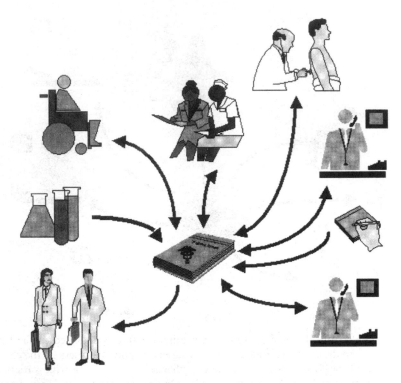

Figure 1.3. Complex processes demanded of the record. As shown in Figures 1.1 and 1.2, the medical record is the incarnation of a complex set of organizational processes, which both gather information to be shared and then distribute that information to those who have valid reasons for accessing it. Paper-based documents are severely limited in meeting the diverse requirements for data collection and information access that are implied by this diagram.

1.1.2   Recurring Issues that Must Be Addressed

There are at least four major issues that have consistently constrained our efforts to build effective patient record systems: (1) the need for standards in the area of clinical terminology; (2) concerns regarding data privacy, confidentiality, and security; (3) challenges of data entry by physicians; and (4) difficulties associated with the integration of record systems with other information resources in the health care setting. The first of these issues is discussed in detail in Chapter 7, and privacy is one of the central topics in Chapter 10. Issues of direct data entry by clinicians are discussed in Chapters 2 and 12 and throughout many other chapters as well. In Section 1.1.3 we examine recent trends in networking and ask how communications are changing the way in which the patient care record can be better integrated with other relevant information resources and clinical processes, which are currently fragmented and poorly coordinated.

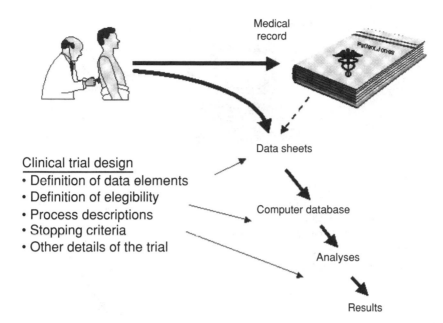

Figure 1.4. Conventional data collection for clinical trials. Although modern clinical trials routinely use computer systems for data storage and analysis, the gathering of research data is often a manual task. Physicians who care for patients enrolled in trials are often asked to fill out special datasheets for later transcription into computer databases. Alternatively, data managers are hired to abstract the relevant data from the traditional paper chart. The trials are generally designed to define data elements that are required and the methods for analysis, but it is common for the process of collecting those data in a structured format to be left to manual processes at the point of patient care.

1.1.3   Integrating the Patient Record with Other Information Resources

Experience has shown that physicians are "horizontal" users of information technology (Greenes and Shortliffe, 1990). Rather than becoming "power users" of a narrowly defined software package, they tend to seek broad functionality across a wide variety of systems and resources. Thus, routine use of computers, and of EHRs, will be most easily achieved if the computing environment offers a critical mass of functionality that makes the system both smoothly integrated and useful for essentially every patient encounter.

With the introduction of networked systems within our health care organizations, there are new opportunities to integrate a wide variety of resources through single clinical workstations (see Chapter 10). The nature of the integration tasks is illustrated in Figure 1.6, in which various workstations are shown at the upper left (machines for use by patients, clinicians, or clerical staff) connected to an enterprise-wide network or **intranet**. In such an environment, diverse clinical, financial, and administrative databases all need to be accessed and integrated, typically by using networks to tie them

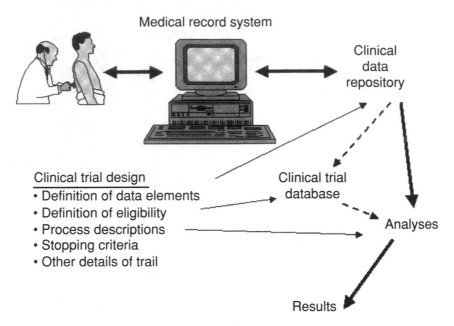

Figure 1.5. Role of electronic health records (EHRs) in supporting clinical trials. With the introduction of computer-based patient record (CPR) systems, the collection of research data for clinical trials can become a by-product of the routine care of the patients. Research data may be analyzed directly from the clinical data repository, or a secondary research database may be created by downloading information from the online patient records. The manual processes in Figure 1.4 are thereby eliminated. In addition, the interaction of the physician with the medical record permits two-way communication, which can greatly improve the quality and efficiency of the clinical trial. Physicians can be reminded when their patients are eligible for an experimental protocol, and the computer system can also remind the clinicians of the rules that are defined by the research protocol, thereby increasing compliance with the experimental plan.

together and a variety of standards for sharing data among them. Thus the clinical data repository has developed as an increasingly common idea. This term refers to a central computer that gathers and integrates clinical data from diverse sources such as the chemistry and microbiology laboratories, the pharmacy, and the radiology department. As is suggested in the diagram, this clinical database can provide the nidus for what will evolve into an EHR as more and more clinical data become available in electronic form and the need for the paper documents shrinks and eventually vanishes.

Another theme in the changing world of health care is the increasing investment in the creation of **clinical guidelines** and **pathways** (see Chapter 20), generally in an effort to reduce practice variability and to develop consensus approaches to recurring management problems. Several government and professional organizations, as well as individual provider groups, have invested heavily in guideline development, often putting an emphasis on using clear evidence from the literature, rather than expert opinion alone,

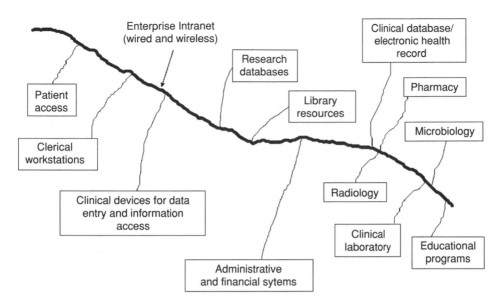

Figure 1.6. Networking the organization. We already live in an era when large hospitals and health care systems have implemented widespread networking technologies that allow diverse systems and users to communicate with one another within their organization. The *enterprise intranet* is a locally controlled network that extends throughout a health care system. It allows specialized workstations to access a wide variety of information sources: educational, clinical, financial, and administrative. An electronic health record (EHR) emerges from such an architecture if a system is implemented that gathers patient-specific data from multiple sources and merges them for ease of access by users such as those illustrated in Figure 1.2. Such systems are often called clinical data repositories, particularly if they do not yet contain the full range of information that would normally occur in a medical record. The enterprise intranet faces challenges of connectivity and integration that are a microcosm of what the larger community experiences in trying to link EHRs and other clinical systems from different organizations.

as the basis for the advice. Despite the success in creating such **evidence-based guidelines**, there is a growing recognition that we need better methods for delivering the decision logic to the point of care. Guidelines that appear in monographs or journal articles tend to sit on shelves, unavailable when the knowledge they contain would be most valuable to practitioners. Computer-based tools for implementing such guidelines, and integrating them with the EHR, present a potential means for making high-quality advice available in the routine clinical setting. Many organizations are accordingly attempting to integrate decision-support tools with their nascent electronic record systems.

Rethinking Common Assumptions

One of the first instincts of software developers is to create an electronic version of an object or process from the physical world. Some familiar notion provides the inspiration for a new software product. Once the software version has been developed, however, human ingenuity and creativity often lead to an evolution that extends the software version far beyond what was initially contemplated. The computer can thus facilitate paradigm shifts in how we think about such familiar concepts.

Consider, for example, the remarkable difference between today's word processors and the typewriter, which was the original inspiration for their development. Although the early word processors were designed largely to allow users to avoid retyping papers each time a minor change was made to a document, the word processors of today bear little resemblance to a typewriter. Consider all the powerful desktop-publishing facilities, integration of figures, spelling correction, grammar aids, etc. Similarly, today's spreadsheet programs bear little resemblance to the tables of numbers that we once created on graph paper. Also consider automatic teller machines (ATMs) and their facilitation of today's worldwide banking in ways that were never contemplated when the industry depended on human bank tellers.

It is accordingly logical to ask what the health record will become after it has been effectively implemented on computer systems and new opportunities for its enhancement become increasingly clear to us. It is unlikely that the computer-based health record a decade from now will bear much resemblance to the antiquated paper folder that still dominates many of our health care environments. One way to anticipate the changes that are likely to occur is to consider the potential role of wide-area networking and the Internet in the record's evolution.

Extending the Record Beyond the Single Institution

In considering ongoing trends in information technology that are likely to make changes inevitable, it would be difficult to start with any topic other than the Internet. The Internet began in 1968 as a U.S. research activity funded by the Advanced Research Projects Agency (ARPA) of the Department of Defense. Initially known as the ARPAnet, the network began as a novel mechanism for allowing a handful of defense-related mainframe computers, located mostly at academic institutions or in the defense industry, to share data files with each other and to provide remote access to computing power at other locations. The notion of electronic mail arose soon thereafter, and machine-to-machine electronic mail exchanges quickly became a major component of the network's traffic. As the technology matured, its value for nonmilitary research activities was recognized, and by 1973 the first medically related research computer had been added to the network (Shortliffe, 1998b, 2000).

During the 1980s, the technology began to be developed in other parts of the world, and the National Science Foundation took over the task of running the principal high-speed **backbone network** in the United States. The first hospitals, mostly academic centers, began to be connected to what had by then become known as the Internet, and in a major policy move it was decided to allow commercial organizations to join the network as well. By April 1995, the Internet in the United States had become a fully commercialized operation, no longer depending on the U.S. government to support even the major backbone connections. Many people point to the Internet as a superb example of the facilitating role of federal investment in promoting innovative technologies. The

Internet is a major societal force that arguably would never have been created if the research and development, plus the coordinating activities, had been left to the private sector.

The explosive growth of the Internet did not occur until the late 1990s, when the World Wide Web (which had been conceived initially by the physics community as a way of using the Internet to share preprints with photographs and diagrams among researchers) was introduced and popularized. The Web is highly intuitive, requires no special training, and provides a mechanism for access to multimedia information that accounts for its remarkable growth as a worldwide phenomenon.

The societal impact of this communications phenomenon cannot be overstated, especially given the international connectivity that has grown phenomenally in the past 15 years. Countries that once were isolated from information that was important to citizens, ranging from consumers to scientists to those interested in political issues, are now finding new options for bringing timely information to the desktop machines of individuals with an Internet connection.

There has accordingly been a major upheaval in the telecommunications industry, with companies that used to be in different businesses now finding that their activities and technologies have merged. In the United States, legislation was passed in 1996 to allow new competition to develop and new industries to emerge. There is ample evidence of the merging of technologies such as cable television, telephone, networking, and satellite communications. High-speed lines into homes and offices are widely available, wireless networking is ubiquitous, and inexpensive mechanisms for connecting to the Internet without using a computer (e.g., using cell phones) have also emerged. The impact on all individuals is likely to be great and hence on our patients and on their access to information and to their health care providers. Medicine cannot afford to ignore these rapidly occurring changes.

1.1.4   *A Model of Integrated Disease Surveillance*[2]

To emphasize the role that the nation's networking infrastructure could play in integrating clinical data and enhancing care delivery, let us envision one model of how disease surveillance, prevention, and care could be influenced by information and communications technology a decade or so from now. Imagine the day when *all* providers, regardless of practice setting (hospitals, emergency rooms, small offices, community clinics, military bases, multispecialty groups, etc.) use EHRs in their medical practices both to assist in patient care and to provide patients with counsel on illness prevention. The full impact of this use of electronic resources will occur when data from all such records are pooled in regional and national surveillance databases (Figure 1.7), mediated through connectivity with the Internet. The challenge, of course, is to find a way to integrate data from such diverse practice settings, especially since it is inevitable that multiple vendors and system developers will be active in the marketplace, competing to provide value-added capabilities that will excite and attract the practitioners for whom their EHR product is intended.

---

[2] This section is adapted from a discussion that originally appeared in (Shortliffe and Sondik, 2004).

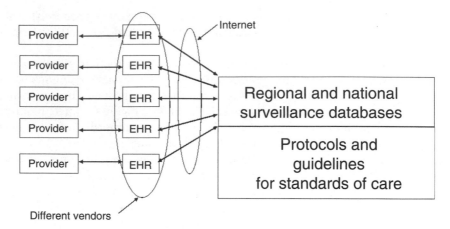

Figure 1.7. A future vision of surveillance databases, in which clinical data are pooled in regional and national repositories through a process of data submission that occurs over the Internet (with attention to privacy and security concerns as discussed in the text). When information is effectively gathered, pooled, and analyzed, there are significant opportunities for feeding back the results of derived insights to practitioners at the point of care.

The practical need to pool and integrate clinical data from such diverse resources and systems emphasizes the practical issues that must be addressed if this vision is to be achieved. Interestingly, most of the potential barriers are logistical, political, and financial rather than technical in nature:

- *Encryption of data*: Concerns regarding privacy and data protection require that Internet transmission of clinical information occur only if those data are **encrypted**, with an established mechanism for identifying and authenticating individuals before they are allowed to decrypt the information for surveillance or research use.
- *HIPAA-compliant policies*: The privacy and security rules that resulted from the 1996 Health Insurance Portability and Accountability Act (HIPAA) do not prohibit the pooling and use of such data (see Chapter 10), but they do lay down policy rules and technical security practices that must be part of the solution in achieving the vision proposed.
- *Standards for data transmission and sharing*: Sharing data over networks requires that all developers of EHRs and clinical databases adopt a single set of standards for communicating and sharing information. The de facto standard for such sharing, **Health Level 7 (HL7),** is widely used but still not uniformly adopted, implemented, or utilized (see Chapter 7).
- *Standards for data definitions*: A uniform "envelope" for digital communication, such as HL7, does not assure that the *contents* of such messages will be understood or standardized. The pooling and integration of data requires the adoption of standards for clinical terminology and for the schemas used to store clinical information in databases (see Chapter 7).

- *Quality control and error checking*: Any system for accumulating, analyzing, and utilizing clinical data from diverse sources must be complemented by a rigorous approach to quality control and error checking. It is crucial that users have faith in the accuracy and comprehensiveness of the data that are collected in such repositories, because policies, guidelines, and a variety of metrics can be derived over time from such information.
- *Regional and national surveillance databases*: Any adoption of the model in Figure 1.7 will require mechanisms for creating, funding, and maintaining the regional and national databases that are involved. The role of state and Federal governments will need to be clarified, and the political issues addressed (including the concerns of some members of the populace that any government role in managing or analyzing their health data may have societal repercussions that threaten individual liberties, employability, etc.).

With the establishment of surveillance databases, and a robust system of Internet integration with EHRs, summary information can flow back to providers to enhance their decision making at the point of care (Figure 1.7). This assumes standards that allow such information to be integrated into the vendor-supplied products that the clinicians use in their practice settings. These may be EHRs or, increasingly, **order-entry systems** that clinicians use to specify the actions that they want to have taken for the treatment or management of their patients. Furthermore, as is shown in Figure 1.7, the databases can help to support the creation of evidence-based guidelines, or clinical research protocols, which can be delivered to practitioners through the feedback process. Thus one should envision a day when clinicians, at the point of care, will receive integrated, non-dogmatic, supportive information regarding:

- Recommended steps for health promotion and disease prevention
- Detection of syndromes or problems, either in their community or more widely
- Trends and patterns of public health importance
- Clinical guidelines, adapted for execution and integration into patient-specific decision support rather than simply provided as text documents
- Opportunities for distributed (community-based) clinical research, whereby patients are enrolled in clinical trials and protocol guidelines are in turn integrated with the clinicians' EHR to support protocol-compliant management of enrolled patients

Implementing the National Health Information Infrastructure

As was previously mentioned, large provider organizations, including hospitals and distributed health systems, routinely use networking technology as the infrastructure on which they build their computer-based communications channels (Figure 1.6). With departmental computer systems (e.g., radiology, clinical laboratory, microbiology, and pharmacy) connected to the network, institutions generally collect and store data in a central clinical data repository. Over time, as this repository becomes more and more comprehensive, it effectively becomes an EHR. Clinicians access the patient data in such repositories using a variety of methods, ranging from tethered workstations installed in offices or nursing stations to handheld wireless devices such as personal digital assistants (PDAs) or tablet computers. Clerical staff members use the same network to enter and access information, and sometimes patients are invited to enter their histories, to access educational materials, or even to review their personal clinical data over such networks. Data may be submitted to research databases, and the users of the network typically have access to library resources or to administrative or financial systems. The integration of such resources within an organization depends on a robust enterprise intranet (Figure 1.6). The implementation and maintenance of an advanced network is one of the fiscal and organizational challenges faced by complex provider institutions.

In the outpatient setting, both small and large networks are becoming commonplace (Figure 1.8). Within an ambulatory practice, physicians and other personnel may have several computers networked together and sharing data from an EHR system. The full utility of the system depends on gateways from these local networks into the Internet because that is where the patients and business associates (such as pharmacies and clinical laboratories) increasingly access and provide information. Several EHR products provide specialized Web interfaces so that patients can access their physician's practice for purposes ranging from appointment scheduling to review of laboratory results and drug lists.

The future vision of Figure 1.7 requires that the surveillance databases that need to be built will depend on the submission of data over the Internet from clinical databases that reside in large organizations (Figure 1.6) and outpatient practice settings (Figure 1.8). Furthermore, the delivery of information to these settings depends on an infrastructure that supports the integration of decision-support elements with the records

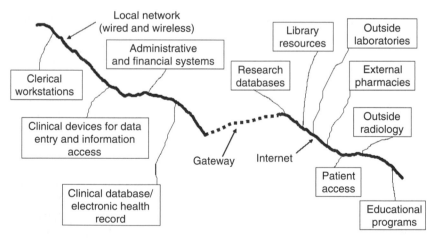

Figure 1.8. Communications networks are increasingly found in outpatient practice settings, including small office practices, but much of their value is enhanced when they are linked through gateways to the Internet and to information resources, organizations, and individuals beyond their own doors.

and order-entry systems used in these same practice environments. *We must tap into these clinical data, as a by-product of routine patient encounters, if we want to create shared research and surveillance databases* (Figure 1.7). If the submission of data for research or surveillance purposes requires an extra step, or special effort by busy clinicians, the process likely will fail, regardless of the good intentions of practitioners. Moreover, this extra step should not be necessary. We can build integrated systems on standards that allow automated data submission and collection via the Internet in a secure, responsible, and confidential manner.

Thus the vision laid out in Figure 1.7 depends on the creation of a **National Health Information Infrastructure (NHII)** (Figure 1.9), which links all practices and practitioners in the country (see Chapter 15 for an extensive discussion), offering them value in terms of access to information, decision support when desired, communication channels with patients and colleagues, and even support for their business operations (e.g., by online submission of invoices to payers that carries the potential for error checking and real-time verification, which will, in turn, greatly shorten the payment cycle for accounts receivable). This idealistic model addresses a large number of the serious problems facing our health care system, ranging from error prevention and reduction in practice variation to reduced administrative costs and enhanced efficiency. The public health system, including disease surveillance, will be only one of the many beneficiaries of such a transition.

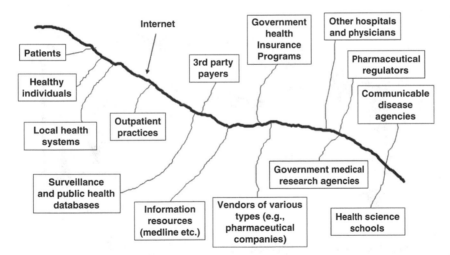

Figure 1.9. Moving beyond the organization. The integrated interconnectivity of all the clinical systems, building on networking technology and standards for data exchange and privacy protection, creates a National Health Information Infrastructure (NHII), which supports clinical care, research, and the public health. The *enterprise Internet* is the integration of an organization's intranet (Figure 1.6, encapsulated in the box here labeled "Local Health System") with the full potential of the worldwide Internet. Both providers and patients increasingly access the Internet for a wide variety of information sources and functions suggested by this diagram (see text).

The Cycle of Information Flow in Clinical Care

The concepts outlined above lead to a composite model of cyclical information flow in the future, as is shown in Figure 1.10. Beginning at the left of the diagram, physicians caring for patients use electronic health records. Information from these records will be forwarded automatically to regional and national registries as well as to research databases (if the patient is enrolled in a community-based clinical trial). The information can be used to develop standards for prevention and treatment, with major guidance from biomedical research. Researchers can draw information either directly from the health records or from the pooled data in registries. The standards for treatment in turn will be translated into protocols, guidelines, and educational materials. This new knowledge and decision-support functionality will be delivered via the NHII back to the clinicians so that the information informs the practice of medicine at the point of care, where it is integrated seamlessly with EHRs and order-entry systems.

Implications for Patients

As the number of Internet users grows, it is not surprising that increasing numbers of patients, as well as healthy individuals, are turning to the Internet for health information (see Figure 1.9). It is a rare North American physician who has not encountered a patient who comes to an appointment armed with a question, or a stack of laser-printed

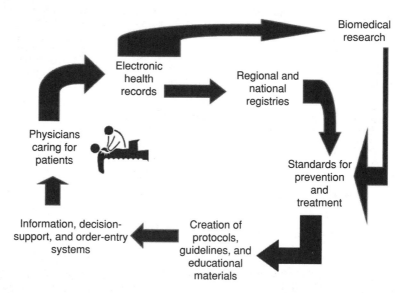

Figure 1.10. The ultimate goal is to create a cycle of information flow, whereby data from distributed electronic health records (EHRs) are automatically submitted to registries and research databases. The resulting new knowledge then can feed back to practitioners at the point of care, using a variety of computer-supported decision support delivery mechanisms.

pages, that arose due to medically related searches on the Web. The companies that provide search engines for the Internet report that medically related sites are among the most popular ones being explored by consumers. As a result, physicians and other care providers must be prepared to deal with information that patients discover on the Web and bring with them when they seek care from clinicians. Some of the information is timely and excellent; in this sense physicians can often learn about innovations from their patients and will need to be increasingly open to the kinds of questions that this enhanced access to information will generate from patients in their practices. On the other hand, much of the health information on the Web lacks peer review or is purely anecdotal. People who lack medical training can be misled by such information, just as they have been in the past by printed information in books and magazines dealing with fad treatments from anecdotal sources. In addition, some sites provide personalized advice, often for a fee, with all the attendant concerns about the quality of the suggestions and the ability to give valid advice based on an electronic mail or Web-based interaction.

In a more positive light, the new communications technologies offer clinicians creative ways to interact with their patients and to provide higher quality care. Years ago medicine adopted the telephone as a standard vehicle for facilitating patient care, and we now take this kind of interaction with patients for granted. If we extend the audio channel to include our visual sense as well, the notion of **telemedicine** emerges (see Chapter 14). Although there are major challenges, which are largely regulatory and fiscal, to be overcome before telemedicine is likely to be widely adopted for direct patient care (Grigsby and Sanders, 1998), there are specialized settings in which it is already proving to be successful and cost-effective (e.g., international medicine, teleradiology, and video-based care of patients in state and federal prisons).

A potentially more practical concept in the short term is to use computers and the Internet as the basis for communication between patients and providers. For example, there has been rapid growth in the use of electronic mail as a mechanism for avoiding "telephone tag" and allowing simple questions to be answered asynchronously (the telephone requires synchronous communication; electronic mail does not). More exploratory, but extremely promising, are communications methods based on the technology of the Web. For example, there are young companies that work with managed care organizations and health care systems to provide Web-based facilities for disease management. Patients log in to a private Web site, provide information about the status of their chronic disease (e.g., blood glucose readings in diabetes), and later obtain feedback from their physician or from disease managers who seek to keep the patients healthy at home, thereby decreasing the need for emergency room or clinic visits.

1.1.4 Requirements for Achieving the Vision

Many of the concepts proposed above depend on the emergence of an Internet with much higher **bandwidth** and **reliability**, decreased **latency**, and financial models that make the applications cost-effective and practical. Major research efforts are underway to address some of these concerns, including the federal **Large-Scale Networking** activity in the United States.[3] In addition, academic institutions have banded together in a consortium designed to create new test beds for high-bandwidth communications in support of research and education. Their initial effort has built on existing federally funded or experimental networks and is known as **Internet 2**.[4] Exploratory efforts that continue to push the state of the art in Internet technology all have significant implications for the future of health care delivery in general and of the computer-based health record in particular (Shortliffe, 1998c).

Education and Training There is a difference between computer literacy (familiarity with computers and their routine uses in our society) and knowledge of the role that computing and communications technology can and should play in our health care system. We are generally doing a poor job of training future clinicians in the latter area and are thereby leaving them poorly equipped for the challenges and opportunities they will face in the rapidly changing practice environments that surround them (Shortliffe, 1995a).

Furthermore, much of the future vision we have proposed here can be achieved only if educational institutions produce a cadre of talented individuals who not only comprehend computing and communications technology but also have a deep understanding of the biomedical milieu and of the needs of practitioners and other health workers. Computer science training alone is not adequate. Fortunately, we have begun to see the creation of formal training programs in biomedical informatics that provide custom-tailored educational opportunities. Many of the trainees are life science researchers, physicians, nurses, pharmacists, and other health professionals who see the career opportunities and challenges at the intersections of biomedicine, information science, computer science, and communications technologies. The demand for such individuals far outstrips the supply, however, both for academic and industrial career pathways (Greenes and Shortliffe, 1990). We need more training programs, expansion of those that already exist, plus support for junior faculty in health science schools who may wish to seek additional training in this area.[5]

Organizational and Management Change Finally, as implied above, there needs to be a greater understanding among health care leaders regarding the role of process reengineering in successful software implementation. Health care provides some of the most complex organizational structures in society, and it is simplistic to assume that off-the-shelf products will be smoothly introduced into a new institution without major analysis, redesign, and cooperative joint-development efforts. Underinvestment and a failure to understand the requirements for process reengineering as part of software implementation, as well as problems with technical leadership and planning, account for many of the frustrating experiences that health care organizations report in their efforts to use computers more effectively in support of patient care and provider productivity.

---

[3] Large-Scale Networking initiative is the successor to the **Next Generation Internet** program, which was active in the 1990s. See http://www.itrd.gov/subcommittee/lsn.html

[4] See www.internet2.org

[5] A directory of some existing training programs is available on the Web at http://www.amia.org/resource/acad&training/f1.html

The vision of the future described here is meant to provide a glimpse of what lies ahead and to suggest the topics that need to be addressed in a book such as this one. Essentially all of the following chapters touch on some aspect of the vision of integrated systems, which extend beyond single institutions. Before embarking on these topics, however, let us emphasize two points. First, the vision presented earlier in this section will become reality only if individual hospitals, academic medical centers, and national coordinating bodies provide the standards, infrastructure, and resources that are necessary. No individual system developer, vendor, or administrator can mandate the standards for connectivity and data sharing implied by an integrated environment such as the one illustrated in Figure 1.9. A national initiative of cooperative planning and implementation for computing and communications resources within single institutions and clinics is required before practitioners will have routine access to information. A uniform environment is required if transitions between resources are to be facile and uncomplicated.

Second, although our vision focused on the clinician's view of integrated information access, other workers in the field have similar needs that can be addressed in similar ways. The academic research community has already made use of much of the technology that needs to be coalesced if the clinical user is to have similar access to data and information.

With this discussion as background, let us now consider the discipline that has led to the development of many of the facilities that need to be brought together in the integrated medical-computing environment of the future. The remainder of this chapter deals with medical computing as a field and with medical information as a subject of study. It provides additional background needed to understand many of the subsequent chapters in this book.

1.2   The Use of Computers in Biomedicine

Biomedical applications of computers is a phrase that evokes different images depending on the nature of one's involvement in the field. To a hospital administrator, it might suggest the maintenance of medical records using computers; to a decision scientist, it might mean the assistance of computers in disease diagnosis; to a basic scientist, it might mean the use of computers for maintaining and retrieving gene-sequencing information. Many physicians immediately think of office-practice tools for tasks such as patient billing or appointment scheduling. The field includes study of all these activities and of a great many others too. More important, it includes the consideration of various external factors that affect the biomedical setting. Unless you keep in mind these surrounding factors, it may be difficult to understand how biomedical computing can help us to tie together the diverse aspects of health care and its delivery.

To achieve a unified perspective, we might consider three related topics: (1) the applications of computers in biomedicine; (2) the concept of medical information (why it is important in medical practice and why we might want to use computers to process it); and (3) the structural features of medicine, including all those subtopics to which computers might be applied. The first of these is the subject of this book. We mention the second and third topics briefly in this and the next chapter, and we provide references in the Suggested Readings section for those students who wish to learn more.

The modern computer is still a relatively young device. Because the computer as a machine is exciting, people may pay a disproportionate amount of attention to it as such—at the expense of considering what the computer can do given the numbers, concepts, ideas, and cognitive underpinnings of a field such as medicine. In recent years, computer scientists, philosophers, psychologists, and other scholars have *collectively* begun to consider such matters as the nature of information and knowledge and how human beings process such concepts. These investigations have been given a sense of timeliness (if not urgency) by the simple existence of the computer. The cognitive activities of clinician begins in practice probably have received more attention over the past two decades than in all previous history (see Chapter 4). Again, the existence of the computer and the possibilities of its extending a clinician's cognitive powers have motivated most of these studies. To develop computer-based tools to assist with decisions, we must understand more clearly such human processes as diagnosis, therapy planning, decision making, and problem solving in medicine.

1.2.1 *Terminology*

Since the 1960s, by which time almost anyone doing serious biomedical computation had access to some kind of computer system, people have been uncertain what name they should use for the biomedical application of computer science concepts. The name *computer science* was itself new in 1960 and was only vaguely defined. Even today, *computer science* is used more as a matter of convention than as an explanation of the field's scientific content.

We use the phrase **medical computer science** to refer to the subdivision of computer science that applies the methods of the larger field to medical topics. As you will see, however, medicine has provided a rich area for computer science research, and several basic computing insights and methodologies have been derived from applied medical-computing research.

The term **information science**, which is occasionally used in conjunction with *computer science*, originated in the field of library science and is used to refer, somewhat generally, to the broad range of issues related to the management of both paper-based and electronically stored information. Much of what information science originally set out to be is now drawing renewed interest under the name **cognitive science**.

Information theory, in contrast, was first developed by scientists concerned about the physics of communication; it has evolved into what may be viewed as a new branch of mathematics. The results scientists have obtained with information theory have illuminated many processes in communications technology, but they have had little effect on our understanding of *human* information processing.

The terms **biomedical computing** or **biocomputation** have been used for a number of years. They are nondescriptive and neutral, implying only that computers are employed for some purpose in biology or medicine. They are often associated with bioengineering applications of computers, however, in which the devices are viewed more as tools for a bioengineering application than as the primary focus of research.

A term originally introduced in Europe is **medical informatics**, which is broader than **medical computing** (it includes such topics as medical statistics, record keeping, and the study of the nature of medical information itself) and deemphasizes the computer while focusing instead on the nature of the field to which computations are applied. Because the term *informatics* became widely accepted in the United States only during the 1990s, **medical information science** had often been used instead in this country; this term, however, may be confused with library science, and it does not capture the broader implications of the European term. As a result, the name *medical informatics* appeared by 2000 to have become the preferred term, even in the United States, although some people dislike the use of what they consider to be an awkward neologism. Indeed, this is the name of the field that we used in the first two editions of this textbook, and it is still heavily used in professional and academic settings. However, especially since the rise of **bioinformatics**, many observers have expressed concern that the adjective "medical" is too focused on physicians and fails to appreciate the relevance of this discipline to other health and life science professionals, although most people in the field do not intend that the word "medical" be viewed as being specifically physician-oriented or even illness-oriented. Thus, the term *health informatics*, or *health care informatics*, has gained some popularity, even though it has the disadvantage of tending to exclude applications to biology (Chapter 22) and, as we will argue shortly, it tends to focus the field's name on an application domain (public health and prevention) rather than the basic discipline and its broad range of applicability.

In the late 1990s, the director of the National Institutes of Health (NIH), Harold Varmus, appointed an advisory group called the Working Group on Biomedical Computing. In June 1999, the group provided a report[6] recommending that the NIH undertake an initiative called the **Biomedical Information Science and Technology Initiative (BISTI)**. With the subsequent creation of another NIH organization called the Bioinformatics Working Group, the visibility of informatics applications in biology was greatly enhanced. Today bioinformatics is a major area of activity at the NIH[7] and in many universities and biotechnology companies around the world. The explosive growth of this field, however, has added to the confusion regarding the naming conventions we have been discussing. In addition, the relationship between *medical informatics* and *bioinformatics* became unclear. As a result, in an effort to be more inclusive and to embrace the biological applications with which many medical informatics groups had already been involved, the name *medical informatics* has gradually given way to **biomedical informatics**. Several academic groups have already changed their names, and a major medical informatics journal (*Computers and Biomedical Research*) was reborn as *The Journal of Biomedical Informatics*.

Despite these concerns, we believe that the broad range of issues in biomedical information management does require an appropriate name and, beginning with this edition, we use the term *biomedical informatics* for this purpose throughout this book. It is becoming the most widely accepted term and should be viewed as encompassing broadly all areas of application in health, clinical practice, and biomedical research. When we speak specifically about computers and their use within biomedical informatics

---

[6] Available at http://www.nih.gov/about/director/060399.html
[7] See http://www.bisti.nih.gov/

activities, we use the terms biomedical computer science (for the methodologic issues) or biomedical computing (to describe the activity itself). Note, however, that biomedical informatics has many other component sciences in addition to computer science. These include the decision sciences, statistics, cognitive science, information science, and even management sciences. We return to this point shortly when we discuss the basic versus applied nature of the field when it is viewed as a basic research discipline.

Although labels such as these are arbitrary, they are by no means insignificant. In the case of new fields of endeavor or branches of science, they are important both in designating the field and in defining or restricting its contents. The most distinctive feature of the modern computer is the generality of its application. The nearly unlimited range of computer uses complicates the business of naming the field. As a result, the nature of computer science is perhaps better illustrated by examples than by attempts at formal definition. Much of this book presents examples that do just this.

Definition: In summary, *we define biomedical informatics as the scientific field that deals with biomedical information, data, and knowledge—their storage, retrieval, and optimal use for problem solving and decision making*. It accordingly touches on all basic and applied fields in biomedical science and is closely tied to modern information technologies, notably in the areas of computing and communication (biomedical computer science). The emergence of biomedical informatics as a new discipline is due in large part to rapid advances in computing and communications technology, to an increasing awareness that the knowledge base of biomedicine is essentially unmanageable by traditional paper-based methods, and to a growing conviction that the process of informed decision making is as important to modern biomedicine as is the collection of facts on which clinical decisions or research plans are made.

1.2.2   Historical Perspective

The modern digital computer grew out of developments in the United States and abroad during World War II, and general-purpose computers began to appear in the marketplace by the mid-1950s (Figure 1.11). Speculation about what might be done with such machines (if they should ever become reliable) had, however, begun much earlier. Scholars at least as far back as the Middle Ages often had raised the question of whether human reasoning might be explained in terms of formal or algorithmic processes.[8] Gottfried Wilhelm von Leibnitz, a seventeenth-century German philosopher and mathematician, tried to develop a calculus that could be used to simulate human reasoning. The notion of a "logic engine" was subsequently worked out by Charles Babbage in the mid nineteenth century.

The first practical application of automatic computing relevant to medicine was Herman Hollerith's development of a punched-card data-processing system for the 1890 U.S. census (Figure 1.12). His methods were soon adapted to **epidemiologic** and public health surveys, initiating the era of electromechanical punched-card data-processing technology, which matured and was widely adopted during the 1920s and

---

[8] An algorithm is a well-defined procedure or sequence of steps for solving a problem.

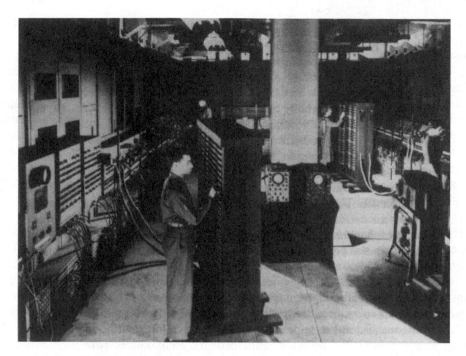

Figure 1.11. The ENIAC. Early computers, such as the ENIAC, were the precursors of today's personal computers (PCs) and handheld calculators. (Photograph courtesy of Unisys Corporation.)

1930s. These techniques were the precursors of the stored program and wholly electronic digital computers, which began to appear in the late 1940s (Collen, 1995).

One early activity in biomedical computing was the attempt to construct systems that would assist a physician in decision making (see Chapter 20). Not all biomedical-

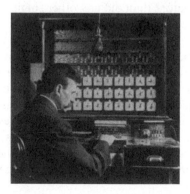

Figure 1.12. Tabulating machines. The Hollerith Tabulating Machine was an early data-processing system that performed automatic computation using punched cards. (Photograph courtesy of the Library of Congress.)

computing programs pursued this course, however. Many of the early ones instead investigated the notion of a total hospital information system (HIS; see Chapter 13). These projects were perhaps less ambitious in that they were more concerned with practical applications in the short term; the difficulties they encountered, however, were still formidable. The earliest work on HISs in the United States was probably that associated with the MEDINET project at General Electric, followed by work at Bolt, Beranek, Newman in Cambridge, Massachusetts, and then at the Massachusetts General Hospital (MGH) in Boston. A number of hospital application programs were developed at MGH by Barnett and his associates over three decades beginning in the early 1960s. Work on similar systems was undertaken by Warner at Latter Day Saints (LDS) Hospital in Salt Lake City, Utah, by Collen at Kaiser Permanente in Oakland, California, by Wiederhold at Stanford University in Stanford, California, and by scientists at Lockheed in Sunnyvale, California.[9]

The course of HIS applications bifurcated in the 1970s. One approach was based on the concept of an integrated or monolithic design in which a single, large, *time-shared computer* would be used to support an entire collection of applications. An alternative was a distributed design that favored the separate implementation of specific applications on smaller individual computers—minicomputers—thereby permitting the independent evolution of systems in the respective application areas. A common assumption was the existence of a single shared database of patient information. The multimachine model was not practical, however, until network technologies permitted rapid and reliable communication among distributed and (sometimes) heterogeneous types of machines. Such distributed HISs began to appear in the 1980s (Simborg et al., 1983).

Biomedical-computing activity broadened in scope and accelerated with the appearance of the *minicomputer* in the early 1970s. These machines made it possible for individual departments or small organizational units to acquire their own dedicated computers and to develop their own application systems (Figure 1.13). In tandem with the introduction of general-purpose software tools that provided standardized facilities to individuals with limited computer training (such as the UNIX operating system and programming environment), the minicomputer put more computing power in the hands of more biomedical investigators than did any other single development until the introduction of the *microprocessor*, a central processing unit (CPU) contained on one or a few chips (Figure 1.14).

Everything changed radically in the late 1970s and early 1980s, when the microprocessor and the *personal computer* (PC) or *microcomputer* became available. Not only could hospital departments afford minicomputers but now individuals also could afford microcomputers. This change enormously broadened the base of computing in our society and gave rise to a new software industry. The first articles on computers in medicine had appeared in clinical journals in the late 1950s, but it was not until the late 1970s that the first advertisements dealing with computers and aimed at physicians began to appear (Figure 1.15). Within a few years, a wide range of computer-based information

---

[9] The latter system was subsequently taken over and further developed by the Technicon Corporation (subsequently TDS Healthcare Systems Corporation). Until recently, the system continued to be part of the suite of products available from Eclipsys, Inc.

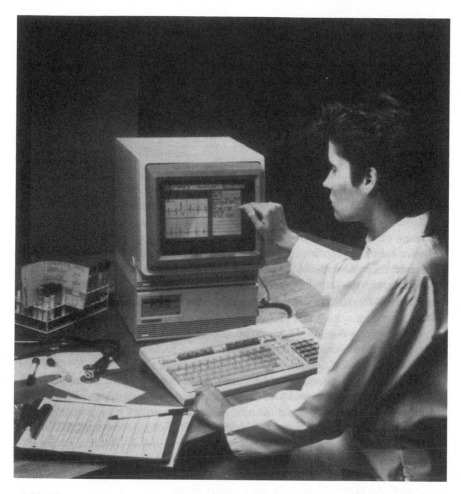

Figure 1.13. Departmental system. Hospital departments, such as the clinical laboratory, were able to implement their own custom-tailored systems when affordable minicomputers became available. Today, these departments often use microcomputers to support administrative and clinical functions. (Photograph courtesy of Hewlett-Packard Company.)

management tools were available as commercial products; their descriptions began to appear in journals alongside the traditional advertisements for drugs and other medical products. Today individual physicians find it practical to employ PCs in a variety of settings, including for applications in patient care or clinical investigation.

The stage is now set with a wide range of hardware of various sizes, types, prices, and capabilities, all of which will continue to evolve in the decades ahead. The trend—reductions in size and cost of computers with simultaneous increases in power (Figure 1.16)—shows no sign of slowing, although scientists are beginning to foresee the ultimate physical limitations to the miniaturization of computer circuits.

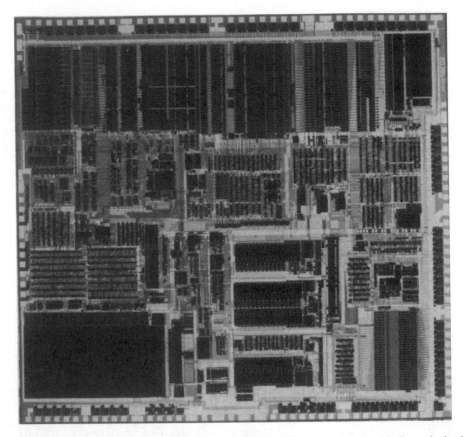

Figure 1.14. Miniature computer. The microprocessor, or "computer on a chip," revolutionized the computer industry in the 1970s. By installing chips in small boxes and connecting them to a computer terminal, engineers produced the personal computer (PC)—an innovation that made it possible for individual users to purchase their own systems.

Progress in biomedical-computing research will continue to be tied to the availability of funding from either government or commercial sources. Because most biomedical-computing research is exploratory and is far from ready for commercial application, the federal government has played a key role in funding the work of the last four decades, mainly through the NIH and the Agency for Health Care Research and Quality (AHRQ). The National Library of Medicine (NLM) has assumed a primary role for biomedical informatics, especially with support for basic research in the field (Figure 1.17). As increasing numbers of applications prove to be cost-effective (see Chapters 6 and 23), it is likely that more development work will shift to industrial settings and that university programs will focus increasingly on fundamental research problems viewed as too speculative for short-term commercialization.

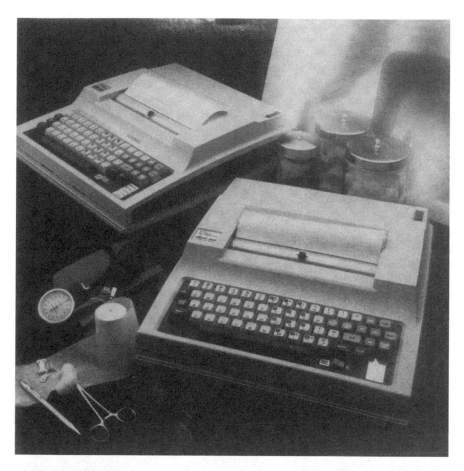

Figure 1.15. Medical advertising. An early advertisement for a portable computer terminal that appeared in general medical journals in the late 1970s. The development of compact, inexpensive peripheral devices and personal computers (PCs) inspired future experiments in marketing directly to clinicians. (Reprinted by permission of copyright holder Texas Instruments Incorporated © 1985.)

1.2.3 Relationship to Biomedical Science and Medical Practice

The exciting accomplishments of biomedical informatics, and the implied potential for future benefits to medicine, must be viewed in the context of our society and of the existing health care system. As early as 1970, an eminent clinician suggested that computers might in time have a revolutionary influence on medical care, on medical education, and even on the selection criteria for health science trainees (Schwartz, 1970). The subsequent enormous growth in computing activity has been met with some trepidation by health professionals. They ask where it will all end. Will health workers gradually be replaced by computers? Will nurses and physicians need to be highly trained in

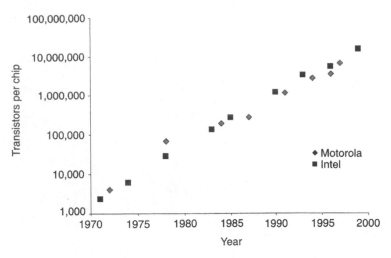

Figure 1.16. Moore's Law. Former Intel chairman Gordon Moore is credited with popularizing the "law" that the size and cost of microprocessor chips will half every 18 months while they double in computing power. This graph shows the exponential growth in the number of transistors that can be integrated on a single microprocessor by two of the major chip manufacturers. (*Source*: San Jose Mercury News, December 1997.)

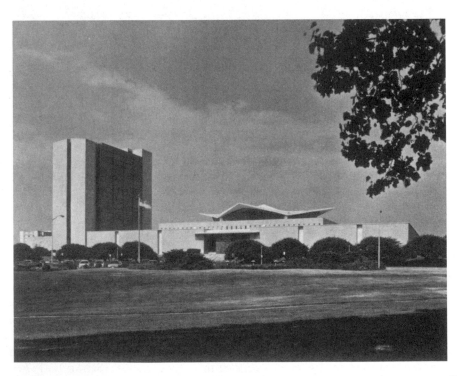

Figure 1.17. The National Library of Medicine (NLM). The NLM, on the campus of the National Institutes of Health (NIH) in Bethesda, Maryland, is the principal biomedical library for the nation (see Chapter 15). It is also a major source of support for research in biomedical informatics. (Photograph courtesy of the National Library of Medicine.)

computer science before they can practice their professions effectively? Will both patients and health workers eventually revolt rather than accept a trend toward automation that they believe may threaten the traditional humanistic values in health care delivery (see Chapter 10) (Shortliffe, 1993)? Will clinicians be viewed as outmoded and backward if they do not turn to computational tools for assistance with information management and decision making (Figure 1.18)?

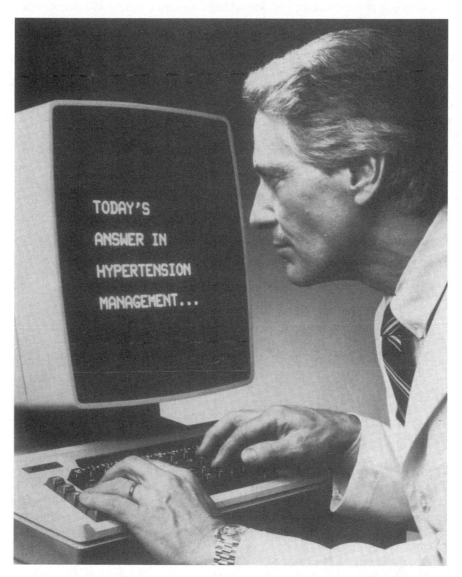

Figure 1.18. Doctor of the future. By the early 1980s, advertisements in medical journals began to use computer equipment as props. The suggestion in this photograph seems to be that an up-to-date physician feels comfortable using computer-based tools in his practice. (Photograph courtesy of ICI Pharma, Division of ICI Americas, Inc.)

Biomedical informatics is intrinsically entwined with the substance of biomedical science. It determines and analyzes the structure of biomedical information and knowledge, whereas biomedical science is constrained by that structure. Biomedical informatics melds the study of biomedical computer science with analyses of biomedical information and knowledge, thereby addressing specifically the interface between computer science and biomedical science. To illustrate what we mean by the "structural" features of medical information and knowledge, we can contrast the properties of the information and knowledge typical of such fields as physics or engineering with the properties of those typical of biomedicine (see Section 1.3).

Biomedical informatics is perhaps best viewed as a basic biomedical science, with a wide variety of potential areas of application (Figure 1.19). The analogy with other **basic sciences** is that biomedical informatics uses the results of past experience to understand, structure, and encode objective and subjective biomedical findings and thus to make them suitable for processing. This approach supports the integration of the findings and their analyses. In turn, the selective distribution of newly created knowledge can aid patient care, health planning, and basic biomedical research.

Biomedical computing is, by its nature, an experimental science. An **experimental science** is characterized by posing questions, designing experiments, performing analyses, and using the information gained to design new experiments. One goal is simply to search for new knowledge, called **basic research**. A second goal is to use this knowledge

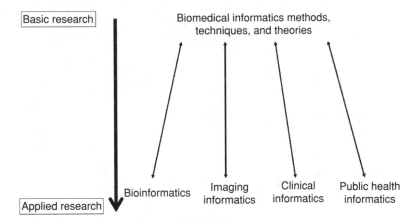

Figure 1.19. Biomedical informatics as basic science. We view the term biomedical informatics as referring to the basic science discipline in which the development and evaluation of new methods and theories are a primary focus of activity. These core concepts and methods in turn have broad applicability in the health and biomedical sciences. The informatics subfields indicated by the names across the bottom of this figure are accordingly best viewed as application domains for a common set of concepts and techniques from the field of biomedical informatics. Note that work in biomedical informatics is motivated totally by the application domains that the field is intended to serve (thus the two-headed arrows in the diagram). Therefore the basic research activities in the field generally result from the identification of a problem in the real world of health or biomedicine for which an informatics solution is sought (see text).

for practical ends, called **applications research**. There is a continuity between these two endeavors (see Figure 1.19). In biomedical informatics, there is an especially tight coupling between the application areas, broad categories of which are indicated at the bottom of Figure 1.19, and the identification of basic research tasks that characterize the scientific underpinnings of the field. Research, however, has shown that there can be a very long period of time between the development of new concepts and methods in basic research and their eventual application in the biomedical world (Balas and Boren, 2000). Furthermore (see Figure 1.20), many discoveries are discarded along the way, leaving only a small percentage of basic research discoveries that have a practical influence on the health and care of patients.

Work in biomedical informatics is inherently motivated by problems encountered in a set of applied domains in biomedicine. The first of these historically has been clinical care (including medicine, nursing, dentistry, and veterinary care), an area of activity that demands patient-oriented informatics applications. We refer to this area as **clinical informatics.**

Closely tied to clinical informatics is **public health informatics** (Figure 1.19), where similar methods are generalized for application to populations of patients rather than to single individuals (see Chapter 15). Thus clinical informatics and public health

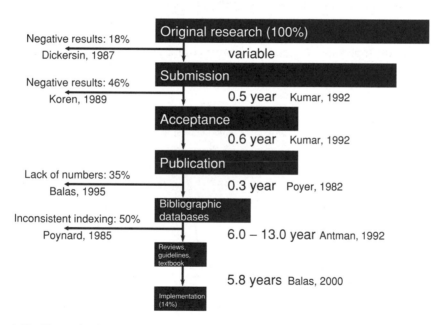

Figure 1.20. Phases in the transfer of research into clinical practice. A synthesis of studies focusing on various phases of this transfer has indicated that it takes an average of 17 years to make innovation part of routine care (Balas and Boren, 2000). Pioneering institutions often apply innovations much sooner, sometimes within a few weeks, but nationwide introduction is usually slow. National utilization rates of specific, well-substantiated procedures also suggests a delay of two decades in reaching the majority of eligible patients. (Courtesy of Dr. Andrew Balas).

informatics share many of the same methods and techniques. Two other large areas of application overlap in some ways with clinical informatics and public health informatics. These include **imaging informatics** (and the set of issues developed around both radiology and other image management and image analysis domains such as pathology, dermatology, and molecular visualization—see Chapters 9 and 18). Finally, there is the burgeoning area of bioinformatics, which at the molecular and cellular levels is offering challenges that draw on many of the same informatics methods as well (see Chapter 22).

As shown in Figure 1.21, there is a spectrum as one moves from left to right across these application domains. In bioinformatics, workers deal with molecular and cellular processes in the application of informatics methods. At the next level, workers focus on tissues and organs, which tend to be the emphasis of imaging informatics work (also called **structural informatics** at some institutions). Progressing to clinical informatics, the focus is on individual patients, and finally to public health, where researchers address problems of populations and of society. Biomedical informatics has important contributions to make across that entire spectrum.

In general, biomedical informatics researchers derive their inspiration from one of the application areas, identifying fundamental methodologic issues that need to be addressed and testing them in system prototypes or, for more mature methods, in actual systems that are used in clinical or biomedical research settings. One important implication of this viewpoint is that the core discipline is identical, regardless of the area of application that a given individual is motivated to address. This argues for unified biomedical informatics educational programs, ones that bring together students with a wide variety of applications interests. Elective courses and internships in areas of specific interest are of course important complements to the core exposures that students

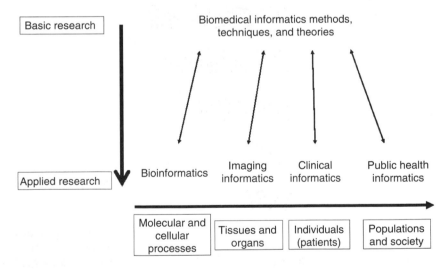

Figure 1.21. Breadth of the biomedical informatics field. The relationship between biomedical informatics as a core scientific discipline and its diverse array of application domains that span biological science, imaging, clinical practice, public health, and others not illustrated (see text).

should receive, but, given the need for teamwork and understanding in the field, it would be counterproductive and wasteful to separate trainees based on the application areas that may interest them.[10]

The scientific contributions of biomedical informatics also can be appreciated through its potential for benefiting the education of health professionals. For example, in the education of medical students, the various cognitive activities of physicians traditionally have tended to be considered separately and in isolation—they have been largely treated as though they are independent and distinct modules of performance. One activity attracting increasing interest is that of formal medical decision making (see Chapter 3). The specific content of this area remains to be defined completely, but the discipline's dependence on formal methods and its use of knowledge and information reveal that it is one aspect of biomedical informatics.

A particular topic in the study of medical decision making is **diagnosis**, which is often conceived and taught as though it were a free-standing and independent activity. Medical students may thus be led to view diagnosis as a process that physicians carry out in isolation before choosing therapy for a patient or proceeding to other modular tasks. A number of studies have shown that this model is oversimplified and that such a decomposition of cognitive tasks may be quite misleading (Elstein et al., 1978; Patel and Groen, 1986). Physicians seem to deal with several tasks at the same time. Although a diagnosis may be one of the first things physicians think about when they see a new patient, patient assessment (diagnosis, management, analysis of treatment results, monitoring of disease progression, etc.) is a process that never really terminates. A physician must be flexible and open-minded. It is generally appropriate to alter the original diagnosis if it turns out that treatment based on it is unsuccessful or if new information weakens the evidence supporting the diagnosis or suggests a second and concurrent disorder. Chapter 4 discusses these issues in greater detail.

When we speak of making a diagnosis, choosing a treatment, managing therapy, making decisions, monitoring a patient, or preventing disease, we are using labels for different aspects of medical care, an entity that has overall unity. The fabric of medical care is a continuum in which these elements are tightly interwoven. Regardless of whether we view computer and information science as a profession, a technology, or a science, there is no doubt about its importance to biomedicine. We can assume computers will be used increasingly in clinical practice, biomedical research, and health science education.

1.2.4   Relationship to Computer Science

During its evolution as an academic entity in universities, computer science followed an unsettled course as involved faculty attempted to identify key topics in the field and to

---

[10] The biomedical informatics training program at Columbia University, for example, was designed with this perspective in mind. Students with interests in clinical, imaging, public health, and biologic applications are trained together and are required to learn something about each of the other application areas. Details of the curriculum can be found at http://www.dbmi.columbia.edu/educ/curriculum/curriculum.html (see also Shortliffe and Johnson, 2002).

find the discipline's organizational place. Many computer science programs were located in departments of electrical engineering, because major concerns of their researchers were computer architecture and design and the development of practical hardware components. At the same time, computer scientists were interested in programming languages and software, undertakings not particularly characteristic of engineering. Furthermore, their work with algorithm design, computability theory,[11] and other theoretical topics seemed more related to mathematics.

Biomedical informatics draws from all of these activities—development of hardware, software, and computer science theory. Biomedical computing generally has not had a large enough market to influence the course of major hardware developments; i.e., computers have not been developed specifically for biomedical applications. Not till the early 1960s (when health-computing experts occasionally talked about and, in a few instances, developed special medical terminals) have people assumed that biomedical-computing applications would use hardware other than that designed for general use.

The question of whether biomedical applications would require specialized programming languages might have been answered affirmatively in the 1970s by anyone examining the MGH Utility Multi-Programming System, known as the **MUMPS** language (Greenes et al., 1970, Bowie and Barnett, 1976), which was specially developed for use in medical applications. For several years, MUMPS was the most widely used language for medical record processing. Under its new name, **M**, it is still in widespread use. New implementations have been developed for each generation of computers. M, however, like any programming language, is not equally useful for all computing tasks. In addition, the software requirements of medicine are better understood and no longer appear to be unique; rather, they are specific to the kind of task. A program for scientific computation looks pretty much the same whether it is designed for chemical engineering or for pharmacokinetic calculations.

How, then, does biomedical informatics differ from biomedical computer science? Is the new discipline simply the study of computer science with a "biomedical flavor"? If you return to the definition of biomedical informatics that we provided in Section 1.2.1, and then refer to Figure 1.19, we believe you will begin to see why biomedical informatics is more than simply the biomedical application of computer science. The issues that it addresses not only have broad relevance to health, medicine, and biology, but the underlying sciences on which biomedical informatics professionals draw are inherently interdisciplinary as well. Thus, for example, successful biomedical informatics research will often draw on, and contribute to, computer science, but it may also be closely related to the decision sciences (probability theory, decision analysis, or the psychology of human problem solving), cognitive science, information sciences, or the management sciences (Figure 1.22). Furthermore, a biomedical informatics researcher will be tightly linked to some underlying problem from the real world of health or biomedicine. As

---

[11] Many interesting problems cannot be computed in a finite time and require heuristics. Computability theory is the foundation for assessing the feasibility and cost of computation to provide the complete and correct results to a formally stated problem.

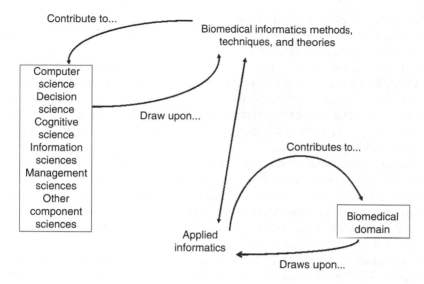

Figure 1.22. Component sciences in biomedical informatics. An informatics application area is motivated by the needs of its associated biomedical domain, to which it attempts to contribute solutions to problems. Thus any applied informatics work draws upon a biomedical domain for its inspiration, and in turn often leads to the delineation of basic research challenges in biomedical informatics that must be tackled if the applied biomedical domain is ultimately to benefit. At the methodologic level, biomedical informatics draws on, and contributes to, a wide variety of component disciplines, of which computer science is only one. As Figures 1.19 and 1.21 show explicitly, biomedical informatics is inherently multidisciplinary, both in its areas of application and in the component sciences on which it draws.

Figure 1.22 illustrates, for example, a biomedical informatics basic researcher or doctoral student will accordingly be motivated by one of the application areas, such as those shown at the bottom of Figures 1.19 and 1.21, but a dissertation worthy of a Ph.D. in the field will usually be identified by a generalizable scientific result that also contributes to one of the component disciplines (Figure 1.22) and on which other scientists can build in the future.

1.2.5   *Relationship to Biomedical Engineering*

If biomedical informatics is a young discipline, by contrast biomedical engineering is a well-established one. Many engineering and medical schools have formal academic programs in the latter subject, often with departmental status and full-time faculty. How does biomedical informatics relate to biomedical engineering, especially in an era when engineering and computer science are increasingly intertwined?

Biomedical engineering departments emerged 35 to 45 years ago, when technology began to play an increasingly prominent role in medical practice. The emphasis in such departments has tended to be research on, and development of, instrumentation (e.g., as discussed in Chapters 17 and 18, advanced monitoring systems, specialized transducers for clinical or laboratory use, and image-enhancement techniques for use in radiology), with an orientation toward the development of medical devices, prostheses,[12] and specialized research tools (Figure 1.23). In recent years, computing techniques have been used both in the design and building of medical devices and in the medical devices themselves. For example, the "smart" devices increasingly found in most specialties are all dependent on microprocessor technology. Intensive care monitors that generate blood pressure records while calculating mean values and hourly summaries are examples of such "intelligent" devices.

The overlap between biomedical engineering and biomedical informatics suggests that it would be unwise for us to draw compulsively strict boundaries between the two fields. There are ample opportunities for interaction, and there are chapters in this book that clearly overlap with biomedical engineering topics—e.g., Chapter 17 on patient-monitoring systems and Chapter 18 on radiology systems. Even where they meet, however, the fields have differences in emphasis that can help you to understand their different evolutionary histories. In biomedical engineering, the emphasis is on medical devices; in biomedical informatics, the emphasis is on biomedical information and

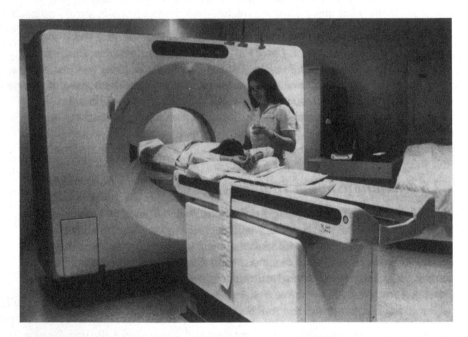

Figure 1.23. Advanced imaging device. Computed tomography (CT) scanners and other imaging devices used in radiology are of interest to both medical computer scientists and biomedical engineers. (Photograph courtesy of Janice Anne Rohn.)

---

[12] Devices that replace body parts—e.g., artificial hips or hearts.

knowledge and on their management with the use of computers. In both fields, the computer is secondary, although both use computing technology. The emphasis in this book is on the informatics end of the spectrum of biomedical computer science, so we shall not spend much time examining biomedical engineering topics.

1.3   The Nature of Medical Information

From the previous discussion, you might conclude that biomedical applications do not raise any unique problems or concerns. On the contrary, the biomedical environment raises several issues that, in interesting ways, are quite distinct from those encountered in most other domains of computer application. Clinical information seems to be systematically different from the information used in physics, engineering, or even clinical chemistry (which more closely resembles chemical applications generally than it does medical ones). Aspects of biomedical information include an essence of uncertainty—we can never know all about a physiological process, and this results in inevitable variability among individuals. These differences raise special problems. It is partly for this reason that some investigators suggest that biomedical computer science differs from conventional computer science in fundamental ways. We shall explore these differences only briefly here; for details, you can consult Blois' book on this subject (see Suggested Readings).

Let us examine an instance of what we will call a *low-level* (or readily formalized) science. Physics is a natural starting point; in any discussion of the hierarchical relationships among the sciences (from the fourth-century BC Greek philosopher Aristotle to the twentieth-century U.S. librarian Melvil Dewey), physics will be placed near the bottom. Physics characteristically has a certain kind of simplicity, or generality. The concepts and descriptions of the objects and processes of physics, however, are necessarily used in all applied fields, including medicine. The laws of physics and the descriptions of certain kinds of physical processes are essential in representing or explaining functions that we regard as medical in nature. We need to know something about molecular physics, for example, to understand why water is such a good solvent; to explain how nutrient molecules are metabolized, we talk about the role of electron-transfer reactions.

Applying a computer (or any formal computation) to a physical problem in a medical context is no different from doing so in a physics laboratory or for an engineering application. The use of computers in various **low-level processes** (such as those of physics or chemistry) is similar and is independent of the application. If we are talking about the solvent properties of water, it makes no difference whether we happen to be working in geology, engineering, or medicine. Such low-level processes of physics are particularly receptive to mathematical treatment, so using computers for these applications requires only conventional numerical programming.

In biomedicine, however, there are other **higher-level processes** carried out in more complex objects such as organisms (one type of which is patients). Many of the important informational processes are of this kind. When we discuss, describe, or record the properties or behavior of human beings, we are using the descriptions of very high-level objects, the behavior of whom has no counterpart in physics or in engineering. The person using computers to analyze the descriptions of these high-level objects and processes encounters serious difficulties (Blois, 1984).

One might object to this line of argument by remarking that, after all, computers are used routinely in commercial applications in which human beings and situations concerning them are involved and that relevant computations are carried out successfully. The explanation is that, in these commercial applications, the descriptions of human beings and their activities have been so highly abstracted that the events or processes have been reduced to low-level objects. In biomedicine, abstractions carried to this degree would be worthless from either a clinical or research perspective.

For example, one instance of a human being in the banking business is the customer, who may deposit, borrow, withdraw, or invest money. To describe commercial activities such as these, we need only a few properties; the customer can remain an abstract entity. In clinical medicine, however, we could not begin to deal with a patient represented with such skimpy abstractions. We must be prepared to analyze most of the complex behaviors that human beings display and to describe patients as completely as possible. We must deal with the rich descriptions occurring at high levels in the hierarchy, and we may be hard pressed to encode and process this information using the tools of mathematics and computer science that work so well at low levels. In light of these remarks, the general enterprise known as **artificial intelligence (AI)** can be aptly described as the application of computer science to high-level, real-world problems.

Biomedical informatics thus includes computer applications that range from processing of very low-level descriptions, which are little different from their counterparts in physics, chemistry, or engineering, to processing of extremely high-level ones, which are completely and systematically different. When we study human beings in their entirety (including such aspects as human cognition, self-consciousness, intentionality, and behavior), we must use these high-level descriptions. We will find that they raise complex issues to which conventional logic and mathematics are less readily applicable. In general, the attributes of low-level objects appear sharp, crisp, and unambiguous (e.g., "length," "mass"), whereas those of high-level ones tend to be soft, fuzzy, and inexact (e.g., "unpleasant scent," "good").

Just as we need to develop different methods to describe high-level objects, the inference methods we use with such objects may differ from those we use with low-level ones. In formal logic, we begin with the assumption that a given proposition must be either true or false. This feature is essential because logic is concerned with the preservation of truth value under various formal transformations. It is difficult or impossible, however, to assume that all propositions have truth values when we deal with the many high-level descriptions in medicine or, indeed, in everyday situations. Such questions as "Was Woodrow Wilson a good president?" cannot be answered with a "yes" or "no" (unless we limit the question to specific criteria for determining the goodness of presidents). Many common questions in biomedicine have the same property.

1.4 Integrating Biomedical Computing and Medical Practice

It should be clear from the previous discussion that biomedical informatics is a remarkably broad and complex topic. We have argued that information management is intrinsic to medical practice and that interest in using computers to aid in information management has grown over the last four decades. In this chapter and throughout the book, we emphasize the myriad ways in which computers are used in biomedicine to ease the burdens of information processing and the means by which new technology promises to change the delivery of health care. The rate at, and degree to, which such changes are realized will be determined in part by external forces that influence the costs of developing and implementing biomedical applications and the ability of clinicians, patients, and the health care system to accrue the potential benefits.

We can summarize several global forces that are affecting biomedical computing and that will determine the extent to which computers are assimilated into medical practice: (1) new developments in computer hardware and software; (2) a gradual increase in the number of professionals who have been trained in both clinical medicine and biomedical informatics; and (3) ongoing changes in health care financing designed to control the rate of growth of medical expenditures (Chapter 23). We touched on the first of these factors in Section 1.2.2, when we described the historical development of biomedical computing and the trend from mainframe computers to microcomputers and PCs. The future view outlined in Section 1.1 similarly builds on the influence that the Internet has provided throughout society during the last decade. The new hardware technologies have made powerful computers inexpensive and thus available to hospitals, to departments within hospitals, and even to individual physicians. The broad selection of computers of all sizes, prices, and capabilities makes computer applications both attractive and accessible. Technological advances in information storage devices are facilitating the inexpensive storage of large amounts of data, thus improving the feasibility of data-intensive applications, such as the all-digital radiology department discussed in Chapter 18. Standardization of hardware and advances in network technology are making it easier to share data and to integrate related information management functions within a hospital or other health care organization.

Computers are increasingly prevalent in all aspects of our lives, whether as an ATM, as the microprocessor in a microwave oven, or as a word processor. Physicians trained in recent years may have used computer programs to learn diagnostic techniques or to manage the therapy of simulated patients. They may have learned to use a computer to search the medical literature, either directly or with the assistance of a specially trained librarian. Simple exposure to computers does not, however, guarantee an eagerness to embrace the machine. Medical personnel will be unwilling to use computer-based systems that are poorly designed, confusing, unduly time-consuming, or lacking in clear benefit (see Chapters 4 and 6).

The second factor is the increase in the number of professionals who are being trained to understand the biomedical issues as well as the technical and engineering ones. Computer scientists who understand biomedicine are better able to design systems responsive to actual needs. Health professionals who receive formal training in biomedical informatics are likely to build systems using well-established techniques while avoiding the past mistakes of other developers. As more professionals are trained in the special aspects of both fields, and as the programs they develop are introduced, health care professionals are more likely to have useful and usable systems available when they turn to the computer for help with information management tasks.

The third factor affecting the integration of computing technologies into health care settings is managed care and the increasing pressure to control medical spending

(Chapter 23). The escalating tendency to apply technology to all patient care tasks is a frequently cited phenomenon in modern medical practice. Mere physical findings no longer are considered adequate for making diagnoses and planning treatments. In fact, medical students who are taught by more experienced physicians to find subtle diagnostic signs by examining various parts of the body nonetheless often choose to bypass or deemphasize physical examinations in favor of ordering one test after another. Sometimes, they do so without paying sufficient attention to the ensuing cost. Some new technologies replace less expensive, but technologically inferior, tests. In such cases, the use of the more expensive approach is generally justified. Occasionally, computer-related technologies have allowed us to perform tasks that previously were not possible. For example, the scans produced with computed tomography or magnetic resonance imaging (see Chapter 18) have allowed physicians to visualize cross-sectional slices of the body for the first time, and medical instruments in intensive care units perform continuous monitoring of patients' body functions that previously could be checked only episodically (see Chapter 17).

Yet the development of expensive new technologies, and the belief that more technology is better, helped to fuel the rapidly escalating health care costs of the 1970s and 1980s, leading to the introduction of managed care and capitation in recent years. Chapter 23 discusses the mechanisms that opened the door to rapid growth in health expenses and the changes in financing and delivery that were designed to curb spending in the new era of cost consciousness. Integrated computer systems potentially provide the means to capture data for detailed cost accounting, to analyze the relationship of costs of care to the benefits of that care, to evaluate the quality of care provided, and to identify areas of inefficiency. Systems that improve the quality of care while reducing the cost of providing that care clearly will be favored. The effect of cost containment pressures on technologies that increase the cost of care while improving the quality are less clear. Medical technologies, including computers, will need to improve the delivery of medical care while either reducing costs or providing benefits that clearly exceed their costs.

Improvements in hardware and software make computers more suitable for biomedical applications. Designers of medical systems must, however, address satisfactorily many logistical and engineering questions before computers can be fully integrated into medical practice. For example, are computer terminals conveniently located? Could handheld devices effectively replace the tethered terminals and workstations of the past? Can users complete their tasks without excessive delays? Is the system reliable enough to avoid loss of data? Can users interact easily and intuitively with the computer? Are patient data secure and appropriately protected from prying eyes? In addition, cost control pressures produce a growing reluctance to embrace expensive technologies that add to the high cost of health care. The net effect of these opposing trends will in large part determine the degree to which computers are integrated into the health care environment.

In summary, rapid advances in computer hardware and software, coupled with an increasing computer literacy of health care professionals and researchers, favor the implementation of effective computer applications in medical practice and life sciences research. Furthermore, in the increasingly competitive health care industry, providers have a greater need for the information management capabilities supplied by computer systems. The challenge is to demonstrate the financial and clinical advantages of these systems.

Suggested Readings

Altman R.B. (1997). Informatics in the care of patients: Ten notable challenges. *Western Journal of Medicine*, 166(6):118–122.
This thoughtful article was written to introduce the concepts of medical informatics to clinicians while explaining a major set of challenges that help to define the goals and research programs for the field.

Blois M.S. (1984). *Information and Medicine: The Nature of Medical Descriptions*. Berkeley, CA: University of California Press.
The author analyzes the structure of medical knowledge in terms of a hierarchical model of information. He explores the ideas of high- and low-level sciences and suggests that the nature of medical descriptions accounts for difficulties in applying computing technology to medicine.

Collen M.F. (1995). *A History of Medical Informatics in the United States: 1950 to 1990*. Bethesda, MD: American Medical Informatics Association, Hartman Publishing.
This comprehensive book traces the history of the field of medical informatics and identifies the origins of the discipline's name (which first appeared in the English-language literature in 1974).

Degoulet P., Phister B., Fieschi, M. (1997). *Introduction to Clinical Informatics*. New York: Springer-Verlag.
This introductory volume provides a broad view of medical informatics and carries the concepts forward with an emphasis on clinical applications.

Elstein A.S., Shulman L.S., Sprafka S.A. (1978). *Medical Problem Solving: An Analysis of Clinical Reasoning*. Cambridge, MA: Harvard University Press.
This classic collection of papers describes detailed studies that have illuminated several aspects of the ways in which expert and novice physicians solve medical problems.

Friedman CP, Altman RB, Kohane IS, McCormick KA, Miller PL, Ozbolt JG, Shortliffe EH, Stormo GD, Szczepaniak MC, Tuck D, Williamson J (2004). Training the next generation of informaticians: The impact of BISTI and bioinformatics. *Journal of American Medical Informatics Association*, 11:167–172.
This important analysis addresses the changing nature of biomedical informatics due to the revolution in bioinformatics and computational biology. Implications for training, as well as organization of academic groups and curriculum development, are discussed.

Institute of Medicine (1991 [revised 1997]). *The Computer-Based Patient Record: An Essential Technology for Health Care,* Washington, DC: National Academy Press.
Institute of Medicine (2002). *Fostering Rapid Advances in Health Care: Learning from System Demonstrations,* Washington, DC: National Academy Press.
National Research Council (1997). *For The Record: Protecting Electronic Health Information,* Washington, DC: National Academy Press.
National Research Council (2000). *Networking Health: Prescriptions for the Internet*, (Washington, DC: National Academy Press.
This set of four reports from branches of the National Academies of Science have had a major influence on health information technology education and policy over the last 15 years.

Institute of Medicine 2000). *To Err is Human: Building a Safer Health System*, Washington, DC: National Academy Press.

Institute of Medicine (2001). *Crossing the Quality Chasm: A New Health Systems for the 21st Century*, Washington, DC: National Academy Press.

Institute of Medicine (2004). *Patient Safety: Achieving a New Standard for Care*, Washington, DC: National Academy Press.

This series of three reports from the Institute of Medicine have outlined the crucial link between heightened use of information technology and the enhancement of quality and reduction in errors in practice. Major programs in patient safety have resulted from these reports, and they have provided motivation for a heightened interest in health care information technology among policy makers, provider organizations, and even patients.

Panel on Transforming Health Care (2001). *Transforming Health Care Through Information Technology* (President's Information Technology Advisory Committee (PITAC), Report to the President), Washington, DC: National Coordinating Office for IT Research and Development, http://www.nitrd.gov/pubs/pitac/pitac-hc-9feb01.pdf

Panel on Transforming Health Care (2004). *Revolutionizing Health Care Through Information Technology* (PITAC, Report to the President), Washington, DC: National Coordinating Office for IT Research and Development, http://www.nitrd.gov/pitac/reports/20040721_hit_report.pdf

These two reports from a Presidential advisory committee provide a provocative view of the future of information technology in health care, making policy recommendations that have guided the White House and Congress in their recent legislative and program announcements.

Shortliffe E. (1993). Doctors, patients, and computers: Will information technology dehumanize health care delivery? *Proceedings of the American Philosophical Society*, 137(3):390–398.

In this paper, the author examines the frequently expressed concern that the introduction of computing technology into health care settings will disrupt the development of rapport between clinicians and patients and thereby dehumanize the therapeutic process. He argues, rather, that computers may have precisely the opposite effect on the relationship between clinicians and their patients.

van Bemmel J.H., Musen, M.A. (1997). *Handbook of Medical Informatics*. Heidelberg, Germany: Springer-Verlag.

This volume provides a comprehensive overview of the field of medical informatics and is an excellent starting reference point for many of the topics in the field.

Questions for Discussion

1. How do you interpret the phrase "logical behavior"? Do computers behave logically? Do people behave logically? Explain your answers.
2. What do you think it means to say that a computer program is "effective"? Make a list of a dozen computer applications with which you are familiar. List the applications in decreasing order of effectiveness, as you have explained this concept. Then, for each application, indicate your estimate of how well human beings perform the same tasks (this will require that you determine what it means for a human being to be effective). Do you discern any pattern? If so, how do you interpret it?
3. Discuss three society-wide factors that will determine the extent to which computers are assimilated into medical practice.

4. Reread the future vision presented in Section 1.1. Describe the characteristics of an integrated environment for managing medical information. Discuss two ways in which such a system could change medical practice.
5. Do you believe that improving the technical quality of health care entails the risk of dehumanization? If so, is it worth the risk? Explain your reasoning.

2
Biomedical Data: Their Acquisition, Storage, and Use

EDWARD H. SHORTLIFFE AND G. OCTO BARNETT

After reading this chapter, you should know the answers to these questions:

- What are medical data?
- How are medical data used?
- What are the drawbacks of the traditional paper medical record?
- What is the potential role of the computer in data storage, retrieval, and interpretation?
- What distinguishes a database from a knowledge base?
- How are data collection and hypothesis generation intimately linked in medical diagnosis?
- What are the meanings of the terms *prevalence*, *predictive value*, *sensitivity*, and *specificity*?
- How are the terms related?
- What are the alternatives for entry of data into a medical database?

2.1 What Are Medical Data?

From earliest times, the ideas of ill health and its treatment have been wedded to those of the observation and interpretation of data. Whether we consider the disease descriptions and guidelines for management in early Greek literature or the modern physician's use of complex laboratory and X-ray studies, it is clear that gathering data and interpreting their meaning are central to the health care process. A textbook on computers in biomedicine will accordingly refer time and again to issues in data collection, storage, and use. This chapter lays the foundation for this recurring set of issues that is pertinent to all aspects of the use of computers in biomedicine, both in the clinical world and in applications related to biology and human genetics.

If data are central to all medical care, it is because they are crucial to the process of *decision making* (as described in detail in Chapters 3 and 4). In fact, simple reflection will reveal that all medical care activities involve gathering, analyzing, or using data. Data provide the basis for categorizing the problems a patient may be having or for identifying subgroups within a population of patients. They also help a physician to decide what additional information is needed and what actions should be taken to gain a greater understanding of a patient's problem or to treat most effectively the problem that has been diagnosed.

It is overly simplistic to view data as the columns of numbers or the monitored wave-forms that are a product of our increasingly technological health care environment. Although laboratory test results and other numeric data are often invaluable, a variety of more subtle types of data may be just as important to the delivery of optimal care: the awkward glance by a patient who seems to be avoiding a question during the medical interview, information about the details of a patient's complaints or about his family or economic setting, the subjective sense of disease severity that an experienced physician will often have within a few moments of entering a patient's room. No physician disputes the importance of such observations in decision making during patient assessment and management, yet the precise role of these data and the corresponding decision criteria are so poorly understood that it is difficult to record them in ways that convey their full mean-ing, even from one physician to another. Despite these limitations, clinicians need to share descriptive information with others. When they cannot interact directly with one another, they often turn to the chart or computer-based record for communication purposes.

We consider a **medical datum** to be any single observation of a patient—e.g., a temper-ature reading, a red blood cell count, a past history of rubella, or a blood pressure read-ing. As the blood pressure example shows, it is a matter of perspective whether a single observation is in fact more than one datum. A blood pressure of 120/80 might well be recorded as a single datum point in a setting where knowledge that a patient's blood pres-sure is normal is all that matters. If the difference between diastolic (while the heart cav-ities are beginning to fill) and systolic (while they are contracting) blood pressures is important for decision making or for analysis, however, the blood pressure reading is best viewed as two pieces of information (systolic pressure = 120 mm Hg, diastolic pressure = 80 mm Hg). Human beings can glance at a written blood pressure value and easily make the transition between its unitary view as a single datum point and the decomposed infor-mation about systolic and diastolic pressures. Such dual views can be much more difficult for computers, however, unless they are specifically allowed for in the design of the method for data storage and analysis. The idea of a *data model* for computer-stored med-ical data accordingly becomes an important issue in the design of medical data systems.

If a medical *datum* is a single observation about a patient, medical *data* are multiple observations. Such data may involve several different observations made concurrently, the observation of the same patient parameter made at several points in time, or both. Thus, a single datum generally can be viewed as defined by four elements:

1. The *patient* in question
2. The *parameter* being observed (e.g., liver size, urine sugar value, history of rheumatic fever, heart size on chest X-ray film)
3. The *value* of the parameter in question (e.g., weight is 70 kg, temperature is 98.6°F, profession is steel worker)
4. The *time* of the observation (e.g., 2:30 A.M. on 14FEB1997[1])

Time can particularly complicate the assessment and computer-based management of data. In some settings, the date of the observation is adequate—e.g., in outpatient

---

[1]Note that it was the tendency to record such dates in computers as "14FEB97" that led to the end-of-century complexities that we called the *Year 2000 problem*. It was shortsighted to think that it was adequate to encode the year of an event with only two digits.

clinics or private offices where a patient generally is seen infrequently and the data collected need to be identified in time with no greater accuracy than a calendar date. In others, minute-to-minute variations may be important—e.g., the frequent blood sugar readings obtained for a patient in diabetic ketoacidosis[2] or the continuous measurements of mean arterial blood pressure for a patient in cardiogenic shock.[3]

It often also is important to keep a record of the circumstances under which a datum was obtained. For example, was the blood pressure taken in the arm or leg? Was the patient lying or standing? Was the pressure obtained just after exercise? During sleep? What kind of recording device was used? Was the observer reliable? Such additional information, sometimes called *modifiers*, can be of crucial importance in the proper interpretation of data. Two patients with the same basic complaint or symptom often have markedly different explanations for their problem, revealed by careful assessment of the modifiers of that complaint.

A related issue is the *uncertainty* in the values of data. It is rare that an observation—even one by a skilled clinician—can be accepted with absolute certainty. Consider the following examples:

- An adult patient reports a childhood illness with fevers and a red rash in addition to joint swelling. Could he or she have had scarlet fever? The patient does not know what his or her pediatrician called the disease nor whether anyone thought that he or she had scarlet fever.
- A physician listens to the heart of an asthmatic child and thinks that he or she hears a heart murmur—but is not certain because of the patient's loud wheezing.
- A radiologist looking at a shadow on a chest X-ray film is not sure whether it represents overlapping blood vessels or a lung tumor.
- A confused patient is able to respond to simple questions about his or her illness, but under the circumstances the physician is uncertain how much of the history being reported is reliable.

As described in Chapters 3 and 4, there are a variety of possible responses to deal with incomplete data, the uncertainty in them, and in their interpretation. One technique is to collect additional data that will either confirm or eliminate the concern raised by the initial observation. This solution is not always appropriate, however, because the *costs* of data collection must be considered. The additional observation might be expensive, risky for the patient, or wasteful of time during which treatment could have been instituted. The idea of *trade-offs* in data collection thus becomes extremely important in guiding health care decision making.

2.1.1 What Are the Types of Medical Data?

The examples in the previous section suggest that there is a broad range of data types in the practice of medicine and the allied health sciences. They range from narrative,

---

[2]Ketoacidosis results from acid production due to poorly controlled blood sugar levels.
[3]Cardiogenic shock is dangerously low blood pressure due to failure of the heart.

textual data to numerical measurements, recorded signals, drawings, and even photographs.

Narrative data account for a large component of the information that is gathered in the care of patients. For example, the patient's description of his or her present illness, including responses to focused questions from the physician, generally is gathered verbally and is recorded as text in the medical record. The same is true of the patient's social and family history, the general review of systems that is part of most evaluations of new patients, and the clinician's report of physical examination findings. Such narrative data were traditionally handwritten by clinicians and then placed in the patient's medical record (Figure 2.1). Increasingly, however, the narrative summaries are dictated and then transcribed by typists who work with word processors to produce printed summaries for inclusion in medical records. The electronic versions of such reports can also easily be integrated into electronic health records (EHRs) and clinical data repositories so that clinicians can access important clinical information even when the paper record is not available. Electronically stored transcriptions of dictated information often include not only patient histories and physical examinations but also other narrative descriptions such as reports of specialty consultations, surgical procedures, pathologic examinations of tissues, and hospitalization summaries when a patient is discharged.

Some narrative data are loosely coded with shorthand conventions known to health personnel, particularly data collected during the physical examination, in which recorded observations reflect the stereotypic examination process taught to all practitioners. It is common, for example, to find the notation "PERRLA" under the eye examination in a patient's medical record. This encoded form indicates that the patient's "Pupils are Equal (in size), Round, and Reactive to Light and Accommodation."[4]

Note that there are significant problems associated with the use of such abbreviations. Many are not standard and can have different meanings depending on the context in which they are used. For example, "MI" can mean "mitral insufficiency" (leakage in one of the heart's valves) or "myocardial infarction" (the medical term for what is commonly called a heart attack). Many hospitals try to establish a set of "acceptable" abbreviations with meanings, but the enforcement of such standardization is often unsuccessful.

Complete phrases have become loose standards of communication among medical personnel. Examples include "mild dyspnea (shortness of breath) on exertion," "pain relieved by antacids or milk," and "failure to thrive." Such standardized expressions are attempts to use conventional text notation as a form of summarization for otherwise heterogeneous conditions that together characterize a simple concept about a patient.

Many data used in medicine take on discrete numeric values. These include such parameters as laboratory tests, vital signs (such as temperature and pulse rate), and certain measurements taken during the physical examination. When such numerical data are interpreted, however, the issue of *precision* becomes important. Can physicians distinguish reliably between a 9-cm and a 10-cm liver span when they examine a patient's abdomen? Does it make sense to report a serum sodium level to two-decimal-place

---

[4]Accommodation is the process of focusing on near objects.

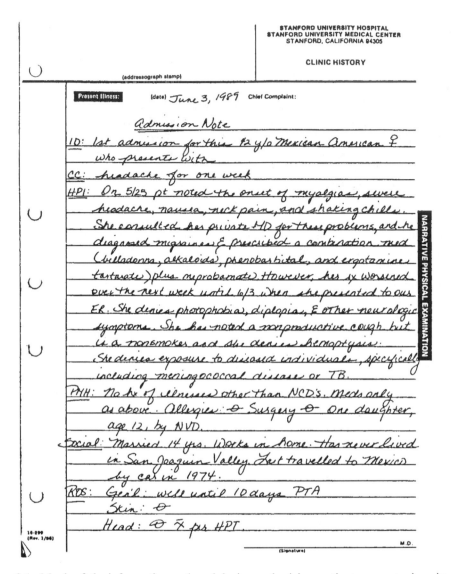

Figure 2.1. Much of the information gathered during a physician–patient encounter is written in the medical record.

accuracy? Is a 1-kg fluctuation in weight from one week to the next significant? Was the patient weighed on the same scale both times (i.e., could the different values reflect variation between measurement instruments rather than changes in the patient)?

In some fields of medicine, analog data in the form of continuous signals are particularly important (see Chapter 17). Perhaps the best-known example is an electrocardiogram (ECG), a tracing of the electrical activity from a patient's heart. When such data are stored in medical records, a graphical tracing frequently is included, with a written interpretation of its meaning. There are clear challenges in determining how such data are best managed in computer storage systems.

Visual images—either acquired from machines or sketched by the physician—are another important category of data. Radiologic images are obvious examples. It also is common for physicians to draw simple pictures to represent abnormalities that they have observed; such drawings may serve as a basis for comparison when they or another physician next see the patient. For example, a sketch is a concise way of conveying the location and size of a nodule in the prostate gland (Figure 2.2).

As should be clear from these examples, the idea of data is inextricably bound to the idea of **data recording**. Physicians and other health care personnel are taught from the outset that it is crucial that they do not trust their memory when caring for patients. They must record their observations, as well as the actions they have taken and the rationales for those actions, for later communication to themselves and other people. A glance at a medical record will quickly reveal the wide variety of data-recording techniques that have evolved. The range goes from hand-written text to commonly understood shorthand notation to cryptic symbols that only specialists can understand; few physicians know how to interpret the data-recording conventions of an ophthalmologist, for example (Figure 2.3). The notations may be highly structured records of brief text or numerical information, hand-drawn sketches, machine-generated tracings of analog signals, or photographic images (of the patient or of his or her radiologic or

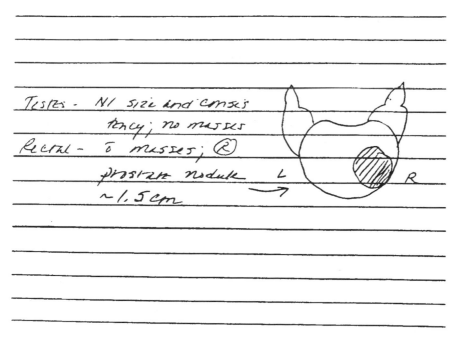

Figure 2.2. A physician's hand-drawn sketch of a prostate nodule. A drawing may convey precise information more easily and compactly than a textual description.

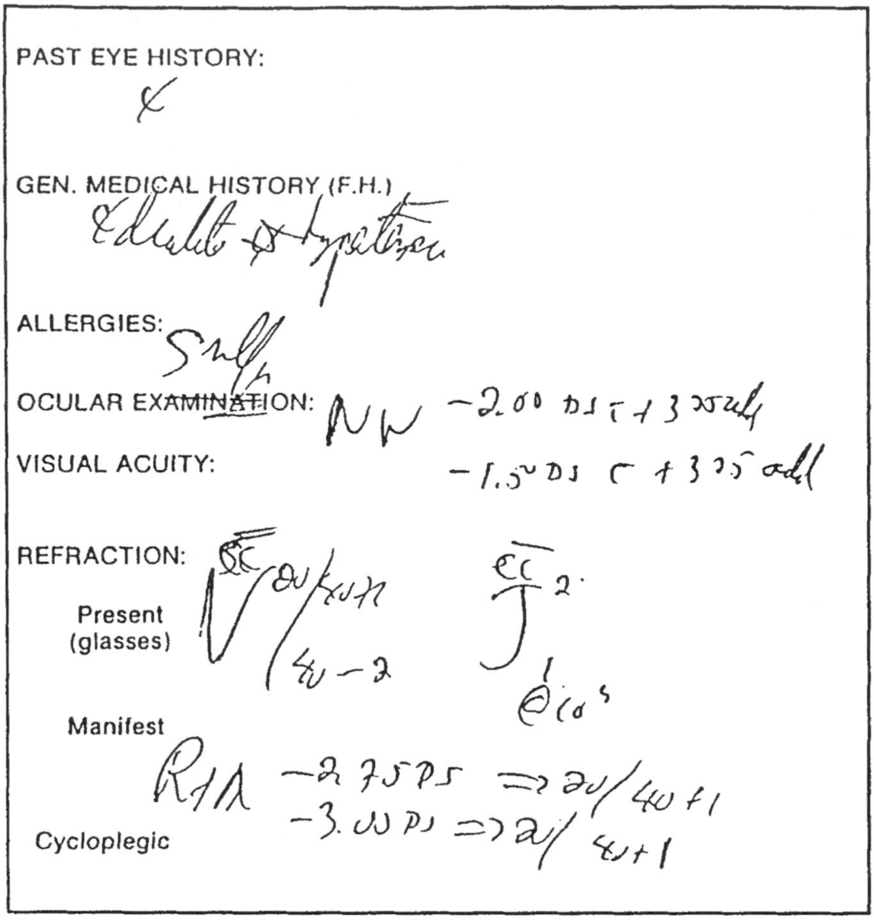
PAST EYE HISTORY:

GEN. MEDICAL HISTORY (F.H.)

ALLERGIES:

OCULAR EXAMINATION:

VISUAL ACUITY:

REFRACTION:

Present (glasses)

Manifest

Cycloplegic

Figure 2.3. An ophthalmologist's report of an eye examination. Most physicians trained in other specialties would have difficulty deciphering the symbols that the ophthalmologist has used.

other studies). This range of data-recording conventions presents significant challenges to the person implementing computer-based medical record systems.

2.1.2 Who Collects the Data?

Health data on patients and populations are gathered by a variety of health professionals. Although conventional ideas of the **healthcare team** evoke images of coworkers treating ill patients, the team has much broader responsibilities than treatment per se; data collection and recording are a central part of its task.

Physicians are key players in the process of data collection and interpretation. They converse with a patient to gather narrative descriptive data on the chief complaint, past illnesses, family and social information, and the system review. They examine the patient, collecting pertinent data and recording them during or at the end of the visit. In addition, they generally decide what additional data to collect by ordering laboratory or radiologic studies and by observing the patient's response to therapeutic interventions (yet another form of data that contributes to patient assessment).

In both outpatient and hospital settings, nurses play a central role in making observations and recording them for future reference. The data that they gather contribute to nursing care plans as well as to the assessment of patients by physicians and by other health care staff. Thus, nurses' training includes instruction in careful and accurate observation, history taking, and examination of the patient. Because nurses typically spend more time with patients than physicians do, especially in the hospital setting, nurses often build relationships with patients that uncover information and insights that contribute to proper diagnosis, to understanding of pertinent psychosocial issues, or to proper planning of therapy or discharge management (Figure 2.4). The role of information systems in contributing to patient care tasks such as care planning by nurses is the subject of Chapter 16.

Various other health care workers contribute to the data-collection process. Office staff and admissions personnel gather demographic and financial information. Physical

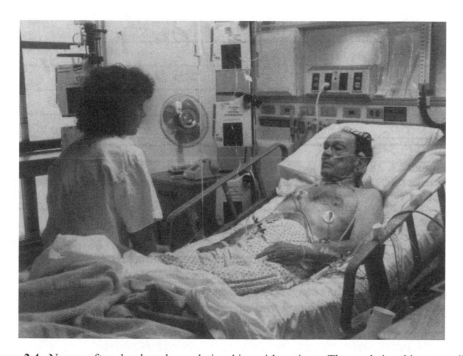

Figure 2.4. Nurses often develop close relationships with patients. These relationships may allow the nurse to make observations that are missed by other staff. This ability is just one of the ways in which nurses play a key role in data collection and recording. (Photograph courtesy of Janice Anne Rohn.)

or respiratory therapists record the results of their treatments and often make suggestions for further management. Laboratory personnel perform tests on biological samples, such as blood or urine, and record the results for later use by physicians and nurses. Radiology technicians perform X-ray examinations; radiologists interpret the resulting data and report their findings to the patients' physicians. Pharmacists may interview patients about their medications or about drug allergies and then monitor the patients' use of prescription drugs. As these examples suggest, many different individuals employed in health care settings gather, record, and make use of patient data in their work.

Finally, there are the technological devices that generate data—laboratory instruments, imaging machines, monitoring equipment in intensive care units, and measurement devices that take a single reading (such as thermometers, ECG machines, sphygmomanometers for taking blood pressure, and spirometers for testing lung function). Sometimes such a device produces a paper report suitable for inclusion in a traditional medical record. Sometimes the device indicates a result on a gauge or traces a result that must be read by an operator and then recorded in the patient's chart. Sometimes a trained specialist must interpret the output. Increasingly, however, the devices feed their results directly into computer equipment so that the data can be analyzed or formatted for electronic storage as well as reported on paper. With the advent of comprehensive EHRs (see Chapter 12), the printing of such data summaries may no longer be required, and all access to information will be through computer workstations.

2.2   Uses of Medical Data

Medical data are recorded for a variety of purposes. They may be needed to support the proper care of the patient from whom they were obtained, but they also may contribute to the good of society through the aggregation and analysis of data regarding populations of individuals. Traditional data-recording techniques and a paper record may have worked reasonably well when care was given by a single physician over the life of a patient. However, given the increased complexity of modern health care, the broadly trained team of individuals who are involved in a patient's care, and the need for multiple providers to access a patient's data and to communicate effectively with one another through the chart, the paper record no longer adequately supports optimal care of individual patients. Another problem occurs because traditional paper-based data-recording techniques have made clinical research across populations of patients extremely cumbersome. Computer-based record keeping offers major advantages in this regard, as we discuss in more detail later in this chapter and in Chapters 12 and 15.

2.2.1   Create the Basis for the Historical Record

Any student of science learns the importance of collecting and recording data meticulously when carrying out an experiment. Just as a laboratory notebook provides a record of precisely what a scientist has done, the experimental data observed, and the rationale for intermediate decision points, medical records are intended to provide a detailed compilation of information about individual patients:

- What is the patient's history (development of a current illness; other diseases that coexist or have resolved; pertinent family, social, and demographic information)?
- What symptoms has the patient reported? When did they begin, what has seemed to aggravate them, and what has provided relief?
- What physical signs have been noted on examination?
- How have signs and symptoms changed over time?
- What laboratory results have been, or are now, available?
- What radiologic and other special studies have been performed?
- What medications are being taken and are there any allergies?
- What other interventions have been undertaken?
- What is the reasoning behind the management decisions?

Each new patient complaint and its management can be viewed as a therapeutic experiment, inherently confounded by uncertainty, with the goal of answering three questions when the experiment is over:

1. What was the nature of the disease or symptom?
2. What was the treatment decision?
3. What was the outcome of that treatment?

As is true for all experiments, one purpose is to learn from experience through careful observation and recording of data. The lessons learned in a given encounter may be highly individualized (e.g., the physician may learn how a specific patient tends to respond to pain or how family interactions tend to affect the patient's response to disease). On the other hand, the value of some experiments may be derived only by pooling of data from many patients who have similar problems and through the analysis of the results of various treatment options to determine efficacy.

Although laboratory research has contributed dramatically to our knowledge of human disease and treatment, especially over the last half century, it is careful observation and recording by skilled health care personnel that has always been of fundamental importance in the generation of new knowledge about patient care. We learn from the aggregation of information from large numbers of patients; thus, the historical record for individual patients is of inestimable importance to clinical research.

2.2.2 Support Communication Among Providers

A central function of structured data collection and recording in health care settings is to assist personnel in providing coordinated care to a patient over time. Most patients who have significant medical conditions are seen over months or years on several occasions for one or more problems that require ongoing evaluation and treatment. Given the increasing numbers of elderly patients in many cultures and health care settings, the care given to a patient is less oriented to diagnosis and treatment of a single disease episode and increasingly focused on management of one or more chronic disorders—possibly over many years.

It was once common for patients to receive essentially all their care from a single provider: the family doctor who tended both children and adults, often seeing the patient over many or all the years of that person's life. We tend to picture such physicians as having especially close relationships with their patients—knowing the family and sharing in many of the patient's life events, especially in smaller communities. Such doctors nonetheless kept records of all encounters so that they could refer to data about past illnesses and treatments as a guide to evaluating future care issues.

In the world of modern medicine, the emergence of subspecialization and the increasing provision of care by *teams* of health professionals have placed new emphasis on the central role of the medical record (Figure 2.5). Now the record not only contains observations by a physician for reference on the next visit but also serves as a communication mechanism among physicians and other medical personnel, such as physical or respiratory therapists, nursing staff, radiology technicians, social workers, or discharge planners. In many outpatient settings, patients receive care over time from a variety of

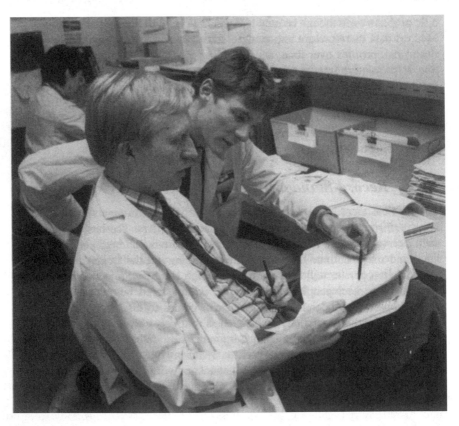

Figure 2.5. One role of the medical record: a communication mechanism among health professionals who work together to plan patient care. (Photograph courtesy of Janice Anne Rohn.)

physicians—colleagues covering for the primary physician, or specialists to whom the patient has been referred, or a managed care organization's case manager. It is not uncommon to hear complaints from patients who remember the days when it was possible to receive essentially all their care from a single physician whom they had come to trust and who knew them well. Physicians are sensitive to this issue and therefore recognize the importance of the medical record in ensuring quality and **continuity of care** through adequate recording of the details and logic of past interventions and ongoing treatment plans. This idea is of particular importance in a health care system, such as ours in the United States, in which chronic diseases rather than care for trauma or acute infections increasingly dominate the basis for interactions between patients and their doctors.

2.2.3   *Anticipate Future Health Problems*

Providing high-quality medical care involves more than responding to patients' acute or chronic health problems. It also requires educating patients about the ways in which their environment and lifestyles can contribute to, or reduce the risk of, future development of disease. Similarly, data gathered routinely in the ongoing care of a patient may suggest that he or she is at high risk of developing a specific problem even though he or she may feel well and be without symptoms at present. Medical data therefore are important in screening for risk factors, following patients' risk profiles over time, and providing a basis for specific patient education or preventive interventions, such as diet, medication, or exercise. Perhaps the most common examples of such ongoing risk assessment in our society are routine monitoring for excess weight, high blood pressure, and elevated serum cholesterol levels. In these cases, abnormal data may be predictive of later symptomatic disease; optimal care requires early intervention before the complications have an opportunity to develop fully.

2.2.4   *Record Standard Preventive Measures*

The medical record also serves as a source of data on interventions that have been performed to prevent common or serious disorders. Sometimes the interventions involve counseling or educational programs (for example, regarding smoking cessation, measures for stopping drug abuse, safe sex practices, and dietary changes to lower cholesterol). Other important preventive interventions include immunizations: the vaccinations that begin in early childhood and may continue throughout life, including special treatments administered when a person will be at particularly high risk (e.g., injections of gamma globulin to protect people from hepatitis, administered before travel to areas where hepatitis is endemic). When a patient comes to his local hospital emergency room with a laceration, the physicians routinely check for an indication of when he most recently had a tetanus immunization. When easily accessible in the record (or from the patient), such data can prevent unnecessary treatments (in this case, an injection) that may be associated with risk or significant cost.

2.2.5   Identify Deviations from Expected Trends

Data often are useful in medical care only when viewed as part of a continuum over time. An example is the routine monitoring of children for normal growth and development by pediatricians (Fig. 2.6). Single data points regarding height and weight may have limited use by themselves; it is the trend in such data points observed over months or years that may provide the first clue to a medical problem. It is accordingly common for such parameters to be recorded on special charts or forms that make the trends easy to discern at a glance. Women who want to get pregnant often keep similar records of body temperature. By measuring temperature daily and recording the values on special charts, women can identify the slight increase in temperature that accompanies ovulation and thus may discern the days of maximum fertility. Many physicians will ask a patient to keep such graphical records so that they can later discuss the data with the patient and include the record in the medical charts for ongoing reference. Such graphs are increasingly created and displayed for viewing by clinicians as a feature of a patient's medical record.

2.2.6   Provide a Legal Record

Another use of medical data, once they are charted and analyzed, is as the foundation for a legal record to which the courts can refer if necessary. The medical record is a legal document; the responsible individual must sign most of the clinical information that is recorded. In addition, the chart generally should describe and justify both the presumed diagnosis for a patient and the choice of management.

We emphasized earlier the importance of recording data; in fact, data do not exist in a generally useful form unless they are recorded. The legal system stresses this point as well. Providers' unsubstantiated memories of what they observed or why they took some action is of little value in the courtroom. The medical record is the foundation for determining whether proper care was delivered. Thus, a well-maintained record is a source of protection for both patients and their physicians.

2.2.7   Support Clinical Research

Although experience caring for individual patients provides physicians with special skills and enhanced judgment over time, it is only by formally analyzing data collected from large numbers of patients that researchers can develop and validate new clinical knowledge of general applicability. Thus, another use of medical data is to support clinical research through the aggregation and statistical analysis of observations gathered from populations of patients (see Section 1.1 and Figures 1.4 and 1.5).

A **randomized clinical trial (RCT)** is a common method by which specific clinical questions are addressed experimentally. RCTs typically involve the random assignment of matched groups of patients to alternate treatments when there is uncertainty about how best to manage the patients' problem. The variables that might affect a patient's course (e.g., age, gender, weight, coexisting medical problems) are measured and recorded. As the study progresses, data are gathered meticulously to provide a record of

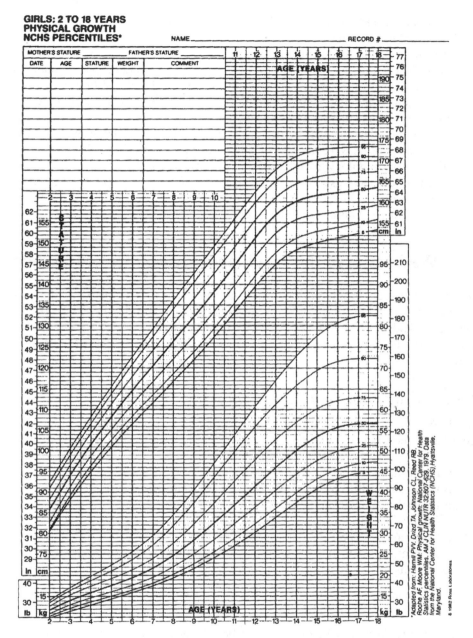

Figure 2.6. A pediatric growth chart. Single datum points would not be useful; it is the changes in values over time that indicate whether development is progressing normally. (*Source*: Reprinted by permission of Ross Laboratories, Columbus, OH 43216.)

how each patient fared under treatment and precisely how the treatment was administered. By pooling such data, sometimes after years of experimentation (depending on the time course of the disease under consideration), researchers may be able to demonstrate a statistical difference among the study groups depending on precise characteristics present when patients entered the study or on the details of how patients were managed. Such results then help investigators to define the standard of care for future patients with the same or similar problems.

Medical knowledge also can be derived from the analysis of large patient data sets even when the patients were not specifically enrolled in an RCT. Much of the research in the field of epidemiology involves analysis of population-based data of this type. Our knowledge of the risks associated with cigarette smoking, for example, is based on irrefutable statistics derived from large populations of individuals with and without lung cancer, other pulmonary problems, and heart disease.

2.3   Weaknesses of the Traditional Medical Record System

The preceding description of medical data and their uses emphasizes the positive aspects of information storage and retrieval in the paper record. All medical personnel, however, quickly learn that use of the medical record is complicated by a bevy of logistical and practical realities that greatly limit the record's effectiveness for its intended uses.

2.3.1   Pragmatic and Logistical Issues

Recall, first, that data cannot effectively serve the delivery of health care unless they are recorded. Their optimal use depends on positive responses to the following questions:

- Can I find the data I need when I need them?
- Can I find the medical record in which they are recorded?
- Can I find the data within the record?
- Can I find what I need quickly?
- Can I read and interpret the data once I find them?
- Can I update the data reliably with new observations in a form consistent with the requirements for future access by me or other people?

All too frequently, the traditional paper record system creates situations in which people answer such questions in the negative. For example:

- The patient's chart may be unavailable when the health care professional needs it. It may be in use by someone else at another location; it may have been misplaced despite the record-tracking system of the hospital, clinic, or office (Figure 2.7); or it may have been taken by someone unintentionally and is now buried on a desk.
- Once the chart is in hand, it might still be difficult to find the information required. The data may have been known previously but never recorded due to an oversight by a physician or other health professional. Poor organization in the chart may lead the

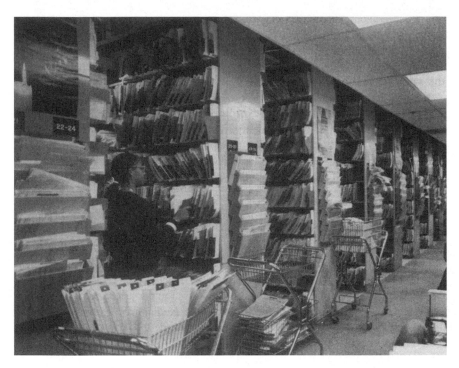

Figure 2.7. A typical storage room for medical records. It is not surprising that charts sometimes are mislaid. (Photograph courtesy of Janice Anne Rohn.)

user to spend an inordinate time searching for the data, especially in the massive paper charts of patients who have long and complicated histories.

- Once the health care professional has located the data, he or she may find them difficult to read. It is not uncommon to hear one physician asking another as they peer together into a chart: "What is that word?" "Is that a two or a five?" "Whose signature is that?" Illegible and sloppy entries can be a major obstruction to effective use of the chart (Figure 2.8).

- When a chart is unavailable, the health care professional still must provide medical care. Thus, providers make do without past data, basing their decisions instead on what the patient can tell them and on what their examination reveals. They then write a note for inclusion in the chart—when the chart is located. In a large institution with thousands of medical records, it is not surprising that such loose notes often fail to make it to the patient's chart or are filed out of sequence so that the actual chronology of management is disrupted in the record.

- When patients who have chronic or frequent diseases are seen over months or years, their records grow so large that the charts must be broken up into multiple volumes. When a hospital clinic or emergency room orders the patient's chart, only the most recent volume typically is provided. Old but pertinent data may be in early volumes that are stored offsite or are otherwise unavailable.

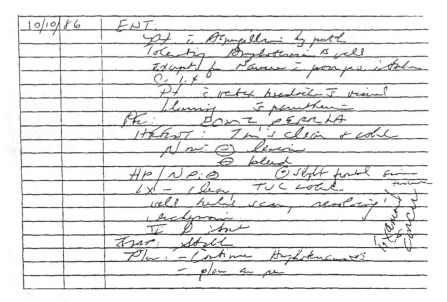

Figure 2.8. Written entries are standard in paper records, yet handwritten notes may be illegible. Notes that cannot be interpreted by other people may cause delays in treatment or inappropriate care.

As described in Chapter 12, computer-based medical record systems offer potential solutions to all these practical problems in the use of the paper record.

2.3.2   Redundancy and Inefficiency

To be able to find data quickly in the chart, health professionals have developed a variety of techniques that provide redundant recording to match alternate modes of access. For example, the result of a radiologic study typically is entered on a standard radiology reporting form, which is filed in the portion of the chart labeled "X-ray." For complicated procedures, the same data often are summarized in brief notes by radiologists in the narrative part of the chart, which they enter at the time of studies because they know that the formal report will not make it back to the chart for 1 or 2 days. In addition, the study results often are mentioned in notes written by the patient's admitting and consulting physicians and by the nursing staff. Although there may be good reasons for recording such information multiple times in different ways and in different locations within the chart, the combined bulk of these notes accelerates the physical growth of the document and, accordingly, complicates the chart's logistical management. Furthermore, it becomes increasingly difficult to locate specific patient data as the chart succumbs to obesity. The predictable result is that someone writes yet another redundant entry, summarizing information that it took hours to track down.

A similar inefficiency occurs because of a tension between opposing goals in the design of reporting forms used by many laboratories. Most health personnel prefer a consistent, familiar paper form, often with color-coding, because it helps them to find information more quickly (Figure 2.9). For example, a physician may know that a urinalysis report form is printed on yellow paper and records the bacteria count halfway down the middle column of the form. This knowledge allows the physician to work backward quickly in the laboratory section of the chart to find the most recent urinalysis sheet and to check at a glance the bacterial count. The problem is that such forms typically store only sparse information. It is clearly suboptimal if a rapidly growing physical chart is filled with sheets of paper that report only a single datum.

2.3.3   Influence on Clinical Research

Anyone who has participated in a clinical research project based on chart review can attest to the tediousness of flipping through myriad medical records. For all the reasons described in Section 1.1 (see Figure 1.4), it is arduous to sit with stacks of patients' charts, extracting data and formatting them for structured statistical analysis, and the process is vulnerable to transcription errors. Observers often wonder how much medical knowledge is sitting untapped in medical records because there is no easy way to analyze experience across large populations of patients without first extracting pertinent data from the paper records.

Suppose, for example, that a physician notices that patients receiving a certain common oral medication for diabetes (call it drug X) seem to be more likely to have significant postoperative hypotension (low blood pressure) than do surgical patients receiving other medications for diabetes. The doctor has based his hypothesis—that drug X influences postoperative blood pressure—on only a few recent observations, however, so he

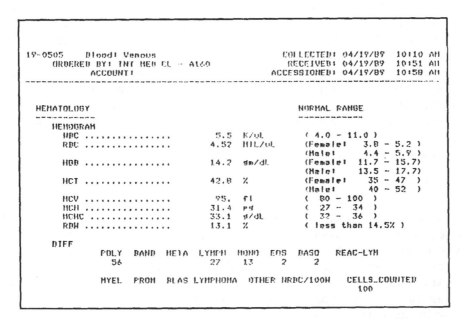

Figure 2.9. Laboratory reporting forms record medical data in a consistent, familiar format.

or she decides to look into existing hospital records to see whether this correlation has occurred with sufficient frequency to warrant a formal investigation. The best way to follow up on his or her theory from existing medical data would be to examine the hospital charts of all patients who have diabetes and also have been admitted for surgery. The task would then be to examine those charts and to note for all patients (1) whether they were taking drug X when admitted and (2) whether they had postoperative hypotension. If the statistics showed that patients receiving drug X were more likely to have low blood pressure after surgery than were similar diabetic patients receiving alternate treatments, a controlled trial (prospective observation and data gathering) might well be appropriate.

Note the distinction between **retrospective chart review** to investigate a question that was not a subject of study at the time the data were collected and **prospective studies** in which the clinical hypothesis is known in advance and the **research protocol** is designed specifically to collect future data that are relevant to the question under consideration. Subjects are assigned **randomly** to different study groups to help prevent researchers— who are bound to be biased, having developed the hypothesis—from unintentionally skewing the results by assigning a specific class of patients all to one group. For the same reason, to the extent possible, the studies are **double blind**; i.e., neither the researchers nor the subjects know which treatment is being administered. Such blinding is of course impractical when it is obvious to patients or physicians what therapy is being given (such as surgical procedures versus drug therapy). Prospective, randomized, double-blind studies are considered the best method for determining optimal management of disease.

Returning to our example, consider the problems in chart review that the researcher would encounter in addressing the postoperative hypotension question retrospectively. First, he would have to identify the charts of interest: the subset of medical records dealing with surgical patients who are also diabetic. In a hospital record room filled with thousands of charts, the task of chart selection can be overwhelming. Medical records departments generally do keep indexes of diagnostic and procedure codes cross-referenced to specific patients (see Section 2.4.1). Thus, it might be possible to use such an index to find all charts in which the discharge diagnoses included diabetes and the procedure codes included major surgical procedures. The researcher might compile a list of patient identification numbers and have the individual charts pulled from the file room for review.

The researcher's next task is to examine each chart serially to find out what treatment the patient was receiving for diabetes at the time of the surgery *and* to determine whether the patient had postoperative hypotension. Finding such information may be extremely time-consuming. Where should the researcher look for it? The admission drug orders might show what the patient received for diabetes control, but it would also be wise to check the medication sheets to see whether the therapy was also administered (as well as ordered) and the admission history to see whether a routine treatment for diabetes, taken right up until the patient entered the hospital, was not administered during the inpatient stay. Information about hypotensive episodes might be similarly difficult to locate. The researcher might start with nursing notes from the recovery room or with the anesthesiologist's datasheets from the operating room, but the patient might not have been hypotensive until after leaving the recovery room and returning to the ward. So the nursing notes from the ward need to be checked too, as well as vital signs sheets, physicians' progress notes, and the discharge summary.

It should be clear from this example that retrospective chart review is a laborious and tedious process and that people performing it are prone to make transcription errors and to overlook key data. One of the great appeals of EHRs is their potential ability to facilitate the chart review process. They obviate the need to retrieve hard copy charts; instead, researchers can use computer-based data retrieval and analysis techniques to do most of the work (finding relevant patients, locating pertinent data, and formatting the information for statistical analyses). Researchers can use similar techniques to harness computer assistance with data management in prospective clinical trials.

2.3.4   The Passive Nature of Paper Records

The traditional manual system has another limitation that would have been meaningless until the emergence of the computer age. A manual archival system is inherently passive; the charts sit waiting for something to be done with them. They are insensitive to the characteristics of the data recorded within their pages, such as legibility, accuracy, or implications for patient management. They cannot take an active role in responding appropriately to those implications.

Increasingly, EHR systems have changed our perspective on what health professionals can expect from the medical chart. Automated record systems introduce new opportunities for dynamic responses to the data that are recorded in them. As described in many of the chapters to follow, computational techniques for data storage, retrieval, and analysis make it feasible to develop record systems that (1) monitor their contents and generate warnings or advice for providers based on single observations or on logical combinations of data; (2) provide automated quality control, including the flagging of potentially erroneous data; or (3) provide feedback on patient-specific or population-based deviations from desirable standards.

2.4   The Structure of Medical Data

Scientific disciplines generally develop a precise terminology or notation that is standardized and accepted by all workers in the field. Consider, for example, the universal language of chemistry embodied in chemical formulae, the precise definitions and mathematical equations used by physicists, the predicate calculus used by logicians, or the conventions for describing circuits used by electrical engineers. Medicine is remarkable for its failure to develop a standardized vocabulary and **nomenclature**, and many observers believe that a true scientific basis for the field will be impossible until this problem is addressed (see Chapter 7). Other people argue that common references to the "art of medicine" reflect an important distinction between medicine and the "hard" sciences; these people question whether it is possible to introduce too much standardization into a field that prides itself in humanism.

The debate has been accentuated by the introduction of computers for data management, because such machines tend to demand conformity to data standards and definitions. Otherwise, issues of data retrieval and analysis are confounded by discrepancies between the meanings intended by the observers or recorders and those intended by the individuals retrieving information or doing data analysis. What is an "upper respiratory infection"? Does it include infections of the trachea or of the mainstem bronchi? How large does the heart have to be before we can refer to "cardiomegaly"? How should we deal with the plethora of disease names based on eponyms (e.g., Alzheimer's disease, Hodgkin's disease) that are not descriptive of the illness and may not be familiar to all practitioners? What do we mean by an "acute abdomen"? Are the boundaries of the abdomen well agreed on? What are the time constraints that correspond to "acuteness" of abdominal pain? Is an "ache" a pain? What about "occasional" cramping?

Imprecision and the lack of a standardized vocabulary are particularly problematic when we wish to aggregate data recorded by multiple health professionals or to analyze trends over time. Without a controlled, predefined vocabulary, data interpretation is inherently complicated, and the automatic summarization of data may be impossible. For example, one physician might note that a patient has "shortness of breath." Later, another physician might note that she has "dyspnea." Unless these terms are designated as synonyms, an automated flowcharting program will fail to indicate that the patient had the same problem on both occasions.

Regardless of arguments regarding the "artistic" elements in medicine, the need for health personnel to communicate effectively is clear both in acute care settings and when patients are seen over long periods. Both high-quality care and scientific progress depend on *some* standardization in terminology. Otherwise, differences in intended meaning or in defining criteria will lead to miscommunication, improper interpretation, and potentially negative consequences for the patients involved.

Given the lack of formal definitions for many medical terms, it is remarkable that medical workers communicate as well as they do. Only occasionally is the care for a patient clearly compromised by miscommunication. If EHRs are to become dynamic and responsive manipulators of patient data, however, their encoded logic must be able to presume a specific meaning for the terms and data elements entered by the observers. This point is discussed in greater detail in Chapter 7, which deals with the multiple efforts to develop health care–computing standards, including a shared, controlled terminology for biomedicine.

2.4.1 Coding Systems

We are used to seeing figures regarding the growing incidences of certain types of tumors, deaths from influenza during the winter months, and similar health statistics that we tend to take for granted. How are such data accumulated? Their role in health planning and health care financing is clear, but if their accumulation required chart review through the process described earlier in this chapter, we would know much less about the health status of the populations in various communities (see Chapter 15).

Because of the needs to know about health trends for populations and to recognize epidemics in their early stages, there are various health-reporting requirements for hospitals (as well as other public organizations) and practitioners. For example, cases of gonorrhea, syphilis, and tuberculosis generally must be reported to local public-health organizations, which code the data to allow trend analyses over time. The Centers for Disease Control and Prevention in Atlanta then pool regional data and report national as well as local trends in disease incidence, bacterial-resistance patterns, etc.

Another kind of reporting involves the coding of all discharge diagnoses for hospitalized patients, plus coding of certain procedures (e.g., type of surgery) that were performed during the hospital stay. Such codes are reported to state and federal health-planning and analysis agencies and also are used internally at the institution for case-mix analysis (determining the relative frequencies of various disorders in the hospitalized population and the average length of stay for each disease category) and for research. For such data to be useful, the codes must be well defined as well as uniformly applied and accepted.

The government publishes a national diagnostic coding scheme called the International Classification of Disease (ICD). Its current version is used by all nonmilitary hospitals in the United States for discharge coding, and must be reported on the bills submitted to most insurance companies (Figure 2.10). Pathologists have developed another widely used diagnostic coding scheme; originally known as Systematized Nomenclature of Pathology (SNOP), it has been expanded to Systematized Nomenclature of Medicine (SNOMED) (Côté and Robboy, 1980; American College of Pathologists, 1982). Another coding scheme developed by the American Medical Association is the Current Procedural Terminology (CPT) (Finkel, 1977). It is similarly widely used in producing bills for services rendered to patients. More details on such schemes are provided in Chapter 7. What warrants emphasis here, however, is the motivation for the codes' development: health care personnel need standardized terms that can support pooling of data for analysis and can provide criteria for determining charges for individual patients.

The historical roots of a coding system reveal themselves as limitations or idiosyncrasies when the system is applied in more general clinical settings. For example, the ICD-9 code was derived from a classification scheme developed for epidemiologic reporting. Consequently, it has more than 50 separate codes for describing tuberculosis infections. SNOMED permits coding of pathologic findings in exquisite detail but only recently has begun to introduce codes for expressing the dimensions of a patient's functional status. In a particular clinical setting, none of the common coding schemes is likely to be completely satisfactory. In some cases, the granularity of the code will be too coarse; on the one hand, a hematologist (person who studies blood diseases) may want to distinguish among a variety of hemoglobinopathies (disorders of the structure and function of hemoglobin) lumped under a single code in ICD. On the other hand, another practitioner may prefer to aggregate many individual codes—e.g., those for active tuberculosis—into a single category to simplify the coding and retrieval of data.

Such schemes cannot be effective unless health care providers accept them. There is an inherent tension between the need for a coding system that is general enough to cover many different patients and the need for precise and unique terms that accurately apply

CHRONIC OBSTRUCTIVE PULMONARY DISEASE AND ALLIED CONDITIONS
(490-496)

490   Bronchitis, not specified as acute or chronic

491   Chronic bronchitis

    491.0 Simple chronic bronchitis
    491.1 Mucopurulent chronic bronchitis
    491.2 Obstructive chronic bronchitis
    491.8 Other chronic bronchitis
    491.9 Unspecified chronic bronchitis

492 Emphysema

    492.0 Emphysematous bleb
    492.8 Other emphysema

493 Asthma

    493.0 Extrinsic asthma
    493.1 Intrinsic asthma
    493.9 Asthma, unspecified

494 Bronchiectasis

495 Extrinsic allergic alveolitis

    495.0 Farmer's lung
    495.1 Bagassosis
    495.2 Bird-fanciers' lung
    495.3 Suberosis
    495.4 Malt workers' lung
    495.5 Mushroom workers' lung
    495.6 Maple bark-strippers' lung
    495.7 "Ventilation" pneumonitis
    495.8 Other specified allergic alveolitis and pneumonitis
        Cheese-washers' lung, Coffee workers' lung, Fish-meal workers' lung,
        Furriers' lung, Grain-handlers' disease or lung, Pituitary snuff-takers'
        disease, Sequoiosis or red-cedar asthma, Wood asthma
    495.9 Unspecified allergic alveolitis and pneumonitis

Figure 2.10. A small subset of the disease categories identified by the Ninth International Classification of Disease, Clinical Modification (ICD-9-CM). (*Source*: Health Care Financing Administration [1980]. *The International Classification of Diseases, 9th Revision, Clinical Modification, ICD-9-CM.* U.S. Department of Health and Human Services, Washington, D.C. DHHS Publication No. [PHS] 80-1260.)

to a specific patient and do not unduly constrain physicians' attempts to describe what they observe. Yet if physicians view the EHR as a blank sheet of paper on which any unstructured information can be written, the data they record will be unsuitable for dynamic processing, clinical research, and health planning. The challenge is to learn how to meet all these needs. Researchers at many institutions have worked for over a decade to develop a unified medical language system (UMLS), a common structure that ties together the various vocabularies that have been created. At the same time, the developers of specific terminologies are continually working to refine and expand their independent coding schemes (Humphreys et al., 1998) (see Chapter 7).

2.4.2   The Data-to-Knowledge Spectrum

A central focus in medical informatics is the information base that constitutes the "substance of medicine." Workers in the field have tried to clarify the distinctions among three terms frequently used to describe the content of computer-based systems: data, information, and knowledge (Blum, 1986b). These terms are often used interchangeably. In this volume, we shall refer to a **datum** as a single observational point that characterizes a relationship.[5] It generally can be regarded as the value of a specific parameter for a particular object (e.g., a patient) at a given point in time. **Knowledge**, then, is derived through the formal or informal analysis (or interpretation) of data. Thus, it includes the results of formal studies and also common sense facts, assumptions, heuristics (strategic rules of thumb), and models—any of which may reflect the experience or biases of people who interpret the primary data. The term **information** is more generic in that it encompasses both organized data and knowledge, although data are not information until they have been organized in some way for analysis or display.

The observation that patient Brown has a blood pressure of 180/110 is a *datum*, as is the report that the patient has had a myocardial infarction (heart attack). When researchers pool and analyze such data, they may determine that patients with high blood pressure are more likely to have heart attacks than are patients with normal or low blood pressure. This data analysis has produced a piece of *knowledge* about the world. A physician's belief that prescribing dietary restriction of salt is unlikely to be effective in controlling high blood pressure in patients of low economic standing (because the latter are less likely to be able to afford special low-salt foods) is an additional personal piece of *knowledge*—a **heuristic** that guides physicians in their decision making. Note that the appropriate interpretation of these definitions depends on the context. Knowledge at one level of abstraction may be considered data at higher levels. A blood pressure of 180/110 mm Hg is a raw piece of data; the statement that the patient has hypertension is an interpretation of that data and thus represents a higher level of knowledge. As input to a diagnostic decision aid, however, the presence or absence of hypertension may be requested, in which case the presence of hypertension is treated as a data item.

A **database** is a collection of individual observations without any summarizing analysis. An EHR system is thus primarily viewed as a database—the place where patient data are stored. A **knowledge base**, on the other hand, is a collection of facts, heuristics, and models that can be used for problem solving and analysis of data. If the knowledge base provides sufficient structure, including semantic links among knowledge items, the computer itself may be able to apply that knowledge as an aid to case-based problem

---

[5]Note that data is a plural term, although it is often erroneously used in speech and writing as though it were singular.

solving. Many decision-support systems have been called *knowledge-based systems*, reflecting this distinction between knowledge bases and databases (see Chapter 20).

2.5   Strategies of Medical Data Selection and Use

It is illusory to conceive of a "complete medical data set." All medical databases, and medical records, are necessarily incomplete because they reflect the selective collection and recording of data by the health care personnel responsible for the patient. There can be marked interpersonal differences in both style and problem solving that account for variations in the way practitioners collect and record data for the same patient under the same circumstances. Such variations do not necessarily reflect good practices, however, and much of medical education is directed at helping physicians and other health professionals to learn what observations to make, how to make them (generally an issue of technique), how to interpret them, and how to decide whether they warrant formal recording.

An example of this phenomenon is the difference between the first medical history, physical examination, and written report developed by a medical student and the similar process undertaken by a seasoned clinician examining the same patient. Medical students tend to work from comprehensive mental outlines of questions to ask, physical tests to perform, and additional data to collect. Because they have not developed skills of selectivity, the process of taking a medical history and performing a physical examination may take more than 1 hour, after which students write extensive reports of what they observed and how they have interpreted their observations. It clearly would be impractical, inefficient, and inappropriate for physicians in practice to spend this amount of time assessing every new patient. Thus, part of the challenge for the neophyte is to learn how to ask only the questions that are necessary, to perform only the examination components that are required, and to record only those data that will be pertinent in justifying the ongoing diagnostic approach and in guiding the future management of the patient.

What do we mean by **selectivity** in data collection and recording? It is precisely this process that often is viewed as a central part of the "art of medicine," an element that accounts for individual styles and the sometimes marked distinctions among clinicians. As is discussed with numerous clinical examples in Chapters 3 and 4, the idea of selectivity implies an ongoing decision-making process that guides data collection and interpretation. Attempts to understand how expert clinicians internalize this process, and to formalize the ideas so that they can better be taught and explained, are central in biomedical informatics research. Improved guidelines for such decision making, derived from research activities in biomedical informatics, not only are enhancing the teaching and practice of medicine but also are providing insights that suggest methods for developing computer-based decision-support tools.

2.5.1   *The Hypothetico-Deductive Approach*

Studies of medical decision makers have shown that strategies for data collection and interpretation may be imbedded in an iterative process known as the **hypothetico-**

deductive approach (Elstein et al., 1978; Kassirer and Gorry, 1978). As medical students learn this process, their data collection becomes more focused and efficient, and their medical records become more compact. The central idea is one of sequential, staged data collection, followed by data interpretation and the generation of hypotheses, leading to hypothesis-directed selection of the next most appropriate data to be collected. As data are collected at each stage, they are added to the growing database of observations and are used to reformulate or refine the active hypotheses. This process is iterated until one hypothesis reaches a threshold level of certainty (e.g., it is proved to be true, or at least the uncertainty is reduced to a satisfactory level). At that point, a management, disposition, or therapeutic decision can be made.

The diagram in Figure 2.11 clarifies this process. As is shown, data collection begins when the patient presents to the physician with some complaint (a symptom or disease). The physician generally responds with a few questions that allow one to focus rapidly on the nature of the problem. In the written report, the data collected with these initial questions typically are recorded as the patient identification, chief complaint, and initial portion of the history of the present illness. Studies have shown that an experienced physician will have an initial set of hypotheses (theories) in mind after hearing the patient's response to the first six or seven questions (Elstein et al., 1978). These hypotheses then serve as the basis for selecting additional questions. As shown in Figure 2.11, answers to these additional questions allow the physician to refine hypotheses about what is the source of the patient's problem. Physicians refer to the set of active hypotheses as the differential diagnosis for a patient; the **differential diagnosis** comprises the set

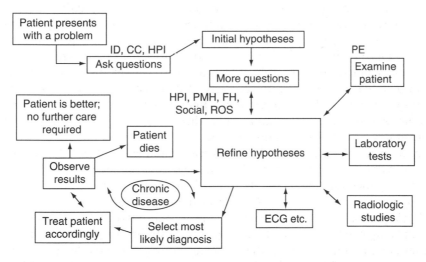

Figure 2.11. A schematic view of the hypothetico-deductive approach. The process of medical data collection and treatment is intimately tied to an ongoing process of hypothesis generation and refinement. See text for full discussion. ID = patient identification; CC = chief complaint; HPI = history of present illness; PMH = past medical history; FH = family history; Social = social history; ROS = review of systems; PE = physical examination.

of possible diagnoses among which the physician must distinguish to determine how best to administer treatment.

Note that the question selection process is inherently heuristic; e.g., it is personalized and efficient, but it is not guaranteed to collect every piece of information that might be pertinent. Human beings use heuristics all the time in their decision making because it often is impractical or impossible to use an exhaustive problem-solving approach. A common example of heuristic problem solving is the playing of a complex game such as chess. Because it would require an enormous amount of time to define all the possible moves and countermoves that could ensue from a given board position, expert chess players develop personal heuristics for assessing the game at any point and then selecting a strategy for how best to proceed. Differences among such heuristics account in part for variations in observed expertise.

Physicians have developed safety measures, however, to help them avoid missing important issues that they might not discover when collecting data in a hypothesis-directed fashion during the history taking for the present illness (Pauker et al., 1976). These measures tend to be focused in four general categories of questions that follow the collection of information about the chief complaint: past medical history, family history, social history, and a brief **review of systems** in which the physician asks some general questions about the state of health of each of the major organ systems in the body. Occasionally, the physician discovers entirely new problems or finds important information that modifies the hypothesis list or modulates the treatment options available (e.g., if the patient reports a serious past drug reaction or allergy).

When physicians have finished asking questions, the refined hypothesis list (which may already be narrowed to a single diagnosis) then serves as the basis for a focused physical examination. By this time, physicians may well have expectations of what they will find on examination or may have specific tests in mind that will help them to distinguish among still active hypotheses about diseases based on the questions that they have asked. Once again, as in the question-asking process, focused hypothesis-directed examination is augmented with general tests that occasionally turn up new abnormalities and generate hypotheses that the physician did not expect on the basis of the medical history alone. In addition, unexplained findings on examination may raise issues that require additional history taking. Thus, the asking of questions generally is partially integrated with the examination process.

When physicians have completed the physical examination, their refined hypothesis list may be narrowed sufficiently that they can undertake specific treatment. It often is necessary to gather additional data, however. Such testing is once again guided by the current hypotheses. The options available include laboratory tests (of blood, urine, other body fluids, or biopsy specimens), radiologic studies (X-ray examinations, nuclear-imaging scans, computed tomography (CT) studies, magnetic resonance scans, sonograms, or any of a number of other imaging modalities), and other specialized tests (electrocardiograms (ECGs), electroencephalograms, nerve conduction studies, and many others). As the results of such studies become available, physicians constantly revise and refine their hypothesis list.

Ultimately, physicians are sufficiently certain about the source of a patient's problem to be able to develop a specific management plan. Treatments are administered, and the patient is observed. Note that the response to treatment is itself a datum point that may affect the hypotheses about a patient's illness. If patients do not respond to treatment, it may mean that their disease is resistant to that therapy and that their physicians should try an alternate approach, or it may mean that the initial diagnosis was incorrect and that physicians should consider alternate explanations for the patient's complaint.

The patient may remain in a cycle of treatment and observation for a long time, as shown in Figure 2.11. This long cycle reflects the nature of chronic-disease management—an aspect of medical care that is accounting for an increasing proportion of the health care community's work (and an increasing proportion of the health care dollar). Alternatively, the patient may recover and no longer need therapy, or he or she may die. Although the process outlined in Figure 2.11 is oversimplified in many regards, it is generally applicable to the process of data collection, diagnosis, and treatment in most areas of medicine.

Note that the hypothesis-directed process of data collection, diagnosis, and treatment is inherently *knowledge-based*. It is dependent not only on a significant fact base that permits proper interpretation of data and selection of appropriate follow-up questions and tests but also on the effective use of heuristic techniques that characterize individual expertise.

Another important issue, addressed in Chapter 3, is the need for physicians to balance financial costs and health risks of data collection against the perceived benefits to be gained when those data become available. It costs nothing but time to examine the patient at the bedside or to ask an additional question, but if the data being considered require, for example, X-ray exposure, coronary angiography, or a CT scan of the head (all of which have associated risks and costs), then it may be preferable to proceed with treatment in the absence of full information. Differences in the assessment of cost-benefit trade-offs in data collection, and variations among individuals in their willingness to make decisions under uncertainty, often account for differences of opinion among collaborating physicians.

2.5.2 *The Relationship Between Data and Hypotheses*

We wrote rather glibly in Section 2.5.1 about the "generation of hypotheses from data"; now we need to ask: What precisely is the nature of that process? As is discussed in Chapter 4, researchers with a psychological orientation have spent much time trying to understand how expert problem solvers evoke hypotheses (Pauker et al., 1976; Elstein et al., 1978; Pople, 1982) and the traditional probabilistic decision sciences have much to say about that process as well. We provide only a brief introduction to these ideas here; they are discussed in greater detail in Chapters 3 and 4.

When an observation evokes a hypothesis (e.g., when a clinical finding makes a specific diagnosis come to mind), the observation presumably has some close association with the hypothesis. What might be the characteristics of that association? Perhaps the finding is almost always observed when the hypothesis turns out to be true. Is that enough to explain hypothesis generation? A simple example will show that such a simple relationship is not enough to explain the evocation process. Consider the hypothesis that a patient is pregnant and the observation that the patient is female. Clearly, all pregnant patients are female. When a new patient is observed to be female, however, the possibility that the patient is pregnant is not immediately evoked. Thus, female gender is a highly *sensitive* indicator of pregnancy (there is a 100 percent certainty that a pregnant patient is female), but it is not a good *predictor* of pregnancy (most females are not pregnant). The idea of **sensitivity**—the likelihood that a given datum will be observed in a patient with a given disease or condition—is an important one, but it will not alone account for the process of hypothesis generation in medical diagnosis.

Perhaps the clinical manifestation seldom occurs unless the hypothesis turns out to be true; is that enough to explain hypothesis generation? This idea seems to be a little closer to the mark. Suppose a given datum is *never* seen unless a patient has a specific disease. For example, a Pap smear (a smear of cells swabbed from the cervix, at the opening to the uterus, treated with Papanicolaou's stain, and then examined under the microscope) with grossly abnormal cells (called class IV findings) is never seen unless the woman has cancer of the cervix or uterus. Such tests are called **pathognomonic**. Not only do they evoke a specific diagnosis but they also immediately prove it to be true. Unfortunately, there are few pathognomonic tests in medicine.

More commonly, a feature is seen in one disease or disease category more frequently than it is in others, but the association is not absolute. For example, there are few disease entities other than infections that elevate a patient's white blood cell count. Certainly it is true, for example, that leukemia can raise the white blood cell count, as can the use of the drug prednisone, but most patients who do not have infections will have normal white blood cell counts. An elevated white count therefore does not *prove* that a patient has an infection, but it does tend to evoke or support the hypothesis that an infection is present. The word used to describe this relationship is **specificity**. An observation is highly specific for a disease if it is generally not seen in patients who do not have that disease. A pathognomonic observation is 100 percent specific for a given disease. When an observation is highly specific for a disease, it tends to evoke that disease during the diagnostic or data-gathering process.

By now, you may have realized that there is a substantial difference between a physician viewing test results that evoke a disease hypothesis and that physician being willing to act on the disease hypothesis. Yet even experienced physicians sometimes fail to recognize that, although they have made an observation that is highly specific for a given disease, it may still be more likely that the patient has other diseases (and does not have the suspected one) unless (1) the finding is pathognomonic or (2) the suspected disease is considerably more common than are the other diseases that can cause the observed abnormality. This mistake is one of the most common errors of intuition that has been identified in the medical decision-making process. To explain the basis for this confusion in more detail, we must introduce two additional terms: *prevalence* and *predictive value*.

The **prevalence** of a disease is simply a measure of the frequency with which the disease occurs in the population of interest. A given disease may have a prevalence of only 5 percent in the general population (1 person in 20 will have the disease) but have a higher prevalence in a specially selected subpopulation. For example, black-lung disease has a low prevalence in the general population but has a much higher prevalence among coal miners, who develop black lung from inhaling coal dust. The task of diagnosis therefore involves updating the probability that a patient has a disease from the **baseline rate** (the prevalence in the population from which the patient was selected) to a post-test probability that reflects the test results. For example, the probability that any given person in the United States has lung cancer is low (i.e., the prevalence of the disease is low), but it is much higher if his or her chest X-ray examination shows a possible tumor. If the patient were a member of the population composed of cigarette smokers in the United States, however, the prevalence of lung cancer would be higher. In this case, the same chest X-ray report would result in an even higher updated probability of lung cancer than it would had the patient been selected from the population of all people in the United States.

The **predictive value (PV)** of a test is simply the post-test (updated) *probability* that a disease is present based on the results of a test. If an observation supports the presence of a disease, the PV will be greater than the prevalence (also called the *pretest risk*). If the observation tends to argue against the presence of a disease, the PV will be lower than the prevalence. For any test and disease, then, there is one PV if the test result is positive and another PV if the test result is negative. These values are typically abbreviated PV^+ (the PV of a positive test) and PV^- (the PV of a negative test).

The process of hypothesis generation in medical diagnosis thus involves both the evocation of hypotheses *and* the assignment of a likelihood (probability) to the presence of a specific disease or disease category. The PV of a positive test depends on the test's sensitivity, specificity, and prevalence. The formula that describes the relationship precisely is:

$$PV^+ = \frac{(\text{sensitivity}) (\text{prevalence})}{(\text{sensitivity}) (\text{prevalence}) + (1 - \text{specificity}) (1 - \text{prevalence})}$$

There is a similar formula for defining PV^- in terms of sensitivity, specificity, and prevalence. Both formulae can be derived from simple probability theory. Note that positive tests with high sensitivity and specificity may still lead to a low post-test probability of the disease (PV^+) if the prevalence of that disease is low. You should substitute values in the PV^+ formula to convince yourself that this assertion is true. It is this relationship that tends to be poorly understood by practitioners and that often is viewed as counterintuitive (which shows that your intuition can misguide you!). Note also (by substitution into the formula) that test sensitivity and disease prevalence can be ignored only when a test is pathognomonic (i.e., when its specificity is 100 percent, which mandates that PV^+ be 100 percent). The PV^+ formula is one of many forms of *Bayes' theorem*, a rule for combining probabilistic data that is generally attributed to the work of Reverend Thomas Bayes in the 1700s. Bayes' theorem is discussed in greater detail in Chapter 3.

2.5.3   *Methods for Selecting Questions and Comparing Tests*

We have described the process of hypothesis-directed sequential data collection and have asked how an observation might evoke or refine the physician's hypotheses about what abnormalities account for the patient's illness. The complementary question is: Given a set of current hypotheses, how does the physician decide what additional data should be collected? This question also has been analyzed at length (Elstein et al., 1978; Pople, 1982) and is pertinent for computer programs that gather data efficiently to assist clinicians with diagnosis or with therapeutic decision making (see Chapter 20). Because understanding issues of test selection and data interpretation is crucial to understanding medical data and their uses, we devote Chapter 3 to these and related issues of medical decision making. In Section 3.6, for example, we shall discuss the use of decision-analytic techniques in deciding whether to treat a patient on the basis of available information or to perform additional diagnostic tests.

2.6   The Computer and Collection of Medical Data

Although this chapter has not directly discussed computer systems, the potential role of the computer in medical data storage, retrieval, and interpretation should be clear. Much of the rest of this book deals with specific applications in which the computer's primary role is data management. One question is pertinent to all such applications: How do you get the data into the computer in the first place?

The need for data entry by physicians has posed a problem for medical-computing systems since the earliest days of the field. Awkward or nonintuitive interactions at computer terminals—particularly ones requiring keyboard typing by the physician—have probably done more to inhibit the clinical use of computers than have any other factor. Doctors, and many other health care staff, tend simply to refuse to use computers because of the awkward interfaces that are imposed.

A variety of approaches have been used to try to finesse this problem. One is to design systems such that clerical staff can do essentially all the data entry and much of the data retrieval as well. Many clinical research systems have taken this approach. Physicians may be asked to fill out structured paper datasheets, or such sheets may be filled out by data abstractors who review patient charts, but the actual entry of data into the database is done by paid transcriptionists.

In some applications, it is possible for data to be entered automatically into the computer by the device that measures or collects them. For example, monitors in intensive care or coronary care units, pulmonary function or ECG machines, and measurement equipment in the clinical chemistry laboratory can interface directly with a computer in which a database is stored. Certain data can be entered directly by patients; there are systems, for example, that take the patient's history by presenting on a computer screen multiple-choice questions that follow a branching logic. The patient's responses to the questions are used to generate electronic or hard copy reports for physicians and also may be stored directly in a computer database for subsequent use in other settings.

When physicians or other health personnel do use the machine themselves, specialized devices often allow rapid and intuitive operator–machine interaction. Most of these devices use a variant of the "point-and-select" approach—e.g., touch-sensitive screens, light pens, and mouse-pointing devices (see Chapter 5). When conventional terminals are used, specialized keypads can be helpful. Designers frequently permit logical selection of items from menus displayed on the screen so that the user does not need to learn a set of specialized commands to enter or review data. Recently we have seen the introduction of handheld tablets with pen-based mechanisms for data entry. Some of the experimental work on pen-based methods for structured clinical data entry is particularly promising (Figure 2.12). **Personal digital assistants (PDAs)** have also begun to

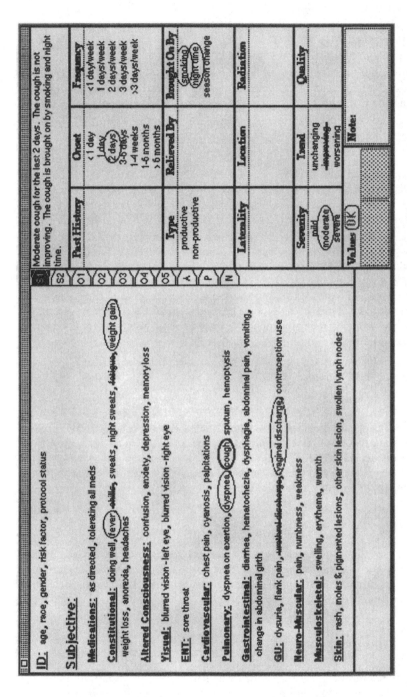

Figure 2.12. The user interface for PEN-Ivory, a prototype system for the entry of progress notes. The left side of the screen represents the encounter form on which the names of medical findings are listed. The right side represents the attributes palette, used to augment findings with specific modifiers (in this case, modifiers refer to "cough," the current entry, which is circled in bold on the encounter form. Users circle, line out, and scratch out words to interact with the system. A text translation of the selected finding and its attributes is displayed at the top right. The page tabs located between the encounter form and the attributes palette are used to move among the pages of the encounter form. (Example screen courtesy of Alex Poon. See also Poon A.D., Fagan L.M., Shortliffe E.H. [1996]. The PEN-Ivory project: Exploring user-interface design for the selection of items from large controlled vocabularies of medicine. *Journal of the American Medical Informatics Association*, 3(2):168–183).

transform both data collection and information access. With the introduction of **wireless networking**, such devices are allowing clinicians to maintain normal mobility (in and out of examining rooms or inpatient rooms) while accessing and entering data that are pertinent to a patient's care.

These issues arise in essentially all application areas, and, because they can be crucial to the successful implementation and use of a system, they warrant particular attention in system design. As more physicians are becoming familiar with computers at home, they will find the use of computers in their practice less of a hindrance. We encourage you to consider human–computer interaction as you learn about the application areas and the specific systems described in later chapters.

Suggested Readings

Campbell J.R., Carpenter P., Sneiderman C., Cohn S., Chute C.G., Warren J. (1997). Phase II evaluation of clinical coding schemes: Completeness, taxonomy, mapping, definitions, and clarity. *Journal of the American Medical Informatics Association*, 4(3):238–251; and Chute C.G., Cohn S., Campbell K.E., Oliver D., Campbell J.R. (1996). The content coverage of clinical classifications. *Journal of the American Medical Informatics Association*, 3(3):224–233.

This pair of articles reports on a detailed study of various systems for coding clinical terminology. The authors attempt to characterize each coding scheme with respect to its ability to express common clinical concepts, demonstrating that none was yet sufficiently robust to encode the complete medical record of a patient.

Patel V.L., Arocha J.F., Kaufman, D.R. (1994). Diagnostic reasoning and medical expertise. *Psychology of Learning and Motivation*, 31:187–252.

This paper illustrates the role of theory-driven psychological research and cognitive evaluation as they relate to medical decision making and the interpretation of clinical data. See also Chapter 4.

Terry K. (2002). Beam it up, doctor: Inexpensive wireless networking technology, now available on PDAs and tablet computers, can connect you with clinical and scheduling data throughout your office. *Medical Economics*, 79(13):34–36.

This article, targeted at practicing clinicians, describes the opportunities for using clinical software on wireless PDAs in outpatient practice settings.

van Bemmel J.H., et al. (Eds.) (1988). Data, information and knowledge in medicine. *Methods of Information in Medicine*, Special issue, 27(3).

This special issue of *Methods of Information in Medicine* contains about 40 articles that were published previously in the journal. It provides a historical perspective on scientific developments in biomedical informatics. The first section presents 10 papers on various aspects of medical data. The remaining sections are devoted to medical systems, medical information and patterns, medical knowledge and decision making, and medical research.

Questions for Discussion

1. You check your pulse and discover that your heart rate is 100 beats per minute. Is this rate normal or abnormal? What additional information would you use in making this

judgment? How does the context in which data are collected influence the interpretation of those data?

2. Given the imprecision of many medical terms, why do you think that serious instances of miscommunication among health care professionals are not more common? Why is greater standardization of terminology necessary if computers rather than humans are to manipulate patient data?

3. Based on the discussion of coding schemes for representing medical information, discuss three challenges you foresee in attempting to construct a standardized medical terminology to be used in hospitals, physicians' offices, and research institutions throughout the United States.

4. How would medical practice change if nonphysicians were to collect all medical data?

5. Consider what you know about the typical daily schedule of a busy clinician. What are the advantages of wireless devices, connected to the Internet, as tools for such clinicians? Can you think of disadvantages as well? Be sure to consider the safety and protection of information as well as workflow and clinical needs.

6. To decide whether a patient has a significant urinary tract infection, physicians commonly use a calculation of the number of bacterial organisms in a milliliter of the patient's urine. Physicians generally assume that a patient has a urinary tract infection if there are at least 10,000 bacteria per milliliter. Although laboratories can provide such quantification with reasonable accuracy, it is obviously unrealistic for the physician explicitly to count large numbers of bacteria by examining a milliliter of urine under the microscope. As a result, one recent article offers the following guideline to physicians: "When interpreting . . . microscopy of . . . stained centrifuged urine, a threshold of one organism per field yields a 95 percent sensitivity and five organisms per field a 95 percent specificity for bacteriuria [bacteria in the urine] at a level of at least 10,000 organisms per ml." (Senior Medical Review, 1987, p. 4)

   a. Describe an experiment that would have allowed the researchers to determine the sensitivity and specificity of the microscopy.

   b. How would you expect specificity to change as the number of bacteria per microscopic field increases from one to five?

   c. How would you expect sensitivity to change as the number of bacteria per microscopic field increases from one to five?

   d. Why does it take more organisms per microscopic field to obtain a specificity of 95 percent than it does to achieve a sensitivity of 95 percent?

3
Biomedical Decision Making: Probabilistic Clinical Reasoning

DOUGLAS K. OWENS AND HAROLD C. SOX

After reading this chapter, you should know the answers to these questions:

- How is the concept of probability useful for understanding test results and for making medical decisions that involve uncertainty?
- How can we characterize the ability of a test to discriminate between disease and health?
- What information do we need to interpret test results accurately?
- What is *expected-value decision making?* How can this methodology help us to understand particular medical problems?
- What are utilities, and how can we use them to represent patients' preferences?
- What is a *sensitivity analysis?* How can we use it to examine the robustness of a decision and to identify the important variables in a decision?
- What are influence diagrams? How do they differ from decision trees?

3.1 The Nature of Clinical Decisions: Uncertainty and the Process of Diagnosis

Because clinical data are imperfect and outcomes of treatment are uncertain, health professionals often are faced with difficult choices. In this chapter, we introduce *probabilistic medical reasoning,* an approach that can help health care providers to deal with the uncertainty inherent in many medical decisions. Medical decisions are made by a variety of methods; our approach is neither necessary nor appropriate for all decisions. Throughout the chapter, we provide simple clinical examples that illustrate a broad range of problems for which probabilistic medical reasoning does provide valuable insight.

As discussed in Chapter 2, medical practice *is* medical decision making. In this chapter, we look at the *process* of medical decision making. Together, Chapters 2 and 3 lay the groundwork for the rest of the book. In the remaining chapters, we discuss ways that computers can help clinicians with the decision-making process, and we emphasize the relationship between information needs and system design and implementation.

The material in this chapter is presented in the context of the decisions made by an individual physician. The concepts, however, are more broadly applicable. Sensitivity and specificity are important parameters of laboratory systems that flag abnormal test results, of patient monitoring systems (Chapter 17), and of information-retrieval systems (Chapter 19). An understanding of what probability is and of how to adjust probabilities after the acquisition of new information is a foundation for our study of clinical consultation systems (Chapter 20). The importance of probability in medical decision making was noted as long ago as 1922:

"[G]ood medicine does not consist in the indiscriminate application of laboratory examinations to a patient, but rather in having so clear a comprehension of the probabilities and possibilities of a case as to know what tests may be expected to give information of value" (Peabody, 1922).

> **Example 1.** You are the director of a large urban blood bank. All potential blood donors are tested to ensure that they are not infected with the human immunodeficiency virus (HIV), the causative agent of acquired immunodeficiency syndrome (AIDS). You ask whether use of the polymerase chain reaction (PCR), a gene-amplification technique that can diagnose HIV, would be useful to identify people who have HIV. The PCR test is positive 98 percent of the time when antibody is present, and negative 99 percent of the time antibody is absent.[1]

If the test is positive, what is the likelihood that a donor actually has HIV? If the test is negative, how sure can you be that the person does not have HIV? On an intuitive level, these questions do not seem particularly difficult to answer. The test appears accurate, and we would expect that, if the test is positive, the donated blood specimen is likely to contain the HIV. Thus, we are shaken to find that, if only one in 1,000 donors actually is infected, the test is more often mistaken than it is correct. In fact, of 100 donors with a positive test, fewer than 10 would be infected. *There would be 10 wrong answers for each correct result.* How are we to understand this result? Before we try to find an answer, let us consider a related example.

> **Example 2.** Mr. James is a 59-year-old man with coronary artery disease (narrowing or blockage of the blood vessels that supply the heart tissue). When the heart muscle does not receive enough oxygen (hypoxia) because blood cannot reach it, the patient often experiences chest pain (angina). Mr. James has twice undergone coronary artery bypass graft (CABG) surgery, a procedure in which new vessels, usually taken from the leg, are grafted onto the old ones such that blood is shunted past the blocked region. Unfortunately, he has again begun to have chest pain, which becomes progressively more severe, despite medication. If the heart muscle is deprived of oxygen, the result can be a heart attack (myocardial infarction), in which a section of the muscle dies.

Should Mr. James undergo a third operation? The medications are not working; without surgery, he runs a high risk of suffering a heart attack, which may be fatal. On the other hand, the surgery is hazardous. Not only is the surgical mortality rate for a third operation higher than that for a first or second one but also the chance that surgery will relieve the chest pain is lower than that for a first operation. All choices in Example 2 entail considerable uncertainty. Furthermore, the risks are grave; an incorrect decision may substantially increase the chance that Mr. James will die. The decision will be difficult even for experienced clinicians.

---

[1] The test sensitivity and specificity used in Example 1 are consistent with initially reported values of the sensitivity and specificity of the PCR test for diagnosis of IIIV, but the accuracy of the test varies across laboratories, and has improved over time (Owens et al., 1996b).

These examples illustrate situations in which intuition is either misleading or inadequate. Although the test results in Example 1 are appropriate for the blood bank, a physician who uncritically reports these results would erroneously inform many people that they had the AIDS virus—a mistake with profound emotional and social consequences. In Example 2, the decision-making skill of the physician will affect a patient's quality and length of life. Similar situations are commonplace in medicine. Our goal in this chapter is to show how the use of probability and decision analysis can help to make clear the best course of action.

Decision making is one of the quintessential activities of the healthcare professional. Some decisions are made on the basis of deductive reasoning or of physiological principles. Many decisions, however, are made on the basis of knowledge that has been gained through collective experience: the clinician often must rely on empirical knowledge of associations between symptoms and disease to evaluate a problem. A decision that is based on these usually imperfect associations will be, to some degree, uncertain. In Sections 3.1.1 through 3.1.3, we examine decisions made under uncertainty and present an overview of the diagnostic process. As Smith (1985, p. 3) said: "Medical decisions based on probabilities are necessary but also perilous. Even the most astute physician will occasionally be wrong."

3.1.1   Decision Making Under Uncertainty

Example 3.   Mr. Kirk, a 33-year-old man with a history of a previous blood clot (thrombus) in a vein in his left leg, presents with the complaint of pain and swelling in that leg for the past 5 days. On physical examination, the leg is tender and swollen to midcalf—signs that suggest the possibility of deep vein thrombosis.[2] A test (ultrasonography) is performed, and the flow of blood in the veins of Mr. Kirk's leg is evaluated. The blood flow is abnormal, but the radiologist cannot tell whether there is a new blood clot.

Should Mr. Kirk be treated for blood clots? The main diagnostic concern is the recurrence of a blood clot in his leg. A clot in the veins of the leg can dislodge, flow with the blood, and cause a blockage in the vessels of the lungs, a potentially fatal event called a *pulmonary embolus*. Of patients with a swollen leg, about one-half actually have a blood clot; there are numerous other causes of a swollen leg. Given a swollen leg, therefore, a physician cannot be sure that a clot is the cause. Thus, the physical findings leave considerable uncertainty. Furthermore, in Example 3, the results of the available diagnostic test are equivocal. The treatment for a blood clot is to administer anticoagulants (drugs that inhibit blood clot formation), which pose the risk of excessive bleeding to the patient. Therefore, physicians do not want to treat the patient unless they are confident that a thrombus is present. But how much confidence *should* be required before

---

[2] In medicine, a *sign* is an objective physical finding (something observed by the clinician) such as a temperature of 101.2°F. A *symptom* is a subjective experience of the patient, such as feeling hot or feverish. The distinction may be blurred if the patient's experience also can be observed by the clinician.

starting treatment? We will learn that it is possible to answer this question by calculating the benefits and harms of treatment.

This example illustrates an important concept: Clinical data are imperfect. The degree of imperfection varies, but all clinical data—including the results of diagnostic tests, the history given by the patient, and the findings on physical examination—are uncertain.

3.1.2 Probability: An Alternative Method of Expressing Uncertainty

The language that physicians use to describe a patient's condition often is ambiguous—a factor that further complicates the problem of uncertainty in medical decision making. Physicians use words such as "probable" and "highly likely" to describe their beliefs about the likelihood of disease. These words have strikingly different meanings to different individuals (Figure 3.1). Because of the widespread disagreement about the meaning of common descriptive terms, there is ample opportunity for miscommunication.

The problem of how to express degrees of uncertainty is not unique to medicine. How is it handled in other contexts? Horse racing has its share of uncertainty. If experienced gamblers are deciding whether to place bets, they will find it unsatisfactory to be told that a given horse has a "high chance" of winning. They will demand to know the odds.

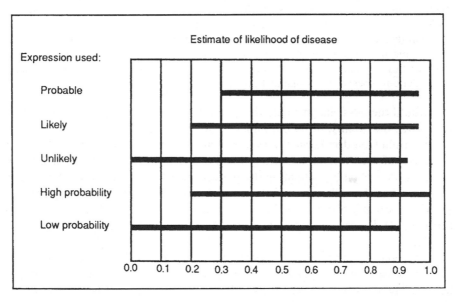

Figure 3.1. Probability and descriptive terms. Different physicians attach different meanings to the same terms. The bars show the wide variation in point probabilities assigned by individual physicians and other health care workers when they were asked to interpret these terms. (*Source*: Bryant G.D., Norman, G.R. [1980]. Expressions of probability: Words and numbers. *New England Journal of Medicine*, 302:411.)

The odds are simply an alternate way to express a probability. The use of probability or **odds** as an expression of uncertainty avoids the ambiguities inherent in common descriptive terms.

3.1.3   Overview of the Diagnostic Process

In Chapter 2, we described the hypothetico-deductive approach, a diagnostic strategy comprising successive iterations of hypothesis generation, data collection, and interpretation. We discussed how observations may evoke a hypothesis and how new information subsequently may increase or decrease our belief in that hypothesis. Here, we review this process briefly in light of a specific example. For the purpose of our discussion, we separate the diagnostic process into three stages.

The first stage involves making an *initial judgment* about whether a patient is likely to have a disease. After an interview and physical examination, a physician intuitively develops a belief about the likelihood of disease. This judgment may be based on previous experience or on knowledge of the medical literature. A physician's belief about the likelihood of disease usually is implicit; he or she can refine it by making an explicit estimation of the probability of disease. This estimated probability, made before further information is obtained, is the **prior probability** or **pretest probability** of disease.

> **Example 4.**   Mr. Smith, a 60-year-old man, complains to his physician that he has pressure-like chest pain that occurs when he walks quickly. After taking his history and examining him, his physician believes there is a high enough chance that he has heart disease to warrant ordering an exercise stress test. In the stress test, an electrocardiogram (ECG) is taken while Mr. Smith exercises. Because the heart must pump more blood per stroke and must beat faster (and thus requires more oxygen) during exercise, many heart conditions are evident only when the patient is physically stressed. Mr. Smith's results show abnormal changes in the ECG during exercise—a sign of heart disease.

How would the physician evaluate this patient? The physician would first talk to the patient about the quality, duration, and severity of his or her pain. Traditionally, the physician would then decide what to do next based on his or her intuition about the etiology (cause) of the chest pain. Our approach is to ask the physician to make his or her initial intuition explicit by estimating the pretest probability of disease. The clinician in this example, based on what he or she knows from talking with the patient, might assess the pretest or prior probability of heart disease as 0.5 (50 percent chance or 1:1 odds; see Section 3.2). We explore methods used to estimate pretest probability accurately in Section 3.2.

After the pretest probability of disease has been estimated, the second stage of the diagnostic process involves gathering more information, often by performing a diagnostic test. The physician in Example 4 ordered a test to reduce the uncertainty about the diagnosis of heart disease. The positive test result supports the diagnosis of heart disease, and this reduction in uncertainty is shown in Figure 3.2a. Although the physician in Example 4 chose the exercise stress test, there are many tests available to diagnose heart disease, and the physician would like to know which test he or she should order next. Some tests reduce uncertainty more than do others (see Figure 3.2b), but may cost more. The more a test reduces uncertainty, the more useful it is. In Section 3.3,

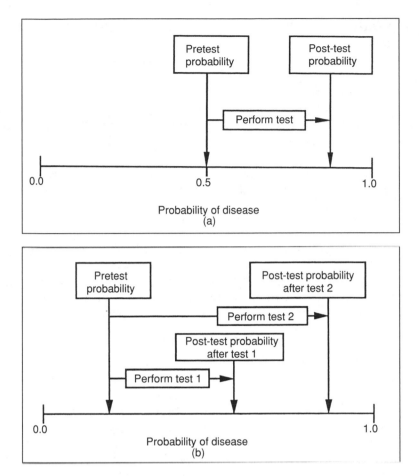

Figure 3.2. The effect of test results on the probability of disease. (a) A positive test result increases the probability of disease. (b) Test 2 reduces uncertainty about presence of disease (increases the probability of disease) more than test 1 does.

we explore ways to measure how well a test reduces uncertainty, expanding the concepts of test sensitivity and specificity first introduced in Chapter 2.

Given new information provided by a test, the third step is to update the initial probability estimate. The physician in Example 4 must ask: "What is the probability of disease given the abnormal stress test?" The physician wants to know the **posterior probability,** or **post-test probability,** of disease (see Figure 3.2a). In Section 3.4, we reexamine Bayes' theorem, introduced in Chapter 2, and we discuss its use for calculating the post-test probability of disease. As we noted, to calculate post-test probability, we must know the pretest probability, as well as the sensitivity and specificity, of the test.[3]

---

[3] Note that pretest and post-test probabilities correspond to the concepts of prevalence and predictive value. The latter terms were used in Chapter 2 because the discussion was about the use of tests for screening *populations* of patients; in a population, the pretest probability of disease is simply that disease's prevalence in that population.

3.2   Probability Assessment: Methods to Assess Pretest Probability

In this section, we explore the methods that physicians can use to make judgments about the probability of disease before they order tests. **Probability** is our preferred means of expressing uncertainty. In this framework, probability (p) expresses a physician's opinion about the likelihood of an event as a number between 0 and 1. An event that is certain to occur has a probability of 1; an event that is certain not to occur has a probability of 0.[4]

The probability of event A is written $p[A]$. The sum of the probabilities of all possible, collectively exhaustive outcomes of a chance event must be equal to 1. Thus, in a coin flip,

$$p[\text{heads}] + p[\text{tails}] = 1.0.$$

The probability of event A and event B occurring together is denoted by $p[A\&B]$ or by $p[A,B]$.

Events A and B are considered **independent** if the occurrence of one does not influence the probability of the occurrence of the other. The probability of two independent events A and B both occurring is given by the product of the individual probabilities:

$$p[A,B] = p[A] \times p[B].$$

Thus, the probability of heads on two consecutive coin tosses is $0.5 \times 0.5 = 0.25$. (Regardless of the outcome of the first toss, the probability of heads on the second toss is 0.5.)

The probability that event A will occur given that event B is known to occur is called the **conditional probability** of event A given event B, denoted by $p[A \mid B]$ and read as "the probability of A given B." Thus a post-test probability is a conditional probability predicated on the test or finding. For example, if 30 percent of patients who have a swollen leg have a blood clot, we say the probability of a blood clot given a swollen leg is 0.3, denoted:

$$p[\text{blood clot} \mid \text{swollen leg}] = 0.3.$$

Before the swollen leg is noted, the pretest probability is simply the prevalence of blood clots in the leg in the population from which the patient was selected—a number likely to be much smaller than 0.3.

Now that we have decided to use probability to express uncertainty, how can we estimate probability? We can do so by either subjective or objective methods; each approach has advantages and limitations.

3.2.1   Subjective Probability Assessment

Most assessments that physicians make about probability are based on personal experience. The physician may compare the current problem to similar problems encountered

---

[4] We assume a Bayesian interpretation of probability; there are other statistical interpretations of probability.

previously and then ask: "What was the frequency of disease in similar patients whom I have seen?"

To make these subjective assessments of probability, people rely on several discrete, often unconscious mental processes that have been described and studied by cognitive psychologists (Tversky and Kahneman, 1974). These processes are termed **cognitive heuristics**.

More specifically, a cognitive heuristic is a mental process by which we learn, recall, or process information; we can think of heuristics as rules of thumb. Knowledge of heuristics is important because it helps us to understand the underpinnings of our intuitive probability assessment. Both naive and sophisticated decision makers (including physicians and statisticians) misuse heuristics and therefore make systematic—often serious—errors when estimating probability. So, just as we may underestimate distances on a particularly clear day (Tversky and Kahneman, 1974), we may make mistakes in estimating probability in deceptive clinical situations. Three heuristics have been identified as important in estimation of probability:

1. *Representativeness.* One way that people estimate probability is to ask themselves: What is the probability that object *A* belongs to class *B*? For instance, what is the probability that this patient who has a swollen leg belongs to the class of patients who have blood clots? To answer, we often rely on the **representativeness** heuristic in which probabilities are judged by the degree to which *A* is representative of, or similar to, *B*. The clinician will judge the probability of the development of a blood clot (thrombosis) by the degree to which the patient with a swollen leg resembles the clinician's mental image of patients with a blood clot. If the patient has all the classic findings (signs and symptoms) associated with a blood clot, the physician judges that the patient is highly likely to have a blood clot. Difficulties occur with the use of this heuristic when the disease is rare (very low prior probability, or prevalence); when the clinician's previous experience with the disease is atypical, thus giving an incorrect mental representation; when the patient's clinical profile is atypical; and when the probability of certain findings depends on whether other findings are present.

2. *Availability.* Our estimate of the probability of an event is influenced by the ease with which we remember similar events. Events more easily remembered are judged more probable; this rule is the **availability** heuristic, and it is often misleading. We remember dramatic, atypical, or emotion-laden events more easily and therefore are likely to overestimate their probability. A physician who had cared for a patient who had a swollen leg and who then died from a blood clot would vividly remember thrombosis as a cause of a swollen leg. The physician would remember other causes of swollen legs less easily, and he or she would tend to overestimate the probability of a blood clot in patients with a swollen leg.

3. *Anchoring and adjustment.* Another common heuristic used to judge probability is **anchoring and adjustment.** A clinician makes an initial probability estimate (the *anchor*) and then adjusts the estimate based on further information. For instance, the physician in Example 4 makes an initial estimate of the probability of heart disease as 0.5. If he or she then learns that all the patient's brothers had died of heart disease, the physician should raise the estimate because the patient's strong family history of

heart disease increases the probability that he or she has heart disease, a fact the physician could ascertain from the literature. The usual mistake is to adjust the initial estimate (the anchor) insufficiently in light of the new information. Instead of raising his or her estimate of prior probability to, say, 0.8, the physician might adjust it to only 0.6.

Heuristics often introduce error into our judgments about prior probability. Errors in our initial estimates of probabilities will be reflected in the posterior probabilities even if we use quantitative methods to derive those posterior probabilities. An understanding of heuristics is thus important for medical decision making. The clinician can avoid some of these difficulties by using published research results to estimate probabilities.

3.2.2   Objective Probability Estimates

Published research results can serve as a guide for more objective estimates of probabilities. We can use the prevalence of disease in the population or in a subgroup of the population, or clinical prediction rules, to estimate the probability of disease.

As we discussed in Chapter 2, the **prevalence** is the frequency of an event in a population; it is a useful starting point for estimating probability. For example, if you wanted to estimate the probability of prostate cancer in a 50-year-old man, the prevalence of prostate cancer in men of that age (5 to 14 percent) would be a useful anchor point from which you could increase or decrease the probability depending on your findings. Estimates of disease prevalence in a defined population often are available in the medical literature.

Symptoms, such as difficulty with urination, or signs, such as a palpable prostate nodule, can be used to place patients into a **clinical subgroup** in which the probability of disease is known. For patients referred to a urologist for evaluation of a prostate nodule, the prevalence of cancer is about 50 percent. This approach may be limited by difficulty in placing a patient in the correct clinically defined subgroup, especially if the criteria for classifying patients are ill-defined. A trend has been to develop guidelines, known as *clinical prediction rules,* to help physicians assign patients to well-defined subgroups in which the probability of disease is known.

Clinical prediction rules are developed from systematic study of patients who have a particular diagnostic problem; they define how physicians can use combinations of clinical findings to estimate probability. The symptoms or signs that make an independent contribution to the probability that a patient has a disease are identified and assigned numerical weights based on statistical analysis of the finding's contribution. The result is a list of symptoms and signs for an individual patient, each with a corresponding numerical contribution to a total score. The total score places a patient in a subgroup with a known probability of disease.

> **Example 5.**   Ms. Troy, a 65-year-old woman who had a heart attack 4 months ago, has abnormal heart rhythm (arrhythmia), is in poor medical condition, and is about to undergo elective surgery.

What is the probability that Ms. Troy will suffer a cardiac complication? Clinical prediction rules have been developed to help physicians to assess this risk (Palda and Detsky, 1997). Table 3.1 lists clinical findings and their corresponding diagnostic weights. We add the diagnostic weights for each of the patient's clinical findings to obtain the total score. The total score places the patient in a group with a defined probability of cardiac complications, as shown in Table 3.2. Ms. Troy receives a score of 20; thus, the physician can estimate that the patient has a 27 percent chance of developing a severe cardiac complication.

Objective estimates of pretest probability are subject to error because of bias in the studies on which the estimates are based. For instance, published prevalences may not apply directly to a particular patient. A clinical illustration is that early studies indicated that a patient found to have microscopic evidence of blood in the urine (microhematuria) should undergo extensive tests because a significant proportion of the patients would be found to have cancer or other serious diseases. The tests involve some risk, discomfort, and expense to the patient. Nonetheless, the approach of ordering tests for

Table 3.1. Diagnostic weights for assessing risk of cardiac complications from noncardiac surgery.

Clinical finding	Diagnostic weight
Age greater than 70 years	5
Recent documented heart attack	
>6 months previously	5
<6 months previously	10
Severe angina	20
Pulmonary edema[a]	
Within 1 week	10
Ever	5
Arrhythmia on most recent ECG	5
>5 PVCs	5
Critical aortic stenosis	20
Poor medical condition	5
Emergency surgery	10

ECG = electrocardiogram; PVCs = premature ventricular contractions on preoperative electrocardiogram.
[a]Fluid in the lungs due to reduced heart function.
(*Source*: Modified from Palda V.A., Detsky A.S. [1997]. Perioperative assessment and management of risk from coronary artery disease. *Annals of Internal Medicine*, 127: 313–318.)

Table 3.2. Clinical prediction rule for diagnostic weights in Table 3.1.

Total score	Prevalence (%) of cardiac complications[a]
0–15	5
20–30	27
>30	60

[a]Cardiac complications defined as death, heart attack, or congestive heart failure.
(*Source*: Modified from Palda V.A., Detsky A.S. [1997]. Perioperative assessment and management of risk from coronary artery disease. *Annals of Internal Medicine*, 127:313 318.)

any patient with microhematuria was widely practiced for some years. A later study, however, suggested that the probability of serious disease in asymptomatic patients with only microscopic evidence of blood was only about 2 percent (Mohr et al., 1986). In the past, many patients may have undergone unnecessary tests, at considerable financial and personal cost.

What explains the discrepancy in the estimates of disease prevalence? The initial studies that showed a high prevalence of disease in patients with microhematuria were performed on patients referred to urologists, who are specialists. The primary care physician refers patients whom he or she suspects have a disease in the specialist's sphere of expertise. Because of this initial screening by primary care physicians, the specialists seldom see patients with clinical findings that imply a low probability of disease. Thus, the prevalence of disease in the patient population in a specialist's practice often is much higher than that in a primary care practice; studies performed with the former patients therefore almost always overestimate disease probabilities. This example demonstrates **referral bias**. Referral bias is common because many published studies are performed on patients referred to specialists. Thus, one may need to adjust published estimates before one uses them to estimate pretest probability in other clinical settings.

We now can use the techniques discussed in this part of the chapter to illustrate how the physician in Example 4 might estimate the pretest probability of heart disease in his or her patient, Mr. Smith, who has pressure-like chest pain. We begin by using the objective data that are available. The prevalence of heart disease in 60-year-old men could be our starting point. In this case, however, we can obtain a more refined estimate by placing the patient in a clinical *subgroup* in which the prevalence of disease is known. The prevalence in a clinical subgroup, such as men with symptoms typical of coronary heart disease, will predict the pretest probability more accurately than would the prevalence of heart disease in a group that is heterogeneous with respect to symptoms, such as the population at large. We assume that large studies have shown the prevalence of coronary heart disease in men with typical symptoms of angina pectoris to be about 0.9; this prevalence is useful as an initial estimate that can be adjusted based on information specific to the patient. Although the prevalence of heart disease in men with typical symptoms is high, 10 percent of patients with this history do not have heart disease.

The physician might use subjective methods to adjust his or her estimate further based on other specific information about the patient. For example, the physician might adjust his or her initial estimate of 0.9 upward to 0.95 or higher based on information about family history of heart disease. The physician should be careful, however, to avoid the mistakes that can occur when one uses heuristics to make subjective probability estimates. In particular, he or she should be aware of the tendency to stay too close to the initial estimate when adjusting for additional information. By combining subjective and objective methods for assessing pretest probability, the physician can arrive at a reasonable estimate of the pretest probability of heart disease.

In this section, we summarized subjective and objective methods to determine the pretest probability, and we learned how to adjust the pretest probability after assessing the specific subpopulation of which the patient is representative. The next step in the diagnostic process is to gather further information, usually in the form of formal diagnostic tests (laboratory tests, X-ray studies, etc.). To help you to understand this step more clearly, we discuss in the next two sections how to measure the accuracy of tests and how to use probability to interpret the results of the tests.

3.3   Measurement of the Operating Characteristics of Diagnostic Tests

The first challenge in assessing any test is to determine criteria for deciding whether a result is normal or abnormal. In this section, we present the issues that you need to consider when making such a determination.

3.3.1   Classification of Test Results as Abnormal

Most biological measurements in a population of healthy people are continuous variables that assume different values for different individuals. The distribution of values often is approximated by the normal (gaussian, or bell-shaped) distribution curve (Figure 3.3). Thus, 95 percent of the population will fall within two standard deviations of the mean. About 2.5 percent of the population will be more than two standard deviations from the mean at each end of the distribution. The distribution of values for ill individuals may be normally distributed as well. The two distributions usually overlap (see Figure 3.3).

How is a test result classified as abnormal? Most clinical laboratories report an "upper limit of normal," which usually is defined as two standard deviations above the mean. Thus, a test result greater than two standard deviations above the mean is

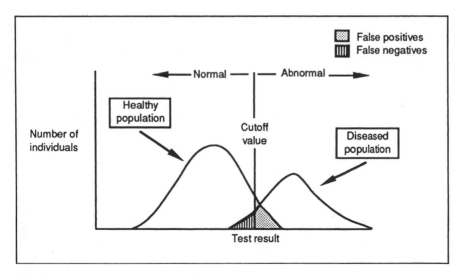

Figure 3.3. Distribution of test results in healthy and diseased individuals. Varying the cutoff between "normal" and "abnormal" across the continuous range of possible values changes the relative proportions of false positives (FPs) and false negatives (FNs) for the two populations.

reported as abnormal (or positive); a test result below that cutoff is reported as normal (or negative). As an example, if the mean cholesterol concentration in the blood is 220 mg/dl, a clinical laboratory might choose as the upper limit of normal 280 mg/dl because it is two standard deviations above the mean. Note that a cutoff that is based on an arbitrary statistical criterion may not have biological significance.

An ideal test would have no values at which the distribution of diseased and nondiseased people overlap. That is, if the cutoff value were set appropriately, the test would be normal in all healthy individuals and abnormal in all individuals with disease. Few tests meet this standard. If a test result is defined as abnormal by the statistical criterion, 2.5 percent of healthy individuals will have an abnormal test. If there is an overlap in the distribution of test results in healthy and diseased individuals, some diseased patients will have a normal test (see Figure 3.3). You should be familiar with the terms used to denote these groups:

- A **true positive** (TP) is a positive test result obtained for a patient in whom the disease is present (the test result correctly classifies the patient as having the disease).
- A **true negative** (TN) is a negative test result obtained for a patient in whom the disease is absent (the test result correctly classifies the patient as not having the disease).
- A **false positive** (FP) is a positive test result obtained for a patient in whom the disease is absent (the test result incorrectly classifies the patient as having the disease).
- A **false negative** (FN) is a negative test result obtained for a patient in whom the disease is present (the test result incorrectly classifies the patient as not having the disease).

Figure 3.3 shows that varying the cutoff point (moving the vertical line in the figure) for an abnormal test will change the relative proportions of these groups. As the cutoff is moved further up from the mean of the normal values, the number of FNs increases and the number of FPs decreases. Once we have chosen a cutoff point, we can conveniently summarize test performance—the ability to discriminate disease from nondisease—in a 2 × 2 **contingency table,** as shown in Table 3.3. The table summarizes the number of patients in each group: TP, FP, TN, and FN. Note that the sum of the first column is the total number of diseased patients, TP+FN. The sum of the second column is the total number of nondiseased patients, FP+TN. The sum of the first row, TP+FP, is the total number of patients with a positive test result. Likewise, FN+TN gives the total number of patients with a negative test result.

A perfect test would have no FN or FP results. Erroneous test results do occur, however, and you can use a 2 × 2 contingency table to define the measures of test performance that reflect these errors.

Table 3.3. A 2 × 2 contingency table for test results.

Results of test	Disease present	Disease absent	Total
Positive result	TP	FP	TP + FP
Negative result	FN	TN	FN + TN
	TP + FN	FP + TN	

TP = true positive; TN = true negative; FP = false positive; FN = false negative.

3.3.2   Measures of Test Performance

Measures of test performance are of two types: measures of agreement between tests or **measures of concordance**, and measures of disagreement or **measures of discordance.** Two types of **concordant test results** occur in the 2×2 table in Table 3.3: TPs and TNs. The relative frequencies of these results form the basis of the measures of concordance. These measures correspond to the ideas of the sensitivity and specificity of a test, which we introduced in Chapter 2. We define each measure in terms of the 2×2 table and in terms of conditional probabilities.

The **true-positive** rate (TPR), or **sensitivity,** is the likelihood that a diseased patient has a positive test. In conditional-probability notation, sensitivity is expressed as the probability of a positive test given that disease is present:

$$p \text{ [positive test|disease]}.$$

Another way to think of the TPR is as a ratio. The likelihood that a diseased patient has a positive test is given by the ratio of diseased patients with a positive test to all diseased patients:

$$\text{TPR} = \frac{\text{number of diseased patients with positive test}}{\text{total number of diseased patients}}.$$

We can determine these numbers for our example from the 2×2 table (see Table 3.3). The number of diseased patients with a positive test is TP. The total number of diseased patients is the sum of the first column, TP+FN. So,

$$\text{TPR} = \frac{\text{TP}}{\text{TP} + \text{FN}}.$$

The **true-negative** rate (TNR), or **specificity,** is the likelihood that a nondiseased patient has a negative test result. In terms of conditional probability, specificity is the probability of a negative test given that disease is absent:

$$p \text{ [negative test|no disease]}.$$

Viewed as a ratio, the TNR is the number of nondiseased patients with a negative test divided by the total number of nondiseased patients:

$$\text{TNR} = \frac{\text{number of nondiseased patients with negative test}}{\text{total number of nondiseased patients}}.$$

From the 2×2 table (see Table 3.3),

$$\text{TNR} = \frac{\text{TN}}{\text{TN} + \text{FP}}.$$

The measures of discordance—**the false-positive** rate (FPR) and the **false-negative** rate (FNR)—are defined similarly. The FNR is the likelihood that a diseased patient has a negative test result. As a ratio,

$$FNR = \frac{\text{number of diseased patients with negative test}}{\text{total number of diseased patients}} = \frac{FN}{FN + TP}.$$

The FPR is the likelihood that a nondiseased patient has a positive test result:

$$FPR = \frac{\text{number of nondiseased patients with positive test}}{\text{total number of nondiseased patients}} = \frac{FP}{FP + TN}.$$

Example 6. Consider again the problem of screening blood donors for HIV. One test used to screen blood donors for HIV antibody is an enzyme-linked immunoassay (EIA). So that the performance of the EIA can be measured, the test is performed on 400 patients; the hypothetical results are shown in the 2×2 table in Table 3.4.[5]

To determine test performance, we calculate the TPR (sensitivity) and TNR (specificity) of the EIA antibody test. The TPR, as defined previously, is:

$$\frac{TP}{TP + FN} = \frac{98}{98 + 2} = 0.98.$$

Thus, the likelihood that a patient with the HIV antibody will have a positive EIA test is 0.98. If the test were performed on 100 patients who truly had the antibody, we would expect the test to be positive in 98 of the patients. Conversely, we would expect two of the patients to receive incorrect, negative results, for an FNR of 2 percent. (You should convince yourself that the sum of TPR and FNR by definition must be 1: TPR+FNR=1.)

And the TNR is:

$$\frac{TN}{TN + FP} = \frac{297}{297 + 3} = 0.99.$$

The likelihood that a patient who has no HIV antibody will have a negative test is 0.99. Therefore, if the EIA test were performed on 100 individuals who had not been infected with HIV, it would be negative in 99 and incorrectly positive in 1. (Convince yourself that the sum of TNR and FPR also must be 1: TNR+FPR=1.)

Table 3.4. A 2×2 contingency table for HIV antibody EIA.

EIA test result	Antibody present	Antibody absent	Total
Positive EIA	98	3	101
Negative EIA	2	297	299
	100	300	

EIA = enzyme-linked immunoassay.

---

[5] This example assumes that we have a perfect method (different from EIA) for determining the presence or absence of antibody. We discuss the idea of *gold-standard tests* in Section 3.3.4. We have chosen the numbers in the example to simplify the calculations. In practice, the sensitivity and specificity of the HIV EIAs are greater than 99 percent.

3.3.3   Implications of Sensitivity and Specificity: How to Choose Among Tests

It may be clear to you already that the calculated values of sensitivity and specificity for a continuous-valued test depend on the particular cutoff value chosen to distinguish normal and abnormal results. In Figure 3.3, note that increasing the cutoff level (moving it to the right) would decrease significantly the number of FP tests but also would increase the number of FN tests. Thus, the test would have become *more* specific but *less* sensitive. Similarly, a lower cutoff value would increase the FPs and decrease the FNs, thereby increasing sensitivity while decreasing specificity. Whenever a decision is made about what cutoff to use in calling a test abnormal, an inherent philosophic decision is being made about whether it is better to tolerate FNs (missed cases) or FPs (nondiseased people inappropriately classified as diseased). The choice of cutoff depends on the disease in question and on the purpose of testing. If the disease is serious and if life-saving therapy is available, we should try to minimize the number of FN results. On the other hand, if the disease in not serious and the therapy is dangerous, we should set the cutoff value to minimize FP results.

We stress the point that sensitivity and specificity are characteristics not of a test per se but rather of the test *and* a criterion for when to call that test abnormal. Varying the cutoff in Figure 3.3 has no effect on the test itself (the way it is performed, or the specific values for any particular patient); instead, it trades off specificity for sensitivity. Thus, the best way to characterize a test is by the range of values of sensitivity and specificity that it can take on over a range of possible cutoffs. The typical way to show this relationship is to plot the test's sensitivity against 1 minus specificity (i.e., the TPR against the FPR), as the cutoff is varied and the two test characteristics are traded off against each other (Figure 3.4). The resulting curve, known as a **receiver-operating characteristic (ROC) curve,** was originally described by researchers investigating methods of electromagnetic-signal detection and was later applied to the field of psychology (Peterson and Birdsall, 1953; Swets, 1973). Any given point along an ROC curve for a test corresponds to the test sensitivity and specificity for a given threshold of "abnormality." Similar curves can be drawn for *any* test used to associate observed clinical data with specific diseases or disease categories.

Suppose a new test were introduced that competed with the current way of screening for the presence of a disease. For example, suppose a new radiologic procedure for assessing the presence or absence of pneumonia became available. This new test could be assessed for trade-offs in sensitivity and specificity, and an ROC curve could be drawn. As shown in Figure 3.4, a test has better discriminating power than a competing test if its ROC curve lies above that of the other test. In other words, test B is more discriminating than test A when its specificity is greater than test A's specificity for any level of sensitivity (and when its sensitivity is greater than test A's sensitivity for any level of specificity).

Understanding ROC curves is important in understanding test selection and data interpretation. Physicians should not necessarily, however, always choose the test with the most discriminating ROC curve. Matters of cost, risk, discomfort, and delay also are

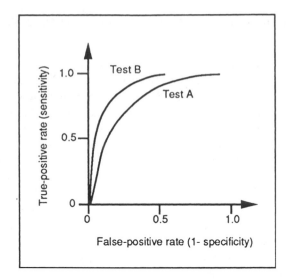

Figure 3.4. Receiver operating characteristic (ROC) curves for two hypothetical tests. Test B is more discriminative than test A because its curve is higher (e.g., the false-positive rate (FPR) for test B is lower than the FPR for test A at any value of true-positive rate (TPR)). The more discriminative test may not always be preferred in clinical practice, however (see text).

important in the choice about what data to collect and what tests to perform. When you must choose among several available tests, you should select the test that has the highest sensitivity and specificity, *provided* that other factors, such as cost and risk to the patient, are equal. The higher the sensitivity and specificity of a test, the more the results of that test will reduce uncertainty about probability of disease.

3.3.4 Design of Studies of Test Performance

In Section 3.3.2, we discussed measures of test performance: a test's ability to discriminate disease from no disease. When we classify a test result as TP, TN, FP, or FN, we assume that we know with certainty whether a patient is diseased or healthy. Thus, the validity of any test's results must be measured against a gold standard: a test that reveals the patient's true disease state, such as a biopsy of diseased tissue or a surgical operation. A **gold-standard test** is a procedure that is used to define unequivocally the presence or absence of disease. The test whose discrimination is being measured is called the **index test**. The gold-standard test usually is more expensive, riskier, or more difficult to perform than is the index test (otherwise, the less precise test would not be used at all).

  The performance of the index test is measured in a small, select group of patients enrolled in a study. We are interested, however, in how the test performs in the broader group of patients in which it will be used in practice. The test may perform differently in the two groups, so we make the following distinction: the **study population** comprises those patients (usually a subset of the clinically relevant population) in whom test discrimination is measured and reported; the **clinically relevant population** comprises those patients in whom a test typically is used.

3.3.5   Bias in the Measurement of Test Characteristics

We mentioned earlier the problem of *referral bias*. Published estimates of disease prevalence (derived from a study population) may differ from the prevalence in the clinically relevant population because diseased patients are more likely to be included in studies than are nondiseased patients. Similarly, published values of sensitivity and specificity are derived from study populations that may differ from the clinically relevant populations in terms of average level of health and disease prevalence. These differences may affect test performance, so the reported values may not apply to many patients in whom a test is used in clinical practice.

> **Example 7.** In the early 1970s, a blood test called the *carcinoembryonic antigen* (CEA) was touted as a screening test for colon cancer. Reports of early investigations, performed in selected patients, indicated that the test had high sensitivity and specificity. Subsequent work, however, proved the CEA to be completely valueless as a screening blood test for colon cancer. Screening tests are used in unselected populations, and the differences between the study and clinically relevant populations were partly responsible for the original miscalculations of the CEA's TPR and TNR. (Ransohoff and Feinstein, 1978)

The experience with CEA has been repeated with numerous tests. Early measures of test discrimination are overly optimistic, and subsequent test performance is disappointing. Problems arise when the TPR and TNR, as measured in the study population, do not apply to the clinically relevant population. These problems usually are the result of bias in the design of the initial studies—notably spectrum bias, test referral bias, or test interpretation bias.

Spectrum bias occurs when the study population includes only individuals who have advanced disease ("sickest of the sick") and healthy volunteers, as is often the case when a test is first being developed. Advanced disease may be easier to detect than early disease. For example, cancer is easier to detect when it has spread throughout the body (metastasized) than when it is localized to, say, a small portion of the colon. In contrast to the study population, the clinically relevant population will contain more cases of early disease that are more likely to be missed by the index test (FNs). Thus, the study population will have an artifactually low FNR, which produces an artifactually high TPR (TPR=1 − FNR). In addition, healthy volunteers are less likely than are patients in the clinically relevant population to have other diseases that may cause FP results;[6] the study population will have an artificially low FPR, and therefore the specificity will

---

[6] Volunteers are often healthy, whereas patients in the clinically relevant population often have several diseases *in addition* to the disease for which a test is designed. These other diseases may cause FP test results. For example, patients with benign (rather than malignant) enlargement of their prostate glands are more likely than are healthy volunteers to have FP elevations of prostate-specific antigen (Meigs et al., 1996), a substance in the blood that is elevated in men who have prostate cancer. Measurement of prostate-specific antigen is often used to detect prostate cancer.

be overestimated (TNR=1 – FPR). Inaccuracies in early estimates of the TPR and TNR of the CEA were partly due to spectrum bias.

Test-referral bias occurs when a positive index test is a criterion for ordering the gold standard test. In clinical practice, patients with negative index tests are less likely to undergo the gold standard test than are patients with positive tests. In other words, the study population, comprising individuals with positive index–test results, has a higher percentage of patients with disease than does the clinically relevant population. Therefore, both TN and FN tests will be underrepresented in the study population. The result is overestimation of the TPR and underestimation of the TNR in the study population.

Test-interpretation bias develops when the interpretation of the index test affects that of the gold standard test or vice versa. This bias causes an artificial concordance between the tests (the results are more likely to be the same) and spuriously increases measures of concordance—the sensitivity and specificity—in the study population. (Remember, the relative frequencies of TPs and TNs are the basis for measures of concordance). To avoid these problems, the person interpreting the index test should be unaware of the results of the gold standard test.

To counter these three biases, you may need to adjust the TPR and TNR when they are applied to a new population. All the biases result in a TPR that is higher in the study population than it is in the clinically relevant population. Thus, if you suspect bias, you should adjust the TPR (sensitivity) downward when you apply it to a new population.

Adjustment of the TNR (specificity) depends on which type of bias is present. Spectrum bias and test interpretation bias result in a TNR that is *higher* in the study population than it will be in the clinically relevant population. Thus, if these biases are present, you should adjust the specificity downward when you apply it to a new population. Test-referral bias, on the other hand, produces a measured specificity in the study population that is *lower* than it will be in the clinically relevant population. If you suspect test referral bias, you should adjust the specificity upward when you apply it to a new population.

3.3.6   Meta-Analysis of Diagnostic Tests

Often, many studies evaluate the sensitivity and specificity of the same diagnostic test. If the studies come to similar conclusions about the sensitivity and specificity of the test, you can have increased confidence in the results of the studies. But what if the studies disagree? For example, by 1995, over 100 studies had assessed the sensitivity and specificity of the PCR for diagnosis of HIV (Owens et al., 1996a, 1996b); these studies estimated the sensitivity of PCR to be as low as 10 percent and to be as high as 100 percent, and they assessed the specificity of PCR to be between 40 and 100 percent. Which results should you believe? One approach that you can use is to assess the quality of the studies and to use the estimates from the highest-quality studies.

For evaluation of PCR, however, even the high-quality studies did not agree. Another approach is to perform a **meta-analysis**: a study that combines quantitatively the estimates from individual studies to develop a **summary ROC curve** (Moses et al., 1993; Owens et al., 1996a, 1996b; Hellmich et al., 1999). Investigators develop a summary ROC curve by using estimates from many studies, in contrast to the type of ROC curve discussed in Section 3.3.3, which is developed from the data in a single study. Summary ROC curves provide the best available approach to synthesizing data from many studies.

Section 3.3 has dealt with the second step in the diagnostic process: acquisition of further information with diagnostic tests. We have learned how to characterize the performance of a test with sensitivity (TPR) and specificity (TNR). These measures reveal the probability of a test result given the true state of the patient. They do not, however, answer the clinically relevant question posed in the opening example: Given a positive test result, what is the probability that this patient has the disease? To answer this question, we must learn methods to calculate the post-test probability of disease.

3.4   Post-test Probability: Bayes' Theorem and Predictive Value

The third stage of the diagnostic process (see Figure 3.2a) is to adjust our probability estimate to take into account the new information gained from diagnostic tests by calculating the post-test probability.

3.4.1   Bayes' Theorem

As we noted earlier in this chapter, a physician can use the disease prevalence in the patient population as an initial estimate of the pretest risk of disease. Once physicians begin to accumulate information about a patient, however, they revise their estimate of the probability of disease. The revised estimate (rather than the disease prevalence in the general population) becomes the pretest probability for the test that they perform. After they have gathered more information with a diagnostic test, they can calculate the post-test probability of disease with Bayes' theorem.

Bayes' theorem is a quantitative method for calculating post-test probability using the pretest probability and the sensitivity and specificity of the test. The theorem is derived from the definition of conditional probability and from the properties of probability (see the Appendix to this chapter for the derivation).

Recall that a conditional probability is the probability that event A will occur given that event B is known to occur (see Section 3.2). In general, we want to know the probability that disease is present (event A), given that the test is known to be positive (event B). We denote the presence of disease as D, its absence as $-$D, a test result as R, and the pretest probability of disease as p[D]. The probability of disease, given a test result, is written p[D| R]. Bayes' theorem is:

$$p[D|R] = \frac{p[D] \times p[R|D]}{p[D] \times p[R|D] + p[-D] \times p[R|-D]}.$$

We can reformulate this general equation in terms of a positive test, (+), by substituting p[D|+] for p[D|R], p[+|D] for p[R|D], p[+|$-$D] for p[R|$-$D], and $1 - p$[D] for p[$-$D]. From Section 3.3, recall that p[+|D]=TPR and p[+|$-$D]=FPR. Substitution provides Bayes' theorem for a positive test:

$$p[D|+] = \frac{p[D] \times \text{TPR}}{p[D] \times \text{TPR} + (1 - p[D]) \times \text{FPR}}.$$

We can use a similar derivation to develop Bayes' theorem for a negative test:

$$p[D|-] = \frac{p[D] \times \text{FNR}}{p[D] \times \text{FNR} + (1 - p[D]) \times \text{TNR}}.$$

Example 8. We are now able to calculate the clinically important probability in Example 4: the post-test probability of heart disease after a positive exercise test. At the end of Section 3.2.2, we estimated the pretest probability of heart disease as 0.95, based on the prevalence of heart disease in men who have typical symptoms of heart disease and on the prevalence in people with a family history of heart disease. Assume that the TPR and FPR of the exercise stress test are 0.65 and 0.20, respectively. Substituting in Bayes' formula for a positive test, we obtain the probability of heart disease given a positive test result:

$$p[D|+] = \frac{0.95 \times 0.65}{0.95 \times 0.65 + 0.05 \times 0.20} = 0.98.$$

Thus, the positive test raised the post-test probability to 0.98 from the pretest probability of 0.95. The change in probability is modest because the pretest probability was high (0.95) and because the FPR also is high (0.20). If we repeat the calculation with a pretest probability of 0.75, the post-test probability is 0.91. If we assume the FPR of the test to be 0.05 instead of 0.20, a pretest probability of 0.95 changes to 0.996.

3.4.2   The Odds-Ratio Form of Bayes' Theorem and Likelihood Ratios

Although the formula for Bayes' theorem is straightforward, it is awkward for mental calculations. We can develop a more convenient form of Bayes' theorem by expressing probability as *odds* and by using a different measure of test discrimination. Probability and odds are related as follows:

$$\text{odds} = \frac{p}{1-p},$$

$$p = \frac{\text{odds}}{1 + \text{odds}}.$$

Thus, if the probability of rain today is 0.75, the odds are 3:1. Thus, on similar days, we should expect rain to occur three times for each time it does not occur.

A simple relationship exists between pretest odds and post-test odds:

$$\text{post} - \text{test odds} = \text{pretest odds} \times \text{likelihood ratio}$$

or

$$\frac{p[D|R]}{p[-D|R]} = \frac{p[D]}{p[-D]} \times \frac{p[R|D]}{p[R|-D]}.$$

This equation is the **odds-ratio form** of Bayes' theorem.[7] It can be derived in a straight-forward fashion from the definitions of Bayes' theorem and of conditional probability that we provided earlier. Thus, to obtain the post-test odds, we simply multiply the pretest odds by the **likelihood ratio** (LR) for the test in question.

The LR of a test combines the measures of test discrimination discussed earlier to give one number that characterizes the discriminatory power of a test, defined as:

$$LR = \frac{p[R \mid D]}{p[R \mid -D]}$$

or

$$LR = \frac{\text{probability of result in diseased people}}{\text{probability of result in nondiseased people}}.$$

The LR indicates the amount that the odds of disease change based on the test result. We can use the LR to characterize clinical findings (such as a swollen leg) or a test result. We describe the performance of a test that has only two possible outcomes (e.g., positive or negative) by two LRs: one corresponding to a positive test result and the other corresponding to a negative test. These ratios are abbreviated LR+ and LR-, respectively.

$$LR^+ = \frac{\text{probability that test is positive in diseased people}}{\text{probability that test is positive in nondiseased people}} = \frac{\text{TPR}}{\text{FPR}}.$$

In a test that discriminates well between disease and nondisease, the TPR will be high, the FPR will be low, and thus LR+ will be much greater than 1. An LR of 1 means that the probability of a test result is the same in diseased and nondiseased individuals; the test has no value. Similarly,

$$LR^- = \frac{\text{probability that test is negative in diseased people}}{\text{probability that test is negative in nondiseased people}} = \frac{\text{FNR}}{\text{TNR}}.$$

A desirable test will have a low FNR and a high TNR; therefore, the LR- will be much less than 1.

Example 9. We can calculate the post-test probability for a positive exercise stress test in a 60-year-old man whose pretest probability is 0.75. The pretest odds are:

$$\text{odds} = \frac{p}{1-p} = \frac{0.75}{1-0.75} = \frac{0.75}{0.25} = 3, \text{ or } 3:1.$$

The LR for the stress test is:

$$LR^+ = \frac{\text{TPR}}{\text{FPR}} = \frac{0.65}{0.20} = 3.25.$$

---

[7] Some authors refer to this expression as the **odds-likelihood form** of Bayes' theorem.

We can calculate the post-test odds of a positive test result using the odds-ratio form of Bayes' theorem:

$$\text{post} - \text{test odds} = 3 \times 3.25 = 9.75 : 1.$$

We can then convert the odds to a probability:

$$p = \frac{\text{odds}}{1 + \text{odds}} = \frac{9.75}{1 + 9.75} = 0.91.$$

As expected, this result agrees with our earlier answer (see the discussion of Example 8).

The odds-ratio form of Bayes' theorem allows rapid calculation, so you can determine the probability at, for example, your patient's bedside. The LR is a powerful method for characterizing the operating characteristics of a test: if you know the pretest odds, you can calculate the post-test odds in one step. The LR demonstrates that a useful test is one that changes the odds of disease. The LRs of many diagnostic tests are available (Sox et al., 1988).

3.4.3   Predictive Value of a Test

An alternative approach for estimation of the probability of disease in a person who has a positive or negative test is to calculate the predictive value of the test. The **positive predictive value** (PV⁺) of a test is the likelihood that a patient who has a positive test result also has disease. Thus, PV⁺ can be calculated directly from a 2×2 contingency table:

$$\text{PV}^+ = \frac{\text{number of diseased patients with positive test}}{\text{total number of patients with a positive test}}$$

From the 2×2 contingency table in Table 3.3,

$$\text{PV}^+ = \frac{\text{TP}}{\text{TP} + \text{FP}} \, .$$

The **negative predictive value** (PV⁻) is the likelihood that a patient with a negative test does not have disease:

$$\text{PV}^- = \frac{\text{number of nondiseased patients with negative test}}{\text{total number of patients with a negative test}}$$

From the 2×2 contingency table in Table 3.3,

$$\text{PV}^- = \frac{\text{TN}}{\text{TN} + \text{FN}} \, .$$

Example 10.   We can calculate the PV of the EIA test from the 2×2 table that we constructed in Example 6 (see Table 3.4) as follows:

$$\text{PV}^+ = \frac{98}{98 + 3} = 0.97.$$

$$\text{PV}^- = \frac{297}{297 + 2} = 0.99.$$

The probability that antibody is present in a patient who has a positive index test (EIA) in this study is 0.97; about 97 of 100 patients with a positive test will have antibody. The likelihood that a patient with a negative index test does not have antibody is about 0.99.

It is worth reemphasizing the difference between PV and sensitivity and specificity, given that both are calculated from the 2 × 2 table and they often are confused. The sensitivity and specificity give the probability of a particular test result in a patient who has a particular disease state. The PV gives the probability of true disease state once the patient's test result is known.

The PV+ calculated from Table 3.4 is 0.97, so we expect 97 of 100 patients with a positive index test actually to have antibody. Yet, in Example 1, we found that less than 1 of 10 patients with a positive test were expected to have antibody. What explains the discrepancy in these examples? The sensitivity and specificity (and, therefore, the LRs) in the two examples are identical. The discrepancy is due to an extremely important and often overlooked characteristic of PV: the PV of a test depends on the *prevalence* of disease in the study population (the prevalence can be calculated as TP + FN divided by the total number of patients in the 2 × 2 table). The PV cannot be generalized to a new population because the prevalence of disease may differ between the two populations.

The difference in PV of the EIA in Example 1 and in Example 6 is due to a difference in the prevalence of disease in the examples. The prevalence of antibody was given as 0.001 in Example 1 and as 0.25 in Example 6. These examples should remind us that the PV+ is not an intrinsic property of a test. Rather, it represents the post-test probability of disease only when the prevalence is identical to that in the 2 × 2 contingency table from which the PV+ was calculated. Bayes' theorem provides a method for calculation of the post-test probability of disease for any prior probability. For that reason, we prefer the use of Bayes' theorem to calculate the post-test probability of disease.

3.4.4 Implications of Bayes' Theorem

In this section, we explore the implications of Bayes' theorem for test interpretation. These ideas are extremely important, yet they often are misunderstood.

Figure 3.5 illustrates one of the most essential concepts in this chapter: The post-test probability of disease increases as the pretest probability of disease increases. We produced Figure 3.5a by calculating the post-test probability after a positive test result for all possible pretest probabilities of disease. We similarly derived Figure 3.5b for a negative test result.

The 45-degree line in each figure denotes a test in which the pretest and post-test probability are equal (LR = 1)—a test that is useless. The curve in Figure 3.5a relates pretest and post-test probabilities in a test with a sensitivity and specificity of 0.9. Note that, at low pretest probabilities, the post-test probability after a positive test result is much higher than is the pretest probability. At high pretest probabilities, the post-test probability is only slightly higher than the pretest probability.

Figure 3.5b shows the relationship between the pretest and post-test probabilities after a negative test result. At high pretest probabilities, the post-test probability after a negative test result is much lower than is the pretest probability. A negative test, however, has little effect on the post-test probability if the pretest probability is low.

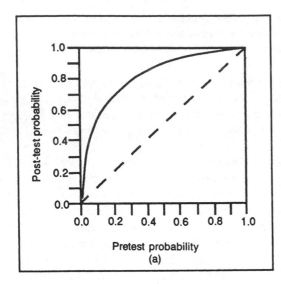

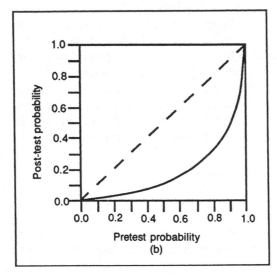

Figure 3.5. Relationship between pretest probability and post-test probability of disease. The dashed lines correspond to a test that has no effect on the probability of disease. Sensitivity and specificity of the test were assumed to be 0.90 for the two examples. (a) The post-test probability of disease corresponding to a *positive* test result (solid curve) was calculated with Bayes' theorem for all values of pretest probability. (b) The post-test probability of disease corresponding to a *negative* test result (solid curve) was calculated with Bayes' theorem for all values of pretest probability. (*Source*: Adapted from Sox, H.C. [1987]. Probability theory in the use of diagnostic tests: Application to critical study of the literature. In Sox H.C. [Ed.], *Common Diagnostic Tests: Use and Interpretation* [pp. 1–17]. Philadelphia: American College of Physicians. Reproduced with permission from the American College of Physicians— American Society of Internal Medicine.)

This discussion emphasizes a key idea of this chapter: the interpretation of a test result depends on the pretest probability of disease. If the pretest probability is low, a positive test result has a large effect, and a negative test result has a small effect. If the pretest probability is high, a positive test result has a small effect, and a negative test result has a large effect. In other words, when the clinician is almost certain of the diagnosis before testing (pretest probability nearly 0 or nearly 1), a confirmatory test has little effect on the posterior probability (see Example 8). If the pretest probability is intermediate or if the result contradicts a strongly held clinical impression, the test result will have a large effect on the post-test probability.

Note from Figure 3.5a that, if the pretest probability is very low, a positive test result can raise the post-test probability into only the intermediate range. Assume that Figure 3.5a represents the relationship between the pretest and post-test probabilities for the exercise stress test. If the clinician believes the pretest probability of coronary artery disease is 0.1, the post-test probability will be about 0.5. Although there has been a large change in the probability, the post-test probability is in an intermediate range, which leaves considerable uncertainty about the diagnosis. Thus, if the pretest probability is low, it is unlikely that a positive test result will raise the probability of disease sufficiently for the clinician to make that diagnosis with confidence. An exception to this statement occurs when a test has a very high specificity (or a large LR$^+$); e.g., HIV antibody tests have a specificity greater than 0.99, and therefore a positive test is convincing. Similarly, if the pretest probability is very high, it is unlikely that a negative test result will lower the post-test probability sufficiently to exclude a diagnosis.

Figure 3.6 illustrates another important concept: test specificity affects primarily the interpretation of a positive test; test sensitivity affects primarily the interpretation of a negative test. In both parts (a) and (b) of Figure 3.6, the top family of curves corresponds to positive test results and the bottom family to negative test results. Figure 3.6a shows the post-test probabilities for tests with varying specificities (TNR). Note that changes in the specificity produce large changes in the top family of curves (positive test results) but have little effect on the lower family of curves (negative test results). That is, an increase in the specificity of a test markedly changes the post-test probability if the test is positive but has relatively little effect on the post-test probability if the test is negative. Thus, if you are trying to *rule in* a diagnosis,[8] you should choose a test with high specificity or a high LR$^+$. Figure 3.6b shows the post-test probabilities for tests with varying sensitivities. Note that changes in sensitivity produce large changes in the bottom family of curves (negative test results) but have little effect on the top family of curves. Thus, if you are trying to exclude a disease, choose a test with a high sensitivity or a high LR$^-$.

3.4.5   Cautions in the Application of Bayes' Theorem

Bayes' theorem provides a powerful method for calculating post-test probability. You should be aware, however, of the possible errors you can make when you use it. Common problems are inaccurate estimation of pretest probability, faulty application of test-performance measures, and violation of the assumptions of conditional independence and of mutual exclusivity.

Bayes' theorem provides a means to adjust an estimate of pretest probability to take into account new information. The accuracy of the calculated post-test probability is

---

[8] In medicine, to *rule in* a disease is to confirm that the patient *does* have the disease; to *rule out* a disease is to confirm that the patient *does not* have the disease. A doctor who strongly suspects that his or her patient has a bacterial infection orders a culture to *rule in* his or her diagnosis. Another doctor is almost certain that his or her patient has a simple sore throat but orders a culture to rule out streptococcal infection (strep throat). This terminology oversimplifies a diagnostic process that is probabilistic. Diagnostic tests rarely, if ever, rule in or rule out a disease; rather, the tests raise or lower the probability of disease.

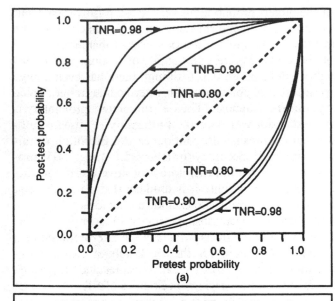

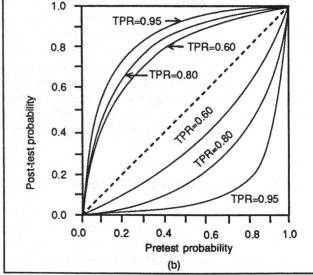

Figure 3.6. Effects of test sensitivity and specificity on post-test probability. The curves are similar to those shown in Figure 3.5 except that the calculations have been repeated for several values of the sensitivity (TPR = true-positive rate) and specificity (TNR = true-negative rate) of the test. (a) The sensitivity of the test was assumed to be 0.90, and the calculations were repeated for several values of test specificity. (b) The specificity of the test was assumed to be 0.90, and the calculations were repeated for several values of the sensitivity of the test. In both panels, the top family of curves corresponds to positive test results, and the bottom family of curves corresponds to negative test results. (*Source*: Adapted from Sox H.C. [1987]. Probability theory in the use of diagnostic tests: Application to critical study of the literature. In Sox H.C. [Ed.], *Common Diagnostic Tests: Use and Interpretation* [pp. 1–17]. Philadelphia: American College of Physicians. Reproduced with permission from the American College of Physicians—American Society of Internal Medicine.)

limited, however, by the accuracy of the estimated pretest probability. Accuracy of estimated prior probability is increased by proper use of published prevalence rates, heuristics, and clinical prediction rules. In a decision analysis, as we shall see, a *range* of prior probability often is sufficient. Nonetheless, if the pretest probability assessment is unreliable, Bayes' theorem will be of little value.

A second potential mistake that you can make when using Bayes' theorem is to apply published values for the test sensitivity and specificity, or LRs, without paying attention to the possible effects of bias in the studies in which the test performance was measured (see Section 3.3.5). With certain tests, the LRs may differ depending on the pretest odds in part because differences in pretest odds may reflect differences in the spectrum of disease in the population.

A third potential problem arises when you use Bayes' theorem to interpret a *sequence* of tests. If a patient undergoes two tests in sequence, you can use the post-test probability after the first test result, calculated with Bayes' theorem, as the pretest probability for the second test. Then, you use Bayes' theorem a second time to calculate the post-test probability after the second test. This approach is valid, however, only if the two tests are conditionally independent. Tests for the same disease are **conditionally independent** when the probability of a particular result on the second test does not depend on the result of the first test, *given* (conditioned on) the disease state. Expressed in conditional probability notation for the case in which the disease is present,

p[second test positive | first test positive and disease present]
= p[second test positive | first test negative and disease present]
= p[second test positive | disease present].

If the conditional independence assumption is satisfied, the post-test odds=pretest odds × LR_1 × LR_2. If you apply Bayes' theorem sequentially in situations in which conditional independence is violated, you will obtain inaccurate post-test probabilities (Gould, 2003).

The fourth common problem arises when you assume that all test abnormalities result from one (and only one) disease process. The Bayesian approach, as we have described it, generally presumes that the diseases under consideration are **mutually exclusive.** If they are not, Bayesian updating must be applied with great care.

We have shown how to calculate post-test probability. In Section 3.5, we turn to the problem of decision making when the outcomes of a physician's actions (e.g., of treatments) are uncertain.

3.5   Expected-Value Decision Making

Medical decision-making problems often cannot be solved by reasoning based on pathophysiology. For example, clinicians need a method for choosing among treatments when the outcome of the treatments is uncertain, as are the results of a surgical operation. You can use the ideas developed in the preceding sections to solve such difficult decision problems. Here we discuss two methods: the decision tree, a method for representing and comparing the expected outcomes of each decision alternative; and the threshold probability, a method for deciding whether new information can change a management decision. These techniques help you to clarify the decision problem and thus to choose the alternative that is most likely to help the patient.

3.5.1   Comparison of Uncertain Prospects

Like those of most biological events, the outcome of an individual's illness is unpredictable. How can a physician determine which course of action has the greatest chance of success?

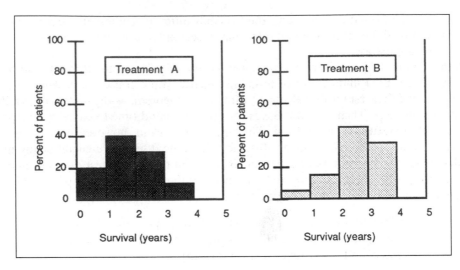

Figure 3.7. Survival after therapy for a fatal disease. Two therapies are available; the results of either are unpredictable.

Example 11.   There are two available therapies for a fatal illness. The length of a patient's life after either therapy is unpredictable, as illustrated by the frequency distribution shown in Figure 3.7 and summarized in Table 3.5. Each therapy is associated with uncertainty: regardless of which therapy a patient receives, he will die by the end of the fourth year, but there is no way to know which year will be the patient's last. Figure 3.7 shows that survival until the fourth year is more likely with therapy B, but the patient might die in the first year with therapy B or might survive to the fourth year with therapy A.

  Which of the two therapies is preferable? This example demonstrates a significant fact: a choice among therapies is a choice among gambles (i.e., situations in which chance determines the outcomes). How do we usually choose among gambles? More often than not, we rely on hunches or on a sixth sense. How should we choose among gambles? We propose a method for choosing called **expected-value decision making:** we characterize each gamble by a number, and we use that number to compare the gambles.[9] In Example 11, therapy A and therapy B are both gambles with respect to dura-

Table 3.5. Distribution of probabilities for the two therapies in Figure 3.7.

Years after therapy	Probability of death	
	Therapy A	Therapy B
1	0.20	0.05
2	0.40	0.15
3	0.30	0.45
4	0.10	0.35

---

[9] Expected-value decision making had been used in many fields before it was first applied to medicine.

tion of life after therapy. We want to assign a measure (or number) to each therapy that summarizes the outcomes such that we can decide which therapy is preferable.

The ideal criterion for choosing a gamble should be a number that reflects preferences (in medicine, often the patient's preferences) for the outcomes of the gamble. **Utility** is the name given to a measure of preference that has a desirable property for decision making: the gamble with the highest utility should be preferred. We shall discuss utility briefly (Section 3.5.4), but you can pursue this topic and the details of decision analysis in other textbooks (see Suggested Readings at the end of this chapter).[10] We use the average duration of life after therapy (survival) as a criterion for choosing among therapies; remember that this model is oversimplified, used here for discussion only. Later, we consider other factors, such as the quality of life.

Because we cannot be sure of the duration of survival for any given patient, we characterize a therapy by the mean survival (average length of life) that would be observed in a large number of patients after they were given the therapy. The first step we take in calculating the mean survival for a therapy is to divide the population receiving the therapy into groups of patients who have similar survival rates. Then, we multiply the survival time in each group[11] by the fraction of the total population in that group. Finally, we sum these products over all possible survival values.

We can perform this calculation for the therapies in Example 11. Mean survival for therapy A $= (0.2 \times 1.0) + (0.4 \times 2.0) + (0.3 \times 3.0) + (0.1 \times 4.0) = 2.3$ years. Mean survival for therapy B $= (0.05 \times 1.0) + (0.15 \times 2.0) + (0.45 \times 3.0) + (0.35 \times 4.0) = 3.1$ years.

Survival after a therapy is under the control of chance. Therapy A is a gamble characterized by an average survival equal to 2.3 years. Therapy B is a gamble characterized by an average survival of 3.1 years. If length of life is our criterion for choosing, we should select therapy B.

3.5.2 Representation of Choices with Decision Trees

The choice between therapies A and B is represented diagrammatically in Figure 3.8. Events that are under the control of chance can be represented by a **chance node.** By convention, a chance node is shown as a circle from which several lines emanate. Each line represents one of the possible outcomes. Associated with each line is the probability of the outcome occurring. For a single patient, only one outcome can occur. Some physicians object to using probability for just this reason: "You cannot rely on population data, because each patient is an individual." In fact, we often *must* use the frequency of the outcomes of many patients experiencing the same event to inform our opinion about what might happen to an individual. From these frequencies, we can make patient-specific adjustments and thus estimate the probability of each outcome at a chance node.

A chance node can represent more than just an event governed by chance. The outcome of a chance event, unknowable for the individual, can be represented by the

---

[10] A more general term for expected-value decision making is expected *utility* decision making. Because a full treatment of utility is beyond the scope of this chapter, we have chosen to use the term *expected value.*

[11] For this simple example, death during an interval is assumed to occur at the end of the year.

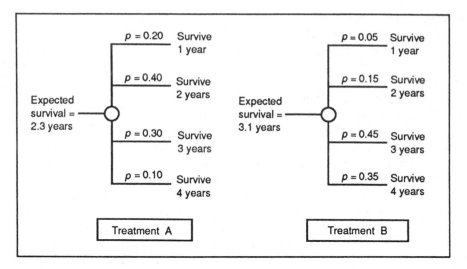

Figure 3.8. A chance-node representation of survival after the two therapies in Figure 3.7. The probabilities times the corresponding years of survival are summed to obtain the total expected survival.

expected value at the chance node. The concept of expected value is important and is easy to understand. We can calculate the mean survival that would be expected based on the probabilities depicted by the chance node in Figure 3.8. This average length of life is called the *expected survival* or, more generally, the *expected value of the chance node*. We calculate the expected value at a chance node by the process just described: we multiply the survival value associated with each possible outcome by the probability that that outcome will occur. We then sum the product of probability times survival over all outcomes. Thus, if several hundred patients were assigned to receive either therapy A or therapy B, the expected survival would be 2.3 years for therapy A and 3.1 years for therapy B.

We have just described the basis of expected-value decision making. The term *expected value* is used to characterize a chance event, such as the outcome of a therapy. If the outcomes of a therapy are measured in units of duration of survival, units of sense of well-being, or dollars, the therapy is characterized by the expected duration of survival, expected sense of well-being, or expected monetary cost that it will confer on, or incur for, the patient, respectively.

To use expected-value decision making, we follow this strategy when there are therapy choices with uncertain outcomes: (1) calculate the expected value of each decision alternative and then (2) pick the alternative with the highest expected value.

3.5.3   Performance of a Decision Analysis

We clarify the concepts of expected-value decision making by discussing an example. There are four steps in decision analysis:

1. Create a decision tree; this step is the most difficult, because it requires formulating the decision problem, assigning probabilities, and measuring outcomes.
2. Calculate the expected value of each decision alternative.
3. Choose the decision alternative with the highest expected value.
4. Use sensitivity analysis to test the conclusions of the analysis.

Many health professionals balk when they first learn about the technique of decision analysis, because they recognize the opportunity for error in assigning values to both the probabilities and the utilities in a decision tree. They reason that the technique encourages decision making based on small differences in expected values that are estimates at best. The defense against this concern, which also has been recognized by decision analysts, is the technique known as *sensitivity analysis*. We discuss this important fourth step in decision analysis in Section 3.5.5.

The first step in decision analysis is to create a **decision tree** that represents the decision problem. Consider the following clinical problem.

> **Example 12.** The patient is Mr. Danby, a 66-year-old man who has been crippled with arthritis of both knees so severely that, while he can get about the house with the aid of two canes, he must otherwise use a wheelchair. His other major health problem is emphysema, a disease in which the lungs lose their ability to exchange oxygen and carbon dioxide between blood and air, which in turn causes shortness of breath (dyspnea). He is able to breathe comfortably when he is in a wheelchair, but the effort of walking with canes makes him breathe heavily and feel uncomfortable. Several years ago, he seriously considered knee replacement surgery but decided against it, largely because his internist told him that there was a serious risk that he would not survive the operation because of his lung disease. Recently, however, Mr. Danby's wife had a stroke and was partially paralyzed; she now requires a degree of assistance that the patient cannot supply given his present state of mobility. He tells his doctor that he is reconsidering knee replacement surgery.
>
> Mr. Danby's internist is familiar with decision analysis. She recognizes that this problem is filled with uncertainty: Mr. Danby's ability to survive the operation is in doubt, and the surgery sometimes does not restore mobility to the degree required by such a patient. Furthermore, there is a small chance that the prosthesis (the artificial knee) will become infected, and Mr. Danby then would have to undergo a second risky operation to remove it. After removal of the prosthesis, Mr. Danby would never again be able to walk, even with canes. The possible outcomes of knee replacement include death from the first procedure and death from a second mandatory procedure if the prosthesis becomes infected (which we will assume occurs in the immediate postoperative period, if it occurs at all). Possible functional outcomes include recovery of full mobility or continued, and unchanged, poor mobility. Should Mr. Danby choose to undergo knee replacement surgery, or should he accept the status quo?

Using the conventions of decision analysis, the internist sketches the decision tree shown in Figure 3.9. According to these conventions, a square box denotes a **decision node,** and each line emanating from a decision node represents an action that could be taken.

According to the methods of expected-value decision making, the internist first must assign a probability to each branch of each chance node. To accomplish this task, the internist asks several orthopedic surgeons for their estimates of the chance of

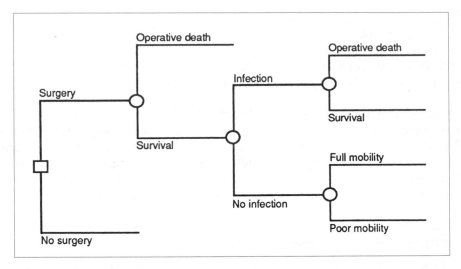

Figure 3.9. Decision tree for knee replacement surgery. The box represents the decision node (whether to have surgery); the circles represent chance nodes.

recovering full function after surgery (p[full recovery]=0.60) and the chance of developing infection in the prosthetic joint (p[infection]=0.05). She uses her subjective estimate of the probability that the patient will die during or immediately after knee surgery (p[operative death]=0.05).

Next, she must assign a value to each outcome. To accomplish this task, she first lists the outcomes. As you can see from Table 3.6, the outcomes differ in two dimensions: length of life (survival) and quality of life (functional status). To characterize each outcome accurately, the internist must develop a measure that takes into account these two dimensions. Simply using duration of survival is inadequate because Mr. Danby values 5 years of good health more than he values 10 years of poor health. The internist can account for this trade-off factor by converting outcomes with two dimensions into outcomes with a single dimension: duration of survival in good health. The resulting measure is called a **quality-adjusted life year** (QALY).[12]

She can convert years in poor health into years in good health by asking Mr. Danby to indicate the shortest period in good health (full mobility) that he would accept in return for his full expected lifetime (10 years) in a state of poor health (status quo). Thus, she asks Mr. Danby: "Many people say they would be willing to accept a shorter life in excellent health in preference to a longer life with significant disability. In your case, how many years with normal mobility do you feel is equivalent in value to 10 years in your current state of disability?" She asks him this question for each outcome. The patient's responses are shown in the third column of Table 3.6. The patient decides that

---

[12] QALYs commonly are used as measures of utility (value) in medical decision analysis and in health policy analysis (see, for example, the discussion of cost-effectiveness analysis in Chapter 8).

Table 3.6. Outcomes for Example 12.

Survival (years)	Functional status	Years of full function equivalent to outcome
10	Full mobility (successful surgery)	10
10	Poor mobility (status quo or unsuccessful surgery)	6
10	Wheelchair-bound (the outcome if a second surgery is necessary)	3
0	Death	0

10 years of limited mobility are equivalent to 6 years of normal mobility, whereas 10 years of wheelchair confinement are equivalent to only 3 years of full function. Figure 3.10 shows the final decision tree—complete with probability estimates and utility values for each outcome.[13]

The second task that the internist must undertake is to calculate the expected value, in healthy years, of surgery and of no surgery. She calculates the expected value at each chance node, moving from right (the tips of the tree) to left (the root of the tree). Let us consider, for example, the expected value at the chance node representing the outcome

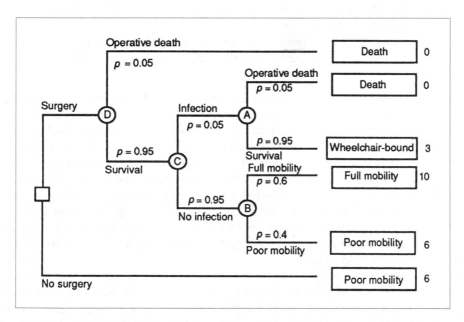

Figure 3.10. Decision tree for knee-replacement surgery. Probabilities have been assigned to each branch of each chance node. The patient's valuations of outcomes (measured in years of perfect mobility) are assigned to the tips of each branch of the tree.

---

[13] In a more sophisticated decision analysis, the physician also would adjust the utility values of outcomes that require surgery to account for the pain and inconvenience associated with surgery and rehabilitation.

of surgery to remove an infected prosthesis (Node A in Figure 3.10). The calculation requires three steps:

1. Calculate the expected value of operative death after surgery to remove an infected prosthesis. Multiply the probability of operative death (0.05) by the QALY of the outcome—death (0 years): $0.05 \times 0 = 0$ QALY.
2. Calculate the expected value of surviving surgery to remove an infected knee prosthesis. Multiply the probability of surviving the operation (0.95) by the number of healthy years equivalent to 10 years of being wheelchair-bound (3 years): $0.95 \times 3 = 2.85$ QALYs.
3. Add the expected values calculated in step 1 (0 QALY) and step 2 (2.85 QALYs) to obtain the expected value of developing an infected prosthesis: $0 + 2.85 = 2.85$ QALYs.

Similarly, the expected value at chance node B is calculated: $(0.6 \times 10) + (0.4 \times 6) = 8.4$ QALYs. To obtain the expected value of surviving knee replacement surgery (Node C), she proceeds as follows:

1. Multiply the expected value of an infected prosthesis (already calculated as 2.85 QALYs) by the probability that the prosthesis will become infected (0.05): $2.85 \times 0.05 = 0.143$ QALYs.
2. Multiply the expected value of never developing an infected prosthesis (already calculated as 8.4 QALYs) by the probability that the prosthesis will not become infected (0.95): $8.4 \times 0.95 = 7.98$ QALYs.
3. Add the expected values calculated in step 1 (0.143 QALY) and step 2 (7.98 QALYs) to get the expected value of surviving knee replacement surgery: $0.143 + 7.98 = 8.123$ QALYs.

The physician performs this process, called **averaging out at chance nodes,** for node D as well, working back to the root of the tree, until the expected value of surgery has been calculated. The outcome of the analysis is as follows. For surgery, Mr. Danby's average life expectancy, measured in years of normal mobility, is 7.7. What does this value mean? It does not mean that, by accepting surgery, Mr. Danby is guaranteed 7.7 years of mobile life. One look at the decision tree will show that some patients die in surgery, some develop infection, and some do not gain any improvement in mobility after surgery. Thus, an individual patient has no guarantees. If the physician had 100 similar patients who underwent the surgery, however, the *average* number of mobile years would be 7.7. We can understand what this value means for Mr. Danby only by examining the alternative: no surgery.

In the analysis for no surgery, the average length of life, measured in years of normal mobility, is 6.0, which Mr. Danby considered equivalent to 10 years of continued poor mobility. Not all patients will experience this outcome; some who have poor mobility will live longer than, and some will live less than, 10 years. The average length of life, however, expressed in years of normal mobility, will be 6. Because 6.0 is less than 7.7, *on average* the surgery will provide an outcome with higher value to the patient. Thus, the internist recommends performing the surgery.

The key insight of expected-value decision making should be clear from this example: given the unpredictable outcome in an individual, the best choice for the individual is the alternative that gives the best result on the average in similar patients. Decision analysis can help the physician to identify the therapy that will give the best results when averaged over many similar patients. The decision analysis is tailored to a specific patient in that both the utility functions and the probability estimates are adjusted to the individual. Nonetheless, the results of the analysis represent the outcomes that would occur *on average* in a population of patients who have similar utilities and for whom uncertain events have similar probabilities.

3.5.4   Representation of Patients' Preferences with Utilities

In Section 3.5.3, we introduced the concept of QALYs, because length of life is not the only outcome about which patients care. Patients' preferences for a health outcome may depend on the length of life with the outcome, on the quality of life with the outcome, and on the risk involved in achieving the outcome (e.g., a cure for cancer might require a risky surgical operation). How can we incorporate these elements into a decision analysis? To do so, we can represent patients' preferences with utilities. The **utility** of a health state is a quantitative measure of the desirability of a health state from the patient's perspective. Utilities are typically expressed on a 0 to 1 scale, where 0 represents death and 1 represents ideal health. For example, a study of patients who had chest pain (angina) with exercise rated the utility of mild, moderate, and severe angina as 0.95, 0.92, and 0.82 (Nease et al., 1995), respectively. There are several methods for assessing utilities.

The **standard-gamble** technique has the strongest theoretical basis of the various approaches to utility assessment, as shown by Von Neumann and Morgenstern and described by Sox et al. (1988). To illustrate use of the standard gamble, suppose we seek to assess a person's utility for the health state of asymptomatic HIV infection. To use the standard gamble, we ask our subject to compare the desirability of asymptomatic HIV infection to those of two other health states whose utility we know or can assign. Often, we use ideal health (assigned a utility of 1) and immediate death (assigned a utility of 0) for the comparison of health states. We then ask our subject to choose between asymptomatic HIV infection and a gamble with a chance of ideal health or immediate death. We vary the probability of ideal health and immediate death systematically until the subject is indifferent between asymptomatic HIV infection and the gamble. For example, a subject might be indifferent when the probability of ideal health is 0.8 and the probability of death is 0.2. At this point of indifference, the utility of the gamble and that of asymptomatic HIV infection are equal. We calculate the utility of the gamble as the weighted average of the utilities of each outcome of the gamble $[(1 \times 0.8) + (0 \times 0.2)]=0.8$. Thus in this example, the utility of asymptomatic HIV infection is 0.8. Use of the standard gamble enables an analyst to assess the utility of outcomes that differ in length or quality of life. Because the standard gamble involves chance events, it also assesses a person's willingness to take risks—called the person's **risk attitude**.

A second common approach to utility assessment is the **time-trade-off** technique (Sox et al., 1988; Torrance and Feeny, 1989). To assess the utility of asymptomatic HIV infection using the time-trade-off technique, we ask a person to determine the length of time in a better state of health (usually ideal health or best attainable health) that he or she would find equivalent to a longer period of time with asymptomatic HIV infection. For example, if our subject says that 8 months of life with ideal health was equivalent to 12 months of life with asymptomatic HIV infection, then we calculate the utility of asymptomatic HIV infection as $8 \div 12 = 0.67$. The time-trade-off technique provides a convenient method for valuing outcomes that accounts for gains (or losses) in both length and quality of life. Because the time trade-off does not include gambles, however, it does not assess a person's risk attitude. Perhaps the strongest assumption underlying the use of the time trade-off as a measure of utility is that people are risk neutral. A **risk-neutral** decision maker is indifferent between the expected value of a gamble and the gamble itself. For example, a risk-neutral decision maker would be indifferent between the choice of living 20 years (for certain) and that of taking a gamble with a 50 percent chance of living 40 years and a 50 percent chance of immediate death (which has an expected value of 20 years). In practice, of course, few people are risk-neutral. Nonetheless, the time-trade-off technique is used frequently to value health outcomes because it is relatively easy to understand.

Several other approaches are available to value health outcomes. To use the **visual analog scale,** a person simply rates the quality of life with a health outcome (e.g., asymptomatic HIV infection) on a scale from 0 to 100. Although the visual analog scale is easy to explain and use, it has no theoretical justification as a valid measure of utility. Ratings with the visual analog scale, however, correlate modestly well with utilities assessed by the standard gamble and time trade-off. For a demonstration of the use of standard gambles, time trade-offs, and the visual analog scale to assess utilities in patients with angina, see Nease et al. (1995). Other approaches to valuing health outcomes include the Quality of Well-Being Scale, the Health Utilities Index, and the EuroQoL (see Gold et al., 1996, ch. 4). Each of these instruments assesses how people value health outcomes and therefore may be appropriate for use in decision analyses or cost-effectiveness analyses.

In summary, we can use utilities to represent how patients value complicated health outcomes that differ in length and quality of life and in riskiness. Computer-based tools with an interactive format are now available for assessing utilities; they often include text and multimedia presentations that enhance patients' understanding of the assessment tasks and of the health outcomes (Sumner et al., 1991; Nease and Owens, 1994; Lenert et al., 1995).

3.5.5   Performance of Sensitivity Analysis

Sensitivity analysis is a test of the validity of the conclusions of an analysis over a wide range of assumptions about the probabilities and the values, or utilities. The probability of an outcome at a chance node may be the best estimate that is available, but there often is a wide range of reasonable probabilities that a physician could use with nearly equal confidence. We use sensitivity analysis to answer this question: Do my conclusions regarding the preferred choice change when the probability and outcome estimates are assigned values that lie within a reasonable range?

The knee-replacement decision in Example 12 illustrates the power of sensitivity analysis. If the conclusions of the analysis (surgery is preferable to no surgery) remain the same despite a wide range of assumed values for the probabilities and outcome

Figure 3.11. Sensitivity analysis of the effect of operative mortality on length of healthy life (Example 12). As the probability of operative death increases, the relative values of surgery versus no surgery change. The point at which the two lines cross represents the probability of operative death at which no surgery becomes preferable. The solid line represents the preferred option at a given probability.

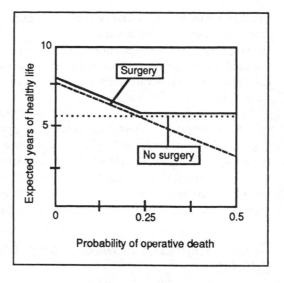

measures, the recommendation is trustworthy. Figures 3.11 and 3.12 show the expected survival in healthy years with surgery and without surgery under varying assumptions of the probability of operative death and the probability of attaining perfect mobility, respectively. Each point (value) on these lines represents one calculation of expected survival using the tree in Figure 3.9. Figure 3.11 shows that expected survival is higher with surgery over a wide range of operative mortality rates. Expected survival is lower with surgery, however, when the operative mortality rate exceeds 25 percent. Figure 3.12 shows the effect of varying the probability that the operation will lead to perfect mobility. The expected survival, in healthy years, is higher for surgery as long as the

Figure 3.12. Sensitivity analysis of the effect of a successful operative result on length of healthy life (Example 12). As the probability of a successful surgical result increases, the relative values of surgery versus no surgery change. The point at which the two lines cross represents the probability of a successful result at which surgery becomes preferable. The solid line represents the preferred option at a given probability.

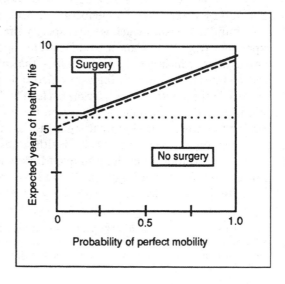

probability of perfect mobility exceeds 20 percent, a much lower figure than is expected from previous experience with the operation. (In Example 12, the consulting orthopedic surgeons estimated the chance of full recovery at 60 percent.) Thus, the internist can proceed with confidence to recommend surgery. Mr. Danby cannot be sure of a good outcome, but he has valid reasons for thinking that he is more likely to do well with surgery than he is without it.

Another way to state the conclusions of a sensitivity analysis is to indicate the range of probabilities over which the conclusions apply. The point at which the two lines in Figure 3.11 cross is the probability of operative death at which the two therapy options have the same expected survival. If expected survival is to be the basis for choosing therapy, the internist and the patient should be indifferent between surgery and no surgery when the probability of operative death is 25 percent.[14] When the probability is lower, they should select surgery. When it is higher, they should select no surgery.

3.5.6 Representation of Long-Term Outcomes with Markov Models

In Example 12, we evaluated Mr. Danby's decision to have surgery to improve his mobility, which was compromised by arthritis. We assumed that each of the possible outcomes (full mobility, poor mobility, death, etc.) would occur shortly after Mr. Danby took action on his decision. But what if we want to model events that might occur in the distant future? For example, a patient with HIV infection might develop AIDS 10 to 15 years after infection; thus, a therapy to prevent or delay the development of AIDS could affect events that occur 10 to 15 years, or more, in the future. A similar problem arises in analyses of decisions regarding many chronic diseases: we must model events that occur over the lifetime of the patient. The decision tree representation is convenient for decisions for which all outcomes occur during a short time horizon, but it is not always sufficient for problems that include events that could occur in the future. How can we include such events in a decision analysis? The answer is to use Markov models (Beck and Pauker, 1983; Sonnenberg and Beck, 1993).

To build a **Markov model,** we first specify the set of health states that a person could experience (e.g., Well, Cancer, and Death in Figure 3.13). We then specify the **transition probabilities,** which are the probabilities that a person will transit from one of these health states to another during a specified time period. This period—often 1 month or 1 year—is the length of the **Markov cycle.** The Markov model then simulates the transitions among health states for a person (or for a hypothetical cohort of people) for a specified number of cycles; by using a Markov model, we can calculate the probability that a person will be in each of the health states at any time in the future.

As an illustration, consider a simple Markov model that has three health states: Well, Cancer, and Death (see Figure 3.13). We have specified each of the transition probabilities in Table 3.7 for the cycle length of 1 year. Thus, we note from Table 3.7 that a person

---

[14] An operative mortality rate of 25 percent may seem high; however, this value is correct when we use QALYs as the basis for choosing treatment. A decision maker performing a more sophisticated analysis could use a utility function that reflects the patient's aversion to risking death.

Figure 3.13. A simple Markov model. The states of health that a person can experience are indicated by the circles; arrows represent allowed transitions between health states.

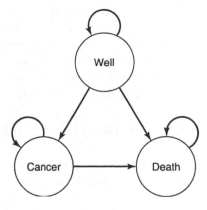

who is in the well state will remain well with probability 0.9, will develop cancer with probability 0.06, and will die from noncancer causes with probability 0.04 during 1 year. The calculations for a Markov model are performed by computer software. Based on the transition probabilities in Table 3.7, the probabilities that a person remains well, develops cancer, or dies from noncancer causes over time is shown in Table 3.8. We can also determine from a Markov model the expected length of time that a person spends in each health state. Therefore, we can determine life expectancy, or quality-adjusted life expectancy, for any alternative represented by a Markov model.

In decision analyses that represent long-term outcomes, the analysts will often use a Markov model in conjunction with a decision tree to model the decision (Owens et al.,

Table 3.7. Transition probabilities for the Markov model in Figure 3.13.

Health state transition	Annual probability
Well to Well	0.9
Well to Cancer	0.06
Well to Death	0.04
Cancer to Well	0.0
Cancer to Cancer	0.4
Cancer to Death	0.6
Death to Well	0.0
Death to Cancer	0.0
Death to Death	1.0

Table 3.8. Probability of future health states for the Markov model in Figure 3.13.

Health state	Probability of health state at end of year						
	Year 1	Year 2	Year 3	Year 4	Year 5	Year 6	Year 7
Well	0.9000	0.8100	0.7290	0.6561	0.5905	0.5314	0.4783
Cancer	0.0600	0.0780	0.0798	0.0757	0.0696	0.0633	0.0572
Death	0.0400	0.1120	0.1912	0.2682	0.3399	0.4053	0.4645

1995, 1997a; Salpeter et al., 1997). The analyst models the effect of an intervention as a change in the probability of going from one state to another. For example, we could model a cancer-prevention intervention (such as screening for breast cancer with mammography) as a reduction in the transition probability from Well to Cancer in Figure 3.13. (See the articles by Beck and Pauker (1983) and Sonnenberg and Beck (1993) for further explanation of the use of Markov models.)

3.6   The Decision Whether to Treat, Test, or Do Nothing

The physician who is evaluating a patient's symptoms and suspects a disease must choose among the following actions:

1. Do nothing further (neither perform additional tests nor treat the patient).
2. Obtain additional diagnostic information (test) before choosing whether to treat or do nothing.
3. Treat without obtaining more information.

When the physician knows the patient's true state, testing is unnecessary, and the doctor needs only to assess the trade-offs among therapeutic options (as in Example 12). Learning the patient's true state, however, may require costly, time-consuming, and often risky diagnostic procedures that may give misleading FP or FN results. Therefore, physicians often are willing to treat a patient even when they are not absolutely certain about a patient's true state. There are risks in this course: the physician may withhold therapy from a person who has the disease of concern, or he may administer therapy to someone who does not have the disease yet may suffer undesirable side effects of therapy.

Deciding among treating, testing, and doing nothing sounds difficult, but you have already learned all the principles that you need to solve this kind of problem. There are three steps:

1. Determine the treatment threshold probability of disease.
2. Determine the pretest probability of disease.
3. Decide whether a test result could affect your decision to treat.

The **treatment threshold probability** of disease is the probability of disease at which you should be indifferent between treating and not treating (Pauker and Kassirer, 1980). Below the treatment threshold, you should not treat. Above the treatment threshold, you should treat (Figure 3.14). Whether to treat when the diagnosis is not certain is a problem that you can solve with a decision tree, such as the one shown in Figure 3.15. You can use this tree to learn the treatment threshold probability of disease by leaving the probability of disease as an unknown, setting the expected value of surgery equal to the expected value for medical (i.e., nonsurgical, such as drugs or physical therapy) treatment, and solving for the probability of disease. (In this example, surgery corresponds to the "treat" branch of the tree in Figure 3.15, and nonsurgical intervention corresponds to the "do not treat" branch.) Because you are indifferent between medical treatment and surgery at this probability, it is the treatment threshold probability. Using

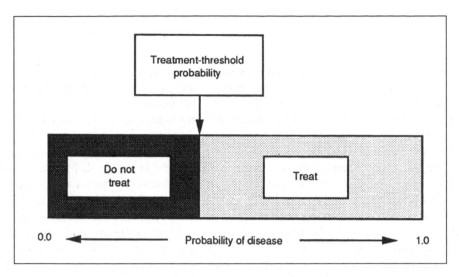

Figure 3.14. Depiction of the treatment threshold probability. At probabilities of disease that are less than the treatment threshold probability, the preferred action is to withhold therapy. At probabilities of disease that are greater than the treatment threshold probability, the preferred action is to treat.

the tree completes step 1. In practice, people often determine the treatment threshold intuitively rather than analytically.

An alternative approach to determination of the treatment threshold probability is to use the equation:

Figure 3.15. Decision tree with which to calculate the treatment threshold probability of disease. By setting the utilities of the *treat* and *do not treat* choices to be equal, we can compute the probability at which the physician and patient should be indifferent to the choice. Recall that $p [-D] = 1 - p [D]$.

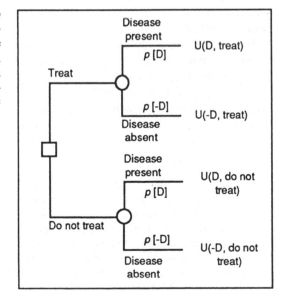

$$p^* = \frac{H}{H + B},$$

where p^* = the treatment threshold probability, H = the harm associated with treatment of a nondiseased patient, and B = the benefit associated with treatment of a diseased patient (Pauker and Kassirer, 1980; Sox et al., 1988). We define B as the difference between the utility (U) of diseased patients who are treated and diseased patients who are not treated (U[D, treat] – U[D, do not treat], as shown in Figure 3.15). The utility of diseased patients who are treated should be greater than that of diseased patients who are not treated; therefore, B is positive. We define H as the difference in utility of nondiseased patients who are not treated and nondiseased patients who are treated (U[–D, do not treat] – U[–D, treat], as shown in Figure 3.15). The utility of nondiseased patients who are not treated should be greater than that of nondiseased patients who are treated; therefore, H is positive. The equation for the treatment threshold probability fits with our intuition: if the benefit of treatment is small and the harm of treatment is large, the treatment threshold probability will be high. In contrast, if the benefit of treatment is large and the harm of treatment is small, the treatment threshold probability will be low.

Once you know the pretest probability, you know what to do in the absence of further information about the patient. If the pretest probability is below the treatment threshold, you should not treat the patient. If the pretest probability is above the threshold, you should treat the patient. Thus you have completed step 2.

One of the guiding principles of medical decision making is this: do not order a test unless it could change your management of the patient. In our framework for decision making, this principle means that you should order a test only if the test result could cause the probability of disease to cross the treatment threshold. Thus, if the pretest probability is above the treatment threshold, a negative test result must lead to a post-test probability that is below the threshold. Conversely, if the pretest probability is below the threshold probability, a positive result must lead to a post-test probability that is above the threshold. In either case, the test result would alter your decision of whether to treat the patient. This analysis completes step 3.

To decide whether a test could alter management, we simply use Bayes' theorem. We calculate the post-test probability after a test result that would move the probability of disease toward the treatment threshold. If the pretest probability is above the treatment threshold, we calculate the probability of disease if the test result is negative. If the pretest probability is below the treatment threshold, we calculate the probability of disease if the test result is positive.

Example 13.   You are a pulmonary medicine specialist. You suspect that a patient of yours has a pulmonary embolus (blood clot lodged in the vessels of the lungs). One approach is to do a radionuclide lung scan, a test in which tiny radioactive particles are injected into a vein. These particles flow into the small vessels of the lung. A scanning device detects the radiation from the particles. The particles cannot go to a part of the lung that is supplied by a vessel that is blocked by a blood clot. Unfortunately, there are other causes of blank areas in the scan so that you cannot be sure that a blood clot is present when there is a blank area. Thus, if the scan is abnormal (shows a blank area), you must perform a definitive test to confirm the diagnosis. Such a test is a pulmonary arteriogram, in which radiopaque dye is injected into the arteries in the lung, and an X-ray image is obtained. The procedure involves further risk, discomfort, and substantial cost to the patient. If the scan is negative, you do no further tests and do not treat the patient.

To decide whether this strategy is correct, you take the following steps:

1. Determine the treatment threshold probability of pulmonary embolus.
2. Estimate the pretest probability of pulmonary embolus.
3. Decide whether a test result could affect your decision to treat for an embolus.

First, assume you decide that the treatment threshold should be 0.10 in this patient. What does it mean to have a treatment threshold probability equal to 0.10? If you could obtain no further information, you would treat for pulmonary embolus if the pretest probability was above 0.10 (i.e., if you believed that there was greater than a 1:10 chance that the patient had an embolus), and would withhold therapy if the pretest probability was below 0.10. A decision to treat when the pretest probability is at the treatment threshold means that you are willing to treat nine patients without pulmonary embolus to be sure of treating one patient who has pulmonary embolus. A relatively low treatment threshold is justifiable because treatment of a pulmonary embolism with blood-thinning medication substantially reduces the high mortality of pulmonary embolism, whereas there is only a relatively small danger (mortality of less than 1 percent) in treating someone who does not have pulmonary embolus. Because the benefit of treatment is high and the harm of treatment is low, the treatment threshold probability will be low, as discussed earlier. You have completed step 1.

You estimate the pretest probability of pulmonary embolus to be 0.05, which is equal to a pretest odds of 0.053. Because the pretest probability is lower than the treatment threshold, you should do nothing unless a positive lung scan result could raise the probability of pulmonary embolus to above 0.10. You have completed step 2.

To decide whether a test result could affect your decision to treat, you must decide whether a positive lung scan result would raise the probability of pulmonary embolism to more than 0.10, the treatment threshold. Lung scans are usually reported as either negative, low probability, or high probability for pulmonary embolism. You review the literature and learn that the LR for a high probability scan is 7.0 to 8.0, and you choose to use the midpoint, 7.5.

A negative lung scan result will move the probability of disease away from the treatment threshold and will be of no help in deciding what to do. A positive result will move the probability of disease toward the treatment threshold and could alter your management decision if the post-test probability were above the treatment threshold. You therefore use the odds-ratio form of Bayes' theorem to calculate the post-test probability of disease if the lung scan result is reported as high probability.

$$\text{Post−test odds} = \text{pretest odds} \times \text{LR}$$
$$= 0.053 \times 7.5 = 0.40.$$

A post-test odds of 0.4 is equivalent to a probability of disease of 0.29. Because the post-test probability of pulmonary embolus is higher than the treatment threshold, a positive lung scan result would change your management of the patient, and you should order the lung scan. You have completed step 3.

This example is especially useful for two reasons: first, it demonstrates one method for making decisions and second, it shows how the concepts that were introduced in this chapter all fit together in a clinical example of medical decision making.

3.7   Alternative Graphical Representations for Decision Models: Influence Diagrams and Belief Networks

In Sections 3.5 and 3.6, we used decision trees to represent decision problems. Although decision trees are the most common graphical representation for decision problems, **influence diagrams** are an important alternative representation for such problems (Nease and Owens, 1997; Owens et al., 1997b).

As shown in Figure 3.16, influence diagrams have certain features that are similar to decision trees, but they also have additional graphical elements. Influence diagrams represent decision nodes as squares and chance nodes as circles. In contrast to decision trees, however, the influence diagram also has arcs between nodes and a diamond-shaped value node. An **arc** between two chance nodes indicates that a probabilistic relationship *may* exist between the chance nodes (Owens et al., 1997b). A **probabilistic relationship** exists when the occurrence of one chance event affects the probability of the occurrence of another chance event. For example, in Figure 3.16, the probability of a positive or negative PCR test result (PCR result) depends on whether a person has HIV infection (HIV status); thus, these nodes have a probabilistic relationship, as indicated by the arc. The arc points from the **conditioning event** to the **conditioned event** (PCR test result is conditioned on HIV status in Figure 3.16). The absence of an arc between two chance nodes, however, always indicates that the nodes are independent or conditionally independent. Two events are **conditionally independent,** given a third event, if the occurrence of one of the events does not affect the probability of the other event conditioned on the occurrence of the third event.

Unlike a decision tree, in which the events usually are represented from left to right in the order in which the events are observed, influence diagrams use arcs to indicate the timing of events. An arc from a chance node to a decision node indicates that the chance event has been observed at the time the decision is made. Thus, the arc from PCR result to Treat? in Figure 3.16 indicates that the decision maker knows the PCR test result (positive, negative, or not obtained) when he or she decides whether to treat. Arcs between decision nodes indicate the timing of decisions: the arc points from an initial decision to subsequent decisions. Thus, in Figure 3.16, the decision maker must decide whether to obtain a PCR test before deciding whether to treat, as indicated by the arc from Obtain PCR? to Treat?

The probabilities and utilities that we need to determine the alternative with the highest expected value are contained in tables associated with chance nodes and the value node (Figure 3.17). These tables contain the same information that we would use in a decision tree. With a decision tree, we can determine the expected value of each alternative by averaging out at chance nodes and folding back the tree (Section 3.5.3). For

Figure 3.16. A decision tree (top) and an influence diagram (bottom) that represent the decisions to test for, and to treat, HIV infection. The structural asymmetry of the alternatives is explicit in the decision tree. The influence diagram highlights probabilistic relationships. HIV = human immunodeficiency virus; HIV+ = HIV infected; HIV− = not infected with HIV; QALE = quality-adjusted life expectancy; PCR = polymerase chain reaction. Test results are shown in quotation marks ("HIV+"), whereas the true disease state is shown without quotation marks (HIV+). (*Source*: Owens D.K., Shachter R.D., Nease R.F. [1997]. Representation and analysis of medical decision problems with influence diagrams. *Medical Decision Making*, 17(3): 241–262. Reproduced with permission.)

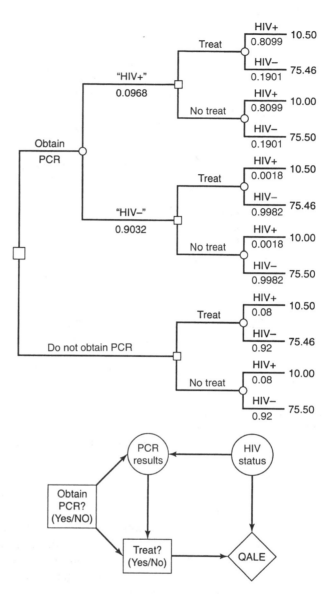

influence diagrams, the calculation of expected value is more complex (Owens et al., 1997b), and generally must be performed with computer software. With the appropriate software, we can use influence diagrams to perform the same analyses that we would perform with a decision tree. Diagrams that have only chance nodes are called **belief networks;** we use them to perform probabilistic inference.

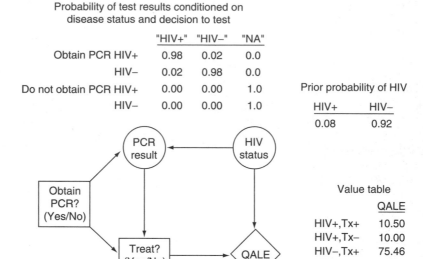

Probability of test results conditioned on
disease status and decision to test

	"HIV+"	"HIV−"	"NA"
Obtain PCR HIV+	0.98	0.02	0.0
HIV−	0.02	0.98	0.0
Do not obtain PCR HIV+	0.00	0.00	1.0
HIV−	0.00	0.00	1.0

Prior probability of HIV

HIV+	HIV−
0.08	0.92

Value table

	QALE
HIV+,Tx+	10.50
HIV+,Tx−	10.00
HIV−,Tx+	75.46
HIV−,Tx	75.50

Figure 3.17. The influence diagram from Figure 3.16, with the probability and value tables associated with the nodes. The information in these tables is the same as that associated with the branches and endpoints of the decision tree in Figure 3.16. HIV = human immunodeficiency virus; HIV+ = HIV infected; HIV− = not infected with HIV; QALE = quality-adjusted life expectancy; PCR = polymerase chain reaction; NA = not applicable; TX+ = treated; TX− = not treated. Test results are shown in quotation marks ("HIV+"), and the true disease state is shown without quotation marks (HIV+). (*Source*: Owens D.K., Shachter R.D., Nease R.F. [1997]. Representation and analysis of medical decision problems with influence diagrams. *Medical Decision Making*, 17: 241–262. Reproduced with permission.)

Why use an influence diagram instead of a decision tree? Influence diagrams have both advantages and limitations relative to decision trees. Influence diagrams represent graphically the probabilistic relationships among variables (Owens et al., 1997b). Such representation is advantageous for problems in which probabilistic conditioning is complex or in which communication of such conditioning is important (such as may occur in large models). In an influence diagram, probabilistic conditioning is indicated by the arcs, and thus the conditioning is apparent immediately by inspection. In a decision tree, probabilistic conditioning is revealed by the probabilities in the branches of the tree. To determine whether events are conditionally independent in a decision tree requires that the analyst compare probabilities of events between branches of the tree. Influence diagrams also are particularly useful for discussion with content experts who can help to structure a problem but who are not familiar with decision analysis. In contrast, problems that have decision alternatives that are structurally different may be easier for people to understand when represented with a decision tree, because the tree shows the structural differences explicitly, whereas the influence diagram does not. The choice of whether to use a decision tree or an influence diagram depends on the problem being analyzed, the experience of the analyst, the availability of software, and the purpose of the analysis. For selected problems, influence diagrams provide a powerful graphical alternative to decision trees.

3.8   The Role of Probability and Decision Analysis in Medicine

You may be wondering how probability and decision analysis might be integrated smoothly into medical practice. An understanding of probability and measures of test performance will prevent any number of misadventures. In Example 1, we discussed a hypothetical test that, on casual inspection, appeared to be an accurate way to screen blood donors for previous exposure to the AIDS virus. Our quantitative analysis, however, revealed that the test results were misleading more often than they were helpful because of the low prevalence of HIV in the clinically relevant population.[15]

The need for knowledgeable interpretation of test results is widespread. The federal government screens civil employees in "sensitive" positions for drug use, as do many companies. If the drug test used by an employer had a sensitivity and specificity of 0.95, and if 10 percent of the employees used drugs, one-third of the positive tests would be FPs. An understanding of these issues should be of great interest to the public, and health professionals should be prepared to answer the questions of their patients.

Although we should try to interpret every kind of test result accurately, decision analysis has a more selective role in medicine. Not all clinical decisions require decision analysis. Some decisions depend on physiologic principles or on deductive reasoning. Other decisions involve little uncertainty. Nonetheless, many decisions must be based on imperfect data, and they will have outcomes that cannot be known with certainty at the time that the decision is made. Decision analysis provides a technique for managing these situations.

For many problems, simply drawing a tree that denotes the possible outcomes explicitly will clarify the question sufficiently to allow you to make a decision. When time is limited, even a "quick and dirty" analysis may be helpful. By using expert clinicians' subjective probability estimates and asking what the patient's utilities might be, you can perform an analysis quickly and learn which probabilities and utilities are the important determinants of the decision. You can spend time in the library or at the bedside getting accurate estimates of these important probabilities and utilities. You can solve other decision problems once and then use the decision trees as often as the need arises by changing the variables to fit the particular patient. Journals such as *Medical Decision Making* contain decision analyses that you can adapt to fit a specific patient. Once you have performed the first quantitative analysis, you often find that some of the variables in the tree have an insignificant effect on the decision. Then, in any further analyses regarding that problem, you will not need to give those variables much attention.

---

[15] We emphasize that blood donors be screened with EIAs rather than with PCR. The sensitivity and specificity of EIAs are greater than 99 percent, and positive EIAs are confirmed with highly specific tests.

Health care professionals sometimes express reservations about decision analysis because the analysis may depend on probabilities that must be estimated, such as the pretest probability. A thoughtful decision maker will be concerned that the estimate may be in error, particularly because the information needed to make the estimate often is difficult to obtain from the medical literature. We argue, however, that uncertainty in the clinical data is a problem for any decision-making method and that the effect of this uncertainty is explicit with decision analysis. The method for evaluating uncertainty is sensitivity analysis: we can examine any variable to see whether its value is critical to the final recommended decision. Thus, we can determine, for example, whether a change in pretest probability from 0.6 to 0.8 makes a difference in the final decision. In so doing, we often discover that it is necessary to estimate only a range of probabilities for a particular variable rather than a precise value. Thus, with a sensitivity analysis, we can decide whether uncertainty about a particular variable should concern us.

The growing complexity of medical decisions, coupled with the need to control costs, has led to major programs to develop clinical practice guidelines. Decision models have many advantages as aids to guideline development (Eddy, 1992): they make explicit the alternative interventions, associated uncertainties, and utilities of potential outcomes. Decision models can help guideline developers to structure guideline-development problems (Owens and Nease, 1993), to incorporate patients' preferences (Nease and Owens, 1994; Owens, 1998a), and to tailor guidelines for specific clinical populations (Owens and Nease, 1997a). In addition, Web-based interfaces for decision models can provide distributed decision support for guideline developers and users by making the decision model available for analysis to anyone who has access to the Web (Sanders et al., 1999).

We have not emphasized computers in this chapter, although they can simplify many aspects of decision analysis (see Chapter 20). MEDLINE and other bibliographic retrieval systems (see Chapter 19) make it easier to obtain published estimates of disease prevalence and test performance. Computer programs for performing statistical analyses can be used on data collected by hospital information systems. Decision analysis software, available for personal computers (PCs), can help physicians to structure decision trees, to calculate expected values, and to perform sensitivity analyses. Researchers continue to explore methods for computer-based automated development of practice guidelines from decision models and use of computer-based systems to implement guidelines (Musen et al., 1996).

Medical decision making often involves uncertainty for the physician and risk for the patient. Most health care professionals would welcome tools that help them make decisions when they are confronted with complex clinical problems with uncertain outcomes. There are important medical problems for which decision analysis offers such aid.

Appendix: Derivation of Bayes' Theorem

Bayes' theorem is derived as follows. We denote the conditional probability of disease, D, given a test result, R, $p[D|R]$. The prior (pretest) probability of D is $p[D]$. The definition of conditional probability is:

$$p[D \mid R] = \frac{p[R, D]}{p[R]}. \tag{3.1}$$

The probability of a test result ($p[R]$) is the sum of its probability in diseased patients and its probability in nondiseased patients:

$$p[R] = p[R, D] + p[R, -D].$$

Substituting into Equation 3.1, we obtain:

$$p[D \mid R] = \frac{p[R, D]}{p[R, D] + p[R, -D]}. \tag{3.2}$$

Again, from the definition of conditional probability,

$$p[R \mid D] = \frac{p[R, D]}{p[D]} \text{ and } p[R \mid -D] = \frac{p[R, -D]}{p[-D]}.$$

These expressions can be rearranged:

$$p[R, D] = p[D] \times p[R \mid D], \tag{3.3}$$

$$p[R, -D] = p[-D] \times p[R \mid -D]. \tag{3.4}$$

Substituting Equations 3.3 and 3.4 into Equation 3.2, we obtain Bayes' theorem:

$$p[D \mid R] = \frac{p[D] \times p[R \mid D]}{p[D] \times p[R \mid D] + p[-D] \times p[R \mid -D]}.$$

Suggested Readings

Gold M.R., Siegel J.E., Russell L.B., Weinstein M.C. (1996). *Cost Effectiveness in Health and Medicine*. New York: Oxford University Press.
This book provides authoritative guidelines for the conduct of cost-effectiveness analyses. Chapter 4 discusses approaches for valuing health outcomes.

Hunink M., Glasziou P., Siegel J., Weeks J., Pliskin J., Einstein A., Weinstein M. (2001). Decision Making in Health and Medicine. Cambridge: Cambridge University Press.
This textbook addresses in detail most of the topics introduced in this chapter.

Nease R.F. Jr., Owens D.K. (1997). Use of influence diagrams to structure medical decisions. *Medical Decision Making*, 17(13):263–275.
Owens D.K., Schacter R.D., Nease R.F. Jr. (1997). Representation and analysis of medical decision problems with influence diagrams. *Medical Decision Making*, 17(3):241–262.
These two articles provide a comprehensive introduction to the use of influence diagrams.

Raiffa H. (1970). *Decision Analysis: Introductory Lectures on Choices Under Uncertainty*. Reading, MA: Addison-Wesley.
This book provides an advanced, nonmedical introduction to decision analysis, utility theory, and decision trees.

Sox H.C. (1986). Probability theory in the use of diagnostic tests. *Annals of Internal Medicine*, 104(1):60–66.
This article is written for physicians; it contains a summary of the concepts of probability and test interpretation.

Sox H.C., Blatt M.A., Higgins M.C., Marton K.I. (1988). *Medical Decision Making*. Boston, MA: Butterworths.
This introductory textbook covers the subject matter of this chapter in greater detail, as well as discussing many other topics. An appendix contains the likelihood ratios of 100 common diagnostic tests.

Tversky A., Kahneman D. (1974). Judgment under uncertainty: Heuristics and biases. *Science*, 185:1124.
This now classic article provides a clear and interesting discussion of the experimental evidence for the use and misuse of heuristics in situations of uncertainty.

Questions for Discussion

1. Calculate the following probabilities for a patient about to undergo CABG surgery (see Example 2):
   a. The only possible, mutually exclusive outcomes of surgery are death, relief of symptoms (angina and dyspnea), and continuation of symptoms. The probability of death is 0.02, and the probability of relief of symptoms is 0.80. What is the probability that the patient will continue to have symptoms?
   b. Two known complications of heart surgery are stroke and heart attack, with probabilities of 0.02 and 0.05, respectively. The patient asks what chance he or she has of having *both* complications. Assume that the complications are conditionally independent, and calculate your answer.
   c. The patient wants to know the probability that he or she will have a stroke given that he or she has a heart attack as a complication of the surgery. Assume that 1 in 500 patients has *both* complications, that the probability of heart attack is 0.05, and that the events are independent. Calculate your answer.
2. The results of a hypothetical study to measure test performance of the PCR test for HIV (see Example 1) are shown in the 2 × 2 table in Table 3.9.
   a. Calculate the sensitivity, specificity, disease prevalence, PV⁺, and PV⁻.
   b. Use the TPR and TNR calculated in part (a) to fill in the 2 × 2 table in Table 3.10. Calculate the disease prevalence, PV⁺, and PV⁻.
3. You are asked to interpret a PCR HIV test in an asymptomatic man whose test was positive when he volunteered to donate blood. After taking his history, you learn that he is an intravenous-drug user. You know that the overall prevalence of HIV infection in your community is 1 in 500 and that the prevalence in intravenous-drug users is 20 times as high as in the community at large.
   a. Estimate the pretest probability that this man is infected with HIV.
   b. The man tells you that two people with whom he shared needles subsequently died of AIDS. Which heuristic will be useful in making a subjective adjustment to the pretest probability in part (a)?

Table 3.9. A 2 × 2 contingency table for the hypothetical study in problem 2.

PCR test result	Gold standard test positive	Gold standard test negative	Total
Positive PCR	48	8	56
Negative PCR	2	47	49
Total	50	55	105

PCR = polymerase chain reaction.

Table 3.10. A 2 × 2 contingency table to complete for problem 2b.

PCR test result	Gold standard test positive	Gold standard test negative	Total
Positive PCR	x	x	x
Negative PCR	100	99,900	x
Total	x	x	x

PCR = polymerase chain reaction.

   c. Use the sensitivity and specificity that you worked out in 2(a) to calculate the post-test probability of the patient having HIV after a positive and negative test. Assume that the pretest probability is 0.10.

   d. If you wanted to increase the post-test probability of disease given a positive test result, would you change the TPR or TNR of the test?

4. You have a patient with cancer who has a choice between surgery or chemotherapy. If the patient chooses surgery, he or she has a 2 percent chance of dying from the operation (life expectancy = 0), a 50 percent chance of being cured (life expectancy = 15 years), and a 48 percent chance of not being cured (life expectancy = 1 year). If the patient chooses chemotherapy, he or she has a 5 percent chance of death (life expectancy = 0), a 65 percent chance of cure (life expectancy = 15 years), and a 30 percent chance that the cancer will be slowed but not cured (life expectancy = 2 years). Create a decision tree. Calculate the expected value of each option in terms of life expectancy.

5. You are concerned that a patient with a sore throat has a bacterial infection that would require antibiotic therapy (as opposed to a viral infection, for which no treatment is available). Your treatment threshold is 0.4, and based on the examination you estimate the probability of bacterial infection as 0.8. A test is available (TPR = 0.75, TNR = 0.85) that indicates the presence or absence of bacterial infection. Should you perform the test? Explain your reasoning. How would your analysis change if the test were extremely costly or involved a significant risk to the patient?

6. What are the three kinds of bias that can influence measurement of test performance? Explain what each one is, and state how you would adjust the post-test probability to compensate for each.

7. How could a computer system ease the task of performing a complex decision analysis? Look at the titles of Chapters 9 through 18 of this text. What role could each kind of system play in the medical-decision process?

8. When you search the medical literature to find probabilities for patients similar to one you are treating, what is the most important question to consider? How should you adjust probabilities in light of the answer to this question?

9. Why do you think physicians sometimes order tests even if the results will not affect their management of the patient? Do you think the reasons that you identify are valid? Are they valid in only certain situations? Explain your answers. See the January 1998 issue of *Medical Decision Making* for articles that discuss this question.

10. Explain the differences in three approaches to assessing patients' preferences for health states: the standard gamble, the time trade-off, and the visual analog scale.

4
Cognitive Science and Biomedical Informatics

Vimla L. Patel and David R. Kaufman

> The future of the telephone...will mean nothing less than a reorganization of society – a state of things in which every individual, however secluded, will have at call every other individual in the community, to the saving of no end of social and business complications, of needless goings to and fro, of disappointments, delays, and a countless host of great and little evils and annoyances which go so far under the present conditions to make life laborious and unsatisfactory. (Heath and Luff, 2000; Scientific American, 1880, p. 16)

After reading this chapter, you should know the answers to these questions:

- How can cognitive science theory meaningfully inform and shape design, development and assessment of health care information systems?
- What are some of the ways in which cognitive science differs from behavioral science?
- What are some of the ways in which we can characterize the structure of knowledge?
- What are the basic components of a cognitive architecture?
- What are some of the dimensions of difference between experts and novices?
- Describe some of the attributes of system usability.
- What are the gulfs of execution and evaluation? What role do these considerations play in system design?
- What is the difference between a textbase and a situation model?
- How can we use cognitive methods to develop and implement clinical practice guidelines for different kinds of clinicians?

4.1 Introduction

Enormous advances in health information technologies and more generally, in computing over the course of the last two decades has begun to permeate diverse facets of clinical practice. The rapid pace of technological developments in the past several years including the Internet, wireless technologies, and handheld devices, to name just a few, afford significant opportunities for supporting, enhancing, and extending user experiences, interactions, and communications (Rogers, 2004). These advances coupled with a growing computer literacy among health care professionals afford the potential for great improvement in health care. Yet many observers note that the health care system is slow to understand information technology and to effectively incorporate it into the work environment (Shortliffe and Blois, 2000). Innovative technologies often produce profound cultural, social, and cognitive changes. These transformations necessitate adaptation at many different levels of aggregation from the individual to the larger institution, sometimes causing disruptions of workflow and user dissatisfaction.

Similar to other complex domains, medical information systems embody ideals in design that often do not readily yield practical solutions in implementation. As computer-based systems infiltrate clinical practice and settings, the consequences often can be felt through all levels of the organization. This impact can have deleterious effects resulting in systemic inefficiencies and suboptimal practices. This can lead to frustrated health care practitioners, unnecessary delays in health care delivery, and even adverse events (Lin et al., 1998; Weinger and Slagle, 2001). In the best-case scenario, mastery of the system necessitates an individual and collective learning curve yielding incremental improvements in performance and satisfaction. In the worst-case scenario, clinicians may revolt and the hospital may be forced to pull the plug on an expensive new technology. How can we manage change? How can we introduce system designs that are more intuitive and coherent with everyday practice?

Cognitive science is a multidisciplinary domain of inquiry devoted to the study of cognition and its role in intelligent agency. The primary disciplines include cognitive psychology, artificial intelligence, neuroscience, linguistics, anthropology, and philosophy. From the perspective of informatics, cognitive science can provide a framework for the analysis and modeling of complex human performance in technology-mediated settings. Cognitive science incorporates basic science research focusing on fundamental aspects of cognition (e.g., attention, memory, early language acquisition) as well as applied research. Applied cognitive research is focally concerned with the development and evaluation of useful and usable cognitive artifacts. **Cognitive artifacts** are human-made materials, devices, and systems that extend people's abilities in perceiving objects, encoding and retrieving information from memory, and problem solving (Gillan and Schvaneveldt, 1999). In this regard, applied cognitive research is closely aligned with the disciplines of **human–computer interaction** (HCI) and human factors. It also has a close affiliation with educational research.

The past couple of decades have produced a cumulative body of experiential and practical knowledge about design and implementation that can guide future initiatives. This practical knowledge embodies the need for sensible and intuitive interfaces, an understanding of workflow, and the need to consult clinicians in advance of implementation. However, experiential knowledge is limited in producing robust generalizations or sound design and implementation principles. There is a need for a theoretical foundation. It is increasingly apparent that biomedical informatics is more than the thin intersection of medicine and computing (Patel and Kaufman, 1998). There is a growing role for the social sciences, including the cognitive and behavioral sciences, in biomedical informatics, particularly as it pertains to HCI and other areas such as information retrieval and decision support. In this chapter, we focus on the foundational role of cognitive science in medical informatics research and practice. Theories and methods from the cognitive sciences can illuminate different facets of design and implementation of information and knowledge-based systems. They can also play a larger role in characterizing and enhancing human performance on a wide range of tasks involving clinicians, patients and healthy consumers of medical information. These tasks may include developing training programs and devising measures to reduce errors or increase efficiency. In this respect, cognitive science represents one of the component basic sciences of biomedical informatics (Shortliffe and Blois, 2001).

4.1.1 Cognitive Science and Biomedical Informatics

How can cognitive science theory meaningfully inform and shape design, development and assessment of health care information systems? We propose that cognitive science can provide insight into principles of system *usability* and *learnability*, the process of medical judgment and decision making, the training of health care professionals, patients and health consumers, as well as the study of collaboration in the workplace.

Precisely how will cognitive science theory and methods make such a significant contribution toward these important objectives? The translation of research findings from one discipline into practical concerns that can be applied to another is rarely a straightforward process (Rogers, 2004). Furthermore, even when scientific knowledge is highly relevant in principle, making that knowledge effective in a design context can still be a significant challenge. In this chapter, we discuss (1) basic cognitive scientific research and theories that provide a foundation for understanding the underlying mechanisms guiding human performance (e.g., findings pertaining to the structure of human memory); (2) research in the area of medical cognition (e.g., studies of medical text comprehension); and (3) applied cognitive research in biomedical informatics (e.g., effects of computer-based clinical guidelines on therapeutic decision making). Each of these areas can differentially contribute to progress in applied medical informatics.

As illustrated in Table 4.1, there are correspondences between basic cognitive science research, medical cognition, and cognitive research in medical informatics along several dimensions. For example, theories of human memory and knowledge organization lend

Table 4.1. Correspondences between cognitive science, medical cognition, and applied cognitive research in medical informatics.

Cognitive science	Medical cognition	Biomedical informatics
Knowledge organization and human memory	Organization of clinical and basic science knowledge	Development and use of medical knowledge bases
Problem solving, heuristics, or reasoning strategies	Medical problem solving and decision making	Medical artificial intelligence, decision-support systems, or medical errors
Perception or attention	Radiologic and dermatologic diagnosis	Medical imaging systems
Text comprehension	Learning from medical texts	Information retrieval, digital libraries, or health literacy
Conversational analysis	Medical discourse	Medical natural language processing
Distributed cognition	Collaborative practice and research in health care	Computer-based provider order-entry systems
Coordination of theory and evidence	Diagnostic and therapeutic reasoning	Evidence-based clinical guidelines
Diagrammatic reasoning	Perceptual processing of patient data displays	Biomedical information visualization

themselves to characterizations of expert clinical knowledge that can then be contrasted with representation of such knowledge in medical systems. Similarly, research in text comprehension has provided a theoretical framework for research in understanding medical texts. This in turn has influenced applied cognitive research on information retrieval from biomedical knowledge sources and research on health literacy.

In this chapter, we propose that cognitive research, theories, and methods can contribute to application in informatics in a number of ways including: (1) seed *basic research findings* that can illuminate dimensions of design (e.g., attention and memory, aspects of the visual system); (2) provide an *explanatory vocabulary* for characterizing how individuals process and communicate health information (e.g., various studies of medical cognition pertaining to doctor–patient interaction); (3) present an *analytic framework* for identifying problems and modeling certain kinds of user interactions; (4) develop and refine *predictive tools* (GOMS methods of analysis, described below); (5) provide *rich descriptive accounts* of clinicians employing technologies in the context of work; and (6) furnish a generative approach for novel designs and productive applied research programs in informatics (e.g., intervention strategies for supporting low literacy populations in health information seeking).

The social sciences are constituted by multiple frameworks and approaches. **Behaviorism** constitutes a framework for analyzing and modifying behavior. It is an approach that has had an enormous influence on the social sciences for most of the twentieth century. Cognitive science partially emerged as a response to the limitations of behaviorism. Section 4.2 contains a brief history of the cognitive and behavioral sciences that emphasizes the points of difference between the two approaches. It also serves to introduce basic concepts in the study of cognition.

4.2   Cognitive Science: The Emergence of an Explanatory Framework

> The search for mind begins in philosophy and philosophy begins in ancient Greece; the first time in history that man recognized that knowledge was not the simple product of human experience, but something that had to be analyzed, externalized, and examined if it were any other phenomena of nature and treated as if it were worthy of study. (Robinson, 1994)

In this section, we sketch a brief history of the emergence of cognitive science in view to differentiate it with competing theoretical frameworks in the social sciences. The section also serves to introduce core concepts that constitute an explanatory framework for cognitive science. Behaviorism is the conceptual framework underlying a particular science of behavior (Zuriff, 1985). This framework dominated experimental and applied psychology as well as the social sciences for the better part of the twentieth century (Bechtel et al., 1998). Behavioral psychology emerged as a discipline at a time when **logical positivism** dominated philosophical thought and the Darwinian theory of evolution was beginning to be a driving force in the biological sciences (Hilgard and Bower, 1975). The guiding principle of logical positivism was that all statements are either analytic (true by logical deduction), verifiable by observation, or meaningless (Smith, 1986). Logical positivists attempted to account for all knowledge without resorting to metaphysics, from the perspective of the "scientific world view." Epistemology was restricted in scope to deal only with matters of justification and validity (Smith, 1986). Darwin's theory of natural selection asserted that species variation, evolution, and survival could be explained by the adaptation of the animal to specific environmental contingencies.

Behaviorism represented an attempt to develop an objective, empirically based science of behavior and more specifically, learning. **Empiricism** is the view that experience is the only source of knowledge (Hilgard and Bower, 1975). Behaviorism endeavored to build a comprehensive framework of scientific inquiry around the experimental analysis of observable behavior. Behaviorists eschewed the study of thinking as an unacceptable psychological method because it was inherently subjective, error-prone, and could not be subjected to empirical validation. Similarly, hypothetical constructs (e.g., mental processes as mechanisms in a theory) were discouraged. All constructs had to be specified in terms of operational definitions so they could be manipulated, measured, and quantified for empirical investigation (Weinger and Slagle, 2001).

Behavioral theories of learning emphasized the correspondence between environmental stimuli and the responses emitted. These studies generally attempted to characterize the changing relationship between stimulus and response under different reinforcement and punishment contingencies. For example, a behavior that was followed by a satisfying state of affairs was more likely to increase the frequency of the act. According to behavior theories, knowledge is nothing more than the sum of an individual's learning history, and transformations of mental states play no part in the learning process.

For reasons that go beyond the scope of this chapter, classical behavioral theories have been largely discredited as a comprehensive unifying theory of behavior. However, behaviorism continues to provide a theoretical and methodological foundation in a wide range of social science disciplines. For example, behaviorist tenets continue to play a central role in public health research. In particular, health behavior research places an emphasis on antecedent variables and environmental contingencies that serve to sustain unhealthy behaviors such as smoking (Sussman, 2001). Applied behaviorism continues to have a significant impact in the mental health treatment. In addition, behavioral research has informed psychometrics and survey research.

Due to the dominance of behaviorism in North American psychology from approximately 1915 to the middle of the century, there was very little research into complex human cognitive processes (Newell and Simon, 1972). Around 1950, there was an increasing dissatisfaction with the limitations and methodological constraints (e.g., the disavowal of unobservables such as mental states) of behaviorism. In addition, developments in logic, information theory, cybernetics, and perhaps most importantly the advent of the digital computer aroused substantial interest in "information processing" (Gardner, 1985).

Newell and Simon (1972) date the beginning of the "cognitive revolution" to the year 1956. They cite Bruner and coworkers' "Study of Thinking," George Miller's influential journal publication "The magic number seven" in psychology, Noam Chomsky's writings on syntactic grammars in linguistics (see Chapter 8), and their own logic theorist program in computer science as the pivotal works. Freed of the restraints imposed by logical positivism, cognitive scientists placed "thought" and "mental processes" at the center of their explanatory framework.

The "computer metaphor" provided a framework for the study of human cognition as the manipulation of "symbolic structures." It also provided the foundation for a model of memory, which was a prerequisite for an information-processing theory (Atkinson and Shiffrin, 1968). The implementation of models of human performance as computer programs provided a measure of objectivity and a *sufficiency test* of a theory, and increased the objectivity of the study of mental processes (Estes, 1975).

There were several influential volumes that established the study of cognition as a central goal of psychology including books by Miller et al. (1986), "Plans, and the Structure of Behavior," and Neisser (1967), "Cognitive Psychology," which attempted a synthesis of the research that had been done into basic mental processes (e.g., perception, attention, and memory processes). Perhaps the most significant landmark publication in the field was Newell and Simon's "Human Problem Solving" (1972). This was the culmination of more than 15 years of work on problem solving and research in artificial intelligence. It was a mature thesis that described a theoretical framework, extended a language for the study of cognition, and introduced protocol-analytic methods that have become ubiquitous in the study of high-level cognition. It laid the foundation for the formal investigation of symbolic information processing (more specifically, problem solving). The development of models of human information processing also provided a foundation for the discipline of HCI and the first formal methods of analysis (Card et al., 1983).

The early investigations of problem solving focused primarily on investigations of experimentally contrived or toy-world tasks such as elementary deductive logic, the Tower of Hanoi (TOH; illustrated in Figure 4.1), and mathematical word problems (Greeno and Simon, 1988). These tasks required very little background knowledge and were well structured, in the sense that all the variables necessary for solving the problem were present in the problem statement. These tasks allowed for a complete description of the task environment; a step-by-step description of the sequential behavior of the subjects' performance; and the modeling of subjects' cognitive and overt behavior in the form of a computer simulation. The TOH, in particular, served as an important test bed for the development of an explanatory vocabulary and framework for analyzing problem-solving behavior.

The TOH is a relatively straightforward task, which consists of three pegs (A, B, and C) and three or more disks which vary in size. The goal is to move the three disks from peg A to peg C one at a time with the constraint that a larger disk can never rest on a smaller one. Problem solving can be construed as *search* in a **problem space**. A problem

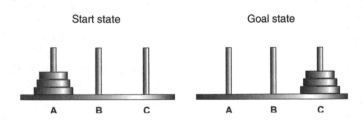

Figure 4.1. Tower of Hanoi (TOH) task illustrating a start state and a goal state.

space has an *initial state*, a *goal state*, and a *set of operators*. Operators are any moves that transform a given state to a successor state. For example, the first move could be to move the small disk to peg B or peg C. In a 3-disk TOH, there are a total of 27 possible states representing the complete problem space. TOH has 3^n states where n is the number of disks. The minimum number of moves necessary to solve a TOH is 2^n-1. Problem solvers will typically maintain only a small set of states at a time.

The search process involves finding a solution strategy that will minimize the number of steps. The metaphor of movement through a problem space provides a means for understanding how individuals can sequentially address the challenges they confront at each stage of a problem and the actions that ensue. We can characterize the problem-solving behavior of the subject at a local level in terms of state transitions or at a more global level in terms of *strategies*. For example, *means–ends analysis* is a commonly used strategy to reduce the difference between the start state and goal state. For example, moving all but the largest disk from peg A to peg B is an interim goal associated with such a strategy.

The most common method of data analysis is known as **protocol analysis** (Newell and Simon, 1972). Protocol analysis refers to a class of techniques for representing verbal **think-aloud protocols** (Greeno and Simon, 1988). Think-aloud protocols are the most common source of data used in studies of problem solving. In these studies, subjects are instructed to verbalize their thoughts as they perform a particular experimental task. Ericsson and Simon (1993) specify the conditions under which verbal reports are acceptable as legitimate data. For example, retrospective think-aloud protocols are viewed as somewhat suspect because the subject has had the opportunity to reconstruct the information in memory and the verbal reports are inevitably distorted. Think-aloud protocols in concert with observable behavioral data such as a subject's actions provide a rich source of evidence to characterize cognitive processes.

Cognitive psychologists and linguists have investigated the processes and properties of language and memory in adults and children for many decades. Early research focused on basic laboratory studies of list learning or the processing of words and sentences (as in a sentence completion task) (Anderson, 1983). Beginning in the early 1970s, van Dijk and Kintsch (1983, summarized) developed an influential method of analyzing the process of text comprehension based on the realization that text can be described at multiple levels of realization from surface codes (e.g., words and syntax) to deeper levels of semantics. Comprehension refers to cognitive processes associated with understanding or deriving meaning from text, conversation, or other informational resources. It involves the processes that people use when trying to make sense of a piece of text, such as a sentence, a book, or a verbal utterance. It also involves the final product of such processes, i.e., the mental representation that the people have of the text (what they have understood).

Comprehension often precedes problem solving and decision making, but is also dependent on perceptual processes that focus attention, the availability of relevant knowledge, and the ability to deploy knowledge in a given context. In fact, some of the more important differences in medical problem solving and decision making arise from differences in knowledge and comprehension. Furthermore, many of the problems associated with decision making are the result of either lack of knowledge or failures to understand the information appropriately.

The early investigations provided a well-constrained artificial environment for the development of the basic methods and principles of problem solving. They also provided a rich explanatory vocabulary (e.g., problem space), but were not fully adequate to account for cognition in knowledge-rich domains of greater complexity and involving uncertainty. In the mid to late 1970s, there was a shift in research to complex "real-life" knowledge-based domains of enquiry (Greeno and Simon, 1988). Problem-solving research was studying performance in domains such as physics (Larkin et al., 1980), medical diagnoses (Elstein et al., 1978), and architecture (Akin, 1982). Similarly the study of text comprehension shifted from research on simple stories to technical and scientific texts in a range of domains including medicine. This paralleled a similar change in artificial intelligence research from "toy programs" to addressing "real-world" problems and the development of expert systems (Clancey and Shortliffe, 1984). The shift to real-world problems in cognitive science was spearheaded by research exploring the nature of expertise. Most of the early investigations on expertise involved laboratory experiments. However, the shift to knowledge-intensive domains provided a theoretical and methodological foundation to conduct both basic and applied research in real-world settings such as the workplace (Vicente, 1999) and the classroom (Bruer, 1993). These areas of application provided a fertile testbed for assessing and extending the cognitive science framework. In recent years, the conventional information-processing approach has come under criticism for its narrow focus on the rational or cognitive processes of the solitary individual. One of the most compelling proposals has to do with a shift from viewing cognition as a property of the solitary individual to viewing it as distributed across groups, cultures, and artifacts. This claim has significant implications for the study of collaborative endeavors and HCI. We explore the concepts underlying distributed cognition in greater detail in a subsequent section. This is discussed in greater depth when we consider the area of medical cognition.

4.3   Human Information Processing

The . . . disregard of physiological and sensory handicaps; of fundamental principles of perception; of basic patterns of motor coordination; of human limitations in the integration of complex motor responses, etc. has led at times to the production of mechanical monstrosities which tax the capabilities of human operators and hinder the integration of man and machine into a system designed for most effective accomplishment of designated tasks. (Fitts, 1951 cited in John, 2003)

Cognitive science serves as a basic science and provides a framework for the analysis and modeling of complex human performance. A computational theory of mind provides the fundamental underpinning for most contemporary theories of cognitive science. The basic premise is that much of human cognition can be characterized as a series of operations or computations on mental representations. *Mental representations* are internal cognitive states that have a certain correspondence with the external world. For example, they may reflect a clinician's hypothesis about a patient's condition after noticing an abnormal gait as the patient entered the clinic. These are likely to elicit further inferences about the patient's underlying condition and may direct the physicians' information-gathering strategies and contribute to an evolving problem representation.

Two interdependent principles by which we can characterize cognitive systems are: (1) architectural theories that endeavor to provide a unified theory for all aspects of cognition and (2) distinction among different kinds of knowledge that is necessary to attain competency in a given domain. Individuals differ substantially in terms of their knowledge, experiences, and endowed capabilities. The architectural approach capitalizes on the fact that we can characterize certain regularities of the human information processing system. These can be either structural regularities (e.g., the existence of, and the relations between, perceptual, attentional, and memory systems and memory capacity limitations) or processing regularities (e.g., processing speed, selective attention, or problem solving strategies). Cognitive systems are characterized functionally in terms of the capabilities they enable (e.g., focused attention on selective visual features), the way they constrain human cognitive performance (e.g., limitations on memory), and their development during the life span. In regard to the life span issue, there is a growing body of literature on cognitive aging and how aspects of the cognitive system such as attention, memory, vision, and motor skill change as functions of aging (Rogers, 2002). This basic science research is of growing importance to informatics as we seek to develop e-health applications for seniors, many of who suffer from chronic health conditions such as arthritis and diabetes. A graphical user interface or, more generally, a Web site designed for younger adults may not be suitable for older adults.

Differences in knowledge organization are a central focus of research into the nature of expertise. Unlike architectural theories, research on knowledge organization embraces a domain-specific focus. In medicine, the expert–novice paradigm has contributed to our understanding of the nature of medical expertise and skilled clinical performance. Cognitive architectures and theories of knowledge organization are presented in Sections 4.3.1 and 4.3.2.

4.3.1 Architectures of Cognition

Fundamental research in perception, cognition, and psychomotor skill over the course of the last 50 years has provided a foundation for design principles in human factors and HCI. The quote by Fitts, a pioneer in cognitive engineering, underscores a ubiquitous complaint that designers routinely violate basic assumptions about the human cognitive system. Although cognitive guidelines have made significant inroads in the design community, there remains a significant gap in applying basic cognitive research (Gillan and Schvaneveldt, 1999). There are invariably challenges in applying basic research and theory to applications. However, there appears to be a growing belief about the need for a more human-centered design and that cognitive research can instrumentally contribute to such an endeavor (Zhang et al., 2002).

Over the course of the last 25 years, there have been several attempts to develop a unified theory of cognition. The goal of such a theory is to provide a single set of mechanisms for all cognitive behaviors from motor skills, language, memory, decision making, problem solving, and comprehension (Newell, 1990). Such a theory provides a means to put together a seemingly disparate voluminous body of human experimental data into a coherent form. Cognitive architecture represents unifying theories of cognition that are embodied in large-scale computer simulation programs. Although there is much plasticity evidenced in human behavior, cognitive processes are bound by biological and physical constraints. Cognitive architectures specify functional rather than biological constraints on human behavior (e.g., limitations on working memory). These constraints reflect the information-processing capacities and limitations of the human cognitive system. Architectural systems embody a relatively fixed permanent structure, which is (more or less) characteristic of all humans and does not substantially vary over an individual's lifetime. It represents a scientific hypothesis about those aspects of human cognition that are relatively constant over time and independent of task (Carroll, 2002).

The ACT-R cognitive architecture developed by Anderson. (1983) represents one of the most comprehensive and widely researched architectural systems. It also represents perhaps the most mature thesis about an integrated information-processing theory. ACT-R has been used to model a wide range of cognitive phenomena pertaining to language, learning, and memory and more recently perception and motor skills. Although ACT-R has been employed mostly to model experimental phenomena, it has been increasingly used as a research tool in HCI. Figure 4.2, modified from Byrne (2003), illustrates the components of the ACT-R/PM architecture. This particular instantiation is intended to be used as a tool to characterize interactive behavior in an HCI context. The objective of this discussion is not to describe this architecture in any detail, but merely to highlight the components of such a system. The architecture consists of a cognitive layer with two long-term memory modules: a procedural memory (modeled as a set of production rules) related to how to execute particular actions (e.g., moving a mouse) and perform various activities and a declarative memory (conceptual knowledge) that contains concepts (medical findings and disorders). The percep-

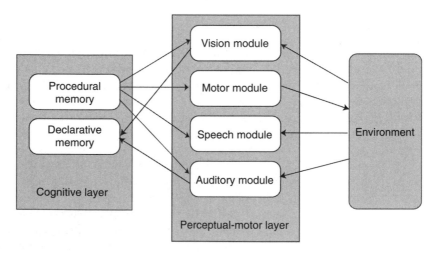

Figure 4.2. Illustration of a cognitive architecture ACT-R/PM. (*Source*: Diagram modified from Byrne [2003]).

tual–motor layer consists of effector (motor and speech) and receptor (vision and auditory), which interact with the world and with the cognitive layer in (relatively) predictable ways.

Human memory is typically divided into at least two structures: long-term memory and short-term or working memory. In this architectural model, working memory is an emergent property of interaction with the environment and not indicated as a separate component. **Long-term memory (LTM)** can be thought of as a repository of all knowledge, whereas **working memory (WM)** refers to the resources needed to maintain information active during cognitive activity (e.g., text comprehension). The information maintained in WM includes stimuli from the environment (e.g., words on a display) and knowledge activated from LTM. In theory, LTM is infinite, whereas WM is limited to 5 to 10 "chunks" of information (a unit of memory that can be retrieved at one time). Problems impose a varying **cognitive load** on WM. This refers to an excess of information that competes for few cognitive resources, creating a burden on WM (Chandler and Sweller, 1991). For example, maintaining a seven-digit phone number in WM is not very difficult. However, to maintain a phone number while engaging in conversation is nearly impossible for most people. Multitasking is one contributing factor for cognitive load. The structure of the task environment, e.g., a crowded computer display, is another contributor. As we discuss later, there are learning situations where the demands can be rather taxing.

The model of a task is *runnable* and produces a sequence of behaviors that can be quantitatively compared to the behaviors produced by humans performing the task (Byrne, 2003). Models based on cognitive architectures can be used to assess a range of performance measures such as error rates, execution times, and learning curves (e.g., trials needed to attain stable performance). Models can even be used to contrast two interfaces and determine which one is more likely to be effective for a particular task.

The use of architectural models necessitates substantial expertise and effort. At present, they exist primarily in academic research laboratories and do not constitute practical tools for applied research. However, cognitive architectures such as SOAR (initially the Model Human Processor) have given rise to formal HCI methods such as GOMS (Goals, Operators, Methods, and Selection Rules; John, 2003). GOMS is a method for describing a task at a very fine level of granularity (such as the keystroke) and the user's knowledge of how to perform the task. The majority of HCI research does not employ an architectural approach. The research is oriented towards descriptive models rather than quantitative predictive models. Nevertheless, architectural theories provide a unifying foundation for understanding patterns of interaction and specifying design principles.

4.3.2   The Organization of Knowledge

Architectural theories specify the structure and mechanisms of memory systems, whereas theories of knowledge organization focus on the content. There are several ways to characterize the kinds of knowledge that reside in LTM and that support decisions and actions. Cognitive psychology has furnished a range of domain-general constructs that accounts for the variability of mental representations needed to engage the external world. Similarly, research in medical cognition, medical artificial intelligence (AI), and medical informatics has developed taxonomies for characterizing the hierarchical nature of medical knowledge.

A central tenet of cognitive science is that humans actively construct and interpret information from their environment. Given that environmental stimuli can take a multitude of forms, the cognitive system needs to adapt corresponding representational forms to capture the essence of these inputs. The power of cognition is reflected in the ability to form abstractions, to represent perceptions, experiences, and thoughts in some medium other than that in which they have occurred without extraneous or irrelevant information (Norman, 1993). Representations enable us to remember, reconstruct, and transform events, objects, images, and conversations absent in space and time from the initial encodings. Representations reflect states of knowledge.

The issue of representation is fundamental to all cognitive research and it would be useful to define it precisely. Palmer (1978) uses the distinction between the *represented world* and the *representing world* to illustrate the ways in which we refer to issues of representation. In psychological research, the represented world refers to the cognitive representations of individuals that are the subject of investigation. The representing world is the means by which we attempt to capture the dimensions of representation selected for inquiry. The function of the representing world is to preserve information about the represented world. There exists a correspondence from objects in the represented world to objects in the representing world (in terms of symbolic structures). If a represented relation **R** holds for ordered pairs of representing objects <x,y>, the representational mapping requires that a corresponding relation, **R′**, holds for each corresponding pair <x′,y′>. So x is a representation of a world y, if some of the relations for objects of x are preserved by relations for corresponding objects of y. For example, a street map is a representation of a city's geography because it (approximately) preserves the spatial relations between different locations. In simple terms, a cognitive representation refers to a correspondence between a mental state and objects out in the physical world. In this section, we are concerned with mental representations. But a similar analysis can be applied to external representations and this is discussed further in a subsequent section.

Propositions are a form of representation that captures the essence of an idea (i.e., semantics) or concept without explicit reference to linguistic content. For example, "hello," "hey," and "what's happening" can typically be interpreted as a greeting containing identical propositional content even though the literal semantics of the phrases may differ. These ideas are expressed as language and translated into speech or text when we talk or write. Similarly, we recover the propositional structure when we read or listen to verbal information. Numerous psychological experiments have demonstrated that people recover the gist of a text or spoken communication (i.e., propositional structure) not the specific words (Anderson, 1985). Studies have also shown the individuals at different levels of expertise will differentially represent a text (Patel and Kaufman, 1998). For example, experts are more likely to selectively encode relevant propositional information that will inform a decision. On the other hand, less-than experts will often remember more information, but much of the recalled information may not be relevant to the decision. Propositional representations constitute an important construct in theories of comprehension, which is discussed later in this chapter.

Propositional knowledge can be expressed using a **predicate calculus** formalism or as a semantic network. The predicate calculus representation is illustrated below. A subject's response is divided into sentences or segments and sequentially analyzed. The formalism includes a head element of a segment and a series of arguments. For example in proposition 1.1, the focus is on a female who has the attributes of being 43 years of age and white. The TEM:ORD or temporal order relation indicates that the events of 1.3 (gastrointestinal (GI) upset) precede the event of 1.2 (diarrhea). The formalism is informed by an elaborate propositional language (Frederiksen, 1975) and was first applied to the medical domain by Patel et al. (1986). The method provides us with a detailed way to characterize the information subjects understood from reading a text, based on their summary or explanations.

Propositional analysis of a think-aloud protocol of a primary care physician

1. 43-year-old white female who developed diarrhea after a brief period of 2 days of GI upset.

1.1	female	ATT: Age (old); DEG: 43 year; ATT: white
1.2	develop	PAT: [she]; THM: diarrhea; TNS: past
1.3	period	ATT: brief; DUR: 2 days; THM: 1.4
1.4	upset	LOC: GI
1.5	TEM:ORD	[1.3], [1.2]

Kintsch's theory suggests that comprehension involves an interaction between what the text conveys and the schemata in LTM (Kintsch, 1988). Comprehension occurs when the reader uses prior knowledge to process the information present in the text. The text information is called the *textbase* (the propositional content of the text). For instance, in medicine the textbase could comprise the representation of a patient problem as written in a patient chart. The situation model is constituted by the textbase representation plus the domain-specific and everyday knowledge that the reader uses to derive a broader meaning from the text. In medicine, the situation model would enable a physician to draw inferences from a patient's history leading to a diagnosis, therapeutic plan, or prognosis (Patel and Groen, 1991). This situation model is typically derived from the general knowledge and specific knowledge acquired through medical teaching, readings (e.g., theories and findings from biomedical research), clinical practice (e.g., knowledge of associations between clinical findings and specific diseases, knowledge of medications or treatment procedures that have worked in the past), and the textbase representation. Like other forms of knowledge representation, the situation model is used to "fit in" the incoming information (e.g., text, perception of the patient). Since the knowledge in LTM differs among physicians, the resulting situation model generated by any two physicians is likely to differ as well. Theories and methods of text comprehension have been widely used in the study of medical cognition and have been instrumental in characterizing the process of guideline development and interpretation. This process is discussed in some detail in a subsequent section.

Schemata represent a higher-level kind of knowledge structure. They can be construed as data structures for representing the generic categories of concepts stored in memory (e.g., fruits, chairs, geometric shapes, and thyroid conditions). There are schemata for concepts underlying situations, events, sequences of actions, etc.

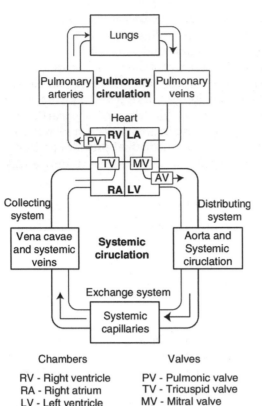

Figure 4.3. Schematic model of circulatory and cardiovascular physiology. The diagram illustrates various structures of the pulmonary and systemic circulation system and the process of blood flow. The illustration is used to exemplify the concept of a mental model and how it could be applied to explaining and predicting physiologic behavior.

Chambers	Valves
RV - Right ventricle	PV - Pulmonic valve
RA - Right atrium	TV - Tricuspid valve
LV - Left ventricle	MV - Mitral valve
LA - Left atrium	AV - Aortic valve

To process information with the use of a schema is to determine which model best fits the incoming information. Schemata have constants (all birds have wings) and variables (chairs can have between one and four legs). The variables may have associated default values (e.g., birds fly), which represent the prototypical circumstance. The frame-based representation in Table 4.2 can be used to model a bird schema.

When a person interprets information, the schema serves as a "filter" for distinguishing relevant and irrelevant information. Schemata can be considered as generic

Table 4.2. Bird schema illustrating slots-values notation.

Type	Animal
Locomotion	Flies,[a] walks, swims
Communication	Sings, squawks
Size	Small,[a] medium, large
Habitat	Trees,[a] lands, water
Food	Insects, seeds, fish

[a]Denotes default value.

knowledge structures that contain slots for particular kinds of propositions. For instance, a schema for myocardial infarction may contain the findings of "chest pain," "sweating," or "shortness of breath," but not the finding of "goiter," which is part of the schema for thyroid disease.

The schematic and propositional representations reflect abstractions and do not necessarily preserve literal information about the external world. Imagine that you are having a conversation at the office about how to rearrange the furniture in your living room. To engage in such a conversation, one needs to be able to construct images of the objects and their spatial arrangement in the room. *Mental images* are a form of internal representation that captures perceptual information recovered from the environment. There is compelling psychological and neuropsychological evidence to suggest that mental images constitute a distinct form of mental representation (Anderson, 1998). Images play a particularly important role in domains of visual diagnosis such as dermatology and radiology.

Mental models are an analog-based construct for describing how individuals form internal models of systems. Mental models are designed to answer questions such as "how does it work?" or "what will happen if I take the following action?". "Analogy" suggests that the representation explicitly shares the structure of the world it represents (e.g., a set of connected visual images of partial road map from your home to your work destination). This is in contrast to an abstraction-based form such as propositions or schemas in which the mental structure consists of either the gist, an abstraction, or a summary representation. However, like other forms of mental representation, mental models are always incomplete, imperfect, and subject to the processing limitations of the cognitive system. Mental models can be derived from perception, language, or from one's imagination (Payne, 2003). *Running* of a model corresponds to a process of mental simulation to generate possible future states of a system from observed or hypothetical state.

For example, when one initiates a Google Search, one may reasonably anticipate that system will return a list of relevant (and less than relevant) Web sites that correspond to the query. Mental models are a particularly useful construct in understanding HCI.

An individual's mental models provide predictive and explanatory capabilities of the function of a physical system. More often the construct has been used to characterize models that have a spatial and temporal context, as is the case in reasoning about the behavior of electrical circuits (White and Frederiksen, 1990). The model can be used to simulate a process (e.g., predict the effects of network interruptions on getting cash from an automatic teller machine (ATM)). Kaufman and coworkers (Kaufman et al., 1996; Patel et al., 1996) characterized clinicians' mental model of the cardiovascular system (specifically, cardiac output). The study characterized the development of understanding the system as a function of expertise. The research also documented various conceptual flaws in subjects' models and how these flaws impacted subjects' predictions and explanations of physiological manifestations. Figure 4.3 illustrates the four chambers of the heart and blood flow in the pulmonary and cardiovascular systems. The claim is that clinicians and medical students have variably robust representations of the structure and function of the system. This model enables prediction and explanation of the effects of perturbations in the system on blood flow and on various clinical measures such as left ventricular ejection fraction.

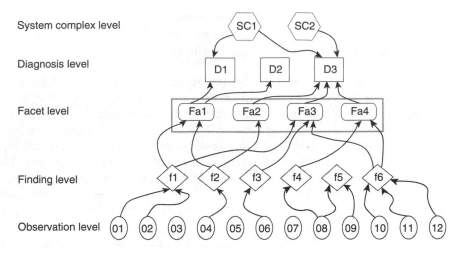

Figure 4.4. Epistemological framework representing the structure of medical knowledge for problem solving.

Conceptual and *procedural* knowledge provide another useful way of distinguishing the functions of different forms of representation. **Conceptual knowledge** refers to one's understanding of domain-specific concepts. **Procedural knowledge** is a kind of knowing related to how to perform various activities. There are numerous technical skills in medical contexts that necessitate the acquisition of procedural knowledge. Conceptual knowledge and procedural knowledge are acquired through different learning mechanisms. Conceptual knowledge is acquired through mindful engagement with materials in a range of contexts (from reading texts to conversing with colleagues). Procedural knowledge is developed as a function of deliberate practice, which results in a learning process known as *knowledge compilation* (Anderson, 1983). However, the development of skills may involve a transition from a declarative or interpretive stage toward increasingly proceduralized stages. For example, in learning to use an electronic health record (EHR) system designed to be used as part of a consultation, a less experienced user will need to attend carefully to every action and input, whereas a more experienced user of this system can more effortlessly interview a patient and simultaneously record patient data (Kushniruk et al., 1996; Patel et al., 2000). Procedural knowledge supports more efficient and automated action, but is often used without conscious awareness.

Procedural knowledge is often modeled in cognitive science and in AI as a *production rule*, which is a condition–action rule that states "if the conditions are satisfied, then execute the specified action" (either an inference or overt behavior). The following example illustrates a simple production rule:

IF the goal is to drive a stick-shift car   CONDITIONS
   and the car is in first gear
   and the car is going more than 10 MPH

THEN shift the car into second gear   ACTIONS

Production rules are a common method for representing knowledge in medical expert systems. The following example is drawn from MYCIN (Davis et al., 1977):

IF the infection is primary bacteremia   CONDITIONS
    and the site of the culture is one of the sterile sites
    and the suspected portal of entry of the organism
    is the gastrointestinal tract

THEN there is suggestive evidence that the identity   ACTIONS
    of the organism is bacteroides

The rule specifies that if the following infection conditions are met, one can draw the inference about the identity of the organism. This method of representation is an effective tool for capturing and formalizing a particular form of knowledge. Cognitive architectures typically employ production rules as a knowledge representation scheme.

Procedural knowledge is rather limited in its generality. A skilled user of one type of EHR system, for instance, will likely exhibit a decrement in performance when using a different system. The extent of this decrease is partly a function of the similarity and differences between the two systems and the kinds of component processes that they employ as well as the user's experience with diverse systems. To take a simple example, pen-based EHR systems engage different motor and perceptual processes than do keyboard-based or touch screen systems.

In addition to differentiating between procedural and conceptual knowledge, one can differentiate **factual knowledge** from conceptual knowledge. Factual knowledge involves merely knowing a fact or set of facts (e.g., risk factors for heart disease) without any in-depth understanding. Facts are routinely disseminated through a range of sources such as pamphlets. The acquisition of factual knowledge alone is not likely to lead to any increase in understanding or behavioral change (Bransford et al., 1999). The acquisition of conceptual knowledge involves the integration of new information with prior knowledge and necessitates a deeper level of understanding. For example, risk factors may be associated in the physician's mind with biochemical mechanisms and typical patient manifestations. This is in contrast to a new medical student who may have largely factual knowledge.

Thus far, we have only considered domain-general ways of characterizing the organization of knowledge. In view to understand the nature of medical cognition, it is necessary to characterize the domain-specific nature of knowledge organization in medicine. Given the vastness and complexity of the domain of medicine, this can be a rather daunting task. Clearly, there is no single way to represent all medical (or even clinical) knowledge, but it is an issue of considerable importance to research in biomedical informatics. Much research has been conducted in medical AI with the aim of developing medical ontologies for use in knowledge-based systems. Patel and Ramoni (1997) address this issue in the context of using empirical evidence from psychological experiments on medical expertise to test the validity of the AI systems. Medical **taxonomies**, **nomenclatures**, and **vocabulary** systems such as UMLS or SNOMED (see Chapter 7) are engaged in a similar pursuit. In our research, we have employed an epistemological framework developed by Evans and Gadd (1989). They proposed a framework that serves to characterize the knowledge used for medical understanding and problem solving, and also for differentiating the levels at which medical knowledge may be organized. This framework represents a formalization of medical knowledge as realized in textbooks and journals, and can be used to provide us with insight into the organization of clinical practitioners' knowledge (see Figure 4.4).

The framework consists of a hierarchical structure of concepts formed by *clinical observations* at the lowest level, followed by *findings*, *facets*, and *diagnoses*. Clinical observations are units of information that are recognized as potentially relevant in the problem-solving context. However, they do not constitute clinically useful facts. Findings comprise observations that have potential clinical significance. Establishing a finding reflects a decision made by a physician that an array of data contains a significant cue or cues that need to be taken into account. Facets consist of clusters of findings that indicate an underlying medical problem or class of problems. They reflect general pathological descriptions such as left ventricular failure or thyroid condition. Facets resemble the kinds of constructs used by researchers in medical AI to describe the partitioning of a problem space. They are interim hypotheses that serve to divide the information in the problem into sets of manageable subproblems and to suggest possible solutions. Facets also vary in terms of their levels of abstraction. Diagnosis is the level of classification that subsumes and explains all levels beneath it. Finally, the systems level consists of information that serves to contextualize a particular problem, such as the ethnic background of a patient.

4.4   Medical Cognition

The study of expertise is one of the principal paradigms in problem-solving research. Comparing experts to novices provides us with the opportunity to explore the aspects of performance that undergo change and result in increased problem-solving skill (Lesgold, 1984). It also permits investigators to develop domain-specific models of competence that can be used for assessment and training purposes.

A goal of this approach has been to characterize expert performance in terms of the knowledge and cognitive processes used in comprehension, problem solving, and decision making, using carefully developed laboratory tasks (Chi and Glaser, 1981; Lesgold et al., 1988) deGroot pioneering research (1965) in chess represents one of the earliest characterizations of expert–novice differences. In one of his experiments, subjects were allowed to view a chessboard for 5 to 10 seconds and were then required to reproduce the position of the chess pieces from memory. The grandmaster chess players were able to reconstruct the mid-game positions with better than 90 percent accuracy, while novice chess players could only reproduce approximately 20 percent of the correct positions. When the chess pieces were placed on the board in a random configuration, not encountered in the course of a normal chess match, expert chess masters' recognition ability fell to that of novices. This result suggests that superior recognition ability is not a function of superior memory, but is a result of an enhanced ability to recognize typical situations (Chase and Simon, 1973). This phenomenon is accounted for by a process known as "chunking." A chunk is any stimulus or patterns of stimuli that has become familiar from repeated exposure and is subsequently stored in memory as a single unit (Larkin et al., 1980). Knowledge-based differences impact on the problem representation and determine the strategies a subject uses to solve a problem. Simon and Simon (1978) compared a novice subject with an expert subject solving textbook physics problems. The results indicated that the expert solved the problem in one quarter of the time required by the novice with fewer errors. The novices solved most of the problems by working *backward* from the unknown problem solution to the givens of the problem statement. The expert worked *forward* from the givens to solve the necessary equations and determine the particular quantities they were asked to solve for. Differences in the directionality of reasoning by levels of expertise has been demonstrated in diverse domains from computer programming (Perkins et al., 1990) to medical diagnoses (Patel and Groen, 1986).

The expertise paradigm spans the range of content domains including physics (Larkin et al., 1980), sports (Allard and Starkes, 1991), music (Sloboda, 1991), and medicine (Patel et al., 1994). Edited volumes (Chi et al., 1988; Ericsson and Smith, 1991; Hoffman, 1992) provide an informative general overview of the area.

This research has focused on differences between subjects varying in levels of expertise in terms of memory, reasoning strategies, and in particular the role of domain-specific knowledge. Among the experts' characteristics uncovered by this research are the following: (1) experts are capable of perceiving large patterns of meaningful information in their domain that novices cannot perceive; (2) they are fast at processing and at the deployment of different skills required for problem solving; (3) they have a superior short-term and long-term memory for materials (e.g., clinical findings in medicine) within their domain of expertise, but not outside their domain; (4) they typically represent problems in their domain at deeper, more principled levels, whereas novices show a superficial level of representation; (5) they spend more time assessing the problem prior to solving it, while novices tend to spend more time working on the solution itself and little time in problem assessment. The critical factor that accounts for the superiority of expert performance has been found to be in the highly interconnected knowledge bases of the expert. (6) Individual experts may differ substantially in terms of exhibiting these kinds of performance characteristics (e.g., superior memory for domain materials).

Usually, someone is designated as an expert based on a certain level of performance, as exemplified by Elo ratings in chess; by virtue of being certified by a professional licensing body, as in medicine, law, or engineering; on the basis of academic criteria, such as graduate degrees; or simply based on years of experience or peer evaluation (Hoffman et al., 1995). The concept of an expert, however, refers to an individual who surpasses competency in a domain (Sternberg and Horvarth, 1999). Although competent performers, for instance, may be able to encode relevant information and generate effective plans of action in a specific domain, they often lack the speed and the flexibility that we see in an expert. A domain expert (e.g., a medical practitioner) possesses an extensive, accessible knowledge base that is organized for use in practice and is tuned to the particular problems at hand. In the study of medical expertise, it has been useful to distinguish different types of expertise. Patel and Groen (1991) distinguished between general and specific expertise, a distinction supported by research indicating differences between subexperts (i.e., expert physicians who solve a case outside their field of specialization) and experts (i.e., domain specialists) in terms of reasoning strategies and organization of knowledge. General expertise corresponds to expertise that cuts across medical subdisciplines (e.g., general medicine). Specific expertise results from detailed experience within a medical subdomain, such as cardiology or endocrinology. An individual may possess both, or only generic expertise. The different levels of expertise are explained in the following definitions that have been modified from Patel and Groen (1991).

Layperson: A person who has only common sense or everyday knowledge of a domain. This is equivalent to a naive person.

Beginner: A person who has the prerequisite knowledge assumed by the domain. Here we distinguish among beginners, depending on the degree and quality of their knowledge. We have identified, for instance, early, intermediate, and advanced beginners.

Novice: A layperson or a beginner. However, the term is mostly used to refer to a beginner or to someone initiated into a domain or a discipline.

Intermediate: Anybody who is above the beginner level but below the subexpert level. As with the beginner or the novice, intermediates are represented by various degrees, depending on their level of training.

Subexpert: A person with a generic knowledge but inadequate specialized knowledge of the domain.

Expert: A person with a specialized knowledge of the domain. We also have made the distinction among medical experts in terms of the nature of their practice, as medical practitioners or medical researchers.

The development of expertise typically follows a somewhat unusual trajectory. It is often assumed that the path from novice to expert goes through a steady process of gradual accumulation of knowledge and fine-tuning of skills. That is, as a person becomes more familiar with a domain, his or her level of performance (e.g., accuracy, quality) gradually increases. However, research has shown that this assumption is often incorrect (Lesgold et al., 1988; Patel et al., 1994). Cross-sectional studies of experts, intermediates, and novices have shown that people at intermediate levels of expertise may perform more poorly than those at lower level of expertise on some tasks. Furthermore, there is a long-standing body of research on learning that has suggested that the learning process involves phases of error-filled performance followed by periods of stable, relatively error-free performance. In other words, human learning does not consist of the gradually increasing accumulation of knowledge and fine-tuning of skills. Rather, it requires the arduous process of continually learning, re-learning, and exercising new knowledge, punctuated by periods of apparent decrease in mastery and declines in performance, which may be necessary for learning to take place. Figure 4.5 presents an illustration of this learning and developmental phenomenon known as the *intermediate effect*.

The intermediate effect has been found in a variety of tasks and with a great number of performance indicators. The tasks used include comprehension and explanation of clinical problems, doctor–patient communication, recall and explanation of laboratory data, generation of diagnostic hypotheses, and problem solving. The performance indicators used have included recall and inference of medical text information, recall and inference of diagnostic hypotheses, generation of clinical findings from a patient in doctor–patient interaction, and requests for laboratory data, among others. The research

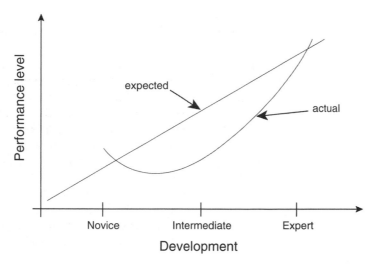

Figure 4.5. Schematic representation of intermediate effect. The straight line gives a commonly assumed representation of performance development by level of expertise. The curved line represents the actual development from novice to expert. The Y-axis may represent any of a number of performance variables such as errors made, concepts recalled, conceptual elaborations, or hypotheses generated in a variety of tasks.

has also identified developmental levels at which the intermediate phenomenon occurs, including senior medical students and residents. It is important to note, however, that in some tasks, the development is *monotonic*. For instance, in diagnostic accuracy, there is a gradual increase, with an intermediate exhibiting higher degree of accuracy than the novice, and the expert demonstrating a still higher degree than the intermediate. Furthermore, when relevance of the stimuli to a problem is taken into account, an appreciable monotonic phenomenon appears. For instance, in recall studies, novices, intermediates, and experts are assessed in terms of the total number of propositions recalled showing the typical nonmonotonic effect. However, when propositions are divided in terms of their relevance to the problem (e.g., a clinical case), experts recall more relevant propositions than intermediates and novices, suggesting that intermediates have difficulty separating what is relevant from what is not.

During the periods when the intermediate effect occurs, a reorganization of knowledge and skills takes place, characterized by shifts in perspectives or a realignment or creation of goals. The intermediate effect is also partly due to the unintended changes that take place as the person reorganizes for intended changes. People at intermediate levels typically generate a great deal of irrelevant information and seem incapable of discriminating what is relevant from what is not. Thus, the intermediate effect can be explained as a function of the learning process, maybe as a necessary phase of learning. Identifying the factors that may be involved in the intermediate effect may help to improve performance during learning (e.g., by designing decision-support systems or intelligent tutoring systems that help the user to focus on relevant information).

There are situations, however, where the intermediate effect disappears. Schmidt and Boshuizew (1993) reported that the intermediate recall phenomenon disappears when short text-reading times are used. Novices, intermediates, and experts given only a short time to read a clinical case (about 30 seconds) recalled the case with increasing accuracy. This suggests that under time-restricted conditions, intermediates cannot engage in extraneous search. In other words, intermediates who are not under time pressure process too much irrelevant information, whereas experts do not. On the other hand, novices lack the knowledge to do much search. Although intermediates may have most of the pieces of knowledge in place, this knowledge is not sufficiently well organized to be efficiently used. Until this knowledge becomes further organized, the intermediate is more likely to engage in unnecessary search.

The intermediate effect is not a one-time phenomenon. Rather, it occurs repeatedly at strategic points in a student's or physician's training that follow periods in which large bodies of new knowledge or complex skills are acquired. These periods are followed by intervals in which there is a decrement in performance until a new level of mastery is achieved.

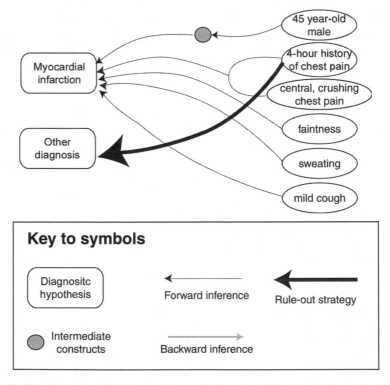

Figure 4.6. Problem interpretation by a novice medical student. The given information from patient problem is represented on the right side of the figure and the new generated information is given on the left side; information in the box represents diagnostic hypotheses. Intermediate hypotheses are represented as solid dark circles (filled). Forward-driven or data-driven inference arrows are shown from left to right (solid dark line). Backward or hypothesis-driven inference arrows are shown from right to left (solid light line). Thick solid dark line represents rule-out strategy.

4.4.1 Expertise in Medicine

The systematic investigation of medical expertise began more than 40 years ago with research by Ledley and Lusted (1959) into the nature of clinical inquiry. They proposed a two-stage model of clinical reasoning involving a hypothesis-generation stage followed by a hypothesis-evaluation stage. This latter stage is most amenable to formal decision-analytic techniques. The earliest empirical studies of medical expertise can be traced to the works of Rimoldi (1961) and Kleinmuntz (1968) who conducted experimental studies of diagnostic reasoning contrasting students with medical experts in simulated problem-solving tasks. The results emphasized the greater ability of expert physicians to selectively attend to relevant information and narrow the set of diagnostic possibilities (i.e., consider fewer hypotheses).

The origin of contemporary research on medical thinking is associated with the seminal work of Elstein et al., (1978) who studied the problem-solving processes of physicians by drawing on then contemporary methods and theories of cognition. This model of problem solving has had a substantial influence on studies of both medical cognition and medical education. They were the first to use experimental methods and theories of cognitive science to investigate clinical competency. Their research findings led to the development of an elaborated model of hypothetico-deductive reasoning, which proposed that physicians reasoned by first generating and then testing a set of hypotheses to account for clinical data (i.e., reasoning from hypothesis to data). First, physicians generated a small set of hypotheses very early in the case, as soon as the first pieces of data became available. Second, they were selective in the data they collected, focusing only on the relevant data. Third, they made use of a hypothetico-deductive method of diagnostic reasoning. The hypothetico-deductive process was viewed as comprising four stages: cue acquisition, hypothesis generation, cue interpretation, and hypothesis evaluation. Attention to initial cues led to the rapid generation of a few select hypotheses. According to the authors, each cue was interpreted as positive, negative, or non-contributory to each hypothesis generated. They were unable to find differences between superior physicians (as judged by their peers) and other physicians (Elstein et al., 1978).

The previous research was largely modeled after early problem-solving studies in knowledge-lean tasks. Medicine is clearly a knowledge-rich domain and a different approach was needed. Feltovich et al. (1984), drawing on models of knowledge representation from medical AI, characterized fine-grained differences in knowledge organization between subjects of different levels of expertise in the domain of pediatric cardiology. For example, novices' knowledge was described as "classically centered," built around the prototypical instances of a disease category. The disease models were described as sparse and lacking cross-referencing between shared features of disease categories in memory. In contrast, experts' memory store of disease models was found to be extensively cross-referenced with a rich network of connections among diseases that can present with similar symptoms. These differences accounted for subjects' inferences about diagnostic cues and evaluation of competing hypotheses.

Patel et al. (1986) studied the knowledge-based solution strategies of expert cardiologists as evidenced by their pathophysiological explanations of a complex clinical problem. The results indicated that subjects who accurately diagnosed the problem employed a forward-oriented (data-driven) reasoning strategy—using patient data to lead toward a complete diagnosis (i.e., reasoning from data to hypothesis). This is in contrast to subjects who misdiagnosed or partially diagnosed the patient problem. They tended to use a backward or hypothesis-driven reasoning strategy. The results of this study presented a challenge to the hypothetico-deductive model of reasoning as espoused by Elstein et al. (1978) that did not differentiate expert-from nonexpert-reasoning strategies.

Patel and Groen (1991) investigated the nature and directionality of clinical reasoning in a range of contexts of varying complexity. The objectives of this research program were both to advance our understanding of medical expertise and to devise more effective ways to teach clinical problem solving. It has been established that the patterns of data-driven and hypothesis-driven reasoning are used differentially by novices and experts. Experts tend to use data-driven reasoning, which depends on the physician's possessing a highly organized knowledge base about the patient's disease (including sets of signs and symptoms). Because of their lack of substantive knowledge or their inability to distinguish relevant from irrelevant knowledge, novices and intermediates use more hypothesis-driven reasoning resulting often in very complex reasoning patterns (see Figures 4.7 & 4.8). The fact that experts and novices reason differently suggests that they might reach different conclusions (e.g., decisions or understandings) when solving medical problems. Similar patterns of reasoning have been found in other domains (Larkin et al., 1980). Due to their extensive knowledge base and the high-level inferences they make, experts typically skip steps in their reasoning.

Although experts typically use data-driven reasoning during clinical performance, this type of reasoning sometimes breaks down and the expert has to resort to hypothesis-driven reasoning. Although data-driven reasoning is highly efficient, it is often error-prone in the absence of adequate domain knowledge, since there are no built-in checks on the legitimacy of the inferences that a person makes. Pure data-driven reasoning is only successful in constrained situations, where one's knowledge of a problem can result in a complete chain of inferences from the initial problem statement to the problem solution, as illustrated in Figure 4.9. In contrast, hypothesis-driven reasoning is slower and may make heavy demands on WM, because one has to keep track of such things as

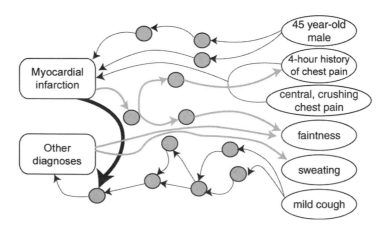

Figure 4.7. Problem interpretation by an intermediate medical student.

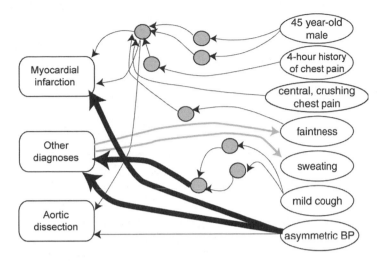

Figure 4.8. Problem interpretation by a senior medical student.

goals and hypotheses. It is, therefore, most likely to be used when domain knowledge is inadequate or the problem is complex. Hypothesis-driven reasoning is usually exemplary of a *weak method* of problem solving in the sense that is used in the absence of relevant prior knowledge and when there is uncertainty about problem solution. In problem-solving terms, strong methods engage knowledge, whereas weak methods refer to general strategies. Weak does not necessarily imply ineffectual in this context.

Studies have shown that the pattern of data-driven reasoning breaks down in conditions of case complexity, unfamiliarity with the problem, and uncertainty (Patel et al., 1990). These conditions include the presence of "loose ends" in explanations, where some particular piece of information remains unaccounted for and isolated from the overall explanation. Loose ends trigger explanatory processes that work by hypothesizing a disease, for instance, and trying to fit the loose ends within it, in a hypothesis-driven reasoning fashion. The presence of loose ends may foster learning, as the person searches for an explanation for them. For instance, a medical student or a physician may encounter a sign or a symptom in a patient problem and look for information that may account for the finding, by searching for similar cases seen in the past, reading a specialized medical book, or consulting a domain expert.

However, in some circumstances, the use of data-driven reasoning may lead to a heavy cognitive load. For instance, when students are given problems to solve while they are training in the use of problem-solving strategies, the situation produces a heavy load on cognitive resources and may diminish students' ability to focus on the task. The reason is that students have to share cognitive resources (e.g., attention, memory) between learning to use the problem-solving method and learning the content of the material. It has been found that when subjects used a strategy based on the use of data-driven reasoning, they were more able to acquire a schema for the problem. In addition, other characteristics associated with expert performance were observed, such as a reduced number of moves to the solution. However, when subjects used a hypothesis-driven reasoning strategy, their problem-solving performance suffered.

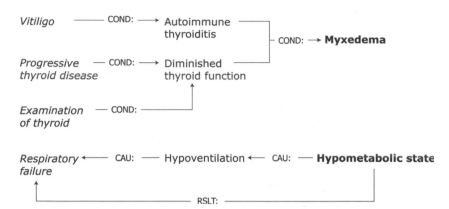

Figure 4.9. Diagrammatic representation of data-driven (top-down) and hypothesis-driven (bottom-up) reasoning. From the presence of vitiligo, a prior history of progressive thyroid disease, and examination of the thyroid (clinical findings on the left side of figure), the physician reasons forward to conclude the diagnosis of myxedema (right of figure). However, the anomalous finding of respiratory failure, which is inconsistent with the main diagnosis, is accounted for as a result of a hypometabolic state of the patient, in a backward-directed fashion. COND = conditional relation; CAU = causal relation; RSLT = resultive relation.

Perceptual diagnosis has also been an active area of inquiry in medical cognition. Studies have investigated clinicians at varying levels of expertise in their ability to diagnose skin lesions presented on a slide. The results revealed a monotonic increase in accuracy as a function of expertise. In a classification task, novices categorized lesions by their surface features (e.g., "scaly lesions"), intermediates grouped the slides according to diagnosis, and expert dermatologists organized the slides according to superordinate categories such as viral infections, which reflected the underlying pathophysiological structure. The ability to abstract the underlying principles of a problem is considered to be one of the hallmarks of expertise, both in medical problem solving and in other domains (Chi et al., 1981). Lesgold et al. (1988) investigated the abilities of radiologists at different levels of expertise, in the interpretation of chest X-ray pictures. The results revealed that the experts were able to rapidly invoke the appropriate schema and initially detect a general pattern of disease, which resulted in a gross anatomical localization and served to constrain the possible interpretations. Novices experienced greater difficulty focusing in on the important structures and were more likely to maintain inappropriate interpretations despite discrepant findings in the patient history.

Recently, Crowley et al. (2003) employed a similar protocol-analytic approach to study difference in expertise in breast pathology. The results suggest systematic differences between subjects at varying levels of expertise corresponding to accuracy of diagnosis, and all aspects of task performance including microscopic search, feature detection, feature identification, and data interpretation. The authors propose a model of visual diagnostic competence that involves development of effective search strategies, fast and accurate recognition of anatomic location, acquisition of visual data interpretation skills, and explicit feature identification strategies that result from a well-organized knowledge base.

The study of medical cognition has been summarized in a series of articles (Patel et al., 1994) and edited volumes (e.g., Evans and Patel, 1989). Other active areas of research include medical text comprehension (discussed in the context of guidelines), therapeutic reasoning, and mental models of physiological systems.

4.5   Human Computer Interaction: A Cognitive Engineering Approach

The history of computing and, more generally, the history of artifacts design are rife with stories of dazzlingly powerful devices with remarkable capabilities that are thoroughly unusable by anyone except for the team of designers and their immediate families. In the *Psychology of Everyday Things*, Norman (1988) describes a litany of poorly designed artifacts ranging from programmable VCRs to answering machines and water faucets that are inherently nonintuitive and very difficult to use. Similarly, there have been numerous innovative and promising medical information technologies that have yielded decidedly suboptimal results and deep user dissatisfaction when implemented in practice. At minimum, difficult interfaces result in steep learning curves and structural inefficiencies in task performance. At worst, problematic interfaces can have serious consequences for patient safety (Lin et al., 1998; Zhang et al., 2002) (see Chapter 9).

Over a decade ago, Nielsen (1993) reported that around 50 percent of the software code was devoted to the user interface, and a survey of developers indicated that, on average, 6 percent of their project budgets were spent on **usability** evaluation. Given the ubiquitous presence of **graphical user interfaces (GUI)**, it is likely that more than 50 percent of code is now devoted to the GUI. On the other hand, usability evaluations have greatly increased over the course of the last 10 years. There have been numerous texts devoted to promoting effective user interface design (Schneiderman, 1992), and the importance of enhancing the user experience has been widely acknowledged by both consumers and producers of information technology (see Chapter 11). Part of the impetus is that usability has been demonstrated to be highly cost-effective. Karat (1994) reported that for every dollar a company invests in the usability of a product, it receives between $10 and $100 in benefits. It is also far more costly to fix a problem after product release than in an early design phase. In our view, usability evaluation of medical information technologies has grown substantially in prominence over the course of the last 10 years. The concept of usability as well as the methods and tools to measure and promote it are now "touchstones in the culture of computing" (Carroll, 2002).

Usability methods have been used to evaluate a wide range of medical information technologies including infusion pumps (Dansky et al., 2001), ventilator management systems, physician-order entry (Ash et al., 2003), pulmonary graph displays (Wachter et al., 2003), information retrieval systems, and research Web environments for clinicians (Elkin et al., 2002). In addition, usability techniques are increasingly used to assess patient-centered environments (Cimino et al., 2000). The methods include observations, focus groups, surveys, and experiments. Collectively, these studies make a compelling case for the instrumental value in such research to improve efficiency, user acceptance, and relatively seamless integration with current workflow and practices.

What do we mean by usability? Nielsen (1993) suggests that usability includes the following five attributes:

1. *learnability*: system should be relatively easy to learn
2. *efficiency*: an experienced user can attain a high level of productivity
3. *memorability*: features supported by the system should be easy to retain once learned
4. *errors*: system should be designed to minimize errors and support error detection and recovery
5. *satisfaction*: the user experience should be subjectively satisfying

These attributes have given rise to various usability evaluation methods such as **heuristic evaluation** (Nielsen, 1994). Heuristic evaluation is a usability inspection method, in which the system is evaluated on the basis of a small set of well-tested design principles such as visibility of system status, user control and freedom, consistency and standards, flexibility and efficiency of use. This methodology embodies a particular philosophy, which emphasizes simplicity and functionality over intricacy of design and presentation. Zhang et al. (2003) employed a modified heuristic evaluation method to test the safety of two infusion pumps. They found numerous usability evaluations in both pumps of varying severity. Their results suggested that one of the pumps was likely to induce more medical errors than the other one.

Even with growth of usability research, there remain formidable challenges to designing and developing usable systems. This is exemplified by the recent events at Cedar Sinai Medical Center, in which a decision was made to suspend use of a computer-based physician-order-entry system just a few months after implementation. Physicians complained that the system, which was designed to reduce medical errors, compromised patient safety, took too much time and was difficult to use (Benko, 2003). To provide another example, we have been working with a mental health computer-based patient record (CPR) system that is rather comprehensive and supports a wide range of functions and user populations (e.g., physicians, nurses, and administrative staff). However, clinicians find it exceptionally difficult and time-consuming to use. The interface is based on a forms metaphor (or template) and is not user- or task-centered. The interface emphasizes completeness of data entry for administrative purposes rather than the facilitation of clinical communication, and is not optimally designed to support patient care (e.g., efficient information retrieval and useful summary reports). In general, the capabilities of this system are not readily usefully deployed to improve human performance. We further discuss issues of EHRs in a subsequent section.

Innovations in technology guarantee that usability and interface design will be a perpetually moving target. In addition, as health information technology reaches out to populations across the digital divide (e.g., seniors and low-literacy patient populations), there is a need to consider new interface requirements. Although evaluation methodologies and guidelines for design yield significant contributions, there is a need for a scientific framework to understand the nature of user interactions. HCI is a multifaceted discipline devoted to the study and practice of usability. HCI has emerged as a central area of both computer science research and development and applied behavioral and social science (Carroll, 2002).

HCI has spawned a professional orientation that focuses on practical matters concerning the integration and evaluation of applications of technology to support human activities. There are also active academic HCI communities that have contributed significant advances to the science of computing. HCI researchers have been devoted to the development of innovative design concepts such as *virtual reality*, *ubiquitous computing*, *multimodal interfaces*, *collaborative workspaces*, and *immersive environments*. HCI research has also been instrumental in transforming the software engineering process toward a more user-centered iterative system development (e.g., rapid prototyping). HCI research has also been focally concerned with the cognitive, social, and cultural dimensions of the computing experience. In this regard, it is concerned with developing analytic frameworks for characterizing how technologies can be used more productively across a range of tasks, settings, and user populations.

Carroll (1997) traces the history of HCI back to the 1970s with the advent of *software psychology*, a behavioral approach to understanding, and furthering software design. Human factors, ergonomics, and industrial engineering research were pursuing some of the same goals along parallel tracks. In the early 1980s, Card et al. (1983) envisioned HCI as a testbed for applying cognitive scientific research and also furthering theoretical development in cognitive science. The GOMS approach to modeling was a direct outgrowth of this initiative. GOMS is a powerful predictive tool, but it is limited in scope to the analysis of routine skills and expert performance. Most medical information technologies such as provider-order-entry systems engage complex cognitive skills.

In recent years, HCI research has begun to "burst at the seams" (Rogers, 2004) with an abundance of new theoretical frameworks, design concepts, and analytical foci. Although we view this as an exciting development, it has also contributed to a certain scientific fragmentation (Carroll, 2003). Our own research is grounded in a cognitive engineering framework, which is an interdisciplinary approach to the development of principles, methods, and tools to assess and guide the design of computerized systems to support human performance (Roth et al., 2002). In supporting performance, the focus is on cognitive functions such as attention, perception, memory, comprehension, problem solving, and decision making. The approach is centrally concerned with the analysis of cognitive tasks and the processing constraints imposed by the human cognitive system.

Models of cognitive engineering are typically predicated on a cyclical pattern of interaction with a system. This pattern is embodied in Norman's seven-stage model of action (1986), illustrated in Figure 4.10. The action cycle begins with a *goal*, e.g., retrieving a patient's health record. The goal is abstract and independent of any system. In this context, let us presuppose that the clinician has access to both a paper record and an electronic record. The second stage involves the formation of an *intention*, which in this case might be to retrieve the record online. The intention leads to the *specification of an action* sequence, which may include logging onto the system (which in itself may necessitate several actions), engaging a search facility to retrieve information, and entering the patient's health record number or some other identifying information. The specification results in *executing an action*, which may necessitate several behaviors. The system responds in some fashion (absence of a response is a response of sort). The user may or may not perceive a change in system state (e.g., system provides no indicators of a wait state). The perceived system response must then be *interpreted* and *evaluated* to

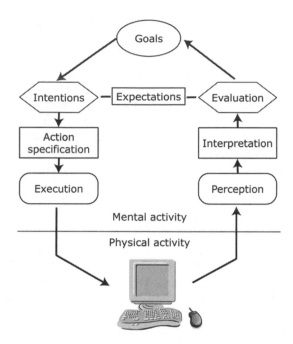

Figure 4.10. Norman's seven-stage model of action.

determine whether the goal has been achieved. This will then determine whether the user has been successful or whether an alternative course of action is necessary.

A complex task will involve substantial nesting of subgoals, involving a series of actions that are necessary before the primary goal can be achieved. To an experienced user, the action cycle may appear to be completely seamless. However, to a novice user, the process may break down at any of the seven stages. There are two primary points at which the action cycle can break down. The *gulf of execution* reflects the difference between the goals and intentions of the user and the kinds of actions enabled by the system. A user may not know the appropriate action sequence or the interface may not provide the prerequisite features to make such sequences transparent. For example, many systems require a goal completion action, such as pressing "Enter," after the primary selection had been made. This is a source of confusion, especially for novice users. The *gulf of evaluation* reflects the degree to which the user can interpret the state of the system and determine how well their expectations have been met. It is sometimes difficult to interpret a state transition and determine whether one has arrived at the right place. Goals that necessitate multiple state or screen transitions are more likely present difficulties for users, especially as they learn the system. Bridging gulfs involves both bringing about changes to the system design and educating users to foster competencies that can be used to make better use of system resources.

Gulfs are partially attributable to differences in the designer's models and the users' mental models. The designer's model is the conceptual model of the system, partially based on an estimation of the user population and task requirements (Norman, 1986). The users' mental models are developed through interacting with similar systems and gaining an understanding of how actions (e.g., clicking on a link) will produce predictable and desired outcomes. Graphical user interfaces that involve direct manipulation of screen objects represent an attempt to reduce the gap between a designer and users' model. The gap is more difficult to narrow in a system of greater complexity that incorporates a wide range of functions, like most medical information technologies.

Norman's theory of action has given rise (or in some case reinforced) the need for sound design principles. For example, the state of a system should be plainly *visible* to the user. There is a need to provide good mappings between the actions (e.g., clicking on a button) and the results of the action as reflected in the state of the system (e.g., screen transitions). Similarly, a well-designed system will provide full and continuous feedback so that the user can understand whether the expectations have been met.

The model has also informed a range of cognitive task-analytic usability evaluation methods such as the cognitive walkthrough (Polson et al., 1992). The study of human performance is predicated on an analysis of both the information-processing demands of a task and the kinds of domain-specific knowledge required to perform it. This analysis is often referred to as cognitive task analysis. The principles and methods that inform this approach can be applied to a wide range of tasks, from the analysis of written guidelines to the investigation of EHR systems. Generic tasks necessitate similar cognitive demands and have a common underlying structure that involves similar kinds of reasoning and patterns of inference. For example, clinical tasks in medicine include diagnostic reasoning, therapeutic reasoning, and patient monitoring and management. Similarly, an admission-order-entry task can be completed using written orders or one of many diverse computer-based order-entry systems. The underlying task of communicating orders in view to admit a patient remains the same. However, the particular implementation will greatly impact the performance of the task. For example, a system may eliminate the need for redundant entries and greatly facilitate the process. On the other hand, it may introduce unnecessary complexity, leading to suboptimal performance.

The **cognitive walkthrough (CW)** is a cognitive task-analytic method that has been applied to the study of usability and learnability of several distinct medical information technologies (Kushniruk et al., 1996). The purpose of a CW is to characterize the cognitive processes of users performing a task. The method involves identifying sequences of actions and goals needed to accomplish a given task. The specific aims of the procedure are to determine whether the user's background knowledge and the cues generated by the interface are likely to be sufficient to produce the correct goal–action sequence required to perform a task. The method is intended to identify potential usability problems that may impede the successful completion of a task or introduce complexity in a way that may frustrate users. The method is performed by an analyst or group of analysts "walking through" the sequence of actions necessary to achieve a goal. Both behavioral or physical actions such as mouse clicks and cognitive actions (e.g., inference needed to carry out a physical action) are coded. The principal assumption underlying this method is that a given task has a specifiable goal–action structure (i.e., the ways in which a user's objectives can be translated into specific actions). As in Norman's model, each action results in a system response (or absence of one), which is duly noted.

The CW method assumes a cyclical pattern of interaction as described previously. The codes for analysis include *goals*, which can be decomposed into a series of *subgoals* and *actions*. For example, opening an Excel spreadsheet (goal) may involve locating an icon or shortcut on one's desktop (subgoal) and double clicking on the application (action). We also characterize the system response (e.g., change in screen, update of values) and attempt to discern potential problems. This is illustrated below in a partial walkthrough of an individual obtaining money from an ATM.

Goal: Obtain $80 cash from Checking Account

1.   **Action:** Enter card (Screen 1)

⇒   **System response:** Enter PIN (Screen 2)

2.   **Subgoal:** Interpret prompt and provide input

3 & 4.   **Actions:** Enter PIN on numeric keypad and hit Enter (press lower white button next to screen)

⇒   **System response:** Do you want a Printed Transaction Record?

         Binary option: Yes or No (Screen 3)

5.   **Subgoal:** Decide whether a printed record is necessary

6.   **Action:** Press button next to No Response

⇒   **System response:** Select Transaction-8 Choices (Screen 4)

7.   **Subgoal:** Choose between Quick Cash and Cash Withdrawal

8.   **Action:** Press button next to Cash Withdrawal

⇒   **System response:** Select Account (Screen 5)

9.   **Action:** Press button next to Checking

⇒   **System response:** Enter dollar amounts in multiples of 20 (Screen 6)

10 & 11. **Action:** Enter $80 on numeric keypad and select Correct

The walkthrough of the ATM reveals that the process of obtaining money from the ATM necessitated a minimum of eight actions, five goals and subgoals, and six screen transitions. In general, it is desirable to minimize the number of actions necessary to complete a task. In addition, multiple screen transitions are more likely to confuse the user. We have employed a similar approach to analyze the complexity of a range of medical information technologies including EHRs, a home telecare system, and infusion pumps used in intensive care settings. The CW process emphasizes the sequential process, not unlike problem solving, involved in completing a computer-based task. The focus is more on the process rather than the content of the displays. In Section 4.5.1, we address the issue of external representations and how they differentially shape task performance.

4.5.1   External Representations

External representations such as images, graphs, icons, audible sounds, texts with symbols (e.g., letter and numbers), shapes, and textures are vital sources of knowledge, means of communication, and cultural transmission. The classical model of information-processing cognition viewed external representations as mere inputs to the mind (Zhang, 1997a). For example, the visual system would process the information in a display, which would serve as input to the cognitive system for further processing (e.g., classifying dermatological lesions), leading to knowledge retrieved from memory and resulting in a decision or action. These external representations served as a stimulus to be internalized (e.g., memorized) by the system. The hard work is then done by the machinery of the mind that develops an internal copy of a slice of the external world and stores it as a mental representation. The appropriate internal representation is then retrieved when needed.

This view has changed considerably in recent years. Norman (1993) argues that external representations play a critical role in enhancing cognition and intelligent behavior. These durable representations (at least those that are visible) persist in the external world and are continuously available to augment memory, reasoning, and computation. Consider a simple illustration involving multidigit multiplication with a pencil and paper. First, imagine calculating 37×93 without any external aids. Unless you are unusually skilled in such computations, the computations exert a reasonably heavy load on WM in relatively short order. One may have to engage in a serial process of calculation and maintain partial products in WM (e.g., 3×37=111). Now consider the use of pencil and paper as illustrated below:

		3	7
×	9	3	
1	1	1	
3	3	3	
3	4	4	1

The individual brings to the task knowledge of the meaning of the symbols (i.e., digits and their place value), arithmetic operators, and addition and multiplication tables (which enable a look-up from memory). The external representations include the positions of the symbols, the partial products of interim calculations, and their spatial relations (i.e., rows and columns). The visual representation, by holding partial results outside the mind, extends a person's WM (Card et al., 1999). Calculations can rapidly become computationally prohibitive without recourse to cognitive aids. The offloading of computations is a central argument in support of distributed cognition, which is the subject of Section 4.5.2.

It is widely understood that not all representations are equal for a given task and individual. The *representational effect* is a well-documented phenomenon in which different representations of a common abstract structure can have a significant effect on reasoning and decision making (Zhang and Norman, 1994). For example, different forms of graphical displays can be more or less efficient for certain tasks. A simple illustration is that Arabic numerals are more efficient for arithmetic (e.g., 37×93) than Roman numerals (XXXVII × XCIII) even though the representations or symbols are isomorphic. Similarly, a digital clock provides an easy readout for precisely determining the time (Norman, 1993). On the other hand, an analog clock provides an interface that enables one to more readily determine time intervals (e.g., elapsed or remaining time) without recourse to calculations. Larkin and Simon (1987) argued that effective displays facilitate problem solving by allowing users to substitute perceptual operations (i.e., recognition processes) for effortful symbolic operations (e.g., memory retrieval and computationally intensive reasoning), and that displays can reduce the amount of time spent searching for critical information. Research has demonstrated that different forms of graphical representations such as graphs, tables, and lists can dramatically change decision-making strategies (Kleinmuntz and Schkade, 1993; Scaife and Rogers, 1996).

Medication prescriptions are an interesting case in point. Chronic illness affects over 100 million individuals in the United States. Many of these individuals suffer from multiple afflictions and must adhere to complex medication regimens. There are various pill organizers and mnemonic devices designed to promote patient compliance. Although these are helpful, prescriptions written by clinicians are inherently hard for patients to follow. The following prescriptions were given to a patient following a mild stroke (Day, 1988 cited in Norman, 1993).

Inderal	−1 tablet 3 times a day
Lanoxin	−1 tablet every A.M.
Carafate	−1 tablet before meals and at bedtime
Zantac	−1 tablet every 12 hours (twice a day)
Quinaglute	−1 tablet 4 times a day
Coumadin	−1 tablet a day

The physician's list is concise and presented in a format whereby a pharmacist can readily fill the prescription. However, the organization by medication does not facilitate a patient's decision of what medications to take at given time of day. Some computation, memory retrieval (e.g., I took my last dose of Lanoxin 6 hours ago), and inference (what medications to bring when leaving one's home for some duration of hours) is necessary to make such a decision. Day proposed an alternative tabular representation (Table 4.3).

In this matrix representation in Table 4.3, the items can be organized by time of day (columns) and by medication (rows). The patient can simply scan the list by either time of day or medication. This simple change in representation can transform a cognitively taxing task into a simpler one that facilitates search (e.g., when do I take Zantac) and computation (e.g., which medications taken at dinner time).

Tables can support quick and easy lookup and embody a compact and efficient representational device. However, a particular external representation is likely to be effective for some populations of users and not others. For example, reading a table

Table 4.3. Tabular representation of medications.

	Breakfast	Lunch	Dinner	Bedtime
Lanoxin	X			
Inderal	X	X	X	
Quinaglute	X	X	X	X
Carafate	X	X	X	X
Zantac		X		X
Coumadin				X

Source: Adapted from Norman (1988).

requires a certain level of numeracy that is beyond the abilities of certain patients with very basic education. Kaufman et al. (2003) conducted a cognitive evaluation of the IDEATel home telemedicine system (Shea et al., 2002; Starren et al., 2002) with a particular focus on (a) system usability and learnability, and (b) the core competencies, skills, and knowledge necessary to productively use the system. The focal point of the intervention is the home telemedicine unit (HTU), which provides the following functions: (1) synchronous videoconferencing with a nurse case manager; (2) electronic transmission of fingerstick glucose and blood pressure readings; (3) e-mail to a physician and nurse case manager; (4) review of one's clinical data; and (5) access to Web-based educational materials. The usability study revealed dimensions of the interface that impeded optimal access to system resources. In addition, we found significant obstacles corresponding to perceptual-motor skills, mental models of the system, and health literacy. One of the most striking findings was the difficulty some patients had dealing with numeric data, especially when they were represented in tabular form. Several patients lacked an abstract understanding of covariation and how it can be expressed as a functional relationship in a tabular format (i.e., cells and rows) as illustrated in Figure 4.11. Others had difficulty establishing the correspondence between the values expressed on the interface of their blood pressure–monitoring device and mathematical representation in tabular format (systolic/diastolic). The familiar monitoring device provided an easy readout and patients could readily make appropriate inferences (e.g., systolic value is higher than usual) and take appropriate measures. However, when interpreting the same values in a table, certain patients had difficulty recognizing anomalous or abnormal results even when these values were rendered as salient by a color-coding scheme. Monitoring glucose and blood pressure values involves discerning patterns over periods of time from days to weeks to even months.

The results suggest that even the more literate patients were challenged to draw inferences over bounded periods of time. They tended to focus on discrete values (i.e., a single reading) in noting whether it was within their normal or expected range. In at least one case, the problems with the representation seemed to be related to the medium of representation rather than the form of representation. One patient experienced considerable difficulty reading the table on the computer display, but maintained a daily diary with very similar representational properties.

Instructions can be embodied in a range of external representations from text to list of procedures to diagrams exemplifying the steps. Everyday nonspecialists are called upon to follow instructions in a variety of application domains (e.g., completing income tax forms, configuring and using a VCR, cooking something for the first time, or inter-

Date	Time	Glucose	Blood pressure
7/23/02	7:20 AM	135	144/82
7/23/02	6:52 PM	163	154/100
7/24/02	6:30 AM	145	161/134
7/24/02	7:08 PM	166	152/88

Figure 4.11. Mapping values between blood pressure monitor and IDEATel table.

preting medication instructions), where correct processing of information is necessary for proper functioning. The comprehension of written information in such cases frequently involves both quantitative and qualitative reasoning, as well as a minimal familiarity with the application domain. This is nowhere more apparent, and critical, than in the case of over-the-counter pharmaceutical labels, the correct understanding of which often demands that the user translate minimal, quantitative formulas into qualitative, and frequently complex, procedures. Medical errors involving the use of therapeutic drugs are amongst the most frequent.

The calculation of dosages for pharmaceutical instructions can be remarkably complex. Consider the following instructions for an over-the-counter cough syrup:

Each teaspoonful (5ml) contains 15 mg of dextromethorphan hydrobromide U.S.P., in a palatable yellow, lemon-flavored syrup.

DOSAGE ADULTS: 1 or 2 teaspoonfuls three or four times daily.
DOSAGE CHILDREN: 1 mg per kg of body weight daily in 3 or 4 divided doses.

If you wish to administer medication to a 22-lb child 3 times a day and wish to determine the dosage (see Figure 4.13), the calculations are as follows:

$$22lbs \div 2.2lbs/kg \times 1mg/kg/day \div 15mg/tsp \div 3doses/day = 2 \div 9tsp/dose$$

Patel et al. (2002) studied 48 lay subjects' response to this problem. The majority of participants (66.5 percent) was unable to correctly calculate the appropriate dosage of cough syrup. Even when calculations were correct, the subjects were unable to estimate the actual amount to administer. There were no significant differences based on cultural or educational background. One of the central problems is that there is a significant mismatch between the designer's conceptual model of the pharmaceutical text and procedures to be followed and the user's mental model of the situation.

Diagrams are tools that we use daily in communication, information storage, planning, and problem solving. Diagrammatic representations are not new devices for communicating ideas. They of course have a long history as tools of science and cultural inventions that augment thinking. For example, the earliest maps, graphical representations of regions of geographical space, date back thousands of years. The phrase "a picture is worth 10,000 words" is believed to be an ancient Chinese proverb (Larkin and Simon, 1987). External representations have always been a vital means for storing, aggregating, and communicating patient data. The psychological study of information displays similarly has a long history dating back to Gestalt psychologists beginning around the turn of the twentieth century. They produced a set of laws of pattern perception for describing how we see patterns in visual images (Ware, 2003). For example, *the law of proximity* states that visual entities that are close together are perceptually grouped. The *law of symmetry* indicates that symmetric objects are more readily perceived.

Advances in graphical user interfaces afford a wide range of novel external representations. Card et al. (1999) define information visualization as "the use of computer-supported, interactive, visual representations of abstract data to amplify cognition." Information visualization of medical data is a vigorous area of research and application

(Starren and Johnson, 2000; Kosara and Miksch, 2002). Medical data can include single data elements or more complex data structures. Representations can also be characterized as either numeric (e.g., laboratory data) or non-numeric information (e.g. symptoms and diseases). Visual representations may be either static or dynamic (changing as additional temporal data becomes available). EHRs need to include a wide range of data representation types, including both numeric and non-numeric (Tang and McDonald, 2001). EHR data representations are employed in a wide range of clinical, research, and administrative tasks by different kinds of users. Medical imaging systems are used for a range of purposes including visual diagnosis (e.g., radiology), assessment and planning, communication, and education and training (Greenes and Brinkley, 2001). The purposes of these representations are to display and manipulate digital images to reveal different facets of anatomical structures in either two or three dimensions. Patient monitoring systems employ static and dynamic (e.g., continuous observations) representations for the presentation of physiological parameters such as heart rate, respiratory rate, and blood pressure (Gardner and Shabot, 2001) (see Chapter 17).

Recently, patient monitoring systems have been the subject of several human factors studies (Lin et al., 1998, 2001; Wachter et al., 2003). Lin et al. (1998) evaluated the interface of a patient-controlled analgesia pump, which had produced several user errors resulting in several patient deaths. They found that the original display introduced substantial cognitive complexity into the task and that a redesigned interface that adhered to human factors principles could lead to significantly faster, easier, and more reliable performance.

Information visualization is an area of great importance in bioinformatics research, particularly in relation to genetic sequencing and alignment. The tools and applications are being produced at a very fast pace. Although there is tremendous promise in such modeling systems, we know very little about what constitutes a usable interface for particular tasks. What sort of competencies or prerequisite skills are necessary to use such representations effectively? There is a significant opportunity for cognitive methods and theories to play an instrumental role in this area.

In general, there have been relatively few cognitive studies characterizing how different kinds of medical data displays impact performance. However, there have been several efforts to develop a typology of medical data representations. Starren and Johnson (2000) proposed a taxonomy of data representations. They characterized five major classes of representation types including list, table, graph, icon, and generated text. Each of these data types has distinct measurement properties (e.g., ordinal scales are useful for categorical data) and is variably suited for different kinds of data, tasks, and users. The authors propose some criteria for evaluating the efficacy of a representation including: (1) latency (the amount of time it takes a user to answer a question based on information in the representation); (2) accuracy; and (3) compactness (the relative amount of display space required for the representation). Further research is needed to explore the cognitive consequences of different forms of external medical data representations. For example, what inferences can be more readily gleaned from a tabular representation versus a line chart? How does configuration of objects in a representation affect latency? We consider some related issues regarding guidelines and EHR interfaces in the following sections.

At present, computational advances in information visualization have outstripped our understanding of how these resources can be most effectively deployed for particular tasks. However, we are gaining a better understanding of the ways in which external representations can amplify cognition. Card et al. (1999) propose six major ways:

1. By increasing the memory
2. By processing resources available to the users (offloading cognitive work to a display)
3. By reducing the search for information (grouping data strategically)
4. By using visual presentations to enhance the detection of patterns
5. By using perceptual attention mechanisms for monitoring (e.g., drawing attention to events that require immediate attention)
6. By encoding information in a manipulable medium (e.g., the user can select different possible views to highlight variables of interest)

4.5.2   Distributed Cognition and Electronic Health Records

In this chapter, we have considered a classical model of information-processing cognition in which mental representations mediate all activity and constitute the central units of analysis. The analysis emphasizes how an individual formulates internal representations of the external world. To illustrate the point, imagine an expert user of a word processor who can effortlessly negotiate tasks through a combination of key commands and menu selections. The traditional cognitive analysis might account for this skill by suggesting that the user has formed an image or schemata of the layout structure of each of eight menus, and retrieves this information from memory each time an action is to be performed. For example, if the goal is to "insert a clip art icon," the user would simply recall that this is subsumed under pictures, which is the ninth item on the "Insert" menu, and then execute the action, thereby achieving the goal. However, there are some problems with this position. Mayes et al. (1988) demonstrated that even highly skilled users could not recall the names of menu headers, yet they could routinely make fast and accurate menu selections. The results indicate that many or even most users relied on cues in the display to trigger the right menu selections. This suggests that the display can have a central role in controlling interaction in graphical user interfaces.

In recent years, the conventional information-processing approach has come under criticism for its narrow focus on the rational or cognitive processes of the solitary individual. In Section 4.5.1, we consider the relevance of external representations to cognitive activity. The emerging perspective of **distributed cognition (DC)** offers a more far-reaching alternative. The distributed view of cognition represents a shift in the study of cognition from being the sole property of the individual to being "stretched" across groups, material artifacts, and cultures (Suchman, 1987; Hutchins, 1995). This viewpoint is increasingly gaining acceptance in cognitive science and HCI research. In the distributed approach to HCI research, cognition is viewed as a process of coordinating distributed internal (i.e., knowledge) and external (e.g., visual displays, manuals) representations. DC has two central points of inquiry: one that emphasizes the inherently social and collaborative nature of cognition (e.g., doctors, nurses, and technical support staff in neonatal care unit jointly contributing to a decision process), and the other that characterizes the mediating effects of technology or other artifacts on cognition.

The DC perspective reflects a spectrum of viewpoints on what constitutes the appropriate unit of analysis for the study of cognition. Let us first consider a more radical departure from the classical model of information processing. Cole and Engestrom (1997) suggest that the natural unit of analysis for the study of human behavior is an activity system, comprising relations among individuals and their proximal, "culturally organized environments." A system consisting of individuals, groups of individuals, and technologies can be construed as a single indivisible unit of analysis. Berg is a leading proponent of the sociotechnical viewpoint within the world of medical informatics. He (1999) argues that "work practices are conceptualized as networks of people, tools, organizational routines, documents and so forth." An emergency ward, outpatient clinic, or obstetrics and gynecology department is seen as an interrelated assembly of humans and things, whose functioning is primarily geared to the delivery of patient care. Berg (1999, p. 89) goes on to emphasize that the "elements that constitute these networks should then not be seen as discrete, well-circumscribed entities with pre-fixed characteristics."

In Berg's view, the study of information systems must reject an approach that segregates individual and collective, human and machine, as well as the social and technical dimensions of information technology. Bowker and Starr (1999) draw on similar theoretical notions in their penetrating analysis of the social construction of classification systems and standards and their unintended consequences. Although there are compelling reasons for adapting a strong socially distributed approach, we have argued for a more moderate perspective in which an individual's mental representations and external representations are both given recognition as instrumental tools in cognition (Patel et al., 2001, 2002). This is consistent with a DC framework that embraces the centrality of external representations as mediators of cognition, but also considers the importance of an individual's internal representations (Perry, 2003).

The mediating role of technology can be evaluated at several levels of analysis from the individual to the organization. Technologies, whether computer-based or artifacts in another medium, transform the ways individuals and groups think. They do not merely augment, enhance, or expedite performance, although a given technology may do all of these things. The difference is not merely one of quantitative change but one that is also qualitative in nature.

In a distributed world, what becomes of the individual? If we adapt a strong socially distributed framework, the individual is part of a larger collective entity. Changes in individual knowledge or competencies are largely secondary concerns and peripheral to the analysis. However, we believe it is important to understand how technologies promote enduring changes in individuals. Salomon et al. (1991) introduce an important distinction in considering the mediating role of technology on individual performance, *the effects with technology* and *the effects of technology*. The former is concerned with the changes in performance displayed by users while equipped with the technology. For example, when using an effective medical information system, physicians should be able to gather information more systematically and efficiently. In this capacity, medical information technologies may alleviate some of the cognitive load associated with a given task and permit them to focus on higher-order thinking skills, such as diagnostic hypothesis generation and evaluation. The effects of technology refer to enduring changes in general cognitive capacities (knowledge and skills) as a consequence of interaction with a technology. This effect is illustrated subsequently in the context of the enduring effects of an EMR system (see Chapter 12). There is a more extended discussion of this in a special issue of *AI in Medicine* on distributed and collaborative cognition (Patel, 1998).

We employed a pen-based EHR system, dossier of clinical information (DCI), in several of our studies (see Kushniruk et al., 1996). Using the pen or computer keyboard, physicians can directly enter information into the EHR such as the patient's chief complaint, past history, history of present illness, laboratory tests, and differential diagnoses. Physicians were encouraged to use the system while collecting data from patients (e.g., during the interview). The DCI system incorporates an extended version of the ICD-9 vocabulary standard (see Chapter 7). The system allows the physician to record information about the patient's differential diagnosis, the ordering of tests, and the prescription of medication. It also provides supporting reference information in the form of an integrated electronic version of the Merck Manual, drug monographs for medications, and information on laboratory tests. The graphical interface provides a highly structured set of resources for representing a clinical problem as illustrated in Figure 4.12.

We have studied the use of this EHR in both laboratory-based research (Kushniruk et al., 1996) and in actual clinical settings (Patel et al., 2000). The laboratory research included a simulated doctor–patient interview. We have observed two distinct patterns of EHR usage in the interactive condition: one in which the subject pursues information from the patient predicated on a hypothesis; and the second which involves the use

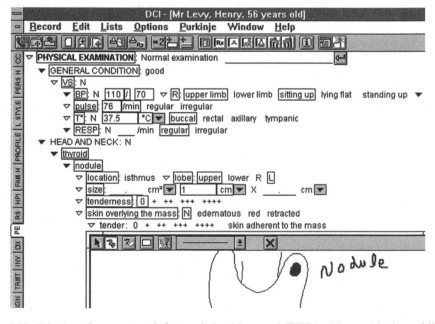

Figure 4.12. Display of a structured electronic health record (EHR) with graphical capabilities.

$$\frac{1 \text{ mg of medicine}}{1 \text{ kg of body weight}} \times 22 \text{ lb} \times \frac{1 \text{ kg}}{2.2 \text{ lb}} \times \frac{1}{\text{total daily dose in milligrams}} = \frac{10}{15} \text{ tsp} = \frac{2}{3} \text{ tsp}$$

$$\frac{2}{3n} \text{ tsp n times daily } (\text{where n} = 3) = \frac{2}{3 \times 3} \text{ tsp, 3 times daily} = \frac{10 \text{ kg}}{15 \times 3 \text{ times daily}} = \frac{2}{9} \text{ tsp, 3 times daily.}$$

Figure 4.13. Calculation of a single dose of an over-the-counter cough syrup for a 22-lb child.

of the EHR display to provide guidance for asking questions to the patient. In the screen-driven strategy, the clinician is using the structured list of findings in the order they appear on the display to elicit information. All experienced users of this system appear to have both strategies in their repertoire.

In general, a screen-driven strategy can enhance performance by reducing the cognitive load imposed by information-gathering goals and allow the physician to allocate more cognitive resources toward testing hypotheses and rendering decisions. On the other hand, this strategy can encourage a certain sense of complacency. We observed both effective as well as counterproductive uses of this screen-driven strategy. A more experienced user consciously used the strategy to structure the information-gathering process, whereas a novice user used it less discriminatingly. In employing this screen-driven strategy, the novice elicited almost all of the relevant findings in a simulated patient encounter. However, the novice also elicited numerous irrelevant findings and pursued incorrect hypotheses. In this particular case, the subject became too reliant on the technology and had difficulty imposing his or her own set of working hypotheses to guide the information-gathering and diagnostic-reasoning processes.

The differential use of strategies is evidence of the mediating effects with technology. Patel et al. (2000) extended this line of research to study the cognitive consequences of using the same EHR system in a diabetes clinic. The study considered the following questions (Patel et al., 2000, p.571):

1. How do physicians manage information flow when using an EHR system?
2. What are the differences in the way physicians organize and represent this information using paper-based and EHR systems?
3. Are there long-term, enduring effects of the use of EHR systems on knowledge representations and clinical reasoning?

One study focused on an in-depth characterization of changes in knowledge organization in a single subject as a function of using the system. The study first compared the contents and structure of 10 matched (for variables such as age and problem type) patient records produced by the physician using the EHR system and paper-based patient records. After having used the system for 6 months, the physician was asked to conduct his next five patient interviews using only hand-written paper records.

The results indicated that the EHRs contained more information relevant to the diagnostic hypotheses. In addition, the structure and content of information was found to correspond to the structured representation of the particular medium. For example, EHRs were found to contain more information about the patient's past medical history, reflecting the query structure of the interface. The paper-based records appear to better preserve the integrity of the time course of the evolution of the patient problem, whereas, this is notably absent from the EHR. Perhaps, the most striking finding is that, after having used the system for 6 months, the structure and content of the physician's paper-based records bear a closer resemblance to the organization of information in the EHR than the paper-based records produced by the physician prior to the exposure to the system. This finding is consistent with the enduring *effects of* technology even in absence of the particular system.

Patel et al (2000) conducted a series of related studies with physicians in the same diabetes clinic. The results of one study replicated and extended the results of the single subject study (reported above) regarding the differential effects of EHRs on paper-based records on represented (recorded) patient information. For example, physicians entered significantly more information about the patients' chief complaint using the EHR. Similarly, physicians represented significantly more information about the history of present illness and review of systems using paper-based records. It is reasonable to assert that such differences are likely to have an impact on clinical decision making. The authors also videotaped and analyzed 20 doctor–patient computer interactions of two physicians varying in their level of expertise. One of the physicians was an intermediate-level user of the EHR and the other was an expert user. The analysis of the physician–patient interactions revealed that the less expert subject was more strongly influenced by the structure and content of the interface. In particular, he was guided by the order of information on the screen when asking the patient questions and recording the responses. This screen-driven strategy is similar to what we documented in a previous study (Kushniruk et al., 1996). Although the expert user similarly used the EHR system to structure his or her questions, he or she was much less bound to the order and sequence of presented information on the EHR screen. This body of research documented both *effects with* and *effects of* technology in the context of EHR use. These include effects on knowledge-organization and information-gathering strategies. The authors conclude that given these potentially enduring effects, the use of a particular EHR will almost certainly have a direct effect on medical decision making.

The above discussed research demonstrates the ways in which information technologies can mediate cognition and even produce enduring changes in how one performs a task. What dimensions of an interface contribute to such changes? What aspects of a display are more likely to facilitate efficient task performance and what aspects are more likely to impede it? Norman (1986) argued that well-designed artifacts could reduce the need for users to remember large amounts of information, whereas poorly designed artifacts increased the knowledge demands on the user and the burden of WM. In the distributed approach to HCI research, cognition is viewed as a process of coordinating distributed internal and external representations and this in effect constitutes an indivisible information-processing system.

How do artifacts in the external world "participate" in the process of cognition? The ecological approach of perceptual psychologist Gibson was based on the analysis of invariant structures in the environment in relation to perception and action. The concept of *affordance* has gained substantial currency in HCI. It has been used to refer to attributes of objects that enable individuals to know how to use them (Rogers, 2004). When the affordance of an object is perceptually obvious, it renders human interactions with objects effortless. For example, one can often perceive the affordance of a door handle (e.g., affords turning or pushing downward to open a door) or a water faucet. On the other hand, there are numerous artifacts in which the affordance is less transparent (e.g., door handles that appear to require being pulled to open a door but actually need to be pushed). External representations constitute affordance in that they can be picked up, analyzed, and processed by perceptual systems alone. According to theories of DC, most cognitive tasks have an internal and external component (Hutchins, 1995), and as a consequence, the problem-solving process involves coordinating information from these representations to produce new information.

One of the appealing features of the DC paradigm is that it can be used to understand how properties of objects on the screen (e.g., links, buttons) can serve as external representations and reduce cognitive load. The distributed resource model proposed by Wright et al. (2000) addresses the question of "what information is required to carry out some task and where should it be located: as an interface object or as something that is mentally represented to the user." The relative difference in the distribution of representations (internal and external) is central in determining the efficacy of a system designed to support a complex task. Wright et al. (2000) were among the first to develop an explicit model for coding the kinds of resources available in the environment and the ways in which they are embodied on an interface.

Horsky et al. (2003) applied the distributed resource model and analysis to a provider-order-entry system. The goal was to analyze specific order-entry tasks such as that involved in admitting a patient and then to identify areas of complexity that may impede optimal recorded entries. The research consisted of two component analyses: a modified CW evaluation based on the distributed resource model and a simulated clinical ordering task performed by seven physicians. The CW analysis revealed that the configuration of resources (e.g., very long menus, complexly configured displays) placed unnecessarily heavy cognitive demands on the user, especially those who were knew to the system. The resources model was also used to account for patterns of errors produced by clinicians. The authors concluded that the redistribution and reconfiguration of resources might yield guiding principles and design solutions in the development of complex interactive systems.

The framework for distributed cognition is still an emerging one in HCI. In our view, it offers a novel and potentially powerful approach for illuminating the kinds of difficulties users encounter and for finding ways to better structuring the interaction by redistributing the resources. The analysis may also provide a window into why technologies sometime fail to reduce errors or even contribute to them.

4.6   Clinical Practice Guidelines

In this section, we illustrate the use of text comprehension methods of analysis in the context of examining the use of clinical practice guidelines (CPG; see Chapter 20). CPGs are aimed at physicians with a wide range of knowledge and experience. A desired result using guidelines is the adoption of best practices, and decreased variability. However, past research on guidelines has found that they are not widely used (Tunis et al., 1994; McAlister et al., 1997). Many reasons have been put forth to account for this situation; among them are the guidelines' lack of integration into workflow and their perceived irrelevance to the actual practice of medicine. Such perception may be due to a mismatch between a guideline's recommended actions and the physician-user's opinion of what should be done for a specific patient in a particular clinical setting. Furthermore, CPGs can be semantically complex, often comprising elaborate collections of prescribed procedures with logical gaps or contradictions that can promote ambiguity and hence frustration on the part of those who attempt to use them. Many CPGs also involve the embedding of procedures within procedures or complicated temporal or causal relations among the various steps in a procedure. An understanding of the semantics of CPGs and of the physician's interpretation of the guideline may help to improve such matching, and ultimately the comprehensibility and usability of CPGs.

The recent interest in clinical guidelines has tended to focus on the creation of the guidelines through a professional consensus process, generally guided by relevant articles from the clinical literature. The successful dissemination of these guidelines has been limited, largely depending on published monographs or articles, which assume that clinicians will read such information and incorporate it into their own practices. We need to be able to identify those aspects of the guidelines where ambiguity arises, leading to differences in interpretation.

The process of interpretation has been investigated extensively in cognitive research. This research suggests that the process of interpretation consists of two components: first, what the text (e.g., literature, guidelines) itself says and, second, what each person interprets from the text. The former conveys the literal or surface meaning of a description, whereas the latter relates to the personal interpretation that each person infers, based on his or her prior knowledge. Even though there may be general agreement as to what the text literally says, there is often great disagreement in terms of the inferences that are generated when that text is ultimately used to support actions. One source of the differences lies in the fact that each person approaches the text with different knowledge and purposes. For instance, studies of medical expertise (Patel et al., 1994) have shown that people presented with the same clinical information differ in the nature and form of the models they construct regarding the patient and the disease.

The representation of a guideline raises issues similar to those in the process of software design, where a designer's conceptual model may or may not be coextensive with the user's mental models. However, guideline represenation is further complicated by the fact that it must reflect the vision of the domain experts who summarized the literature and conceptualized the problem. The representation of a guideline should reflect the intentions of these people who generate the guideline in the first place. On the one hand, any two interpretations generated from the same guideline should be equivalent in terms of the information that is inferred and the facility with which the information is inferred (Zhang, 1997b). By investigating the guideline development process, one can attempt to maximize the equivalence among interpretations by several decision makers, which can be done by identifying processes or problems that may be shown to generate ambiguity (Patel et al., 1998). On the other hand, guidelines should allow for flexibility in interpretation, such that patient- or context-specific information can be included in the recommendation without violating the guideline. By investigating the actual process of guideline development we can uncover those aspects that remain implicit because of the familiarity of the guideline designers with the subject matter of the guideline or their knowledge of the procedures employed. This implicit knowledge can be brought to the surface by cognitive methods, as it may be unknown to end users of the guidelines (such as practicing physicians). This implicit knowledge can be made more explicit and incorporated into the guideline procedures.

Although one long-term goal of guideline development may be the automation of such processes, there are many translation steps that occur before the computer-mediated guideline can be made available to a clinician. Figures 4.15 and 4.16 present the various steps in the development process, which can be categorized by the location at which such translations occur. The first step is the generation of the paper guidelines at authoring institutions, such as the American College of Physicians (ACP), which involves evidence-based consensus development, generally through examination of reports in the scientific literature. The second step is the translation of the paper guidelines into an algorithmic form to be easily used by physicians. The third step in the process is to translate the paper-based guideline into computer-based representations. The fourth step is the implementation of the computer-based representations in clinical institutions. The final step is the end user's (e.g., a clinician's) interpretation of the guideline as it is represented in the guideline applications in specific clinical settings.

From the methodological perspective, our research team has focused on the development and refinement of a theoretical and methodological framework for the use of cognitive analysis to support the representation of biomedical knowledge and the design of clinical systems, using clinical practice guidelines. A hypothesis underlying such development is that propositional and semantic analyses, when used as part of the system development process, can improve the validity, usability, and comprehension of the resulting biomedical applications. The framework is based on a large body of research on the study of how people mentally represent information and subsequently use it for

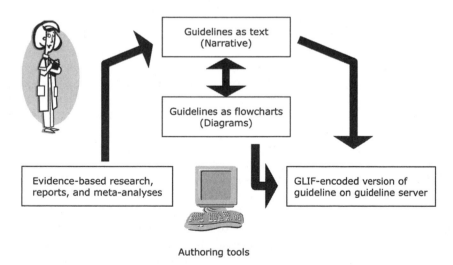

Authoring tools

Figure 4.14. Process of guideline creation.

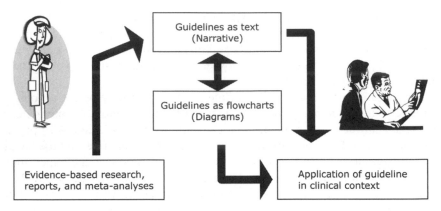

Figure 4.15. Process of guideline encoding.

solving problems and making decisions in health domains (Patel et al., 2002). This research draws on the study of memory and the study of comprehension. Of particular relevance is research devoted to investigating the comprehension and memory of language, expressed verbally or in text. In addition, research on how contextual variables affect performance is informative because these psychological processes are influenced by situational variables. One important factor limiting the acceptance and use of CPGs may be the mismatch between a guideline's recommended actions and the physician-user's mental models of what seems appropriate in a given case.

Figure 4.16 presents the methodological steps that we discuss in this section of the chapter. Beginning at the bottom with the thoughts and ideas that an individual brings to a design or problem-solving task, people express those notions using spoken language or written text. In the case of CPGs, the written documents have tended to be the basis for direct manual encoding of the logic into a computer-based representation.

Comprehension is an essential step in design, problem solving, and decision making, since one needs to have a firm understanding of an issue before effective decisions are made or problems are solved successfully. Although some texts, such as CPGs, are designed to provide a plan of action, an inadequate understanding could lead to errors in nonroutine situations. Comprehension involves the construction of a mental representation of some aspects of the external world (i.e., an external representation, such as a CPG). As discussed previously, mental representations have been expressed symbolically in various forms, including propositions, production rules, schemas, and mental images (Zhang and Norman, 1994). In the field of comprehension, however, it has been found that propositions are an empirically adequate representational form for investigating text understanding.

In the cognitive processing of written discourse, the reader generates meaning from the text itself by transforming the information in the written text into some semantic form or conceptual message. This interpretation of meaning is "filtered through" the person's prior knowledge about the text message. Understanding, then, may be regarded as a process whereby readers attempt to infer the knowledge structure of a writer through the text, based on what they already know. The reader's own knowledge base is

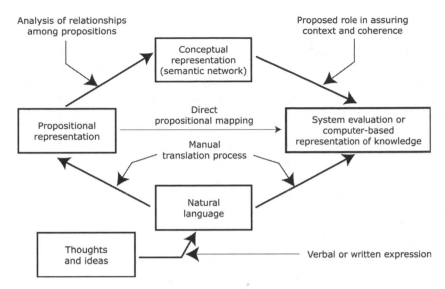

Figure 4.16. An outline of the process of translation from internal representations (mental models) into natural and computer-representable languages. It shows the use of cognitive and semantic methods of analysis (thick arrows) to develop a conceptual model of an individual's knowledge or understanding. The thin arrows show typical pathways for developing computer representations, uninformed by cognitive analysis. This model may be used to guide the computer-based representation of knowledge or the evaluation of a system's adequacy as reflected in a user's mental models during problem solving.

used as a source of "data structures" from which inferences are drawn (Frederiksen, 1975). Thus, the final product of discourse processing consists of what the text "says" and whatever prior knowledge and experiences the users "attach" to the text. In this sense, the reader constructs a cognitive model of the situation described in the text. It is, then, from the interaction between the textbase and the situation model that the conceptual representation emerges (Patel and Arocha, 1995). This representation varies greatly from reader to reader as prior knowledge and experiences differ. Many processes are involved in the interaction between the text and prior knowledge, including linguistic and cognitive strategies as well as attitudes, interests, plans, and goals. Given that interpretation depends on knowledge and that the aim of guidelines is to decrease variation in clinical practice (regardless of a user's background clinical knowledge), analyses of CPGs and the ways in which they are interpreted may be an important addition to the guideline development process (Patel et al., 2001). This can help to identify sources of incorrect inferences (e.g., inferences that are based upon ambiguous text or are affected adversely by inadequate prior knowledge).

The techniques of propositional and semantic analysis that captures the semantics of language can be used to identify ambiguous areas in the text that lead to such misunderstanding (Patel and Groen, 1986). Propositional analysis is a method of semantic analysis developed in cognitive science (Kintsch, 1988), for the representation of linguistic information, which we have used extensively in the domain of biomedicine (Patel et al., 1994). In particular, propositional analysis is a formal method for investigating representation of meaning in memory. Propositions are assumed to reflect units of thought, and their analysis provides a technique for identifying and classifying such units. The usefulness of the notion of propositions is that propositional representations provide ways of explicitly representing ideas and their interrelations. A proposition is an idea underlying a piece of text (whether the text be a phrase, a sentence, or a paragraph), which corresponds to the unit of the mental representation of symbolic information in human memory.

Propositional and semantic analyses provide information on the coherence and comprehensibility of text. Through these analyses, verbal protocols may be examined for the generation of inferences and the directionality of reasoning (i.e., whether from data to hypothesis generation or from hypothesis to data collection). Generation of accurate inferences is very important in discourse comprehension. Subjects' transcribed protocol can be analyzed for inferences when they are asked to read a text and are then asked to recall what they have read. By specifying the propositional structure both of the text and of the subject's "recall" one can determine which parts of the subject's recall are straightforward recapitulations of the text (recall) and which are modifications (inferences). Because a propositional representation is a list, it is difficult to visualize the whole structure of someone's understanding of a text. Hence the next step in the analytical process is creation of a semantic network that provides a picture of the whole conceptual representation at any desired level of detail. Semantic networks are graphs consisting of a non-empty set of nodes and a set of links connecting such nodes (Sowa, 1983, 2000). Nodes may represent clinical findings, hypotheses, or steps in a procedure, whereas links may represent directed connections between nodes. One can think of semantic networks as being complementary to propositional representations, making it possible to visualize the relational structure of the propositions in their totality. Within this structure, propositions that describe attribute information form the nodes of the network (these are the semantic structures), and those that describe relational information form the links (the logical structures). Therefore the nodes define the content of the network, and the links define the structure of the network. Thus, the semantic network conveys two types of information: conceptual (i.e., the concepts used) and structural (i.e., how the concepts relate to one another).

4.6.1 Methods of Cognitive Analysis Using CPG as Illustration

We use a series of examples as illustration of how a cognitive theory and its methods are used in analysis of CPGs. In particular, we investigate clinical decision making as a function of expertise both without and with the use of CPGs, presented in both diagrammatic (algorithms) and textual formats (written guidelines). In the literature on the use of CPGs, there is no mention of expertise as a factor in determining use of guidelines in clinical practice. Cognitive studies have shown that experts solve problems in diagnosis and management based on their practical knowledge of diseases and patients and rarely make use of evidence from purely scientific studies in supporting their decisions. One of the ways that CPGs are being promoted is through the growing reliance on evidence-based medicine. The assumption here is that practitioners will incorporate the latest available evidence and that this information is sufficient for improving practice. The availability of the evidence, however, may not be enough. Indeed, a second factor likely to affect the use of CPGs that is seldom mentioned is the format of guideline presentation. Guidelines are typically presented in text and diagrammatic (algorithm) forms. Text guidelines consist of the description of a procedure together with supporting information for the procedure, usually in the form of scientific evidence from clinical studies. The diagrammatic guidelines are presented as algorithms depicting the procedures to follow and the conditions of applicability of each procedure.

As we have discussed in this chapter, research in cognition has demonstrated that various forms of presentation of information have different effects on cognition, where they serve the purpose of aiding the organization of problem-solving activity (Koedinger and Anderson, 1992) and facilitate the making of inferences (Larkin and Simon, 1987). As discussed previously, in domains such as medicine, the representation effect can have a profound influence on decisions. The same data presented in two distinct formats (e.g., different diagrammatic representations) may lead to different decisions (Cole and Stewart, 1994; Elting, Martin, Cantor, and Rubenstein, 1999). This underscores the need to investigate how the different modalities of information presentation affect the interpretation and use of CPGs. Like most guidelines, these are directed at primary care physicians (PCPs), who are usually the first and frequently the principal medical contact points for patients. Theoretically, diagrammatic representations of a CPG could organize all the relevant information into a manageable form, and therefore, would aid in decision making. We investigated the impact of (1) text-based and (2) algorithm-based practice guidelines on performance of specialists and PCPs during clinical decision making. Data were collected using clinical scenarios and a think-aloud paradigm, both with (primed) and without (spontaneous) the use of the guidelines. The two guidelines used in the study were management of diabetes and screening for thyroid disease. The results showed that both experts and nonexperts used guidelines as reminders during the problem-solving process, and that nonexperts used guidelines during the learning process as an aid to knowledge reorganization. These results were obtained irrespective of whether the guideline was algorithm- or text-based. The subjects of the study expressed their desire to use guidelines that provide faster access to pertinent information. While algorithms (flowcharts) can be read faster, they are often too rigid and not as complete as the text-based guidelines. Figure 4.17 gives the total number of tests as a function of expertise for both spontaneous and primed problem-solving situations with CPGs. Without the guideline, PCPs requested more information about the patient than did the experts. Many of the PCPs'questions were not directly relevant to thyroid dysfunction (e.g., questions about depression or divorce). In addition, PCPs asked for a greater number of tests than did endocrinologists. Of these tests, only 45 percent were specific to thyroid dysfunction. Experts asked for fewer tests, most of which were specific to thyroid dysfunction. Guidelines helped the PCPs in separating relevant information from irrelevant ones, thus constraining their search space. This process-oriented analysis was instrumental in elucidating differences in performance between experts and general practitioners in the use of guidelines. These results provided insight into how guidelines can be fine-tuned for different users and purposes.

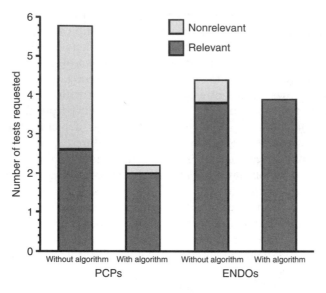

Figure 4.17. Total number of tests requested that are relevant and nonrelevant to thyroid disease as a function of expertise during spontaneous problem solving (without the help of any diagrammatic guideline) and during primed problem solving (when diagrammatic guideline support was added) by primary care physicians (PCPs) and endocrinologists (ENDOs).

These empirical results, coupled with design principles from cognitive science, formed an essential part of the evolutionary development process of GLIF3 (a guideline encoding language) and improved the validity, usability, and comprehension of the resulting knowledge representations.

The current research relates to the Guideline Interchange Format (GLIF), a representational language developed by the InterMed Collaboratory (Ohno-Machado et al., 1998). The principle mandate of the InterMed Collaboratory was to develop a sharable computer-interpretable guideline representation format (GLIF), and shared infrastructural software, tools, and system components that will facilitate and support the development of diverse, institution-specific applications (Friedman and Wyatt, 1997b; Ohno-Machado et al., 1998). Specifically, GLIF allows for a formal specification of medical concepts and data, decision and eligibility criteria, and medical actions. This will enable structuring the mapping of terms used in guideline encoding into the codes used by different institutional CPRs, thus facilitating the sharability of encoded guidelines.

For GLIF-encoded guidelines to be implemented successfully in different institutions, the information contained in the guidelines must be encoded in a manner that ensures representational flexibility and interpreted in accordance with its intended meaning. If the shared information encoded in guidelines is represented in a manner such that it is too general or specific, the guidelines may not be useful in a given context. Furthermore, the users of guidelines may interpret them at different levels of abstraction, leading to different representations. GLIF-encoded guidelines will be interpreted differently depending on the level of expertise of the user, where the guidelines must be flexible enough to accommodate such differences. Thus, the encoding of guidelines in GLIF involves a fine balance between the flexibility of the guideline, so that it may be used for a wide variety of purposes in a wide variety of settings, and the inclusion of details necessary for informational and computational equivalence. In one of our studies, we compare the original GLIF2 with the updated version GLIF3. Differing in both content and structure, the representations developed in GLIF3 were found to contain a greater level of representational detail and less ambiguity than those developed in GLIF2. GLIF3 was found to be more robust than GLIF2 for representing content and logical structure of the clinical guidelines studied. The nature of problems identified was different in the two guidelines studied: one designed for the pharmacological treatment of depression (Snow et al. 2000) and another used in the screening for thyroid disease (Helfand and Redfern, 1998). During the encoding of the thyroid guideline, the subject experienced problems due to lack of information, and lack of clarity where information that is required is specified using vague or ambiguous statements in the original guideline. During the encoding of the depression guideline, the subject experienced one problem due to lack of clarity. Thus, the problems related to the original guidelines that the subject experienced were mostly due to a lack of information in the guidelines that did not allow information to be specified in as much detail as needed. For example, this included the need for knowing exact values from the materials for encoding normal ranges for FT4 tests in the thyroid guideline.

When the guidelines are not used effectively by practitioners, one cannot exclude several possible sources of the problem. We typically try to use post hoc "trouble-shooting" techniques to figure out the source of errors or nonacceptance, which provides some measure of insight into the problem. However, given that there are complex processes involved, it is very difficult to be precise about the nature of the problem in "after the fact" analyses. In addition, such analyses are subject to hindsight bias. We have proposed a formative, proactive analysis of the processes in guideline development and use—one that is based on theories from cognition and comprehension. Detailed analyses of the description of the CPG development process can also help us to contextualize and interpret the errors that arise during use. The identification and categorization of the errors can be used to inform the guideline development cycle. Such feedback of information can allow designers either to improve the clarity and accuracy of the information to be delivered or to tailor it to the characteristics of specific users. This cognitive approach gives us a methodological tool that allows us to compare how the meaning intended by the guideline designer is interpreted and understood by the users. Furthermore, we can identify points of misunderstanding and errors that can have consequences for the appropriate implementation of CPGs.

4.7 Conclusion

Theories and methods from the cognitive sciences can shed light on a range of issues pertaining to the design and implementation of health information technologies. They can also serve an instrumental role in understanding and enhancing the performance of clinicians and patients as they engage in a range of cognitive tasks pertaining to matters of health. In our view, the potential scope of applied cognitive research in biomedical informatics is very broad. Significant inroads have been made in areas such as EHRs and CPGs. However, there are promising areas of future cognitive research that remain largely uncharted. These include understanding how various visual representations or graphical forms mediate reasoning in bioinformatics and developing ways to bridge the digital divide to facilitate health information seeking in disadvantaged patient populations. These are only a few of the cognitive challenges related to harnessing the potential of cutting-edge technologies in order to improve health care.

Suggested Readings

Bechtel W., Graham G., Balota D.A. (1998). A companion to cognitive science. Malden, MA: Blackwell.
This edited volume provides a comprehensive introduction to cognitive science. The volume is divided into short and comprehensible chapters.

Carroll J.M. (2003). HCI Models, Theories, and Frameworks: Toward a Multidisciplinary Science. San Francisco, CA: Morgan Kaufmann.
An up-to-date edited volume on recent cognitive approaches to HCI.

Evans D.A., Patel V.L. (1989). Cognitive Science in Medicine. Cambridge, MA: MIT Press.
The first (and only) book devoted to cognitive issues in medicine. This multidisciplinary volume contains chapters by many of the leading figures in the field.

Gardner H. (1985). The Mind's New Science: A History of the Cognitive Revolution. New York: Basic Books.
A historical introduction to cognitive science that is very well written and engaging. The chapters cover developments in the emergence of the field as well as developments in each of the sub-disciplines such as psychology, linguistics, and neuroscience.

Norman D.A. (1993). Things That Make Us Smart: Defending Human Attributes in the Age of the Machine. Reading, MA: Addison-Wesley.
This book addresses significant issues in human–computer interaction in a very readable and entertaining fashion.

Patel V.L., Kaufman D.R., Arocha J.F. (2000). Conceptual change in the biomedical and health sciences domain. In R. Glaser (Ed.), Advances in Instructional Psychology: Educational Design and Cognitive Science (5th ed., Vol.5, pp.329–392, xvi+404pp.). Mahwah, NJ, US: Lawrence Erlbaum.
This chapter provides a detailed discussion of theories, methods, and research findings as they pertain to conceptual knowledge in the biomedical and health sciences.

Patel V.L., Kaufman D.R., Arocha J.F. (2002). Emerging paradigms of cognition in medical decision-making. Journal of Biomedical Informatics, 35, 52–75.
This relatively recent article summarizes new directions in decision-making research. The authors articulate a need for alternative paradigms for the study of medical decision-making.

Questions for Discussion

1. What are some of the assumptions of the distributed cognition framework? What implications does this approach have for the evaluation of electronic medical record systems?
2. Explain the difference between the *effects of technology* and the *effects with technology*. How can each of these effects contribute to improving patient safety and reducing medical errors?

3. Explain the significance of the representational effect. What considerations need to be taken into account in developing representations for different populations of users and for different tasks?

4. The use of electronic medical records (EMR) has been shown to differentially affect clinical reasoning relative to paper charts. Briefly characterize the effects they have on reasoning, including those that persist after the clinician ceases to use the system. Speculate about the potential impact of EMRs on patient care.

5. A large urban hospital is planning to implement a provider order entry system. You have been asked to advise them on system usability and to study the cognitive effects of the system on performance. Discuss the issues involved and suggests some of the steps you would take to study system usability.

6. What steps are involved in the process of translating internal representations (mental models) into natural and computer-representable languages and expressing them in a guideline format?

7. The development of expertise has been characterized as a "non-monotonic" process. Explain the nature of this development process using some of the findings in relation to a) diagnostic reasoning and b) memory for clinical information.

5
Essential Concepts for Biomedical Computing

GIO WIEDERHOLD AND THOMAS C. RINDFLEISCH

After reading this chapter, you should know the answers to these questions:

- How are medical data stored and manipulated in a computer?
- Why does a computer system have both memory and storage?
- How can data be entered into a computer accurately and efficiently?
- How can information be displayed clearly?
- What are the functions of a computer's operating system?
- What advantages does using a database management system provide over storing and manipulating your own data directly?
- How do local area networks facilitate data sharing and communication within health care institutions?
- How can the confidentiality of data stored in distributed computer systems be protected?
- How is the Internet used for medical applications?

5.1 Computer Architectures

Health professionals encounter computers in many settings. In more and more hospitals, physicians and nurses can order drugs and laboratory tests, review test results, and record medical observations using a hospital information system. Most hospitals and outpatient clinics have computers to help them manage financial and administrative information. Many physicians in private practice have purchased personal computers to allow them to access and search the medical literature, to communicate with colleagues, and to help their office staff with tasks such as billing and word processing. Nearly every one reads and writes e-mails, and surfs the Net for information or purchases.

Computers differ in speed, storage capacity, and cost; in the number of users that they can support; in the ways that they are interconnected; and in the types of application programs that they can run. On the surface, the differences among computers can be bewildering, and, as we discuss in Chapter 6, the selection of appropriate software and hardware is crucial to the success of a computer system. Despite these differences, however, most computers use the same basic mechanisms to store and process information and to communicate with the outside world. At the conceptual level, the similarities among machines greatly outweigh the differences. In this chapter, we discuss the fundamental concepts related to computer hardware and software, including data acquisition, security, and communications relevant to medical computing. We assume that you have already used some type of personal computer (PC) but have not been concerned with its internal workings. Our aim is to give you the background necessary for understanding the technical aspects of the applications discussed in later chapters. If you already have an understanding of how computers work, you may want to skim this chapter.

5.1.1 Hardware

Early computers were expensive to purchase and operate. Only large institutions could afford to acquire a computer and to develop its software. In the 1960s, the development of integrated circuits (ICs) on silicon chips resulted in dramatic increases in computing power per dollar. Since that time, computer hardware has become smaller, faster, and more reliable. Every year more powerful computers have cost less than less capable models from the year before. At the same time, standard software packages have been developed that remove much of the burden of routine operations and writing the infrastructure of applications. The result is that computers are ubiquitous today.

General-purpose computers are classified into three types: servers, workstations, and personal computers (PCs). This distinction reflects several parameters but primarily relates to style of usage:

1. **Servers** are computers that share their resources with other computers and support the activities of many users simultaneously within an enterprise (e.g., admissions staff, pharmacy, and billing). Major servers are midsized or larger **mainframe** computers that are operated and maintained by professional computing personnel. A single mainframe might handle the information-processing needs of a large hospital or at least handle the large, shared databases and the data-processing tasks for activities such as billing and report generation. Smaller servers may exist in a laboratory or a group practice to carry out information-processing tasks similar to those run on mainframes. Such servers may be maintained by staff within that unit.
2. **Personal computers** are at the other end of the spectrum: they are relatively inexpensive single-user machines. They help users with tasks such as preparing letters and documents, creating graphics for oral presentations, and keeping track of expenses and income. They also provide access to services on the Internet—e.g., sending and receiving e-mails, searching for and displaying information, and collaborating with colleagues. The information stored on PCs is most often regarded as private and usually is not accessed by more than one user. PCs may take the form of desktop machines, portable laptop machines, tablets, or handheld machines.
3. **Workstations** are machines of moderate size and cost. Most have more processing capacity than PCs, so they can perform more demanding computing tasks, such as image processing or system modeling and simulation. They are characterized by having only a small number of users (typically only one) at any given time, by interacting effectively with servers, by integrating information from diverse sources, and by responding to requests from other workstations. Multiple workstations in an enterprise may be connected into a network that makes integrated services available.

The boundaries between these categories of computers are not sharp. PCs are often powerful enough to function as workstations, and large workstations can be configured to act as servers. All types of computers can also be equipped for special tasks, such as the patient-monitoring tasks discussed in Chapter 17 and the three-dimensional modeling of anatomical regions discussed in Chapter 18. In these roles, the computers may be workstations for the specialists or servers for the larger community. Computers (e.g., handheld devices or PCs) that are not used for processing, but only for accessing servers and workstations are referred to as **terminals**.

Most modern computers have similar organizations and basic **hardware** (physical equipment) structures. The most common **computer architectures** follow the principles expressed by John von Neuman in 1945. Figure 5.1 illustrates the configuration of a simple **von Neuman machine** in which the computer is composed of one or more

- **Central processing units (CPUs)** that perform computation
- **Computer memories** that store programs and data that are being used actively by a CPU
- **Storage devices**, such as **magnetic disks** and tapes, and **optical disks**, that provide long-term storage for programs and data
- **Input** and **output** devices, such as keyboards, pointing devices, video displays, and laser printers, that facilitate user interactions
- **Communication** equipment, such as modems and network interfaces, that connect computers to each other and to broader networks of computers
- **Data buses** that are electrical pathways that transport encoded information between these subsystems

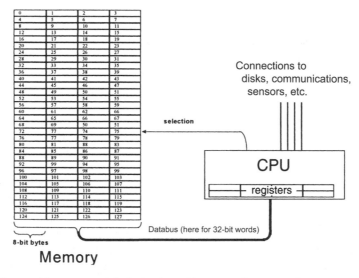

Figure 5.1. The von Neuman model: the basic architecture of most modern computers. The computer comprises a single central processing unit (CPU), an area for memory, and a data bus for transferring data between the two.

Machines designed with other than von Neuman architectures are possible but remain relatively uncommon. PCs and workstations typically have only one CPU. In more sophisticated machines, when more processing power is required to solve complex problems, multiple CPUs and memories may be interconnected to support **parallel processing**. The challenge then is for the software to distribute the computation across these units to gain a proportionate benefit.

Central Processing Unit

Although complete computer systems appear to be complex, the underlying principles are simple. A prime example is a processing unit itself. Here simple components can be carefully combined to create systems with impressive capabilities. The structuring principle is that of *hierarchical organization*: primitive units (electronic switches) are combined to form basic units that can store letters and numbers, add digits, and compare values with one another. The basic units are assembled into **registers** capable of storing and manipulating text and large numbers. These registers in turn are assembled into the larger functional units that make up the central component of a computer: the CPU. Physically a CPU may be a single chip or may be composed of a number of chips placed onto a circuit board. Some high-performance computers use chips that contain multiple CPUs.

The logical atomic element for all digital computers is the *binary digit* or **bit**. Each bit can assume one of two values: 0 or 1. An electronic switch that can be set to either of two states stores a single bit value. (Think of a light switch that can be either on or off.) These primitive units are the building blocks of computer systems. Sequences of bits (implemented as sequences of switches) are used to represent larger numbers and other kinds of information. For example, four switches can store 2^4, or 16, values. Because each unit can have a value of either 0 or 1, there are 16 combinations of 4-bit values: 0000, 0001, 0010, 0011, 0100, 0101, 0110, and so on, up to 1111. Thus, 4 bits can represent any decimal value from 0 to 15; e.g., the sequence 0101 is the **binary** (base 2) representation of the decimal number 5—namely, $0 \times 2^3 + 1 \times 2^2 + 0 \times 2^1 + 1 \times 2^0 = 5$. A byte is a sequence of 8 bits; it can take on 2^8 or 256 values.

Groups of bits and bytes can represent not only decimal integers but also fractional numbers, general characters (upper-case and lower-case letters, digits, and punctuation marks), instructions to the CPU, and more complex data types such as pictures, spoken language, and the content of a medical record. Figure 5.2 shows the **American Standard Code for Information Interchange (ASCII)**, a convention for representing 95 common characters using 7 bits. These 7 bits are commonly placed into an 8-bit unit, a byte, which is the common way of transmitting and storing these characters. The eighth bit may be used for formatting information (as in a word processor) or for additional special characters (such as currency and mathematical symbols or characters with diacritic marks), but its use is not covered by the ASCII base standard. Not all characters seen on a keyboard can be encoded and stored as ASCII. The Delete and Arrow keys are often dedicated to edit functions, and the Control, Escape, Function, and Alt keys are used to modify other keys or to interact directly with programs. For foreign languages a standard called **Unicode** represents characters needed for other languages using 16 bits; ASCII is a small subset of Unicode.

Character	Binary code	Character	Binary code	Character	Binary code
blank	010 0000	@	100 0000	`	110 0000
!	010 0001	A	100 0001	a	110 0001
"	010 0010	B	100 0010	b	110 0010
#	010 0011	C	100 0011	c	110 0011
$	010 0100	D	100 0100	d	110 0100
%	010 0101	E	100 0101	e	110 0101
&	010 0110	F	100 0110	f	110 0110
'	010 0111	G	100 0111	g	110 0111
(	010 1000	H	100 1000	h	110 1000
)	010 1001	I	100 1001	i	110 1001
*	010 1010	J	100 1010	j	110 1010
+	010 1011	K	100 1011	k	110 1011
,	010 1100	L	100 1100	l	110 1100
-	010 1101	M	100 1101	m	110 1101
.	010 1110	N	100 1110	n	110 1110
/	010 1111	O	100 1111	o	110 1111
0	011 0000	P	101 0000	p	111 0000
1	011 0001	Q	101 0001	q	111 0001
2	011 0010	R	101 0010	r	111 0010
3	011 0011	S	101 0011	s	111 0011
4	011 0100	T	101 0100	t	111 0100
5	011 0101	U	101 0101	u	111 0101
6	011 0110	V	101 0110	v	111 0110
7	011 0111	W	101 0111	w	111 0111
8	011 1000	X	101 1000	x	111 1000
9	011 1001	Y	101 1001	y	111 1001
:	011 1010	Z	101 1010	z	111 1010
;	011 1011	[	101 1011	{	111 1011
<	011 1100	\	101 1100	|	111 1100
=	011 1101	]	101 1101	}	111 1101
>	011 1110	^	101 1110	~	111 1110
?	011 1111	–	101 1111	null	111 1111

Figure 5.2. The American Standard Code for Information Interchange (ASCII) is a standard scheme for representing alphanumeric characters using 7 bits. The upper-case and lower-case alphabet, the decimal digits, and common punctuation characters are shown here with their ASCII representations.

The CPU works on data that it retrieves from memory, placing them in working registers. By manipulating the contents of its registers, the CPU performs the mathematical and logical functions that are basic to information processing: addition, subtraction, and comparison ("is greater than," "is equal to," "is less than"). In addition to registers that perform computation, the CPU also has registers that it uses to store instructions—a computer program is a set of such instructions—and to control processing. In essence, a computer is an instruction follower: it fetches an instruction from memory and then executes the instruction, which usually is an operation that requires the retrieval, manipulation, and storage of data into memory or registers. The processor performs a simple loop, fetching and executing each instruction of a program in sequence. Some instructions can direct the processor to begin fetching instructions from a different place in memory or point in the program. Such a transfer of control provides flexibility in program execution.

Memory

The computer's working memory stores the programs and data currently being used by the CPU. Working memory has two parts: **read-only memory (ROM)** and **random-access memory (RAM)**.

ROM, or fixed memory, is permanent and unchanging. It can be read, but it cannot be altered or erased. It is used to store a few crucial programs that do not change and that must be available at all times. One such predefined program is the **bootstrap** sequence, a set of initial instructions that is executed each time the computer is started. ROM also is used to store programs that must run quickly—e.g., the graphics programs that run the Macintosh interface.

More familiar to computer users is RAM, often just called **memory**. RAM can be both read and written into. It is used to store the programs, control values, and data that are in current use. It also holds the intermediate results of computations and the images to be displayed on the screen. RAM is much larger than ROM. Its size is one of the primary parameters used to describe a computer. For example, we might speak of a 256-**megabyte** PC. A megabyte is 2^{20} or 1,048,576 bytes. (A **kilobyte** is 2^{10} or 1024 bytes, and a **gigabyte** is 2^{30} or 1,073,741,824 bytes.) A 256-megabyte memory can store 268,445,456 bytes of information, but thinking of "mega" as meaning a "million" (decimal) is adequate in practice.

A sequence of bits that can be accessed by the CPU as a unit is called a **word**. The **word size** is a function of the computer's design; it typically is an even number of bytes. Early PCs had word sizes of 8 or 16 bits; newer, faster computers have 32-bit or 64-bit word sizes that allow processing of larger chunks of information at a time. The bytes of memory are numbered in sequence—say from 0 to 268,445,455 for a 256-megabyte computer. The CPU accesses each word in memory by specifying the sequence number, or address, of its starting byte.

The computer's memory is relatively expensive, being specialized for fast read–write access; therefore, it is limited in size. It is also **volatile**: its contents are changed when the next program runs, and memory contents are not retained when power is turned off. For many medical applications we need to store more information than can be held in memory, and we want to save all that information for a long time. To save valuable programs, data, or results we place them into long-term storage.

Long-Term Storage

Programs and data that must persist over long periods are stored on storage devices, often magnetic disks, which provide peristent storage for less cost per unit than memory. The needed information is loaded from such storage into working memory whenever it is used. Conceptually, storage can be divided into two types: (1) **active storage** is used to store data that have long-term validity and that may need to be retrieved with little delay (in a few seconds or less), e.g., the medical record of a patient who currently is being treated within the hospital; and (2) **archival storage** is used to store data for documentary or legal purposes, e.g., the medical record of a patient who has been discharged.

Computer storage also provides a basis for the sharing of information. Whereas memory is dedicated to an executing program, data written on storage in file systems or in **databases** is available to other users who can access the computer's storage devices. Files and databases complement direct communication among computer users and have the advantage that the writers and readers need not be present at the same time in order to share information.

Magnetic disks are the most common medium for active storage. A disk storage unit, like the one shown in Figure 5.3, consists of one or more disks (either fixed or removable), a drive system to rotate the disk, moveable read–write heads to access the data, a mechanism to position the read–write head over the disk's surface, and associated electronics. Several disks may be stacked in a disk drive, and typically both surfaces of a disk can be written on. The read–write heads are mounted on arms so that they can access most of the surface. Each magnetic disk is a round, flat plate of magnetizable material. The disk spins beneath its read–write head; as it spins, data can be copied from or to the disk surface by the read–write head. Writing places a sequence of magnetized

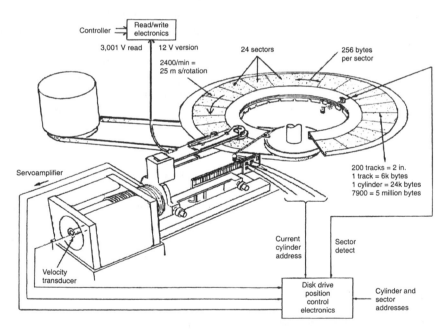

Figure 5.3. A typical magnetic disk drive. Drive parameters—such as number of tracks, data density along the tracks, rotation speed, and seek time across tracks—improve continually with technology advances. (*Source*: Drawing courtesy of Hewlett-Packard.)

domains on the disk's surface along circular tracks. Reading detects the presence or absence of magnetization along those tracks.

Retrieval of data from magnetic disks is relatively slow and has not improved as much as other aspects of storage, such as cost and capacity. Whereas the CPU can quickly access any data element in RAM by addressing the memory location directly, it must access externally stored data in two time-consuming steps. First, it must mechanically position the read–write head over the track that stores the data. Second, it must search through that track sequentially, following the track as the disk rotates. Once the read–write head has been positioned correctly, blocks of data can be transferred rapidly. Whereas data in memory can be accessed in microseconds or less, access times for data stored on disk are typically on the order of 0.1 second.

The disks themselves can be either **hard disks** or **floppy disks**. Floppy disks can be removed from their drive units and are inexpensive relative to hard disks. They are useful for local archiving of data and for shipping of data through the mail. Floppy disks may hold one megabyte or more. Hard disks are typically fixed in the units and often hold 1 or more gigabytes.

When data or programs have to be moved from one computer to another, newer kinds of portable or removable storage devices are handy. Common types are **memory sticks** or **flash cards**. Such technology is popular because of its use in digital cameras, and it is also used in many other applications like cell phones, electronic voting machines, and deep-space-imaging missions. At least four different standards are in use: Flash cards (about 8×5 cm), CompactFlash cards (about 3.5×4 cm), SD cards (about 2.25×4 cm), and memory sticks (about 2×5 cm). Economical readers and adaptors for such devices connect to the Universal Serial Bus (USB) ports available on desktops and laptops, so that one can accommodate the variety of formats with a modest amount of effort. Flash memory devices are available economically that hold more than 1 gigabyte of data.

A common medium for archival storage is **magnetic tape**, which is a ribbon of plastic covered with magnetizable material. Like the disk drive, a tape drive has a read–write head that places or detects magnetized domains along the tracks of the tape. Magnetic tape is still the least expensive medium for storing information, but retrieval of data archived on tape is slow. An operator (either human or robotic) must locate the tape and physically mount it on a tape drive—a procedure that can take minutes or hours. The tape then must be scanned linearly from the beginning until the information of interest is located.

A wide variety of tape formats exist. Early tapes were mounted on reels. Tape cartridges that hold tens of gigabytes of data fit in the palm of your hand. Archiving data on tape has the risk that the contents may become corrupted over the years unless they are refreshed regularly. Also, older tape formats may become obsolete, and the devices needed for retrieval from those formats may disappear. Converting large archives to newer formats is a major undertaking.

Optical disk storage (in the forms of **compact disks (CDs)**, or **digital versatile disks** or **digital video disks (DVDs)**) is one of the most convenient means for long-term storage. A large quantity of data can be stored on each optical disk—currently somewhat under 1 gigabyte per CD and up to 17 gigabytes for two-sided DVDs. The short wavelength of light permits a much higher density of data-carrying spots on the surface than magnetic techniques. A semiconductor laser reads data by detecting reflections from the disk; data are written by the laser, which is set at a higher intensity to alter the reflectivity. **Compact disk read-only memory (CD-ROM)** is used for prerecorded information, such as large programs to be distributed and for distributing full-text literature, storing permanent medical records, and archiving digitized X-ray images (see Chapter 18). DVD technology, similar to CDs but with yet higher densities, provides about 25 times more capacity per disk and is taking over where data requirements are massive, as for storage of images, speech, and video.

Hardware for writing onto CDs and DVDs is now available at commodity prices. CD writing capability is routinely delivered with new PCs. Such systems can record data once but allow reading of those data as often as desired. Such a disk is called a CD-R. Rewritable CDs (CD-RWS) are also available. Their slow access time and slow writing speed limit their use mainly to archiving. A major obstacle to overcome is the lack of a fast and economical means for indexing and searching the huge amount of information that can be stored. Similar options exist for DVDs, although the industry is still grappling with differences in recording and data organization standards. The choices of storage devices and media have major effects on the performance and cost of a computer system. Data that are needed rapidly must be kept in more expensive active storage—typically hard disks. Less time-critical data can be archived on less expensive media, which have longer access times. Because data are often shared, the designer must also consider who will want to read the data and how the data will be read. People can share by copying the data and physically transporting the copy to a destination with a compatible drive unit. Floppy disks, FLASH cards, CDs, or DVDs are all convenient for transport. An alternative to physical transport is remote access to persistent storage by means of communication networks; the practice of sending files using file transfer programs or as attachments to e-mail messages is often more convenient than physical exchanges of files. Compatibility of storage devices becomes less important, but the capabilities of the communication networks and their protocols are crucial (see later discussion on Internet communication).

Input Devices

Data and user-command entry remain the most costly and awkward aspects of medical data processing. Certain data can be acquired automatically; e.g., many laboratory instruments provide electronic signals that can be transmitted to computers directly, and many diagnostic radiology instruments produce output in digital form. Furthermore, redundant data entry can be minimized if data are shared among computers over networks or across direct interfaces. For example, if a clinic's computer can acquire data from a laboratory computer directly, clinic personnel will not have to reenter into the computer-based medical record the information displayed on printed reports of laboratory test results. Many types of data are, however, still entered into the medical record manually by data entry clerks or by other health care personnel. The most common instrument for data entry is the typewriter-style **keyboard** associated with a **video display terminal (VDT)**. As an operator types characters on the keyboard, they are sent to the computer and are echoed back for viewing on the **display monitor**. A **cursor** indicates the current position on the screen. Most programs allow the cursor to be moved with a **pointing device**, often a **mouse**, so that making insertions and corrections is convenient. Although most clerical personnel are comfortable with this mode of data entry, some health professionals lack typing skills and are not motivated to learn them. Thus, systems developers have experimented with a variety of alternative input devices that minimize or eliminate the need to type.

With the pointer, a user can *select* an item displayed on the screen by moving the cursor on the screen and then clicking on a button. With a **touch screen**, a user can select items simply by touching the screen—when the user's finger or a stylus touches the screen, it identifies a position in the grid that crosses the screen, indicating the item of interest. Alternatively, a **light pen**, a **track ball**, or a **joystick** can be used to point to the screen, but these devices are mainly used in specialized settings. There are also three-dimensional pointing devices, where the indicator is held in front of the screen, and a three-dimensional display provides feedback to the user. Some three-dimensional pointing devices used in medical training virtual-reality environments also provide computer-controlled force or **tactile feedback**, so that a user can experience the resistance, for example, of a simulated needle being inserted for venupuncture or a simulated scalpel making a surgical incision.

Often, pointers are used in conjunction with **menus**, listing items that users can select among (Figure 5.4). Thus, users can select data simply by clicking on relevant items rather than by typing characters. By listing or highlighting only valid options, menus also facilitate coding and can enforce the use of a standardized vocabulary. To deal with a large number of choices, menus are arranged hierarchically; e.g., to order a treatment, a physician might first select *drug order* from a menu of alternative actions, then the appropriate *drug class* from a submenu, and finally an individual drug from the next submenu. If there are still many alternatives, the drug list might be partitioned further; e.g., the drugs might be grouped alphabetically by name. Menu selection is efficient; an experienced user can select several screens per second. Typing a drug name is more time consuming and carries the risk of misspelling. Menu design is still an art. An excess of displayed choices slows down the user—displaying more than seven entries demands careful reading. Also, if the system designer's concepts do not match those of the user, the latter can get lost in the hierarchy and be frustrated. Finally, there is evidence that users who use a mouse for extensive periods may be subject to repetitive-stress wrist injury, especially when keyboards and pointers are placed on conventional desks or tables, rather than at elbow height.

Graphical output can be used to create interesting and attractive interfaces to programs. For example, the input screens of the ONCOCIN system, intended to provide physicians with advice on cancer treatment protocols, look just like the paper flowcharts that physicians have used for years. Physicians enter patient data into the database directly by using a mouse to select values from menus (Figure 5.5). In addition, graphics open the door for intuitive data entry—e.g., the use of images to record information and the use of **icons** to specify commands. Physicians can use images to indicate the location of an injury, the size of a tumor, the area to be covered by radiation therapy, and so on (Figure 5.6). Because of the imprecision of medical language, a graphical indication of the affected body parts can be a valuable supplement to coded or textual

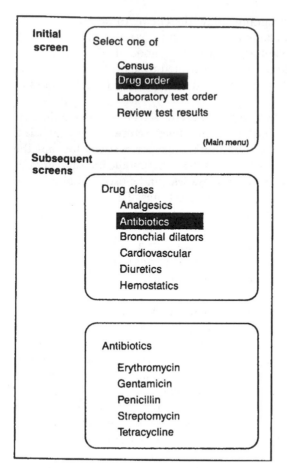

Figure 5.4. Initial and subsequent screens of a menu-driven order-entry system. The highlighted entry indicates which item was selected (with a mouse, light pen, or finger) to display the subsequent screen.

descriptions. Graphical interfaces and flowsheets are now commonplace in commercial clinical information systems, and image libraries are being incorporated to support the documentation process.

Using icons for selection again requires designing the interface carefully. Icons must be distinctive and intuitive. Having hundreds of icons on a screen is not helpful, and having many similar icons is even less so. Icons are often labeled with brief texts and may also show longer explanations that appear on the screen when the cursor is held over them. Techniques suitable for occasional users are typically inefficient for frequent users, but users often move from familiar tasks to unfamiliar ones and vice versa, and switching modes explicitly is awkward.

Much medical information is available as narrative text—e.g., physician-transcribed visit notes, hospital discharge summaries, and the medical literature. **Text-scanning devices** can scan lines or entire pages of typeset text and convert each character into its ASCII code by a process known as optical character recognition (OCR). These devices reduce the need to retype information that previously was typed, but they can only less

Lymphoma Flow Sheet										326
Mass / X-ray										
Disease Activity										

Hematology									
WBC x 1000	8.6	9.0	1.5	4.2	9.0	3.6	5.6	3.3	?
% polys	71	93	29						
% lymphs			43						
PCV	29.6	32.9	33.7	33.6	30.9	31.6	28.4	29.3	
Hemoglobin	10.1	11.1	11.3	11.6	10.4	10.5	9.4	9.9	?
Platelets x 1000	562	511	516	592	436	255	500	345	?
Sed. Rate	100								
% total granulocytes	75	93	39	82.6	83.4	90.3	80.3	70.1	?
Granulocytes	6.45		.585		7.506		4.4968		

Chemotherapy	
Radiotherapy	
Symptom Review	
Toxicity	?
Physical Examination	
Chemistry	?
To order: Labs and Procedures	
To order: Nuclear Medicine and Tomography	
Scheduling	

Time	Day	28	03	10	17	24	30	7	14	21
	Month	May	Jun	Jun	Jun	Jun	Jun	Jul	Jul	Jul
	Year	87	87	87	87	87	87	87	87	87

Numerical menu: 7 8 9 erase / 4 5 6 n/a / 1 2 3 clear / 0 abort / done

Figure 5.5. The data-entry screen of the ONCOCIN consultation system. The screen is a computer-based representation of the familiar paper flowchart on which physicians normally record information regarding their cancer patients. The physician can enter the platelet count into the database by selecting digits from the numerical menu displayed in the upper right corner of the figure. Only the hematology section of the flowchart currently is visible. The physician can view data on disease activity, chemotherapies, and so on by selecting from the alternative section headings. (*Source*: Courtesy of Stanford Medical Informatics, Stanford University.)

Figure 5.6. Images can be used to provide an alternate means of entering data. Rather than describing the location of a tumor in words, a physician using the ONCOCIN consultation system can indicate the location of a lesion by selecting regions on a torso. In this figure, the physician has indicated involvement of the patient's liver. (*Source*: Courtesy of Stanford Medical Informatics, Stanford University.)

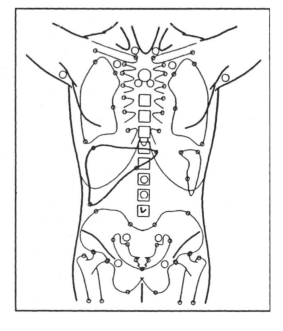

reliably capture handwritten information. Even with typed material, scanners often have error rates of several percent, so the scanned material must be reviewed carefully if it is important. Having to make corrections greatly reduces the benefits of automatic scanning.

Most physicians are comfortable dictating their notes; therefore, researchers have investigated the possibility of using voice input for data entry. The simplest method for capturing voice data is to record messages directly from a microphone. The voice signal then is encoded in digital form (see Section 5.2), identified as a voice message, and stored and transmitted with the other computer data. When the data are retrieved, the message is simply played back through a speaker. Search and indexing are, however, not enabled in that case. With automatic speech recognition, the digitized voice signals are matched to the patterns of a vocabulary of known words, and in some cases using grammar rules to allow recognition of more general legal sentence structures. The speech input is then stored as ASCII-coded text. Currently, systems exist that can interpret sequences of discrete words, and there are successful systems that can recognize continuous speech in which the sounds run together. This technology is improving in flexibility and reliability, but error rates are sufficiently high that review of the resulting text is advisable. Without review the text is still useful for creating indexes for search, but then the source material must be referenced and remain available.

In neither case does the computer truly understand the content of the messages with existing computer technology. This same lack of understanding applies to the processing of most textual data, which are entered, stored, retrieved, and printed without any analysis of their meaning.

Output Devices

The *presentation* of results, or of the **output**, is the complementary step in the processing of medical data. Many systems compute information that is transmitted to health care providers and is displayed immediately on local PCs so that action can be taken. Another large volume of output consists of reports, which are printed or simply are kept available to document the actions taken. Chapter 12 describes various reports and messages that are commonly used to present patient information. Here we describe the devices that are used to convey these outputs.

Most immediate output appears at its destination on a display screen, such as the **cathode-ray tube (CRT)** display or the flat-panel **liquid crystal display (LCD)** of a PC, often in color. Important findings may be highlighted on the screen in boldface type, by an intense color, or by a special icon. PCs include at least rudimentary sound capability, so if results require urgent attention, a sound such as a ringing bell may alert personnel to the data's arrival. More routinely, results are placed in storage and are automatically retrieved when an authorized provider accesses the patient's record.

When entering or reviewing data, users can edit the data displayed on the screen before releasing them for persistent storage. Graphical output is essential for summarizing and presenting the information derived from voluminous data. Most computers have the ability to produce graphical output, but specific health care information systems differ greatly in their capabilities to display trend lines, images, and other graphics.

A graphics screen is divided into a grid of picture elements called **pixels**. One or more bits in memory represent the output for each pixel. In a black-and-white monitor, the value of each pixel on the screen is associated with the level of intensity, or **gray scale**. For example, 2 bits can distinguish 2^2 or 4 display values per pixel: black, white, and two intermediate shades of gray. For color displays, the number of bits per pixel determines the **contrast** and **color resolution** of an image. Three sets of multiple bits are necessary to specify the color of pixels on color graphics monitors, giving the intensity for red, green, and blue components of each pixel color, respectively. For instance, three sets of 2 bits per pixel provide 2^6 or 64 color mixtures. The number of pixels per square inch determines the **spatial resolution** of the image (Figure 5.7). As we discuss in Chapter 18,

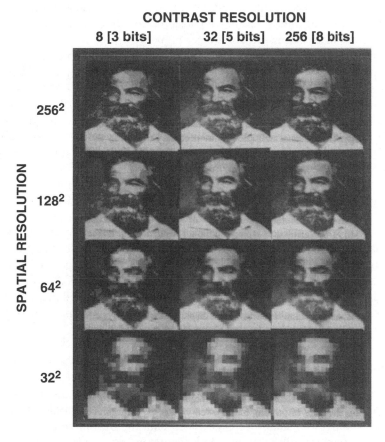

Figure 5.7. Demonstration of how varying the number of pixels and the number of bits per pixel affects the spatial and contract resolution of a digital image. The image in the upper right corner was displayed using a 2563256 array of pixels, 8 bits per pixel; the subject (Walt Whitman) is easily discernible. (*Source*: Reproduced with permission from Price R.R., James A.E. [1982]. Basic principles and i°nstrumentation of digital radiography. In Price R.R., et al. (Eds.), *Digital Radiography: A Focus on Clinical Utility*. Orlando, FL: WB Saunders.)

both parameters determine the requirements for storing images. A display with good spatial resolution requires about 1600×1200 pixels. LCD color projectors are readily available so that the output of a workstation can also be projected onto a screen for group presentations.

Much diagnostic information is produced in image formats that can be shown on graphics terminals. Examples are ultrasound observations, magnetic resonance images (MRIs), computed tomography (CT) scans, etc. High-resolution displays can display digitally encoded X-ray images. Computer processing can add value to such image output, as described in Chapter 18.

For portability and traditional filing, output is *printed* on paper. Printing information is slower than is displaying it on a screen, so printing is best done in advance of need. In a clinic, relevant portions of various patient records may be printed on high-volume printers the night before scheduled visits. For presentations the availability of high-quality LCD projectors has almost entirely replaced use of slides and viewgraphs, allowing rapid production of dynamic presentations.

Laser printers use an electromechanically controlled laser beam to generate an image on a xerographic surface, which is then used to produce paper copies, just as is done in a copier. Laser printers permit the user to select from a variety of fonts and to produce graphics that match closely the look of visual displays. Their resolution is often better than that of displays, allowing up to 600 dots (pixels) per inch (commercial typesetting equipment may have a resolution of several thousand dots per inch). Whenever the resolution of printers and visual terminals differs, output displays should be designed with care to make both forms of output equally acceptable.

Color printing with laser technology is becoming more common, as prices drop. Color **ink-jet printers** are inexpensive and still dominate the market, but the ink cartridges raise the cost under high use. Liquid ink is sprayed on paper by a head that moves back and forth for each line of pixels. Ink-jet printers have lower resolution than laser printers and are relatively slow, especially at high resolution. To avoid blotting of the ink droplets, coated paper is used for output at more than 200 pixels per inch. Because they are inexpensive, color ink-jet printers can be placed close to PCs, and the color can enhance readers' comprehension of clinical results. Ink-jet printers that produce images of photographic quality are also readily available. Here the base colors are merged while being sprayed so that true color mixes are placed on the paper.

Local Data Communications

Information can be shared most effectively by allowing access for all authorized participants whenever and wherever they need it. Transmitting data electronically among applications and computer systems facilitates such sharing by minimizing delays and by supporting interactive collaborations. Videoconferencing is also supported on PCs. Transmitting paper results in a much more passive type of information sharing. As we describe in Chapter 13, data communication and integration are critical functions of health care information systems. Modern computing and communications are deeply intertwined.

Computer systems used in health care are specialized to fulfill the diverse needs of health professionals in various areas, such as physicians' offices, laboratories, pharmacies, intensive care units, and business offices. Even if their hardware is identical, their content will differ, and some of that content must be shared with other applications in the health care organization. Over time, the hardware in the various areas will also diverge—e.g., imaging departments will require more capable displays and larger storage, other areas will use more processor power, and still others will serve more users. Demand for growth and funding to accommodate change occurs at different times. Communication among diverse systems bridges the differences in computing environments.

Communication can occur via telephone lines, dedicated or shared wires, fiber-optic cables, infrared, or radio waves. In each case different communication interfaces must be attached to the computer, different conventions or communication protocols must be obeyed, and a different balance of performance and reliability can be expected.

A traditional method for communicating computer information is to use the existing dial-up telephone system. A sending computer dials a receiving computer, and, when the connection is established, a **modem** (modulator-demodulator) converts the digital data from a computer to analog signals in the voice range. The tones are transmitted over the telephone lines. At the receiver, the tones are reconverted to the original digital form by another modem and are placed into the computer memory. The receiver can return responses to the sender, sending results or requests for more data. Thus, a conversation takes place between computers. When the conversation is complete, the modems disconnect and the telephone line is released.

As technologies improved, modems supported increasing transmission speeds, or **bit rates**. The overall bit rate of a communication link is a combination of the rate at which signals (or symbols) can be transmitted and the efficiency with which digital information (in the form of bits) is encoded in the symbols. Frequently the term **baud** is used to indicate the signal transmission speed—one baud corresponds to one signal per second. At lower speeds, bits were encoded one per signal, so the baud rate and bit rate were similar. At higher speeds, more complex methods are used to encode bits in the channel signals. Thus, a 56,000 bit per second (bps) modem may use a signal rate of only 8,000 baud and an encoding that transmits up to 8 bits per signal. For graphics information, speeds of more than 500,000 bps are desirable.

Digital telephone services are widely available now. **Digital Subscriber Line (DSL)** and the earlier **Integrated Services Digital Network (ISDN)** allow relatively high-speed network communications using conventional telephone wiring (twisted pairs). Currently, they allow sharing of data and voice transmission up to a total rate of 1.5 to 9 **megabits** per second (Mbps), depending on the distance from a local telephone office. Their error rate, and the cost of dealing with errors, is lower as well, because of the use of sophisticated digital encoding. A special modem and interface unit is required, at a cost similar to a capable dial-up modem. The rates charged by the telephone companies for DSL/ISDN lines also differ from those for dial-up lines. In remote areas digital services may be unavailable, but the telephone companies are broadening access to digital services, including over wireless telephone channels. Transmission for rapid distribution of information can occur via cable modems using television cable or direct satellite broadcast. These alternatives have a very high capacity, but that capacity is then shared by all subscribers. Also for both DSL and digital cable services, transmission speeds are often asymmetrical, with relatively low-speed service (typically on the order of 100 kilobits per second) used to communicate back to the data source. This design choice is rationalized by the assumption that most users *receive* more data than they *send*, for example, in downloading and displaying graphics, images, and video, while typing relatively compact commands uplink to make this happen. This assumption breaks down if users generate large data objects on their personal machine that then have to be sent uplink to other users. In this case it may be more cost-effective in terms of user time to purchase a symmetric communication service.

Frame Relay is a network protocol designed for sending digital information over shared, **wide-area networks (WANs)**. It transmits variable-length messages or packets of information efficiently and inexpensively over dedicated lines that may handle aggregate speeds up to 45 Mbps. **Asynchronous Transfer Mode (ATM)** is a protocol designed for sending streams of small, fixed-length cells of information (each 53 bytes long) over very high-speed dedicated connections—most often digital optical circuits. The underlying optical transmission circuit sends cells synchronously and supports multiple ATM circuits. The cells associated with a given ATM circuit are queued and processed asynchronously with respect to each other in gaining access to the multiplexed (optical) transport medium. Because ATM is designed to be implemented by hardware switches, information bit rates over 10 gigabits per second (Gbps) are possible today, and even higher speeds are expected in the future.

For communication needs within an office, a building, or a campus, installation of a **local-area network** (LAN) allows local data communication without involving the telephone company or **network access provider**. Such a network is dedicated to linking multiple computer nodes together at high speeds to facilitate the sharing of resources—data, software, and equipment—among multiple users. Users working at individual workstations can retrieve data and programs from network **file servers**: computers dedicated to storing local files, both shared and private. The users can process information locally and then save the results over the network to the file server or send output to a fast, shared printer.

There are a variety of **protocols** and technologies for implementing LANs, although the differences should not be apparent to the user. Typically data are transmitted as messages or **packets** of data; each packet contains the data to be sent, the network addresses of the sending and receiving nodes, and other control information. LANs are limited to operating within a geographical area of at most a few miles and often are restricted to a specific building or a single department. Separate remote LANs may be connected by **bridges**, routers, or switches (see below), providing convenient communication between machines on different networks. The telecommunication department of a health care organization often takes responsibility for implementing and linking multiple LANs to form an enterprise network. Important services provided by such network administrators include integrated access to WANs, specifically to the Internet (see later discussion on Internet communication), service reliability, and security.

Early LANs used coaxial cables as the communication medium because they could deliver reliable, high-speed communications. With improved communication signal–processing technologies, however, **twisted-pair wires** (Cat-5 and better quality) have become the standard. Twisted-pair wiring is inexpensive and has a high **bandwidth** (capacity for information transmission) of at least 100 Mbps. Twisted-pair wiring is susceptible to electrical interference, although less so than dial-up telephone connections. An alternate medium, **fiber-optic cable**, offers the highest bandwidth (over 1 billion bps or 1 Gbps) and a high degree of reliability because it uses light waves to transmit information signals and is not susceptible to electrical interference. Fiber-optic cable is used in LANs to increase transmission speeds and distances by at least one order of magnitude over twisted-pair wire. In addition, fiber-optic cable is lightweight and easy to install. Splicing and connecting into optical cable is more difficult than into twisted-pair wire, however, so inhouse delivery of networking services to the desktop is still easier using twisted-pair wires. Fiber-optic cable and twisted-pair wires are often used in a complementary fashion—fiber-optic cable for the high-speed, shared backbone of an enterprise network or LAN and twisted-pair wires extending out from side-branch hubs to bring service to the workplace.

When coaxial cable installations are in place (e.g., in closed circuit television or in cable television services), LANs using coaxial cable can transmit signals using either broadband or baseband technology. **Broadband** is adapted from the technology for transmitting cable television. A broadband LAN can transmit multiple signals simultaneously, providing a unified environment for sending computer data, voice messages, and images. Cable modems provide the means for encoding and decoding the data, and each signal is sent within an assigned frequency range (channel). **Baseband** is simpler and is used in most LAN installations. It transmits digital signals over a single set of wires, one packet at a time, without special encoding as a television signal.

Messages also can be transmitted through the air by radio, microwave, infrared, satellite signal, or line-of-sight laser-beam transmission, but these modes have limited application. Users in a hospital or clinic can use radio signals from portable devices to communicate with their workstations or with servers that contain clinical data and thus can gain entry to the LANs and associated services. Hospitals have many instruments that generate electronic interference, and often have reinforced concrete walls, so that radio transmission may not be reliable over long distances. Cellular telephone services are widespread, especially in urban areas, and can be used for data communications. Such services typically only provide low bandwidth though and are still expensive for extended use. In many medical settings the use of cellular or similar radio technologies is prohibited for fear of interference with patient pacemakers or delicate instruments.

Rapid data transmission is supported by LANs. Many LANs still operate at 10 Mbps, but 100-Mbps networks are becoming more cost-effective with commercial technology. Even at 10 Mbps, the entire contents of this book could be transmitted in a few seconds. Multiple users and high-volume data transmissions such as video will congest a LAN and its servers, however, so the effective transmission speed seen by each user may be much lower. When demand is high, multiple LANs can be installed. Gateways, routers, and switches shuttle packets among these networks to allow sharing of data between computers as though the machines were on the same LAN. A **router** or a **switch** is a special device that is connected to more than one network and is equipped to forward packets that originate on one network segment to machines that have addresses on another network. **Gateways** perform routing and can also translate packet formats if the two connected networks run different communication protocols.

Internet Communication

External routers can also link the users on a LAN to a **regional network** and then to the **Internet**. The Internet is a WAN that is composed of many regional and local networks interconnected by long-range **backbone links**, including international links. The Internet and the regional networks, begun by the National Science Foundation in the mid-1980s, included a relatively small number of regional networks to provide coverage for metropolitan or larger areas (Quarterman, 1990). Regional and national networking services are now provided by many commercial communications companies, and users get access to the regional networks through their institutions or privately by paying an **Internet service provider** (ISP), who in turn gets WAN access through a network access provider (NAP). There are other WANs besides the Internet, some operated by demanding commercial users, and others by parts of the federal government, such as the Department of Defense, the National Aeronautics and Space Administration, and the Department of Energy. Nearly all countries have their own networks so that information can be transmitted to most computers in the world. Gateways of various types connect all these networks, whose capabilities may differ. It is no longer possible to show the Internet map on a single diagram, but to illustrate the principle of hierarchical geographical interconnections still being used, we show a simplified diagram of the Internet from circa 1995 (Figure 5.8).

All Internet participants agree on many conventions called **Internet standards**. The most fundamental is the protocol suite referred to as the **Transmission Control Protocol/Internet Protocol (TCP/IP)**. Data transmission is always by structured packets, and all machines are currently identified by a standard for 32-bit IP addresses. **Internet addresses** consist of a sequence of four 8-bit numbers, each ranging from 0 to 255—most often written as a dotted sequence of numbers: a.b.c.d. Although IP addresses are not assigned geographically (the way ZIP codes are), the first number identifies a region, the second a local area, the third a local net, and the fourth a specific computer. Computers that are permanently linked into the Internet may have a fixed IP address assigned, whereas users whose machines reach the Internet by dialing into an ISP or making a wireless connection only when needed, may get a temporary address that persists just during a session. The Internet is in the process of changing to a protocol (IPv6) that supports 64-bit IP addresses, because the worldwide expansion of the Internet and proliferation of networked individual computer devices is exhausting the old 32-bit address space. While the changeover is complex, much work has gone into making this transition transparent to the user.

Because 32-bit (or 64-bit) numbers are difficult to remember, computers on the Internet also have names assigned. Multiple names may be used for a given computer that performs distinct services. The names can be translated to IP addresses—e.g., when they are used to designate a remote machine—by means of a hierarchical name management system called the **Domain Name System** (DNS). Designated computers, called **name-servers**, convert a name into an IP address before the message is placed on the network; routing takes place based on only the numeric IP address. Names are also most often expressed as dotted sequences of name segments, but there is no correspondence between the four numbers of an IP address and the parts of a name. The Internet is

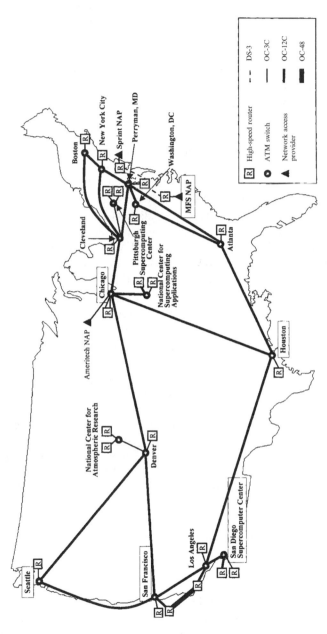

Figure 5.8. The very high-speed Backbone Network Service (vBNS) developed by the National Science Foundation around 1995 as a successor to the NSFNet is an example of hierarchical Internet architecture in general use today—cross-country backbones connected to gateways into regional network providers. The vBNS was itself a transitional experimental network that established the engineering and applications principles for practical very high-speed communications services in support of research and education institutions throughout the United States. The circles at junctions of cross-country lines are high-speed Asynchronous Transfer mode (ATM) switches. The routers are network access providers (NAPs), which supply network connectivity for regional Internet service providers (ISPs) and connections to other networks. DC-3 = Digital Signal level 3 (T3) line at 44.736 Mbps; OC-3C = Optical Carrier 3 synchronous optical transmission line at 155.52 Mbps; OC-12C = Optical Carrier 12 synchronous optical transmission line at 622.08 Mbps; OC-48 = Optical Carrier 48 synchronous optical transmission line at 2.488 Gbps. (*Source:* MCI-Worldcom.)

growing rapidly; therefore, periodic reorganizations of parts of the network are common. Numeric IP addresses may have to change, but the logical name for a resource can stay the same and the (updated) DNS can take care of keeping the translation up to date. This overall process is governed today by the **Internet Corporation for Assigned Names and Numbers (ICANN)**. Three conventions are in use for composing Internet names from segments:

1. *Functional convention*: Under the most common convention for the United States, names are composed of hierarchical segments increasing in specificity from right to left, beginning with one of the top-level domain-class identifiers—e.g., *computer.institution.class* (smi.stanford.edu) or *institution.class* (whitehouse.gov). Initially the defined top-level domain classes were .com, .edu, .gov, .int, .mil, .org, and .net (for commercial, educational, government, international organizations, military, non-profit, and ISP organizations, respectively). As Internet use has grown, more classes are being added—seven more have become fully operational in 2002 (.aero, .biz, .coop, .info, .museum, .name, and .pro). This list will likely grow further in the future. Note that these *functional* top-level domain names (or classes) have three or more characters. Name hierarchies can be as deep as desired, but simplicity helps users to remember the names. Other conventions have evolved as well: www is often used as a prefix to name the **World Wide Web (WWW)** services on a computer (e.g., www.nlm.nih.gov) (see Section 5.1.2 for network communications).

2. *Geographic convention*: Names are composed of hierarchical segments increasing in specificity from right to left and beginning with a two-character top-level country domain identifier—e.g., institution.town.state.country (cnri.reston.va.us or city.palo-alto.ca.us). Many countries outside of the United States use a combination of these conventions, such as csd.abdn.ac.uk, for the Computer Science Department at the University of Aberdeen (an academic institution in the United Kingdom). Note that the case of an IP address is ignored, although additional fields, such as file names used to locate Web content resources, may be case-sensitive.

3. *Attribute list address (X.400) convention*: Names are composed of a sequence of attribute-value pairs that specifies the components needed to resolve the address—e.g., /C=GB/ADMD=BT/PRMD=AC/O=Abdn/OU=csd/, which is equivalent to the address csd.abdn.ac.uk. This convention derives from the X.400 address standard that is used mainly in the European community. It has the advantage that the address elements (e.g., /C for Country name, /ADMD for Administrative Management Domain name, and /PRMD for Private Management Domain name) are explicitly labeled and may come in any order. Country designations differ as well. However, this type of address is generally more difficult for humans to understand and has not been adopted broadly in the Internet community.

An institution that has many computers may provide a service whereby all its communications (e.g., incoming e-mails) go to a single address, e.g., stanford.edu or aol.com, and then local tables are used to direct each message to the right computer or individual. Such a scheme insulates outside users from internal naming conventions and changes, and can allow dynamic machine selection for the service in order to distribute loading. Such a central site can also provide a firewall—a means to attempt to keep viruses and unsolicited and unwanted connections or messages (spam) out. The nature of attacks on networks and their users is such that constant vigilance is needed at these service sites to prevent system and individual intrusions.

The routing of packets of information between computers on the Internet is the basis for a rich array of information services. Each such service—be it resource naming, electronic mail, file transfer, remote computer log in, World Wide Web, or another service—is defined in terms of sets of protocols that govern how computers speak to each other. These worldwide intercomputer-linkage conventions allow global sharing of information resources, as well as personal and group communications. The Web's popularity and growing services continues to change how we deal with people, form communities, make purchases, entertain ourselves, and perform research. The scope of all these activities is more than we can cover in this book, so we restrict ourselves to topics important to health care. Even with this limitation, we can only scratch the surface of many topics.

5.1.2   Software

All the functions performed by the hardware of a computer system—data acquisition from input devices, transfer of data and programs to and from working memory, computation and information processing by the CPU, formatting and presentation of results—are directed by computer programs, or software.

Programming Languages

In our discussion of the CPU in Section 5.1, we explained that a computer processes information by manipulating words of information in registers. Instructions that tell the processor which operations to perform also are sequences of 0s and 1s, a binary representation called **machine language** or **machine code**. Machine-code instructions are the only instructions that a computer can process directly. These binary patterns, however, are difficult for people to understand and manipulate. People think best symbolically. Thus, a first step toward making programming easier and less error prone was the creation of an assembly language. **Assembly language** replaces the sequences of bits of machine-language programs with words and abbreviations meaningful to humans; a programmer instructs the computer to LOAD a word from memory, ADD an amount to the contents of a register, STORE it back into memory, and so on. A program called an **assembler** translates these instructions into binary machine-language representation before execution of the code. There is a one-to-one correspondence between instructions in assembly and machine languages. To increase efficiency, we can combine sets of assembly instructions into **macros** and thus reuse them. An assembly-language programmer must consider problems on a hardware-specific level, instructing the computer to transfer data between registers and memory and to perform primitive operations, such as incrementing registers, comparing characters, and handling all processor exceptions (Figure 5.9).

On the other hand, the problems that the users of a computer wish to solve are real-world problems on a higher conceptual level. They want to be able to instruct the

```
Assembly-language program:


              ORG  0          /Origin of program is location 0
              LDA A           /Load operand from location A
              ADD B           /Add operand from location B
              STA C           /Store sum in location C
              HLT             /Halt
        A,    DEC  3          /Location A contains decimal 3
        B,    DEC  15         /Location B contains decimal 15
        C,    DEC  0          /Location C contains decimal 0
              END             /End of program



Machine-language program:

        Location            Instruction code

           0            0010 0000 0000 0100
           1            0001 0000 0000 0101
          10            0011 0000 0000 0110
          11            0111 0000 0000 0001
         100            0000 0000 0000 0011
         101            0000 0000 0000 1111
         110            0000 0000 0000 0000
```

Figure 5.9. An assembly-language program and a corresponding machine-language program to add two numbers and to store the result.

computer to perform tasks such as to retrieve the latest serum creatinine test result, to monitor the status of hypertensive patients, or to compute a patient's current account balance. To make communication with computers more understandable and less tedious, computer scientists developed higher-level, user-oriented **symbolic-programming languages**.

Using a higher-level language, such as one of those listed in Table 5.1, a programmer defines variables to represent higher-level entities and specifies arithmetic and symbolic operations without worrying about the details of how the hardware performs these operations. The details of managing the hardware are hidden from the programmer, who can specify with a single statement an operation that may translate to tens or hundreds of machine instructions. A compiler is used to translate automatically a high-level program into machine code. Some languages are interpreted instead of compiled. An **interpreter** converts and executes each statement before moving to the next statement, whereas a compiler translates all the statements at one time, creating a binary program, which can subsequently be executed many times. MUMPS (M) is an interpreted language, LISP may either be interpreted or compiled, and FORTRAN routinely is compiled before execution. Hundreds of languages have been developed—we discuss here only a few that are important from a practical or conceptual level.

Each statement of a language is characterized by **syntax** and **semantics**. The syntactic rules describe how the statements, declarations, and other language constructs are written—they define the language's grammatical structure. Semantics is the meaning given to the various syntactic constructs. The following sets of statements (written in Pascal, FORTRAN, COBOL, and LISP) all have the same semantics:

```
C:= A+B          C:= A+B          LN IS "The value       (SETQ C
PRINTF (c)       WRITE 10,        is NNN.FFF"            (PLUS A B))
no layout        6 c 10           ADD A TO B, GIVING C   (format file
choice           FORMAT           MOVE C TO LN           6 "The value
                 ("The value      WRITE LN               is ~5,2F" C)
                 is F5.2")
```

They instruct the computer to add the values of variables A and B, to assign the result to variable C, and to write the result onto a file. Each language has a distinct syntax for indicating which operations to perform. Regardless of the particular language in which a program is written, in the end, the computer manipulates sequences of 0s and 1s within its registers.

Computer languages are tailored to handle specific types of computing problems, as shown in Table 5.1, although all these languages are sufficiently flexible to deal with nearly any type of problem. Languages that focus on a simple, general computational infrastructure, such as C or Java have to be augmented with large collections of libraries of procedures, and learning the specific libraries takes more time than does learning the language itself. Languages also differ in usability. A language meant for education and highly reliable programs will include features to make it foolproof, by way of checking that the types of values, such as integers, decimal numbers, and strings of characters, match throughout their use—this is called **type checking**. Such features may cause programs to be slower in execution, but more reliable. Without type checking, smart programmers can instruct the computers to perform some operations more efficiently than is possible in a more constraining language.

Sequences of statements are grouped into *procedures*. Procedures enhance the clarity of larger programs and also provide a basis for reuse of the work by other programmers. Large programs are in turn mainly sequences of invocations of such procedures, some coming from libraries (such as format in LISP) and others written for the specific application. These procedures are called with *arguments*—e.g., the medical record number of a patient—so that a procedure to retrieve a value, such as the patient's age: age(number). An important distinction among languages is how those arguments are transmitted. Just giving the value in response to a request is the safest method. Giving the name provides the most information to the procedure, and giving the reference (a pointer to where the value is stored) allows the procedure to go back to the source, which can be efficient but also allows changes that may not be wanted. Discussions about languages often emphasize these various features, but the underlying concern is nearly always the trade-off of protection versus power.

Table 5.1. Distinguishing features of 12 common programming languages.

Programming language	First year	Primary application domain	Type	Operation	Type checks	Procedure call method	Data management method
FORTRAN	1957	Mathematics	Procedural	Compiled	Little	By reference	Simple files
COBOL	1962	Business	Procedural	Compiled	Yes	By name	Formatted files
Pascal	1978	Education	Procedural	Compiled	Strong	By name	Record files
Smalltalk	1976	Education	Object	Interpreted	Yes	By defined methods	Object persistence
PL/1	1965	Math, business	Procedural	Compiled	Coercion	By reference	Formatted files
Ada	1980	Math, business	Procedural	Compiled	Strong	By name	Formatted files
Standard ML	1989	Logic, math	Functional	Compiled	Yes	By value	Stream files
MUMPS (M)	1962	Data handling	Procedural	Interpreted	No	By reference	Hierarchical files
LISP	1964	Logic	Functional	Either	No	By value	Data persistence
C	1976	Data handling	Procedural	Compiled	Little	By reference	Stream files
C++	1986	Data handling	Hybrid	Compiled	Yes	By reference	Object files
JAVA	1995	Data display	Object	Either	Strong	By value	Object classes

Programmers work in successively higher levels of abstraction by writing, and later invoking, standard procedures in the form of functions and subroutines. Built-in functions and subroutines create an environment in which users can perform complex operations by specifying single commands. Tools exist to combine related functions for specific tasks—e.g., to build a forms interface that displays retrieved data in a certain presentation format.

Specialized languages can be used directly by nonprogrammers for well-understood tasks, because such languages define additional procedures for specialized tasks and hide yet more detail. For example, users can search for, and retrieve data from, large databases using the Structured Query Language (SQL) of database management systems (discussed later in this section). With the help of statistical languages, such as SAS or SPSS, users can perform extensive statistical calculations, such as regression analysis and correlation. Other users may use a spreadsheet program, such as Lotus 1-2-3 or Excel, to record and manipulate data with formulas in the cells of a spreadsheet matrix. In each case, the physical details of the data storage structures and the access mechanisms are hidden from the user. Each of these programs provides its own specialized language for instructing a computer to perform desired high-level functions.

The end users of a computer may not even be aware that they are programming if the language is so natural that it matches their needs in an intuitive manner. Moving icons on a screen and dragging and dropping them into boxes or onto other icons is a form of programming supported by many layers of interpreters and compiler-generated code. If the user saves a **script** (a keystroke-by-keystroke record) of the actions performed for later reuse, then he or she has created a program. Some systems allow such scripts to be viewed and edited for later updates and changes; e.g., there is a macro function available in the the Microsoft Excel spreadsheet and the Microsoft Word text editor.

Even though many powerful languages and packages handle these diverse tasks, we still face the challenge of incorporating multiple functions into a larger system. It is easy to envision a system where a Web browser provides access to statistical results of data collected from two related databases. Such interoperation is not yet simple, however, and people must have programming expertise to resolve the details of incompatibilities among the specialized tools.

Data Management

Data provide the infrastructure for recording and sharing information. Data become information when they are organized to affect decisions, actions, and learning (see Chapter 2). Accessing and moving data from the points of collection to the points of use are among the primary functions of computing in medicine. These applications must deal with large volumes of varied data and manage them, for *persistence*, on external storage. The mathematical facilities of computer languages are based on common principles and are, strictly speaking, equivalent. The same conceptual basis is not available for data management facilities. Some languages allow only internal structures to be made persistent; in that case, external library programs are used for handling storage.

Handling data is made easier if the language supports moving structured data from internal memory to external, persistent storage. Data can, for instance, be viewed as a *stream*, a model that matches well with data produced by some instruments, by TCP connections over the Internet, or by a ticker tape. Data can also be viewed as *records*, matching well with the rows of a table (Figure 5.10); or data can be viewed as a *hierarchy*, matching well with the structure of a medical record, including patients, their visits, and their findings during a visit.

If the language does not directly support the best data structure to deal with an application, additional programming must be done to construct the desired structure out of the available facilities. The resulting extra layer, however, typically costs money and introduces inconsistencies among applications trying to share information.

Operating Systems

Users interact with the computer through an **operating system (OS)**: a program that supervises and controls the execution of all other programs and that directs the operation of the hardware. The OS is software that is included with a computer system and it manages the resources, such as memory, storage, and devices, for the user. Once started, the **kernel** of the OS resides in memory at all times and runs in the background. It assigns the CPU to specific tasks, supervises other programs running in the computer, controls communication among hardware components, manages the transfer of data from input devices to output devices, and handles the details of file management such as the creation, opening, reading, writing, and closing of data files. In shared systems, it allocates the resources of the system among the competing users. The OS insulates users from much of the complexity of handling these processes. Thus, users are able to concentrate on higher-level problems of information management. They do get involved in specifying which programs to run and in giving names to the directory structures and files that are to be made persistent. These names provide the links to the user's work from one session to another. Deleting files that are no longer needed and archiving those that should be kept securely are other interactions that users have with the OS.

Programmers can write **application programs** to automate routine operations that store and organize data, to perform analyses, to facilitate the integration and communication of information, to perform bookkeeping functions, to monitor patient status, to aid in education—in short, to perform all the functions provided by medical

Record Number	Name	Sex	Date of Birth
22-546-998	Adams, Clare	F	11Nov1998
62-847-991	Barnes, Tanner	F	07Dec1997
47-882-365	Clark, Laurel	F	10May1998
55-202-187	Davidson, Travis	M	10Apr2000

Figure 5.10. A simple patient data file containing records for four pediatric patients. The key field of each record contains the medical record number that uniquely identifies the patient. The other fields of the record contain demographic information.

computing systems (see Chapter 6). These programs are then filed by the OS and are available to its users when needed.

PCs typically operate as **single-user systems**, whereas servers are **multiuser systems**. Workstations can handle either approach, although they often give a single-user preference. In a *multiuser* system, all users have simultaneous access to their **jobs**; users interact through the OS, which switches resources rapidly among all the jobs that are running. Because people work slowly compared with computer CPUs, the computer can respond to multiple users, seemingly at the same time. Thus, all users have the illusion that they have the full attention of the machine, as long as they do not make very heavy demands. Such shared resource access is important where databases must be shared, as we discuss below in Database Management Systems. When it is managing sharing, the OS spends resources for queuing, switching, and requeuing jobs. If the total demand is too high, the overhead increases disproportionately and slows the service for everyone. High individual demands are best allocated to workstations, which can be nearly as powerful as servers and which dedicate all resources to a primary user.

Because computers need to perform a variety of services, several application programs reside in main memory simultaneously. **Multiprogramming** permits the effective use of multiple devices; while the CPU is executing one program, another program may be receiving input from external storage, and another may be generating results on the laser printer. In **multiprocessing** systems, several processors (CPUs) are used by the OS within a single computer system, thus increasing the overall processing power. Note, however, that multiprogramming does not necessarily imply having multiple processors.

Memory may still be a scarce resource, especially under multiprogramming. When many programs and their data are active simultaneously, they may not all fit in the physical memory on the machine at the same time. To solve this problem, the OS will partition users' programs and data into **pages**, which can be kept in temporary storage on disk and are brought into main memory as needed. Such a storage allocation is called **virtual memory**. Virtual memory can be many times the size of real memory, so users can allocate many more pages than main memory can hold. Also individual programs and their data can use more memory than is available on a specific computer. Under virtual memory management, each address referenced by the CPU goes through an address mapping from the **virtual address** of the program to a physical address in main memory (Figure 5.11). When a memory page is referenced that is not in physical storage, the CPU creates space for it by swapping out a little-used page to secondary storage and bringing in the needed page from storage. This mapping is handled automatically by the hardware on most machines but still creates significant delays, so the total use of virtual memory must be limited to a level that permits the system to run efficiently.

A large collection of **system programs** is generally associated with the kernel of an OS. These programs include utility programs, such as **graphical user interface** (GUI) routines; **text editors** and **graphic editors**; compilers to handle programs written in higher-level languages; **debuggers** for newly created programs; communication software; diagnostic programs to help maintain the computer system; and substantial libraries of standard routines (such as for listing and viewing files, starting and stopping programs, and checking on system status). Modern libraries include tools such as sorting programs and programs to perform complex mathematical functions and routines to present and

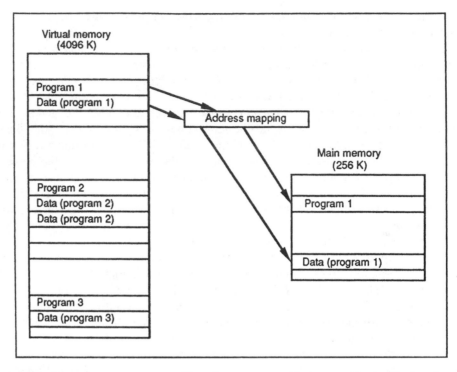

Figure 5.11. Virtual-memory system. Virtual memory provides users with the illusion that they have many more addressable memory locations than there are in real memory—in this case, more than five times as much. Programs and data stored on peripheral disks are swapped into main memory when they are referenced; logical addresses are translated automatically to physical addresses by the hardware.

manipulate windows that access a variety of application programs, handle their point-and-click functions, allow a variety of fonts, and the like. The storage demands of these libraries are increasing—a few hundred megabytes for system programs is not unusual on PCs, and workstations and servers may have several times those requirements. Not all system programs will ever be used by a user, but determining what is needed and deleting the rest is more work than most users want to undertake.

Database Management Systems

Throughout this book, we emphasize the importance to good medical decision making of timely access to relevant and complete data from diverse sources. Computers provide the primary means for organizing and accessing these data; however, the programs to manage the data are complex and are difficult to write. Database technology supports the integration and organization of data and assists users with data entry, long-term storage, and retrieval. Programming data management software is particularly difficult when multiple users share data (and thus may try to access data simultaneously), when they must search through voluminous data rapidly and at unpredictable times, and when the relationships among data elements are complex. For health care applications, it is important that the data be complete and virtually error-free. Furthermore, the need for long-term reliability makes it risky to entrust a medical database to locally written programs. The programmers tend to move from project to project, computers will be replaced, and the organizational units that maintain the data may be reorganized.

Not only the individual data values but also their meanings and their relationships to other data must be stored. For example, an isolated data element (e.g., the number 99.7) is useless unless we know that that number represents a human's body temperature in degrees Fahrenheit and is linked to other data necessary to interpret its value—the value pertains to a particular patient who is identified by a unique medical record number, the observation was taken at a certain time (02:35, 7Feb2000) in a certain way (orally), and so on. To avoid loss of descriptive information, we must keep together clusters of related data throughout processing. These relationships can be complex; e.g., an observation may be linked not only to the patient but also to the person recording the observation, to the instrument that he used to acquire the values, and to the physical state of the patient (refer to Chapter 2).

The meaning of data elements and the relationships among those elements are captured in the structure of the database. **Databases** are collections of data, typically organized into fields, records, and files (see Figure 5.10), as well as descriptive meta data. The **field** is the most primitive building block; each field represents one data element. For example, the database of a hospital's registration system typically has fields such as the patient's identification number, name, date of birth, gender, admission date, and admitting diagnosis. Fields are usually grouped together to form **records**. A record is uniquely identified by one or more **key fields**—e.g., patient identification number and observation time. Records that contain similar information are grouped in **files**. In addition to files about patients and their diagnoses, treatments, and drug therapies, the database of a health care information system will have separate files containing information about charges and payments, personnel and payroll, inventory, and many other topics. All these files relate to one another: they may refer to the same patients, to the same personnel, to the same services, to the same set of accounts, and so on.

Meta data describes where in the record specific data are stored, and how the right record can be located. For instance, a record may be located by searching and matching patient ID in the record. The meta data also specifies where in the record the digits representing the birthdate are located and how to convert the data to the current age. When the structure of the database changes—e.g., because new fields are added to a record—the meta data must be changed as well. When data are to be shared, there will be continuing requirements for additions and reorganizations to the files and hence the meta data. The desire for **data independence**—i.e., keeping the applications of one set of users independent from changes made to applications by another group—is the key reason for using a database management system for shared data.

A **database management system (DBMS)** is an integrated set of programs that helps users to store and manipulate data easily and efficiently. The conceptual (logical) view of a database provided by a DBMS allows users to specify what the results should be without worrying too much about how they will be obtained; the DBMS handles the details of managing and accessing data. A crucial part of a database kept in a DBMS is the **schema**, containing the needed meta data. A schema is the machine-readable definition of the contents and organization of the records of all the data files. Programs are insulated by the DBMS from changes in the way that data are stored, because the programs access data by field name rather than by address. The schema file of the DBMS must be modified to reflect changes in record format, but the application programs that use the data do not need to be altered. A DBMS also provides facilities for entering, editing, and retrieving data. Often, fields are associated with lists or ranges of valid values; thus, the DBMS can detect and request correction of some data-entry errors, thereby improving database integrity.

Users retrieve data from a database in either of two ways. Users can query the database directly using a query language to extract information in an ad hoc fashion—e.g., to retrieve the records of all male hypertensive patients aged 45 to 64 years for inclusion in a retrospective study. Figure 5.12 shows the syntax for such a query using SQL. Query formulation can be difficult, however; users must understand the contents and underlying structure of the database to construct a query correctly. Often, database programmers formulate the requests for health professionals.

To support occasional use, **front-end applications** to database systems can help a user retrieve information using a menu based on the schema. Certain applications, such as a drug order–entry system, will use a database system without the pharmacist or ordering physician being aware of the other's presence. The medication-order records placed in the database by the physician create communication transactions with the pharmacy; then, the pharmacy application creates the daily drug lists for the patient care units.

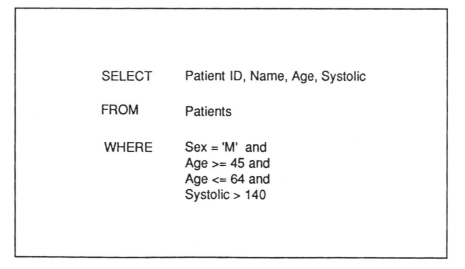

```
SELECT      Patient ID, Name, Age, Systolic

FROM        Patients

WHERE       Sex = 'M'  and
            Age >= 45 and
            Age <= 64 and
            Systolic > 140
```

Figure 5.12. An example of a simple database query written in Structured Query Language (SQL). The program will retrieve the records of males whose age is between 45 and 64 years and whose systolic blood pressure is greater than 140 mm Hg.

Some database queries are routine requests—e.g., the resource utilization reports used by health care administrators and the end-of-month financial reports generated for business offices. Thus, DBMSs often also provide an alternative, simpler means for formulating such queries, called **report generation**. Users specify their data requests on the input screen of the report-generator program. The report generator then produces the actual query program using information stored in the schema, often at predetermined intervals. The reports are formatted such that they can be distributed without modification. The report-generation programs can extract header information from the schema. Routine report generation should, however, be periodically reviewed in terms of its costs and benefits. Reports that are not read are a waste of computer, natural, and people resources. A reliable database will be able to provide needed and up-to-date information when that information is required.

Many DBMSs support multiple **views**, or models, of the data. The data stored in a database have a single physical organization, yet different user groups can have different perspectives on the contents and structure of a database. For example, the clinical laboratory and the finance department might use the same underlying database, but only the data relevant to the individual application area are available to each group. Basic patient information will be shared; the existence of other data is hidden from groups that do not need them. Application-specific descriptions of a database are stored in such **view schemas**. Through the views, a DBMS controls access to data, as discussed in Section 5.3. Thus, a DBMS facilitates the integration of data from multiple sources and avoids the expense of creating and maintaining multiple files containing redundant information. At the same time, it accommodates the differing needs of multiple users. The use of database technology, combined with communications technology (see the following discussion on Software for Network Communications), will enable health care institutions to attain the benefits both of independent, specialized applications and of large integrated databases.

Database design and implementation has become a highly specialized field. Most medical applications use standard products from established vendors. An introduction to the topic is provided by Garcia-Molina et al. (2002). Wiederhold's book (1981) discusses the organization and use of databases in health care settings.

Software for Network Communications

The ability of computers to communicate with each other over local and remote networks brings tremendous power to computer users. Internet communications make it possible to share data and resources among diverse users and institutions around the world. Network users can access shared patient data (such as a hospital's medical records) or nationwide databases (such as bibliographic databases of scientific literature or genomics databases describing what is known about the biomolecular basis of life and disease). Networks make it possible for remote users to communicate with one another and to collaborate. In this section, we introduce the important concepts that allow you to understand network technology.

Network power is realized by means of a large body of communications software. This software handles the physical connection of each computer to the network, the internal preparation of data to be sent or received over the network, and the interfaces between the network data flow and applications programs. There are now tens of millions of computers of different kinds on the Internet and hundreds of programs in each machine that service network communications. Two key ideas make it possible to manage the complexity of network software: *network service stacks* and *network protocols*. These strategies allow communication to take place between any two machines on the Internet, ensure that application programs are insulated from changes in the network infrastructure, and make it possible for users to take advantage easily of the rapidly growing set of information resources and services. The **network stack** serves to organize communications software *within* a machine. Because the responsibilities for network communications are divided into different levels, with clear interfaces between the levels, network software is made more modular. The four-level network stack for TCP/IP is shown in Figure 5.13, which also compares that stack to the seven-level stack defined by the International Standards Organization.

At the lowest level—the Data Link and Physical Transport level—programs manage the physical connection of the machine to the network, the physical-medium packet formats, and the means for detecting and correcting errors. The Network level implements the IP method of addressing packets, routing packets, and controlling the timing and sequencing of transmissions. The Transport level converts packet-level communications into several services for the Application level, including a reliable serial byte stream

ISO Level	TCP/IP Service Level
5–7	Applications: SMTP, FPT, TELNET, DNS, ...
4	Transport: TCP and UDP
3	Network: IP (including ICMP, ARP, and RARP)
1–2	Data link and Physical transport: (Ethernet, Token Rings, Wireless, ...)

Figure 5.13. TCP/IP network service level stack and corresponding levels of the Open Systems Interconnection (OSI) Reference model developed by the International Standards Organization (ISO). Each level of the stack specifies a progressively higher level of abstraction. Each level serves the level above and expects particular functions or services from the level below it. SMTP = Simple Mail Transport Protocol; FTP = File Transfer Protocol; DNS = Domain Name System; TCP = Transmission Control Protocol; UDP = User Datagram Protocol; IP = Internet Protocol; ICMP = Internet Control Message Protocol; ARP = Address Resolution Protocol; RARP = Reverse Address Resolution Protocol.

(TCP), a transaction-oriented User Datagram Protocol (UDP), and newer services such as real-time video.

The Application level is where programs run that support electronic mail, file sharing and transfer, Web posting, downloading, browsing, and many other services. Each layer communicates with only the layers directly above and below it and does so through specific interface conventions. The network stack is machine- and OS-dependent—because it has to run on particular hardware and to deal with the OS on that machine (filing, input–output, memory access, etc.). But its layered design serves the function of modularization. Applications see a standard set of data-communication services and do not each have to worry about details such as how to form proper packets of an acceptable size for the network, how to route packets to the desired machine, how to detect and correct errors, or how to manage the particular network hardware on the computer. If a computer changes its network connection from a **Token Ring** to an **Ethernet** network, or if the **topology** of the network changes, the applications are unaffected. Only the lower level Data Link and Network layers need to be updated.

Internet protocols are shared conventions that serve to standardize communications *between* machines—much as, for two people to communicate effectively, they must agree on the syntax and meaning of the words they are using, the style of the interaction (lecture versus conversation), a procedure for handling interruptions, and so on. Protocols are defined for every Internet service (such as routing, electronic mail, and Web access) and establish the conventions for representing data, for requesting an action, and for replying to a requested action. For example, protocols define the format conventions for e-mail addresses and text messages (RFC822), the attachment of multimedia content (Multipurpose Internet Mail Extensions (MIME)), the delivery of e-mail messages (Simple Mail Transport Protocol (SMTP)), the transfer of files (File Transfer Protocol (FTP)), connections to remote computers (Telnet), the formatting of Web pages (Hypertext Markup Language (HTML)), the exchange of routing information, and many more. By observing these protocols, machines of different types can communicate openly and can interoperate with each other. When requesting a Web page from a server using the Hypertext Transfer Protocol (HTTP), the client does not have to know whether the server is a UNIX machine, a Windows machine, or a mainframe running VMS—they all appear the same over the network if they adhere to the HTTP protocol. The layering of the network stack is also supported by protocols. As we said, within a machine, each layer communicates with only the layer directly above or below. Between machines, each layer communicates with only its peer layer on the other machine, using a defined protocol. For example, the SMTP application on one machine communicates with only an SMTP application on a remote machine. Similarly, the Network layer communicates with only peer Network layers, for example, to exchange routing information or control information using the Internet Control Message Protocol (ICMP).

We briefly describe four of the basic services available on the Internet: electronic mail, FTP, Telnet, and access to the World Wide Web.

1. *Electronic mail*: Users send and receive messages from other users via electronic mail, mimicking use of the postal service. The messages travel rapidly: except for queuing delays at gateways and receiving computers, their transmission is nearly instanta-

neous. Electronic mail was one of the first protocols invented for the Internet (around 1970, when what was to become the Internet was still called the **ARPANET**). A simple e-mail message consists of a **header** and a **body**. The header contains information formatted according to the RFC822 protocol, which controls the appearance of the date and time of the message, the address of the sender, addresses of the recipients, the subject line, and other optional header lines. The body of the message contains free text. The user addresses the e-mail directly to the intended reader by giving the reader's account name or a personal alias followed by the IP address of the machine on which the reader receives mail—e.g., JohnSmith@IP.address. If the body of the e-mail message is encoded according to the MIME standard it may also contain arbitrary multimedia information, such as drawings, pictures, sound, or video. Mail is sent to the recipient using the SMTP standard. It may either be read on the machine holding the addressee's account or it may be downloaded to the addressee's PC for reading using either the Post Office Protocol (POP) or the Internet Mail Access Protocol (IMAP). Some mail protocols allow the sender to specify an acknowledgment to be returned when the mail has been deposited or has been read. Electronic mail has become an important communication path in health care, allowing asynchronous, one-way, communications between participants. Requests for services, papers, meetings, and collaborative exchanges are now largely handled by electronic mail (Lederberg, 1978).

It is easy to broadcast electronic mail by sending it to a **mailing list** or a specific **list-server**, but electronic mail etiquette conventions dictate that such communications be focused and relevant. **Spamming**, which is sending e-mail solicitations or announcements to broad lists, is annoying to recipients, but is difficult to prevent. Conventional e-mail is sent in clear text over the network so that anyone observing network traffic can read its contents. Protocols for encrypted e-mail, such as Privacy-Enhanced Mail (PEM) or encrypting attachments, are also available, but are not yet widely deployed. They ensure that the contents are readable by only the intended recipients.

2. *File Transfer Protocol* (FTP): FTP facilitates sending and retrieving large amounts of information—of a size that is uncomfortably large for electronic mail. For instance, programs and updates to programs, complete medical records, papers with many figures or images for review, and the like are best transferred via FTP. FTP access requires several steps: (1) accessing the remote computer using the IP address; (2) providing user identification to authorize access; (3) specifying the name of a file to be sent or fetched using the file-naming convention at the destination site; and (4) transferring the data. For open sharing of information by means of FTP sites, the user identification is by convention "anonymous" and the requestor's e-mail address is used as the password.

3. *Telnet*: Telnet allows a user to log in on a remote computer. If the log-in is successful, the user becomes a fully qualified user of the remote system, and the user's own machine becomes a relatively passive terminal. The smoothness of such a terminal emulation varies depending on the differences between the local and remote computers. Many Telnet programs emulate well-known terminal types, such as the VT100, which are widely supported and minimize awkward mismatches of character-use conventions. Modest amounts of information can be brought into the user's machine by

copying data displayed in the terminal window into a local text editor or other program (i.e., by copying and pasting).

4. *World Wide Web* (WWW): Web **browsing** facilitates user access to remote information resources made available by Web servers. The user interface is typically a **Web browser** that understands the basic World Wide Web protocols. The **Universal Resource Locator** (URL) is used to specify *where a resource is located* in terms of the protocol to be used, the domain name of the machine it is on, and the name of the information resource within the remote machine. The **HyperText Markup Language (HTML)** describes *what the information should look like when displayed*. These formats are oriented toward graphic displays, and greatly exceed the capabilities associated with Telnet character-oriented displays. HTML supports conventional text, font settings, headings, lists, tables, and other display specifications. Within HTML documents, highlighted **buttons** can be defined that point to other HTML documents or services. This **hypertext** facility makes it possible to create a web of cross-referenced works that can be navigated by the user. HTML can also refer to subsidiary documents that contain other types of information—e.g., graphics, equations, images, video, speech— that can be seen or heard if the browser has been augmented with **helpers** or **plug-ins** for the particular format used. Browsers, such as Netscape Navigator or Internet Explorer, also provide choices for downloading the presented information so that no separate FTP tasks need to be initiated. The **HyperText Transfer Protocol (HTTP)** is used to communicate between browser clients and servers and to retrieve HTML documents. Such communications can be **encrypted** to protect sensitive contents of interactions (e.g., credit card information or patient information) from external view using protocols such as **Secure Sockets Layer (SSL)**.

HTML documents can also include small programs written in the Java language, called **applets**, which will execute on the user's computer when referenced. Applets can provide animations and also can compute summaries, merge information, and interact with selected files on the user's computer. The Java language is designed such that operations that might be destructive to the user's machine environment are blocked, but downloading remote and untested software still represents a substantial security risk (see Section 5.3).

The HTML captures many aspects of document description from predefined markup related to the appearance of the document on a display to markup related to internal links, scripts, and other semantic features. To separate appearance-related issues from other types of markup, to provide more flexibility in terms of markup types, and to work toward more open, self-defining document descriptions, a more powerful markup framework, called **eXtensible Markup Language** (XML), has emerged. XML (and its related markup protocols) is discussed in more detail in Chapter 19.

A **client–server** interaction is a generalization of the four interactions we have just discussed, involving interactions between a client (requesting) machine and a server (responding) machine. A client–server interaction, in general, supports collaboration between the user of a local machine and a remote computer. The server provides information and computational services according to some protocol, and the user's computer—the client—generates requests and does complementary processing (such as displaying HTML documents and images). A common function provided by servers is database access. Retrieved information is transferred to the client in response to requests, and then the client may perform specialized analyses on the data. The final results can be stored locally, printed, or mailed to other users.

5.2   Data Acquisition and Signal Processing

A prominent theme of this book is that capturing and entering data into a computer manually is difficult, time-consuming, error-prone, and expensive. **Real-time acquisition** of data from the actual source by direct electrical connections to instruments can over-come these problems. Direct acquisition of data avoids the need for people to measure, encode, and enter the data manually. Sensors attached to a patient convert biological signals—such as blood pressure, pulse rate, mechanical movement, and electrocardio-gram (ECG)—into electrical signals, which are transmitted to the computer. Tissue density can be obtained by scanning of an X-ray transmission. The signals are sampled periodically and are converted to digital representation for storage and processing. Automated data-acquisition and signal-processing techniques are particularly impor-tant in patient-monitoring settings (see Chapter 17). Similar techniques also apply to the acquisition and processing of human voice input.

Most naturally occurring signals are **analog signals**—signals that vary continuously. The first bedside monitors, for example, were wholly analog devices. Typically, they acquired an analog signal (such as that measured by the ECG) and displayed its level on a dial or other continuous display (see, e.g., the continuous signal recorded on the ECG strip shown in Figure 17.4).

The computers with which we work are **digital computers**. A digital computer stores and processes values in discrete values taken at discrete points and at discrete times. Before computer processing is possible, analog signals must be converted to digital units. The conversion process is called **analog-to-digital conversion (ADC)**. You can think of ADC as *sampling* and *rounding*—the continuous value is observed (sampled) at some instant and is rounded to the nearest discrete unit (Figure 5.14). You need 1 bit to distinguish between two levels (e.g., on or off); if you wish to discriminate among four levels, you need 2 bits (because $2^2=4$), and so on.

Two parameters determine how closely the digital data represent the original analog signal: the precision with which the signal is recorded and the frequency with which the signal is sampled. The **precision** is the degree to which a digital estimate of a signal matches the actual analog value. The number of bits used to encode the digital estimate and their correctness determines precision; the more bits, the greater the number of lev-els that can be distinguished. Precision also is limited by the accuracy of the equipment that converts and transmits the signal. Ranging and calibration of the instruments, either manually or automatically, is necessary for signals to be represented with as much accuracy as possible. Improper ranging will result in loss of information. For example, a change in a signal that varies between 0.1 and 0.2 volts will be undetectable if the instrument has been set to record changes between −2.0 and 2.0 in 0.5-volt increments (Figure 5.15 shows another example of improper ranging).

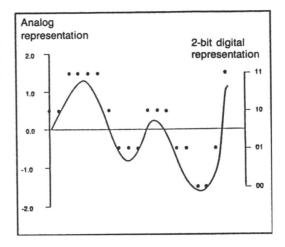

Figure 5.14. Analog-to-digital conversion (ADC). ADC is a technique for transforming continuous-valued signals to discrete values. In this example, each sampled value is converted to one of four discrete levels (represented by 2 bits).

The **sampling rate** is the second parameter that affects the correspondence between an analog signal and its digital representation. A sampling rate that is too low relative to the rate with which a signal changes value will produce a poor representation (Figure 5.16). On the other hand, oversampling increases the expense of processing and storing the data. As a general rule, you need to sample at least twice as frequently as the highest-frequency component that you need to observe in a signal. For instance, looking at an ECG, we find that the basic contraction repetition frequency is at most a few per second, but that the **QRS wave** within each beat (see Section 17.5) contains useful frequency components on the order of 150 cycles per second, i.e., the QRS signal rises and

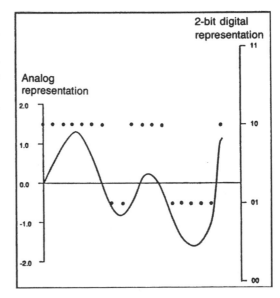

Figure 5.15. Effect on precision of ranging. The amplitude of signals from sensors must be ranged to account, for example, for individual patient variation. As illustrated here, the details of the signal may be lost if the signal is insufficiently amplified. On the other hand, overamplification will produce clipped peaks and troughs.

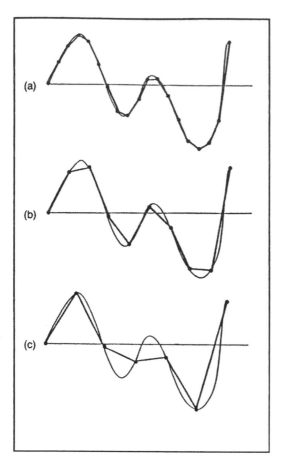

Figure 5.16. The greater the sampling rate is, the more closely the sampled observations will correspond to the underlying analog signal. The sampling rate in (a) is highest; that in (b) is lower; and that in (c) is the lowest. When the sampling rate is very low (as in c), the results of the analog-to-digital conversion (ADC) can be misleading. Note the degradation of the quality of the signal from (a) to (c). (Figure 17.5 illustrates the effects of varying sampling rate on the quality of an electrocardiogram (ECG) signal.)

falls within a much shorter interval than the basic heart beat. Thus, the ECG data-sampling rate should be at least 300 measurements per second. The rate calculated by doubling the highest frequency is called the **Nyquist frequency**. The ideas of sampling and signal estimation apply just as well to spatially varying signals (like images) with the temporal dimension replaced by one or more spatial dimensions.

Another aspect of signal quality is the amount of **noise** in the signal—the component of the acquired data that is not due to the specific phenomenon being measured. Primary sources of noise include random fluctuations in a signal detector or electrical or magnetic signals picked up from nearby devices and power lines. Once the signal has been obtained from a sensor, it must be transmitted to the computer. Often, the signal is sent through lines that pass near other equipment. En route, the analog signals are susceptible to electromagnetic interference. Inaccuracies in the sensors, poor contact between sensor and source (e.g., the patient), and disturbances from signals produced by processes other than the one being studied (e.g., respiration interferes with the ECG) are other common sources of noise.

Three techniques, often used in combination, minimize the amount of noise in a signal before its arrival in the computer:

1. *Shielding*, *isolation*, and *grounding* of cables and instruments carrying analog signals all reduce electrical interference. Often, two twisted wires are used to transmit the signal—one to carry the actual signal and the other to transmit the ground voltage at the sensor. At the destination, a differential amplifier measures the difference. Most types of interference affect both wires equally; thus, the difference should reflect the true signal. The use of glass fiber-optic cables, instead of copper wires, for signal transmission eliminates interference from electrical machinery, because optical signals are not affected by relatively slow electrical or magnetic fields.

2. For robust transmission over long distances, analog signals can be *converted* into a frequency-modulated representation. An FM signal represents changes of the signal as changes of frequency rather than of amplitude. **Frequency modulation (FM)** reduces noise greatly, because interference directly disturbs only the amplitude of the signal. As long as the interference does not create amplitude changes near the high carrier frequency, no loss of data will occur during transmission.

   Conversion of analog signals to digital form provides the most robust transmission. The closer to the source the conversion occurs, the more reliable the data become. Digital transmission of signals is inherently less noise-sensitive than is analog transmission: interference rarely is great enough to change a 1 value to a 0 value or vice versa. Furthermore, digital signals can be coded, permitting detection and correction of transmission errors. Placing a microprocessor near the signal source is now the most common way to achieve such a conversion. The development of **digital signal processing (DSP)** chips—also used for computer voice mail and other applications—facilitates such applications.

3. **Filtering algorithms** can be used to reduce the effect of noise. Usually, these algorithms are applied to the data once they has been stored in memory. A characteristic of noise is its relatively random pattern. Repetitive signals, such as an ECG, can be integrated over several cycles, thus reducing the effects of random noise. When the noise pattern differs from the signal pattern, Fourier analysis can be used to filter the signal; a signal is decomposed into its individual components, each with a distinct period and amplitude. (The article by Wiederhold and Clayton [1985] in the Suggested Readings explains *Fourier analysis* in greater detail.) Unwanted components of the signal are assumed to be noise and are eliminated. Some noise (such as the 60-cycle interference caused by a building's electrical circuitry) has a regular pattern. In this case, the portion of the signal that is known to be caused by interference can be filtered out.

Once the data have been acquired and cleaned up, they typically are processed to reduce their volume and to abstract information for use by interpretation programs. Often, the data are analyzed to extract important parameters, or features, of the signal—e.g., the duration or intensity of the ST segment of an ECG. The computer also can analyze the shape of the waveform by comparing one part of a repetitive signal to another, e.g., to detect ECG beat irregularities, or by comparing a waveform to models of known patterns, or templates. In **speech recognition**, the voice signals can be compared with stored profiles of spoken words. Further analysis is necessary to determine the meaning or importance of the signals—e.g., to allow automated ECG-based cardiac diagnosis or to respond properly to the words recognized in a spoken input.

5.3   Data and System Security

Medical records contain much information about us. These documents and databases include data ranging from height and weight measurements, blood pressures, and notes regarding bouts with the flu, cuts, or broken bones to information about topics such as fertility and abortions, emotional problems and psychiatric care, sexual behaviors, sexually transmitted diseases, human immunodeficiency virus (HIV) status, substance abuse, physical abuse, and genetic predisposition to diseases. Some data are generally considered to be mundane, others highly sensitive. Within the medical record, there is much information about which any given person may feel sensitive. As discussed in Chapter 10 health information is considered to be confidential, and access to such information must be controlled because disclosure could harm us, for example, by causing social embarrassment or prejudice, by affecting our insurability, or by limiting our ability to get and hold a job. Medical data also must be protected against loss. If we are to depend on electronic medical records for care, they must be available whenever and wherever we need care, and the information that they contain must be accurate and up to date. Orders for tests or treatments must be validated to ensure that they are issued by authorized providers. The records must also support administrative review and provide a basis for legal accountability. These requirements touch on three separate concepts involved in protecting health care information.

Privacy refers to the desire of a person to control disclosure of personal health and other information. **Confidentiality** applies to information—in this context, the ability of a person to control the release of his or her personal health information to a care provider or information custodian under an agreement that limits the further release or use of that information. **Security** is the protection of privacy and confidentiality through a collection of policies, procedures, and safeguards. Security measures enable an organization to maintain the integrity and availability of information systems and to control access to these systems' contents. Health privacy and confidentiality are discussed further in Chapter 10.

Concerns about, and methods to provide, security are part of most computer systems, but health care systems are distinguished by having especially complex considerations for the use and release of information. In general, the security steps taken in a health care information system serve five key functions (National Research Council, 1997):

1. **Availability** ensures that accurate and up-to-date information is available when needed at appropriate places.
2. **Accountability** helps to ensure that users are responsible for their access to, and use of, information based on a documented need and right to know.
3. **Perimeter** definition allows the system to control the boundaries of trusted access to an information system, both physically and logically.

4. **Role-limited access** enables access for personnel to only that information essential to the performance of their jobs and limits the real or perceived temptation to access information beyond a legitimate need.
5. **Comprehensibility and control** ensures that record owners, data stewards, and patients can understand and have effective control over appropriate aspects of information confidentiality and access.

The primary approach to ensuring availability is to protect against loss of data by redundancy—performing regular system backups. Because hardware and software systems will never be perfectly reliable, information of long-term value is copied onto archival storage, and copies are kept at remote sites to protect the data in case of disaster. For short-term protection, data can be written on duplicate storage devices. If one of the storage devices is attached to a remote processor, additional protection is conferred. Critical medical systems must be prepared to operate even during environmental disasters. Therefore, it is also important to provide secure housing and alternative power sources for CPUs, storage devices, network equipment, etc. It is also essential to maintain the integrity of the information system software to ensure availability. Backup copies provide a degree of protection against software failures; if a new version of a program damages the system's database, the backups allow operators to roll back to the earlier version of the software and database contents.

Unauthorized software changes—e.g., in the form of **viruses** or **worms**—are also a threat. A virus may be attached to an innocuous program or data file, and, when that program is executed or data file is opened, several actions take place:

1. The viral code copies itself into other files residing in the computer.
2. It attaches these files to outgoing messages, to spread itself to other computers.
3. The virus may collect email addresses to further distribute its copies.
4. The virus may install other programs to destroy or modify other files, often to escape detection.
5. A program installed by a virus may record keystrokes with passwords or other sensitive information, or perform other dilaterious actions.

A software virus causes havoc with computer operations, even if it does not do disabling damage, by disturbing operations and system access and by producing large amounts of Internet traffic as it repeatedly distributes itself. To protect against viruses, all programs loaded onto the system should be checked against known viral codes and for unexpected changes in size or configuration. It is not always obvious that a virus program has been imported. For example, a word-processing document may include macros that help in formatting the document. Such a macro can also include viral codes, however, so the document can be infected. Spreadsheets, graphical presentations, and so on are also subject to infection by viruses.

Accountability for use of medical data can be promoted both by surveillance and by technical controls. Most people working in a medical environment are highly ethical. In addition, knowledge that access to, and use of, data records are being watched, through scanning of access **audit trails**, serves as a strong impediment to abuse.

Technical means to ensure accountability include two additional functions: *authentication* and *authorization*.

1. The user is **authenticated** through a positive and unique identification process, such as name and password combination.
2. The authenticated user is **authorized** within the system to perform only certain actions appropriate to his or her role in the health care system—e.g., to search through certain medical records of only patients under his or her care.

Authentication and authorization can be performed most easily within an individual computer system, but, because most institutions operate multiple computers, it is necessary to coordinate these access controls consistently across all the systems. Enterprise-wide access-control standards and systems are available and are being deployed now much more extensively than even a few years ago.

Perimeter definition requires that you know who your users are and how they are accessing the information system. For health care providers within a small physician practice, physical access can be provided with a minimum of hassle using simple name and password combinations. If a clinician is traveling or at home and needs remote access to a medical record, however, greater care must be taken to ensure that the person is who he or she claims to be and that communications containing sensitive information are not observed inappropriately. But where is the boundary for being considered a trusted insider? Careful control of where the network runs and how users get outside access is necessary. Most organizations install a firewall to define the boundary: all sharable computers of the institution are located within the firewall. Anyone who attempts to access a shared system from the outside must first pass through the firewall, where strong authentication and protocol access controls are in place. Having passed this authentication step, the user can then access enabled services within the **firewall** (still limited by the applicable authorization controls). Even with a firewall in place, it is important for enterprise system administrators to monitor and ensure that the firewall is not bypassed—e.g., a malicious intruder could install a modem on an inside telephone line, install or use surreptitiously a wireless base station, or load unauthorized software. **Virtual Private Network (VPN)** technologies offer a powerful way to let bona fide users access information resources remotely. Using a client–server approach, an encrypted communication link is negotiated between the user's client machine and an enterprise server. This approach protects all communications and uses strong authentication to identify the user. No matter how secure the connection is, however, sound security ultimately depends on responsible users and care that increasingly portable computers (laptops, tablets, or handheld devices) are not lost or stolen so that their contents are accessible by unauthorized people.

Strong authentication and authorization controls depend on cryptographic technologies. **Cryptographic encoding** is a primary tool for protecting data that are stored and are transmitted over communication lines. Two kinds of cryptography are in common use— secret-key cryptography and public-key cryptography. In **secret-key cryptography**, the same key is used to encrypt and to decrypt information. Thus, the key must be kept secret, known to only the sender and intended receiver of information. In **public-key**

cryptography, two keys are used, one to encrypt the information and a second to decrypt it. Because two keys are involved, only one need be kept secret. The other one can be made publicly available. This arrangement leads to important services in addition to the exchange of sensitive information, such as digital signatures (to certify authorship), content validation (to prove that the contents of a message have not been changed), and nonrepudiation (to ensure that an order or payment for goods received cannot be disclaimed). Under either scheme, once data are encrypted, a key is needed to decode and make the information legible and suitable for processing.

Keys of longer length provide more security, because they are harder to guess. Because powerful computers can help intruders to test millions of candidate keys rapidly, single-layer encryption with keys of 56-bit length (the length prescribed by the 1975 **Data Encryption Standard (DES)**) are no longer considered secure, and keys of 128 bits are routine. If a key is lost, the information encrypted with the key is effectively lost as well. If a key is stolen, or if too many copies of the key exist for them to be tracked, unauthorized people may gain access to information. Holding the keys in **escrow** by a trusted party can provide some protection against loss.

Cryptographic tools can be used to control authorization as well. The authorization information may be encoded as digital **certificates**, which then can be validated with a certification authority and checked by the services so that the services do not need to check the authorizations themselves. Centralizing authentication and authorization functions simplifies the coordination of access control, allows for rapid revocation of privileges as needed, and reduces the possibility of an intruder finding holes in the system. A central authentication or authorization server must itself be guarded and managed with extreme care, however, so that enterprise-wide access-control information is not stolen.

Role-limited access control is based on extensions of authorization schemes. Even when overall system access has been authorized and is protected, further checks must be made to control access to specific data within the record. A medical record is most often not partitioned according to external access criteria, and the many different collaborators in health care all have diverse needs for, and thus rights to, the information collected in the medical record. Examples of valid access privileges include the following:

- *Patients*: the contents of their own medical records
- *Community physicians*: records of their patients
- *Specialty physicians*: records of patients referred for consultations
- *Public health agencies*: incidences of communicable diseases
- *Medical researchers*: anonymous records or summarization of data for patient groups approved by an **Institutional Review Board (IRB)**.
- *Billing clerks*: records of services, with supporting clinical documentation as required by insurance companies
- *Insurance payers*: justifications of charges

Different types of information kept in medical records have different rules for release, as determined by state and federal law (such as provisions of the new Health Insurance Portability and Accountability Act (HIPAA); see Chapter 7) and as set by institutional policy following legal and ethical considerations. For instance, the medical record of a patient who has heart problems might include notations that the patient also had a positive HIV test result, which should not be revealed to health services researchers conducting an unrelated outcomes study. Based on institutional policy, such notations might be masked before release of records for research purposes. Depending on the study design, the patients' names and other identifying information might also be masked.

To protect the confidentiality of medical records against inappropriate release to collaborators, the records should be inspected before release, but such checking requires more resources than most health care institutions are able to devote. Increasingly, under HIPAA requirements, resources are being devoted to system security and ensuring confidentiality of health care data; often, however, such resources are used to resolve problems after a violation is reported (National Research Council, 1997). Even minimal encryption is rarely used because of the awkwardness of current tools for handling the keys and accessing the data. To respond to these new requirements, we need better, easier to use, and more transparent tools to protect privacy and the confidentiality of health information (Sweeney, 1996; Wiederhold et al., 1996).

5.4 Summary

As we have discussed in this chapter, the synthesis of large-scale information systems is accomplished through the careful construction of hierarchies of hardware and software. Each successive layer is more abstract and hides many of the details of the preceding layer. Simple methods for storing and manipulating data ultimately produce complex information systems that have powerful capabilities. Communication links that connect local and remote computers in arbitrary configurations, and the security mechanisms that span these systems, transcend the basic hardware and software hierarchies. Thus, without worrying about the technical details, users can access a wealth of computational resources and can perform complex information management tasks, such as storing and retrieving, communicating, and processing information.

Suggested Readings

Garcia-Molina H., Ullman J.D., Widom J.D. (2002). *Database Systems: The Complete Book.* Englewood Cliffs, NJ: Prentice-Hall.
The first half of the book provides in-depth coverage of databases from the point of view of the database designer, user, and application programmer. It covers the latest database standards SQL:1999, SQL/PSM, SQL/CLI, JDBC, ODL, and XML, with broader coverage of SQL than most other texts. The second half of the book provides in-depth coverage of databases from the point of view of the DBMS implementer. It focuses on storage structures, query processing, and transaction management. The book covers the main techniques in these areas with broader coverage of query optimization than most other texts, along with advanced topics including multidimensional and bitmap indexes, distributed transactions, and information-integration techniques.

Hennessy J.L., Patterson D.A. (1996). *Computer Architecture: A Quantitative Approach* (2nd ed.). San Francisco: Morgan Kaufmann.
This technical book provides an in-depth explanation of the physical and conceptual underpinnings of computer hardware and its operation. It is suitable for technically oriented readers who want to understand the details of computer architecture.

McDonald C.J. (Ed.). (1987). *Images, Signals, and Devices* (M.D. Computing: Benchmark Papers). New York: Springer-Verlag.
The second in a series of Benchmark Papers from M.D. Computing, this volume introduces the use of computers in bioengineering. It contains articles on imaging and monitoring, including overviews of technologies such as computed tomography.

McDonald C.J. (Ed.). (1987). *Tutorials* (M.D. Computing: Benchmark Papers). New York: Springer-Verlag.
The third in a series of Benchmark Papers, this volume contains 17 tutorials originally published in M.D. Computing, including articles on computer hardware, local-area networks, operating systems, and programming languages. The collection will be of interest to computing novices who wish to understand how computers work or who would like to learn elementary programming skills.

National Research Council. (1997). *For the Record: Protecting Electronic Health Information.* Washington, DC: National Academy Press.
This report documents an extensive study of current security practices in US health care settings and recommends significant changes. It sets guidelines for policies, technical protections, and legal standards for acceptable access to, and use of, health care information. It is well suited for lay, medical, and technical readers who are interested in an overview of this complex topic.

Tanenbaum A. (1996). *Computer Networks* (3rd ed.). Englewood Cliffs, NJ: Prentice-Hall.
The heavily revised edition of a classic textbook on computer communications, this book is well organized, clearly written, and easy to understand. The introductory chapter describes network architectures and the International Standards Organization's Open Systems Interconnection (OSI) reference model. Each of the remaining chapters discusses in detail a layer of the OSI model.

Wiederhold G. (1981). *Databases for Health Care.* New York: Springer-Verlag.
This book uses a health care perspective to introduce the concepts of database technology. Although dated in some respects, the book describes the structures and functions of databases and discusses the scientific and operational issues associated with their use, including the problems of missing data and the conflict between data sharing and data confidentiality.

Wiederhold G., Clayton P.D. (1985). *Processing biological data in real time. M.D. Computing,* 2(6):16–25.
This article discusses the principles and problems of acquiring and processing biological data in real time. It covers much of the material discussed in the signal-processing section of this chapter and it provides more detailed explanations of analog-to-digital conversion and Fourier analysis.

Questions for Discussion

1. Why do computer systems use magnetic disks to store data and programs rather than keeping the latter in main memory where they could be accessed much more quickly?

2. What are four considerations in deciding whether to keep data in active versus archival storage?
3. Explain how an operating system insulates users from hardware changes.
4. Discuss the advantages and disadvantages of individual workstations linked in a LAN versus shared access to mainframe computers.
5. Define the terms data independence and database schema. How do database management systems facilitate data independence?
6. Why have so many different computer languages been developed?
7. How can you prevent inappropriate access to electronic medical record information? How can you detect that such inappropriate access might have occurred?

6
System Design and Engineering in Health Care

GIO WIEDERHOLD AND EDWARD H. SHORTLIFFE

After reading this chapter, you should know the answers to these questions:

- What key functions do medical computer systems perform?
- Why is communication between medical personnel and computing personnel crucial to the successful design and implementation of a health information system?
- What are the trade-offs between purchasing a turnkey system and developing a custom-designed system?
- What resources are available remotely for medical computer systems?
- What design features most heavily affect a system's acceptance by health professionals?
- Why do systems in health care, once implemented and installed successfully, have a long lifetime?

6.1 How Can a Computer System Help in Health Care?

In Chapter 5, we introduced basic concepts related to computer and communications hardware and software. In this chapter, we show how information systems created from these components can be used by health professionals to support health care delivery. We describe the basic functions performed by health information systems and discuss important considerations in system design, implementation, and evaluation. You should keep these concepts in mind as you read about the various medical computing applications in the chapters that follow. Think about how each system meets (or fails to meet) the needs of its users and about the practical reasons why certain systems have been accepted for routine use in patient care whereas other systems have failed to make the transition from the research environment to the real world.

At a minimum, a system's success depends on the selection of adequate hardware and sufficient data-storage, and data-transmission capabilities. More crucial is the software, which defines how data are obtained, organized, and processed to yield information. The technical issues related to specific hardware and software choices are beyond the scope of this book. Instead, we provide a general introduction to practical issues in the design and implementation of systems. In particular, we stress the importance of designing systems that not only meet users' requirements for information but also fit smoothly into users' everyday routines. There are many types of users of a health care information system, and often it is necessary to consider each, one at a time.

There are *health care professionals*, for whom the quality of the results is paramount, but who are invariably pressed for time. There are *administrators*, who have to make personnel and financial decisions that are crucial to institutional well-being. There are *clerical personnel*, who enter and retrieve much of the data. Some systems also provide for direct interaction by *patients*. In addition, there are *operational personnel* who maintain the system and ensure its reliability. Initially there are professional system *designers*, *implementers*, and *integrators*, but their numbers and availability decrease as the systems move into routine operation. Before the system is turned over to users, there must be adequate documentation and training. For instance, clerks require clear procedures for their interaction with the system so that errors are minimized. A central theme of this chapter is the importance of communication between health care and computing professionals in defining problems and developing solutions that can be implemented within an institution. With this perspective, we explore the factors that create a need for automation and discuss important considerations in the design, development, and evaluation of health information systems.

A problem in moving systems from their originators, the computing experts, to health care personnel is that their education and experience has too often emphasized different scientific principles. The formality of computing is evidenced in rules that can be applied to many instances, and hence provide consistency and efficiency. Practice in health care focuses on individual instances, one at a time. Some of those will require deep and unique considerations. Much learning in health care stems from examples, and flexibility is expected when a new case differs in some crucial ways. For a computing expert, adapting to a very flexible approach can lead to an explosion of rules, and impossibly complex software. One role of this book is to help in mutual understanding of the isues on both sides, leading to an appreciation of the value of obtaining training and expertise at the intersection of biomedicine and computing.

6.1.1   What Is a System?

Until now, we have referred informally to *health information systems* and *computer systems*. What do we mean when we refer to a *system*? In the most general sense, a **system** is an organized set of procedures for accomplishing a task. It is described in terms of (1) the problem to be solved; (2) the data and knowledge required to address the problem; and (3) the internal process for transforming the available **input** into the desired **output** (Figure 6.1). When we talk about systems in this book, we usually mean *computer-based* (or just *computer*) systems. A **computer system** combines both manual and automated processes; people and machines work in concert to manage and use information. A computer system has these components:

- **Hardware**: The physical equipment, including processing units (e.g., the central processing unit (CPU)), data-storage devices, comunication equipment, terminals, and printers
- **Software**: The computer programs that direct the hardware to carry out the automated processes—i.e., to respond to user requests and schedules, to process input data, to store some data for long periods, and to communicate informative results to the users; at times the software will prompt the users to perform manual processes

Figure 6.1. A computer system applies locally defined and general procedures to produce results from new input data, from stored data, and from information obtained from remote external sources.

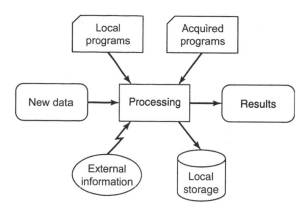

- **Customers**: The users who interact with the software and hardware of the system, issue requests, and use the results or forward them to others; there will be other users who are concerned with providing input, system operations, backup, and maintenance

The role of a computer is, broadly speaking, the conversion of data into information. Every piece of data must be supplied by a person, by another computer system, or by data collection equipment, as seen in patient monitoring (see Chapter 17). Information that is output is delivered to health care professionals or becomes input to another computer system. In other words, a medical computer system is a module within the overall health care delivery system.

The overall health care system not only determines the need for the computer system (e.g., which data must be processed and which reports must be generated) but also the requirements for the system's operation (e.g., the degree of reliability and responsiveness to requests for information). Acquisition and operation of a computer system has implications for the organization of an institution. Who controls the information? Who is responsible for the accuracy of the data? How will the system be financed?

The installation of a computer system has sociological consequences as well. The introduction of a new system alters the work routines of health care workers. Furthermore, it may affect the traditional roles of health care workers and the existing relationships among groups of individuals—e.g., between physicians and nurses, between nurses and patients, and between physicians and patients. Important ethical and legal questions that arise include the confidentiality of patient information, the appropriate role of computers in patient care (especially in medical decision making), and the responsibility of developers and users for ensuring the correct operation of the system (see Chapter 10). Although the technical challenges in system development must be met, organizational factors are crucial determinants of the success of a computer system within the institution. These factors can differ greatly among institutions and can make the transfer of a well-functioning system to another site difficult.

6.1.2   *Functions of a Computer System*

Computers have been used in every aspect of health care delivery, from the simple processing of business data, to the collection and interpretation of physiological data, to the education of physicians and nurses. Each chapter in Unit II of this book describes an important area for the application of computers in biomedicine. The unique characteristics of each problem area create special requirements for system builders to address. The motivation for investing in these applications, however, is the computer's ability to help health professionals in some aspect of information management. We identify eight topics that define the range of basic functions that may be provided by medical computer systems:

1. Data acquisition and presentation
2. Record keeping and access
3. Communication and integration of information
4. Surveillance
5. Information storage and retrieval
6. Data analysis
7. Decision support
8. Education

These functions are detailed in the discussions of each of the types of health care and biomedical applications addressed in Chapters 12 through 22. Any system will assist its users with several of those functions. In hospital information systems (Chapter 13) most of these functions will be performed, but typically within multiple departments by a variety of computing systems. Those systems must, in turn, communicate with each other (Webster, 1988). Although decision support is a primary function for only two categories of applications, essentially all uses of computers in medicine will support decision making by the variety of staff that uses them.

Data Acquisition

The amount of data needed to describe the state of even a single person is huge. Health professionals require assistance with data acquisition to deal with the data that must be collected and processed.. One of the first uses of computers in a medical setting was the automatic analysis of specimens of blood and other body fluids by instruments that measure chemical concentrations or that count cells and organisms. These systems then present the results of such analyses in a clear form. Signalling when results are outside the expected range alerts the health care staff. Computer-based patient-monitoring systems that collect physiological data directly from patients were another early application of computing technology (see Chapter 17). Such systems ensure that vital signs, electrocardiograms (ECGs), and other indicators of patient status are measured frequently and consistently. More recently, researchers have developed medical imaging applications as described in Chapters 9 and 18, including computed tomography (CT), magnetic resonance imaging (MRI), and digital subtraction angiography. The calculations for these computationally intensive applications cannot be performed manually; the computers collect and manipulate millions of individual observations.

Early computer-based medical instruments and measurement devices that perform data acquisition provided their results only to human beings. Today, most instruments supply data directly into the patient record, although the interfaces are still awkward and poorly standardized (see Chapter 7). Computer-based systems that acquire information, such as one's health history, from patients are also data-acquisition systems; they free health professionals from the need to collect and enter routine demographic and history information.

Record Keeping

Given the data-intensive nature of health care delivery, it is no surprise that collecting and keeping records is a primary function of many medical computer systems. Computers are well suited to performing tedious and repetitive data-processing tasks, such as collecting and tabulating data, combining related data, and formatting and producing reports. They are particularly useful for processing large volumes of data. Automated billing is a natural application of computers in health care settings, and was typically the first component installed when a hospital, clinic, or private practice decided to use computer technology. Unfortunately, the level of documentation required for performing billing is inadequote for treating patients.

Individual departments within a hospital also have their own computer systems and maintain their own records. For instance, clinical laboratories use computer-based information systems to keep track of orders and specimens and to report test results; most pharmacy and radiology departments use computers to perform analogous functions. Their systems may connect to outside services (e.g., pharmacy systems are typically connected to one or more drug distributors) so that ordering and delivery are rapid and local inventories can be kept small. By automating processing in areas such as these, health care facilities are able to speed up services, reduce direct labor costs, and minimize the number of errors.

Computer systems acquired by hospital departments are often obtained from specialized vendors. Such vendors contribute their experience in serving clinical laboratories, pharmacy operations, or other areas. They will supply their customers with updates when capabilities improve or regulations change. Sometimes the services may actually be operated remotely at a vendor's site. Unfortunately, this diversity makes it difficult to integrate the information from the disparate systems into a coherent whole, a problem addressed in Chapter 13.

Communication and Integration

In hospitals and other large-scale health care institutions, myriad data are collected by multiple health professionals who work in a variety of settings; each patient receives care from a host of providers—nurses, physicians, technicians, pharmacists, and so on. Communication among the members of the team is essential for effective health care delivery. Data must be available to decision makers when and where they are needed, independent of when and where they were obtained. Computers help by storing, transmitting, sharing, and displaying those data. As we describe in Chapters 2 and 12, the patient record is the primary vehicle for communication of clinical information. The limitation of the traditional paper-based patient record is the concentration of information in a single location, which prohibits simultaneous entry and access by multiple people. Hospital information systems (HISs) (see Chapter 13) and EHR systems (Chapter 12) allow distribution of many activities, such as admission, appointment, and resource scheduling; review of laboratory test results; and inspection of patient records to the appropriate sites.

Information necessary for specific decision-making tasks is rarely available within a single computer system. Clinical systems are installed and updated when needed, available, and affordable. Furthermore, in many institutions, inpatient, outpatient, and financial activities are supported by separate organizational units. Patient treatment decisions require inpatient and outpatient information. Hospital administrators must integrate clinical and financial information to analyze costs and to evaluate the efficiency of health care delivery. Similarly, clinicians may need to review data collected at other health care institutions, or they may wish to consult published biomedical information. Communication networks that permit sharing of information among independent computers and geographically distributed sites are now widely available. Actual integration of the information they contain requires additional software, adherence to standards, and operational staff to keep it all working as technology and systems evolve.

Surveillance

Timely reactions to data are crucial for quality in health care, especially when a patient has unexpected problems. Data overload, created by the ubiquity of information technology, is as detrimental to good decision making as is data insufficiency. Data indicating a need for action may be available but are easily overlooked by overloaded health professionals. Surveillance and monitoring systems can help people cope with all the data relevant to patient management by calling attention to significant events or situations, for example, by reminding doctors of the need to order screening tests and other preventive measures (see Chapters 12 and 20) or by warning them when a dangerous event or constellation of events has occurred.

Laboratory systems routinely identify and flag abnormal test results. Similarly, when patient-monitoring systems in intensive care units detect abnormalities in patient status, they sound alarms to alert nurses and physicians to potentially dangerous changes. A pharmacy system that maintains computer-based drug-profile records for patients can screen incoming drug orders and warn physicians who order a drug that interacts with another drug that the patient is receiving or a drug to which the patient has a known allergy or sensitivity. By correlating data from multiple sources, an integrated clinical information system can monitor for complex events, such as interactions among patient diagnosis, drug regimen, and physiological status (indicated by laboratory test results). For instance, a change in cholesterol level can be due to prednisone given to an arthritic patient and may not indicate a dietary problem.

Surveillance also extends beyond the health care setting. Appearances of new infectious diseases, unexpected reactions to new medications, and environmental effects should be monitored. Thus the issue of data integration has a national or global scope (see the discussion of the National Health Information Infrastructure in Chapter 1 and Chapter 15 that deals with public health informatics).

Information Storage and Retrieval

Storage and retrieval of information is essential to all computer systems. Storage enables sharing of information with people who are not available at the same time. Storage must be well organized and indexed so that information recorded in an EHR system can be easily retrieved. Here the variety of users must be considered. Getting cogent recent information about a patient entering the office differs from the needs that a researcher will have in accessing the same data. The query interfaces provided by EHR and clinical research systems assist researchers in retrieving pertinent records from the huge volume of patient information. As we discuss in Chapter 19, bibliographic retrieval systems are an essential component of health information services.

Data Analysis

Raw data as acquired by computer systems are detailed and voluminous. Data analysis systems must aid decision makers by reducing and presenting the intrinsic information in a clear and understandable form. Presentations should use graphs to facilitate trend analysis and compute secondary parameters (means, standard deviations, rates of change, etc.) to help spot abnormalities. Clinical research systems have modules for performing powerful statistical analyses over large sets of patient data. The researcher, however, should have insight into the methods being used. For clinicians, graphics are essential for interpretation of data and results.

Decision Support

In the end, all the functions described here support decision making by health professionals. The distinction between decision-support systems and systems that monitor events and issue alerts is not clear-cut; the two differ primarily in the degree to which they interpret data and recommend patient-specific action. Perhaps the best-known examples of decision-support systems are the clinical consultation systems or event-monitoring systems that use population statistics or encode expert knowledge to assist physicians in diagnosis and treatment planning (see Chapter 20). Similarly, some nursing information systems help nurses to evaluate the needs of individual patients and thus assist their users in allocating nursing resources. In Chapter 20, we discuss computer-based systems that use algorithmic, statistical, or artificial-intelligence (AI) techniques to provide advice about patient care.

Education

Rapid growth in biomedical knowledge and in the complexity of therapy management has produced an environment in which students cannot learn all they need to know during training—they must learn how to learn and must make a lifelong educational commitment. Today, physicians and nurses have available a broad selection of computer programs designed to help them to acquire and maintain the knowledge and skills they need to care for their patients. The simplest programs are of the drill-and-practice variety; more sophisticated programs can help students to learn complex problem-solving skills, such as diagnosis and therapy management (see Chapter 21). Computer-aided instruction provides a valuable means by which health professionals can gain experience and learn from mistakes without endangering actual patients. Clinical decision-support systems and other systems that can explain their recommendations also perform an educational function. In the context of real patient cases, they can suggest actions and explain the reasons for those actions.

6.1.3 *Identifying and Analyzing the Need for a Computer System*

The first step in the introduction of computers into health care settings is to identify a clinical, administrative, or research need—an inadequacy or inefficiency in the delivery of health care. The decision to acquire or replace a computer system may be motivated by a desire to improve the *quality* of care, to lower the *cost* of care, to improve *access* to care, or to collect the information needed to document and evaluate the health care delivery process itself. A new computer-based system may correct defects in the old system, for example, by reading bar codes on containers to reduce the level of drug-administration errors. Other computer systems can provide functions not possible with a manual system—e.g., allow integrated access to patient records. In some cases, a computer system simply duplicates the capabilities of the prior system but at lower maintenance cost.

The sophistication of medical computer systems has increased substantially since their inception, when computers were first applied to the problems of health care delivery. The developers of new systems make progress by building on lessons learned from past operations, emulating the successes, and trying to avoid the mistakes of earlier systems. As the discipline has matured, researchers and users have gained a better understanding of the types of problems computer systems can solve and the requirements for system success.

Clearly, computers facilitate many aspects of health care delivery. Operating a computer system, however, is not a panacea; an information system cannot aid in decision making, for example, if critical information is not available or if health professionals do not know how to apply the information once they have it. Similarly, a computer will not transform a poorly organized process into one that operates smoothly—automating a defective approach makes matters worse, not better.

Communication with other system components is today viewed as crucial. Performing local tasks in a unit of the hospital better but not communicating the results with other units just creates more work and delays. A careful workflow analysis before attempting computer-based improvements allows system developers and health care personnel to clarify the requirements for change and may identify correctable deficiencies in current systems (Leymann and Roller, 2000).

Ideally, we first recognize a *need*, and then search for techniques to address it. At times, this logical sequence has been inverted; the development of new hardware or computing methodologies may motivate system developers and marketeers to apply innovative technology in a medical context. Development driven by technology often fails to deal with clinical realities. The adoption of any new system requires users to learn and to adjust to a new routine, and, given the time constraints under which health professionals operate, users may be unwilling to discard a working system unless they perceive a clear reason to change.

Once health professionals have recognized a need for a computer system, the next step is to identify the function or combination of functions that fulfills that need. There usually are many possible solutions to a broadly defined problem. A precise definition of the problem narrows the range of alternative solutions. Is the problem one of access to data? Do health professionals have the data they need to make informed decisions? Is the problem an inability to analyze and interpret data? As we explained in the previous section, computer systems perform a variety of functions, ranging from simply displaying relevant information to aiding actively in complex decision making.

The natural temptation is to minimize this important first step of problem definition and to move directly to the solution phase. This approach is dangerous, however, and it may result in the development of an unacceptable system. Consider, for example, a situation in which physicians desire improved access to patient data. Health care personnel may seek assistance from technologists to implement a specific technical solution to the perceived problem. They may request that each patient's complete medical history be stored in a computer. When that is achieved, however, they may find that the relevant information is hidden among the many irrelevant data and is more tedious to access than before. If the system developers had analyzed the problem carefully, they might have realized that the raw medical data simply were too voluminous to be informative. A more appropriate solution would include integration, filtering and ranking so that only easy-to-read summaries with essential information are displayed.

The development of information systems requires a substantial commitment in terms of labor, money, and time. Once health professionals have clearly defined the need for a system, the question of value inevitably arises. Scarce resources devoted to this project are unavailable for other potential projects. The administrator of a health care institution who works within a fixed budget must decide whether to invest in a computer system or to spend the money in other ways—e.g., an institutional decision maker may prefer to purchase new laboratory equipment or to expand the neonatal intensive care unit.

To assess the value of a health information system relative to competing needs, the administrator must estimate the costs and benefits attributable to the system. Some benefits are relatively easy to quantify. If admission clerks can process each admission twice as fast using the new system as they could using the old one, an institution needs fewer clerks to perform the same amount of work—a measurable savings in labor costs. Many benefits, however, are less easily quantified. For example, how can we quantify the benefits due to reduced patient mortality and morbidity, increased patient satisfaction, or reduced stress and fatigue among the staff? In Chapter 11 we introduce cost–benefit and cost-effectiveness analyses—two methodologies that can help decision makers to assess the worth of a computer system relative to alternative investments.

6.2   Understanding Health Information Systems

Whether they aim to produce a comprehensive information system for a 500-bed hospital, a patient record system for a small clinic, or a simple billing program for a physician in private practice, system developers should follow the same basic process. In the initial phase of system development, the primary task is to define the problem. The goal is to produce a clear and detailed statement of the system's objectives—i.e., what the system will do and what conditions it must meet if it is to be accepted by its users. The systems analysts also must establish the relative priorities of multiple, sometimes conflicting, goals—e.g., low cost, high efficiency, easy maintenance, and high reliability.

We frame the discussion of this section in terms of institutional system planning and development. Many of the same issues, however, apply to the development of smaller systems as well, albeit on a correspondingly smaller scale of complexity. Since a variety of systems exist in this world, the first step is to assess the use of computers in similar settings. Creating a detailed list of candidate functions is the first task (Webster, 1988). These functions can then by ranked by local importance.

Ideally, a commercial system exists that provides all the essential functions. If there is none, priorities may be reviewed, and systems may be adapted or augmented. Excessive adaptations diminish the benefits of a commercial choice, since now maintenance responsibilities devolve onto the hospital or clinic. Sometimes it is necessary to design a system to handle new requirements and novel functions. After acquisition or development of a system, the next step is to establish the system within the organization. Major activities at this stage include training users, installing and testing the system, and, finally, evaluating and maintaining the operational system on an ongoing basis.

Maintenance is a demanding task. It invoves correcting errors, ongoing adaptions to growth, new hardware, new communication capabilities, new standards, and new professional regulations. Long-lived systems also require ongoing perfection of interfaces, performance, and linkages to other sources (Pigoski, 1997). Over the lifetime of a computer system these tasks exceed by a factor of two to five the original acquisition costs. Many software suppliers will provide most maintenance services for 15 to 30 percent of the purchase price annually. If those services are performed well, they are more than worth the price.

6.2.1   An Illustrative Case Study

In addition to identifying functional requirements, a **requirements analysis** must be sensitive to the varying needs and probable concerns of the system's intended users. These human aspects of computer system design often have been overlooked, and the results can be devastating. Consider, for example, the following hypothetical case, which embodies many of the issues that are the subject of this chapter.[1]

A major teaching hospital purchased and installed a large computer system that assists physicians with ordering drugs and laboratory tests, the clinical laboratories with reporting laboratory test results, head nurses with creating nursing schedules, and the admissions staff with monitoring hospital occupancy. Personnel access the system using workstations located in each nursing unit. There also are printers associated with each unit so that the computer can generate reports for the patient charts (which continue to be paper-based) and worksheets used by the hospital staff. This information system depends on a large, dedicated computer, which is housed in the hospital complex and is supported by several full-time personnel. It has modules to assist hospital staff with both administrative and clinical duties. The following four modules are the primary subsystems used in patient care.

1. *The pharmacy system*: With this component of the information system, physicians order drugs for their patients; the requests are displayed immediately in the hospital pharmacy. Pharmacists then fill the prescriptions and affix computer-printed labels to each bottle. The drugs are delivered to the ward by a pneumatic-tube system. The computer keeps a record of all drugs administered to each patient and warns physicians about possible drug interactions at the time that new prescriptions are ordered.
2. *The laboratory system*: With this component, physicians order laboratory tests for their patients. The requests are displayed in the clinical laboratory, and worksheets are created to assist laboratory personnel in planning blood-drawing schedules and performing tests. As soon as test results are available, health professionals can display them on the screen of any workstation, and paper summaries are printed on the wards for inclusion in the patients' charts.
3. *The bed-control system*: The admissions office of the hospital, in conjunction with the various ward administrators, uses this component to keep track of the location of patients within the hospital. When patients are transferred to another ward, the computer is notified so that physicians, telephone operators, and other personnel can locate them easily. The system also is used to identify patients whose discharge has been ordered; thus, the system aids the admissions office in planning bed assignments for new patients.
4. *The diagnosis system*: To help physicians reach correct diagnoses for their patients, this component provides a clinical consultation program. Physicians enter their patient's signs and symptoms and can combine them with laboratory test results and X-ray examination results. The system then suggests a list of likely diagnoses.

[1] This case study is adapted from Shortliffe E.H. (1984) Coming to terms with the computer. In Reiser S.J., Anbar M. (Eds.), *The Machine at the Bedside: Strategies for Using Technology in Patient Care* (pp. 235–239). Cambridge, UK: Cambridge University Press. It is used here with permission from Cambridge University Press.

Despite the new capabilities provided by the system, after 3 months of use it received mixed reviews about its effectiveness. Most of the people who raised concerns were involved in patient care. A consulting expert was called in to assess the computer system's strengths and weaknesses. She interviewed members of the hospital staff and noted their responses.

One nurse said: I like the system a lot. I found it hard to get used to at first (I never have been a very good typist), but once I got the hang of it, I found that it simplified much of my work. The worst problem has turned out to be dealing with doctors who don't like the system; when they get annoyed, they tend to take it out on us, even though we're using the system exactly as we've been trained to do. For instance, I can't log onto the computer as a physician to log verbal orders in someone else's name, and that makes some of the doctors furious. The only time I personally get annoyed with the computer is when I need to get some work done and the other nurses are using all the ward workstations. They ought to have a few more machines available.

One medical resident was less than enthusiastic about the new clinical system: I wish they'd rip the darn thing out! It is totally unrealistic in terms of the kinds of things it asks us to do or won't allow us to do. Did the guys who built it have any idea what it is like to practice medicine in a hospital like this? For example, the only way we used to be able to keep our morning ward rounds efficient was to bring the chart rack with us and to write orders at the bedside. With the new system, we have to keep sending someone back to the ward workstation to log orders for a patient. What's worse, they won't let the medical student order drugs, so we have to send an intern. Even the nurses aren't allowed to log orders in our name—something to do with the "legality" of having all orders entered by a licensed physician—but that was never a problem with paper order sheets as long as we eventually countersigned the orders. Some of the nursing staff are doing everything by the book now, and sometimes they seem to be obstructing efficiency rather than aiding it. And the designers were so hung up on patient confidentiality that we have a heck of a time cross-covering patients on other services at night. The computer won't let me write orders on any patient who isn't "known" to be mine, so I have to get the other physicians' passwords from them when they sign out to me at night. And things really fall apart when the machine goes down unexpectedly. Everything grinds to a halt, and we have to save our management plans on paper and transcribe them into the system when it finally comes up. I should add that the system always seems to be about three hours late in figuring out about patient transfers. I'm forever finding that the computer still thinks a patient is on the first floor when I know he's been transferred to the intensive care unit.

In addition, the "diagnosis system" is a joke. Sure, it can generate lists of diseases, but it doesn't really understand what the disease processes are, can't explain why it thinks one disease is more likely than another, and is totally unable to handle patients who have more than one simultaneous disease. I suppose the lists are useful as memory joggers, but I no longer even bother to use that part of the system.

And by the way, I still don't really know what all those options on the screen mean. We had a brief training session when they first installed the system, but now we're left to fend for ourselves. Only a couple of the house staff seem to know how to make the system do what they want reliably. What's the best part of the system? I guess it is the decrease in errors in orders for drugs and lab tests and the improved turnaround time on those orders—but I'm not sure the improvement is worth the hassle. How often do I use the system? As rarely as possible!

A hospital pharmacist said: The system has been a real boon to our pharmacy operation. Not only can we fill new orders promptly because of the improved communication but also the system prints labels for the bottles and has saved us the step of typing them ourselves. Our inventory control also is much improved; the system produces several useful reports that help us to anticipate shortages and to keep track of drugs that are about to expire. The worst thing about the system, from my point of view, is the effect it has had on our interaction with the medical staff. We used to spend some of our time consulting with the ward teams about drug interactions, for example. You know, we'd look up the relevant articles and report back at ward rounds the next day. Now our role as members of the ward teams has been reduced by the system's knowledge about drugs. Currently, a house officer finds out about a potential drug interaction at the moment she is ordering a treatment, and the machine even gives references to support the reported incompatibility.

One member of the hospital's computing staff expressed frustration: Frankly, I think the doctors have been too quick to complain about this system. It has been here for only three months, and we're still discovering problems that will take some time to address. What bothers me is the gut reaction many of them seem to have; they don't even want to give the system a chance. Every hospital is a little different, and it is unrealistic to expect any clinical system to be right for a new institution on the first day. There has to be a breaking-in period. We're trying hard to respond to the complaints we've heard through the grapevine. We hope that the doctors will be pleased when they see that their complaints are being attended to and new features are being introduced.

This example, although hypothetical, does not exaggerate the kinds of reactions that computer systems sometimes have evoked in clinical settings. Developers of real-world systems have encountered similar problems after introducing their systems into real clinical settings. This example was inspired in part by the experience of one of the authors (E.H. Shortliffe) with a pharmacy system that was implemented in several teaching wards of the hospital where he served his medical internship. The initial version of the system failed to account for key aspects of the way in which health professionals practiced medicine. All drug orders had to be entered into the computer, and, because the terminals were located at the nursing stations, physicians could no longer complete their orders at the bedside. They either had to return to the nursing station after seeing each patient or had to enter all the orders after completing patient rounds. Furthermore, physicians personally had to enter the orders. The system did not allow them to countersign orders entered by nurses or medical students. The inflexibility of the system forced physicians to alter their practice patterns. The physicians objected loudly, and the system was subsequently removed. Although the system was later redesigned to remedy the earlier problems, it was never fully reimplemented because of persistent negative bias caused by the failure of the earlier version.

In another instance, the introduction of a new blood bank system at a large institution instigated disputes between physicians and nurses over responsibility for the entry of blood orders. In this case, the system was designed to encourage direct order entry but also allowed nurses to enter orders. Given the option, physicians continued to write paper orders and relied on nurses for order entry. Nurses, however, balked at performing this task, which they perceived as being the physicians' responsibility. Even seemingly trivial matters can cause problems. At the same institution, for example, objection by surgeons was one factor in the decision to use passwords rather than machine-readable identification cards to control system access; surgeons typically do not carry personal belongings when wearing surgical garb and thus would have been unable to log onto the system (Gardner, 1989).

These cases help to emphasize the importance of responsiveness to detailed needs of the intended *users* and of awareness of different users' varying constraints and motivations when a system is intended to meet both clinical and administrative goals. The key considerations suggested by the scenario include (1) analyzing where the system is to fit into the existing workflow; (2) deciding what to purchase from a commercial system vendor and what to develop internally; (3) designing for the actual customers; (4) involving those customers throughout the development; and (5) planning for subsequent changes. We discuss these topics in detail in Section 6.3.

6.2.2   *Involving Customers During Development*

Although the central focus of this chapter is *computer*-based information systems, it is important to realize that people are the critical component of these systems (see Chapter 4). People identify the need for systems; people select, develop, implement, and evaluate the systems; and, eventually, people operate and maintain the systems. A successful system must take into account both the needs of the intended users and the constraints under which these users function.

Even the most perceptive and empathetic developer cannot anticipate all the needs of all types of customers. Thus, the success of a system depends on interaction between health and technical personnel as well as among the heath care professionals. Effective communication among the participants in designing a system, however, is potentially difficult because these people are likely to have widely varying background, education, experience, and styles of interaction. Appointing a wide variety of personnel to a large design committee is likely to be ineffective as well, because committees are best suited for forging compromise solutions, whereas computer systems can and should serve a precise set of objectives.

A major barrier to communication is attributable to a difference between the health care and more formal scientific paradigms. In Chapter 1, we discussed the ways in which clinical information differs from the information used in the basic sciences (recall the difference between low-level and high-level sciences discussed in Section 1.3), and we examined reasons why biomedical informatics differs from basic computer science. In medical practice, as in other human tasks, we expect that a person who can deal with a certain type of problem can, with little incremental effort, extrapolate to handle similar and related problems. In the formal mathematical sciences, however, the ability to solve problems can depend critically on what appear to be small, but fundamental differences in basic assumptions.

The rigor of the mathematical approach also is reflected in computer systems so that computer systems will never be as flexible as people are. Although it is easy to imagine that a computer program that deals with one class of problems embodies sufficient concepts to deal with other (seemingly) similar problems, the work required to adapt or extend the program often costs as much as the original development and sometimes much more. Occasionally, adaptation is impossible. For health care professionals the difficulty of altering some aspects of software is hard to appreciate, because these people interact mainly with human beings rather than with seemingly smart machines.

Empathy for the differences in the two approaches to problem solving can minimize certain problems. Health information specialists—people trained in both computer science and health science—can facilitate communication and mediate discussions. They can ease the process of specifying accurately and realistically the need for a system and of designing workable solutions to satisfy those needs. One objective of this book is to provide basic material for people who serve in this intermediary role.

6.3   Developing and Implementing Systems in Health Care

The initial task is to circumscribe what a new system in a health care setting should encompass. Will the new system replace all existing computing capabilities, or will it provide new functions, or will it replace some existing systems? If it replaces an existing system, the current functions being provided can be enumerated and the data requirements specified. For new functions additional data will be needed, and if some older functions can be omitted, the input requirements might actually be less. Sometimes a new system may replace parts of multiple existing processes, making the task of defining its functions and data requirements yet harder. Studying related services at other sites will help. Relying only on vendor presentations is risky. In Section 6.3.2 methods to chart those considerations are presented.

6.3.1   System Acquisition Alternatives

There are vendors willing to sell systems for any task that a health care institution may require. For most tasks some vendor will have a system already designed and ready to be adapted to your specifications. The actual functions and data requirements of a system acquired from a vendor may, however, differ from what was envisaged. The manner in which desired functions are provided will also differ among vendors. Demonstrations by vendors to customers can provide insights, and the feedback obtained may well change the expectations that were specified initially. Some desired features may turn out to be costly to implement and maintain, and compromises are likely.

Some required services can be obtained by contracting for them remotely. Searches for published information are best performed over the Internet (Chapter 19). Some services, such as managing supply inventories, may be jointly supported by in-house staff and external contractors. We address remote operations in Section 6.3.4.

For essential operations, a health care institution must control its own systems. We focus on the software requirements because the selection of hardware is primarily determined by the requirements that software imposes.

Commercial Off-the-Shelf Software

Much software is available off the shelf from commercial companies. The selection is widest for the more general needs, such as financial management—general ledger, accounts payable, and general accounts receivable. For health care institutions the selection is more limited or may require adaptation to the institution. For instance, financial receivables in health care—largely based on mixes of insurance, government, and private payments—have more complexity than standard business systems allow. Several software companies that serve the health care industry provide appropriate software. The major concern becomes ensuring smooth interaction among software packages obtained from different vendors. Following the emerging standards for remote services is helpful.

Once an organization has decided to acquire a new computer system, it faces the choice of buying a commercial system or building a system in-house. The primary trade-off between purchasing a **turnkey system**—a vendor-supplied system that requires only installation and "the turn of a key" to make it operational—and developing a **custom-designed system** is one of compatibility with the conventions in the institution versus expense, delay, and ongoing maintenance. Substantial new systems take years to design and develop. A vendor-supplied system usually is less expensive than is a custom-designed system, because the vendor can spread the costs of development and subsequent maintenance over multiple clients. A compromise is to custom-tailor a vendor system to the needs that are particular to one's institution, but the costs for changes not foreseen by the vendor will be disproportionally high. The maintenance costs for computer systems is on the order of 15 to 30 percent per year, and custom-tailoring greatly increases those costs. If an institution can find a commercial system that approximately meets its needs, it should purchase that system, even it has to change its own methods somewhat.

If no available commercial system for some function is adequate, the institution may choose to build its own system or to make do with the current system; the option of keeping the current system should always be considered as one of the possible alternatives. Building an entire system for all functions in a health care institution is not a viable option today. Before embarking on in-house development of any software system, administrators must assess whether the institution possesses the resources and expertise necessary for long-term success. For example, do in-house staff have the knowledge and experience to manage development and implementation of a new system? Can subsystems and components be obtained so that the local effort is minimized? Can outside consultants and technical staff be hired to assist? Who will maintain the system if it is installed successfully? In Section 6.3.3, we describe the development process, mainly to show its complexity.

Turnkey systems include all the hardware, software, and technical support necessary to operate the system. They should become operational rapidly, and most delays will be due to integration of the system with existing services. Unfortunately, the functions supplied by a turnkey system rarely match an institution's information management needs. The system may not perform all the desired functions, may provide superfluous features, or may require some reorganization and modification of responsibilities and established workflows within the institution. It is also important to consider carefully the reputation of the vendor and the terms of the contract and to answer questions such as "What is the extent of the support and maintenance?" and "To what extent can the system be parameterized to the institution (e.g., selecting interchange standards to other systems in the institution, handling local billing policies, and dealing with multiple pharmacies)?"

Technology Transfer

Attractive innovations in health care services are typically demonstrated in a research setting. Subsequent adopters should not underestimate the difficulty of transferring novel technology to a working environment. One rule of thumb we accept is that the work needed to develop an academically successful demonstration of a new computing technology is one-seventh of the work required to transform the demonstration into a practical system. Professional experience is needed to validate that the new system works under all conditions encountered in a clinical practice and that the system can recover from mechanical failures. If new linkages are needed to other systems, yet more work is needed, and if those systems have to be adapted, even slightly, arrangements with their owners and vendors have to be made. Even though changes required for integration may be minor, understanding and validating changes to other systems incur a high cost. During integration, computing personnel must modify the existing system, develop and check interfaces, and retrain the various types of users. The effect is that the time and cost already estimated must be multiplied by a further factor of three or four. The difficulty of software technology transfer has been a significant obstacle to the growth of medical computing.

6.3.2   Specifying Information Processes

In the health care environment, the major portion of computing deals with data rather than complex algorithms. Most data are obtained from patients, laboratories, health care personnel, and insurance providers. The data then are transmitted, stored, transformed, summarized, and analyzed to help health professionals, managers, and patients to plan actions and interventions. Certain data must be archived for legal purposes. To understand the task that a system, or subsystem, performs, it is best to consider the **data flow**.

Data Flow

A graphical representation called the **data-flow diagram** (DFD) provides a succinct way to understand the objectives of a system. It represents the sources of data, the processes for transforming the data, and the points in the system where long-term or short-term data storage is required, and the destinations where reports are generated or where results from queries are presented. The DFD in Figure 6.2a is a model of a simple laboratory information system. It illustrates the flow of laboratory test orders and results, as well as the basic functions of the proposed system: (1) creation of specimen collection schedules; (2) analysis of results; (3) reporting of test results; and (4) performance

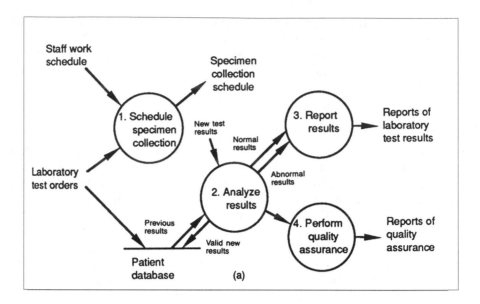

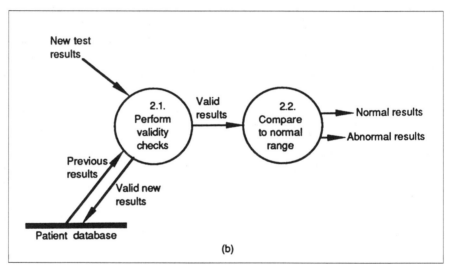

Figure 6.2. A data-flow diagram (DFD) that graphically represents the processes and data flows within a laboratory information system. (a) *Bubbles* depict processes (or functions), *vectors* depict data flows, and *straight lines* depict databases. (b) Often, DFDs are layered to show greater detail within higher-level processes. This second-level DFD decomposes the process of analyzing test results into two lower-level processes. Note that the net inputs and outputs of this DFD match the inputs and outputs of the higher-level process shown in part (a).

of quality-assurance activities. The designer can describe each higher-level process in the DFD by creating a more detailed DFD (Figure 6.2b).

The initial DFD is often based on an analysis of current workflow activities and processes. That approach helps people to identify outputs that are not obvious or that are needed only for rare cases—e.g., for investigation of infrequent infections. It is easy to overlook information needs that are informally obtained. Many informal mechanisms for communication and storage disappear when computers are used to collect and store data. Health professionals trade much valuable information in hallways and at nursing stations; e.g., they will discuss a baffling case to help develop new insights and approaches. Some crucial information never enters the formal record but is noted on scraps of paper or stored in people's memories. System designers must take care to allow support of such mechanisms, perhaps by having unconstrained note fields with the records. Once all needed outputs are indicated on the DFD, analysts can trace back to ensure that all required inputs are available in the flow. The absence of even minor functions can produce errors in health care delivery and will be perceived as a failure of the system, leading to resistance by the customers. Recall from the hypothetical case, for example, the friction between physicians and nurses that arose when the new system failed to allow for verbal orders. Often, technologists discount resistance as an unwillingness to keep up with progress, but they should interpret it as a signal that something is wrong with the new system. When such requirements arise later, they should be accepted as part of routine maintenance, since not all future requirements can be foreseen.

Using the clear graphical representation of the DFD helps the intended users to recognize aberrations and to provide feedback to the system designers. A DFD in which everything seems to connect to everything else is not helpful for analysis or implementation. Complex data flows should first be simplified so that the implementation is straightforward. If the result is still complex, a good layout can help. Major data flows should go left to right, minor flows should be shown in lighter colors, and special cases can use overlays. The final DFD can differ greatly from the initial one.

Data Storage

Most of the data and information that is documented in a DFD is stored in databases. Database software is large and crucial to reliable operations. Alternate database management systems will differ in scale and cost, and many vendors support several choices. An institution may already have made commitments to some database system vendor. It is best to limit the variety of such complex software and to share its maintenance costs. It is hence wise to ensure that the databases that come with commercial software are open—i.e., documented, set up, and maintained in a stable manner so that foreign applications can extract and contribute data to them.

Most business software today depends on relational databases. Such databases provide a means for exchanging information among software components that are otherwise independent. A vendor's schema must be adaptable, so that it can specify all the data that the software will exchange. Once health care databases are widely accessible, serious issues about access to, and release of, private medical data arise, as discussed in Chapter 10.

Further software components may need to be written to interact with an accessible database, but the database schema constrains the design of the programs while simplifying the implementation choices. The standards associated with the relational approach also simplify exchange of data over communication links, so redundant effort in data entry and result reporting can be avoided.

For health records systems, off-the-shelf software has not been easy to adapt. Clinical patient information is too complex to be easily and efficiently mapped into relational databases, so the benefits of open databases and component-based transaction services are just being realized in the core of medical applications. This means that many health care institutions have to deal with databases for medical functions that are not easy to access. For off-the-shelf systems even minor changes may require contractual negotiations with a vendor.

6.3.3   Building a New Software System

If the institution is prepared to build a computer system to meet some specific needs, system developers can employ a variety of software-engineering tools to organize and manage the development process. Although major efforts are rare in today's health care settings, it is useful to understand this process for interacting with vendors or enthusiastic innovators. Software system development tools include formal techniques for system analysis, methodologies of **structured programming**, and testing methods. They are supplemented by methods for managing the project and metrics for assessing the performance of the product and of the software development process itself. The field of **software engineering** had its beginnings in the late 1960s and early 1970s. As the systems being developed grew more complex, teams of programmers, analysts, and managers replaced individual programmers who had worked in isolation. Reuse of existing modules became important (Boehm, 1999). Many software prototypes are still developed in isolation but must be moved to a comprehensive setting before they can be marketed and distributed.

In the 1980s, the cost of hardware (which previously had dominated the total cost of a system) declined rapidly. The largest system cost now is software maintenance, an aspect rarely considered when building prototypes. More recently, standard software components have become available so that new approaches to the creation of systems are opening up. There is no single right way to implement computer systems in health care.

Software Lifecycle

Figure 6.3 depicts the classic **waterfall model** of any engineering development process from requirements analysis through specification, design, implementation, testing, and maintenance. Specialists may be engaged for each of the phases. The tasks of one phase should be completed and documented before the next phase is tackled so that the specialists for the next phase are presented with a complete specification. As Figure 6.3 suggests, problems found in a later phase require feedback to earlier phases and can cause expensive rework. If the work delegated to future phases is well understood, the

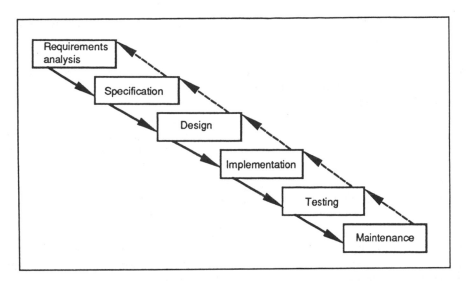

Figure 6.3. The waterfall model represents the traditional system-development process. It recognizes six sequential phases, each with feedback to the earlier phase.

waterfall model can work well. If the specifications challenge later phases, the risk of cost overruns and even failure is great. For instance, specifying X-ray images to be displayed at every terminal within one-tenth of a second requires extensive resources, and, if their cost becomes intolerable, the entire design might have to be revised.

Although the waterfall model conveys a clear view of the software life cycle, the delays inherent in such a phased development process make this methodology inappropriate for innovative applications. It is hard to obtain adequate specifications when you are developing an application for inexperienced customers. They will not see the product until the testing phase and cannot provide feedback until that time. If it takes years to complete the first four phases of the process, even good specifications are likely to have become obsolete—the organizations and their information sources and needs will have changed. It typically takes a second implementation to get a smoothly operating system.

Requirements for some health care systems are presented in Section 6.1.2, but just listing the requirements is insufficient for phase 2. The requirements have to be quantified: where is the information needed, by whom, in what form, within what context, how fast, how often, and how reliable should it be? High reliability can mean that redundant storage and processing has to be included in the design. A single program for a single user can be built without explicit attention to phases 2 and 3, but a large project requires a more careful approach.

In the **specification phase**, the general system requirements are analyzed and formalized. Systems analysts specify the intended behavior precisely and concisely—the specific functions the system must accomplish, the data it will require, the results it will produce, the performance requirements for speed and reliability, and so on. They answer questions such as "What are the sources of necessary information?" and "What are the viable mechanisms for communication in the current system?" Here the DFD becomes an important tool.

Once the functional specification has been produced and validated against the requirements specified by the prospective users, it is expanded into a design that can be implemented. The initial task is to partition the system into manageable modules. All but the smallest systems are partitioned into subsystems, subsystems into smaller components, and so on, until the whole has been decomposed into manageable components (Figure 6.4). A single module should not require more than a few implementors and not take more than a few months to write and test. Any subsystem should also have few data flows into and out of it, as determined by the DFD. Simplicity allows subsequent testing to cover all cases. Notice in Figure 6.4, for example, that an HIS can be viewed as a hierarchy of nested and interrelated subsystems. In general, a subsystem has strong internal linkages relative to its linkages with the external world.

As part of the design, the hardware needed now and in the future is determined; frequently more hardware can simplify the design and its implementation. For instance, copying data to locations close to a critical customer can improve response time and availability in case of communication problems.

In the **implementation phase**, the subsystems are created in-house or are obtained from public or commercial sources. Even good design specifications cannot cover all the details at the module level. For a good implementation, the module programmers must understand the health care setting. If the system does not function suitably for the end users—namely, if they find the output wrong or not sufficiently helpful—costly rework will be needed after the technical testing phase. Such problems might be caused because

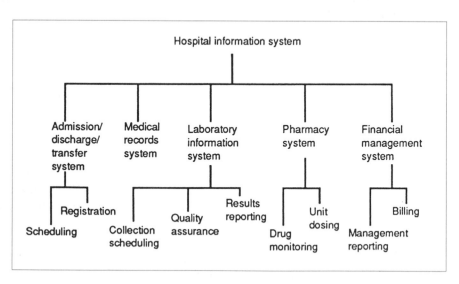

Figure 6.4. A hospital information system comprises interrelated subsystems that serve individual departments. In turn, each subsystem comprises multiple functional components.

the implementation was wrong, the design did not foresee performance problems, the specification was imprecise, or requirements were incomplete or became obsolete. If the errors are due to earlier phases, making the corrections becomes more costly.

In practice, the implementation phase will acquire as many readymade components as can be found and will put them together into a system. The components are selected to match the specifications, and less detailed design takes place. Analysts can visit sites where the components are used, and customers can see sample results early on. Early feedback to the design phase can occur. Because available components will rarely match requirements precisely, compromises in specifications will have to be made, although many vendors will try to create adaptable components that match the needs of many institutions. If some components fail to meet the needs of the customer, the vendor may be induced to improve them, or staff may decide to build some components in-house, raising the subsequent maintenance costs.

When all the components are ready, **system integration** takes place. Mistakes in partitioning, missing data flows, and incomplete interface specification become apparent. For large systems, built by many people, this is the riskiest phase. Even competent people may interpret specifications and design documents differently; some interface or data organization differences make integration impossible without redesign.

Testing of the system has to be planned carefully. Subsystems are tested by their developers, because customers probably will not be able to test incomplete functions. Because testing implies the discovery of failure points, this phase has to start slowly to allow for repair of errors so as to avoid frustration by the testers—especially when real customers begin to do testing. It is in this phase that we find out whether the hypothetical requirements, stated initially, are adequate. If they are not, major rework may be needed. Testing takes as long as implementation. Many new systems are abandoned at this point.

If the system, after testing by builders and customers, is accepted for routine use, the **maintenance phase** starts. Ongoing changes in requirements will necessitate changes in the system. In theory, the same cycle should be followed for any substantial changes, but the original large staff rarely remains available, and thus the adjustments may be made haphazardly. Because software systems often remain in place for 10 to 20 years, the maintenance phase, costing perhaps 25 percent per year, requires a greater financial commitment over time than the original development phases required.

Alternative Methodologies

To obtain early results and reduce the risk of failure, a software development group may follow alternative methodologies. In the **spiral model**, the group generates a simple prototype system by performing the four initial phases rapidly (Boehm, 1998). The result is presented to the customers, who assess it and expand and modify the requirements. Then a second cycle ensues (Figure 6.5). After a few cycles, the prototype is made operational; the operational prototype will require some maintenance, but any significant changes have to wait for yet another iteration of the spiral. Ideally, each cycle takes 3 to 6 months, so the patience of the customers is not exhausted. In the spiral model, the staff is expected to remain intact for many iterations so that essential knowledge is not lost, because little time is spent on documentation.

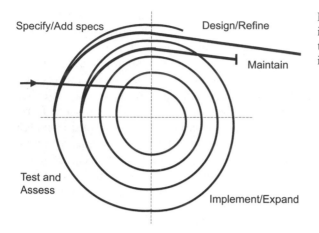

Specify/Add specs   Design/Refine

Maintain

Test and
Assess

Implement/Expand

Figure 6.5. The spiral model of implementation. Rapid iterations lead to system cycles that can be assessed incrementally by the customers.

The spiral model methodology also entails substantial risks:

1. The initial prototype is so minimal that the result is not of sufficient interest to the users, and no meaningful feedback ensues; for instance, a system may not permit access to actual patient data.
2. The system does not attain sufficient functionality after several cycles, so it cannot be placed into service; for instance, laboratory results are not yet automatically included in a patient's record.
3. An acceptable small system cannot be scaled to the next level on a standard cycle because of an overly simplified initial design decision, so major rework is needed; for example, no means exist for out-of-queue processing, so stat (emergency) laboratory tests cannot be given priority.

Developers have experimented with other software engineering methodologies, but all require that developers and customers perform similar tasks. For instance, by assessing which components are likely to be hard and risky to build and giving them more attention, the team can reduce implementation risks while accelerating delivery. This *water sluice* methodology avoids a problem of the spiral model in which, to satisfy the cyclic time constraints, the easy processes are done first. Making correct assessments requires considerable experience.[1] "See http://www.db.stanford.edu/~burback/watersluice/node34.html".

Business Objects

Object-oriented programming focuses on the specification of small, reusable data structures and associated methods, called *objects*. For instance, a *visit object* may be defined as a component of a patient record with methods as *schedule*, *check-in*, *record findings*, *issue orders*, etc. The visit object must have well-defined interactions with other objects of concern to the system, such as *patient*, *doctor*, *nurse*, *clinic*, or *pharmacy*. Given a suite of suitable objects, this approach allows rapid composition of software modules.

Libraries of such business objects are becoming available. Programmers must have substantial experience to define objects of sufficient competence and generality while allowing for their many interactions, as required in health care systems.

For complex data, the object-oriented approach may be best. All the data related to major concepts in the information systems is brought together and is accessed via methods that isolate the complexity of the data structures from the programs that use the data. Programming languages that enable object-oriented programming are listed in Table 5.1. The design of object classes to support a specific business domain is a complex task, but there are standard libraries of defined objects. If these libraries are used, the programming task is reduced to prescribing the sequence and content of the interactions among these objects—e.g., patients, their problems, and their visits.

Standard object libraries for some domains are now available—e.g., presentation graphics, telecommunications, and business finance. Many organizations are defining and implementing collections of business objects for a variety of other areas. However, if multiple groups enter a single topic area without common standards (see Chapter 7), their products will not interoperate, and it will take some time before dominant library products emerge. If multiple libraries are needed for a project, an interchange format for data is needed as well. Having a standard database can provide the required storage, but such a database must be capable of holding the data organized in object formats.

Summary

As we indicated in Section 6.3.1, few health care organizations have the resources to see major software system developments through to a successful completion. If a modest computer system development effort can address problems specific to some health care setting, however, it may be worthwhile to undertake a local effort. There are still problems that require novel solutions and technology not available from most vendors of health care systems. Many problems in health care are poorly structured and may require methods based on AI. Such an effort will typically be established as a subsystem in the institutional network and be initially isolated from daily operational responsibilities. The subsystem will depend on available complementary system resources, such as an existing patient-admitting system. Using the spiral approach, experience can be gathered from local customers that outsiders would not be able to supply. It is still essential to ensure reliability, security, and data confidentiality, as discussed in Chapter 10. A new subsystem, no matter how beneficial, is likely to be rejected if it entails risks to the routine services of health care delivery, patients' confidence, or cost accounting.

6.3.4   Incorporating Remote Services

Our health care systems do not operate in isolation. Within major institutions, there will be several distinct computer systems, such as in the laboratory, in physician offices, and in account billing. Outside of the institution, there are other organizations that use computer systems, such as drug and linen suppliers, laboratories that do outsourced work, insurance companies, public health service agencies, and the National Institutes of Health (NIH), including the National Library of Medicine (NLM). The capabilities of modern networks, as introduced in Chapter 5, enable direct linkages to all these systems, and greatly reduce paper copies and manual transcription of information. The interfaces are diverse, however, unless standards are adopted, as discussed in Chapter 7. Even when standard interfaces are agreed on at one point in time, technology eventually renders them obsolete. Nonetheless, the ability to interact with remote services is essential, and the cost of maintaining interfaces is less than that of transcribing the information by hand or of entering it manually into the home system (see Section 6.3.5). External services require different business arrangements depending on whether they are **informational services** (informal, broad public access) or **business services** (contractual, user access only).

Information on the World Wide Web

For informational systems accessed via the World Wide Web, the Hypertext Markup Language (HTML) dominates Web services. A **markup language** identifies items of the contents. The term *hyper* refers to the capability of references in an HTML document to link to other documents through a Universal Resource Locator (URL), which identifies files at remote locations, such as http://www.dlib.org. The HTML focuses on the presentation of information and allows the definition of text, headings, tables, images, or even program fragments that provide dynamic displays, using the Java language (see Chapter 5). This information is interpreted by a **browser**, which provides the most suitable presentation for display. Browsers deal well with inconsistencies, errors, or novel specifications, providing the most reasonable presentation. The utility of these tools for health care information is presented in Chapter 19.

For business services, the inherent flexibility of the Web and HTML is also a liability. There is no guarantee of completeness of the information or of consistency of content. Many standards have been developed for data interchange; each typically is created for a specific domain, as discussed in Chapter 7. To allow data–quality interchange on the Web, the eXtensible Markup Language (XML) has been widely adopted. Rather than focusing on presentation formats, it specifies contents through extensive use of tags. The meaning of the tags is specified for specific domains (Connolly, 1997). The **XML format** provides a common syntactic technical infrastructure and allows sharing of software tools. A variety of efforts are underway that are specific to health care, as described in Chapter 7, which will enable easier integration of remote services.

6.3.5   *Designing for Effectiveness*

A system's success depends not only on whether it meets the users' informational needs but also on how it interacts with those users. There are many types of users, ranging from technical specialists to people who only require easy-to-use information services. The resident's complaints in the hypothetical example illustrated an important point: the disruption of effective and established routines and the inconvenience often associated with computer information systems can cause users to work around the system and thus to fail to share its capabilities. Studies of the attitudes of health care personnel regarding computer-based clinical consultation systems have shown that successful programs not only must provide expert-level advice but also must be integrated into the daily routines of physicians and other users (Friedman and Gustafson, 1977; Teach and Shortliffe, 1981; Detmer and Friedman, 1994). Computer-based information systems should acknowledge the hectic schedules of health professionals and should demystify and simplify the mechanics of the human–computer interface (HCI). By involving users in system design, developers can avoid many of the impediments to widespread success.

The following parameters of computer systems are among the most important to consider during system design:

- *Quality and style of interface*: From a customer's point of view, a system's interface is the system. To be effective, interfaces must have clear presentations, avoid unnecessary detail, and provide a consistent interaction. Since users will have many interaction points with computers, consistency is a global issue. Menus, graphics, and consistent use of color all help to make systems more attractive and simpler to learn and use. Today, clicking on a mouse is ubiquitous, but requires that users are settled in front of the screen. Traditionally physicians were reluctant to type at a keyboard; furthermore, sitting down and starting an interaction is awkward in many health care settings. Thus, system developers have experimented with a number of alternative devices for interaction, including light pens and touch screens. Researchers are investigating speech recognition and natural language understanding. These technologies are now available for limited vocabulary, but not yet as natural and easy as talking with human beings. Mobile devices such as personal digital assistants (PDAs) and laptops have opened up major new opportunities for interaction between clinical systems and their users. In systems that perform decision support and offer advice about patient care, the style of communication is particularly important. Is the system too terse or too verbose? Does it project a helpful attitude or does it seem pedantic or judgmental? Can it justify its recommendations?
- *Convenience*: Customers must have convenient access to the system. The number and placement of workstations and printers are important considerations if the system is to be assimilated into users' routines. For example, if an EHR system is intended to replace the traditional patient record, it must be accessible wherever and whenever health professionals need to look up patient data—in the physician's office, in the nursing station, possibly at the bedside, and so on. Sufficient workstations should be available that users do not have to wait to use the system, even during times of peak use. Logging in must be rapid. Convenience is a major reason for the growth in interest in mobile devices, especially given the highly mobile nature of health workers in clinical environments.
- *Speed and response*: System developers must choose hardware and communication methods that have sufficient capacity to handle customers' demands for information during peak hours, whether through wired or wireless connections. The software must allow users timely access to the data in the form they need. Minor errors in formulating information requests must be easily undone. Health professionals are understandably reluctant to use systems that are hostile, tedious, or unduly time-consuming.
- *Reliability*: In the event of hardware or software failure, health personnel must resort to manual procedures. Redundant hardware and frequent data backup can minimize the loss of time and data.

- *Security*: The confidentiality of medical data is an important issue in the design of health information systems (see Chapter 10). The system should be easily accessible to authorized personnel, yet it should not release information to unauthorized users. These conflicting goals are difficult to achieve. The most common compromise solution is to assign an account with a password to each user, and sometimes a physical token (*cryptocard* with a second password that changes frequently) or **biometric identifier** (such as the user's thumbprint). Variable access to the data then can be controlled for individual users or for classes of users. Certain operations may be restricted to particular workstations. For example, the ability to modify patient charges is best restricted to financial personnel working from workstations located in the accounting office. Medical notes are hard to classify and may require filtering before they can be released to outsiders (Wiederhold et al., 1996).
- *Integration*: The integration of information from independent systems eliminates some of the difficulties and enhances the benefits of using computer systems. If, for example, a laboratory system and a pharmacy system are independent and incompatible, health professionals must access two separate systems (possibly from different workstations) to view a single patient's data. If the two systems need to share data, people will have to collect output from the first and reenter it into the second system. The development of local-area networks (LANs) has provided the infrastructure to allow exchange of information among independent systems and has reduced the need for redundant entry and storage of critical information (a waste of time and a source of errors). Standards, such as those based on XML, reduce the cost of acquiring and maintaining software for integration. The ensuing collaboration will help in developing common terminologies and reduce misunderstandings.

Technological progress is enabling the introduction of effective systems in health care. While the path is difficult and often frustrating, there is no doubt that health care has come to depend on computing and data processing as core capabilities in modern care-delivery environments.

6.3.6   Planning for Change

Many health information systems—particularly custom-designed systems—take a long time to develop. This delay is risky; it is hard for the medical establishment to perceive what is being done by the system development staff, and the development staff receives no feedback on the correctness of the assumptions on which they are basing their design. The involvement of users through demonstrations and training sessions and the incremental installation of the system can build the enthusiasm and support of users and can provide computing personnel an invaluable means for evaluating progress.

Visiting similar sites can provide the insights that are needed to develop judgments about new systems or proposed improvements. **Prototypes**—working models that exhibit the essential features of the system under development—facilitate communication between computing personnel and users. Users develop a realistic idea of what the system will look like, how it will work, and what it will do. Developers receive feedback and can modify the system in response to users' comments, thus improving the likelihood that the final system will be deemed acceptable. A good prototype provides a realistic demonstration of the method of interaction with the system and should be able to deal with most of the common varieties of data input. Much simplification is possible when reliability and data permanence can be ignored, as they can be in a prototype system that is intended only for demonstration and discussion.

Formal training courses also can help to dispel the mystery of a new system. Without adequate reinforcement, however, people are apt to forget what they learn. A training program for a new system should start slowly and extend over the period of its implementation so that surprises are minimized. When some subsystem installation is imminent, health professionals should receive specific and intensive training in its use. Experience with windows and mouse interfaces shows that intuitive metaphors allow users to experiment and explore the system's capabilities and reduce the need for formal training. The feedback provided to the developers during successive phases helps to ensure that problems will not be repeated or multiplied as the system nears completion.

Training is simplified if part of the system is operational. Customers can see real examples of the system in action and thus are less likely to develop overly ambitious expectations. Because those parts of the system that are installed first usually are less problematic, the initial phase is likely to be a success. The attitude generated by initial success can enhance the acceptance of the system in other areas, including those areas that inherently are more difficult to address using computer-based techniques. In hospitals, for instance, computer systems often are used first in the admissions office, where the applications are relatively straightforward, and later are expanded for use on medical wards, where the user community is particularly diverse and demanding.

6.4 Summary

A variety of software and information services are available for health care applications, ranging from turnkey systems, covering many of the needs of an institution, through major subsystems for hospital departments and large Web-based services that require only remote access to databases and to object libraries that are helpful for building local applications. Unfortunately, composing an effective and economical system that is fully sufficient for the financial, clinical, and ancillary needs in health care is nearly impossible. Today, most health care institutions are faced with the choice of either committing to a major vendor, and accepting that vendor's complete system or a subset thereof, or dealing with a variety of purchased, adapted, and in-house developed subsystems that overlap and have gaps. Gaps often require human transcription and replicated data input. The maintenance of the systems requires ongoing efforts to keep them up to date as operational and clinical requirements and processes change.

Information systems development is a political as well as a technical process. Health institutions, just like all other organizations, are composed of different groups of individuals, and often these groups have conflicting priorities, objectives, and values. The technical issues are generally complex and difficult; careful implementation processes can conflict with urgent needs. Risks are rife in internal software development, in acquiring vendors' software, and in their integration. Health administrators, physicians, nurses, ancillary personnel, and patients have diverse needs that the computer system must accommodate. Information systems can alter relationships among these people—they affect patterns of communication, perceived influence, authority, and control. A strategy for implementation must recognize and deal with these political forces. A new system should disrupt the organizational infrastructure as little as possible. The article by Keen (1981) (listed in the Suggested Readings) discusses the political aspects of system development and implementation in greater detail.

Suggested Readings

Anderson J.G., Jay S.J. (Eds.). (1987). *Use and Impact of Computers in Clinical Medicine.* New York: Springer-Verlag.
This collection of papers presents research on the factors that affect the adoption, diffusion, and utilization of clinical information systems in hospitals. It includes chapters on the attitudes of health professionals toward computers and the probable effects of clinical systems on aspects of medical practice, such as the role of physicians, relations between doctors and patients, and the organization of the health care delivery system.

Blum B. (1992). *Software Engineering: A Holistic Approach.* New York: Oxford University Press.
This philosophical but unbiased textbook on software engineering was written by a practioner who has had substantial experience developing clinical applications. It covers the system-development process, data-flow diagrams, and structured coding techniques.

Boehm B. (1999). Managing Software Productivity and Reuse. *IEEE Computer,* 31(9):111–113.
Making modules reusable, at some additional costs, reduces subsequent development costs.

Boehm B., Egyed A., Kwan J., Port D., Shah A., Madachy, R. (1998). Using the WinWin Spiral Model: A case study. *IEEE Computer,* 31(7):33–44.
This brief note introduces the WinWin Spiral Model, mainly in relation to student projects. The WinWin Spiral Model has two add-ons to the classic spiral model: (1) analysis at the beginning of each spiral cycle and (2) process anchor points. A risk of using the spiral model is that methods used initally may not scale to the eventual requirements.

Booch G. (1994). *Object-Oriented Design with Applications* (2nd ed.). Redwood City, CA: Benjamin-Cummings.
This is an introduction to object-oriented programming, by one of its chief proponents and tool builders.

Keen P.G.W. (1981). Information systems and organizational change. *Communications of the ACM,* 24:24.
This paper emphasizes the pluralistic nature of organizations. It discusses the changes in patterns of communication, influence, and control that often occur when new information systems are implemented, and it suggests strategies for minimizing social inertia and resistance.

Leymann, F. and Roller D. (2000). *Production Workflow: Concepts and Techniques.* Englewood Cliffs, NJ: Prentice-Hall.
This book illustrates the principles of linking computing and manual tasks for smooth interaction.

Monson-Haefel, R. (1999). *Enterprise JavaBeans*. Cambridge, MA: O'Reilly & Associates.
JavaBeans is a technology to define business objects that can be composed to assemble rapidly an analyzable and maintainable data-processing system.

Pigoski, T.M. (1997). *Practical Software Maintenance: Best Practices for Managing Your Software Investment*. Los Alamitos, CA: IEEE Computer Society Press.
A basic reference for computer software maintenance. Corrections are 20 to 25 percent of the effort, adaptations 40 to 60 percent, and perfection consumes the remainder.

Reiser S.J., Anbar M. (Eds.). (1984). *The Machine at the Bedside: Strategies for Using Technology in Patient Care*. Cambridge, UK: Cambridge University Press.
This book discusses the theory and use of health care technologies—such as intensive care, diagnostic imaging, and electronic fetal monitoring—in the context of legal, ethical, economic, and social concerns. It contains 23 case studies that depict the benefits and limitations of using these technologies.

Shlaer S., Mellor S.J. (1992). *Object Life Cycles, Modeling the World in States*. Englewood Cliffs, NJ: Prentice-Hall.
This influential textbook was developed by protagonists of the object-oriented software development approach.

Webster, J. G. (1988) (Ed.). *Encyclopedia of Medical Devices and Instrumentation*. New York: Wiley.
This reference includes many technical definitions, including an extensive description of hospital information systems, listing over 200 functions that such a system might provide.

Questions for Discussion

1. Reread the hypothetical case in Section 6.2.1.
   a. What are three primary benefits of the clinical system? What are three primary disadvantages?
   b. Do you think that the benefits of the system outweigh the disadvantages? Are there adequate noncomputer-based solutions to the problems with which the system was designed to help? If so, what are they?
   c. How would you change the system in your institution or in one you have read about? Among the topics you might address are the effects of the system on hospital routine, computer reliability, and terminal availability and the adequacy of user training programs.
2. Describe an outpatient clinic's billing system in terms of inputs, outputs, and processes. Sketch a simple data-flow diagram that represents your model of the system.
3. Discuss the inherent tension between protecting the confidentiality of patient records and providing health professionals with rapid and convenient access to clinical information. What level of system security do you think provides an appropriate balance between these conflicting goals?
4. Discuss three barriers to technology transfer among health care institutions.
5. Explain the difference between outcome and process measures of system performance. Identify two outcome and two process parameters that you might use to

evaluate the performance of a clinical consultation system that assists physicians in diagnosing disease. Describe an experiment that you could perform to evaluate the effect of the system on one of these parameters. What potential difficulties can you foresee in conducting your experiment? What can you do to compensate for these difficulties?

6. In what three ways is the use of a clinical consultation system similar to the use of human consultants or static sources of health information such as textbooks? In what three ways is it different?

7
Standards in Biomedical Informatics

W. Edward Hammond and James J. Cimino

After reading this chapter, you should know the answers to these questions:

- Why are standards important in biomedical informatics?
- What data standards are necessary to be able to exchange data seamlessly among systems?
- What organizations are active in standards development?
- What aspects of biomedical information management are supported today by standards?
- What is the process for creating consensus standards?
- What factors and organizations influence the creation of standards?

7.1 The Idea of Standards

Ever since Eli Whitney developed interchangeable parts for rifle assembly, standards have been created and used to make things or processes work more easily and economically—or, sometimes, to work at all. A standard can be defined in many physical forms, but essentially it comprises a set of rules and definitions that specify how to carry out a process or produce a product. Sometimes, a standard is useful because it provides a way to solve a problem that other people can use without having to start from scratch. Generally, though, a standard is useful because it permits two or more disassociated people to work in some cooperative way. Every time you screw in a light bulb or play a music cassette, you are taking advantage of a standard. Some standards make things work more easily. Some standards evolve over time,[1] others are developed deliberately.

The first computers were built without standards, but hardware and software standards quickly became a necessity. Although computers work with values such as 1 or 0, and with "words" such as 10101100, humans need a more readable language (see Chapter 5). Thus, standard character sets, such as ASCII and EBCDIC, were developed. The first standard computer language, COBOL, was written originally to simplify program development but was soon adopted as a way to allow sharing of code and

---

[1]The current standard for railroad-track gauge originated with Roman chariot builders, who set the axle length based on the width of two horses. This axle length became a standard as road ruts developed, requiring that the wheels of chariots—and all subsequent carriages—be the right distance apart to drive in the ruts. When carriage makers were called on to develop railway rolling stock, they continued to use the same axle standard.

development of software components that could be integrated. As a result, COBOL was given official standard status by the American National Standards Institute (ANSI).[2] In like manner, hardware components depend on standards for exchanging information to make them as interchangeable as were Whitney's gun barrels.

A 1987 technical report from the International Standards Organization (ISO) states that "any meaningful exchange of utterances depends upon the prior existence of an agreed upon set of semantic and syntactic rules" (International Standards Organization, 1987). In biomedical informatics, where the emphasis is on collection, manipulation, and transmission of information, standards are greatly needed but have only recently begun to be available. At present, the standards scene is evolving so rapidly that any description is inevitably outdated within a few months. This chapter emphasizes the need for standards in general, standards development processes, current active areas of standards development, and key participating organizations that are making progress in the development of usable standards.

7.2   The Need for Health Informatics Standards

Standards are generally required when excessive diversity creates inefficiencies or impedes effectiveness. The health care environment has traditionally consisted of a set of loosely connected, organizationally independent units. Patients receive care across primary, secondary, and tertiary care settings, with little bidirectional communication and coordination among the services. Patients are cared for by one or more primary physicians, as well as by specialists. There is little coordination and sharing of data between inpatient care and outpatient care. Both the system and patients, by choice, create this diversity in care. Within the inpatient setting, the clinical environment is divided into clinical specialties that frequently treat the patient without regard to what other specialities have done. Ancillary departments function as detached units, performing their tasks as separate service units, reporting results without follow-up about how those results are used or whether they are even seen by the ordering physician. Reimbursement requires patient information that is often derived through a totally separate process, based on the fragmented data collected in the patient's medical record and abstracted specifically for billing purposes. The resulting set of diagnosis and procedure codes often correlates poorly with the patient's original information (Jollis et al., 1993).

Early hospital information systems (HISs) for billing and accounting purposes were developed on large, monolithic mainframe computers (see Chapter 13); they followed a pattern of diversity similar to that seen in the health care system itself. As new functions were added in the 1970s, they were implemented on mainframe computers and were managed by a data processing staff that usually was independent of the clinical and even of the administrative staff. The advent of the minicomputer supported the development of departmental systems, such as those for the clinical laboratory, radiology department, or pharmacy. This model of the central mainframe coupled with

---

[2]Interestingly, medical informaticians were responsible for the second ANSI standard language: MUMPS (now known as M).

independent minicomputer-based departmental systems is still common in installed systems today. Clinical systems, as they have developed, continue to focus on dedicated departmental operations, and clinical-specialty systems thus do not permit the practicing physician to see a unified view of the patient.

There are many pressures on health care information systems to change the status quo such that data collected for a primary purpose can be reused in a multitude of ways. Newer models for health care delivery, such as integrated delivery networks, health maintenance organizations (HMOs), and preferred provider organizations (PPOs), have increased the need for coordinated, integrated, and consolidated information (see Chapters 13 and 23), even though the information comes from disparate departments and institutions. Various management techniques, such as continuous quality improvement and case management, require up-to-date, accurate abstracts of patient data. Post hoc analyses for clinical and outcomes research require comprehensive summaries across patient populations. Advanced tools, such as clinical workstations (Chapter 12) and decision-support systems (Chapter 20), require ways to translate raw patient data into generic forms for tasks as simple as summary reporting and as complex as automated medical diagnosis. All these needs must be met in the existing setting of diverse, interconnected information systems—an environment that cries out for implementation of standards.

One obvious need is for standardized identifiers for individuals, health care providers, health plans, and employers so that such participants can be recognized across systems. Choosing such an identifier is much more complicated than simply deciding how many digits the identifier should have. Ideal attributes for these sets of identifiers have been described in a publication from the American Society for Testing and Materials (ASTM) (American Society for Testing and Materials, 1999). The identifier must include a check digit to ensure accuracy when the identifier is entered by a human being into a system. A standardized solution must also determine mechanisms for issuing identifiers to individuals, facilities, and organizations; for maintaining databases of identifying information; and for authorizing access to such information (also see Chapter 13).

The Centers for Medicare and Medicaid Services (CMS), formerly known as the Health Care Financing Administration (HCFA), has defined a National Provider Identifier (NPI) that has been proposed as the national standard. This number is a seven-character alphanumeric base identifier plus a one-character check digit. No meaning is built into the number, each number is unique and is never reissued, and alpha characters that might be confused with numeric characters (e.g., 0, 1, 2, 4, and 5 can be confused with O, I or L, Z, Y, and S) have been eliminated. CMS has also defined a Payor ID for identifying health care plans. The Internal Revenue Service's employer identification number has been adopted as the Employer Identifier.

The most controversial issue is identifying each individual or patient. Many people consider assignment and use of such a number to be an invasion of privacy and are concerned that it could be easily linked to other databases. Public Law 104-191, passed in August 1996 (see Section 7.3.3), required that Congress formally define suitable identifiers. Pushback by privacy advocates and negative publicity in the media resulted in Congress declaring that this issue would not be moved forward until privacy legislation was in place and implemented (see Chapter 10). The Department of Health and Human Services has recommended the identifiers discussed above, except for the person identifier.

A hospital admissions system records that a patient has the diagnosis of diabetes mellitus, a pharmacy system records that the patient has been given gentamicin, a laboratory system records that the patient had certain results on kidney function tests, and a radiology system records that a doctor has ordered an X-ray examination for the patient that requires intravenous iodine dye. Other systems need ways to store these data, to present the data to clinical users, to send warnings about possible disease–drug interactions, to recommend dosage changes, and to follow the patient's outcome. A standard for coding patient data is nontrivial when one considers the need for agreed-on definitions, use of qualifiers, differing (application-specific) levels of granularity in the data, and synonymy, not to mention the breadth and depth that such a standard would need to have.

The inclusion of medical knowledge in clinical systems is becoming increasingly important and commonplace. Sometimes, the knowledge is in the form of simple facts such as the maximum safe dose of a medication or the normal range of results for a laboratory test. Much medical knowledge is more complex, however. It is challenging to encode such knowledge in ways that computer systems can use (see Chapter 2), especially if one needs to avoid ambiguity and to express logical relations consistently. Thus the encoding of clinical knowledge using an accepted standard would allow many people and institutions to share the work done by others. One standard designed for this purpose is the Arden Syntax, discussed in Chapter 20.

Because the tasks we have described require coordination of systems, methods are needed for transferring information from one system to another. Such transfers were traditionally accomplished through custom-tailored point-to-point interfaces, but this technique has become unworkable as the number of systems and the resulting permutations of necessary connections have grown. A current approach to solving the multiple-interface problem is through the development of messaging standards. Such messages must depend on the preexistence of standards for patient identification and data encoding.

Although the technical challenges are daunting, methods for encoding patient data and shipping those data from system to system are not sufficient for developing practical systems. Security must also be addressed before such exchanges can be allowed to take place. Before a system can divulge patient information, it must ensure that requesters are who they say they are and that they are permitted access to the requested information (see Chapter 5). Although each clinical system can have its own security features, system builders would rather draw on available standards and avoid reinventing the wheel. Besides, the secure exchange of information requires that interacting systems use standard technologies. Fortunately, many researchers are busy developing such standards.

7.3   Standards Undertakings and Organizations

It is helpful to separate our discussion of the general process by which standards are created from our discussion of the specific organizations and the standards that they produce. The process is relatively constant, whereas the organizations form, evolve, merge, and are disbanded. Let us consider, for purposes of illustration, how a standard might be developed for sending laboratory data in electronic form from one computer system to another in the form of a message.

7.3.1   The Standards Development Process

There are four ways in which a standard can be produced:

1. *Ad hoc method*: A group of interested people and organizations (e.g., laboratory-system and hospital-system vendors) agree on a standard specification. These specifications are informal and are accepted as standards through mutual agreement of the participating groups. An example produced by this method is the American College of Radiology/National Electrical Manufacturers Association (ACR/NEMA) DICOM standard for medical imaging.
2. *De facto method*: A single vendor controls a large enough portion of the market to make its product the market standard. An example is Microsoft's Windows.
3. *Government-mandate method*: A government agency, such as CMS or the National Institute for Standards and Technology (NIST) creates a standard and legislates its use. An example is CMS's UB92 insurance-claim form.
4. *Consensus method*: A group of volunteers representing interested parties works in an open process to create a standard. Most health care standards are produced by this method. An example is the Health Level 7 (HL7) standard for clinical-data interchange (Figure 7.1).

The process of creating a standard proceeds through several stages (Libicki, 1995). It begins with an *identification stage*, during which someone becomes aware that there exists a need for a standard in some area and that technology has reached a level that can support such a standard. For example, suppose there are several laboratory systems sending data to several central hospital systems—a standard message format would allow each laboratory system to talk to all the hospital systems without specific point-to-point interface programs being developed for each possible laboratory-to-laboratory or laboratory-to-hospital combination. If the time for a standard is ripe, then several individuals can be identified and organized to help with the *conceptualization stage*, in which the characteristics of the standard are defined. What must the standard do? What is the scope of the standard? What will be its format?

In the laboratory system example above, one key discussion would be on the scope of the standard. Should the standard deal only with the exchange of laboratory data, or should the scope be expanded to include other types of data exchange? Should the data elements being exchanged be sent with a tag identifying the data element, or should the data be defined positionally? In the ensuing *discussion stage*, the participants will begin to create an outline that defines content, to identify critical issues, and to produce a time line. In the discussion, the pros and cons of the various concepts are discussed. What will be the specific form for the standard? For example, will it be message based? Will the data exchange be based on a query or on a trigger event? Will the standard define the message content, the message syntax, the terminology, and the network protocol, or will the standard deal with a subset of these issues?

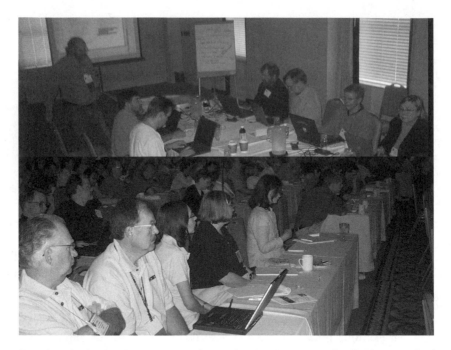

Figure 7.1. Standards development meetings. The development of effective standards often requires the efforts of dedicated volunteers, working over many years. Work is often done in small committee meetings and then presented to a large group to achieve consensus. Here we see meetings of the HL7 Vocabulary Technical Committee (top) and an HL7 plennary meeting (bottom). See Section 7.5.2 for a discussion on HL7.

The participants are generally well informed in the domain of the standard, so they appreciate the needs and problems that the standard must address. Basic concepts are usually topics for heated discussion; subsequent details may follow at an accelerated pace. Many of the participants will have experience in solving problems to be addressed by the standard and will protect their own approaches. The meanings of words are often debated. Compromises and loosely defined terms are often accepted to permit the process to move forward. For example, the likely participants would be vendors of competing laboratory systems and vendors of competing HISs. All participants would be familiar with the general problems but would have their own proprietary approach to solving them. Definitions of basic concepts normally taken for granted, such as what constitutes a test or a result, would need to be clearly stated and agreed on.

The writing of the draft standard is usually the work of a few dedicated individuals—typically people who represent the vendors in the field. Other people then review that draft; controversial points are discussed in detail and solutions are proposed and finally accepted. Writing and refining the standard is further complicated by the introduction of people new to the process who have not been privy to the original discussions and who want to revisit points that have been resolved earlier. The balance between moving forward and being open is a delicate one. Most standards-writing groups have adopted an **open policy**: Anyone can join the process and can be heard. Most standards development organizations—certainly those by accredited groups— support an open balloting process. A draft standard is made available to all interested parties, inviting comments and recommendations. All comments are considered. Negative ballots must be addressed specifically. If the negative comments are persuasive, the standard is modified. If they are not, the issues are discussed with the submitter in an attempt to convince the person to remove the negative ballot. If neither of these efforts is successful, the comments are sent to the entire balloting group to see whether the group is persuaded to change its vote. The resulting vote then determines the content of the standard. Issues might be general, such as deciding what types of laboratory data to include (pathology? blood bank?), or specific, such as deciding the specific meanings of specific fields (do we include the time the test was ordered? specimen drawn? test performed?).

A standard will generally go through several versions on its path to maturity. The first attempts at implementation are frequently met with frustration as participating vendors interpret the standard differently and as areas not addressed by the standard are encountered. These problems may be dealt with in subsequent versions of the standard. Backward compatibility is a major concern as the standard evolves. How can the standard evolve, over time, and still be economically responsible to both vendors and users? An implementation guide is usually produced to help new vendors profit from the experience of the early implementers.

A critical stage in the life of a standard is *early implementation*, when acceptance and rate of implemention are important to success. This process is influenced by accredited standards bodies, by the federal government, by major vendors, and the marketplace. The maintenance and promulgation of the standard are also important to ensure widespread availability and continued value of the standard. Some form of conformance testing is ultimately necessary to ensure that vendors adhere to the standard and to protect its integrity.

Producing a standard is an expensive process in terms of both time and money. Vendors and users must be willing to support the many hours of work, usually on company time; the travel expense; and the costs of documentation and distribution. In the United States, the production of a consensus standard is voluntary, in contrast to in Europe, where most standards development is funded by governments.

An important aspect of standards is *conformance*, a concept that covers compliance with the standard and also usually includes specific agreements among users of the standard who affirm that specific rules will be followed. A conformance document identifies specifically what data elements will be sent, when, and in what form. Even with a perfect standard, a conformance document is necessary to define business relationships between two or more partners.

A second important concept is *certification*. The use of most standards is enhanced by a certification process in which a neutral body certifies that a vendor's product, in fact, does comply and conform with the standard.

7.3.2 *Information Standards Organizations*

Sometimes, standards are developed by organizations that need the standard to carry out their principal functions; in other cases, coalitions are formed for the express purpose of developing a particular standard. The latter organizations are discussed later, when we examine the particular standards developed in this way. There are also *standards organizations* that exist for the sole purpose of fostering and promulgating standards. In some cases, they include a membership with expertise in the area where the standard is needed. In other cases, the organization provides the rules and framework for standard development but does not offer the expertise needed to make specific decisions for specific standards, relying instead on participation by knowledgeable experts when a new standard is being studied.

This section describes in some detail several of the best known **standards development organizations** (SDOs). Our goal has been to familiarize you with the names or organizational and historical aspects of the most influential health-related standards groups. For a detailed understanding of an organization or the standards it has developed, you will need to refer to current primary resources. Many of the organizations maintain Web sites with excellent current information on their status.

American National Standards Institute

ANSI is a private, nonprofit membership organization founded in 1918. It originally served to coordinate the U.S. voluntary census standards systems. Today, it is responsible for approving official *American National Standards*. ANSI membership includes over 1,100 companies; 30 government agencies; and 250 professional, technical, trade, labor, and consumer organizations.

ANSI does not write standards; rather, it assists standards developers and users from the private sector and from government to reach consensus on the need for standards. It helps them to avoid duplication of work, and it provides a forum for resolution of differences. ANSI administers the only government-recognized system for establishing American National Standards. ANSI also represents U.S. interests in international standardization. ANSI is the U.S. voting representative in the ISO and the International Electrotechnical Commission (IEC). There are three routes for a standards development body to become ANSI approved so as to produce an American National Standard: Accredited Organization; Accredited Standards Committee (ASCs); and Accredited Canvass.

An organization that has existing organizational structure and procedures for standards development may be directly accredited by ANSI to publish American National Standards, provided that it can meet the requirements for due process, openness, and consensus. HL7 (discussed in Section 7.5.2) is an example of an ANSI Accredited Organization.

ANSI may also create internal ASCs to meet a need not filled by an existing Accredited Organization. ASC X12 (discussed in Section 7.5.2) is an example of such a committee.

The final route, Accredited Canvass, is available when an organization does not have the formal structure required by ANSI. Through a canvass method that meets the criterion of balanced representation of all interested parties, a standard may be approved as an American National Standard. ASTM (discussed below) creates its ANSI standards using this method.

European Committee for Standardization Technical Committee 251

The European Committee for Standardization (CEN) established, in 1991, Technical Committee 251 (TC 251—not to be confused with ISO TC 215 described below) for the development of standards for health care informatics. The major goal of TC 251 is to develop standards for communication among independent medical information systems so that clinical and management data produced by one system could be transmitted to another system. The organization of TC 251 parallels efforts in the United States through various working groups. These groups similarly deal with data interchange standard, medical record standards, code and terminology standards, imaging standards, and security, privacy and confidentiality. Both Europe and the United States are making much effort toward coordination in all areas of standardization. Draft standards are being shared. Common solutions are being accepted as desirable. Groups are working together at various levels toward a common goal. CEN TC 251 is organized into four working groups:

- Information models
- Terminology
- Security, safety and quality
- Technology for interoperability

Within each working group, project teams are formed to work on specific projects. The teams consist mostly of "consultants" who are paid by the European Union. There has been very little vendor involvement in the development of these standards; that omission has created some reluctance in the acceptance of certain standards by the vendors. CEN also develops standards for specific applications, for example, a standard for transmitting drug prescriptions.

CEN has made major contributions to data standards in health care. One important CEN pre-standard ENV 13606 on the electronic health record (EHR) is being advanced by CEN as well as significant input from Australia and the OpenEHR Foundation. There is an increasing cooperation among the CEN participants and several of the U.S. standards bodies. CEN standards may be published through the ISO as part of the Vienna Agreement.

International Standards Organization Technical Committee 215—Health Informatics

In 1989, interests in the European Committee for Standardization (CEN) and the United States led to the creation of Technical Committee (TC) 215 for Health Information within ISO. In the initial meeting in Orlando in August 1989, the technical committee formed four (subsequently six) working groups:

- Working Group 1—Health Records and Modeling Coordination
- Working Group 2—Messaging and Communications
- Working Group 3—Health Concept Representation
- Working Group 4—Security
- Working Group 5—Smart Cards (formed in 1999)
- Working Group 6—ePharmacy and Medicines (formed in 2003)

TC 215 now meets once in a year and follows rather rigid procedures to create ISO standards. Twenty-four countries are active participants in the TC with another 20 countries acting as observers. While the actual work is done in the working groups, the balloting process is very formalized—one vote for each participating country. For most work there are a defined series of steps, beginning with a New Work Item Proposal and getting five countries to participate; a Working Document, a Committee Document; a Draft International Standard, a Final Draft International Standard (FDIS); and finally an International Standard. This process, if fully followed, takes several years to produce an International Standard. Under certain conditions, a fast track to FDIS is permitted. Technical Reports and Technical Specifications are also permitted.

The United States has been assigned the duties of Secretariat, and those duties were originally assigned to ASTM. In 2003, the Health Care Information and Management Society (HIMSS) assumed the duties of Secretariat. HIMSS also serves as the U.S. Technical Advisory Group Administrator, which represents the U.S. position in ISO.

A recent change in ISO policy is permitting standards developed by other bodies to move directly to become ISO standards. Originally, CEN and ISO developed an agreement, called the Vienna Agreement, that would permit CEN standards to move into ISO for parallel development and be balloted in each organization. In 2000, a new process was added with the Institute of Electrical and Electronics Engineers (IEEE—see Section 7.5.2) called the ISO/IEEE Pilot Project in which IEEE standards could be moved directly to ISO (and in this case to TC 215, WG2) for approval as ISO standards. Although working out the actual procedures has been painful, the process is now functional. ISO approval of standards is very important since a number of countries have laws that require the use of ISO standards if they exist (including the United States).

American Society for Testing and Materials

ASTM was founded in 1898 and chartered in 1902 as a scientific and technical organization for the development of standards for characteristics and performance of materials. The original focus of ASTM was standard test methods. The charter was subsequently broadened in 1961 to include products, systems, and services, as well as materials. ASTM is the largest nongovernment source of standards in the United States. It has over 30,000 members who reside in over 90 different countries. ASTM is a charter member of ANSI. ASTM technical committees are assigned 12 ISO committee and subcommittee secretariats and have over 50 assignments to serve as Technical Advisory Groups (TAGs) for developing U.S. positions on international standards. ASTM Committee E31 on Computerized Systems is responsible for the development of the medical information standards. Table 7.1 shows the domains of its various subcommittees.

Table 7.1. ASTM E31 subcommittees.

Subcommittee	Medical information standard
E31.01	Controlled Vocabularies for Health Care Informatics
E31.10	Pharmaco-Informatics Standards
E31.11	Electronic Health Record Portability
E31.13	Clinical Laboratory Information Management Systems
E31.14	Clinical Laboratory Instrument Interface
E31.16	Interchange of Electrophysiological Waveforms and Signals
E31.17	Access, Privacy, and Confidentiality of Medical Records
E31.19	Electronic Health Record Content and Structure
E31.20	Data and System Security for Health Information
E31.21	Health Information Networks
E31.22	Health Information Transcription and Documentation
E31.23	Modeling for Health Informatics
E31.24	Electronic Health Record System Functionality
E31.25	XML for Document Type Definitions in Health care
E31.26	Personal (Consumer) Health Records
E31.28	Electronic Health Records

Health Care Informatics Standards Board

Responding to a request by CEN TC 251 to identify a single American organization that represents the standards work in the United States, ANSI formed a Health Care Informatics Standards Planning Panel (HISPP) in January 1992. This panel had a balanced representation from standards development groups, health care vendors, government agencies, and health care providers.

One of the charter goals of the HISPP was to coordinate the work of the message-standards group for health care data interchange and health care informatics to achieve the evolution of a unified set of nonredundant, nonconflicting standards that is compatible with ISO and non-ISO communications environments. In addition, a balanced subcommittee of the planning panel was formed to interact with and to provide input to CEN TC 251 in a coordinated fashion and to explore avenues of international standards development. A second subcommittee, with the specific objective of coordinating HISPP activities with TC 251, met in November 1992 and agreed to basic rules in the distribution of working documents (once approved by HISPP) to TC 251.

As work progressed and more organizations became actively interested in health care standards, ANSI and the members of HISPP recognized the need for a permanent body to coordinate the health care standards activities. The ANSI Board was petitioned to form a Health Care Informatics Board. In December 1995, the HISPP was dissolved and the Health Care Informatics Standards Board (HISB) was created.

The scope of the HISB includes standards for:

1. Health care models and electronic health care records
2. Interchange of health care data, images, sounds, and signals within and between organizations and practices
3. Health care codes and terminology

4. Communication with diagnostic instruments and health care devices
5. Representation and communication of health care protocols, knowledge, and statistical databases
6. Privacy, confidentiality, and security of medical information
7. Additional areas of concern or interest with regard to health care information

A major contribution of the HISB has been the creation and maintenance of an Inventory of Health Care Information Standards pertaining to the Health Insurance Portability and Accountability Act of 1996 (discussed in Section 7.3.3; see also Chapter 10).

Health Care Information and Management Systems Society

The Health Care Information and Management Systems Society (HIMSS) is a health care industry membership organization focused on providing leadership for the optimal use of health care information technology and management systems for the betterment of human health. HIMSS was founded in 1961 with offices in Chicago, Washington, D.C., and other locations across the country, HIMSS represents more than 13,000 individual members and some 150 member corporations that employ more than 1 million people. HIMSS shapes and directs health care public policy and industry practices through its advocacy, educational and professional development initiatives designed to promote information and management systems' contributions to quality patient care.

Computer-Based Patient Record Institute

The Computer-Based Patient Record Institute (CPRI) was an active proponent of standards activities after its inception in 1992. Although not a standards developer, CPRI made major contributions in the area of content of the computer-based patient record; security, privacy, and confidentiality; the universal health identifier; and terminology. In 2002, CPRI merged into HIMSS.

Integrating the Healthcare Enterprise

The goal of the Integrating the Healthcare Enterprise (IHE) initiative is to stimulate integration of health care information resources. While information systems are essential to the modern health care enterprise, they cannot deliver full benefits if they operate using proprietary protocols or incompatible standards. Decision makers need to encourage comprehensive integration among the full array of imaging and information systems.

IHE is sponsored jointly by the Radiological Society of North America (RSNA) and the HIMSS. Using established standards and working with direction from medical and information technology professionals, industry leaders in health care information and imaging systems cooperate under IHE to agree upon implementation profiles for the transactions used to communicate images and patient data within the enterprise. Their incentive for participation is the opportunity to demonstrate that their systems can operate efficiently in standards-based, multi-vendor environments with the functionality of real HISs. Moreover, IHE enables vendors to direct product development resources toward building increased functionality rather than redundant interfaces.

National Quality Forum

The National Quality Forum (NQF) is a private, not-for-profit membership organization created to develop and implement a national strategy for health care quality measurement and reporting. The mission of the NQF is to improve American health care through endorsement of consensus-based national standards for measurement and public reporting of health care performance data that provide meaningful information about whether care is safe, timely, beneficial, patient-centered, equitable and efficient.

National Institute of Standards and Technology

The National Institute of Standards and Technology (NIST) is a nonregulatory federal agency within the U.S. Department of Commerce. Its mission is to develop and promote measurement, standards, and technology to enhance productivity, facilitate trade, and improve the quality of life. In health care, NIST is providing measurement tools, manufacturing assistance, research and development support and quality guidelines as an effort to contain health care costs without compromising quality. Specifically, NIST has contributed measurement reference standards for clinical laboratories (for example, measurement standards for measuring cholesterol), mammography calibrations, micronutrients measurement quality assurance standards and others.

Workgroup for Electronic Data Interchange

The Workgroup for Electronic Data Interchange (WEDI) was formed in 1991 as a broad health care coalition to promote greater health care electronic commerce and connectivity in response to a challenge by then-Secretary of Health and Human Services Louis Sullivan. The challenge was to bring together industry leaders to identify ways to reduce administrative costs in health care through thoughtful implementation of Electronic Data Interchange (EDI).

Specifically, the goals of WEDI are:

- To define, prioritize, and reach consensus on critical issues affecting the acceptance of electronic commerce by the health care community
- To serve as a primary resource for identifying and removing obstacles that impede implementation of electronic commerce
- To educate and promote action by providing information resources on the benefits and effective use of electronic commerce, and on the implementation products and services available

WEDI incorporated as a formal organization in 1995. It has developed action plans to promote EDI standards, architectures, confidentiality, identifiers, health cards, legislation, and publicity. WEDI is one of the four organizations named specifically in the Health Insurance Portability and Accountability Act of 1996 (HIPAA) law to be consulted in the development of health care standards that would be selected to meet HIPAA requirements.

7.3.3   *Health Insurance Portability and Accountability Act of 1996*

The HIPAA was signed into law on August 21, 1996. The administrative-simplification portion of HIPAA requires that the Secretary of Health and Human Services (HHS) adopt standards for the electronic transmission of specific administrative transactions. These standards will apply to health plans, health care clearinghouses, and health care providers who transmit any health information in electronic form; Figure 7.2 shows the kinds of transactions covered. Recommendations made thus far include the use of X12N standards for health claims, the National Council for Prescription Drug Programs (NCPDP) for prescription reimbursement, and HL7 for claims attachments.

7.4   Coded Terminologies, Terminologies, and Nomenclatures

As discussed in Chapter 2, the capture, storage, and use of clinical data in computer systems is complicated by lack of agreement on terms and meanings. The many terminologies discussed in this section have been developed to ease the communication of coded medical information.

1. The Secretary must adopt standards for transactions, and data elements for such transactions, to enable health information to be exchanged electronically that are appropriate for financial and administrative transactions consistent with the goals of improving the operation of the health care system and reducing costs, including:
   a. Health Claims or equivalent encounter information
   b. Health Claims Attachments
   c. Enrollment and Disenrollment in a Health Plan
   d. Eligibility For a Health Plan
   e. Health Care Payment and Remittance Advice
   f. Health Plan Premium Payments
   g. First Report of Injury
   h. Health Claim Status
   i. Referral Certification and Authorization
   j. Coordination of Benefits
2. The Secretary shall adopt standards providing for a unique health identifier for each individual, employer, health plan, and health care provider for use in the health care system.
3. The Secretary shall adopt standards for code sets for appropriate data elements for financial and administrative transactions.
4. The Secretary shall adopt security standards that . . . specify procedures for the electronic transmission and authentication of signatures.

Figure 7.2. Requirements of the Health Insurance Portability and Accountability Act of 1996. These requirements define the first round of standards required to meet the immediate needs of the health care community.

7.4.1   Motivation for Controlled Terminologies

The encoding of medical information is a basic function of most clinical systems. Standards for such encoding can serve two purposes. First, they can save system developers from reinventing the wheel. For example, if an application allows caregivers to compile problem lists about their patients, using a standard terminology saves developers from having to create their own. Second, using commonly accepted standards can facilitate exchange of data among systems. For example, if a central database is accepting clinical data from many sources, the task is greatly simplified if each source is using the same coding scheme. System developers often ignore available standards and continue to develop their own solutions. It is easy to believe that the developers have resisted adoption of standards because it is too much work to understand and adapt to any system that was "not invented here." The reality, however, is that the available standards are often inadequate for the needs of the users (in this case, system developers). As a result, no standard terminology enjoys the wide acceptance sufficient to facilitate the second function: exchange of coded clinical information.

In discussing coding systems, the first step is to clarify the differences among a **terminology**, a **vocabulary**, and a **nomenclature**. These terms are often used interchangeably by creators of coding systems and by authors discussing the subject. Fortunately, although there are few accepted standard terminologies, there is a generally accepted standard *about* terminology: ISO Standard 1087 (Terminology—Vocabulary). Figure 7.3 lists the various definitions for these terms. For our purposes, we consider the currently available standards from the viewpoint of their being terminologies.

The next step in the discussion is to determine the basic use of the terminology. In general, there are two different levels relevant to medical data encoding: abstraction and representation. **Abstraction** entails examination of the recorded data and then selection of items from a terminology with which to label the data. For example, a patient might be admitted to the hospital and have a long and complex course; for the purposes of

---

- **Object:** Any part of the perceivable or conceivable world
- **Name:** Designation of an object by a linguistic expression
- **Concept:** A unit of thought constituted through abstraction on the basis of properties common to a set of objects
- **Term:** Designation of a defined concept in a special language by a linguistic expression
- **Terminology:** Set of terms representing the system of concepts of a particular subject field
- **Nomenclature:** System of terms that is elaborated according to preestablished naming rules
- **Dictionary:** Structured collection of lexical units, with linguistic information about each of them
- **Vocabulary:** Dictionary containing the terminology of a subject field

Figure 7.3. Terminologic terms, adapted from ISO Standard 1087. Terms not defined here—such as definition, lexical unit, and linguistic expression—are assumed by the Standard to have common meanings.

billing, however, it might be relevant that the patient was diagnosed only as having had a myocardial infarction. Someone charged with abstracting the record to generate a bill might then reduce the entire set of information to a single code. **Representation**, on the other hand, is the process by which as much detail as possible is coded. Thus, for medical record example, the representation might include codes for each physical finding noted, laboratory test performed, and medication administered.

When we discuss a controlled terminology, we should consider the domain of discourse. Virtually any subject matter can be coded, but there must be a good match with any standard selected for the purpose. For example, a terminology used to code disease information might be a poor choice for coding entries on a problem list because it might lack items such as "abdominal pain," "cigarette smoker," or "health maintenance."

The next consideration is the content of the standard itself. There are many issues, including the degree to which the standard covers the terminology of the intended domain; the degree to which data are coded by assembly of terms into descriptive phrases (postcoordination) versus selection of a single, precoordinated term; and the overall structure of the terminology (list, strict hierarchy, multiple hierarchy, semantic network, and so on). There are also many qualitative issues to consider, including the availability of synonyms and the possibility of redundant terms (i.e., more than one way to encode the same information).

Finally, we should consider the methods by which the terminology is maintained. Every standard terminology must have an ongoing maintenance process, or it will become obsolete rapidly. The process must be timely and must not be disruptive to people using an older version of the terminology. For example, if the creators of the terminology choose to rename a code, what happens to the data previously recorded with that code?

7.4.2   Specific Terminologies

With these considerations in mind, let us survey some of the available controlled terminologies. People often say, tongue in cheek, that the best thing about standards is that there are so many from which to choose. We give introductory descriptions of a few current and common terminologies. New terminologies appear annually, and existing proprietary terminologies often become publicly available. When reviewing the following descriptions, try to keep in mind the background motivation for a development effort. All these standards are evolving rapidly, and one should consult the Web sites or other primary sources for the most recent information.

International Classification of Diseases and Its Clinical Modifications

One of the best known terminologies is the *International Classification of Diseases* (ICD). First published in 1893, it has been revised at roughly 10-year intervals, first by the Statistical International Institute and later by the World Health Organization (WHO). The *Ninth Edition* (ICD-9) was published in 1977 (World Health Organization, 1977) and the *Tenth Edition* (ICD-10) in 1992 (World Health Organization, 1992). The coding system consists of a *core classification* of three-digit codes that are the minimum required for reporting mortality statistics to WHO. A fourth digit (in the first decimal place) provides an additional level of detail; usually .0 to .7 are used for more specific forms of the core term, .8 is usually "other," and .9 is "unspecified." Terms are arranged in a strict hierarchy, based on the digits in the code. For example, bacterial pneumonias are classified as shown in Figures 7.4 and 7.5. In addition to diseases, ICD includes

```
003 Other salmonella infections
       003.2 Localized salmonella infections
               003.22 Salmonella pneumonia *
020 Plague
       020.3 Primary pneumonic plague
       020.4 Secondary pneumonic plague
       020.5 Pneumonic plague, unspecified
021 Tularemia
       021.2 Pulmonary tularemia *
022 Anthrax
       022.1 Pulmonary anthrax
481 Pneumococcal pneumonia
482 Other bacterial pneumonia
       482.0 Pneumonia due to Klebsiella pneumoniae
       482.1 Pneumonia due to Pseudomonas
       482.2 Pneumonia due to Hemophilus influenzae
       482.3 Pneumonia due to Streptococcus
               482.30 Pneumonia due to Streptococcus, unspecified *
               482.31 Pneumonia due to Group A Streptococcus *
               482.32 Pneumonia due to Group B Streptococcus *
               482.39 Other streptococcal pneumonia *
       482.4 Pneumonia due to Staphylococcus
               482.40 Pneumonia due to Staphylococcus, unspecified *
               482.41 Pneumonia due to Staphylococcus aureus *
               482.49 Other Staphylococcus pneumonia *
       482.8 Pneumonia due to other specified bacteria
               482.81 Pneumonia due to anaerobes *
               482.82 Pneumonia due to Escherichia coli *
               482.83 Pneumonia due to other Gram-negative bacteria *
               482.84 Legionnaires' disease *
               482.89 Pneumonia due to other specified bacteria *
       482.9 Bacterial pneumonia, unspecified
483 Pneumonia due to other specified organism
       483.0 Mycoplasma pneumoniae *
484 Pneumonia in infectious diseases classified elsewhere *
       484.3 Pneumonia in whooping cough *
       484.5 Pneumonia in anthrax *
```

Figure 7.4. Examples of codes in ICD-9 and ICD-9-CM (*) showing how bacterial pneumonia terms are coded. Tuberculosis terms, pneumonias for which the etiologic agent is not specified, and other intervening terms are not shown. Note that some terms, such as "Salmonella Pneumonia" were introduced in ICD-9-CM as a children of organism-specific terms, rather than under 482 (other bacterial pneumonia).

A01 Typhoid and paratyphoid fevers
    A01.0 Typhoid Fever
        A01.03 Typhoid Pneumonia *
A02 Other salmonella infection
    A02.2 Localized salmonella infections
        A02.22 Salmonella pneumonia *
A20 Plague
    A20.2 Pneumonic plague
A22 Anthrax
    A22.1 Pulmonary anthrax
A37 Whooping cough
    A37.0 Whooping cough due to *Bordetella pertussis*
        A37.01 Whooping cough due to *Bordetella pertussis* with pneumonia *
    A37.1 Whooping cough due to *Bordetella parapertussis*
        A37.11 Whooping cough due to *Bordetella parapertussis* with pneumonia *
    A37.8 Whooping cough due to other Bordetella species
        A37.81 Whooping cough due to other Bordetella species with pneumonia *
    A37.9 Whooping cough, unspecified
        A37.91 Whooping cough, unspecified species with pneumonia *
A50 Congenital syphilis
    A50.0 Early congenital syphilis, symptomatic
        A50.04 Early congenital syphilitic pneumonia *
A54 Gonococcal infection
    A54.8 Other gonococcal infection
        A54.84 Gonococcal pneumonia *
J13 Pneumonia due to *Streptococcus pneumoniae*
J14 Pneumonia due to *Hemophilus influenzae*
J15 Bacterial pneumonia, not elsewhere classified
    J15.0 Pneumonia due to *Klebsiella pneumoniae*
    J15.1 Pneumonia due to Pseudomonas
    J15.2 Pneumonia due to staphylococcus
        J15.20 Pneumonia due to staphylococcus, unspecified *
        J15.21 Pneumonia due to *Staphylococcus aureus* *
        J15.29 Pneumonia due to other staphylococcus *
    J15.3 Pneumonia due to streptococcus, group B
    J15.4 Pneumonia due to other streptococci
    J15.5 Pneumonia due to *Escherichia coli*
    J15.6 Pneumonia due to other aerobic Gram-negative bacteria
    J15.7 Pneumonia due to *Mycoplasma pneumoniae*
    J15.8 Other bacterial pneumonia
    J15.9 Bacterial pneumonia, unspecified
P23 Congenital pneumonia
    P23.2 Congenital pneumonia due to staphylococcus
    P23.3 Congenital pneumonia due to streptococcus, group B
    P23.4 Congenital pneumonia due to *Escherichia coli*
    P23.5 Congenital pneumonia due to Pseudomonas
    P23.6 Congenital pneumonia due to other bacterial agents

Figure 7.5. Examples of codes in ICD-10 and ICD-10-CM (*) showing how bacterial pneumonia terms are coded. Tuberculosis terms, pneumonias for which the etiologic agent is not specified, and other intervening terms are not shown. Note that ICD-10 classifies Mycoplasma pneumoniae as a bacterium, while ICD-9 does not. Also, neither ICD-10 nor ICD-10-CM have a code for "Melioidosis Pneumonia," but ICD-10-CM specifies that the code A24.1 Acute and fulminating melioidosis (not shown) should be used.

several "families" of terms for medical-specialty diagnoses, health status, disablements, procedures, and reasons for contact with health care providers.

ICD-9 was generally been perceived as inadequate for the level of detail desired for statistical reporting in the United States (Kurtzke, 1979). In response, the U.S. National Center for Health Statistics published a set of **clinical modifications** (CM) (Commission on Professional and Hospital Activites, 1978). **ICD-9-CM**, as it is known, is compatible with ICD-9 and provides extra levels of detail in many places by adding fourth-digit and fifth-digit codes. Figure 7.4 shows a sample of additional material. Most of the diagnoses assigned in the United States are coded in ICD-9-CM, allowing compliance with international treaty (by conversion to ICD-9) and supporting billing requirements (by conversion to diagnosis-related groups or DRGs). A clinical modification for ICD-10 is presently under review; examples are shown in Figure 7.5.

Diagnosis-Related Groups

Another U.S. creation for the purpose of abstracting medical records is the DRGs, developed initially at Yale University for use in prospective payment in the Medicare program (3M Health Information System, updated annually). In this case, the coding system is an abstraction of an abstraction; it is applied to lists of ICD-9-CM codes that are themselves derived from medical records. The purpose of DRG coding is to provide a relatively small number of codes for classifying patient hospitalizations while also providing some separation of cases based on severity of illness. The principal bases for the groupings are factors that affect cost and length of stay. Thus, a medical record containing the ICD-9-CM primary diagnosis of pneumococcal pneumonia (481) might be coded with one of 18 codes (Figure 7.6), depending on associated conditions and procedures; additional codes are possible if the pneumonia is a secondary diagnosis.

International Classification of Primary Care

The World Organization of National Colleges, Academies and Academic Associations of General Practitioners/Family Physicians (WONCA) publishes the *International Classification of Primary Care* (ICPC) with the WHO, the lastest version of which is *ICPC-2*, published in 1988. ICPC-2 is a classification of some 1400 diagnostic concepts that are partially mapped into ICD-9. ICPC-2 contains all 380 concepts of the *International Classification of Health Problems in Primary Care* (ICHPPC), Third Edition, including reasons for an encounter. ICPC provides seven axes of terms and a structure to combine them to represent clinical encounters. Although the granularity of the terms is generally larger than that of other classification schemes (e.g., all pneumonias are coded as R81), the ability to represent the interactions of the concepts found in a medical record is much greater through the **postcoordination** of atomic terms. In postcoordination, the coding is accomplished through the use of multiple codes as needed to describe the data. Thus, for example, a case of bacterial pneumonia would be coded in ICPC as a combination of the code R81 and the code for the particular test result that identifies the causative agent. This method is in contrast to the **precoordination** approach in which every type of pneumonia is assigned its own code.

Respiratory disease w/ major chest operating room procedure, no major complication or comorbidity	75
Respiratory disease w/ major chest operating room procedure, minor complication or comorbidity	76
Respiratory disease w/ other respiratory system operating procedure, no complication or comorbidity	77
Respiratory infection w/ minor complication, age greater than 17	79
Respiratory infection w/ no minor complication, age greater than 17	80
Simple Pneumonia w/ minor complication, age greater than 17	89
Simple Pneumonia w/ no minor complication, age greater than 17	90
Respiratory disease w/ ventilator support	475
Respiratory disease w/ major chest operating room procedure and major complication or comorbidity	538
Respiratory disease, other respiratory system operating procedure and major complication	539
Respiratory infection w/ major complication or comorbidity	540
Respiratory infection w/ secondary diagnosis of bronchopulmonary dysplasia	631
Respiratory infection w/ secondary diagnosis of cystic fibrosis	740
Respiratory infection w/ minor complication, age not greater than 17	770
Respiratory infection w/ no minor complication, age not greater than 17	771
Simple Pneumonia w/ minor complication, age not greater than 17	772
Simple Pneumonia w/ no minor complication, age not greater than 17	773
Respiratory infection w/ primary diagnosis of tuberculosis	798

Figure 7.6. Diagnosis-related group codes assigned to cases of bacterial pneumonia depending on co-occurring conditions or procedures (mycobacterial disease is not shown here except as a co-occurring condition). "Simple Pneumonia" codes are used when the primary bacterial pneumonia corresponds to ICD-9 code 481, 482.2, 482.3, or 482.9, and when there are only minor or no complications. The remaining ICD-9 bacterial pneumonias (482.0, 482.1, 482.2, 482.4, 482.8, 484, and various other codes such as 003.22) are coded as "Respiratory Disease" or "Respiratory Infection." Cases in which pneumonia is a secondary diagnosis may also be assigned other codes (such as 798), depending on the primary condition.

Current Procedural Terminology

The American Medical Association developed the *Current Procedural Terminology* (CPT) in 1966 (American Medical Association, updated annually) to provide a precoordinated coding scheme for diagnostic and therapeutic procedures that has since been adopted in the United States for billing and reimbursement. Like the DRG codes, CPT codes specify information that differentiates the codes based on cost. For example, there are different codes for pacemaker insertions, depending on whether the leads are "epicardial, by thoracotomy" (33200), "epicardial, by xiphoid approach" (33201), "transvenous, atrial" (33206), "transvenous, ventricular" (33207), or "transvenous, atrioventricular (AV) sequential" (33208). CPT also provides information about the reasons for a procedure. For example, there are codes for arterial punctures for "withdrawal of blood for diagnosis" (36600), "monitoring" (36620), "infusion therapy" (36640), and "occlusion therapy" (75894). Although limited in scope and depth (despite containing over 8000 terms), CPT-4 is the most widely accepted nomenclature in the United States for reporting physician procedures and services for federal and private insurance third-party reimbursement.

Diagnostic and Statistical Manual of Mental Disorders

The American Psychiatric Association published its *Diagnostic and Statistical Manual of Mental Disorders*(DSM-IV), Fourth Edition, in 1994 (American Psychiatric Association, 1994), revised in 1996 (DSM-IV-R). The DSM nomenclature provides definitions of psychiatric disorders and includes specific diagnostic criteria. Thus, it is used not only for coding patient data but also as a tool for assigning diagnoses. Each edition of DSM has been coordinated with corresponding editions of ICD; DSM-IV is coordinated with ICD-10 and contains over 450 terms.

Read Clinical Codes

The Read Clinical Codes comprise a set of terms designed specifically for use in coding electronic medical records. Developed by James Read in the 1980s (Read and Benson, 1986; Read, 1990), the first version was adopted by the British National Health Service (NHS) in 1990. Version 2.0 was developed to meet the needs of hospitals for cross-mapping their data to ICD-9. Version 3.0 (NHS Centre for Coding and Classification, 1994a) was developed to support not only medical record summarization but also patient-care applications directly. Whereas previous versions of the Read Codes were organized in a strict hierarchy, Version 3.0 took an important step by allowing terms to have multiple parents in the hierarchy, i.e., the hierarchy became that of a directed acyclic graph. Version 3.1 added the ability to make use of term modifiers through a set of templates for combining terms in specific, controlled ways so that both precoordination and postcoordination are used. Finally, the NHS undertook a series of "clinical terms" projects that expanded the content of the Read Codes to ensure that the terms needed by practitioners are represented in the Codes (NHS Centre for Coding and Classification, 1994b).

SNOMED Clinical Terms and Its Predecessors

Drawing from the New York Academy of Medicine's *Standard Nomenclature of Diseases and Operations* (SNDO) (New York Academy of Medicine, 1961), the College of American Pathologists (CAP) developed the *Standard Nomenclature of Pathology* (SNOP) as a multiaxial system for describing pathologic findings (College of American Pathologists, 1971) through postcoordination of topographic (anatomic), morphologic, etiologic, and functional terms. SNOP has been used widely in pathology systems in the United States; its successor, the *Systematized Nomenclature of Medicine* (SNOMED) has evolved beyond an abstracting scheme to become a comprehensive coding system.

Largely the work of Roger Côté and David Rothwell, SNOMED was first published in 1975, was revised as SNOMED II in 1979, and then greatly expanded in 1993 as the *Systematized Nomenclature of Human and Veterinary Medicine—SNOMED*

International (Côté et al., 1993). Each of these version was **multi-axial**; coding of patient information was accomplished through the postcoordination of terms from multiple axes to represent complex terms that did not exist as single codes in SNOMED. In 1996, SNOMED changed from a multi-axial structure to a more logic-based structure called a *Reference Terminology* (Spackman et al., 1997; Campbell et al., 1998), intended to support more sophisticated data encoding processes and resolve some of the problems with earlier version of SNOMED (see Figure 7.7). In 1999, CAP and the NHS announced an agreement to merge their products into a single terminology called *SNOMED Clinical Terms* (SNOMED-CT) (Spackman, 2000), containing terms for over 344,000 concepts (see Figure 7.8).

Despite the broad coverage of SNOMED-CT, it continues to allow users to create new, ad hoc terms through postcoordination of existing terms. While this increases the

Concept: Bacterial pneumonia
  Concept Status Current
  Fully defined by ...
    Is a
      Infectious disease of lung
      Inflammatory disorder of lower respiratory tract
      Infective pneumonia
      Inflammation of specific body organs
      Inflammation of specific body systems
      Bacterial infectious disease
    Causative agent:
      Bacterium
    Pathological process:
      Infectious disease
    Associated morphology:
      Inflammation
    Finding site:
      Lung structure
    Onset:
      Subacute onset
      Acute onset
      Insidious onset
      Sudden onset
    Severity:
      Severities
    Episodicity:
      Episodicities
    Course:
      Courses
  Descriptions:
    Bacterial pneumonia (disorder)
    Bacterial pneumonia
  Legacy codes:
    SNOMED: DE-10100
    CTV3ID: X100H

Figure 7.7. Description-logic representation of the SNOMED-CT term "Bacterial Pneumonia." The "Is a" attributes define bacterial pneumonia's position in SNOMED-CT's multiple hierarchy, while attributes such as "Causative Agent" and "Finding Site" provide definitional information. Other attributes such as "Onset" and "Severities" indicate ways in which bacterial pneumonia can be postcoordinated with others terms, such as "Acute Onset" or any of the descendants of the term "Severities." "Descriptions" refers to various text strings that serve as names for the term, while "Legacy Codes" provide backward compatibility to SNOMED and Read Clinical Terms.

Pneumonia
  Bacterial pneumonia
    Proteus pneumonia
    Legionella pneumonia
    Anthrax pneumonia
    Actinomycotic pneumonia
    Nocardial pneumonia
    Meningococcal pneumonia
    Chlamydial pneumonia
      Neonatal chlamydial pneumonia
      Ornithosis
        Ornithosis with complication
        Ornithosis with pneumonia
    Congenital bacterial pneumonia
      Congenital staphylococcal pneumonia
      Congenital group A hemolytic streptococcal pneumonia
      Congenital group B hemolytic streptococcal pneumonia
      Congenital *Escherichia coli* pneumonia
      Congenital pseudomonal pneumonia
    Chlamydial pneumonitis in all species except pig
      Feline pneumonitis
    Staphylococcal pneumonia
    Pulmonary actinobacillosis
    Pneumonia in Q fever
    Pneumonia due to Streptococcus
      Group B streptococcal pneumonia
      Congenital group A hemolytic streptococcal pneumonia
      Congenital group B hemolytic streptococcal pneumonia
      Pneumococcal pneumonia
        Pneumococcal lobar pneumonia
        AIDS with pneumococcal pneumonia
    Pneumonia due to Pseudomonas
      Congenital pseudomonal pneumonia
    Pulmonary tularemia
    Enzootic pneumonia of calves
    Pneumonia in pertussis
    AIDS with bacterial pneumonia
    Enzootic pneumonia of sheep
    Pneumonia due to *Klebsiella pneumoniae*
    Hemophilus influenzae pneumonia
    Porcine contagious pleuropneumonia
    Pneumonia due to pleuropneumonia-like organism
    Secondary bacterial pneumonia
  Pneumonic plague
    Primary pneumonic plague
    Secondary pneumonic plague
  Salmonella pneumonia
    Pneumonia in typhoid fever
  Infective pneumonia
    Mycoplasma pneumonia
      Enzootic mycoplasmal pneumonia of swine
  Achromobacter pneumonia
  Bovine pneumonic pasteurellosis
  Corynebacterial pneumonia of foals
  Pneumonia due to *Escherichia coli*
  Pneumonia due to *Proteus mirabilis*

expressivity, users must be careful not to be *too* expressive because there are few rules about how the postcoordination coding should be done, the same expression might end up being represented differently by different coders. For example, "acute appendicitis" can be coded as a single disease term, as a combination of a modifier ("acute") and a disease term ("appendicitis"), or as a combination of a modifier ("acute"), a morphology term ("inflammation") and a topography term ("vermiform appendix"). Users must therefore be careful when postcoordinating terms, not to recreate a meaning that is satisfied by a single code. The description logic, such as the example in Figure 7.7, can help guide users when selecting modifiers.

Galen

In Europe, a consortium of universities, agencies, and vendors, with funding from the Advanced Informatics in Medicine initiative (AIM), has formed the GALEN project to develop standards for representing coded patient information (Rector et al., 1995). GALEN is developing a reference model for medical concepts using a formalism called Structured Meta Knowledge (SMK). In SMK, terms are defined through relationships to other terms, and grammars are provided to allow combinations of terms into sensible phrases. The reference model is intended to allow representation of patient information in a way that is independent of the language being recorded and of the data model used by an electronic medical record system. The GALEN developers are working closely with CEN TC 251 (see Section 7.3.2) to develop the content that will populate the reference model with actual terms. In 2000, an open source foundation called OpenGALEN (www.opengalen.org) was developed, which distributes their reference model free of charge and works with software vendors and terminology developers to support its extension and use.

Logical Observations, Identifiers, Names, and Codes

An independent consortium, led by Clement J. McDonald and Stanley M. Huff, has created a naming system for tests and observations. Originally called *Laboratory Observations, Identifiers, Names and Codes* (LOINC), the system has been extended to include nonlaboratory observations (vital signs, electrocardiograms, and so on), so

---

Figure 7.8. Examples of codes in SNOMED -CT, showing some of the hierarchical relationships among bacterial pneumonia terms. Tuberculosis terms and certain terms that are included in SNOMED-CT for compatability with other terminologies are not shown. Note that some terms such as "Congenital group A hemolytic streptococcal pneumonia" appear under multiple parent terms, while other terms, such as "Congenital staphylococcal pneumonia" are not listed under all possible parent terms (e.g., it is under "Congenital pneumonia" but not under "Staphylococcal pneumonia"). Some terms, such as "Pneumonic plague" and "Mycoplasma pneumonia" are not classified under Bacterial Pneumonia, althogh the causative agents in their descriptions ("Yersinia pestis" and "Myocplasma pneumoniae", respectively) are classified under "Bacterium", the causative agent of Bacterial pneumonia.

Logical has replaced *Laboratory* to reflect the change (Huff, 1998). Figure 7.9 shows some typical fully specified names for common laboratory tests. The standard specifies structured coded semantic information about each test, such as the substance measured and the analytical method used. Using this system, a person can code new names for new tests, which can be recognized by other users of the coded information; however, officially recognized names (such as those in the Figure 7.9) are given more compact LOINC codes. The LOINC committee is collaborating with CEN to coordinate their work with the similar EUCLIDES work in Europe (EUCLIDES Foundation International, 1994).

Nursing Terminologies

Nursing organizations and research teams have been extremely active in the development of standard coding systems for documenting and evaluating nursing care. One review counted a total of 12 separate projects active worldwide (Coenen et al., 2001), including coordination with SNOMED and LOINC. These projects have arisen because general medical terminologies fail to represent the kind of clinical concepts needed in nursing care. For example, the kinds of problems that appear in a physician's problem list (such as "myocardial infarction" and "diabetes mellitus") are relatively well represented in many of the terminologies that we have described, but the kinds of problems that appear in a nurse's assessment (such as "activity intolerance" and "knowledge deficit related to myocardial infarction") are not. Preeminent nursing terminologies include the North American Nursing Diagnosis Association (NANDA) codes, the Nursing Interventions Classification (NIC), the Nursing Outcomes Classification (NOC), the Georgetown Home Health Care Classification (HHCC), and the Omaha System (which covers problems, interventions, and outcomes).

Despite the proliferation of standards for nursing terminologies, gaps remain in the coverage of this domain (Henry and Mead, 1997). Recently, the International Council of Nurses and the International Medical Informatics Association Nursing Informatics Special Interest Group have worked together to develop an ISO standard for a reference terminology model that attempts to identify and formally represent the distinguishing characteristics of nursing diagnoses and actions (International Standards Organization, 2003).

Drug Codes

A variety of public and commercial terminologies have been developed to represent terms used for prescribing, dispensing and administering drugs. The *WHO Drug Dictionary* is an international classification of drugs that provides proprietary drug names used in different countries, as well as all active ingredients and the chemical substances, with Chemical Abstract numbers. Drugs are classified according to the *Anatomical-Therapeutic-Chemical* (ATC) classification, with cross-references to manufacturers and reference sources. The current dictionary contains 25,000 proprietary drug names, 15,000 single ingredient drugs, 10,000 multiple ingredient drugs, and 7,000 chemical substances. The dictionary now covers drugs from 34 countries and grows at a rate of about 2,000 new entries per year.

Blood glucose	GLUCOSE:MCNC:PT:BLD:QN:
Plasma glucose	GLUCOSE:MCNC:PT:PLAS:QN:
Serum glucose	GLUCOSE:MCNC:PT:SER:QN:
Urine glucose concentration	GLUCOSE:MCNC:PT:UR:QN:
Urine glucose by dip stick	GLUCOSE:MCNC:PT:UR:SQ:TEST STRIP

Glucose tolerance test at
    2 hours
	GLUCOSE^2H POST 100 G GLUCOSE PO:
	    MCNC:PT:PLAS:QN:

Ionized whole blood calcium	CALCIUM.FREE:SCNC:PT:BLD:QN:
Serum or plasma ionized calcium	CALCIUM.FREE:SCNC:PT:SER/PLAS:QN:
24-hour calcium excretion	CALCIUM.TOTAL:MRAT:24H:UR:QN:
Whole blood total calcium	CALCIUM.TOTAL:SCNC:PT:BLD:QN:
Serum or plasma total calcium	CALCIUM.TOTAL:SCNC:PT:SER/PLAS:QN:
Automated hematocrit	HEMATOCRIT:NFR:PT:BLD:QN: AUTOMATED COUNT
Manual spun hematocrit	HEMATOCRIT:NFR:PT:BLD:QN:SPUN
Urine erythrocyte casts	ERYTHROCYTE CASTS:ACNC:PT:URNS:SQ: MICROSCOPY.LIGHT

Erythrocyte MCHC	ERYTHROCYTE MEAN CORPUSCULAR HEMOGLOBIN
	    CONCENTRATION:MCNC:PT:RBC:QN:AUTOMATED
	    COUNT

Erythrocyte MCH	ERYTHROCYTE MEAN CORPUSCULAR
	    HEMOGLOBIN:MCNC:PT:RBC:QN: AUTOMATED
	    COUNT

Erythrocyte MCV	ERYTHROCYTE MEAN CORPUSCULAR VOLUME:ENTVOL:PT:RBC:QN:AUTOMATED COUNT
Automated Blood RBC	ERYTHROCYTES:NCNC:PT:BLD:QN: AUTOMATED COUNT
Manual blood RBC	ERYTHROCYTES:NCNC:PT:BLD:QN: MANUAL COUNT
ESR by Westergren method	ERYTHROCYTE SEDIMENTATION RATE:VEL:PT:BLD:QN:WESTERGREN
ESR by Wintrobe method	ERYTHROCYTE SEDIMENTATION RATE:VEL:PT:BLD:QN:WINTROBE

Figure 7.9. Examples of common laboratory test terms as they are encoded in LOINC. The major components of the fully specified name are separated here by ":" and consist of the substance measured, the property (e.g., MCNC = mass concentration; SCNC = substance concentration; NFR = numeric fraction; and NCNC = number concentration), the time (PT = point in time), the specimen, and the method (SQ = semiquantitative; QN = quantitative; QL = qualitative).

The *National Drug Codes* (NDC), produced by the U.S. Food and Drug Administration (FDA), is applied to all drug packages. It is widely used in the United States, but it is not as comprehensive as the WHO codes. The FDA designates part of the code based on drug manufacturer, and each manufacturer defines the specific codes for their own products. As a result, there is no uniform class hierarchy for the codes, and codes may be reused at the manufacturer's discretion. Due in part to the inadequacies of the NDC codes, pharmacy information systems typically purchase proprietary terminologies from knowledge base vendors. These terminologies map to NDC, but provide additional information about therapeutic classes, allergies, ingredients, and forms.

The need for standards for drug terminologies has led to a collaboration between the FDA, the U.S. National Library of Medicine (NLM), the Veterans Administration (VA), and the pharmacy knowledge base vendors that is producing a representational model for drug terms called *RxNorm*. The NLM is providing RxNorm to the public as part of the Unified Medical Language System (UMLS) (see below) to support mapping between NDC codes, the VA's *National Drug File* (VANDF) and various proprietary drug terminologies (Nelson, 2002). RxNorm curently contains 14,000 terms.

Medical Subject Headings

The *Medical Subject Headings* (MeSH), maintained by the NLM (National Library of Medicine, updated annually), is the terminology by which the world medical literature is indexed. MeSH arranges terms in a structure that breaks from the strict hierarchy used by most other coding schemes. Terms are organized into hierarchies and may appear in multiple places in the hierarchy (Figure 7.10). Although it is not generally used as a direct coding scheme for patient information, it plays a central role in the UMLS.

Bioinformatics Terminologies

For the most part, the terminologies discussed above fail to represent the levels of detail needed by biomolecular researchers. This has become a more acute problem with the

Figure 7.10. Partial tree structure for the Medical Subject Headings showing pneumonia terms. Note that terms can appear in multiple locations, although they may not always have the same children, implying that they have somewhat different meanings in different contexts. For example, Pneumonia means "lung inflammation" in one context (line 3) and "lung infection" in another (line 16).

```
Respiratory Tract Diseases
    Lung Diseases
        Pneumonia
            Bronchopneumonia
            Pneumonia, Aspiration
                Pneumonia, Lipid
            Pneumonia, Lobar
            Pneumonia, Mycoplasma
            Pneumonia, Pneumocystis carinii
            Pneumonia, Rickettsial
            Pneumonia, Staphylococcal
            Pneumonia, Viral
        Lung Diseases, Fungal
            Pneumonia, Pneumocystis carinii
Respiratory Tract Infections
    Pneumonia
        Pneumonia, Lobar
        Pneumonia, Mycoplasma
        Pneumonia, Pneumocystis carinii
        Pneumonia, Rickettsial
        Pneumonia, Staphylococcal
        Pneumonia, Viral
    Lung Diseases, Fungal
        Pneumonia, Pneumocystis carinii
```

advent of bioinformatics and the sequencing of organism genomes (see Chapter 22). As in other domains, researchers have been forced to develop their own terminologies. As these researchers have begun to exchange information, they have recognized the need for standard naming conventions as well as standard ways of representing their data with terminologies. Prominent efforts to unify naming systems include the Gene Ontology (GO) (Harris et al., 2004) and the National Cancer Institute's caCORE framework (Covitz et al., 2003]. However, terminology standards alone are not sufficient for information sharing. In addition, work is under way to develop standard ways of using these terminologies to encode data. Two early efforts are the Distributed Annotation System (DAS) (Dowell et al., 2001), for representing genetic sequences, and the Minimal Information About a Microarray Experiment (MIAME) (Brazma et al., 2001) for representing results of microarray experiments (see Chapter 22).

Unified Medical Language System

In 1986, Donald Lindberg and Betsy Humphreys, at the NLM, began consulting contractors to identify ways to construct a resource that would bring together and disseminate controlled medical terminologies. An experimental version of the *UMLS* was first published in 1989 (Humphreys, 1990); the UMLS has been updated annually since then. Its principal component is the Metathesaurus, which contains over one million terms collected from over 100 different sources (including many of those that we have discussed), and attempts to relate synonymous and similar terms from across the different sources (Figure 7.11). Figure 7.12 lists the preferred names for all pneumonia concepts in the Metathesaurus; Figure 7.13 shows how like terms are grouped into concepts and are tied to other concepts through semantic relationships.

Interchange Registration of Coding Schemes

To accommodate the many coding schemes that are in use (and are likely to persist) in health care applications today, the CEN Project Team PT 005 has defined a draft standard that describes procedures for international registration of coding schemes used in health care (Health Care Financial Management Association, 1992). The protocol specifies the allocation of a unique six-character *Health Care Coding Scheme Designator* (HCD) to each registered coding scheme. A code value can then be assigned an unambiguous meaning in association with an HCD.

7.5   Data-Interchange Standards

The recognition of the need to interconnect health care applications led to the development and enforcement of **data-interchange standards**. The conceptualization stage began in 1980 with discussions among individuals in an organization called the American Association for Medical Systems and Informatics (AAMSI). In 1983, an AAMSI task force was established to pursue those interests in developing standards. The discussions were far ranging in topics and focus. Some members wanted to write

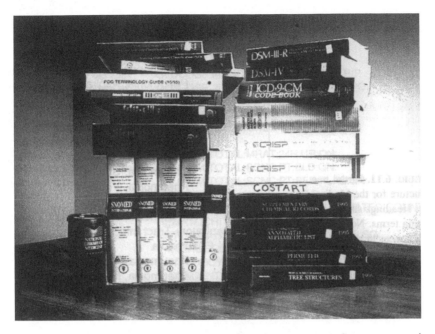

Figure 7.11. Sources for the UMLS. The Unified Medical Language System, comprises contributed terminologies from a large number of sources, including all the text compendia shown here. (*Source*: Courtesy National Library of Medicine and Lexical Technology, Inc.)

standards for everything, including a standard medical terminology, standards for HISs, standards for the computer-based patient record, and standards for data interchange. Citing the need for data interchange between commercial laboratories and health care providers, the task force agreed to focus on data-interchange standards for clinical laboratory data. Early activities were directed mainly toward increasing interest of AAMSI members in working to create health care standards.

The development phase was multifaceted. The AAMSI task force became subcommittee E31.11 of the ASTM and developed and published ASTM standard 1238 for the exchange of clinical-laboratory data. Two other groups—many members of which had participated in the earlier AAMSI task force—were formed to develop standards, each with a slightly different emphasis: HL7 and Institute of Electrical and Electronics Engineering (IEEE) Medical Data Interchange Standard. The American College of Radiology (ACR) joined with the National Electronic Manufacturers Association (NEMA) to develop a standard for the transfer of image data. Two other groups developed related standards independent of the biomedical informatics community: (1) ANSI X12 for the transmission of commonly used business transactions, including health care claims and benefit data, and (2) National Council for Prescription Drug Programs (NCPDP) for the transmission of third-party drug claims. Development was further complicated by the independent creation of standards by several groups in Europe, including EDIFACT.

```
C0004626: Pneumonia, Bacterial
C0023241: Legionnaires' Disease
C0032286: Pneumonia due to other specified bacteria
C0032308: Pneumonia, Staphylococcal
C0152489: Salmonella pneumonia
C0155858: Other bacterial pneumonia
C0155859: Pneumonia due to Klebsiella pneumoniae
C0155860: Pneumonia due to Pseudomonas
C0155862: Pneumonia due to Streptococcus
C0155865: Pneumonia in pertussis
C0155866: Pneumonia in anthrax
C0238380: PNEUMONIA, KLEBSIELLA AND OTHER GRAM NEGATIVE BACILLI
C0238381: PNEUMONIA, TULAREMIC
C0242056: PNEUMONIA, CLASSIC PNEUMOCOCCAL LOBAR
C0242057: PNEUMONIA, FRIEDLAENDER BACILLUS
C0275977: Pneumonia in typhoid fever
C0276026: Hemophilus influenzae pneumonia
C0276039: Pittsburgh pneumonia
C0276071: Achromobacter pneumonia
C0276080: Pneumonia due to Proteus mirabilis
C0276089: Pneumonia due to Escherichia coli
C0276523: AIDS with bacterial pneumonia
C0276524: AIDS with pneumococcal pneumonia
C0339946: Pneumonia with tularemia
C0339947: Pneumonia with anthrax
C0339952: Secondary bacterial pneumonia
C0339953: Pneumonia due to Escherichia coli
C0339954: Pneumonia due to proteus
C0339956: Typhoid pneumonia
C0339957: Meningococcal pneumonia
C0343320: Congenital pneumonia due to staphylococcus
C0343321: Congenital pneumonia due to group A hemolytic streptococcus
C0343322: Congenital pneumonia due to group B hemolytic streptococcus
C0343323: Congenital pneumonia due to Escherichia coli
C0343324: Congenital pneumonia due to pseudomonas
C0348678: Pneumonia due to other aerobic Gram-negative bacteria
C0348680: Pneumonia in bacterial diseases classified elsewhere
C0348801: Pneumonia due to streptococcus, group B
C0349495: Congenital bacterial pneumonia
C0349692: Lobar (pneumococcal) pneumonia
C0375322: Pneumococcal pneumonia {Streptococcus pneumoniae pneumonia}
C0375323: Pneumonia due to Streptococcus, unspecified
C0375324: Pneumonia due to Streptococcus Group A
C0375326: Pneumonia due to other Streptococcus
C0375327: Pneumonia due to anaerobes
C0375328: Pneumonia due to Escherichia coli
C0375329: Pneumonia due to other Gram-negative bacteria
C0375330: Bacterial pneumonia, unspecified
```

Figure 7.12. Some of the bacterial pneumonia concepts in the Unified Medical Language System Metathesaurus.

```
Bacterial pneumonia
    Source:    CSP93/PT/2596-5280; DOR27/DT/U000523;
               ICD91/PT/482.9; ICD91/IT/482.9
    Parent:    Bacterial Infections; Pneumonia; Influenza with Pneumonia
    Child:     Pneumonia, Mycoplasma
    Narrower:  Pneumonia, Lobar; Pneumonia, Rickettsial; Pneumonia,
               Staphylococcal; Pneumonia due to Klebsiella pneumoniae;
               Pneumonia due to Pseudomonas; Pneumonia due to Hemophilus
               influenzae
    Other:     Klebsiella pneumoniae, Streptococcus pneumoniae

Pneumonia, Lobar
    Source:    ICD91/IT/481; MSH94/PM/D011018; MSH94/MH/D011018;
               SNM2/RT/M-40000; ICD91/PT/481; SNM2/PT/D-0164;
               DXP92/PT/U000473; MSH94/EP/D011018;
               INS94/MH/D011018;INS94/SY/D011018
    Synonym:   Pneumonia, diplococcal
    Parent:    Bacterial Infections; Influenza with Pneumonia
    Broader:   Bacterial Pneumonia; Inflammation
    Other:     Streptococcus pneumoniae
    Semantic:  inverse-is-a: Pneumonia
               has-result: Pneumococcal Infections

Pneumonia, Staphylococcal
    Source:    ICD91/PT/482.4; ICD91/IT/482.4; MSH94/MH/D011023;
               MSH94/PM/D011023; MSH94/EP/D011023; SNM2/PT/D-017X;
               INS94/MH/D011023; INS94/SY/D011023
    Parent:    Bacterial Infections; Influenza with Pneumonia
    Broader:   Bacterial Pneumonia
    Semantic   inverse-is-a: Pneumonia; Staphylococcal Infections

Pneumonia, Streptococcal
    Source:    ICD91/IT/482.3
    Other:     Streptococcus pneumoniae

Pneumonia due to Streptococcus
    Source:    ICD91/PT/482.3
    ATX:       Pneumonia AND Streptococcal Infections AND NOT Pneumonia, Lobar
    Parent:    Influenza with Pneumonia

Pneumonia in Anthrax
    Source:    ICD91/PT/484.5; ICD91/IT/022.1; ICD91/IT/484.5
    Parent:    Influenza with Pneumonia
    Broader:   Pneumonia in other infectious diseases classified elsewhere
    Other:     Pneumonia, Anthrax

Pneumonia, Anthrax
    Source:    ICD91/IT/022.1; ICD91/IT/484.5
    Other:     Pneumonia in Anthrax
```

Figure 7.13. Some of the information available in the Unified Medical Language System about selected pneumonia concepts. Concept's preferred names are shown in italics. Sources are identifiers for the concept in other terminologies. Synonyms are names other than the preferred name. ATX is an associated Medical Subject Heading expression that can be used for Medline searches. The remaining fields (Parent, Child, Broader, Narrower, Other, and Semantic) show relationships among concepts in the Metathesaurus. Note that concepts may or may not have hierarchical relations to each other through Parent–Child, Broader–Narrower, and Semantic (is-a and inverse-is-a) relations. Note also that Pneumonia, Streptococcal and Pneumonia due to Streptococcus are treated as separate concepts, as are Pneumonia in Anthrax and Pneumonia, Anthrax.

7.5.1   General Concepts and Requirements

The purpose of a data-interchange standard is to permit one system, the **sender**, to transmit to another system, the **receiver**, all the data required to accomplish a specific communication, or **transaction set**, in a precise, unambiguous fashion. To complete this task successfully, both systems must know what format and content is being sent and must understand the words or terminology, as well as the delivery mode. When you order merchandise, you fill out a form that includes your name and address, desired items, quantities, colors, sizes, and so on. You might put the order form in an envelope and mail it to the supplier at a specified address. There are standard requirements, such as where and how to write the receiver's (supplier's) address, your (the sender's) address, and the payment for delivery (the postage stamp). The receiver must have a mailroom, a post office box, or a mailbox to receive the mail.

A communications model, called the Open Systems Interconnection (OSI) reference model (ISO 7498-1), has been defined by the ISO (see Chapter 5 and the discussion of software for network communications). It describes seven levels of requirements or specifications for a communications exchange: physical, data link, network, transport, session, presentation, and application (Stallings, 1987a; Tanenbaum, 1987; Rose, 1989). Level 7, the application level, deals primarily with the semantics or data-content specification of the transaction set or message. For the data-interchange standard, HL7 requires the definition of all the data elements to be sent in response to a specific task, such as the admission of a patient to a hospital. In many cases, the data content requires a specific terminology that can be understood by both sender and receiver. For example, if a physician orders a laboratory test that is to be processed by a commercial laboratory, the ordering system must ensure that the name of the test on the order is the same as the name that the laboratory uses. When a panel of tests is ordered, both systems must share a common understanding of the panel composition. This terminology understanding is best ensured through use of a terminology table that contains both the test name and a unique code. Unfortunately, several code sets exist for each data group, and none are complete. An immediate challenge to the medical-informatics community is to generate one complete set. In other cases, the terminology requires a definition of the domain of the set, such as what are the possible answers to the data parameter "ethnic origin."

The sixth level, presentation, deals with what the syntax of the message is, or how the data are formatted. There are both similarities and differences at this level across the various standards bodies. Two philosophies are used for defining syntax: one proposes a *position-dependent* format; the other uses a *tagged-field* format. In the position-dependent format, the data content is specified and defined by position. For example, the sixth field, delimited by "m," is the gender of the patient and contains an M, F, or U or is empty. A tagged-field representation is "SEX=M."

The remaining OSI levels—session, transport, network, data link, and physical—govern the communications and networking protocols and the physical connections made to the system. Obviously, some understanding at these lower levels is necessary before a linkage between two systems can be successful. Increasingly, standards groups are defining scenarios and rules for using various protocols at these levels, such as TCP/IP (see Chapter 5). Much of the labor in making existing standards work lies in these lower levels.

Typically, a transaction set or message is defined for a particular event, called a **trigger event**. The message is composed of several data segments; each data segment consists of one or more data fields. Data fields, in turn, consist of data elements that may be one of several data types. The message must identify the sender and the receiver, the message number for subsequent referral, the type of message, special rules or flags, and any security requirements. If a patient is involved, a data segment must identify the patient, the circumstances of the encounter, and additional information as required. A reply from the receiving system to the sending system is mandatory in most circumstances and completes the communications set.

It is important to understand that the sole purpose of the data-interchange standard is to allow data to be sent from the sending system to the receiving system; the standard does not in any manner constrain the application system that uses those data. Application independence permits the data-interchange standard to be used for a wide variety of applications. However, the standard must ensure that it accommodates all data elements required by the complete application set.

7.5.2   Specific Data-Interchange Standards

As health care increasingly depends on the connectivity within an institution, an enterprise, an integrated delivery system, a geographic system, or even a national integrated system, the ability to interchange data in a seamless manner becomes critically important. The economic benefits of data-interchange standards are immediate and obvious. Consequently, it is in this area of health care standards that most effort has been expended. All of the SDOs in health care have some development activity in data-interchange standards.

In the following sections we summarize many of the current standards for data-interchange. Examples are provided to give you a sense of the technical issues that arise in defining a data-exchange standard, but details are beyond the scope of this book. For more information, consult the primary resources or the Web sites for the relevant organizations.

Digital Imaging and Communications in Medicine (DICOM)[3]

With the introduction of computed tomography and other digital diagnostic imaging modalities, people needed a standard method for transferring images and associated information between devices, manufactured by different vendors, that display a variety of digital image formats. ACR formed a relationship with the NEMA in 1983 to develop such a standard for exchanging radiographic images, creating a unique professional/vendor group. The purposes of the ACR/NEMA standard were to promote a generic digital-image communication format, to facilitate the development and expansion of picture-archiving and communication systems (PACSs; see Chapter 18), to allow

---

[3] DICOM began as a standards-development effort of the American College of Radiology/National Electronic Manufacturers Association (ACR/NEMA) and was thus initially known as the ACR/NEMA standard.

the creation of diagnostic databases for remote access and to enhance the ability to integrate new equipment with existing systems. Later the group became an international organization with ACR becoming just a member organization. NEMA still manages the organization in the United States.

Version 1.0 of the DICOM standard, published in 1985, specified a hardware interface, a data dictionary, and a set of commands. This standard supported only point-to-point communications. Version 2.0, published in 1988, introduced a message structure that consisted of a command segment for display devices, a new hierarchy scheme to identify an image, and a data segment for increased specificity in the description of an image (e.g., the details of how the image was made and of the settings).

In the DICOM standard, individual units of information, called data elements, are organized within the data dictionary into related groups. Groups and elements are numbered. Each individual data element, as contained within a message, consists of its group-element tag, its length, and its value. Groups include command, identifying, patient, acquisition, relationship, image presentation, text, overlay, and pixel data.

The latest version of DICOM is Version 3.0. It incorporates an object-oriented data model and adds support for ISO standard communications. DICOM provides full networking capability; specifies levels of conformance; is structured as a nine-part document to accommodate evolution of the standard; introduces explicit information objects for images, graphics, and text reports; introduces service classes to specify well-defined operations across the network; and specifies an established technique for identifying uniquely any information object. DICOM also specifies image-related management information exchange, with the potential to interface to HISs and radiology information systems. An updated Version 3.0 is published annually.

The general syntax used by DICOM in representing data elements includes a data tag, a data length specification, and the data value. That syntax is preserved over a hierarchical nested data structure of items, elements, and groups. Data elements are defined in a data dictionary and are organized into groups. A data set consists of the structured set of attributes or data elements and the values related to an information object. Data-set types include images, graphics, and text. A multivendor demonstration of DICOM Version 3.0 was first demonstrated at the RSNA meeting in Chicago in November 1992.

The protocol architecture for DICOM Version 3.0 is shown in Figure 7.14, which illustrates the communication services for a point-to-point environment and for a networked environment, identifies the communication services and the upper-level protocols necessary to support communication between DICOM Application Entities. The upper-layer service supports the use of a fully conformant stack of OSI protocols to achieve effective communication. It supports a wide variety of international standards-based network technologies using a choice of physical networks such as Ethernet, FDDI, ISDN, X.25, dedicated digital circuits, and other local area network (LAN) and wide area network (WAN) technologies. In addition, the same upper-layer service can be used in conjunction with TCP/IP transport protocols. DICOM is now producing a number of standards including structured reports and Web access to, and presentation of, DICOM persistent objects.

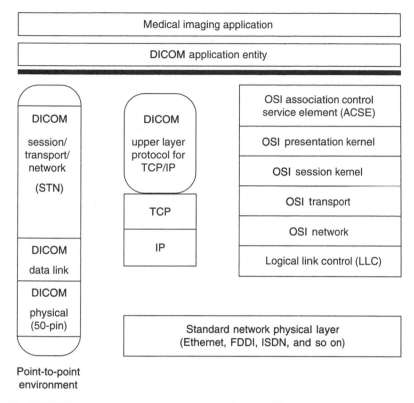

Figure 7.14. DICOM communications-protocol architecture illustrating the different approaches to dealing with the OSI reference model communication levels.

ASTM International

ASTM was founded in 1898 and chartered in 1902 as a scientific and technical organization for the development of standards for characteristics and performance of materials. The original focus of ASTM was standard test methods. The charter was subsequently broadened in 1961 to include products, systems, and services, as well as materials. ASTM is the largest nongovernment source of standards in the United States. It has over 30,000 members who reside in over 90 different countries. ASTM is a charter member of ANSI. ASTM technical committees are assigned 12 ISO committee and subcommittee secretariats and have over 55 assignments to serve as TAGs for developing U.S. positions on international standards. ASTM Committee E31 on Health care Informatics was established in 1970 and is responsible for the development of standards related to the architecture, content, portability, format, security, and communications.

In 1984, the first ASTM health care data-interchange standard was published: E1238, Standard Specification for Transferring Clinical Observations Between Independent Systems. This standard is used in large commercial and reference clinical laboratories in the United States and has been adopted by a consortium of French laboratory system vendors who serve 95 percent of the laboratory volume in France. The ASTM E1238 standard is message based; it uses position-defined syntax and is similar to the HL7 standard (see next section). An example of the ASTM 1238 standard describing a message transmitted between a clinic and a commercial clinical laboratory is shown in Figure 7.15. Related data-interchange standards include E1467 (from Subcommittee E31.16), Specification for Transferring Digital Neurophysiological Data Between Independent Computer Systems. Another important ASTM standard is E1460, Defining and Sharing Modular Health Knowledge Bases (Arden Syntax for Medical Logic Modules; see Chapter 20). In 1998, ownership of the Arden Syntax was transferred to HL7, where it will be developed by the Arden Syntax and Clinical Decision Support Technical Committee. New activities of ASTM include work toward the establishment of a standard for the Continuity of Care Record (CCR) that will enable health care providers to base future care on relevant and timely patient information.

Health Level 7

An ad hoc standards group was formed in March 1987 as a result of efforts to develop an integrated HIS by interconnecting function-specific systems. That group adopted the name **HL7** to reflect the application (seventh) level of the OSI reference model.[4] The original primary goal of HL7 was to provide a standard for the exchange of data among hospital computer applications that eliminated, or substantially reduced, the hospital-specific interface programming and program maintenance that was required at that time. The standard was designed to support single, as well as batch, exchanges of transactions among the systems implemented in a wide variety of technical environments.

H|~^\&|95243|HAMMO001|COMMUNITY AND FAMILY MEDICINE|BOX 2914^DUKE
UNIVERSITY MEDICAL CENTER^DURHAM^NC|919-684-6721||SMITHKLINE
CLINICAL LABS|TEST MESSAGE|D|2|199401170932<cr>

P|1|999-99-9999|||GUNCH^MODINE^SUE||19430704|F|
RT 1, BOX 97^ZIRCONIA^NC^27401||704-982-
1234||DOCTOR^PRIMARY^A^^DR.<cr>

OBR|1|101||80018^CHEM 18|R||||N|||||M D&PRIMARY&A&DR.<cr>

OBR|2|102||85025^AUTO CBC|R||||N||||| MD&PRIMARY&A&DR.

Figure 7.15. An example of a message in the ASTM 1238 format. The message consists of the header segment, H, the patient segment, P, and general order segments, OBR. Primary delimiters are the vertical bars (|); secondary delimiters are the carets (^). Note the similarities of this message to the HL7 message in Figure 7.4.

---

[4] See http://www.hl7.org for current information on HL7 and its evolution.

Today, HL7 has over 500 organizational members and over 2,200 individual members; HL7 is the most widely implemented health care data-messaging standard and is in use at over 1,500 health care facilities.

The standard was built on existing production protocols—particularly ASTM 1238. The HL7 standard is message based and uses an event trigger model that causes the sending system to transmit a specified message to the receiving unit, with a subsequent response by the receiving unit. Messages are defined for various trigger events. Version 1.0 was published in September 1987 and served mainly to define the scope and format of standards. Version 2.0, September 1988, was the basis for several data-interchange demonstrations involving more than 10 vendors. Version 2.1, June 1990, was widely implemented in the United States and abroad. In 1991, HL7 became a charter member of ANSI; on June 12, 1994, it became an ANSI-accredited Standard Developers Organization (SDO). Version 2.2 was published in December 1994 and on February 8, 1996, it was approved by ANSI as the first health care data-interchange American National Standard. Version 2.3, March 1997, considerably expanded the scope by providing standards for the interchange of data relating to patient administration (admission, discharge, transfer, and outpatient registration), patient accounting (billing), order entry, clinical-observation data, medical information management, patient and resource scheduling, patient-referral messages, patient-care messages that support communication for problem-oriented records, adverse-event reporting, immunization reporting, and clinical trials, as well as a generalized interface for synchronizing common reference files. Version 2.4, which became an ANSI standard in October 2000 introduced conformance query profiles and added messages for laboratory automation, appliccation management, and personnel management. ANSI recently approved the HL7 Version 2.0 Extensible Markup Language (XML) Encoding Syntax. The XML capability of HL7 v2.xml makes messages Web-enabled. Version 2.5, which is more consistent and supports more functionality than any other previous version, became an ANSI standard in 2003.

Figure 7.16 illustrates the exchange that occurs when a patient is transferred from the operating room (which uses a system called DHIS) to the surgical intensive-care unit (which uses a system called TMR). Note the similarity between these messages and the ASTM example.

Version 3.0 of the standard (currently in the ballot process) is object oriented and based on a **Reference Information Model** (RIM) being developed by HL7. The RIM has evolved from a number of commercial and academic health care data models, and it accommodates the data elements defined in the current Version 2.x HL7 standard.

This RIM is a collection of subject areas, scenarios, classes, attributes, use cases, actors, trigger events, interactions, and so on that depict the information needed to specify HL7 messages. In this sense it is more than a data-interchange standard, seeking to merge standards notions that include terminology and representation as well as data exchange. The stated purpose of the RIM is to provide a model for the creation of message specifications and messages for HL7. The RIM was approved as an ANSI standard in 2003, and has been introduced as an ISO standard. HL7 has also introduced a V3 suite of standards including V3 Abstract Data Types; Clinical Data Architecture, Release 2; and Context Management Standard (CCOW).

```
MSH|^~&\|DHIS|OR|TMR|SICU|199212071425|password|ADT|16603529|P|2.1<cr>

EVN|A02|199212071425||<cr>

PID|||Z99999^5^M11||GUNCH^MODINE^SUE|RILEY|19430704 |F||C|RT. 1, BOX
97^ZIRCONIA^NC^27401 |HEND|(704)982-1234|(704)983-1822||S|C||245-33-
9999<cr>

PV1|1|I|N22^2204|||OR^03|0940^DOCTOR^HOSPITAL^A||| SUR|||||A3<cr>

OBR|7|||93000^EKG REPORT|R|199401111000|199401111330|||RMT||||19940111
11330|?|P030||||||199401120930|||||||88-126666|A111|VIRANYI^ANDREW<cr>

OBX|1|ST|93000.1^VENTRICULAR RATE(EKG)||91|/MIN|60-100<cr>

OBX|2|ST|93000.2^ATRIAL RATE(EKG)||150|/MIN|60-100<cr>

  . . .

OBX|8|ST|93000&IMP^EKG DIAGNOSIS|1|^ATRIAL FIBRILATION<cr>
```

Figure 7.16. An example of an HL7 ADT transaction message. This message includes the Message Heading segment, the EVN trigger definition segment, the PID patient-identification segment, the PV1 patient-visit segment, the OBR general-order segment, and several OBX results segments.

Institute of Electrical and Electronics Engineers

IEEE is an international organization that is a member of both ANSI and ISO. Through IEEE, many of the world's standards in telecommunications, electronics, electrical applications, and computers have been developed. There were two major IEEE standards projects in health care. IEEE P1157, MEDIX, was organized in November 1987 to draft a standard for the exchange of data between hospital computer systems. The MEDIX committee, in formation, was committed to developing a standard set of hospital-system interface transactions based on the ISO standards for all seven layers of the OSI reference model. Its work has produced a family of documents that defines the communications models for medical data interchange among diverse systems. As events developed, the work of the MEDIX committee was informally merged into HL7 activities.

IEEE 1073, Standard for Medical Device Communications, has produced a family of documents that defines the entire seven-layer communications requirements for the **Medical Information Bus** (MIB). The MIB is a robust, reliable communication service designed for bedside devices in the intensive care unit, operating room, and emergency room (see Chapter 20 for further discussion of the MIB in patient-monitoring settings). These standards have been harmonized with work in CEN, and the results are being released as ISO standards.

The National Council for Prescription Drug Programs

NCPDP is an ANSI-accredited SDO and is a trade organization. Its mission is to create and promote data-interchange standards for the pharmacy services sector of the health care industry and to provide information and resources that educate the industry. Currently, NCPDP has developed three ANSI-approved standards: a telecommunication standard (Version 3.2 and Version 7.0), a SCRIPT standard (Version 5.0), and a manufacturer rebate standard (Version 3.01). The telecommunication standard provides a standard format for the electronic submission of third-party drug claims. The standard was developed to accommodate the eligibility verification process at the point of sale and to provide a consistent format for electronic claims processing. Primarily pharmacy providers, insurance carriers, third-party administrators, and other responsible parties use the standard. This standard addresses the data format and content, transmission protocol, and other appropriate telecommunication requirements. Version 5.1 (September, 1999) of this standard is one of the transactions standards required for use by HIPAA.

Version 1.0, released in 1988, used formats with fixed fields only. Version 2.0 added only typographic corrections to the Version 1.0 standard. The major thrust of the changes in Versions 3.0 and 3.1, in 1989, was the change from fixed-field transactions to a hybrid or variable format in which the fields can be tailored to the required content of the message. The current release is Version 3.2 (February, 1992). It introduces the fixed-length Recommended Transaction Data Sets (RTDS), which define three different message types, and a separate Data Dictionary format. The Data Dictionary defines permissible values and default values for fields contained in the specification. An online, real-time version was developed in 1996.

The standard uses defined separator characters at a group and a field level. The telecommunications specifications for sending two prescriptions includes three required sections (Transaction Header; Group Separator, First-Claim Information; and Group Separator, Second-Claim Information [R]) and three optional sections (Header Information, First-Claim Information, and Second-Claim Information [O]). The NCPDP communication standard is used in more than 60 percent of the nation's total prescription volume.

The SCRIPT Standard and Implementation Guide was developed for transmitting prescription information electronically between prescribers and providers. The stardard, which adheres to EDIFACT syntax requirements and utilizes ASC X12 data types where possible, addresses the electronic transmission of new prescriptions, prescription refill requests, prescription fill status notifications, and cancellation notifications.

ANSI X12

ASC X12, an independent organization accredited by ANSI, has developed message standards for purchase-order data, invoice data, and other commonly used business documents. The subcommittee X12N has developed a group of standards related to providing claim, benefits, and claim payment or advice. The specific standards that strongly relate to the health care industry are shown in Table 7.2.

Table 7.2. ANSI X12N standards.

Code	Title	Purpose
148	First Report of Injury, Illness or Incident	Facilitates the first report of an injury, incident, or illness
270	Health-Care Eligibility/Benefit Inquiry	Provide for the exchange of eligibility information and for response to individuals in a health care plan
271	Health-Care Eligibility/Benefit Information	
275	Patient Information	Supports the exchange of demographic, clinical, and other patient information to support administrative reimbursement processing as it relates to the submission of health-care claims for both health-care products and services
276	Health-Care Claim Status Request	Queries the status of a submitted claim and reports the status of a submitted claim
277	Health-Care Claim Status Notification	
278	Health-Care Service Review Information	Provides referral certification and authorization Provides referral certification and authorization
811	Consolidated Service Invoice/Statement	Facilitate health-plan premium billing and payment
820	Payment Order/Remittance Advice	
IHCLME	Interactive Health-Care Claim/Encounter	Supports administrative reimbursement processing as it relates to the submission of health-care claims for both health-care products and services in an interactive environment
IHCE/BI	Interactive Health-Care Eligibility/ Benefit Inquiry	Provide for the exchange of eligibility information and for response to individuals within a health plan
IHCE/BR	Interactive Health-Care Eligibility/ Benefit Response	

The X12 standards define commonly used business transactions in a formal, structured manner called *transaction sets*. A transaction set is composed of a transaction-set header control segment, one or more data segments, and a transaction-set trailer control segment. Each segment is composed of a unique segment ID; one or more logically related simple data elements or composite data structures, each preceded by a data element separator; and a segment terminator. Data segments are defined in a data segment directory; data elements are defined in a data element directory; composite data structures are defined in a composite data structure directory; control segments and the binary segment are defined in a data segment directory.

A sample 835 Interchange Document is shown in Figure 7.17. This standard is similar to ASTM and HL7 in that it uses labeled segments with positionally defined components.

There are several additional organizations that either create standards related to health care or have influence on the creation of standards.

```
ST*835*0001<n/l>
BPR*X*3685*C*ACH*CTX*01*122000065*DA*296006596*IDNUMBER*
SUPPLECODE*01*134999883*DA*867869899*940116<n/l>
TRN*1*45166*IDNUMBER<n/l>
DTM*009*940104<n/l>
N1*PR*HEALTHY INSURANCE COMPANY<n/l>
N3*1002 WEST MAIN STREET<n/l>
N4*DURHAM*NC*27001<n/l>
N1*PE*DUKE MEDICAL CENTER<n/l>
N3*2001 ERWIN ROAD<n/l>
N4*DURHAM*NC*27710<n/l>
CLP*078189203*1*6530*4895*CIN<n/l>
CAS*PR*1*150<n/l>
CAS*PR*2*550<n/l>
NM1*15*IAM*A*PATIENT<n/l>
REF*1K*942238493<n/l>
DTM*232*940101<n/l>
DTM*233*940131<n/l>
SE*22*0001<n/l>
```

Figure 7.17. An example of ANSI X12 Interchange Document (Standard 835). This message is derived from a batch process, business-document orientation to a data-interchange model. The example does not include the control header or the functional-group header. The first line identifies the segment as a transaction-set header (ST). The last line is the transaction-set trailer (SE). The leading alphanumeric characters are tags that identify data content. For example, DTM is a date/time reference; N3 is address information; and BPR is the beginning segment for payment order/remittance advice.

American Dental Association

In 1983, the American Dental Association (ADA) committee MD 156, became an ANSI-accredited committee responsible for all specifications for dental materials, instruments, and equipment. In 1992, a Task Group of the ASC MD 156 was established to initiate the development of technical reports, guidelines, and standards on electronic technologies used in dental practice. Five working groups promote the concept of a dental computer-based clinical workstation and allow the integration of different software and hardware components into one system. Areas of interest include digital radiography, digital intraoral video cameras, digital voice-text-image transfer, periodontal probing devices, and CAD/CAM. Proposed standards include Digital Image Capture in Dentistry, Infection Control in Dental Informatics, Digital Data Formats for Dentistry, Construction and Safety for Dental Informatics, Periodontal Probe Standard Interface, Computer Oral Health Record, and Specification for the Structure and Content of the Computer-Based Patient Record.

Uniform Code Council

The Uniform Code Council (UCC) is an ANSI-approved organization that defines the universal product code. Standards include specifications for the printing of machine-readable representations (bar codes).

Health Industry Business Communications Council

The Health Industry Business Communications Council (HIBCC) has developed the Health Industry Bar Code (HIBC) Standard, composed of two parts. The HIBC Supplier Labeling Standard describes the data structures and bar code symbols for bar coding of health care products. The HIBCC Provider Applications Standard describes data structures and bar code symbols for bar coding of identification data in a health care provider setting. HIBCC also issues and maintains Labeler Identification Codes that identify individual manufacturers. The HIBCC administers the Health Industry Number System, which provides a unique identifier number and location information for every health care facility and provider in the United States The HIBCC also administers the Universal Product Number Repository, which identifies specific products and is recognized internationally.

The Electronic Data Interchange for Administration, Commerce, and Transport

The EDI for Administration, Commerce, and Transport (EDIFACT) is a set of international standards, projects, and guidelines for the electronic interchange of structured data related to trade in goods and services between independent computer-based information systems (National Council for Prescription Drug Programs Data Dictionary, 1994). The standard includes application-level syntax rules, message design guidelines, syntax implementation guidelines, data element dictionary, code list, composite data-elements dictionary, standard message dictionary, uniform rules of conduct for the interchange of trade data by transmission, and explanatory material.

The basic EDIFACT (ISO 9735) syntax standard was formally adopted in September 1987 and has undergone several updates. In addition to the common syntax, EDIFACT specifies standard messages (identified and structured sets of statements covering the requirements of specific transactions), segments (the groupings of functionally related data elements), data elements (the smallest items in a message that can convey data), and code sets (lists of codes for data elements). The ANSI ASC X12 standard is similar in purpose to EDIFACT, and work is underway to coordinate and merge the two standards.

EDIFACT is concerned not with the actual communications protocol but rather with the structuring of the data that are sent. EDIFACT is independent of the machine, media, system, and application and can be used with any communications protocol or with physical magnetic tape.

Data Interchange Standards for Bioinformatics

As discussed in Chapter 22, significant work is under way to compile large databases of genomic and proteonomic information. XML has proven particularly attractive as a method for representing this information to support interchange among databases, including the Systems Biology Markup Language (SBML) (Hucka et al., 2003), the Tissue Microarray Data Exchange (TMA-DE) (Berman et al., 2003), and the Microarray and Gene Expression Markup Language (MAGE-ML) (Spellman et al., 2002).

7.6   Today's Reality and Tomorrow's Directions

7.6.1   The Interface: Standards and Workstations

Much of the early work in creating standards for data exchange was in the area of exchanging data between distributed systems, most often in the background and unsolicited. As the online use of information systems by professional users increases, and as the need to bring in data from distributed systems escalates, data-interchange standards requirements will expand to support a request mode, which will allow specific data elements from disparate sources to be integrated at the desktop.

Much of the work to date on data-interchange standards will certainly be useful in connecting health professionals' workstations to the rest of the world. We must recognize, however, that data-messaging standards have thus far focused primarily on exchanging medical data in a way that is largely driven by the desired function—to support an admission, test ordering, or results reporting. Only casual work has been done in developing standards for queries from users to such data sources. Queries will tend to return many more data than the workstations need unless new standards are developed. Should queries for workstations be based on the de facto database query standard, SQL (see Chapter 5)? If so, what modifications will be required to support queries from workstations while building on other ideas of data exchange?

User queries will need to identify the patient and either request or transmit data elements to other components of the distributed environment. Query methods will be required to support a variety of scenarios: a single test value with date and time, a set of vital signs, a problem list, a list of allergies, a complete data set for an outpatient encounter, a complete data set for a hospitalization, current drugs, or a complete patient record. Invariably, each such exchange of data must control and pass along the patient's rights and wishes regarding access to and use of the data (see Chapter 10).

Standardized access to knowledge systems and bibliographic systems must support scripting and data-entry mechanisms to ensure that a data system can properly and accurately provide a response. Workstations typically permit cut and paste from one module to another; the data representation must thus accommodate a standard linkage to enable user-directed transfer between systems. The global use of decision-support systems will require high-speed query and response for the typically large number of data elements required to execute the decision logic, as well as high computational speeds to process the information and to provide an acceptable real-time response on the workstation.

Patient information will be retrieved not only by patient name or identification number but also by patient characteristics. For example, a physician at a workstation may ask for data on all patients who have coronary artery disease with more than three-vessel involvement, who have had a myocardial infarction (heart attack), who are diabetic, who were treated surgically, and who have lived more than 5 years. The underlying system must use a variety of standards to translate this query into a manageable task, returning the correct data and preserving access constraints.

How good are the standards that are available today? What do users have to do to incorporate today's operational versions of standards into systems that they are implementing? First, much negotiation is necessary among vendors who are interfacing systems. There are two reasons for this need. Different parts of the various standards have different levels of maturity. For example, in HL7, the ADT version of the standard is defined more completely than is the observation-reporting section, when the latter is used to transmit complete clinical data. Most of the standards are not complete, except for their support of some well-defined documents such as insurance-claim forms. Standards are only now beginning to use an object-oriented model of the data to minimize ambiguity and to ensure completeness. Vendors may interpret the use of a data field differently, depending on their perspective or orientation. A billing vendor may understand the meaning of a field entirely differently from a clinical system vendor. The incompleteness of the standards—for example, in managing a complex set of trigger events—may lead one vendor to make assumptions not obvious to another vendor. The issue of optionality creates confusion and requires negotiation among vendors for a well-structured interface. Terminology standards also are not adequate for seamless interfaces. The second problem faced by vendors lies in the lower levels of the OSI reference model. Most of the standards bodies are now addressing the lower levels by defining strategies and rules for the lower-level protocols, most frequently using TCP/IP rather than pure OSI protocols.

From a user's perspective, the problem lies in how closely the vendor's implementation adheres to the standard. In many cases, the vendor defines standard compliance loosely, and the user purchases a system that cannot be easily interfaced. The only solution to this problem is certification by some agency—an unpopular task at best. Legal concerns and the difficulty of certifying compliance to the standards are obstacles that must be overcome.

Do today's standards reduce costs? The answer depends on the vendor. Some vendors charge little or nothing for standard interfaces, others charge the same as they do for custom interfaces. Over time, however, the cost of the interface will be driven down considerably by the users. In the case of imaging standards, the standards are necessary to develop the market for displaying images in a variety of settings.

7.6.2   Future Directions

The 2000 Institute of Medicine (IOM) publication *To Err is Human* (Institute of Medicine, 2000) noted that the U.S. medical system may be responsible for as many as 98,000 deaths per year due to medical error. A second 2001 IOM publication *Crossing the Quality Chasm* (Institute of Medicine, 2001), noted the poor quality of health care in the U.S. The IOM subsequently formed a Patient Safety Task Force that published a report *Patient Safety: Achieving a New Standard for Care* (Institute of Medicine, 2003) in which the data standards required for health are identified and the status of health data standards are discussed. The eHealth Initiative and the Markle Foundation created a public–private collaborative to report on the requirements, gaps and status of data standards for health. Their final report, *The Data Standards Working Group: Report and*

Recommendations, June 5, 2003[5] made recommendations for adoption of specific standards and on additional standards that need to be created. As part of the eGov initiative, the federal government established the Consolidated Health Informatics (CHI) inititative to establish a portfolio of existing clinical terminologies and messaging standards enabling federal agencies to build interoperable federal health data systems. Over 20 departments/agencies are participating in the CHI including HHS, VA, DOD, SSA, GSA and NIST. Todate the CHI has adopted a number of standards from several standards developer organizations that are discussed in this chapter. In June 2003, HHS empowered the IOM and HL7 to create functional standards for the EHR. At the recommendation of the National Committee for Vital and Health Statistics, HHS established an initiative for creating a National Health Care Informatics Infrastructure that will have as its goals improving patient safety and quality, rapidly detecting bioterrorism and other health threats, and enhancing the efficiency of the health care system (see Chapter 1).

The General Accounting Office reported in a study from the early 1990s that several hundred standards would be required by the health care industry (United States General Accounting Office, 1993). Other authors have estimated the numbers to be in the thousands. We believe that the most probable need will be 20 to 30 standards. One problem in trying to standardize everything is the conflict between a standard and the opportunity for a vendor to use creativity in a product to enhance sales. Standards should not stifle creativity but rather encourage it. For example, standardization of the screen displays for an EHR system is unlikely to occur, because individual vendors have different beliefs about the best designs. On the other hand, it is likely that components of the displays may be standardized. The use of the mouse (e.g., single and double clicks, right and left clicks) needs to be standardized in function. The use of visual objects also needs to be (and can be) standardized. It is likely that icons that represent functions also will be standardized in time.

At the present time, standards do not exist to support fully the requirements of health-professional workstations. A standard is necessary whenever someone other than the originator of the data must understand and use the data received electronically. For seamless electronic interchange of clinical data, standard formats need to be defined to include all types of data representation—images, signals and waveforms, sound and voice, and video, including motion video. Other candidate issues where the definition of standards would be helpful include specifying the location of data (in terms of both physical location and database characteristics) and defining the rules for the retention of data and for tighter coupling of data.

Core data sets for health care specialty groups and defined health care scenarios are likely candidates for standardization. The Centers for Disease Control and Prevention, for example, has defined a set of standard codes for the emergency department. Forms, such as discharge summaries, operative notes, and so on, can be exchanged meaningfully between organizations if they use a standard format. Decision-support algorithms and clinical guidelines will be more widely used and accepted if they go through a consensus standardization process.

---

[5] Available on the Web at http://www.marklc.org/downloadable_assets/dswg_report.pdf.

The future of messaging standards seems bright. The prevailing attitude in all the existing standards groups—in Europe and in the United States—favors developing workable standards so that we can solve new problems. Participants favor working together; proprietary and "not-invented-here" concerns are minimal. The willingness to separate data content from syntax is important. The development of a common, global data model is critical. Definitions of terminology, coding, and standard data structures are approaching reality. Clearly, the goals of "plug and play" have not yet been realized, but they may be obtainable within the next few years.

Suggested Readings

Abbey L.M., Zimmerman J. (Eds.) (1991). *Dental Informatics: Integrating Technology into the Dental Environment*. New York: Springer-Verlag.
This text demonstrates that the issues of standards extend throughout the areas of application of biomedical informatics. The standards issues discussed in this chapter for clinical medicine are shown to be equally pertinent for dentistry.

Chute C.G. (2000). Clinical classification and terminology: some history and current observations. *Journal of the American Medical Informatics Association*, 7(3):298–303.
This article reviews the history and current status of controlled terminologies in health care.

Cimino J.J. (1998). Desiderata for controlled medical vocabularies in the twenty-first century. *Methods of Information in Medicine*, 37(4–5):394–403.
This article enumerates a set of desirable characteristics for controlled terminologies in health care.

Henchley, A. (2003). *Understanding Version 3. A primer on the HL7 Versison 3 Communication Standard*. Munich, Germany: Alexander Moench Publishing Co.
Easily readable overview of HL7 Version 3 messaging standard.

Henderson, M. (2003). *HL7 Messaging*. Silver Spring, MD: OTech Inc.
Description of HL6 V2 wirh examples. Available from HL7.

Institute of Medicine (2003). *Patient Safety: Achieving a New Standard for Care*. Washington, D.C.: National Academy Press.
Discusses approaches to the standardization of collection and reporting of patient data.

Stallings W. (1987b). *Handbook of Computer-Communications Standards*. New York: Macmillan.
This text provides excellent details on the Open Systems Interconnection mode of the International Standards Organization.

Stallings W. (1997). *Data and Computer Communications*. Englewood Cliffs, NJ: Prentice-Hall.
This text provides details on communications architecture and protocols and on local and wide area networks.

Questions for Discussion

1. What are the five possible approaches to accelerating the creation of standards?
2. Define five health care standards, not mentioned in the chapter, that might also be needed?

3. What role should the government play in the creation of standards?
4. At what level might a standard interfere with a vendor's ability to produce a unique product?
5. Define a hypothetical standard for one of the areas mentioned in the text for which no current standard exists. Include the conceptualization and discussion points. Specifically state the scope of the standard.

8
Natural Language and Text Processing in Biomedicine

CAROL FRIEDMAN AND STEPHEN B. JOHNSON

After reading this chapter, you should know the answers to these questions:

- Why is natural language processing (NLP) important?
- What are the potential uses for NLP in the biomedical domain?
- What forms of knowledge are used in NLP?
- What are the principal techniques of NLP?
- What are the challenges for NLP in the clinical domain?
- What are the challenges for NLP in the biological domain?

8.1 Motivation for NLP

Natural language is the primary means of human communication. In biomedical areas, knowledge and data are disseminated in written form through articles in the scientific literature, technical and administrative reports, and patient charts used in health care (Johnson, 2000). Information is also disseminated verbally through scientific interactions in conferences, lectures, and consultations, although, in this chapter we focus on the written form. Increasingly, computers are being employed to facilitate this process of collecting, storing, and distributing biomedical information. *Textual data* are now widely available in an electronic format, through the use of transcription services, word processing, and speech recognition technology (see Chapter 5). Important examples include articles published in the biomedical literature (see Chapter 19) and reports describing particular processes of patient care (e.g., radiology reports and discharge summaries; see Chapter 12).

While the ability to access and review *narrative data* is highly beneficial to researchers, clinicians, and administrators, the information is not in a form amenable to further computer processing, for example, storage in a structured database to enable subsequent retrievals. Narrative text is difficult to access reliably because the variety of expression is vast; many different words can be used to denote a single concept and an enormous variety of grammatical structures can be used to convey equivalent information. At present, the most significant impact of the computer in medicine is seen in processing **structured data**, information represented in a regular, predictable form. This information is often numeric in nature (e.g., measurements recorded in a scientific study) or made up of discrete data elements (e.g., elements selected from a predefined list of biomedical terms, such as the names of diseases or genes). The techniques of NLP provide a means to bridge the gap between textual and structured data, allowing humans to interact using familiar natural language while enabling computer applications to process data effectively.

8.2   Applications of NLP

NLP has a wide range of potential applications in the biomedical domain. NLP enables a new level of functionality for health care and research-oriented applications that would not be otherwise possible. NLP methods can help manage large volumes of text (e.g., patient reports or journal articles) by extracting relevant information in a timely manner. Some text-processing tasks are currently performed by humans, for example, human coders identify diagnoses and procedures in patient documents for billing purposes, and database curators extract genomic information on organisms from the literature. However, it is generally not feasible to perform these tasks manually because they are too costly and too time consuming. For example, an automated system could process enormous numbers of patient reports to detect medical errors, whereas it would not be possible for experts to check such large volumes. Because automated systems are based on rules determined by experts, it is possible to incorporate the best and most current knowledge into the rules. Such systems are generally more consistent and objective than humans. Another significant advantage of NLP is the ability to standardize information occurring in documents from diverse applications and institutions, representing the information uniformly with common output structure and vocabulary.

The following are important applications of NLP technology in biomedicine:

- **Information extraction** locates and structures important information in text, usually without performing a complete analysis. This is the most common application in biomedicine, and is the primary focus of this chapter. The technique may be limited to the identification of isolated terms in text (e.g., medications or proteins), which can then be mapped to canonical or standardized forms. A slightly more complex application may search for recognizable patterns in text, such as names of people or places, dates, and numerical expressions. More sophisticated techniques identify and represent the relations among the terms within a sentence. Such advanced methods are necessary for reliable retrieval of information in patient documents and the biomedical literature because the correct interpretation of a biomedical term typically depends on its relation with other terms. For example, `fever` has different interpretations in `no fever, high fever, fever lasted 2 days,` and `check for fever`.[1] In the biomolecular domain, an important use of this technology involves extracting interactions from individual journal articles, and then subsequently combining them in order to automatically generate pathways. Figure 8.1 is an example of a pathway in the form of a graph that was created by extracting some interactions from one journal article in *Cell* (Maroto et al., 1997).

---

[1]The natural language processing literature typically connotes narrative text in *italics*; however, in this chapter we will depict text from narrative reports using Courier font to distinguish it from important informatics terms that are italicized throughout this book.

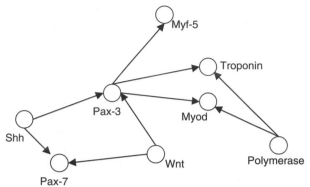

Figure 8.1. A graph showing interactions that were extracted from an article. A vertex represents a gene or protein, and an edge represents the interaction. The arrow represents the direction of the interaction so that the agent is represented by the outgoing end of the arrow and the target by the incoming end.

- **Information retrieval** helps users to access documents in very large collections, such as the scientific literature. This is a crucial application in biomedicine, due to the explosion of information available in electronic form. The essential goal of information retrieval is to match a user's query against the collection and return the most similar documents. Because matching is approximate, the process is usually iterative, requiring several rounds of refinement. The most basic form of *indexing* isolates simple words and terms. More advanced approaches use methods similar to those employed in information extraction, identifying complex noun phrases and determining their relationships in order to improve the accuracy of retrieval. For example, it is important to distinguish between a journal article that discusses the use of a drug to treat a medical condition from an article that discusses a medical condition being a side effect of a drug.

- **Text generation** formulates natural language sentences from a given source of information, usually structured data. These techniques can be used to generate text from a structured database, such as summarizing trends and patterns in laboratory data. Another important application is the generation of small summaries from large texts. This may involve summarization of a single document (e.g., a single clinical report such as a discharge summary), or of multiple documents (e.g., multiple journal articles).

- **User interfaces** (see Chapter 12) enable humans to communicate more effectively with computer systems. Tools that facilitate data entry are an important application in biomedicine. Data can be captured by keyboard (e.g., using templates or macros) or by speech recognition technology that enables users to enter words directly into computer systems by speaking. Additional examples (somewhat less common) include issuing commands or querying a database using natural language.

- **Machine translation** converts text in one language (e.g., English) into another (e.g., Spanish). These applications are important in multilingual environments in which human translation is too expensive or time consuming. Examples include translating medication instructions to assist patients, translating consent forms to enroll diverse subjects in a study, and translating journal articles to reach an international audience.

8.3   Knowledge Used in NLP

While current linguistic theories differ in certain details, there is broad consensus that linguistic knowledge consists of multiple levels: *morphology* (parts of words), *lexicography* (words and terms), *syntax* (phrases and sentences), *semantics* (words, phrases and sentences), and *pragmatics* (paragraphs and documents). Human language processing may appear deceptively simple, because we are not conscious of the effort involved in learning and using language. However, a long process of acculturation is necessary to attain proficiency in speaking, reading, and writing, with further intensive study to master the language of biological science or medicine. The sections below briefly describe the nature of the knowledge in each of these levels.

Morphology concerns the combination of **morphemes** (roots, prefixes, suffixes) to produce words. **Free morphemes** can occur as separate words, while **bound morphemes** cannot, e.g., de-in detoxify, -tion in creation, -s in dogs. **Inflectional morphemes** express grammatically required features or indicate relations between different words in the sentence, but do not change the basic syntactic category, thus big, bigg-er, bigg-est are all adjectives. **Derivational morphemes** change the part of speech or the basic meaning of a word, thus -ment added to a verb forms a noun (judg-ment); re-activate means activate again. Compared with other languages, English does not exhibit complex morphology, and therefore many NLP systems for general English do not incorporate morphological knowledge. However, biomedical language has a very rich morphological structure especially for chemicals (e.g., Hydroxy-nitro-di-hydro-thym-ine) and procedures (hepatico-cholangio-jejuno-stom-y). Recognizing morphemes enables an NLP system to handle words much more flexibly, especially in dealing with new words. However, determining the correct separation can be difficult. In the previous chemical example, the first split must be made after hydr- (because the -o- is part of -oxy) while the fifth split occurs after hydro-. In the procedure example, the system must distinguish stom (mouth) from tom (cut) in -stom.

Lexicography concerns the categorization of **lexemes**, the words and atomic terms of the language. Each lexeme belongs to one or more *parts of speech* in the language, such as noun (e.g., chest), adjective (e.g., mild), or tensed verb (e.g., improves), which are the elementary components of the English grammar. Lexemes may also have *subcategories*, depending on the basic part of speech, which are usually expressed by inflectional morphemes. For example, nouns have number (e.g., plural or singular as in legs, leg), person (e.g., first, second, third as in I, you, he, respectively), and case (e.g., subjective, objective, possessive as in I, me, my, respectively). Lexemes can consist of more than one word as in foreign phrases (ad hoc), prepositions (along with), and idioms (follow up, on and off). Biomedical lexicons tend to contain many multiword lexemes, e.g., lexemes in the clinical domain include congestive heart failure and diabetes mellitus, and in the biomolecular domain include the gene named ALL1-fused gene from chromosome 1q.

Syntax concerns the *structure* of the phrases and sentences. Lexemes combine (according to their parts of speech) in well-defined ways to form phrases such as noun phrases (e.g., severe chest pain), adjectival phrases (e.g., painful to touch), or verb phrases (e.g., `has increased`). Each phrase generally consists of a main part of speech and modifiers, e.g., nouns are frequently modified by adjectives while verbs are frequently modified by adverbs. The phrases then combine in well-defined ways to form sentences (`he complained of severe chest pain`). General English imposes many restrictions on the formation of sentences, e.g., every sentence requires a subject, and count nouns (like `cough`) require an article (e.g., `a` or `the`). Clinical language is often *telegraphic*, relaxing many of these restrictions to achieve a highly compact form. For example, clinical language allows all of the following as sentences: `the cough worsened; cough worsened; cough`. Because the community widely uses and accepts these alternate forms, they are not considered ungrammatical but constitute a **sublanguage** (Kittredge and Lehrberger 1982; Grishman and Kittredge, 1986; Friedman, 2002). There is a wide variety of sublanguages in the biomedical domain, each exhibiting specialized content and linguistic forms.

Semantics concerns the *meaning* or *interpretation* of words, phrases, and sentences. Each word has one or more meanings or *word senses* (e.g., `capsule`, as in `renal capsule` or as in `vitamin B12 capsule`), and the meanings of the words combine to form a meaningful sentence, as in `there was thickening in the renal capsule`). Representing the semantics of general language is an extremely difficult problem, and an area of active research. Biomedical sublanguages are easier to interpret than general languages because they exhibit highly restrictive semantic patterns that can be represented more easily (Harris et al., 1989, 1991; Sager et al., 1987). Sublanguages tend to have a relatively small number of **semantic types** (e.g., medication, gene, disease, body part, or organism) and a small number of **semantic patterns**: medication-treats-disease, gene-interacts with-gene.

Pragmatics concerns how sentences combine to form *discourse* (paragraphs, documents, dialogues, etc.), and studies how this context affects the interpretation of the meaning of individual sentences. For example, in a mammography report, `mass` generally denotes `breast mass`, in a radiological report of the chest it denotes `mass in lung` whereas in a religious journal it is likely to denote a ceremony. Similarly, in a health care setting, `he drinks heavily` is assumed to be referring to alcohol and not water. Another pragmatic consideration is the interpretation of pronouns and other referential expressions (`there`, `tomorrow`). For example, in `An infiltrate was noted in right upper lobe; it was patchy`, `it` refers to `infiltrate` and not `lobe`. Other linguistic devices are used to link sentences together, for example to convey a complex temporal sequence of events.

8.4   NLP Techniques

NLP involves three major tasks: (1) representing the various kinds of linguistic knowledge discussed in Section 8.3, (2) using the knowledge to carry out the applications described in Section 8.2, and (3) acquiring the necessary knowledge in computable form. The field of computer science provides a number of formalisms that can be used to represent the knowledge (task 1). These include symbolic or logical formalisms (e.g., **finite state machines** and **context-free grammars**) and statistical formalisms (e.g., **Markov**

models and **probabilistic context-free grammars**). The use of these representations to analyze language is generally called **text parsing**, while their use to create language is called **text generation**. Traditionally, the acquisition of linguistic knowledge (task 3) has been performed by trained linguists, who manually construct linguistically based rule systems, or grammars. This process is extremely time intensive. Increasingly, there is interest in using methods of machine learning to acquire the knowledge with less effort from linguists. However, machine learning generally requires the creation of training data, which also requires extensive manual annotation.

Most NLP systems are designed with separate modules that handle different functions. The modules typically coincide with the linguistic levels described in Section 8.3. In general, the output from lower levels serves as input to higher levels. For example, the result of lexical analysis is input to syntactic analysis, which in turn is input to semantic analysis. Each system packages these processing steps somewhat differently. At each stage of processing, the module for that stage regularizes the data in some aspect while preserving the informational content as much as possible.

8.4.1   Morphology

The first step in processing generally consists of reading the electronic form of a text (usually it is initially one large string), and separating it into individual units called tokens (the process is called **tokenization**), which include morphemes, words (really morpheme sequences), numbers, symbols (e.g., mathematical operators), and punctuation. The notion of what constitutes a word is far from trivial. The primary indication of a word in general English is the occurrence of white space before and after a word; however, there are many exceptions. A word may be followed by certain punctuation marks without an intervening space, such as by a period, comma, semicolon, or question mark, or may have a "-" in the middle. In biomedicine, periods and other punctuation marks can be part of words (e.g., q.i.d. meaning four times a day in the clinical domain or M03F4.2A, a gene name that includes a period), and are used inconsistently, thereby complicating the tokenization process. Chemical and biological names often include parentheses, commas, and hyphens, for example (w)adh-2.

Symbolic approaches to tokenization are based on pattern matching. Patterns are conveniently represented by the formalism known as a **regular expression** or equivalently, a **finite state automata** (Jurafsky and Martin, 2000, pp. 21–52). For example, the following regular expression will identify the tokens contained in the sentence patient's wbc dropped to 12:

$$[\text{a-z}]+(\text{'s})? \mid [\text{0-9}]+ \mid [\text{.}]$$

The vertical bar (|) separates alternative expressions, which in this case specify three different kinds of tokens (alphabetic, numeric, and punctuation). Expressions in square brackets represent a range or choice of characters. The expression [a-z] indicates a lower case letter, while [0-9] indicates a digit. The plus sign denotes one or more occurrences of an expression. The question mark indicates an optional expression (apostrophe -s). Finally [.] indicates a period. This regular expression is very limited, because it does not deal with capital letters (e.g., `Patient`), numbers with a decimal point (`3.4`), or abbreviations terminated by a period (`mg.`).

More complex regular expressions can handle many of the morphological phenomena described above. However, situations that are locally ambiguous are more challenging. For example, in the sentence "`5 mg. given.`" the period character is used in two different ways: (1) to signal an abbreviation, and (2) to terminate the sentence. There is also the significant issue that we may not have anticipated all the possible patterns. Probabilistic methods such as Markov models provide a more robust solution. Markov models can be represented as a table (**transition matrix**). For this simple example, the table might appear as shown in Table 8.1. The rows represent the current symbol in the sentence, and the columns represent the words that can follow. Each cell indicates the probability that a given word can follow another.

In mathematical notation this can be written as P(following|current). The probability of a given sequence of tokens can be approximated by multiplying the probabilities of the individual transitions. Thus,

$$P(5 \text{ mg. given}) = P(mg.|5)P(given|mg.)P(given|.) = 0.9 \times 0.9 \times 0.7 = 0.567$$
$$P(5 \text{ mg. given}) = P(mg|5)P(.|mg)P(given|mg)P(.|given) = 0.8 \times 0.4 \times 0.8 \times 0.7 = 0.1792$$

To find the best tokenization of a given sequence of characters, it is necessary to determine all possible ways of dividing the tokens and then to select the one that yields the maximum probability. For long sequences, a more efficient method known as the **Viterbi algorithm** is used, which considers only a small proportion of the possible sequences (Jurafsky and Martin 2000, pp. 177–180). In practice, the transition matrix would be very large to accommodate the wide range of possible tokens found in biomedical text. The transition probabilities are typically estimated from training sets in which linguists have verified the correct tokenization. However, for accuracy, it is important that the training set be typical for the intended text and that the training set is sufficiently large.

8.4.2 Lexicography

Once text is tokenized, an NLP system needs to perform **lexical look up** to identify the words or multiword terms known to the system, and determine their categories and canonical forms. Many systems carry out tokenization on complete words and perform lexical look up immediately afterwards. This requires that the lexicon contains all the possible combinations of morphemes. Each lexical entry assigns a word to one or more parts of speech, and a canonical form. For example, `abdominal` is an adjective where the canonical form is `abdomen`, and `activation` is a noun that is the nominal form

Table 8.1. Transition probabilities for morphemes.

	5	mg	mg.	given	.
5	0.1	0.8	0.9	0.4	0.6
mg	0.3	0.1	0.1	0.9	0.4
mg.	0.3	0.1	0.1	0.9	0.2
given	0.7	0.6	0.6	0.2	0.7
.	0.6	0.4	0.4	0.8	0.1

of the verb `activate`. A few systems perform morphological analysis during tokenization. In that case, the lexicon only needs entries for roots, prefixes, and suffixes, with additional entries for irregular forms. For example, the lexicon would contain entries for the roots `abdomen` (with variant `abdomin-`) the adjective suffix `-al`, and `activat-`, verb suffix `-e`, and noun suffix `-ion`.

Lexical look up is not straightforward because a word may be associated with more than one part of speech. For example, `stay` may be a noun (as in `her hospital stay`) or a verb (as in `refused to stay`). Without resolution, these ambiguities could cause inaccuracies in parsing and interpretation, and must be addressed in subsequent stages of processing, using syntactic and semantic information. Alternatively, various methods for **part of speech tagging** may be used to resolve ambiguities by considering the surrounding words. For example, when `stay` follows `the` or `her` it is usually tagged as a noun, but after `to` it is usually tagged as a verb. A symbolic approach to this problem is the use of transformation rules that change the part of speech tag assigned to a word based on previous or following tags. The meaning of some part of speech tags are provided in Table 8.2.

The following are the rules that might be applied to clinical text.

Change NN to VB if the previous tag is TO
Change NN to JJ if the following tag is NN
Change IN to TO if the following tag is VB

Examples of applying these rules are shown in Table 8.3.

Table 8.2. Meanings of part of speech tags.

Tag	Meaning
NN	Singular noun
NNS	Plural noun
NNP	Proper noun singular
IN	Preposition
VB	Infinitive verb
VBD	Past-tense verb
VBG	Progressive verb form
VBN	Past participle
VBZ	Present-tense verb
JJ	Adjective
DT	Article
PP$	Possessive pronoun

Table 8.3. Application of transformation rules to part of speech tags.

Before rule application	After rule application
total/NN hip/NN replacement/NN	total/JJ hip/NN replacement/NN
a/DT total/NN of/IN four/NN units/NNS	(no change)
refused/VBD to/TO stay/NN	refused/VBD to/TO stay/VB
her/PP$ hospital/NN stay/NN	(no change)
unable/JJ to/IN assess/VB	unable/JJ to/TO assess/VB
allergy/NN to/IN penicillin/NN	(no change)

Rules for part of speech tagging can be created by hand or constructed automatically using **transformation-based learning**, based on a sample corpus where the correct parts of speech have been manually annotated (Jurafsky and Martin 2000, pp. 307–312). Statistical approaches to part of speech tagging are based on Markov models (as described above for morphology). The transition matrix specifies the probability of one part of speech following another (see Table 8.4):

The following sentence shows the correct assignment of part of speech tags: `Rheumatology/NN consult/NN continued/VBD to/TO follow/VB patient/NN`.

This assignment is challenging for a computer, because `consult` can be tagged VB (`Orthopedics asked to consult`), `continued` can be tagged VBN (`penicillin was continued`), and `to` can be tagged IN. However, probabilities can be calculated for these sequences using the matrix in Table 8.4 (these were estimated from a large corpus of clinical text). By multiplying the transitions together, a probability for each sequence can be obtained (as described above for morphology), and is shown in Table 8.5. Note that the correct assignment has the highest probability.

8.4.3   Syntax

Many NLP systems perform some type of **syntactic analysis**. A **grammar** specifies how the words combine into well-formed structures, and consists of rules where categories combine with other categories or structures to produce a well-formed structure with underlying relations. Generally, words combine to form phrases consisting of a head word and modifiers, and phrases form sentences or clauses. For example, in English there are noun phrases (NP) that contain a noun and optionally left and right modifiers,

Table 8.4. Transition probabilities for part of speech tags.

	NN	VB	VBD	VBN	TO	IN
NN	0.34	0.00	0.22	0.02	0.01	0.40
VB	0.28	0.01	0.02	0.27	0.04	0.39
VBD	0.12	0.01	0.01	0.62	0.05	0.19
VBN	0.21	0.00	0.00	0.03	0.11	0.65
TO	0.02	0.98	0.00	0.00	0.00	0.00
IN	0.85	0.00	0.02	0.05	0.00	0.08

Table 8.5. Probabilities of alternative part of speech tag sequences.

Part of speech tag sequence	Probability
NN NN VBD TO VB NN	0.001149434
NN NN VBN TO VB NN	0.000187779
NN VB VBN TO VB NN	0.000014194
NN NN VBD IN VB NN	0.000005510
NN NN VBN IN VB NN	0.000001619
NN VB VBD TO VB NN	0.000000453
NN VB VBN IN VB NN	0.000000122
NN VB VBD IN VB NN	0.000000002

such as definite articles, adjectives, or prepositional phrases (i.e., `the patient, lower extremities, pain in lower extremities, chest pain`), and verb phrases (VP), such as `had pain, will be discharged,` and `denies smoking.`

Simple phrases can be represented using **regular expressions** (as shown above for tokenization). In this case, syntactic categories are used to match the text instead of characters. A regular expression (using the tags defined in Table 8.2) for a simple noun phrase (i.e., a noun phrase that has no modifiers on the right side) is:

DT? JJ* NN* (NN|NNS)

This structure specifies a simple noun phrase as consisting of an optional determiner (i.e., `a, the, some, no`), followed by zero or more adjectives, followed by zero or more singular nouns, and terminated by a singular or plural noun. For example, the above regular expression would match the noun phrase `no/AT usual/JJ congestive/JJ heart/NN failure/NN symptoms/NNS` but would not match `heart/NN the/AT unusual/JJ`, because in the above regular expression `the` cannot occur in the middle of a noun phrase.

Some systems perform partial parsing using regular expressions. These systems determine local phrases, such as simple noun phrases (i.e., noun phrases without right adjuncts) and simple adjectival phrases, but do not determine relations among the phrases. These systems tend to be robust because it is easier to recognize isolated phrases than it is to recognize complete sentences, but typically they lose some information. For example, in `amputation below knee`, the two noun phrases `amputation` and `knee` would be extracted, but the relation `below` might not be.

More complex structures can be represented by **context-free grammars** (Jurafsky and Martin 2000, pp. 325–344). A complete noun phrase cannot be handled using a regular expression because it contains nested structures, such as nested prepositional phrases or nested relative clauses. A very simple grammar of English is shown in Figure 8.2.

Context-free rules use part of speech tags (see Table 8.2) and the operators found in regular expressions, for optionality (?), repetition (*), and alternative (|). The difference is that each rule has a nonterminal symbol on the left side (S, NP, VP, PP), which consists of a rule that specifies a sequence of grammar symbols (nonterminal, and terminal) on the right side. Thus, the S (sentence) rule contains an NP followed by a VP. Additionally, other rules may refer to these symbols or to the atomic parts of speech. Thus, the NP rule contains PP, which in turn contains NP.

Applying the grammar rules to a given sentence is called parsing, and if the grammar rules can be satisfied, the grammar yields a nested structure that can be represented

```
S     → NP  VP .
NP    → DT? JJ* (NN|NNS) CONJN* PP*  |  NP and NP
VP    → (VBZ|VBP) NP? PP*
PP    → IN NP
CONJN → and (NN|NNS)
```

Figure 8.2. A simple syntactic context-free grammar of English. A sentence is represented by the rule S, a noun phrase by the rule NP, a verb phrase by VP, and a prepositional phrase by PP. Terminal symbols in the grammar, which correspond to syntactic parts of speech, are underlined in the figure.

graphically as a **parse tree**. For example, the sentence the patient had pain in
lower extremities would be assigned the parse tree shown in Figure 8.3.

Alternatively, brackets can be used to represent the nesting of phrases instead of a
parse tree. Subscripts on the brackets specify the type of phrase or tag:

[$_S$ [$_{NP}$ [$_{DT}$ the] [$_{NN}$ patient]] [$_{VP}$ [$_{VBD}$ had]
[$_{NP}$ [$_{NN}$ pain] [$_{PP}$ [$_{IN}$ in] [$_{NP}$ [$_{JJ}$ lower] [$_{NNS}$ extremities]]]]]]

The following shows an example of a parse in the biomolecular domain for the sentence
Activation of Pax-3 blocks Myod phosphorylation:

[$_S$ [$_{NP}$ [$_{NN}$ Activation] [$_{PP}$ [$_{IN}$ of] [$_{NP}$ [$_{NN}$ Pax-3]]]]
[$_{VP}$ [$_{VBZ}$ blocks] [$_{NP}$ [$_{NNP}$ Myod] [$_{NN}$ phosphorylation]]]]

Grammar rules generally give rise to many possible structures for a parse tree (structural ambiguity). If a word has more than one part of speech, the choice of part of
speech for the word can result in different structures for the sentence. For example, when
swallowing occurs before a noun, it can be an adjective (JJ) that modifies the noun,
or a verb (VBG) that takes the noun as an object:

```
Swallowing/JJ evaluation/NN showed/VBD no/DT dysphagia/NN
Swallowing/VBG food/NN showed/VBD no/DT dysphagia/NN
```

Additionally, the sequence of alternative choices of rules in the grammar can yield
different groupings of phrases. For example, sentence 1a below corresponds to a parse
based on the grammar rules shown in Figure 8.2, where the VP rule contains a PP (e.g.,
denied in the ER) and the NP rule contains only a noun (e.g., pain). Sentence 1b

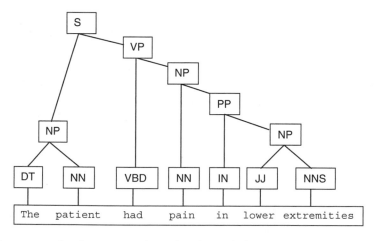

Figure 8.3. A parse tree for the sentence the patient had pain in lower extremities according to the
context-free grammar shown in Figure 8.2. Notice that the terminal nodes in the tree correspond
to the syntactic categories of the words in the sentence.

corresponds to the same atomic sequence of syntactic categories but the parse is different because the VP rule contains only a verb (e.g., `denied`) and the NP contains a noun followed by a PP (e.g., `pain in the abdomen`). Prepositions and conjunctions are also a frequent cause of ambiguity. In 2a, the NP consists of a conjunction of the head nouns so that the left adjunct (e.g., `pulmonary`) is distributed across both nouns (i.e., this is equivalent to an interpretation `pulmonary edema` and `pulmonary effusion`), whereas in 2b the left adjunct `pulmonary` is attached only to `edema` and is not related to `effusion`. In 3a, the NP in the prepositional phrase PP contains a conjunction (i.e., this is equivalent to `pain in hands` and `pain in feet`) whereas in 3b two NPs are also conjoined but the first NP consists of `pain in hands` and the second consists of `fever`.

1a. `Denied [ pain] [ in the ER]`
1b. `Denied [ pain [ in the abdomen]]`

2a. `Pulmonary [ edema and effusion]`
2b. `[ Pulmonary edema] and anemia`

3a. `Pain in [ hands and feet]`
3b. `[ Pain in hands] and fever`

More complex forms of ambiguity do not exhibit differences in parts of speech or in grouping, but require determining deeper syntactic relationships. For example, when a verb ending in `-ing` is followed by `of`, the following noun can be either the subject or object of the verb.

```
Feeling of lightheadedness improved.
Feeling of patient improved.
```

Statistical approaches provide one method of addressing ambiguity. The essential idea is to exploit the fact that some choices in the grammar are more likely than others. This can be represented using a **probabilistic context-free grammar**, which associates a probability with each choice in a rule (Jurafsky and Martin 2000, pp. 448–458). The grammar above can be annotated with probabilities for each choice by placing a numerical superscript after each symbol. The number indicates the probability of including the given category in the parse tree. For example, the probability of having a determiner (DT) is 0.9, while not having one has a probability of 0.1. The probability of a present tense verb (VBZ) is 0.4, while a past tense verb (VBD) is 0.6.

$$S \rightarrow NP\ VP.$$
$$NP \rightarrow DT?^{.9}\ JJ*^{.8}\ (NN|^{.6}\ NNS)\ PP*^{.8}$$
$$VP \rightarrow (VBZ|^{.4}\ VBD)\ NP?^{.9}\ PP*^{.7}$$
$$PP \rightarrow IN\ NP$$

The probability of a given parse tree is the product of the probabilities of each grammar rule used to make it. For example, there are two ways to parse `X-ray shows` patches in lung using this grammar (shown below). The first interpretation in which shows is modified by lung has probability 3.48×10^{-8}, while the second interpretation in which patches is modified by lung has probability 5.97×10^{-8}.

$$[_S [_{NP} \text{NN } 0.1 \times 0.2 \times 0.6 \times 0.2] [_{VP} \text{VBZ } [_{NP} \text{NN } 0.1 \times 0.2 \times 0.6 \times 0.2] [_{PP} \text{IN } [_{NP} \text{NN } 0.1 \times 0.2 \times 0.6 \times 0.2]] 0.4 \times 0.9 \times 0.7]]$$

$$[_S [_{NP} \text{NN } 0.1 \times 0.2 \times 0.6 \times 0.2] [_{VP} \text{VBZ } [_{NP} [_{PP} \text{IN } [_{NP} \text{NN } 0.1 \times 0.2 \times 0.6 \times 0.2] \text{NN } 0.1 \times 0.2 \times 0.6 \times 0.8] 0.4 \times 0.9 \times 0.3]]$$

8.4.4 Semantics

Semantic analysis involves steps analogous to those described above for syntax. First, semantic interpretations must be assigned to individual words. Then, these are combined into larger semantic structures (Jurafsky and Martin 2000, pp. 510–512). Semantic information about words is generally maintained in the lexicon. A **semantic type** is usually a broad class that includes many instances while a **semantic sense** distinguishes individual word meanings (Jurafsky and Martin 2000, pp. 592–601). For example, aspirin, ibuprofen and Motrin all have the same semantic type (medication), ibuprofen and Motrin have the same semantic sense (they are synonymous), which is distinct from the sense of aspirin (a different drug).

A lexicon may be created manually by a linguist, or be derived from external knowledge sources, such as the **Unified Medical Language System** (UMLS) (Lindberg et al., 1993; see Chapter 7) or GenBank (Benson et al., 2003). While external sources can save a substantial effort, the types and senses provided may not be appropriate for the text being analyzed. Narrow categories may be too restrictive, and broad categories may introduce ambiguities. Morphological knowledge can be helpful in determining semantic types in the absence of lexical information. For example, in the clinical domain, suffixes like – itis and -osis indicate diseases, while -otomy and ectomy indicate procedures. However, such techniques cannot determine the specific sense of a word.

As with parts of speech, many words have more than one semantic type, and the NLP system must determine which of these is intended in the given context. For example, growth can be either an abnormal physiologic process (e.g., for a tumor) or a normal one (e.g., for a child). The word left can indicate laterality (pain in left leg) or an action (patient left hospital). This problem is much harder than syntactic disambiguation because there is no well-established notion of word sense, different lexicons recognize different distinctions, and the space of word senses is substantially larger than that of syntactic categories. Words may be ambiguous within a particular domain, across domains, or with a general English word. Abbreviations are notoriously ambiguous. For example, the abbreviation MS may denote multiple sclerosis or mitral stenosis or it may denote the general English usage (i.e., as in Ms White). The ambiguity problem is particularly troublesome in the biomolecular domain because gene symbols in many model organism databases consist of three letters, and are ambiguous with other English words, and also with different gene symbols of different model organisms. For example, nervous and to are English words that are also the names of genes. When writing about a specific organism, authors use

alias names, which may correspond to different genes. For example, in articles associated with the mouse, according to the Mouse Genome Database (MGD) (Blake et al.,
2003), authors may use the term `fbp1` to denote three different genes.

Semantic disambiguation of **lexemes** can be performed using the same methods
described above for syntax. Rules can assign semantic types using contextual knowledge
of other nearby words and their types. For example, `discharge from hospital`
and `discharge from eye` can be disambiguated depending on whether the noun
following `discharge` is an institution or a body location. As illustrated in Table 8.6, a
rule may change the hospitalization action sense (e.g., HACT) that denotes `dis-`
`charge` to the body substance sense `discharge` (e.g., BSUB) if the following semantic category is a body part (e.g., PART).

Statistical approaches, such as Markov models, can be used to determine the most
likely assignment of semantic types (Jurafsky and Martin 2000, pp. 636–645). As with
methods for morphology and syntax, large amounts of training data are required to
provide sufficient instances of the different senses for each ambiguous word. This is
extremely labor intensive because a linguist must manually annotate the corpus,
although in certain cases automated annotation is possible.

Larger semantic structures consisting of **semantic relations** can be identified using
regular expressions, which specify patterns of semantic types. The expressions may be
semantic and look only at the semantic categories of the words in the sentence. This
method may be applied in the biomolecular domain to identify interactions between
genes or proteins. For example, the regular expression

[GENE|PROT] MFUN [GENE|PROT]

will match sentences consisting of very simple gene or protein interactions (e.g., `Pax-`
`3/GENE activated/MFUN Myod/GENE`). In this case, the elements of the pattern
consist of semantic classes: GENE (gene), molecular function (MFUN), and **PROT**
(protein). This pattern is very restrictive because any deviation from the pattern will
result in a failed match. Regular expressions that skip over parts of the sentence when
trying to find a match are much more robust, and can be used to detect relevant patterns
for a broader variety of text, thus incurring some loss of specificity and precision while
achieving increased sensitivity. For example, the regular expression

[GENE|PROT] .* MFUN .* [GENE|PROT]

can be satisfied by skipping over intermediate tags in the text. The dot (.) matches
any tag, and the asterisk (*) allows for an arbitrary number of occurrences. For
example, using the above expression, the interaction, `Pax-3 activated Myod` would

Table 8.6. Application of transformation rules to semantic tags. HACT denotes an action (e.g.,
admission, discharge), PART denotes a body part (e.g., *eye, abdomen*), and BSUB denotes a body
substance (e.g., *sputum*).

Before rule application	After rule application
*Discharge/HACT from hospital/*HORG	(no change)
Discharge/HACT from eye/PART	*Discharge/BSUB from eye/PART*

be obtained for the sentence `Pax-3/GENE, only when activated/MFUN by Myod/GENE, inhibited/MFUN phosphorylation/MFUN`. In this example, the match does not capture the information correctly because the relation `only when` was skipped. The correct interpretation of the individual interactions in this sentence should be `Myod activated Pax-3`, and `Pax-3 inhibited phosphorylation`. Note that the simple regular expression shown above does not provide for the latter pattern (i.e., GENE-MFUN-MFUN), for the connective relation, or for the passive structure.

An alternate method of processing sentences with regular expressions, which is currently the most widely employed in general English because it is very robust, uses **cascading finite state automata (FSA)** (Hobbs et al., 1996). In this technique, a series of different FSAs are employed so that each performs a special tagging function. The tagged output of one FSA becomes the input to a subsequent FSA. For example, one FSA may perform tokenization and lexical look up, another may perform partial parsing to identify syntactic phrases, such as noun phrases and verb phrases, and the next may determine semantic relations. In that case, the patterns for the semantic relations will be based on a combination of syntactic phrases and their corresponding semantic classes, as shown below. The pattern for biomolecular interactions might then be represented using a combination of tags:

$$NP_{[GENE | PROT]} \quad .^* \quad VP_{MFUN} \quad .^* \quad NP_{[GENE | PROT]}$$

The advantage of cascading FSA systems is that they are relatively easy to adapt to different information extraction tasks because the FSAs that are domain independent (tokenizing and phrasal FSAs) remain the same while the domain-specific components (semantic patterns) change with the domain and or the extraction task. These types of systems have been used to extract highly specific information, such as detection of terrorist attacks, identification of joint mergers, and changes in corporation management (Sundheim 1991, 1992, 1994, 1996; Chinchor 1998). However, they may not be accurate enough for clinical applications.

More complex semantic structures can be recognized using a **semantic grammar** that is a context-free grammar based on semantic categories. As shown in Figure 8.4, a simple grammar for clinical text might define a clinical sentence as a Finding, which consists of optional degree information and optional change information followed by a symptom.

```
S  →        Finding .
Finding  → DegreePhrase?  ChangePhrase? SYMP
ChangePhrase  → NEG? CHNG
DegreePhrase  → DEGR | NEG
```

Figure 8.4. A simple semantic context-free grammar for the English clinical domain. A sentence S consists of a FINDING, which consists of an optional DEGREEPHRASE, an optional CHANGEPHRASE and a Symptom. The DEGREEPHRASE consists of a degree type word or a negation type word; the CHANGEPHRASE consists of an optional negation type word followed by a change type word. The terminal symbols in the grammar correspond to semantic parts of speech and are underlined.

This is particularly effective for domains where the text is very compact, and where typical sentences consist primarily of noun phrases because the subject (i.e., `patient`) and verb have been omitted. For example, `increased/CHNG tenderness/SYMP` is a typical sentence in the clinical domain where both the subject and verb are omitted. For the simple grammar illustrated in Figure 8.4, the parsed sentence would be a **FINDING** that consists of a **CHANGEPHRASE** (e.g., `increased`) followed by a **SYMPTOM** (e.g., `tenderness`). Note that ambiguity is possible in this grammar because a sentence such as `No/NEG increased/CHNG tenderness/SYMP` could be parsed in two ways. In the incorrect parse shown in Figure 8.5, the **DEGREEPHRASE** (e.g., `no`) and the **CHANGEPHRASE** (e.g., `increased`) both modify `tenderness`, whereas in the correct parse (see Figure 8.6) only the **CHANGEPHRASE** (e.g., `no increased`) modifies `tenderness`, and within the **CHANGEPHRASE**, no modifies **CHANGE** (e.g., `increased`); in this case only the change information is negated but not the symptom.

NLP systems can handle more complex language structures by integrating syntactic and semantic structures into the grammar (Friedman et al., 1994). In that case, the grammar would be similar to that shown in Figure 8.4, but the rules would also include syntactic structures. Additionally, the grammar rule may also specify the representational output form, which represents the underlying interpretation of the relations. For example, in Figure 8.4, the rule for FINDING would specify an output form denoting that SYMP is the primary finding and the other elements are the modifiers.

More comprehensive syntactic structures can be recognized using a broad-coverage context-free grammar of English, which is subsequently combined with a semantic

Figure 8.5. A parse tree for the sentence no increased tenderness according to the grammar shown in Figure 8.4. In this interpretation, which is incorrect, no and increased each modify tenderness.

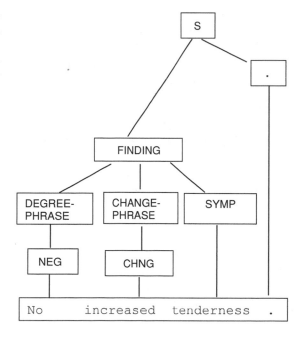

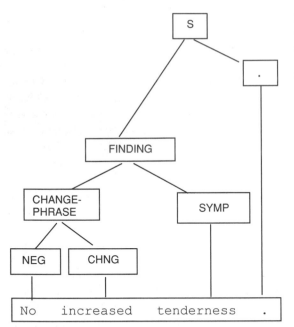

Figure 8.6. Another parse tree for the sentence no increased tenderness according to the grammar shown in Figure 8.4. This shows the correct interpretation because no modifies increased, which modifies tenderness.

component (Sager et al., 1987). After the syntactic structures are recognized, they are followed by syntactic rules that regularize the structures. For example, passive sentences, such as the chest X-ray was interpreted by a radiologist, would be transformed to the active form (e.g., a radiologist interpreted the chest X-ray). Another set of semantic rules would then operate on the regularized syntactic structures to interpret their semantic relations.

8.4.5   *Pragmatics*

Syntactic and semantic components of NLP systems evaluate each sentence in isolation. Complete analysis of a text (e.g., a clinical note or journal article) requires analysis of relationships between sentences and larger units of discourse, e.g., paragraphs and sections (Jurafsky and Martin, 2000, pp. 669–696). One of the most important mechanisms in language for creating linkages between sentences is the use of **referential expressions**, which include pronouns (he, she, her, himself), proper nouns (Dr. Smith, Atlantic Hospital), and noun phrases modified by the definite article or a demonstrative (the left breast, this medication, that day, these findings).

Each referential expression has a unique **referent** that must be identified in order to make sense of the text. The following text contains several examples. The proper noun Dr. Smith refers to the physician treating the patient. In clinical text, proper nouns can also refer to patients, family members, and departments and patient care institutions. In scientific discourse, proper nouns typically refer to scientists and research institutions. In the first two sentences, his and he refer to the patient, while he refers to the physician in the fourth sentence. There are several definite noun phrases (e.g., the epithelium, the trachea, and the lumen), which have to be resolved. In this case, the referents are parts of the patient's body.

His laboratory values on admission were notable for a chest X-ray showing a right upper lobe pneumonia. He underwent upper endoscopy with dilatation. It was noted that his respiratory function became compromised each time the balloon was dilated. Subsequently, Dr. Smith saw him in consultation. He performed a bronchoscopy and verified that there was an area of tumor. It had not invaded the epithelium or the trachea. But it did partially occlude the lumen.

Automatic resolution of referential expressions can draw on both syntactic and semantic information in the text. Syntactic information for resolving referential expressions includes:

- *Agreement* of syntactic features between the referential phrase and potential referents
- *Recency* of potential referents (nearness to referential phrase)
- *Syntactic position* of potential referents (e.g., subject, direct object, object of preposition)
- The *pattern of transitions* of topics across the sentences

Syntactic features that aid in resolution include such distinctions as singular/plural, animate/inanimate, and subjective/objective/possessive. For example, pronouns in the above text carry the following features: he (singular, animate, subjective), his (singular, animate, possessive), and it (singular, inanimate, subjective/objective). Animate pronouns (he, she, her) almost always refer humans. The inanimate pronoun it usually refers to things (e.g., it had not invaded), but sometimes does not refer to anything when it occurs in "cleft" constructions: it was noted, it was decided to and it seemed likely that.

Referential expressions are usually very close to their referents in the text. In it had not invaded, the pronoun refers to the immediately preceding noun phrase area of tumor. The pronoun in it did partially occlude has the same referent, but in this case there are two intervening nouns: epithelium or trachea. Thus, a rule that assigns pronouns to the most recent noun would work for the first case, but not for the second.

The syntactic position of a potential referent is an important factor. For example, a referent in subject position is a more likely candidate than the direct object, which in turn is more likely than an object of a preposition. In the fifth sentence of the text above, the pronoun he could refer to the patient or to the physician. The proper noun Dr. Smith is the more likely candidate, because it is the subject of the preceding sentence.

Centering theory accounts for reference by noting how the center (focus of attention) of each sentence changes across the discourse (Grosz et al., 1995). In the above text, the patient is the center of the first three sentences, the physician is the center of the fourth and fifth sentence, and the area of tumor is the center of the last sentence. In this approach, resolution rules attempt to minimize the number of changes in centers. Thus, in the above text it is preferable to resolve he in sentence five as the physician rather than the patient because it results in smoother transition of centers.

Semantic information for resolving referential expressions involves consideration of the semantic type of the expression, and how it relates to potential referents (Hahn et al., 1999).

- Semantic type is the same as the potential referent.
- Semantic type is a subtype of the potential referent.
- Semantic type has a close semantic relationship with the potential referent.

For example, in the following text, the definite noun phrase the density must be resolved. If the phrase a density occurred previously, this would be the most likely referent. Instead, the phrase a spiculated nodule is selected since nodule and density have closely related semantic types. In the previous text, the noun phrase the balloon is also definite and requires resolution. Since there is no previous noun of similar type, it is necessary to establish a semantic relationship with a preceding noun. The word dilation is the best candidate because a balloon is a medical device used by that procedure.

The patient's gynecologist palpated a mass in the left breast on September 10, 1995. The patient had a mammogram, which showed a spiculated nodule at the two to three o'clock position in the left breast, which was not present in 1994. There were also microcalcifications medial and inferior to the density.

Temporal expressions are another important linguistic mechanisms for connecting the events in a discourse (Sager et al., 1987, pp. 175–194). For example, in the above text the mammogram occurs after the palpation event, and we are told that the nodule was not present before the palpation. There are many different kinds of temporal expressions. The dates in the above example locate an event at a point or interval in time. Other examples include at 7:30am, on Tuesday, August 1, 2003, in Fall 1998. Additional expressions can be used to position an event relative to a position in time, e.g., yesterday, this morning, last summer, and two years ago, a few days before admission, several weeks later and since age 12.

In the absence of temporal expressions, time in a narrative tends to flow forward. This rule enables one to determine that the mammogram occurred at or after the palpation in the above text. Temporal conjunctions (e.g., before, after, while, and when) are used to directly relate two events in time. Temporal modifiers are used to specify the duration of an event (e.g., 4 hours, all week, half a year), and frequency (e.g., twice, every hour, and 1 pack per day).

8.5   Challenges of Clinical Language

NLP is challenging for general language, but there are issues that are particularly germane in the clinical domain, which are discussed below.

Good performance: If the output of an NLP system is to be used to help manage and improve the quality of clinical care and to facilitate research, it must have high enough sensitivity, accuracy, and specificity for the intended clinical applications. Different applications require varying levels of performance; however, generally, the performance should not be significantly worse than that of medical experts or the model organism database curators. This requirement means that before an application involving NLP can be used for a practical application, it would have to be evaluated so that the adequacy of performance can be measured. Additionally, since there is typically a trade-off between sensitivity and specificity, a system should be flexible to maximize the appropriate measure that is needed by the application.

Recovery of implicit information: Many health care reports are very compact and often omit information that can be assumed by other experts. An automated system may need to capture the implicit information in order to perform a particular task, necessitating that either the NLP system itself or the application using the output of the NLP system contains enough medical knowledge to make the appropriate inferences that are necessary in order to capture implicit information. For example, in one evaluation study we performed, medical experts when reading the sentence in an obstetrical report she had been ruptured times 25 1/2 hours inferred that rupture meant rupture of membranes because they related their domain knowledge to the context.

Intraoperability: In order to be functional in a clinical environment, an NLP system has to be seamlessly integrated into a clinical information system, and generate output that is in a form usable by other components of the system. This generally means that:

- The system will have to handle many different interchange formats (i.e., Extensible Markup Language (XML), HL7).
- The system will have to handle different formats that are associated with the different types of reports. Some reports often contain tables with different types of configurations. For example, Figure 8.7 shows portions of a cardiac catheterization report. Some of the sections contain text (i.e., procedures performed, comments, general conclusions), some consist of structured fields (i.e., height, weight) that are separated from each other by white space, and some consist of tabular data (i.e., pressure). The structured fields are easy for a human to interpret but are problematic for a general NLP program, because white space and indentation rather than linguistic structures determine the format of the table.
- The NLP system has to generate output that can be stored in an existing clinical repository. However, the output often has complex and nested relations, and it may be complicated or impossible to map the output to the database schema without substantial loss of information. Depending on the database schema loss of information may be unavoidable. An alternative approach would involve designing a complex database that can store nested data and data with a wide range of modifiers to accompany the NLP system. Such a database has been in use at Columbia Presbyterian Medical Center (CPMC) since the early 1990s (Friedman et al., 1990; Johnson et al., 1991), and has been critical for the effective use of NLP technology at CPMC.
- The underlying clinical information system may require a controlled vocabulary for data that are used for subsequent automated applications. This necessitates that the output of the NLP system be mapped to an appropriate controlled vocabulary;

```
Procedures performed: Right Heart Catheterization
Pericardiocentesis

Complications: None
Medications given during procedure: None
Hemodynamic data
Height (cm.): 180                 Weight (kg): 74.0
Body surface area (sq. m   93): 1.   Hemoglobin (gm/dl):
Heart rate:  102


Pressure (mmHg)
Sys    Dias   Mean   Sat

RA             14     13     8
RV             36     9      12
PA             44     23     33     62%
PCW    25     30     21


Conclusions: Postoperative cardiac transplant
Abnormal hemodynamics
Pericardial effusion
Successful pericardiocentesis
General comments:
1600cc of serosanguinous fluid were drained from the pericardial sac with
improvement in hemodynamics.
```

Figure 8.7. A portion of an actual cardiac catheterization report.

sometimes the vocabulary is homegrown and sometimes it is a standard vocabulary, such as the UMLS (Lindberg et al., 1993), *Systematized Nomenclature of Medicine* (SNOMED) (Côté, et al., 1993), or *International Classification of Diseases* (ICD-9), ninth edition (World Health Organization, 1990). Since natural language is very expressive and varied, most likely, there will be important terms that will have no corresponding controlled vocabulary concept, and a method for handling this type of situation will have to be designed. Additionally, the NLP system has to be capable of mapping to different controlled vocabularies, depending on the application.

Interoperability: NLP systems are time consuming and difficult to develop, and in order to be operational for multiple institutions and diverse applications, they would minimally have to generate output containing a controlled vocabulary. It would be ideal if the controlled vocabulary were one of the "standard" vocabularies. Otherwise, explicit definitions of the controlled vocabulary terms would be needed for each institution or application. In addition to a controlled vocabulary, a standard representational model for medical language is needed in order to represent important relations, such as negation, certainty, severity, change, and temporal information that are associated with the clinical terms. Since there is no standardized language model currently, an understanding of the model generated by each NLP is necessary in order for automated applications to use NLP output appropriately. An effort to merge different representational models of medical language to create a widely used model for medical language was undertaken by a large number of researchers called *The Canon group* (Evans et al., 1994). That effort resulted in a common model for radiological reports of the chest (Friedman et al., 1995), but the model was not actually utilized by the different researchers.

Training sets for development: Development of NLP systems is based on analysis (manual or automated) of samples of the text to be processed. In the clinical domain, this means that large collections of online patient records in textual form must be available for training the NLP systems. This is very problematic because many NLP researchers do not have direct ties to clinical information systems. Access to online patient records is confidential, requires the approval of **institutional review boards** (IRB), and generally necessitates removal of identifying information. Removal of identifying information from structured fields is straightforward; however, identifying information occurring in the text itself, such as names, addresses, phone numbers, unique characteristics (i.e., Mayor of New York) make this task extremely difficult. Ideally, for transferability among different health care institutions, data from a large number of different institutions is desirable so that the NLP system is not trained for a particular institution, but because of patient confidentiality, the data is difficult, if not impossible, to obtain. The problem is slightly different when processing the literature. For example, the abstracts can be obtained through the Medline database and are available to the public. Additionally, Pubmed Central (Wheeler et al., 2002) and other electronic journals provide full text articles.

Evaluation: Evaluation of an NLP system is critical but difficult in the health care domain because of the difficulty of obtaining a **gold standard** and because it is difficult to share the data across institutions. A fuller discussion on evaluation of NLP systems can be found in (Friedman et al., 1997; Hripcsak and Wilcox, 2002). Generally, there is no gold standard available that can be used to evaluate the performance of an NLP system. Therefore, for each evaluation, recruitment of subjects who are medical experts is generally required to obtain a gold standard for a test set. There are several ways an evaluation can be carried out. One way involves having experts determine if all the information and relations are correctly extracted and encoded based on the test set of text reports. Obtaining a gold standard for this type of evaluation is very time consuming and costly, since medical experts would have to structure and encode the information in the reports manually. For example, in a study that was performed associated with SNOMED encoding, it took a physician who was experienced in coding 60 hours to encode all the clinical information in one short emergency room report (Lussier et al., 2001).

Another way to carry out an evaluation would be to evaluate performance of a clinical application that uses the output generated by an NLP system. This type of evaluation would not only evaluate the information and relations captured by the system, but would also evaluate the accessibility and practical utility of the structured information for use with other clinical applications. An advantage of this type of evaluation is that it is generally easier for experts to provide a gold standard for this type of evaluation because they would not have to encode all the information in the report, but would only be required to detect particular clinical conditions in the reports. This is a much less time-consuming task than encoding all the data, and generally does not necessitate special training because medical experts routinely read patient reports and interpret the information in them. To perform this type of evaluation, knowledge engineering skills as well as clinical expertise would be required in order to formulate the queries that will be needed to retrieve the appropriate information generated by the NLP system, and to make the appropriate inferences. Formulation of the query can be relatively straightforward or complex depending on the particular task. For example, to determine whether a patient experienced a change in mental status based on information in the discharge summary, many different terms associated with that concept must be searched for, such as `hallucinating, confusion, Alzheimer's disease, decreased mental status`. In addition, over 24 different modifier concepts, such as `rule out, at risk for, family history, negative, previous admission for`, and `work up` may modify the relevant terms, signifying that the change in mental status should be disregarded because the modifiers denote that the patient did not currently experience a change in mental status, but may have in the past, a family member may have experienced it, or a work up was being performed.

When evaluating a particular application using NLP output, the performance measurements would be associated with the particular application, and performance would constitute the performance of both the NLP system and the automated query. For example, if the NLP system correctly extracted the finding `confusion` from the report but the query did not include that condition, there could be a loss of sensitivity; similarly, if the query did not filter out modifier conditions, such as `negative`, there could be a loss of precision. When analyzing results for this type of evaluation study, it would be important to determine whether errors occurred within the NLP system or by the query that retrieved the reports. Additionally, it would be important to ascertain how to fix the error and how much effort would be involved. In the above examples, simple corrections would be involved: one correction would involve adding a new term, `confusion`, to the query; the second would involve adding a modifier term to the filter. Corrections to the NLP system could involve adding entries to a lexicon, which is also very straightforward. However, a more complex change would involve revising the grammar rules.

In order to obtain a better understanding of the underlying methods used by different NLP systems, an evaluation effort that is carried out by a third party, in which NLP systems can participate, is needed to allow for comparison of performance across the different systems. In the general English domain, this was accomplished for a number of years by the Message Understanding Conferences (Sundheim, 1991, 1992, 1994, 1996; Chinchor, 1998), which were supported with funding from DARPA. These inter-system evaluations not only allowed for comparison of systems but also substantially fostered the growth, improvement, and understanding of NLP systems in the general English domain. Presently, similar efforts are occurring for NLP systems in the biological community, as evidenced by the KDD Challenge, the TREC Genomics Track, the BioCreAtIvE Assessment of Information Extraction systems in Biology (e.g., the following web sites are associated with NLP evaluation efforts within the bioinformatics community—http://www.biostat.wisc. edu/~craven/kddcup/, http://ir.ohsu.edu/genomics/, and http://www.pdg.cnb.uam.es/ BioLINK/BioCreative. eval.html).

Determining types of information to capture: Determining which information an NLP system should capture is an important decision. Some NLP systems may process partial information in the report, such as admission diagnoses or chief complaints, but not the complete report. Other NLP systems may be highly specialized and may also include expert medical knowledge (i.e., knowledge to determine whether a patient has community-acquired pneumonia).

Granularity of the information: NLP systems may capture the clinical information at many different levels of granularity. One level of coarse granularity consists of classification of reports. For example, several systems (Aronow et al., 1999) classified reports as positive or negative for specific clinical conditions, such as breast cancer. Another level of granularity, which is useful for information retrieval and indexing, captures relevant terms by mapping the information to a controlled vocabulary, such as the UMLS (Aronson et al., 2001; Nadkarni et al., 2001), but modifier relations are not captured. A more specific level of granularity also captures positive and negative modification (Mutalik et al., 2001; Chapman et al., 2001), but not other types of modification (e.g., severity, time of event, duration, and frequency). An even more specific level of granularity captures all modifiers associated with the term, facilitating reliable retrieval.

Expressiveness versus ease of access: Natural language is very expressive. There are often several ways to express a particular medical concept and also numerous ways to express modifiers of the concept. For example, severity information may be expressed in more than 200 different expressions, with terms such as `faint`, `mild`, `borderline`, `1+`, `3rd degree`, `severe`, `extensive`, and `mild to moderate`. These modifiers make it more complex to retrieve reports based on NLP-structured output since such a wide variety has to be accounted for. In addition, nesting of information also adds complexity. For example, a change type of modifier, such as `improvement` (as in `no improvement in pneumonia`), would be represented using nesting: the change modifier `improvement` would modify `pneumonia` and the negation modifier, `no`, would modify `improvement`. In this situation, a query that detects changes concerned with `pneumonia` would have to look for primary findings associated with pneumonia, filter out cases not associated with a current episode, look for a change modifier of the finding, and, if there is one, make sure there is no negation modifier on the change modifier. Another form of representation would facilitate retrieval by flattening the nesting. In this case, some information may be lost but ideally only the information that is not critical. For example, `slightly improved` may not be clinically different from `improved` depending on the application. Since this type of information is fuzzy and imprecise, the loss of information may not be significant. However, the loss of a modifier `no` would be significant, and those cases should be handled specially.

Heterogeneous formats: There is no standardized structure for clinical reports, or for the format of the text within the report. Frequently, there is no period (i.e., ".") to demarcate the end of a sentence, but a new line or a tabular format is used instead. This is easy for humans to manually interpret but difficult for computers. In addition, the sections and subsections of the reports are not standardized. For example, in CPMC, there are many different section headers for reporting diagnostic findings (e.g., Diagnosis, Diagnosis on admission, Final Diagnosis, Preoperative Diagnosis, and Medical Diagnosis). In addition, section headers are frequently omitted or several sections are merged into one. For example, past clinical history and family history may be reported in the history of present illness section. In addition, there is a lack of uniformity for specifying subsections. For example, surgical pathology reports often refer to findings for different specimens, which are mentioned throughout the report, but are not uniformly identified (e.g., the same specimen may be called `specimen A, slide A`, or just `A` within the same report).

Lack of a standardized set of domains: Knowledge of the domain being processed is important for NLP systems since a domain provides context that is often needed by the NLP system. For example, knowledge of the domain would facilitate recovery of implicit information (e.g., `mass` in a mammogram denotes `mass in breast`), or to resolve an ambiguous word or abbreviation (e.g., `pvc` in a chest X-ray denotes `pulmonary vascular congestion` whereas in an electrocardiogram it denotes `premature ventricular complexes`). Currently, there are no standard domains for naming different types of clinical documents. For example, at CPMC, there is a domain called `cardiology report`, which can correspond to an echocardiogram, catheterization diagnostic report, electrocardiography report, or stress test. Additionally, although individual radiology reports are coded, the different areas within radiology (e.g., abdomen, musculoskeletal system, etc.) have not been classified.

Large number of different clinical domains: There are a large number of different clinical domains, and a lexicon has to be developed for each domain. Each domain may be associated with its own lexicon but maintaining separate lexicons would be inefficient and error prone, since there is a significant amount of overlap among the terms. However, if one lexicon is maintained for all the domains, ambiguity increases because more terms become associated with multiple senses. For example, the term `discharge` may refer to `discharge from institution`, `discharge from eye`, or `electrical discharge from lead` (seen in a few electrocardiogram reports).

Interpreting clinical information: The interpretations of the findings may vary according to the type of report. For example, when retrieving information from the `Diagnosis Section` of a discharge summary, the interpretation will generally be more straightforward than when extracting information from radiological reports. Radiological reports generally do not contain definitive diagnoses, but contain a continuum of findings that range from patterns of light (e.g., `patchy opacity`), to descriptive findings (e.g., `focal infiltrate`) to interpretations and diagnoses (e.g., `pneumonia`). In some types of clinical reports, the descriptive findings may be expressed without further interpretation (e.g., a finding `pneumonia` may not be present in a radiological report; instead, findings consistent with `pneumonia`, such as `consolidation` or `infiltrate` may occur), or the interpretation may be included along with the descriptive findings. Therefore, in order to use an NLP system to detect pneumonia based on chest X-ray findings, the NLP system or application using the system would have to contain medical knowledge. The knowledge needed to detect a particular condition may be quite complex. In order to develop such a component, machine learning techniques could be used that involve collecting training instances, which would then be used to develop rules automatically (Wilcox and Hripcsak, 1999) or to train a Bayesian network (Christensen et al., 2002), but this may be costly since performance is impacted by sample size (McKnight et al., 2002), and, for many conditions, a large number of instances would have to be obtained for satisfactory performance. An alternative would involve manually writing the rules by observing the target terms that the NLP system can generate along with sample output. For that situation, the rules will generally consist of combinations of **Boolean operators** (e.g., `and`, `or`, and `not`) and findings. For example, a rule, which detects a comorbidity of neoplastic disease based on information in a discharge summary, could consist of a Boolean combination of over 200 terms (Chuang et al., 2002).

Compactness of text: Generally, clinical reports are very compact, contain abbreviations, and often omit punctuation marks. Some abbreviations will be well known but others may be defined uniquely. An example of a typical resident sign-out note, which is full of abbreviations and missing punctuation, is shown in Figure 8.8. Lack of punctuation means that sentence boundaries are poorly delineated, thereby making it more difficult for NLP systems because they generally depend on recognition of well-defined sentences. Abbreviations cause problems because they are highly ambiguous and not well defined.

Interpretation depends on context: Contextual information must be included in the findings since it often affects the interpretation. The section of the report and the type of report is important for the interpretation. For example, `pneumonia` in the Clinical Information Section of a chest X-ray report may mean `rule out pneumonia` or `patient has pneumonia`, whereas the occurrence of `pneumonia` in the Diagnosis Section is not ambiguous. Similarly, `history of asthma` in the Family History Section does not mean that the patient has asthma.

Rare events: Natural language systems require a sufficient number of training examples, which are needed to refine or test the system. Certain occurrences of interest, such as medical errors and adverse events, are not always reported frequently. Thus, it may be difficult to find a large number of reports necessary for training and testing an NLP system for certain applications. For those cases, terminological knowledge sources may be helpful for providing lexical knowledge related to rare terms that may occur in text associated with the events of interest.

Occurrence of typographic and spelling errors: Clinical reports occasionally contain typographic errors, which may cause the system to lose information or to misinterpret information. Automated correction of spelling errors is difficult and could create additional errors. For example, a typographic error `hyprtension` will cause a loss of clinical information; it is not trivial to correct this error automatically without additional knowledge because it may refer to `hypertension` or `hypotension`. A particularly serious error could involve substitution of a similar sounding medical term. For

---

Admit 10/23
71 yo woman h/o DM, HTN, Dilated CM/CHF, Afib s/p embolic event, chronic diarrhea, admitted with SOB. CXR pulm edema. Rx'd Lasix.
All: none
Meds Lasix 40mg IVP bid, ASA, Coumadin 5, Prinivil 10, glucophage 850 bid, glipizide 10 bid, immodium prn
Hospitalist = Smith PMD = Jones Full Code, Cx >101

Figure 8.8. An example of a resident sign-out note.

example, the drug `Evista` may be misspelled `E-Vista`, which is a different drug. This type of error is troublesome not only for automated systems but also for medical experts when reading the information manually.

Limited availability of electronic records: Not all clinical documents are in electronic form. At many hospitals daily clinical notes (such as nursing notes and progress notes) are recorded in the paper chart but are not available online; however, the information they contain is critical for patient care. NLP systems must have the documents available electronically in textual form in order to process them. A scanner could be used to obtain the documents in electronic form as image files, but then **optical character recognition** (OCR) technology would have to be used to obtain textual versions of the documents. However, OCR technology is generally not accurate enough for this purpose, especially since human experts often find the documents difficult to read.

8.6   Challenges for Biological Language Processing

Dynamic nature of domain: The biomolecular domain is very dynamic, continually creating new names for biomolecular entities and withdrawing older names. For example, for the week ending July 20, 2003, the Mouse Genome Informatics Web site (Blake et al., 2003) reported 104 name changes, representing changes related only to the mouse organism. If the other organisms being actively sequenced were also considered, the number of name changes during that week would be much larger.

Ambiguous nature of biomolecular names: Short symbols consisting of two to three letters are frequently used that correspond to names of biomolecular entities. Since the number of different combinations consisting of only a few letters is relatively small, it is highly likely that this would lead to names that correspond to different meanings. For example, `to`, which is a very frequent English word, corresponds to two different Drosophila genes and to the mouse gene `tryptophan 2,3-dioxygenase`. Another situation that contributes to the amount of ambiguity in gene names is that the different model organism groups name genes and other entities independently of each other, leading to names which are the same but which represent different entities. The ambiguity problem is actually worse if the entire biomedical domain is considered. For example, `cad` represents over 11 different biomolecular entities in Drosophila and the mouse but it also represents the clinical concept `coronary artery disease`. Another contributing factor to the ambiguity problem is due to the different naming conventions for the organisms. These conventions were not developed for NLP purposes but for consistency within the individual databases. For example, Flybase states that "Gene names must be concise. They should allude to the gene's function, mutant phenotype or other relevant characteristic. The name must be unique and not have been used previously for a Drosophila gene." This rule is fairly loose and leads to ambiguities.

Large number of biomolecular entities: The number of entities in this domain is very large. For example, there are about 70,000 genes when considering only humans, fly, mouse, and worm, and the number of corresponding proteins is over 100,000. Additionally, there are over 1 million species as well as a large number of cell lines and small molecules. Having such a large number of names means the NLP system has to keep a very large knowledge base of names or be capable of dynamically recognizing the type by considering the context. When entities are dynamically recognized without use of a knowledge source, it would be very difficult to identify them within an established nomenclature system.

Variant names: Names are created within the model organism database communities, but they are not always exactly the same as the names used by authors when writing articles. There are many ways authors may vary the names (particularly long names), which leads to difficulties in name recognition. This is also true in the medical domain, but the problem is exacerbated in the biomolecular domain because of the frequent use of punctuation, and other special types of symbols. Some of the more common types of variations are due to punctuation and use of blanks (`bmp-4, bmp 4, bmp4`), numerical variations (`syt4, syt IV`), variations containing Greek letters (`iga, ig alpha`), and word order differences (`phosphatidylinositol 3-kinase, catalytic, alpha polypeptide, catalytic alpha polypeptide phosphatidylinositol 3-kinase`).

Nesting of names: The names of many biomolecular entities are long and contain substrings that are also names. For example, `caspase recruitment domain 4` and `caspase` both correspond to gene names; if a variant form of `caspase recruitment domain 4` occurs in an article and the entire name is not recognized by the NLP system, the substring `caspase` would be recognized in error.

Lack of a standard nomenclature: The different model organism communities have different nomenclatures, each of which are standard for a particular organism. Each of the communities maintains a database that names the entities, provide unique identifiers, and list synonyms and preferred forms. However, each community maintains different databases that have different schemas and taxonomies; therefore, an NLP system has to obtain the knowledge needed from a diverse set of resources. Although Gene Ontology (GO) (Gene Ontology Consortium, 2003) is a consortium that aims to produce a uniform controlled vocabulary that can be applied to all organisms (even as knowledge of gene and protein roles in cells accumulates and changes), it applies only to biological functions, processes, and structures.

Heterogeneity of the text: Many abstracts can be obtained from Medline. These are easy to process because they can be obtained in the form of plain text. However, a substantial portion of biomolecular information occurs only in the full journal articles, which have different file formats. They may occur as Portable Document Format (PDF), Hypertext Markup Language (HTML), or XML files, which must first be converted to plain text. PDF file formats cannot be easily converted to text; although there is software that is commercially available to perform the conversion, it is currently error prone. Additionally, HTML files are suitable for presentation of the file in a browser, but cannot be relied on for specifying the semantics of the information. For example, it may be possible to recognize a section such as "**Introduction**" because it is enclosed in a tag consisting of a large bold font. An additional problem is that some of the important information may be in a figure which is in graphic format, and therefore not accessible as text. For example, in chemical journals, the names of chemical compounds often appear as a single letter followed by the full name and the diagram. In the text of the article, the single letter appears in place of the name, causing a loss of information. An additional problem is that the journals are often available only through subscriptions, which can be costly.

Complexity of the language: The structure of the biological language is very challenging. In clinical text, the important information is typically expressed as noun phrases, which consists of descriptive information such as findings and modifiers. In biomolecular text, the important information usually consists of interactions and relations, which are expressed as verbs or noun phrases that are frequently highly nested. Verb phrases are generally more complex structures than noun phrases. The arguments of a verb are important to capture as well as the order of the arguments (e.g., `Raf-1 activates Mek-1` has a different meaning than `Mek-1 activates Raf-1`). A typical sentence usually contains several nested interactions. For example, the sentence `Bad phosphorylation induced by interleukin-3 (IL-3) was inhibited by specific inhibitors of phosphoinositide 3-kinase (PI 3-kinase)` consists of four interactions (and also two parenthesized expressions specifying abbreviated forms). The interaction and the arguments are illustrated in Table 8.7. The nested relations can be illustrated more clearly as a tree (see Figure 8.9). Notice that the arguments of some interactions are also interactions (i.e., the second argument of

Table 8.7. Nested interactions extracted from the sentence *Bad phosphorylation induced by interleukin-3 (IL-3) was inhibited by specific inhibitors of phosphoinositide 3-kinase (PI 3-kinase).* A "?" denotes that the argument was not present in the sentence.

Interaction	Argument 1 (agent)	Argument 2 (target)	Interaction id
Phosphorylate	?	Bad	1
Induce	Interleukin-3	1	2
Inhibit	?	Phosphoinositide 3-kinase	3
Inhibit	3	1	4

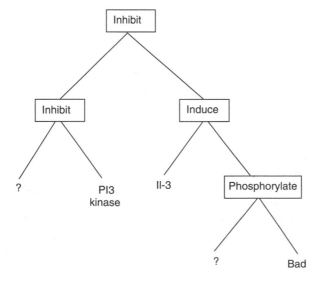

Figure 8.9. A tree showing the nesting of biomolecular interactions that are in the sentence Bad phosphorylation induced by interleukin-3 (IL-3) was inhibited by specific inhibitors of phosphoinositide 3-kinase (PI 3-kinase).

induce is `phosphorylate`). Also note that an argument which is not specified in the sentence is represented by a "?".

Multidisciplinary nature: In order for NLP researchers to work on biological text to extract the appropriate information, they need some knowledge of the domain. This is a big challenge because the understanding requires knowledge of biology, chemistry, physics, mathematics, and computer science.

8.7   Biomedical Resources for NLP

A number of controlled vocabularies provide terminological knowledge for NLP systems in the biomedical domain:

- UMLS (including the Metathesaurus, Semantic Network, the Specialist Lexicon; see Chapter 7)—can be used as a knowledge base and source for a medical lexicon. The Specialist Lexicon provides detailed syntactic knowledge for words and phrases, and includes a comprehensive medical vocabulary. It also provides a set of tools to assist in NLP, such as a lexical variant generator, an index of words corresponding to UMLS terms, a file of derivational variants (e.g., `abdominal, abdomen`), spelling variants (e.g., `fetal, foetal`), and a set of neoclassical forms (e.g., `heart, cardio`). The UMLS Metathesaurus provides the concept identifiers, and the Semantic Network specifies the semantic categories for the concepts. The UMLS also contains the terminology associated with various languages (e.g., French, German, Russian).
- Other controlled vocabularies (e.g., SNOMED, ICD-9, *Laboratory Observations, Identifiers, Names and Codes* (LOINC)) can also be used as sources of lexical knowledge for NLP. These vocabularies are also valuable as multilingual resources. For example, SNOMED was used as a lexical resource for French (Zweigenbaum and Courtois, 1998), and ICD was used as a resource for development of an interlingua (Baud et al., 1998).
- Biological databases. These include Model Organism Databases, such as Mouse Genome Informatics (Blake et al., 2003), the Flybase Database (Flybase Consortium, 2003), the WormBase Database (Todd et al., 2003), and the `Saccharomyces` Database (Issel-Tarver et al., 2001), as well as more general databases GenBank (Benson et al., 2003), Swiss-Prot (Boeckmann et al., 2003), LocusLink (Pruitt et al., 2001).
- GENIA corpus (Ohta et al., 2002). This corpus currently contains over 2,500 abstracts taken from Medline, which are related to transcription factors in human blood cells. It has over 100,000 hand-annotated terms marked with syntactic and semantic information appropriate for the biological domain, and is valuable for use as a gold standard for evaluation and training data for machine learning techniques. It also has an accompanying ontology.

Acknowledgments

The material in this chapter is derived in part from work sponsored by the U.S. Government for the National Academies. Any opinions, findings, conclusions, or recommendations expressed in the material are those of the authors and do not necessarily reflect the views of the U.S. Government, or the National Academies.

Suggested Readings

Allen J. (1995). *Natural Language Understanding* (2nd ed.). Redwood City, CA: Benjamin Cummings.
This textbook, which is intended for computer scientists and computational linguists, provides a description of the theories and techniques used in natural language understanding. The focus is on the use of symbolic rule-based methods, and syntactic, semantic, and discourse levels of processing.

Charniak E. (1993). *Statistical Language Learning*. Cambridge: MIT Press.
This is the first textbook covering statistical language processing, which is intended for computer scientists. It is brief, but it is clearly written.

Friedman C. (Ed.) (2002). Special issue: Sublanguage. *Journal of Biomedical Informatics*, 35(4).
This special issue on sublanguage includes six articles by leading researchers on current work in sublanguage processing in the biomedical domain.

Harris Z., Gottfried M., Ryckmann T., Mattick Jr. P., Daladier A., Harris T.N., Harris S. (1989). *The Form of Information in Science: Analysis of an Immunology Sublanguage*. Reidel, Dordrecht: Boston Studies in the Philosophy of Science.
This book offers an in-depth description of methods for analyzing the languages of biomedical science. It provides detailed descriptions of linguistic structures found in science writing and the mapping of the information to a compact formal representation. The book includes an extensive analysis of 14 full-length research articles from the field of immunology, in English and in French.

Jurafsky D., Martin J.H. (2000). *Speech and Language Processing: An Introduction to Natural Language Processing, Computational Linguistics and Speech Recognition*. New York: Prentice-Hall.
This is an excellent textbook, which comprehensively covers in-depth methods in natural language processing, computational linguistics, and speech recognition. The natural language-processing methods include symbolic and statistical models, and also covers a broad range of practical applications.

Manning C.D., Schütze H. (1999). *Foundations of Statistical Natural Language Processing*. Cambridge: MIT Press.
This textbook contains a comprehensive introduction to statistical natural language processing, and includes the theories and algorithms needed for building statistical NLP systems.

Sager N., Friedman C., Lyman M.S. (1987). *Medical Language Processing: Computer Management of Narrative Data*. New York: Addison-Wesley.
This book describes early techniques used by the Linguistic String Project, a pioneering language processing effort in the biomedical field, explaining how biomedical text can be automatically analyzed and the relevant content summarized.

Questions for Discussion

1. Develop a regular expression to regularize the tokens in lines 4–9 of the cardiac catheterization report shown in Figure 8.7 (`Complications` through `Heart Rate`).

2. Create a lexicon for the last seven lines of the cardiac catheterization report shown in Figure 8.7 (`Conclusions` through the last sentence). For each word, determine all the parts of speech that apply, using the tags in Table 8.2. Which words have more than one part of speech? Choose eight clinically relevant words in that section of the report, and suggest appropriate semantic categories for them that would be consistent with the SNOMED axes and with the UMLS semantic network.

3. Using the grammar in Figure 8.3, draw all possible parse trees for each of the sample sentences 1a, 2a, and 3a discussed in Section 8.4.3. For each sentence, indicate which parse represents the correct structure.

4. Using the grammar in Figure 8.3, draw a parse tree for the last sentence of cardiac catheterization report shown in Figure 8.7.

5. Using the grammar in Figure 8.4, draw parse trees for the following sentences: `no increase in temperature; low grade fever; marked improvement in pain; not breathing`. (Hint: some lexemes have more than one word.)

6. Identify all the referential expressions in the text below and determine the correct referent for each. Assume that the computer attempts to identify referents by finding the most recent noun phrase. How well does this resolution rule work? Suggest a more effective rule.

```
The patient went to receive the AV fistula on December 4.
However, he refuses transfusion. In the operating room it was
determined upon initial incision that there was too much edema
to successfully complete the operation and the incision was
closed with staples. It was well tolerated by the patient.
```

9
Imaging and Structural Informatics

JAMES F. BRINKLEY AND ROBERT A. GREENES

9.1 Introduction

As is evident to anyone who has had an X-ray, a magnetic resonance imaging (MRI) exam, or a biopsy, images play a central role in the health care process. In addition, images play important roles in medical communication and education, as well as in research. In fact much of our recent progress, particularly in diagnosis, can be traced to the availability of increasingly sophisticated images that not only show the structure of the body in incredible detail but also show the function.

Although there are many **imaging modalities**, images of all types are increasingly being converted to or initially acquired in digital form. This form is more or less the same across all imaging modalities. It is therefore amenable to common image-processing methodologies for enhancement, analysis, display, and storage.

Because of the ubiquity of images in biomedicine, the increasing availability of images in digital form, the rise of high-powered computer hardware and networks, and the commonality of image-processing solutions, digital images have become a core data type that must be considered in many biomedical informatics applications. Therefore, this chapter is devoted to a basic understanding of this core data type and many of the image-processing operations that can be applied to it. Chapter 18, on the other hand, describes the integration of images and image processing in various applications, particularly those in radiology since radiology places the greatest demands on imaging methods.

The topics covered by this chapter and Chapter 18 are generally part of biomedical imaging informatics (Kulikowski, 1997), a subfield of biomedical informatics that has arisen in recognition of the common issues that pertain to all image modalities and applications once the images are converted to digital form. By trying to understand these common issues, we can develop general solutions that can be applied to all images, regardless of the source.

The common tasks addressed by imaging informatics can be roughly classified as **image generation, image manipulation, image management**, and **image integration**. Image generation is the process of generating the images and converting them to digital form if they are not intrinsically digital. Image manipulation uses preprocessing and post-processing methods to enhance, visualize, or analyze the images. Image management includes methods for storing, transmitting, displaying, retrieving, and organizing images. Image integration is the combination of images with other information needed for interpretation, management, and other tasks. Because radiology places the greatest demand on image management, and because radiology represents the primary application of imaging methods, Chapter 18 is primarily concerned with the latter two tasks whereas this chapter concentrates on the former two.

A major purpose of image processing is to extract information about the structure of the body. As such, imaging informatics overlaps **structural informatics**, which is the study of methods for representing, organizing, and managing diverse sources of information about the physical organization of the body and other physical structures, both for its own sake, and as a means for organizing other information (Brinkley, 1991). Many of the topics in this chapter therefore have to do with how to represent, extract, and characterize the anatomic information that is present in images.

The examples for this chapter, particularly those for three-dimensional and functional imaging, are primarily taken from brain imaging, which is part of the growing field of **neuroinformatics** (Koslow and Huerta, 1997). We choose brain imaging because: (1) brain imaging is a strong area of interest of one of the authors (JB), (2) the national Human Brain Project (HBP) (Human Brain Project, 2003) is generating substantial results in the area of brain imaging, (3) a large portion of current medical imaging work is in brain imaging, and (4) some of the most advanced image-related work in informatics is currently being done in this area. Thus, in addition to introducing the concepts of digital images and image processing, this chapter represents an intersection of many of the concepts in imaging informatics, structural informatics, and neuroinformatics.

We first introduce basic concepts of digital images, and then describe methods for imaging the structure of the body in both two dimensions and three dimensions. We then describe two-dimensional and three-dimensional methods for processing structural images, primarily as a means for visualizing, extracting, and characterizing anatomy. The chapter ends with a discussion of methods for imaging the function of the body, virtually all of which involve mapping or registering the functional data onto the structural representations extracted using the techniques described in earlier sections.

9.2   Basic Concepts

9.2.1   Digital Images

A **digital image** typically is represented in a computer by a two-dimensional array of numbers (a **bit map**). Each element of the array represents the intensity of a small square area of the picture, called a **pixel**. If we consider the image of a volume, then a three-dimensional array of numbers is required; each element of the array in this case represents a volume element, called a **voxel**.

We can store any image in a computer in this manner, either by converting it from an analog to a digital representation or by generating it directly in digital form. Once an image is in digital form, it can be handled just like all other data. It can be transmitted over communications networks, stored compactly in databases on magnetic or optical media, and displayed on graphics monitors. In addition, the use of computers has created an entirely new realm of capabilities for image generation and analysis; images can be computed rather than measured directly. Furthermore, digital images can be manipulated for display or analysis in ways not possible with film-based images.

9.2.2   *Imaging Parameters*

All images can be characterized by several parameters of image quality. The most useful of these parameters are spatial resolution, contrast resolution, and temporal resolution. These parameters have been widely used to characterize traditional X-ray images; they also provide an objective means for comparing images formed by digital imaging modalities.

- **Spatial resolution** is related to the sharpness of the image; it is a measure of how well the imaging modality can distinguish points on the object that are close together. For a digital image, spatial resolution is generally related to the number of pixels per image area.
- **Contrast resolution** is a measure of the ability to distinguish small differences in intensity, which in turn are related to differences in measurable parameters such as X-ray attenuation. For digital images, the number of bits per pixel is related to the contrast resolution of an image.
- **Temporal resolution** is a measure of the time needed to create an image. We consider an imaging procedure to be a real-time application, if it can generate images concurrent with the physical process it is imaging. At a rate of at least 30 images per second, it is possible to produce unblurred images of the beating heart.

Other parameters that are specifically relevant to medical imaging are the degree of invasiveness, the dosage of ionizing radiation, the degree of patient discomfort, the size (portability) of the instrument, the ability to depict physiologic function as well as anatomic structure, and the availability and cost of the procedure at a specific location.

A perfect imaging modality would produce images with high spatial, contrast, and temporal resolution; it would be low in cost, portable, free of risk, painless, and noninvasive; it would use nonionizing radiation; and it would depict physiologic functions as well as anatomic structure.

9.3   Structural Imaging

Imaging the structure of the body has been and continues to be the major application of medical imaging, although, as described in Section 9.6, functional imaging is a very active area of research. The development of the various structural imaging modalities can be seen partly as a search for the perfect imaging modality; a primary reason for the proliferation of modalities is that no single modality satisfies all the desiderata. Another reason for the proliferation of image-generation methods is that progress has occurred in parallel in four main areas, and researchers have developed new methods quickly by combining elements from each of these areas. The four areas of development are energy source, reconstruction method, higher dimensionality, and contrast agents.

9.3.1 Energy Source

Light

The earliest medical images used **light** to create photographs, either of gross anatomic structures or, if a microscope was used, of histologic specimens. Light is still an important source for creation of images, and in fact optical imaging has seen a resurgence of late for areas such as molecular imaging (Weissleder and Mahmood, 2001) and imaging of brain activity on the exposed surface of the cerebral cortex (Pouratian et al., 2003). Visible light, however, does not allow us to see more than a short distance beneath the surface of the body.

X-Rays

X-rays were first discovered in 1895 by Wilhelm Conrad Roentgen, who was awarded the 1901 Nobel Prize in Physics for this achievement. The discovery caused worldwide excitement, especially in the field of medicine; by 1900, there were already several medical radiological societies. Thus, the foundation was laid for a new branch of medicine devoted to imaging the structure and function of the body (Kevles, 1997).

Film-based **radiography** is the primary modality used in radiology departments today, although this emphasis is changing rapidly as digital or **computed radiography (CR)** services are installed. We produce a typical X-ray image by projecting an X-ray beam— one form of ionizing radiation—from an X-ray source through a patient's body (or other object) and onto an X-ray-sensitive film. Because an X-ray beam is differentially absorbed by the various body tissues, the X-rays produce shadows on the radiographic film. The resultant **shadowgraph** is a superposition of all the structures traversed by each beam. **Digital radiography (DR)** applies the same techniques, but nonfilm detectors are used. In a technique known as CR, a latent image is recorded on a specially coated cassette that is scanned by a computer to capture the image in digital form; in other techniques, detectors capture the data directly in digital form. Although the images obtained by these techniques may be printed subsequently on film, they do not need to be.

Both film and fluoroscopic screens were used initially for recording X-ray images, but the fluoroscopic images were too faint to be used clinically. By the 1940s, however, television and image-intensifier technology were used to produce clear real-time fluorescent images. Today, a standard procedure for many types of examinations is to combine real-time television monitoring of X-ray images with the creation of selected higher resolution film images. Until the early 1970s, film and **fluoroscopy** were the only X-ray modalities available.

Traditional X-ray images have high spatial resolution and medium cost. Furthermore, they can be generated in real time (fluoroscopy) and can be produced using portable instruments. Their limitations are their relatively poor contrast resolution, their use of ionizing radiation, and their inability to depict physiologic function. Alternate imaging principles have been applied to increase contrast resolution, to eliminate exposure to X-ray radiation, and so on. For example, in nuclear-medicine imaging, a **radioactive isotope** is chemically attached to a biologically active compound (such as iodine) and then is injected into the patient's peripheral circulation. The compound collects in the specific body compartments or organs (such as the thyroid), where it is stored or processed by the body. The isotope emits radiation locally, and the radiation is measured using a special detector. The resultant nuclear-medicine image depicts the level of radioactivity that was measured at each point. Because the counts are inherently digital, computers have been used to record them. Multiple images also can be processed to obtain dynamic information, such as the rate of arrival or of disappearance of isotope at particular body sites.

Ultrasound

Another common energy source is **ultrasound** (echosonography), which developed out of research performed by the Navy during World War II. **Ultrasonography** uses pulses of high-frequency sound waves rather than ionizing radiation to image body structures. As each sound wave encounters tissues in a patient's body, a portion of the wave is reflected and a portion continues. The time required for the echo to return is proportional to the distance into the body at which it is reflected; the amplitude (intensity) of a returning echo depends on the acoustical properties of the tissues encountered and is represented in the image as brightness. The system constructs two-dimensional images by displaying the echoes from pulses of multiple adjacent one-dimensional paths. Such images can be stored in digital memories or recorded on videotape and then displayed as television (raster-display) images.

Nuclear Magnetic Resonance

Creation of images from **magnetism** grew out of **nuclear magnetic resonance (NMR) spectroscopy**, a technique that has long been used in chemistry to characterize chemical compounds. Many atomic nuclei within the body have a net magnetic moment, so they act like tiny magnets. When a small chemical sample is placed in an intense, uniform magnetic field, these nuclei line up in the direction of the field, spinning around the axis of the field with a frequency dependent on the type of nucleus, on the surrounding environment, and on the strength of the magnetic field.

If a radio pulse of a particular frequency is applied at right angles to the stationary magnetic field, those nuclei with rotation frequency equal to that of the radiofrequency pulse resonate with the pulse and absorb energy. The higher energy state causes the nuclei to change their orientation with respect to the fixed magnetic field. When the radiofrequency pulse is removed, the nuclei return to their original aligned state, emitting a detectable radiofrequency signal as they do so. Characteristic parameters of this signal—such as intensity, duration, and frequency shift away from the original pulse—are dependent on the density and environment of the nuclei.

In the case of traditional NMR spectroscopy, different molecular environments cause different frequency shifts (called chemical shifts), which we can use to identify the particular compounds in a sample. In the original NMR method, however, the signal is not localized to a specific region of the sample, so it is not possible to create an image. Creation of images from NMR signals known as MRI had to await the development of computer-based reconstruction techniques, which represent one of the most spectacular applications of computers in medicine.

9.3.2   Reconstruction Methods

Reconstruction techniques were first applied to X-ray images aimed at addressing the problem of superposition of structures in standard projection imaging. An X-ray image at a given point represents the total attenuation due to all the overlaid structures traversed by a beam as that beam passes through the body; shadows cast by surrounding structures may obscure the object that the clinician wishes to visualize. **Contrast radiography**—the use of radiopaque contrast material to highlight the areas of interest (e.g., stomach, colon, urinary tract)—was used as early as 1902 to address this problem. The first clinical experiments with **angiography**—imaging of blood vessels performed by the injection of opacifying agents into the bloodstream—were conducted in 1923.

The desire to separate superimposed structures also led to the development of a variety of analog tomographic techniques. In these methods, the X-ray source and detector were moved in opposite arcs, thereby causing a thin tomographic (planar) section to remain in focus while other planes were blurred. This method, however, exposes the patient to a relatively high X-ray dose because the blurred areas are exposed continuously.

Mathematical methods for reconstructing images from projections were first developed by Radon in 1917 and later were improved by other researchers. These methods were used in the 1950s and 1960s to solve scientific problems in many fields, including radio astronomy and electron microscopy. In the late 1960s, Cormack used the techniques to reconstruct phantoms (objects with known shape) using X-rays. In the early 1970s, Hounsfield led a team at the London-based EMI Corporation, which developed the first commercially viable computed tomography (CT) scanner.

Instead of depicting a directly measurable parameter (the absorption of X-ray beams as they pass through the body), CT mathematically reconstructs an image from X-ray-attenuation values that have been measured from multiple angles. As a result, it is possible to view cross-sectional slices through the body rather than two-dimensional projections of superimposed structures. Thus, CT images provide a precise mapping of the internal structures of the body in three-dimensional space—a function not provided by standard X-ray images. They also greatly improve contrast resolution.

In the basic CT imaging technique, the patient is placed between an X-ray-sensitive detector and an X-ray source that produces a collimated (pencil-like) beam. The measured difference between the source and detector X-ray intensities represents the amount of X-ray attenuation due to the tissues traversed by the beam; this measured attenuation is a superposition, or **projection**, of the attenuations of all the individual tissue elements traversed by the beam. In the simplest reconstruction method, called **back-projection**, the measured intensity is distributed uniformly over all the pixels traversed by the beam. For example, if the measured attenuation is 20, and 10 pixels were traversed, then the CT number of each of the 10 pixels is incremented by 2 units.

The attenuation measured from a single projection is not sufficient to reconstruct an image. The same back-projection computation, however, can be applied to the attenuations measured from multiple projections. The source and detector are rotated about the patient, and the X-ray attenuation is measured along each path. Because each pixel is traversed by multiple projection paths, its computed attenuation is the sum of the contributions from each path. The total sum provides a reasonable first approximation of the X-ray attenuation of the individual pixel. The image is further refined using a mathematical edge-enhancement technique called **convolution**. In effect, convolution removes shadows that result from the back projection, thus sharpening the blurry image.

The development of the CT scanner dramatically improved our ability to visualize adjacent structures; for the first time, physicians were able to see inside a living human being clearly, but noninvasively. This ability led to a revolution in medicine almost as great as the one occasioned by the invention of X-ray imaging. As a result, Cormack and Hounsfield were awarded the 1979 Nobel Prize in Medicine.

After the invention of the CT scanner, this basic method of reconstruction from projections was applied to other energy sources, including magnetism (MRI), ultrasound (ultrasound-transmission tomography), and variants of nuclear-medicine imaging called **positron-emission tomography (PET)** and single-photon-emission computed tomography (SPECT).

The most dramatic example of reconstruction from projections other than CT is MRI, which is based on NMR (Oldendorf, 1991). As described in the previous section, NMR takes advantage of magnetic properties of nuclei to characterize the distribution and chemical environment of nuclei within a chemical sample. To create an image using these parameters, we need a way to restrict this sample to a small volume within a larger tissue. With this restriction, the parameters of the NMR signal from each small tissue volume can be mapped to voxel intensities depicting different tissue characteristics.

The restriction to a small sample volume is accomplished by taking advantage of the fact that the resonant frequency of atomic nuclei varies with the magnetic field. If the field can be made different for each small tissue volume, then a radiofrequency pulse with a given frequency will excite only those nuclei in the small volume that have the resonant frequency of that pulse. The basic method uses electromagnetic coils to superimpose a varying magnetic field on a large fixed magnetic field, thereby setting up a gradient in the magnetic field.

This gradient is changed electronically, setting the location of the sample volume. For example, we use one gradient to set the plane of section (the z direction, although the orientation of this section may be arbitrary with respect to the patient), and a second gradient sets a line within a single section (the x,y plane). As in CT, the signal detected along this line is a summation of the signals from all voxels along the line. Therefore, the x,y gradient is electronically rotated, rotating the plane of section and generating additional lines within a given plane. The same reconstruction techniques developed for CT then reconstruct the values for the individual voxels within the given plane. Because there are many different parameters that can be measured for each sampled voxel, many different types of images can be constructed, many of which are still being developed.

9.3.3   *Higher Dimensionality*

Most routine images in radiology are still two-dimensional. Because the body is a three-dimensional object that changes over time, however, there will always be a drive to create three-dimensional time-varying images. In recent years, advances in digital hardware have provided the storage and throughput to manage large time-varying voxel-based data sets. Reconstruction modalities—such as CT, PET, and MRI—all are either inherently three-dimensional or can be made three-dimensional by acquisition of a series of closely spaced parallel slices (see Section 9.5). Thus, the only drawbacks of these techniques are the time and expense required to acquire a series of parallel slices, both of which are becoming smaller.

Ultrasound images, on the other hand, cannot be acquired as parallel slices because sound does not pass through bone or air. For this reason, we usually obtain three-dimensional ultrasound information by attaching a three-dimensional locating device to the transducer. The locator gives the position and orientation of the slice plane in space. Before the availability of hardware that could store large numbers of volume data, the ultrasound images were first processed in two dimensions to extract relevant anatomy as two-dimensional contours or regions; the two-dimensional contours were converted to three-dimensional contours based on the location information and then were displayed with vector graphics (Brinkley et al., 1978). Such an approach was useful for quantitation, but did not provide a realistic three-dimensional view of the object.

9.3.4 Contrast Agents

As noted above, one of the major motivators for development of new imaging modalities is the desire to increase contrast resolution. We have already discussed the use of radiologic contrast agents and reconstruction techniques as examples of highly successful attempts to increase contrast resolution among the different energy sources. In addition, histologic staining agents such as hematoxylin and eosin (H&E) have been used for years to enhance contrast in tissue sections, and magnetic contrast agents such as gadolinium have been introduced to enhance contrast in MR images.

Although these methods have been very successful, they generally are somewhat nonspecific. In recent years, advances in molecular biology have led to the ability to design contrast agents that are highly specific for individual molecules. In addition to radioactively tagged molecules used in nuclear medicine, molecules are tagged for imaging by magnetic resonance and optical energy sources. Tagged molecules are imaged in two dimensions or three dimensions, often by application of reconstruction techniques developed for clinical imaging. Tagged molecules have been used for several years *in vitro* by such techniques as immunocytochemistry (binding of tagged antibodies to antigen) (Van Noorden, 2002) and *in situ* hybridization (binding of tagged nucleotide sequences to DNA or RNA) (King et al., 2000). More recently, methods have been developed to image these molecules in the living organism, thereby opening up entirely new avenues for understanding the functioning of the body at the molecular level.

9.3.5 New and Emerging Structural Imaging Methods

Many new imaging techniques have been developed in recent years. Most of these techniques can be seen as a combination of an energy source, a computer-based processing or reconstruction technique, increased dimensionality due to advances in digital hardware, and, increasingly, use of molecular contrast agents. The remainder of this section describes a few examples of these techniques.

At the gross anatomic level, **charge-coupled device (CCD) cameras** can be used to convert existing film-based equipment to units that can produce images in digital form. Storage phosphor, or CR, systems replace film by substituting a reusable phosphor plate in a standard film cassette. The exposed plate is processed by a reader system that scans the image into digital form, erases the plate, and packages the cassette for reuse. An important advantage of CR systems is that the cassettes are of standard size, so they can be used in any equipment that holds film-based cassettes (Horii, 1996). More recently, CR uses CCD arrays to capture the image directly.

Many new modalities are being developed based on magnetic resonance. For example, *magnetic resonance arteriography* (MRA) and *magnetic resonance venography* (MRV) image blood flow (Lee, 2003), and *diffusion tensor imaging* (DTI) is increasingly being used to image white matter fiber tracts in the brain (Figure 9.1) (Le Bihan et al., 2001).

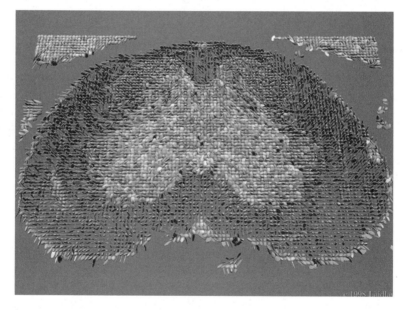

Figure 9.1. Diffusion tensor image (DTI) of the mouse spinal cord. At each pixel the DTI technique outputs a 3 × 3 diffusion tensor describing the measured diffusion of water in each of the six principle directions in three-dimensional space. In gray matter, the diffusion is generally uniform (isotropic) in all directions, but in white matter diffusion is reduced in the direction perpendicular to the fibers. Thus, DTI is used to visualize white matter fiber tracts. Since each pixel (or voxel in three-dimensions) is described by a 3 × 3 matrix, visualization techniques from computer graphics are needed in order to represent the information at each pixel. In this figure, the diffusion tensors are represented by ellipsoids with axes along the principle directions of the diffusion tensor. Photograph courtesy of David Laidlaw (Ahrens et al., 1998), http://www.gg.caltech.edu/~dhl/images.html.

Ultrasound machines have essentially become specialized computers with attached peripherals, with active development of three-dimensional imaging. The ultrasound transducer now often sweeps out a three-dimensional volume rather than a two-dimensional plane, and the data are written directly into a three-dimensional array memory, which is displayed using volume or **surface-based rendering** techniques (Figure 9.2) (Ritchie et al., 1996).

At the microscopic level, the *confocal microscope* uses electronic focusing to move a two-dimensional slice plane through a three-dimensional tissue slice placed in a microscope. The result is a three-dimensional voxel array of a microscopic, or even submicroscopic, specimen (Wilson, 1990; Paddock, 1994). At the electron microscopic level *electron tomography* generates three-dimensional images from thick electron-microscopic sections using techniques similar to those used in CT (Perkins et al., 1997).

At the molecular level tagged molecules are increasingly introduced into the living organism, and imaged with optical, radioactive or magnetic energy sources, often using reconstruction techniques and often in three dimensions. The combination of these various methods with highly specific tagged molecules has given rise to the field of **molecular imaging** (Weissleder and Mahmood, 2001; Massoud and Gambhir, 2003), which in addition to functional brain imaging (Section 9.6) represents some of the most exciting new developments in biomedical imaging. It is now becoming possible to combine gene sequence information, gene expression array data, and molecular imaging to determine not only which genes are expressed but also where they are expressed in the organism. These capabilities will become increasingly important in the **post-genomic era** for determining exactly how genes generate both the structure and function of the organism.

9.4   Two-Dimensional Image Processing

The rapidly increasing number and types of digital images has created many opportunities for image processing, since one of the great advantages of digital images is that

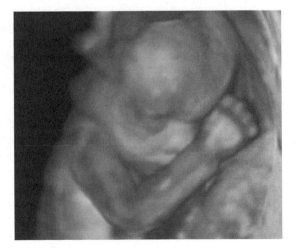

Figure 9.2. Three-dimensional ultrasound image of a fetus, *in utero*. The ultrasound probe sweeps out a three-dimensional volume rather than the conventional two-dimensional plane. The volume can be rendered directly using volume-rendering techniques, or as in this case, fetal surfaces can be extracted and rendered using surface-rendering techniques. Photograph courtesy of Per Perm, "GE Healthcare", http://www. gemedicalsystems.com/rad/us/education/ msucme3d.html.

they can be manipulated just like any other kind of data. This advantage was evident from the early days of computers, and success in processing satellite and spacecraft images generated considerable interest in biomedical image processing, including automated image analysis for interpretation. Beginning in the 1960s, researchers devoted a large amount of work to this end, with the hope that eventually much of radiographic image analysis could be automated.

One of the first areas to receive attention was automated interpretation of chest X-ray images, because, previously, most patients admitted to a hospital were subjected to routine chest X-ray examinations. (This practice is no longer considered cost effective except for selected subgroups of patients.) Subsequent research, however, confirmed the difficulty of completely automating radiographic image interpretation, and much of the initial enthusiasm has long ago worn off. Currently, there is less emphasis on completely automatic interpretation and more on systems that aid the user, except in specialized areas such as brain imaging.

9.4.1   Basic Concepts in Two-Dimensional Image Processing

Digital image manipulation, or **image processing**, generally involves the transformation of one or more input images either into one or more output images or into some abstract representation of the contents of the input images. For example, the intensity values can be modified to improve contrast resolution, or a set of terms (*pleural effusion, lung nodule*) can be attached to specific regions of interest.

Images can be enhanced to permit human viewing, to show views not present in the original images, to flag suspicious areas for closer examination by the clinician, to quantify the size and shape of an organ, and to prepare the images for integration with other information. Most of these applications require one or more of the four basic image-processing steps: global processing, segmentation, feature detection, and classification. These steps are generally performed in order, although later steps may feed back to earlier ones, and not all steps are required for each application. Most steps generalize from two-dimensional to three-dimensional images, but three-dimensional images give rise to additional image-processing opportunities and challenges that are discussed in Section 9.5.

Global processing involves computations on the entire image, without regard to specific local content. The purpose is to enhance an image for human visualization or for further analysis by the computer. A simple but important example is *gray-scale windowing* of CT images. The CT scanner generates pixel values (Hounsfield numbers, or CT numbers) in the range of −1,000 to +3,000. Humans, however, cannot distinguish more than about 100 shades of gray. To appreciate the full precision available with a CT image, the operator can adjust the midpoint and the range of the displayed CT values. By changing the level and width (i.e., intercept and slope of the mapping between pixel value and displayed gray scale or, roughly, the brightness and contrast) of the display, radiologists enhance their ability to perceive small changes in contrast resolution within a subregion of interest.

Segmentation involves the extraction of regions of interest (ROIs) from the overall image. The ROIs usually correspond to anatomically meaningful structures, such as organs or parts of organs. The structures may be delineated by their borders, in which case **edge-detection techniques** (such as edge-following algorithms) are used, or by their composition on the image, in which case **region-detection techniques** (such as texture analysis) are used (Haralick and Shapiro, 1992). Neither of these techniques has been completely successful; regions often have discontinuous borders or nondistinctive internal composition. Furthermore, contiguous regions often overlap. These and other complications make segmentation the most difficult subtask of the medical image-analysis problem. Because segmentation is difficult for a computer, it is often performed manually by a human operator or through a combination of automated and operator-interactive approaches. It therefore remains a major bottleneck that prevents more widespread application of image-processing techniques.

Feature detection is the process of extracting useful parameters from the segmented regions. These parameters may themselves be informative—for example, the volume of the heart or the size of the fetus. They also may be used as input into an automated **classification** procedure, which determines the type of object found. For example, small round regions on chest X-ray images might be classified as tumors, depending on such features as intensity, perimeter, and area.

Mathematical models often are used to aid in the performance of image-analysis subtasks. In classic pattern-recognition applications, the subtasks of global processing, segmentation, feature detection, and classification usually are performed sequentially. People, however, appear to perform pattern-recognition iteratively. For example, radiologists can perceive faint images and can trace discontinuous borders, in part because they know which features they are searching for. Many researchers have applied artificial intelligence techniques to imitate such interaction among subtasks. The computer is programmed with some of the higher-level anatomic knowledge that radiologists use when they interpret images. Thus, high-level organ models provide feedback to guide the lower-level process of segmentation.

The nature of the application determines which of these subtasks is performed, the choice of technique for each subtask, and the relative order of the subtasks. Because image understanding is an unsolved problem, and because many applications are possible, there is a wealth of image-processing techniques that can be applied to digital images.

9.4.2 *Examples of Two-Dimensional Image Processing*

Although completely automated image-analysis systems are still in the future, the widespread availability of digital images, combined with image management systems such as picture archiving and communication systems (PACS; Chapter 18) and powerful workstations, has led to many applications of image-processing techniques. In general, routine techniques are available on the manufacturer's workstations (e.g., an MR console or an ultrasound machine), whereas more advanced image-processing algorithms are available as software packages that run on independent workstations.

The primary uses of two-dimensional image processing in the clinical environment are for image enhancement, screening, and quantitation. Software for such image processing is primarily developed for use on independent workstations. Several journals are devoted to medical image processing (e.g., *IEEE Transactions on Medical Imaging,*

Journal of Digital Imaging, Neuroimage), and the number of journal articles is rapidly increasing as digital images become more widely available. We describe just a few examples of image-processing techniques in the remainder of this section.

Image enhancement uses global processing to improve the appearance of the image either for human use or for subsequent processing by computer. All manufacturers' consoles and independent image-processing workstations provide some form of image enhancement. We have already mentioned CT windowing. Another technique is **unsharp masking**, in which a blurred image is subtracted from the original image to increase local contrast and to enhance the visibility of fine-detail (high-frequency) structures. **Histogram equalization** spreads the image gray levels throughout the visible range to maximize the visibility of those gray levels that are used frequently. **Temporal subtraction** subtracts a reference image from later images that are registered to the first. A common use of temporal subtraction is digital-subtraction angiography (DSA) in which a background image is subtracted from an image taken after the injection of contrast material.

Screening uses global processing, segmentation, feature detection, and classification to determine whether an image should be flagged for careful review by a radiologist or pathologist. In such an approach, the computer is allowed to flag a reasonable number of normal images (false positives) as long as it misses very few abnormal images (false negatives). If the number of flagged images is small compared with the total number of images, then automated screening procedures can be economically viable. Screening techniques have been applied successfully to mammography images for identifying mass lesions and clusters of microcalcifications, to chest X-rays for small cancerous nodules, and to Papanicolaou (Pap) smears for cancerous or precancerous cells (Giger and MacMahon, 1996), as well as to many other images (Figure 9.3; see also Color Plate I).

Quantitation uses global processing and segmentation to characterize meaningful regions of interest. For example, heart size, shape, and motion are subtle indicators of heart function and of the response of the heart to therapy (Clarysse et al., 1997). Similarly, fetal head size and femur length, as measured on ultrasound images, are valuable indicators of fetal well-being (Brinkley, 1993b). Although the literature describes a wealth of automatic or semiautomatic techniques for segmenting images of the heart or of the fetus, the most common clinical scenario continues to be manual outlining by trained technicians. This situation should change, however, as semiautomatic techniques (those that let the user correct segmentation errors by the computer) become widely available on independent workstations that are custom-tailored for particular applications.

9.5   Three-Dimensional Image Processing

The growing availability of three-dimensional and higher dimensionality structural and functional images (Section 9.3.3) leads to exciting opportunities for realistically observing the structure and function of the body. Nowhere have these opportunities been more widely exploited than in brain imaging. Therefore, this section concentrates on three-dimensional brain imaging, with the recognition that many of the methods developed for the brain have been or will be applied to other areas as well.

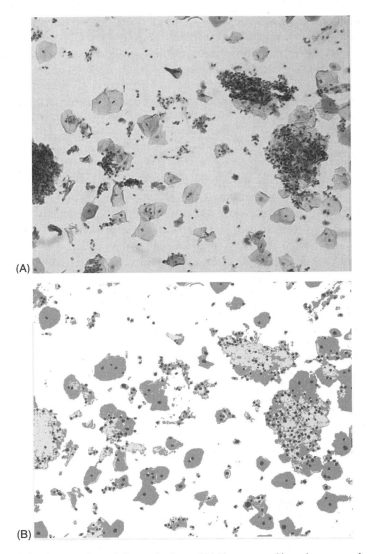

Figure 9.3. Automated screening of Papanicolaou (PAP) smears. Since large numbers of PAP smears are acquired routinely, there is a need to reduce the cost and potential errors associated with purely manual interpretation. (A) Raw microscopic image of cervical cells. (B) Segmented image. The program has segmented the cells and nuclei from the raw image, prior to feature detection and classification based on the features. Abnormally classified cells are flagged for review by the human operator. Photograph courtesy of Peter Locht, Visible Diagnostics, http://www.imm.dtu.dk/visiondag/VD03/medicinsk/pl.pdf.

The basic two-dimensional image-processing operations of global processing, segmentation, feature detection, and classification generalize to higher dimensions, and are usually part of any image-processing application. However, three-dimensional and higher dimensionality images give rise to additional informatics issues, which include image **registration** (which also occurs to a lesser extent in two dimensions), *spatial* representation of anatomy, *symbolic* representation of anatomy, integration of spatial and symbolic anatomic representations in *atlases*, anatomic *variation*, and *characterization* of anatomy. All but the first of these issues deal primarily with anatomic structure, and therefore could be considered part of the field of structural informatics. They could also be thought of as being part of imaging informatics and neuroinformatics.

The following sections discuss these additional informatics issues.

9.5.1   Registration

As noted previously, three-dimensional image volume data are represented in the computer by a three-dimensional volume array, in which each *voxel* (volume element, analogous to the pixel in two dimensions) represents the image intensity in a small volume of space. In order to accurately depict anatomy, the voxels must be accurately registered (or located) in the three-dimensional volume (*voxel registration*), and separately acquired image volumes from the same subject must be registered with each other (*volume registration*).

Voxel Registration

Technologies such as CT, MRI, MRV, MRA, and confocal microscopy (Section 9.3) are inherently three-dimensional; the scanner generally outputs a series of image slices that can easily be reformatted as a three-dimensional volume array, often following alignment algorithms that compensate for any patient motion during the scanning procedure. For this reason, almost all CT and MR manufacturers' consoles contain some form of three-dimensional reconstruction and visualization capabilities.

As noted in Section 9.3.3, two-dimensional images can be converted to three-dimensional volumes by acquiring a set of closely spaced parallel sections through a tissue or whole specimen. In this case the problem is how to align the sections with each other. For whole sections (either frozen or fixed), the standard method is to embed a set of thin rods or strings in the tissue prior to sectioning, to manually indicate the location of these *fiducials* on each section, then to linearly transform each slice so that the corresponding fiducials line up in three dimensions (Prothero and Prothero, 1986). A popular current example of this technique is the Visible Human, in which a series of transverse slices were acquired, then reconstructed to give a full three-dimensional volume (Spitzer and Whitlock, 1998).

It is difficult to embed fiducial markers at the microscopic level, so intrinsic tissue landmarks are often used as fiducials, but the basic principle is similar. However, in this case tissue distortion may be a problem, so nonlinear transformations may be required. For example, Fiala and Harris (2001) have developed an interface that allows the user to indicate, on electron-microscopy sections, corresponding centers of small organelles such as mitochondria. A nonlinear transformation (warp) is then computed to bring the landmarks into registration.

An approach being pursued (among other approaches) by the National Center for Microscopy and Imaging Research (http://ncmir.ucsd.edu/) combines reconstruction from thick serial sections with electron tomography (Soto et al., 1994). In this case the tomographic technique is applied to each thick section to generate a three-dimensional digital slab, after which the slabs are aligned with each other to generate a three-dimensional volume. The advantages of this approach over the standard serial section method are that the sections do not need to be as thin, and fewer of them need be acquired.

An alternative approach to three-dimensional voxel registration from two-dimensional images is stereo-matching, a technique developed in computer vision that acquires multiple two-dimensional images from known angles, which finds corresponding points on the images, and uses the correspondences and known camera angles to compute three-dimensional coordinates of pixels in the matched images. The technique is being applied to the reconstruction of synapses from electron micrographs by a HBP collaboration between computer scientists and biologists at the University of Maryland (Agrawal et al., 2000).

Volume Registration

A related problem to that of aligning individual sections is the problem of aligning separate image volumes from the same subject, i.e., *intrasubject* alignment. Because different image modalities provide complementary information, it is common to acquire more than one kind of image volume on the same individual. This approach has been particularly useful for brain imaging because each modality provides different information. For example, PET (Section 9.3.2) provides useful information about function, but does not provide good localization with respect to anatomy. Similarly, MRV and MRA (Section 9.3.5) show blood flow but do not provide the detailed anatomy visible with standard MRI. By combining images from these modalities with MRI, we can show functional images in terms of the underlying anatomy, thereby providing a common neuroanatomic framework.

In our own (JB) HBP work, we acquire an MRI volume dataset depicting cortical anatomy, an MRV volume depicting veins, and an MRA volume depicting arteries (Modayur et al., 1997; Hinshaw et al., 2002). By "fusing" these separate modalities into a single common frame of reference (anatomy, as given by the MRI dataset), it is possible to gain information that is not apparent from one of the modalities alone. In our case the fused datasets are used to generate a visualization of the brain surface as it appears at neurosurgery, in which the veins and arteries provide prominent landmarks (Figure 9.9).

The primary problem to solve in **multimodality image fusion** is volume registration—that is, the alignment of separately acquired image volumes. In the simplest case, separate image volumes are acquired during a single sitting. The patient's head may be immobilized, and the information in the image headers may be used to rotate and resample the image volumes until all the voxels correspond.

However, if the patient moves, or if examinations are acquired at different times, other registration methods are needed. When intensity values are similar across modalities, registration can be performed automatically by intensity-based optimization methods (Woods et al., 1992; Collins et al., 1994). When intensity values are not similar (as is the case with MRA, MRV, and MRI), images can be aligned to templates of the same modalities that are already aligned (Woods et al., 1993; Ashburner and Friston,

1997). Alternatively, landmark-based methods can be used. The landmark-based methods are similar to those used to align serial sections, but in this case the landmarks are three-dimensional points. The Montreal Register Program (MacDonald, 1993) (which can also do nonlinear registration, as discussed in Section 9.5.5) is an example of such a program.

9.5.2   *Spatial Representation of Anatomy*

The reconstructed and registered three-dimensional image volumes can be visualized directly using **volume rendering** techniques (Foley et al., 1990; Lichtenbelt et al., 1998) (Figure 9.2) which project a two-dimensional image directly from a three-dimensional voxel array by casting rays from the eye of the observer through the volume array to the image plane. Because each ray passes through many voxels, some form of segmentation (usually simple thresholding) often is used to remove obscuring structures. As workstation memory and processing power have advanced, volume rendering has become widely used to display all sorts of three-dimensional voxel data—ranging from cell images produced by confocal microscopy to three-dimensional ultrasound images, or to brain images created from MRI or PET.

Volume images can also be given as input to image-based techniques for warping the image volume of one structure to other, as described in Section 9.5.5. However, more commonly the image volume is processed in order to extract an explicit *spatial* (or quantitative) representation of anatomy. Such an explicit representation permits improved visualization, quantitative analysis of structure, comparison of anatomy across a population, and mapping of functional data. It is thus a component of most research involving three-dimensional image processing.

Extraction of spatial representations of anatomy, in the form of three-dimensional surfaces or volume regions, is accomplished by a three-dimensional generalization of the segmentation techniques discussed in Section 9.4.1. As in the two-dimensional case, fully automated segmentation is an unsolved problem, as attested to by the number of papers about this subject in *IEEE Transactions on Medical Imaging*. However, because of the high quality of MRI brain images, a great deal of progress has been made in recent years for brain imaging in particular; in fact, several software packages do a credible job of automatic segmentation, particularly for normal macroscopic brain anatomy in cortical and subcortical regions (Collins et al., 1995; Friston et al., 1995; Subramaniam et al., 1997; Dale et al., 1999; MacDonald et al., 2000; Brain Innovation B.V., 2001; FMRIDB Image Analysis Group, 2001; Van Essen et al., 2001; Hinshaw et al., 2002). The HBP-funded Internet Brain Segmentation Repository (Kennedy, 2001) is developing a repository of segmented brain images to use in comparing these different methods.

Popular segmentation and reconstruction techniques include reconstruction from serial sections, region-based methods, edge-based methods, model- or knowledge-based methods, and combined methods.

Reconstruction from Serial Sections

The classic approach to extracting anatomy is to manually or semiautomatically trace the contours of structures of interest on each of a series of aligned image slices, then to

tile a surface over the contours (Prothero and Prothero, 1982). The tiled surface usually consists of an array of three-dimensional points connected to each other by edges to form triangular facets. The resulting three-dimensional *surface mesh* is then in a form where it can be further analyzed or displayed using standard three-dimensional surface rendering techniques such as those applied in the computer-generated film industry (Foley, 2001).

Neither fully automatic contour tracing nor fully automatic tiling has been satisfactorily demonstrated in the general case. Thus, semiautomatic contour tracing followed by semiautomatic tiling remains the most common method for reconstruction from serial sections, and reconstruction from serial sections itself remains the method of choice for extracting microscopic three-dimensional brain anatomy (Fiala and Harris, 2001).

Region-Based and Edge-Based Segmentation

This and the following sections primarily concentrate on segmentation at the macroscopic level.

In region-based segmentation, voxels are grouped into contiguous regions based on characteristics such as intensity ranges and similarity to neighboring voxels (Shapiro and Stockman, 2001). A common initial approach to region-based segmentation is to first classify voxels into a small number of tissue classes such as gray matter, white matter, cerebrospinal fluid, and background, then to use these classifications as a basis for further segmentation (Choi et al., 1991; Zijdenbos et al., 1996). Another region-based approach is called region growing, in which regions are grown from seed voxels manually or automatically placed within candidate regions (Davatzikos and Bryan, 1996; Modayur et al., 1997). The regions found by any of these approaches are often further processed by mathematical morphology operators (Haralick, 1988) to remove unwanted connections and holes (Sandor and Leahy, 1997).

Edge-based segmentation is the complement to region-based segmentation; intensity gradients are used to search for and link organ boundaries. In the two-dimensional case, contour-following methods connects adjacent points on the boundary. In the three-dimensional case, isosurface-following or marching-cubes (Lorensen and Cline, 1987) methods connect border voxels in a region into a three-dimensional surface mesh.

Both region-based and edge-based segmentation are essentially low-level techniques that only look at local regions in the image data.

Model- and Knowledge-Based Segmentation

The most popular current method for medical image segmentation, for the brain as well as other biological structures, is the use of **deformable models**. Based on pioneering work called "Snakes" by Kass et al. (1987), deformable models have been developed for both two dimensions and three dimensions. In the two-dimensional case the deformable model is a contour, often represented as a simple set of linear segments or a *spline*, which is initialized to approximate the contour on the image. The contour is then deformed according to a cost function that includes both intrinsic terms limiting how much the contour can distort, and extrinsic terms that reward closeness to image borders. In the three-dimensional case, a three-dimensional surface (often a triangular mesh) is deformed in a similar manner. There are several examples of HBP-funded work that use deformable models for brain segmentation (Davatzikos and Bryan, 1996; Dale et al., 1999; MacDonald et al., 2000; Van Essen et al., 2001).

An advantage of deformable models is that the cost function can include knowledge of the expected anatomy of the brain. For example, the cost function employed in the method developed by MacDonald (MacDonald et al., 2000) includes a term for the expected thickness of the brain cortex. Thus, these methods can become somewhat knowledge-based, where knowledge of anatomy is encoded in the cost function.

An alternative knowledge-based approach explicitly records shape information in a geometric constraint network (GCN) (Brinkley, 1992), which encodes local shape variation based on a training set. The shape constraints define search regions on the image in which to search for edges. Found edges are then combined with the shape constraints to deform the model and reduce the size of search regions for additional edges (Brinkley, 1985, 1993a). One potential advantage of this sort of model over a pure deformable model is that knowledge is explicitly represented in the model, rather than implicitly represented in the cost function.

Combined Methods

Most brain segmentation packages use a combination of methods in a sequential pipeline. For example, in our own recent work (JB) we first use a GCN model to represent the overall cortical "envelope", excluding the detailed gyri and sulci (Hinshaw et al., 2002). The model is semiautomatically deformed to fit the cortex, then used as a mask to remove noncortex such as the skull. Isosurface following is then applied to the masked region to generate the detailed cortical surface. The model is also used on aligned MRA and MRV images to mask out noncortical veins and arteries prior to isosurface following. The extracted cortical, vein, and artery surfaces are then rendered to produce a composite visualization of the brain as seen at neurosurgery (Figure 9.9).

MacDonald et al. (2000) describe an automatic multiresolution surface deformation technique called anatomic segmentation using proximities (ASP), in which an inner and outer surface are progressively deformed to fit the image, where the cost function includes image terms, model-based terms, and proximity terms. Dale et al. (1999) describe an automated approach that is implemented in the FreeSurfer program (Fischl et al., 1999). This method initially finds the gray-white boundary, then fits smooth gray-white (inner) and white-CSF (outer) surfaces using deformable models. Van Essen et al. (2001) describe the SureFit program, which finds the cortical surface midway between the gray-white boundary and the gray-CSF boundary. This mid-level surface is created from probabilistic representations of both inner and outer boundaries that are determined using image intensity, intensity gradients, and knowledge of cortical topography. Other software packages also combine various methods for segmentation (Davatzikos and Bryan, 1996; Brain Innovation B.V., 2001; FMRIDB Image Analysis Group, 2001; Sensor Systems Inc., 2001; Wellcome Department of Cognitive Neurology, 2001).

9.5.3   Symbolic Representation of Anatomy

Given segmented anatomic structures, whether at the macroscopic or microscopic level, and whether represented as three-dimensional surface meshes or extracted three-dimensional regions, it is often desirable to attach labels (names) to the structures. If the names are drawn from a controlled terminology they can be used as an index into a database of segmented structures, thereby providing a qualitative means for comparing structures from multiple subjects.

If the terms in the vocabulary are organized into symbolic qualitative models (**ontologies**) of anatomic concepts and relationships, they can support systems that manipulate and retrieve segmented structures in "intelligent" ways. If the anatomic ontologies are linked to other ontologies of physiology and pathology, they can provide increasingly sophisticated knowledge about the *meaning* of the various images and other data that are increasingly becoming available in online databases. It is our belief that this kind of knowledge (by the computer, as opposed to the scientist) will be required in order to achieve the seamless integration of all forms of imaging and nonimaging data.

At the most fundamental level, *Nomina Anatomica* (International Anatomical Nomenclature Committee, 1989) and its successor, *Terminologia Anatomica* (Federative Committee on Anatomical Terminology, 1998) provide a classification of officially sanctioned terms that are associated with macroscopic and microscopic anatomical structures. This canonical term list, however, has been substantially expanded by synonyms that are current in various fields, and has also been augmented by a large number of new terms that designate structures omitted from *Terminologia Anatomica*. Many of these additions are present in various controlled terminologies (e.g., MeSH (National Library of Medicine, 1999), SNOMED (Spackman et al., 1997), Read Codes (Schultz et al., 1997), GALEN (Rector et al., 1993)). Unlike *Terminologia* these vocabularies are entirely computer-based, and therefore lend themselves for incorporation in computer-based applications.

The most complete primate *neuroanatomical* terminology is *NeuroNames*, developed by Bowden and Martin at the University of Washington (Bowden and Martin, 1995). *NeuroNames*, which is included as a knowledge source in the National Library of Medicine's Unified Medical Language System (UMLS; see Chapter 7) (Lindberg et al., 1993), is primarily organized as a part-of hierarchy of nested structures, with links to a large set of ancillary terms that do not fit into the strict part-of hierarchy. Other neuroanatomical terminologies have also been developed (Paxinos and Watson, 1986; Swanson, 1992; Bloom and Young, 1993; Franklin and Paxinos, 1997). A challenge for biomedical informatics is either to come up with a single consensus terminology or to develop Internet tools that allow transparent integration of distributed but commonly agreed-on terminology, with local modifications.

Classification and ontology projects to date have focused primarily on arranging the terms of a particular domain in hierarchies. As we noted with respect to the evaluation of *Terminologia Anatomica* (Rosse, 2000), insufficient attention has been paid to the relationships between these terms. *Terminologia*, as well as anatomy sections of the controlled medical terminologies, mix *-is a-* and *-part of-*relationships in the anatomy segments of their hierarchies. Although such heterogeneity does not interfere with using these term lists for keyword-based retrieval, these programs will fail to support higher-level knowledge (reasoning) required for knowledge-based applications.

In our own Structural Informatics Group at the University of Washington we (JB and co-workers) are addressing this deficiency by developing a *Foundational Model of Anatomy* (FMA), (Figure 9.4) which we define as a comprehensive symbolic description of the structural organization of the body, including anatomical concepts, their preferred names and synonyms, definitions, attributes, and relationships (Rosse et al., 1998; Rosse and Mejino, 2003).

The FMA is being implemented in Protégé-2000, a frame-based knowledge acquisition system developed at Stanford (Musen, 1998; Mejino et al., 2001). In Protégé anatomical concepts are arranged in class–subclass hierarchies, with inheritance of defining attributes along the *is-a* link, and other relationships (e.g., parts, branches, spatial adjacencies) represented as additional slots in the frame. The FMA currently consists of over 70,000 concepts, represented by about 100,000 terms, and arranged in over 1.2 million links using 110 types of relationships. These concepts represent structures at all levels: macroscopic (to 1 mm resolution) cellular, and macromolecular. Brain

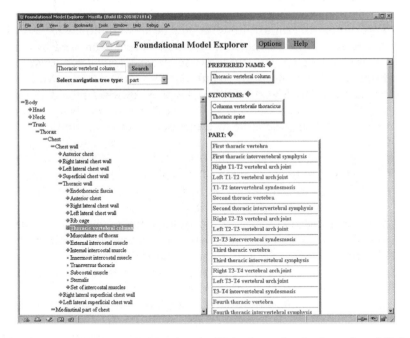

Figure 9.4. The Foundational Model Explorer, a Web viewer for the frame-based University of Washington Foundational Model of Anatomy (FMA). The left panel shows a hierarchical view along the part of link. Hierarchies along other links, such as is-a, branch-of, tributary-of, can also be viewed in this panel. The right hand panel shows the detailed local and inherited attributes (slots) associated with a selected structure, in this case the thoracic vertebral column. See also Figure 9.5. Photograph courtesy of the Structural Informatics Group, University of Washington.

structures have been added by integrating *NeuroNames* with the FMA as a *Foundational Model of Neuroanatomy* (FMNA) (Martin et al., 2001).

Our belief is that the FMA will prove useful for symbolically organizing and integrating biomedical information, particularly that obtained from images. But in order to answer nontrivial queries in neuroscience and other basic science areas, and to develop "smart tools" that rely on deep knowledge, additional ontologies must also be developed, among other things, for physiologic functions mediated by neurotransmitters, and pathologic processes and their clinical manifestations, as well as for the radiologic appearances with which they correlate. The relationships that exist between these concepts and anatomical parts of the body must also be explicitly modeled. Next-generation informatics efforts that link the FMA and other anatomical ontologies with separately developed functional ontologies will be needed in order to accomplish this type of integration.

9.5.4   Atlases

Spatial representations of anatomy, in the form of segmented regions on two-dimensional or three-dimensional images, or three-dimensional surfaces extracted from image volumes, are often combined with symbolic representations to form digital atlases. A digital atlas (which for this chapter refers to an atlas created from three-dimensional image data taken from real subjects, as opposed to artists' illustrations) is generally created from a single individual, which therefore serves as a "canonical" instance of the species. Traditionally, atlases have been primarily used for education, and most digital atlases are used the same way.

As an example in two dimensions, the Digital Anatomist Interactive Atlases (Sundsten et al., 2000) were created by outlining ROIs on two-dimensional images (many of which are snapshots of three-dimensional scenes generated by reconstruction from serial sections) and labeling the regions with terminology from the FMA. The atlases, which are available on the Web, permit interactive browsing where the names of structures are given in response to mouse clicks; dynamic creation of "pin diagrams", in which selected labels are attached to regions on the images; and dynamically generated quizzes, in which the user is asked to point to structures on the image (Brinkley et al., 1997).

As an example in three dimensions, the Digital Anatomist Dynamic Scene Generator (DSG, Figure 9.5; see also Color Plate II) creates interactive three-dimensional atlases "on-the-fly" for viewing and manipulation over the Web (Brinkley et al., 1999; Wong et al., 1999). In this case the three-dimensional scenes generated by reconstruction from serial sections are broken down into three-dimensional "primitive" meshes, each of which corresponds to an individual part in the FMA. In response to commands such as "display the branches of the coronary arteries" the DSG looks up the branches in the FMA, retrieves the three-dimensional model primitives associated with those branches, determines the color for each primitive based on its type in the FMA is-a hierarchy, renders the assembled scene as a two-dimensional snapshot, then sends it to a Web-browser, where the user may change the camera parameters, add new structures, or select and highlight structures. The complete scene may also be downloaded for viewing in a VRML browser.

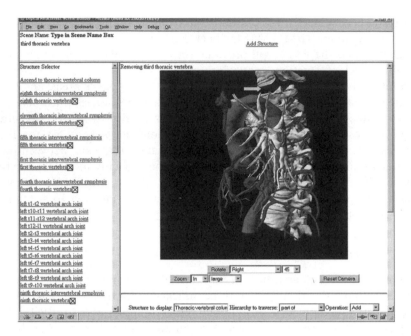

Figure 9.5. The Digital Anatomist Dynamic Scene Generator (see text). This-scene was created by requesting the following structures from the scene generator server: the parts of the aorta, the branches of the ascending aorta, the tributaries of the right atrium, the branches of the tracheo-bronchial tree, and the parts of the thoracic vertebral column. The server was then requested to rotate the camera 45 degrees, and to provide the name of a structure selected with the mouse, in this case the third thoracic vertebra. The selected structure was then hidden (note the gap indicated by the arrow). The left frame shows a partial view of the FMA part of hierarchy for the thoracic vertebral column. Checked structures are associated with three-dimensional "primitive" meshes that were loaded into the scene. Photograph courtesy of the Structural Informatics Group, University of Washington.

An example of a three-dimensional brain atlas created from the Visible Human is Voxelman (Hohne et al., 1995), in which each voxel in the Visible Human head is labeled with the name of an anatomic structure in a "generalized voxel model" (Hohne et al., 1990), and highly detailed three-dimensional scenes are dynamically generated. Several other brain atlases have also been developed primarily for educational use (Johnson and Becker, 2001; Stensaas and Millhouse, 2001).

In keeping with the theme of anatomy as an organizing framework, atlases have also been developed for integrating functional data from multiple studies (Bloom and Young, 1993; Toga et al., 1994, 1995; Swanson, 1999; Fougerousse et al., 2000; Rosen et al., 2000; Martin and Bowden, 2001). In their original published form these atlases permit manual drawing of functional data, such as neurotransmitter distributions, onto hard-copy printouts of brain sections. Many of these atlases have been or are in the process of being converted to digital form. The Laboratory of Neuroimaging (LONI) at UCLA has been particularly active in the development and analysis of digital atlases (Toga, 2001b), and the Caltech HBP has released a Web-accessible three-dimensional mouse atlas acquired with micro-MR imaging (Dhenain et al., 2001).

The most widely used human brain atlas is the Talairach atlas, based on postmortem sections from a 60-year-old woman (Talairach and Tournoux, 1988). This atlas introduced a proportional coordinate system (often called "Talairach space") which consists of 12 rectangular regions of the target brain that are piecewise affine transformed to corresponding regions in the atlas. Using these transforms (or a simplified single affine transform based on the anterior and posterior commissures), a point in the target brain can be expressed in Talairach coordinates, and thereby related to similarly transformed points from other brains. Other human brain atlases have also been developed (Hohne et al., 1992; Caviness et al., 1996; Drury and Van Essen, 1997; Schaltenbrand and Warren, 1977; Van Essen and Drury, 1997).

9.5.5 *Anatomic Variation*

Brain information systems often use atlases as a basis for mapping functional data onto a common framework, much like geographic information systems (GISs) use the earth as the basis for combining data. However, unlike GISs, brain information systems must deal with the fact that no two brains are exactly alike, especially in the highly folded human cerebral cortex. Thus, not only do brain-imaging researchers have to develop methods for representing individual brain anatomy, they must also develop methods for relating the anatomy of multiple brains. Only by developing methods for relating multiple brains will it be possible to generate a common anatomic frame of reference for organizing neuroscience data. Solving this problem is currently a major focus of work in the HBP and in imaging informatics in general.

Two general approaches for quantitatively dealing with anatomic variation can be defined: (1) warping to a **template atlas**, and (2) **population-based atlases**. Variation can also be expressed in a qualitative manner, as described in the section on qualitative classification.

Warping to a Template Atlas

The most popular current quantitative method for dealing with anatomic variation is to deform or warp an individual target brain to a single brain chosen as a template. If the template brain has been segmented and labeled as an atlas (Section 9.5.4), and if the registration of the target brain to the template is exact, then the target brain will be automatically segmented, and any data from other studies that are associated with the template brain can be automatically registered with the target brain by inverting the warp (Christensen et al., 1996; Toga and Thompson, 2001). Such a procedure could be very useful for surgical planning, for example, since functional areas from patients whose demographics match that of the surgical patient could be superimposed on the patient's anatomy (Kikinis et al., 1996).

The problem, of course, comes with the word "exact". Since no two brains are even topologically alike (sulci and gyri are present in one brain that are not present in another), it is impossible to completely register one brain to another. Thus, the research problem, which is very actively being pursued by many HBP researchers (Toga and Thompson, 2001), is how to register two brains as closely as possible. Methods for doing this can be divided into volume-based warping and surface-based warping.

Volume-based warping. Pure volume-based registration directly registers two image volumes, without the preprocessing segmentation step. Whereas intra (single)-patient registration (see Section 9.5.1) establishes a linear transformation between two datasets, inter (multiple)-patient registration establishes a nonlinear transformation (warp) that relates voxels in one volume to corresponding voxels in the other volume. Because of the great variability of the cerebral cortex pure volume-based registration is best suited for subcortical structures rather than the cortex. As in the linear case there are two basic approaches to nonlinear volume registration: *intensity-based* and *landmark-based*, both of which generally use either physically based approaches or minimization of a cost function to achieve the optimal warp.

The intensity-based approach uses characteristics of the voxels themselves, generally without the segmentation step, to nonlinearly align two image volumes (Gee et al., 1993; Collins et al., 1995; Christensen et al., 1996; Kjems et al., 1999). Most start by removing the skull, which often must be done manually.

The *landmark-based* approach is analogous to the two-dimensional case; the user manually indicates corresponding points in the two datasets (usually with the aid of three orthogonal views of the image volumes). The program then brings the corresponding points into registration while carrying along the intervening voxel data. The Montreal Register program (MacDonald, 1993) can do nonlinear three-dimensional warps, as can the 3-D Edgewarp program (Bookstein and Green, 2001), which is a generalization of the 2-D Edgewarp program developed by Bookstein (1989).

A variation of landmark-based warping matches curves or surfaces rather than points, then uses the surface warps as a basis for interpolating the warp for intervening voxels (Thompson and Toga, 1996; Davatzikos, 1997).

Surface-based warping. Surface-based registration is primarily used to register two cortical surfaces. The surface is first extracted using techniques described in Section 9.5.2, then image-based or other functional data are "painted" on the extracted surface where they are carried along with whatever deformation is applied to the surface. Since the cortical surface is the most variable part of the brain, yet the most interesting for many functional studies, considerable research is currently being done in the area of surface-based registration (Van Essen et al., 1998).

It is very difficult if not impossible to match two surfaces in their folded up state, or to visualize all their activity. (The cerebral cortex gray matter can be thought of as a two-dimensional sheet that is essentially crumpled up to fit inside the skull). Therefore, much effort has been devoted to "reconfiguring" (Van Essen et al., 2001) the cortex so that it is easier to visualize and register (Figure 9.6). A prerequisite for these techniques is that the segmented cortex must be topologically correct. The programs FreeSurfer (Dale et al., 1999), Surefit (Van Essen et al., 2001), ASP (MacDonald et al., 2000), and others all produce surfaces suitable for reconfiguration.

Common reconfiguration methods include *inflation, expansion to a sphere,* and *flattening. Inflation* uncrumples the detailed gyri and sulci of the folded surface by partially

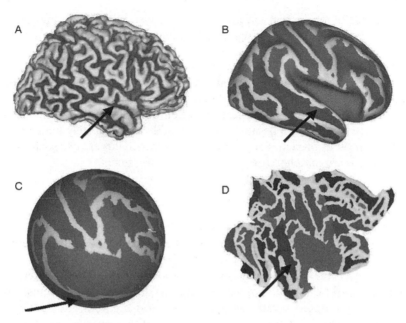

Figure 9.6. Brain surface reconfiguration using the Caret software suite developed by the David Van Essen laboratory at Washington University (Van Essen et al., 2001). The brain surface is first segmented (A), then inflated (B), expanded to a sphere (C), and flattened (D). At all stages any structural or functional data painted on the surface are carried along with the reconfiguration. In this case the brain sulci are painted onto the surface. The arrows point to the superior temporal sulcus in each configuration. Photograph courtesy of the SUMS database at Washington University (Van Essen, 2002), http://brainmap.wustl.edu:8081/sums/directory.do?dir_id=636032.

blowing the surface up like a balloon (Fischl et al., 1999; Brain Innovation B.V., 2001; Van Essen et al., 2001). The resulting surface looks like a lissencephalic (smooth) brain, in which only the major lobes are visible, and the original sulci are painted on the surface as darker intensity curves. These marks, along with any functional data, are carried along in the other reconfiguration methods as well.

Expansion to a sphere further expands the inflated brain to a sphere, again with painted lines representing the original gyri and sulci. At this point it is simple to define a surface-based coordinate system as a series of longitude–latitude lines referred to a common origin. This spherical coordinate system permits more precise quantitative comparison of different brains than three-dimensional Talairach coordinates because it respects the topology of the cortical surface. The surface is also in a form where essentially two-dimensional warping techniques can be applied to deform the gyri and sulci marked on the sphere to a template spherical brain.

The third approach is to *flatten* the surface by making artificial cuts on the inflated brain surface, then spreading out the cut surface on at two-dimensional plane while minimizing distortion (Fischl et al., 1999; Hurdal et al., 2000; Van Essen et al., 2001). Since it is impossible to eliminate distortion when projecting a sphere to a plane, multiple methods of projection have been devised, just as there are multiple methods for projecting the earth's surface (Toga and Thompson, 2001). In all cases, the resulting flat map, like a two-dimensional atlas of the earth, is easier to visualize than a three-dimensional representation since the entire cortex is seen at once. Techniques for warping one cortex to another are applicable to flat maps as well as spherical maps, and the warps can be inverted to map pooled data on the individual extracted cortical surface.

The problem of warping any of these reconfigured surfaces to a template surface is still an active area of research because it is impossible to completely match two cortical surfaces. Thus, most approaches are hierarchical, in which larger sulci such as the lateral and central sulcus are matched first, followed by minor sulci.

Population-Based Atlases

The main problem with warping to a template atlas is deciding which atlas to use as a template. Which brain should be considered the "canonical" brain representing the population? As noted previously, the widely used Talairach atlas is based on a 60-year-old woman. The Visible Human male was a 38-year-old convict and the female was an older women. What about other populations such as different racial groups? These considerations have prompted several groups to work on methods for developing brain atlases that encode variation among a population, be it the entire population or selected subgroups. The International Consortium for Brain Mapping (ICBM), a collaboration among several brain mapping institutions spearheaded at UCLA (http://www.loni.ucla.edu/ICBM), is collecting large numbers of normal brain-image volumes from collaborators around the world (Mazziotta et al., 2001). To date several thousand brain-image volumes, many with DNA samples for later correlation of anatomy with genetics, are stored on a massive file server. As data collection continues methods are under development for combining these data into population-based atlases.

A good high-level description of these methods can be found in a review article by Toga and Thompson (2001). In that article three main methods are described for developing population-based atlases: *density-based*, *label-based*, and *deformation-based* approaches.

In the *density-based* method, a set of brains is first transformed to Talairach space by linear registration. Corresponding voxels are then averaged, yielding an "average" brain that preserves the major features of the brain but smoothes out the detailed sulci and gyri (Figure 9.7; see also Color Plate III). The Montreal average brain, which is an average of 305 normal brains (Evans et al., 1994), is constructed in this way. Although not detailed enough to permit precise comparisons of anatomic surfaces, it is nevertheless useful as a coarse means for relating multiple functional sites. For example, in our own work (JB) we have mapped cortical language sites from multiple patients onto the average brain, allowing a rough comparison of their distribution for different patient subclasses (Martin et al., 2000).

In the *label-based* approach, a series of brains are segmented, and then linearly transformed to Talairach space. A probability map is constructed for each segmented structure, such that at each voxel the probability can be found that a given structure is present at that voxel location. This method has been implemented in the Talairach Demon, an Internet server and Java client, developed by Fox et al. as part of the ICBM project

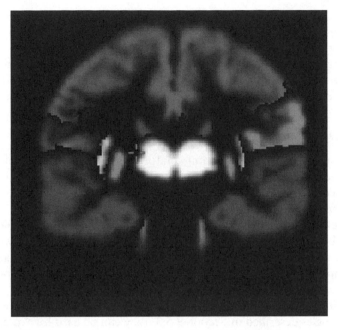

Figure 9.7. Probabilistic brain atlas, coronal section. Individual MRI image volumes from 53 subjects were linearly aligned, and each subject's lobes and deep nuclei were manually delineated. These delineations were averaged across the subjects and used to create probability maps for the likelihood of finding the specified lobe or nuclei at a given voxel position. Each structure is depicted in a different color in the color version of this image. The intensity of the color is proportional to the probability of finding that structure at the specified location. Photograph courtesy of Arthur Toga, Laboratory for Neuro Imaging, UCLA. http://www.loni.ucla.edu/NCRR/NCRR.Probabilistic.html.

(Lancaster et al., 2000). A Web user inputs one or more sets of Talairach coordinates, and the server returns a list of structure probabilities for those coordinates.

In the *warp-based* method, the statistical properties of deformation fields produced by nonlinear warping techniques (see Section 9.5.5) are analyzed to encode anatomic variation in population subgroups (Christensen et al., 1996; Thompson and Toga, 1997). These atlases can then be used to detect abnormal anatomy in various diseases.

9.5.6   Characterization of Anatomy

The main reason for finding ways to represent anatomy is to examine the relationship between structure and function in both health and disease. For example, how does the branching pattern of the dendritic tree influence the function of the dendrite? Does the pattern of cortical folds influence the distribution of language areas in the brain? Does the shape of the corpus callosum relate to a predisposition to schizophrenia?

Can subtle changes in brain structure be used as a predictor for the onset of Alzheimer's disease? These kinds of questions are becoming increasingly possible to answer with the availability of the methods described in the previous sections. However, in order to examine these questions, methods must be found for characterizing and classifying the extracted anatomy. Both qualitative and quantitative approaches are being developed.

Qualitative Classification

The classical approach to characterizing anatomy is for the human biologist to group individual structures into various classes based on perceived patterns. This approach is still widely used throughout science since the computer has yet to match the pattern-recognition abilities of the human brain.

An example classification at the cellular level is the 60 to 80 morphologic cell types that form the basis for understanding the neural circuitry of the retina (which is an outgrowth of the brain) (Dacey, 1999). At the macroscopic level, Ono has developed an atlas of cerebral sulci that can be used to characterize an individual brain based on sulcal patterns (Ono et al., 1990).

If these and other classifications are given systematic names and are added to the symbolic ontologies described in Section 9.5.3, they can be used for "intelligent" indexing and retrieval, after which quantitative methods can be used for more precise characterization of structure–function relationships.

Quantitative Classification

Quantitative characterization of anatomy is often called *morphometrics* (Bookstein, 1997) or *computational neuroanatomy* (Ascioli, 1999). Quantitative characterization permits more subtle classification schemes than are possible with qualitative methods, leading to new insights into the relation between structure and function, and between structure and disease (Toga, 2001a; Toga and Thompson, 2001).

For example, at the ultrastructural level, *stereology*, which is a statistical method for estimating from sampled data the distribution of structural components in a volume (Weibel, 1979), is used to estimate the density of objects such as synapses in image volumes reconstructed from serial electron micrographs (Fiala and Harris, 2001).

At the cellular level Ascoli et al. are engaged in the L-neuron project, which attempts to model dendritic morphology by a small set of parameterized generation rules, where the parameters are sampled from distributions determined from experimental data (Figure 9.8) (Ascioli, 1999). The resulting dendritic models capture a large set of dendritic morphologic classes from only a small set of variables. Eventually, the hope is to generate virtual neural circuits that can simulate brain function.

At the macroscopic level landmark-based methods have shown changes in the shape of the corpus callosum associated with schizophrenia that are not obvious from visual inspection (DeQuardo et al., 1999). Probabilistic atlas-based methods are being used to characterize growth patterns and disease-specific structural abnormalities in diseases such as Alzheimer's and schizophrenia (Thompson et al., 2001). As these techniques

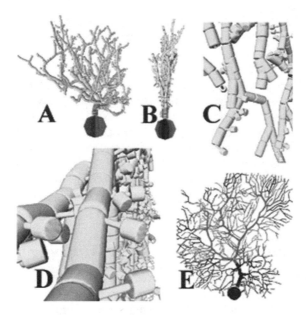

Figure 9.8. The L-neuron project. The branching pattern of a given population of neurons is modeled by a small set of parameters measured from experimental data. These parameters are used to generate synthetic neurons (A to D) that look very similar to experimentally reconstructed neurons (E). The virtual cell displayed in panels A to D was created with only 11 lines of stochastic rules to resemble the real 2107-compartment Purkinje cell shown in panel E. (A) Front view; (B) side view; (C) detail on dendritic branches; (D) detail on dendritic spines. Photograph courtesy of Georgio Ascioli, George Mason University, http://www.krasnow.gmu.edu/ascoli/CNG/index.htm. (Reprinted from Ascoli, GA. Progress and Perspectives in Computational Neuroanatomy. Anat Rec. 257(6): 195-207. Copyright © 1999, Wiley. Reprinted by Permission of Wiley-Liss Inc., A Subsidiary of John Wiley & Sons, Inc.)

become more widely available to the clinician, they should permit earlier diagnosis and hence potential treatment for these debilitating diseases.

9.6   Functional Imaging

Many imaging techniques not only show the structure of the body but also the function. For imaging purposes, function can be inferred by observing changes of structure over time. In recent years this ability to image function has greatly accelerated. For example, ultrasound and angiography are widely used to show the functioning of the heart by depicting wall motion, and ultrasound doppler can image both normal and disturbed blood flow (Mehta et al., 2000). **Molecular imaging** (Section 9.3.5) is increasingly able to depict the expression of particular genes superimposed on structural images, and thus can also be seen as a form of functional imaging.

A particularly profound application of functional imaging is the understanding of cognitive activity in the brain. It is now routinely possible to put a normal subject in a scanner, to give the person a cognitive task, such as counting or object recognition, and to observe which parts of the brain light up. This unprecedented ability to observe the functioning of the living brain opens up entirely new avenues for exploring how the brain works.

Functional brain-imaging modalities can be classified as *image-based* or *nonimage-based*. In both cases it is taken as axiomatic that the functional data must be mapped to the individual subject's anatomy, where the anatomy is extracted from structural images using techniques described in the previous sections. Once mapped to anatomy, the functional data can be integrated with other functional data from the same subject, and with functional data from other subjects whose anatomy has been related to a template or probabilistic atlas. Techniques for generating, mapping, and integrating functional data are part of the field of Functional Brain Mapping, which has become very active in the last few years, with several conferences (Organization for Human Brain Mapping, 2001) and journals (Fox, 2001; Toga et al., 2001) devoted to the subject.

9.6.1   Image-Based Functional Brain Mapping

Image-based functional data generally come from scanners that generate relatively low-resolution volume arrays depicting spatially localized activation. For example, PET (Heiss and Phelps, 1983; Aine, 1995) and magnetic resonance spectroscopy (MRS) (Ross and Bluml, 2001) reveal the uptake of various metabolic products by the functioning brain; and **functional magnetic resonance imaging (fMRI)** reveals changes in blood oxygenation that occur following neural activity (Aine, 1995). The raw intensity values generated by these techniques must be processed by sophisticated statistical algorithms to sort out how much of the observed intensity is due to cognitive activity and how much is due to background noise.

As an example, one approach to fMRI imaging is the boxcar paradigm applied to language mapping (Corina et al., 2000). The subject is placed in the MRI scanner and told to silently name objects shown at 3-second intervals on a head-mounted display. The actual objects ("on" state) are alternated with nonsense objects ("off" state), and the fMRI signal is measured during both the on and the off states. Essentially the voxel values at the off (or control) state are subtracted from those at the on state. The difference values are tested for significant difference from nonactivated areas, then expressed as *t*-values. The voxel array of *t*-values can be displayed as an image.

A large number of alternative methods have been and are being developed for acquiring and analyzing functional data (Frackowiak et al., 1997). The output of most of these techniques is a low-resolution three-dimensional image volume in which each voxel value is a measure of the amount of activation for a given task. The low-resolution volume is then mapped to anatomy by linear registration to a high-resolution structural MR dataset, using one of the linear registration techniques described in Section 9.5.1.

Many of these and other techniques are implemented in the SPM program (Friston et al., 1995), the AFNI program (Cox, 1996), the Lyngby toolkit (Hansen et al., 1999), and several commercial programs such as Medex (Sensor Systems Inc., 2001), and BrainVoyager (Brain Innovation B.V., 2001). The FisWidgets project at the University of Pittsburgh is developing a set of Java wrappers for many of these programs that allow customized creation of graphical user interfaces in an integrated desktop environment

COLOR PLATE I

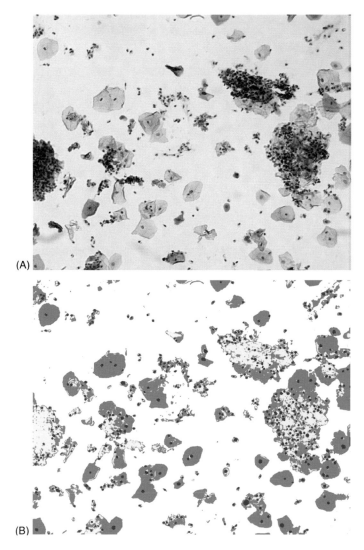

Figure 9.3. Automated screening of Papanicolaou (PAP) smears. Since large numbers of PAP smears are acquired routinely, there is a need to reduce the cost and potential errors associated with purely manual interpretation. (A) Raw microscopic image of cervical cells. (B) Segmented image. The program has segmented the cells and nuclei from the raw image, prior to feature detection and classification based on the features. Abnormally classified cells are flagged for review by the human operator. Photograph courtesy of Peter Locht, Visible Diagnostics, http://www.imm.dtu.dk/visiondag/VD03/medicinsk/pl.pdf.

COLOR PLATE II

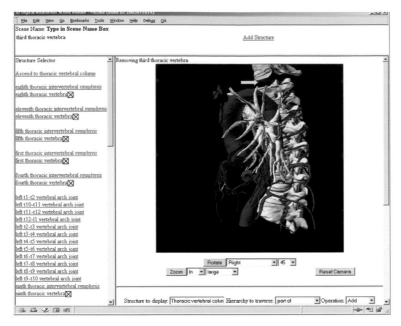

Figure 9.5. The Digital Anatomist Dynamic Scene Generator (see text). This-scene was created by requesting the following structures from the scene generator server: the parts of the aorta, the branches of the ascending aorta, the tributaries of the right atrium, the branches of the tracheo-bronchial tree, and the parts of the thoracic vertebral column. The server was then requested to rotate the camera 45 degrees, and to provide the name of a structure selected with the mouse, in this case the third thoracic vertebra. The selected structure was then hidden (note the gap indicated by the arrow). The left frame shows a partial view of the FMA part of hierarchy for the thoracic vertebral column. Checked structures are associated with three-dimensional "primitive" meshes that were loaded into the scene. Photograph courtesy of the Structural Informatics Group, University of Washington.

COLOR PLATE III

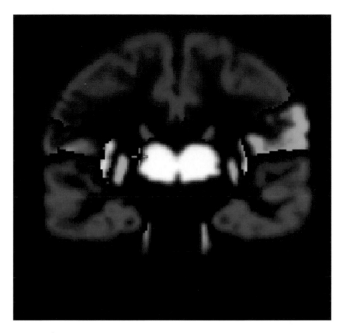

Figure 9.7. Probabilistic brain atlas, coronal section. Individual MRI image volumes from 53 subjects were linearly aligned, and each subject's lobes and deep nuclei were manually delineated. These delineations were averaged across the subjects and used to create probability maps for the likelihood of finding the specified lobe or nuclei at a given voxel position. Each structure is depicted in a different color in the color version of this image. The intensity of the color is proportional to the probability of finding that structure at the specified location. Photograph courtesy of Arthur Toga, Laboratory for Neuro Imaging, UCLA. http://www.loni.ucla.edu/NCRR/NCRR.Probabilistic.html.

COLOR PLATE IV

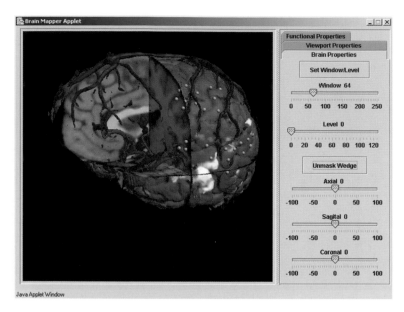

Figure 9.9. Remote visualization of integrated structural and functional brain data mapped onto a single patient's brain. MRI, MRV (veins), and MRA (arteries) brain-image volumes are acquired and registered, then segmented to generate the cortical surface, arteries, and brains. fMRI data representing areas of language processing are registered to the structural volumes, then projected to the surface as the light-colored regions. Cortical stimulation mapping (CSM) data (small spheres) acquired during neurosurgery are also registered to the patient's anatomy. The integrated data are rendered on a visualization server, which can be accessed from a web browser using a simple Java applet. Photograph courtesy of the Structural Informatics Group, University of Washington.

(Cohen, 2001). A similar effort (VoxBox) is underway at the University of Pennsylvania (Kimborg and Aguirre, 2002).

9.6.2 Nonimage-Based Functional Mapping

In addition to the image-based functional methods there are an increasing number of techniques that do not directly generate images. The data from these techniques are generally mapped to anatomy, and then displayed as functional overlays on anatomic images.

For example, cortical stimulation mapping (CSM) is a technique for localizing functional areas on the exposed cortex at the time of neurosurgery (Figure 9.9; see also Color Plate IV). In our own work (JB) the technique is used to localize cortical language areas so that they can be avoided during the resection of a tumor or epileptic focus (Ojemann et al., 1989). Following removal of a portion of the skull (craniotomy) the patient is awakened and asked to name common images shown on slides. During this

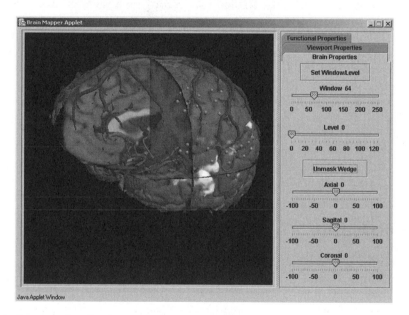

Figure 9.9. Remote visualization of integrated structural and functional brain data mapped onto a single patient's brain. MRI, MRV (veins), and MRA (arteries) brain-image volumes are acquired and registered, then segmented to generate the cortical surface, arteries, and brains. fMRI data representing areas of language processing are registered to the structural volumes, then projected to the surface as the light-colored regions. Cortical stimulation mapping (CSM) data (small spheres) acquired during neurosurgery are also registered to the patient's anatomy. The integrated data are rendered on a visualization server, which can be accessed from a web browser using a simple Java applet. Photograph courtesy of the Structural Informatics Group, University of Washington.

time the surgeon applies a small electrical current to each of a set of numbered tags placed on the cortical surface. If the patient is unable to name the object while the current is applied the site is interpreted as essential for language and is avoided at surgery. In this case, the functional-mapping problem is how to relate these stimulation sites to the patient's anatomy as seen on an MRI scan.

Our approach, which we call visualization-based mapping (Modayur et al., 1997; Hinshaw et al., 2002), is to acquire image volumes of brain anatomy (MRI), cerebral veins (MRV), and cerebral arteries (MRA) prior to surgery, to segment the anatomy, veins, and arteries from these images, and to generate a surface-rendered three-dimensional model of the brain and its vessels that matches as closely as possible the cortical surface as seen at neurosurgery. A visual-mapping program then permits the user to drag numbered tags onto the rendered surface such that they match those seen on the intraoperative photograph. The program projects the dragged tags onto the reconstructed surface, and records the x-y-z image-space coordinates of the projections, thereby completing the mapping.

The real goal of functional neuroimaging is to observe the actual electrical activity of the neurons as they perform various cognitive tasks. fMRI, MRS, and PET do not directly record electrical activity. Rather, they record the results of electrical activity, such as (in the case of fMRI) the oxygenation of blood supplying the active neurons. Thus, there is a delay from the time of activity to the measured response. In other words these techniques have relatively poor temporal resolution (Section 9.2.2). **Electroencephalography (EEG)** or **magnetoencephalography (MEG)**, on the other hand, are more direct measures of electrical activity since they measure the electromagnetic fields generated by the electrical activity of the neurons. Current EEG and MEG methods involve the use of large arrays of scalp sensors, the output of which are processed in a similar way to CT in order to localize the source of the electrical activity inside the brain. In general this "source-localization problem" is under-constrained, so information about brain anatomy obtained from MRI is used to provide further constraints (George et al., 1995).

9.7   Conclusions

This chapter focuses on methods for processing images in biomedicine, with an emphasis on brain imaging and the extraction and characterization of anatomic structure, both for its own sake, and as a substrate on which to map function. Other than the interest and expertise of the authors, an important reason to concentrate on brain imaging is that a large part of the most advanced image-processing work is currently in this area. As these techniques develop, and as new imaging modalities increasingly become available for imaging other and more detailed body regions, the techniques will increasingly be applied in all areas of biomedicine. For example, the development of molecular-imaging methods is analogous to functional-brain imaging, in that functional data, in this case from gene expression rather than cognitive activity, are mapped to an anatomic substrate. Since the same basic principles apply in both functional-brain mapping and molecular imaging, the same techniques apply: spatial and symbolic representation of anatomy, dealing with anatomic variation, characterization of anatomy, visualization, and multimodality image fusion.

Thus, these general methods will increasingly be applied to diverse areas of biomedicine. As they are applied, and as imaging modalities continue to proliferate, an increasing demand will be placed on methods for managing the images and for storing and accessing them. At the same time, imaging will continue to play an increasing role in integrated biomedical information systems. These two subjects, management of images, and integration in biomedical applications, are the subjects of Chapter 18.

Questions for Discussion

1. What is the general principle that underlies computed axial tomography (CT)? What are the advantages of CT images over conventional X-ray images?
2. Explain the general principle underlying magnetic resonance imaging (MRI)? What are the advantages of this method compared to older methods of imaging?
3. Explain the differences among contrast, spatial, and temporal resolution.
4. Describe the four standard image-processing steps, and suggest how these might be applied by an image-analysis program looking for abnormal cells in a PAP smear.
5. What is the segmentation step in image analysis? Why is it so difficult to perform? Give two examples of ways by which current systems avoid the problem of automatic segmentation. Give an example of how knowledge about the problem to be solved (e.g., local anatomy) could be used in future systems to aid in automatic segmentation.
6. What additional informatics issues arise when going from two-dimensional to three-dimensional image processing? What are the three-dimensional versions of two-dimensional image-processing operations such as region growing and edge finding?
7. What is a three-dimensional brain atlas? What are the methods for registering a patient image volume to that atlas? What is the use of a brain atlas?
8. Give some example techniques for imaging the function of the brain.

Suggested Readings

Brinkley J.F. (1991). Structural informatics and its applications in medicine and biology. *Academic Medicine*, 66(10):589–591.
Short introduction to the field.

Brinkley J.F., Rosse C. (2002). Imaging and the Human Brain Project: A review. *Methods of Information in Medicine*, 41:245–260.
Review of image processing work related to the brain. Much of the brain-related material for this chapter was taken from this article.

Potchen E.J. (2000). Prospects for progress in diagnostic imaging. *Journal of Internal Medicine*, 247(4):411–424.
Nontechnical description of newer imaging methods such as cardiac MRI, diffusion tensor imaging, fMRI, and molecular imaging. Current and potential use of these methods for diagnosis.

Robb R.A. (2000). *Biomedical Imaging, Visualization, and Analysis*. New York: Wiley-Liss.
Overview of biomedical imaging modalities and processing techniques.

Rosse C., Mejino J.L.V. (2003). A reference ontology for bioinformatics: The Foundational Model of Anatomy. *Journal of Bioinformatics*, 36(6):478–500.
Description and principles behind a large symbolic ontology of anatomy.

Shapiro L.G., Stockman G.C. (2001). *Computer Vision*. Upper Saddle River, NJ: Prentice-Hall. Detailed description of many of the representations and methods used in image processing. Not specific to medicine, but most of the methods are applicable to medical imaging.

10
Ethics and Health Informatics: Users, Standards, and Outcomes

Kenneth W. Goodman and Randolph A. Miller

After reading this chapter, you should know the answers to these questions:

- Why is ethics important to informatics?
- What are the leading ethical issues that arise in health care informatics?
- What are examples of appropriate and inappropriate uses and users for health-related software?
- Why does the establishment of standards touch on ethical issues?
- Why does system evaluation involve ethical issues?
- What challenges does informatics pose for patient and provider confidentiality?
- How can the tension between the obligation to protect confidentiality and that to share data be minimized?
- How might computational health care alter the traditional provider–patient relationship?
- What ethical issues arise at the intersection of informatics and managed care?
- What are the leading issues in the debate over governmental regulation of health care computing tools?

10.1 Ethical Issues in Health Informatics

More and more the tendency is towards the use of mechanical aids to diagnosis; nevertheless, the five senses of the doctor do still, and must always, play the preponderating part in the examination of the sick patient. Careful observation can never be replaced by the tests of the laboratory. The good physician now or in the future will never be a diagnostic robot. (The surgeon Sir William Arbuthnot Lane writing in the November 1936 issue of *New Health*)

Human values should govern research and practice in the health professions. Health care informatics, like other health professions, encompasses issues of appropriate and inappropriate behavior, of honorable and disreputable actions, and of right and wrong. Students and practitioners of the health sciences, including informatics, share an important obligation to explore the moral underpinnings and ethical challenges related to their research and practice.

Although ethical questions in medicine, nursing, human subjects research, psychology, social work, and affiliated fields continue to evolve, the key issues are generally well known. Major questions in bioethics have been addressed in numerous professional, scholarly, and educational contexts. Ethical matters in health informatics are, in general, less familiar, even though certain of them have received attention for decades (Szolovits and Pauker, 1979; Miller et al., 1985; de Dombal, 1987). Indeed, informatics now constitutes a source of some of the most important and interesting ethical debates in all the health professions.

People often assume that the confidentiality of electronically stored patient information is the primary source of ethical attention in informatics. Although confidentiality and privacy are indeed of vital importance and significant concern, the field is rich with other ethical issues, including the appropriate selection and use of informatics tools in clinical settings; the determination of who should use such tools; the role of system evaluation; the obligations of system developers, maintainers, and vendors; and the use of computers to track clinical outcomes to guide future practice. In addition, informatics engenders many important legal and regulatory questions.

To consider ethical issues in health care informatics is to explore a significant intersection among several professions—health care delivery and administration, applied computing, and ethics—each of which is a vast field of inquiry. Fortunately, growing interest in bioethics and computer-related ethics has produced a starting point for such exploration. An initial ensemble of guiding principles, or ethical criteria, has emerged to orient decision making in health care informatics. These criteria are of practical utility to health informatics.

10.2   Health-Informatics Applications: Appropriate Use, Users, and Contexts

Application of computer-based technologies in the health professions can build on previous experience in adopting other devices, tools, and methods. Before they perform most health-related interventions (e.g., genetic testing, prescription of medication, surgical and other therapeutic procedures), clinicians generally evaluate appropriate evidence, standards, presuppositions, and values. Indeed, the very evolution of the health professions entails the evolution of evidence, of standards, of presuppositions, and of values.

To answer the clinical question, "What should be done in this case?" we must pay attention to a number of subsidiary questions, such as:

1. What is the problem?
2. What am I competent to do?
3. What will produce the most desirable results?
4. What will maintain or improve patient care?
5. How strong are my beliefs in the accuracy of my answers to questions 1 through 4?

Similar considerations determine the appropriate use of informatics tools.

10.2.1   The Standard View of Appropriate Use

Excitement often accompanies initial use of computer-based tools in clinical settings. Based on the uncertainties that surround any new technology, however, scientific evidence counsels caution and prudence. As in other clinical areas, evidence and reason determine the appropriate level of caution. For instance, there is considerable evidence that electronic laboratory information systems improve access to clinical data when compared with manual, paper-based test-result distribution methods. To the extent that such systems improve care at an acceptable cost in time and money, there is an obligation to use computers to store and retrieve clinical laboratory results. There is less evidence, however, that existing (circa 2006) **clinical expert systems** can improve patient care in typical practice settings at an acceptable cost in time and money.

Clinical expert systems (see Chapter 20) are intended to provide decision support for diagnosis and therapy in a more detailed and sophisticated manner than that provided by simple reminder systems (Duda and Shortliffe, 1983). Creation of expert systems and maintenance of related knowledge bases still involve leading-edge research and development. It is also important to recognize that humans are still superior to electronic systems in understanding patients and their problems, in efficient collection of pertinent data across the spectrum of clinical practice, in the interpretation and representation of data, and in clinical synthesis. Humans may always be superior at these tasks, although such a claim must be subjected to empirical testing from time to time.

What has been called the standard view of computer-assisted clinical diagnosis (Miller, 1990) holds in part that human cognitive processes, being more suited to the complex task of diagnosis than machine intelligence, should not be overridden or trumped by computers. The standard view states that when adequate (and even exemplary) decision-support tools are developed, they should be viewed and used as supplementary and subservient to human clinical judgment. They should take this role because the clinician caring for the patient knows and understands the patient's situation and can make compassionate judgments better than computer programs; they are also the individuals whom the state licenses, and specialty boards accredit, to practice medicine, surgery, nursing, pharmacy, or other health-related activities. Corollaries of the standard view are that: (1) practitioners have an obligation to use any computer-based tool responsibly, through adequate user training and by developing an understanding of the system's abilities and limitations; and (2) practitioners must not abrogate their clinical judgment reflexively when using computer-based decision aids. Because the skills required for diagnosis are in many respects different from those required for the acquisition, storage, and retrieval of laboratory data, there is no contradiction in urging extensive use of electronic laboratory information systems, but cautious or limited use (for the time being) of expert diagnostic decision-support tools.

The standard view addresses one aspect of the question, "How and when should computers be used in clinical practice?" by capturing important moral intuitions about error avoidance and evolving standards. Error avoidance and the benefits that follow from it shape the obligations of practitioners. In computer-software use, as in all other areas of clinical practice, good intentions alone may be insufficient to insulate recklessness from culpability. Thus, the standard view may be seen as a tool for both error avoidance and ethically optimized action.

Ethical software use should be evaluated against a broad background of evidence for actions that produce favorable outcomes. Because informatics is a science in extraordinary ferment, system improvements and evidence of such improvements are constantly emerging. Clinicians have an obligation to be familiar with this evidence after attaining minimal acceptable levels of familiarity with informatics in general and with the clinical systems they use in particular.

10.2.2   Appropriate Users and Educational Standards

Efficient and effective use of health care informatics systems requires training, experience, and education. Indeed, such requirements resemble those for other tools used in health care and in other domains. Inadequate preparation in the use of tools is an invitation to catastrophe. When the stakes are high and the domain large and complex—as is the case in the health professions—education and training take on moral significance.

Who should use a health care–related computer application? Consider expert decision-support systems as an example. An early paper on ethical issues in informatics noted that potential users of such systems include physicians, nurses, physicians' assistants, paramedical personnel, students of the health sciences, patients, and insurance and government evaluators (Miller et al., 1985). Are members of all these groups appropriate users? We cannot answer the question until we are clear about the precise intended use for the system (i.e., the exact clinical questions the system will address). The appropriate level of training must be correlated with the question at hand. At one end of an appropriate-use spectrum, we can posit that medical and nursing students should employ decision-support systems for educational purposes; this assertion is relatively free of controversy once it has been verified that such tools convey accurately a sufficient quantity and quality of educational content. But it is less clear that patients, administrators, or managed-care gatekeepers, for example, should use expert decision-support systems for assistance in making diagnoses, in selecting therapies, or in evaluating the appropriateness of health professionals' actions. To the extent that some systems present general medical advice in hypermedia format, such as might occur with Dr. Spock's print-based child care primer, use by laypersons may be condoned. There are additional legal concerns related to negligence and product liability, however, when health-related products are sold directly to patients rather than to licensed practitioners and when such products give patient-specific counsel rather than general clinical advice.

Suitable use of a software program that helps a user to suggest diagnoses, to select therapies, or to render prognoses must be plotted against an array of goals and best practices for achieving those goals, including consideration of the characteristics and requirements of individual patients. For example, the multiple interconnected inferential strategies required for arriving at an accurate diagnosis depend on knowledge of facts; experience with procedures; and familiarity with human behavior, motivation, and values. **Diagnosis** is a process rather than an event (Miller, 1990), so even well-validated diagnostic systems must be used appropriately in the overall context of patient care.

To use a diagnostic decision-support system, the clinician must be able to recognize when the computer program has erred, and, when it is accurate, what the output means and how it should be interpreted. This ability requires knowledge of both the diagnostic sciences and the software applications and their limitations. After assigning a diagnostic label, the clinician must communicate the diagnosis, prognosis, and implications to a patient and must do so in ways both appropriate to the patient's educational background and conducive to future treatment goals. It is not enough to be able to tell patients that they have cancer, human immunodeficiency virus (HIV), diabetes, or heart disease and simply to hand over a number of prescriptions. The care provider must also offer context when available, comfort when needed, and hope as appropriate. The reason many jurisdictions require pretest and posttest HIV counseling, for instance, is not to vex busy health professionals but rather to ensure that comprehensive, high-quality care—rather than just diagnostic labeling—has been delivered.

This discussion points to the following set of ethical principles for appropriate use of decision-support systems:

1. A computer program should be used in clinical practice only after appropriate evaluation of its efficacy and the documentation that it performs its intended task at an acceptable cost in time and money.
2. Users of most clinical systems should be health professionals who are qualified to address the question at hand on the basis of their licensure, clinical training, and experience. Software systems should be used to augment or supplement, rather than to replace or supplant, such individuals' decision making.
3. All uses of informatics tools, especially in patient care, should be preceded by adequate training and instruction, which should include review of all available forms of previous product evaluations.

Such principles and claims should be thought of as analogous to other standards or rules in clinical medicine and nursing.

10.2.3 Obligations and Standards for System Developers and Maintainers

Users of clinical programs must rely on the work of other people who are often far removed from the context of use. Users depend on the developers and maintainers of a system and must trust evaluators who have validated a system for clinical use. Health care software applications are among the most complex tools in the technological armamentarium. Although this complexity imposes certain obligations on end users, it also commits a system's developers, designers, and maintainers to adhere to reasonable standards and, indeed, to acknowledge their moral responsibility for doing so.

Ethics, Standards, and Scientific Progress

The very idea of a **standard of care** embodies a number of complex assumptions linking ethics, evidence, outcomes, and professional training. To say that a nurse or physician must adhere to a standard is to say, in part, that they ought not to stray from procedures that have been shown or are generally believed to work better than other procedures. Whether a procedure or device "works better" than another can be difficult to determine. Such determinations in the health sciences constitute progress and indicate that we know more than we used to know. Criteria for evidence and proof are applied. Evidence from randomized controlled trials is preferable to evidence from uncontrolled retrospective studies, and verification by independent investigators is required before the most recent reports are put into common practice.

People who develop, maintain, and sell health care computing systems and components have obligations that parallel those of system users. These obligations include holding patient care as the leading value. The Hippocratic injunction primum non nocere (first do no harm) applies to developers as well as to practitioners. Although this principle is easy to suggest and, generally, to defend it invites subtle, and sometimes overt, resistance from people who hold profit or fame as primary motivators. To be sure, quests for fame and fortune often produce good outcomes and improved care, at least eventually. Even so, that approach fails to take into account the role of intention as a moral criterion.

In medicine, nursing, and psychology, a number of models of the **professional–patient relationship** place trust and advocacy at the apex of a hierarchy of values. Such a stance cannot be maintained if goals and intentions other than patient well-being are (generally) assigned primacy. The same principles apply to people who produce and attend to health care information systems. Because these systems are health care systems—and are not devices for accounting, entertainment, real estate, and so on—and because the domain is shaped by pain, vulnerability, illness, and death, it is essential that the threads of trust run throughout the fabric of clinical system design and maintenance.

System purchasers, users, and patients must trust developers and maintainers to recognize the potentially grave consequences of errors or carelessness, trust them to care about the uses to which the systems will be put, and trust them to value the reduced suffering of other people at least as much as they value their own personal gain. We emphatically do not mean to suggest that system designers and maintainers are blameworthy or unethical if they hope and strive to profit from their diligence, creativity, and effort. Rather, we suggest that no amount of financial benefit for a designer can counterbalance bad outcomes or ill consequences that result from recklessness, avarice, or inattention to the needs of clinicians and their patients.

Quality standards should stimulate scientific progress and innovation while safeguarding against system error and abuse. These goals might seem incompatible, but they are not. Let us postulate a standard that requires timely updating and testing of knowledge bases that are used by decision-support systems. To the extent that database accuracy is needed to maximize the accuracy of inferential engines, it is trivially clear how such a standard will help to prevent decision-support mistakes. Furthermore, the standard should be seen to foster progress and innovation in the same way that any insistence on best possible accuracy helps to protect scientists and clinicians from pursuing false leads, or wasting time in testing poorly wrought hypotheses. It will not do for database maintainers to insist that they are busy doing the more productive or scientifically stimulating work of improving knowledge representation, say, or database design. Although such tasks are important, they do not supplant the tasks of updating and testing tools in their current configuration or structure. Put differently, scientific and technical standards are perfectly able to stimulate progress while taking a cautious or even conservative stance toward permissible risk in patient care.

This approach has been described as "progressive caution." "Medical informatics is, happily, here to stay, but users and society have extensive responsibilities to ensure that we use our tools appropriately. This might cause us to move more deliberately or slowly than some would like. Ethically speaking, that is just too bad" (Goodman, 1998b).

System Evaluation as an Ethical Imperative

Any move toward "best practices" in health informatics is shallow and feckless if it does not include a way to measure whether a system performs as intended. This and related measurements provide the ground for quality control and, as such, are the obligations of system developers, maintainers, users, administrators, and perhaps other players (see Chapter 11).

> Medical computing is not merely about medicine or computing. It is about the introduction of new tools into environments with established social norms and practices. The effects of computing systems in health care are subject to analysis not only of accuracy and performance but of acceptance by users, of consequences for social and professional interaction, and of the context of use. We suggest that system evaluation can illuminate social and ethical issues in medical computing, and in so doing improve patient care. That being the case, there is an ethical imperative for such evaluation. (Anderson and Aydin, 1998)

To give a flavor of how a comprehensive evaluation program can ethically optimize implementation and use of an informatics system, consider these ten criteria for system scrutiny (Anderson and Aydin, 1994):

1. Does the system work as designed?
2. Is it used as anticipated?
3. Does it produce the desired results?
4. Does it work better than the procedures it replaced?
5. Is it cost effective?
6. How well have individuals been trained to use it?
7. What are the anticipated long-term effects on how departments interact?
8. What are the long-term effects on the delivery of medical care?
9. Will the system have an impact on control in the organization?
10. To what extent do effects depend on practice setting?

Another way to look at this important point is that people use computer systems. Even the finest system might be misused, misunderstood, or mistakenly allowed to alter or erode previously productive human relationships. Evaluation of health information systems in their contexts of use should be taken as a moral imperative. Such evaluations require consideration of a broader conceptualization of "what works best" and must look toward improving the overall health care delivery system rather than only that system's technologically based components. These higher goals entail the creation of a corresponding mechanism for ensuring institutional oversight and responsibility (Miller and Gardner, 1997a, 1997b).

10.3   Privacy, Confidentiality, and Data Sharing

Some of the greatest challenges of the Information Age arise from placing computer applications in health care settings while upholding traditional principles. One challenge involves balancing two competing values: (1) free access to information, and (2) protection of patients' **privacy** and **confidentiality**.

Only computers can manage the vast amount of information generated during clinical encounters and other health care transactions; at least in principle, such information should be easily available to health professionals so that they can care for patients effectively. Yet, making this information readily available creates opportunities for access by extraneous individuals. Access may be available to curious health care workers who do not need the information to fulfill job-related responsibilities, and, even more worrisome, to other people who might use the information to harm patients physically, emotionally, or financially. Seemingly, clinical system administrators must therefore choose between either improving care through use of computer systems or protecting confidentiality by restricting use of computer systems. Fortunately, it is a mistake to view these objectives as incompatible.

10.3.1   Foundations of Health Privacy and Confidentiality

Privacy and confidentiality are necessary for people to mature as individuals, to form relationships, and to serve as functioning members of society. Imagine what would happen if the local newspaper produced a daily account detailing everyone's actions, meetings, and conversations. It is not that most people have terrible secrets to hide but rather that the concepts of solitude, intimacy, and the desire to be left alone make no sense without the expectation that our actions and words will be kept private and held in confidence.

The terms *privacy* and *confidentiality* are not synonymous. Privacy generally applies to people, including their desire not to suffer eavesdropping, whereas confidentiality is best applied to information. One way to think of the difference is as follows. If someone follows you and spies on you entering an acquired immunodeficiency syndrome (AIDS) clinic, your privacy is violated; if someone sneaks into the clinic and looks at your health care record, your record's confidentiality is breached. In discussions of the electronic health care record, the term privacy may also refer to individuals' desire to restrict the disclosure of personal data (National Research Council, 1997).

There are several important reasons to protect privacy and confidentiality. One is that privacy and confidentiality are widely regarded as *rights* of all people, and such protections help to accord them respect. On this account, people do not need to provide a justification for keeping their health data secret; privacy and confidentiality are entitlements that a person does not need to earn, to argue for, or to defend. Another reason is more practical: protecting privacy and confidentiality benefits both individuals and society. Patients who know that their health care data will not be shared inappropriately are more comfortable disclosing those data to clinicians. This trust is vital for the successful physician–patient or nurse–patient relationship, and it helps practitioners to do their jobs.

Privacy and confidentiality protections also benefit public health. People who fear disclosure of personal information are less likely to seek out professional assistance, increasing the risks that contagion will be spread and maladies will go untreated. In addition, and sadly, people still suffer discrimination, bias, and stigma when certain health data do fall into the wrong hands. Financial harm may occur if insurers are given unlimited access to family members' records, or access to patients' genetic-testing results, because some insurers might be tempted to increase the price of insurance for individuals at higher risk of illness.

The ancient idea that physicians should hold health care information in confidence is therefore applicable whether the data are written on paper, etched in stone, or embedded in silicon. The obligations to protect privacy and to keep confidences fall to system designers and maintainers, to administrators, and, ultimately, to the physicians, nurses, and other people who elicit the information in the first place. The upshot for all of them is this: protection of privacy and confidentiality is not an option, a favor, or a helping hand offered to patients with embarrassing health care problems; it is a duty that does not vary with the malady or the data-storage medium.

Some sound clinical practice and public-health traditions run counter to the idea of absolute confidentiality. When a patient is hospitalized, it is expected that all appropriate (and no inappropriate) employees of the institution—primary-care physicians, consultants, nurses, therapists, and technicians—will be given access to the patient's medical records, when it is in the interest of patient care to do so. In most communities of the United States, the contacts of patients who have active tuberculosis or certain sexually transmitted diseases are routinely identified so that they may receive proper medical attention; the public interest is protected because the likelihood is decreased that they will transmit an infection unknowingly to other people. In addition, it is essential for health care researchers to be able to pool data from patient cases that meet specified conditions to determine the natural history of the disease and the effects of various treatments. Examples of benefits from such pooled data analyses range from the ongoing results generated by regional collaborative chemotherapy trials to the discovery, more than two decades ago, of the appropriateness of shorter lengths of stay for patients with myocardial infarction (McNeer et al., 1975). Most recently, the need for robust **syndromic surveillance** has been asserted as necessary for adequate bioterrorism preparedness.

10.3.2 Electronic Clinical and Research Data

Access to electronic patient records holds extraordinary promise for clinicians and for other people who need timely, accurate patient data. Institutions that are not using computer-based patient records may be falling behind, a position that may eventually become blameworthy. On the other hand, systems that make it easy for clinicians to access data also make it easy for other people to access it. Failure to prevent inappropriate access is at least as wrong as failure to provide adequate and appropriate access. It might therefore seem that the computer-based patient record imposes contradictory burdens on system overseers and users.

In fact, there is no contradiction between the obligation to maintain a certain standard of care (in this case, regarding minimal levels of computer use) and ensuring that such a technical standard does not imperil the rights of patients. Threats to confidentiality and privacy are fairly well known. They include economic abuses, or discrimination by third-party payers, employers, and others who take advantage of the burgeoning market in health data; insider abuse, or record snooping by hospital or clinic workers who are not directly involved in a patient's care but examine a record out of curiosity, for blackmail, and so on; and malevolent hackers, or people who, via networks or other means, copy, delete, or alter confidential information (National Research Council, 1997). Indeed, the National Research Council has noted problems arising from widespread dissemination of information throughout the health care system—dissemination that often occurs without explicit patient consent. Health care providers, third-party payers, managers of pharmaceutical benefits programs, equipment suppliers, and oversight organizations collect large amounts of patient-identifiable health information for use in managing care, conducting quality and utilization reviews, processing claims, combating fraud, and analyzing markets for health products and services (National Research Council, 1997).

The proper approach to such challenges is one that will ensure both that appropriate clinicians and other people have rapid, easy access to patient records and that other people do not have access. Is that another contradictory burden? No. There are several ways to restrict inappropriate access to electronic records. They are generally divided into technological methods and institutional or policy approaches (Alpert, 1998):

- Technological methods: Computers can provide the means for maximizing their own security, including authenticating users, by making sure that users are who they say they are; prohibiting people without a professional need from accessing health information; and using audit trails, or logs, of people who do inspect confidential records so that patients and other people can review the logs.
- Policy approaches: The National Research Council has recommended that hospitals and other health care organizations create security and confidentiality committees and establish education and training programs. These recommendations parallel an approach that has worked well elsewhere in hospitals for matters ranging from infection control to bioethics.

Such recommendations are all the more important when health data are accessible through networks. The rapid growth of **integrated delivery networks (IDNs)** (see Chapter 13) and the National Health Information Infrastructure (NHII), for example, illustrates the need not to view health data as a well into which one drops a bucket but rather as an irrigation system that makes its contents available over a broad—sometimes an *extremely* broad—area. It is not yet clear whether privacy and confidentiality protections that are appropriate in hospitals will be valid in a networked environment. System developers, users, and administrators are obliged to identify appropriate measures. There is no excuse for failing to make ethics a top priority throughout the data storage and sharing environment.

Electronic Data and Human Subjects Research

The use of patient information for **clinical research** and for quality assessment raises interesting ethical challenges. The presumption of a right to confidentiality seems to include the idea that patient records are inextricably linked to patient names or to other identifying data. In an optimal environment, then, patients can monitor who is looking at their records. But if all unique identifiers have been stripped from the records, is there any sense in talking about confidentiality?

The benefits to **public health** loom large in considering record-based research. A valuable benefit of the electronic health care record is the ability to access vast numbers of patient records to determine the incidence and prevalence of various maladies, to track the efficacy of clinical interventions, and to plan efficient resource allocation (see Chapter 14). Such research and planning would, however, impose onerous or intractable burdens if informed, or valid consent had to be obtained from every patient whose record was represented in the sample. To cite confidentiality as an impediment to all such research is to stand on ceremony that not only fails to protect patients but also forecloses on potentially beneficial scientific investigations.

A more practical course is to establish safeguards that optimize the research ethically. This goal can be reached via a number of paths. The first is to establish mechanisms to anonymize the information in individual records or to decouple the data contained in the records from any unique patient identifier. This task is not always straightforward. A specific job description ("this 30-year-old starting quarterback of the Wildcats professional football team was admitted with a shattered collarbone"), or a rare disease diagnosis coupled with demographic data, or a nine-digit postal code may act as a surrogate unique identifier; that is, detailed information can serve as a data fingerprint that picks out an individual patient even though the patient's name, Social Security number, or other (official) unique identifier has been removed from the record.

Such challenges point to a second means of optimizing database research ethically, the use of institutional panels, such as **medical record committees** or institutional review boards. Submission of database research to appropriate institutional scrutiny is one way to make the best use of more or less anonymous electronic patient data. Competent panel members should be educated in the research potential of electronic health care records, as well as in ethical issues in epidemiology and public health. Scrutiny by such committees could also ethically optimize internal research for quality control, outcomes monitoring, and so on (Goodman, 1998b; Miller and Gardner, 1997a, 1997b).

Challenges in Bioinformatics

Safeguards are increasingly likely to be challenged as genetic information makes its way into the health care record (see Chapter 22). The risks of bias, discrimination, and social stigma increase dramatically as **genetic data** become available to clinicians and investigators. Indeed, genetic information "goes beyond the ordinary varieties of medical information in its predictive value" (Macklin, 1992). Genetic data also may be valuable to people predicting outcomes, allocating resources, and the like (Table 10.1). In addition, genetic data are rarely associated with only a single person; they may provide information about relatives, including relatives who do not want to know about their genetic makeup or maladies as well as relatives who would love dearly to know more about their kin's genome. There is still much work to be done in sorting out and addressing the

Table 10.1. Correlation of clinical findings with genetic data.[a]

Syndrome	Number of signs	Clinical findings
Atkin-Flaitz	3	Short stature, obesity, hypertelorism
Young-Hughes	2	Short stature, obesity
Vasquez	2	Short stature, obestity
Stoll	2	Short stature, obesity
Simpson-Golabi-Behemel	2	Obesity, hypertelorism
Otopalato-Digital	2	Short stature, hypertelorism
FG	2	Short stature, hypertelorism
Chudley	2	Short stature, obesity
Borjeson	2	Short stature, obesity
Albright Hereditary Osteodystrophy	2	Short stature, obesity
Aarskog	2	Short stature, hypertelorism

[a]Databases with genetic information can be used to help correlate clinical findings with diagnoses of genetic maladies. Here are the results of a "Make Diagnosis" query based on short stature, obesity, and hypertelorism (abnormally large distance between paired organs, especially eyes) performed on the X-Linked Recessive Mental Retardation Database at the University of Miami.
(*Source*: Division of Genetics, Department of Pediatrics, University of Miami School of Medicine.)

ethical issues related to electronic storage, sharing, and retrieval of genetic data (Goodman, 1996).

Bioinformatics offers excellent opportunities to increase our knowledge of genetics, genetic diseases, and public health. These opportunities, however, are accompanied by responsibilities to attend to the ethical issues raised by methods, applications, and consequences.

10.4   Social Challenges and Ethical Obligations

The expansion of **evidence-based medicine** and, in the United States, of managed care places a high premium on the tools of health informatics. The need for data on clinical outcomes is driven by a number of important social and scientific factors. Perhaps the most important among these factors is the increasing unwillingness of governments and insurers to pay for interventions and therapies that do not work or that do not work well enough to justify their cost.

Health informatics helps clinicians, administrators, third-party payers, governments, researchers, and other parties to collect, store, retrieve, analyze, and scrutinize vast amounts of data. Such tasks may be undertaken not for the sake of any individual patient but rather for cost analysis and review, quality assessment, scientific research, and so forth. These functions are important, and if computers can improve their quality or accuracy, then so much the better. Challenges arise when intelligent machines are mistaken for decision making surrogates or when institutional or public policy recommends or demands that computer output stand proxy for human cognition.

10.4.1   Informatics and Managed Care

Consider the extraordinary utility of **prognostic scoring systems** or machines that use physiologic and mortality data to compare new critical-care patients with thousands of previous patients (Knaus et al., 1991). Such systems allow hospitals to track the performance of their critical-care units by, say, comparing the previous year's outcomes to this year's or by comparing one hospital to another. If, for instance, patients with a particular profile tend to survive longer than their predecessors, then it might be inferred that **critical care** has improved. Such scoring systems can be useful for internal research and for quality management (Figure 10.1).

Now suppose that most previous patients with a particular physiologic profile have died in critical-care units; this information might be used to identify ways to improve care of such patients—or it might be used in support of arguments to contain costs by denying care to subsequent patients fitting the profile.

An argument in support of such a nonresearch application might be that decisions to withdraw or withhold care are often and customarily made on the basis of subjective and fragmented evidence; so it is preferable to make such decisions on the basis of objective data of the sort that otherwise underlie sound clinical practice. Such

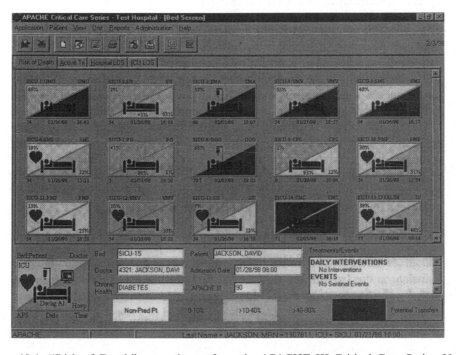

Figure 10.1. "Risk of Death" screen image from the APACHE III Critical Care Series. Using APACHE, clinicians in the intensive-care units are able to monitor critical events and required interventions, and administrators are able to manage the units' staffing based on the acuity of the patients on the units. (*Source*: Courtesy of APACHE Medical Systems, Inc.)

outcomes data are precisely what fuels the engines of managed care, wherein health professionals and institutions compete on the basis of cost and outcomes (see Chapter 23). Why, people may argue, should society, or a managed-care organization, or an insurance company pay for critical care when there is objective evidence that such care will not be efficacious? Contrarily, consider the effect of denying care to such patients on the basis of future scientific insights. Scientific progress is often made by noticing that certain patients do better under certain circumstances, and investigation of such phenomena leads to better treatments. If all patients meeting certain criteria were denied therapy on the basis of a predictive tool, it would become a self-fulfilling prophecy for a much longer time that all such patients would not do well.

Now consider use of a decision-support system to evaluate, review, or challenge decisions by human clinicians; indeed, imagine an insurance company using a diagnostic expert system to determine whether a physician should be reimbursed for a particular procedure. If the expert system has a track record for accuracy and reliability, and if the system "disagrees" with the human's diagnosis or treatment plan, then the insurance company can contend that reimbursement for the procedure would be a mistake. After all, why pay a provider for doing a procedure that is not indicated, at least according to the computer?

In the two examples just offered (a prognostic scoring system is used to justify termination of treatment to conserve resources, and a diagnostic expert system is used to deny a physician reimbursement for procedures deemed inappropriate), there seems to be justification for adhering to the computer output. There are, however, three reasons why it is problematic to use clinical computer programs to guide policy or practice in these ways:

1. As we saw earlier with the standard view of computational diagnosis (and, by easy extension, prognosis), human cognition is still superior to machine intelligence. The act of rendering a diagnosis or prognosis is not merely a statistical operation performed on uninterpreted data. Rather, identifying a malady and predicting its course requires understanding a complex ensemble of causal relations, interactions among a large number of variables, and having a store of salient background knowledge.
2. Decisions about whether to treat a given patient are often value laden and must be made relative to treatment goals. In other words, it might be that a treatment will improve the quality of life but not extend life, or vice versa (Youngner, 1988). Whether such treatment is appropriate cannot be determined scientifically or statistically (Brody, 1989).
3. Applying computational operations on aggregate data to individual patients runs the risk of including individuals in groups they resemble but to which they do not actually belong. Of course, human clinicians run this risk all the time—the challenge of inferring correctly that an individual is a member of a set, group, or class is one of the oldest problems in logic and in the philosophy of science. The point is that computers have not solved this problem, yet, and allowing policy to be guided by simple or unanalyzed correlations constitutes a conceptual error.

The idea is not that diagnostic or prognostic computers are always wrong—we know that they are not—but rather there are numerous instances in which we do not know whether they are right. It is one thing to allow aggregate data to guide policy; doing so is just using scientific evidence to maximize good outcomes. But it is altogether different to require that a policy disallow individual **clinical judgment** and expertise.

Informatics can contribute in many ways to health care reform. Indeed, computer-based tools can help to illuminate ways to reduce costs, to optimize clinical outcomes, and to improve care. Scientific research, quality assessment, and the like are, for the most part, no longer possible without computers. But it does not follow that the insights from such research apply in all instances to the myriad variety of actual clinical cases at which competent human clinicians excel.

10.4.2 Effects of Informatics on Traditional Relationships

Patients are often sick, scared, and vulnerable. Treating illness, easing fear, and respecting vulnerability are among the core obligations of physicians and nurses. The growth of health informatics should be seen as posing exciting challenges to complement these traditional duties and the relationships that the duties govern. We have pointed out that medical decisions are shaped by nonscientific considerations. This point is important when we assess the effects of informatics on human relationships. Thus:

> The practice of medicine or nursing is not exclusively and clearly scientific, statistical, or procedural, and hence is not, so far, computationally tractable. This is not to make a hoary appeal to the "art and science" of medicine; it is to say that the science is in many contexts inadequate or inapplicable: Many clinical decisions are not exclusively medical—they have social, personal, ethical, psychological, financial, familial, legal, and other components; even art might play a role. (Miller and Goodman, 1998)

Professional–Patient Relationships

If computers, databases, and networks can improve physician–patient or nurse–patient relationships, perhaps by improving communication, then we shall have achieved a happy result. If reliance on computers impedes the abilities of health professionals to establish trust and to communicate compassionately, however, or further contributes to the dehumanization of patients (Shortliffe, 1994), then we may have paid too dearly for our use of these machines.

Suppose that a physician uses a decision-support system to test a diagnostic hypothesis or to generate differential diagnoses, and suppose further that a decision to order a particular test or treatment is based on that system's output. A physician who is not able to articulate the proper role of computational support in his decision to treat or test will risk alienating those patients who, for one reason or another, will be disappointed, angered, or confused by the use of computers in their care. To be sure, the physician might just withhold this information from patients, but such deception carries its own threats to trust in the relationship.

Patients are not completely ignorant about the processes that constitute human decision making. What they do understand, however, may be subverted when their doctors and nurses use machines to assist delicate cognitive functions. We must ask whether patients should be told the accuracy rate of decision machines—when they have yet to be given comparable data for humans. Would such knowledge improve the informed-consent process, or would it "constitute another befuddling ratio that inspires doubt more than it informs rationality?" (Miller and Goodman, 1998).

To raise such questions is consistent with promoting the responsible use of computers in clinical practice. The question whether computer use will alienate patients is an empirical one; it is a question for which we have inadequate data to answer. (Do patients respond well to e-mail messages from their doctors, or do they not?) To address the question now anticipates potential future problems. We must ensure that the exciting potential of health informatics is not subverted by our forgetting that the practice of medicine, nursing, and allied professions is deeply human and fundamentally intimate and personal.

Consumer Health Informatics

The growth of the World Wide Web and the commensurate evolution of clinical and health resources on the Internet also raise issues for professional–patient relationships. **Consumer health informatics**—technologies focused on patients as the primary users—makes vast amounts of information available to patients. There is also, however, misinformation—even outright falsehoods and quackery—posted on some sites (see Chapter 14). If physicians and nurses have not established relationships based on trust, the erosive potential of apparently authoritative Internet resources can be great. Physicians accustomed to newspaper-inspired patient requests for drugs and treatments can expect everincreasing demands that are informed by Web browsing. The following issues will gain in ethical importance over the next decade:

- Peer review: How and by whom is the quality of a Web site to be evaluated? Who is responsible for the accuracy of information communicated to patients?
- Online consultations: There is yet no standard of care for online medical consultations. What risks do physicians and nurses run by giving advice to patients whom they have not met or examined? This question is especially important in the context of **telemedicine** or **remote-presence health care**, the use of video teleconferencing, image transmission, and other technologies that allow clinicians to evaluate and treat patients in other than face-to-face situations (see Chapter 24).
- Support groups: Internet support groups can provide succor and advice to the sick, but there is a chance that someone who might benefit from seeing a physician will not do so because of comforts and information otherwise attained, and that her not doing so will lead to bad consequences. How should this problem be addressed?

That a resource is touted as worthwhile does not mean that it is. We lack evidence to illuminate the utility of consumer health informatics and its effects on professional–patient relationships. Such resources should not be ignored, and they often are useful for improving health. But we insist that here—as with decision support, appropriate use and users, evaluation, and privacy and confidentiality—there is an ethical imperative to proceed with caution. Informatics, like other health technologies, will thrive if our enthusiasm is open to greater evidence and is wed to deep reflection on human values.

10.5   Legal and Regulatory Matters

The use of clinical computing systems in health care raises a number of legal and regulatory questions.

10.5.1   Difference Between Law and Ethics

As might be anticipated, ethical and legal issues often overlap. Ethical considerations apply in attempts to determine what is good or meritorious and which behaviors are desirable or correct in accordance with higher principles. Legal principles are generally derived from ethical ones but deal with the practical regulation of morality or behaviors and activities. Many legal principles deal with the inadequacies and imperfections in human nature and the less-than-ideal behaviors of individuals or groups. **Ethics** offers conceptual tools to evaluate and guide moral decision making. Laws directly tell us how to behave (or not to behave) under various specific circumstances and prescribe remedies or punishments for individuals who do not comply with the law. Historical precedent, matters of definition, issues related to detectability and enforceability, and evolution of new circumstances affect legal practices more than they influence ethical requirements.

10.5.2   Legal Issues in Health Care Informatics

Major legal issues related to the use of software applications in clinical practice and in biomedical research include liability under tort law; potential use of computer applications as expert witnesses in the courtroom; legislation governing privacy and confidentiality; and copyrights, patents, and intellectual property issues.

Liability Under Tort Law

In the United States and in many other nations, principles of tort law govern situations in which harm or injuries result from the manufacture and sale of goods and services (Miller et al., 1985). Because there are few, if any, U.S. legal precedents directly involving harm or injury to patients resulting from use of clinical software applications (as opposed to a small number of well-documented instances where software associated with medical devices has caused harm), the following discussion is hypothetical. The principles involved are, however, well established with voluminous legal precedents outside the realm of clinical software.

A key legal distinction is the difference between products and services. **Products** are physical objects, such as stethoscopes, that go through the processes of design, manufacture, distribution, sale, and subsequent use by purchasers. **Services** are intangible activities provided to consumers at a price by (presumably) qualified individuals.

The practice of clinical medicine has been deemed a service through well-established legal precedents. On the other hand, clinical software applications can be viewed as either goods (software programs designed, tested, debugged, placed on diskettes or other media, and distributed physically to purchasers) or services (applications that provide advice to practitioners engaged in a service such as delivering health care). There are few legal precedents to determine unequivocally how software will be viewed by the courts, and it is possible that clinical software programs will be treated as goods under some circumstances and as services under others.

Two ideas from tort law potentially apply to the clinical use of software systems: (1) the **negligence theory**, and (2) **strict product liability**. Providers of goods and services are expected to uphold the standards of the community in producing goods and delivering services. When individuals suffer harm due to substandard goods or services, they may sue the service providers or goods manufacturers to recover damages. **Malpractice** litigation in health care is based on negligence theory.

Because the law views delivery of health care as a service (provided by clinicians), it is clear that negligence theory will provide the minimum legal standard for clinicians who use software during the delivery of care. Patients who are harmed by clinical practices based on imperfect software applications may sue the health care providers for negligence or malpractice, just as patients may sue attending physicians who rely on the imperfect advice of a human consultant (Miller et al., 1985). Similarly, a patient might sue a practitioner who has not used a decision-support system when it can be shown that use of the decision-support system is part of the current standard of care, and that use of the program might have prevented the clinical error that occurred (Miller, 1989). It is not clear whether the patients in such circumstances can also sue the software manufacturers, as it is the responsibility of the licensed practitioner, and not of the software vendor, to uphold the standard of care in the community through exercising sound clinical judgment. Based on a successful malpractice suit against a clinician who used a clinical software system, it might be possible for the practitioner to sue the manufacturer or vendor for negligence in manufacturing a defective clinical software product, but cases of this sort have not yet been filed. If there were such suits, it might be difficult for a court to discriminate between instances of improper use of a blameless system and proper use of a less than perfect system.

In contrast to negligence, strict product liability applies only to harm caused by defective products and is not applicable to services. The primary purpose of strict product liability is to compensate the injured parties rather than to deter or punish negligent individuals (Miller et al., 1985). For strict product liability to apply, three conditions must be met:

1. The product must be purchased and used by an individual.
2. The purchaser must suffer physical harm as a result of a design or manufacturing defect in the product.
3. The product must be shown in court to be "unreasonably dangerous" in a manner that is the demonstrable cause of the purchaser's injury.

Note that negligence theory allows for adverse outcomes. Even when care is delivered in a competent, caring, and compassionate manner, some patients with some illnesses will not do well. Negligence theory protects providers from being held responsible for all individuals who suffer bad outcomes. As long as the quality of care has met the standards, the practitioner should not be found liable in a malpractice case (Miller et al., 1985). Strict product liability, on the other hand, is not as forgiving or understanding.

No matter how good or exemplary are a manufacturer's designs and manufacturing processes, if even one in ten million products is defective, and that one product defect is the cause of a purchaser's injury, then the purchaser may collect damages (Miller et al., 1985). The plaintiff needs to show only that the product was unreasonably dangerous and that its defect led to harm. In that sense, the standard of care for strict product liability is 100 percent perfection. To some extent, appropriate product labeling (e.g., "Do not use this metal ladder near electrical wiring") may protect manufacturers in certain strict product liability suits in that clear, visible labeling may educate the purchaser to avoid "unreasonably dangerous" circumstances. Appropriate labeling standards may benefit users and manufacturers of clinical expert systems (Geissbuhler and Miller, 1997).

Health care programs sold to clinicians who use them as decision-support tools in their practices are likely to be treated under negligence theory as services. When advice-giving clinical programs are sold directly to patients, however, and there is less opportunity for intervention by a licensed practitioner, it is more likely that the courts will treat them as products, using strict product liability, because the purchaser of the program is more likely to be the individual who is injured if the product is defective.

Privacy and Confidentiality

The ethical basis for privacy and confidentiality in health care is discussed in Section 10.3.1. It is unfortunate that the legal state of affairs for privacy and confidentiality of electronic health records is at present chaotic (as it is for written records, to some extent). This state of affairs has not significantly changed in the three decades since it was described in a classic *New England Journal of Medicine* article (Curran et al., 1969).

However, a key U.S. law, the Health Insurance Portability and Accountability Act (HIPAA), became effective in 2002, prompting significant change—especially with the April 2003 application of the law's privacy standards. A major impetus for the law was that the process of "administrative simplification," prized for its potential to increase efficiency and reduce costs, would also pose threats to patient privacy and confidentiality. Coming against a backdrop of a variety of noteworthy cases in which patient data were improperly—and often embarrassingly—disclosed, the law was also seen as a badly needed tool to restore confidence in the ability of health professionals to protect confidentiality. While the law has been accompanied by debate both on the adequacy of its measures and the question whether compliance was unnecessarily burdensome, it nevertheless establishes the first nationwide privacy protections. At its core, it embodies the idea that individuals should control disclosure of their health data. Among its provisions, the law requires that patients be informed about their privacy rights; that uses of "protected health information" not needed for treatment, payment or operations be limited to exchanges of the "minimum necessary" amount of information; and that all employees in "covered entities" be educated about privacy (see Web sites by the U.S. Government, http://aspe.hhs.gov/admnsimp; Georgetown University, http://www.healthprivacy.org; or the University of Miami, http://privacy.med.miami.edu, for overviews).

Copyright, Patents, and Intellectual Property

Intellectual property protection afforded to developers of software programs, biomedical knowledge bases, and World Wide Web pages remains an underdeveloped area of law. Although there are long traditions of copyright and patent protections for non-electronic media, their applicability to computer-based resources is not clear. **Copyright law** protects intellectual property from being copied verbatim, and **patents** protect specific methods of implementing or instantiating ideas. The number of lawsuits in which one company claimed that another copied the functionality of its copyrighted program (i.e., its "look and feel") has grown, however, and it is clear that copyright law does not protect the "look and feel" of a program beyond certain limits. Consider, for example, the unsuccessful suit in the 1980s by Apple Computer, Inc., against Microsoft, Inc., over the "look and feel" of Microsoft Windows as compared with the Apple Macintosh interface (which itself resembled the earlier Xerox Alto interface).

It is not straightforward to obtain copyright protection for a list that is a compilation of existing names, data, facts, or objects (e.g., the telephone directory of a city), unless you can argue that the result of compiling the compendium creates a unique object (e.g., a new organizational scheme for the information) (Tysyer, 1997). Even when the compilation is unique and copyrightable, the individual components, such as facts in a database, may not be copyrightable. That they are not copyrightable has implications for the ability of creators of biomedical databases to protect database content as intellectual property. How many individual, unprotected facts can someone copy from a copyright-protected database before legal protections prevent additional copying?

A related concern is the intellectual-property rights of the developers of materials made available through the World Wide Web. Usually, information made accessible to the public that does not contain copyright annotations is considered to be in the public domain. It is tempting to build from the work of other people in placing material on the Web, but copyright protections must be respected. Similarly, if you develop potentially copyrightable material, the act of placing it on the Web, in the public domain, would allow other people to treat your material as not protected by copyright. Resolution of this and related questions may await workable commercial models for electronic publication on the World Wide Web, whereby authors could be compensated fairly when other people use or access their materials. Electronic commerce should eventually provide copyright protection and revenue similar to the age-old models that now apply to paper-based print media; for instance, to use printed books and journals, you must generally borrow them from a library or purchase them.

10.5.3   *Regulation and Monitoring of Computer Applications in Health Care*

In 1996, the U.S. **Food and Drug Administration (FDA)** announced that it would hold public meetings to discuss new methods and approaches to regulating clinical software systems as medical devices. In response, a consortium of professional organizations related to health care information (the American Medical Informatics Association, the Center for Health Care Information Management, the Computer-Based Patient Record

Institute, the American Health Information Management Association, the Medical Library Association, the Association of Academic Health Science Libraries, and the American Nurses Association) drafted a position paper published in both summary format and as a longer discussion with detailed background and explanation (Miller and Gardner, 1997a, 1997b). The position paper was subsequently endorsed by the boards of directors of all the organizations (except the Center for Health Care Information Management) and by the American College of Physicians Board of Regents.

The recommendations from the consortium include these:

- Recognition of four categories of clinical system risks and four classes of monitoring and regulatory actions that can be applied based on the level of risk in a given setting.
- Local oversight of clinical software systems, whenever possible, through the creation of autonomous **software oversight committees**, in a manner partially analogous to the institutional review boards that are federally mandated to oversee protection of human subjects in biomedical research. Experience with prototypical software-oversight committees at pilot sites should be gained before any national dissemination.
- Adoption by health care-information system developers of a code of good business practices.
- Recognition that budgetary, logistic, and other constraints limit the type and number of systems that the FDA can regulate effectively.
- Concentration of FDA regulation on those systems posing highest clinical risk, with limited opportunities for competent human intervention, and FDA exemption of most other clinical software systems.

The recommendations for combined local and FDA monitoring are summarized in Table 10.2.

10.6 Summary and Conclusions

Ethical issues are important to health informatics. An initial ensemble of guiding principles, or ethical criteria, has emerged to orient decision making:

1. Specially trained humans remain, so far, best able to provide health care for other humans. Hence, computer software should not be allowed to overrule a human decision.
2. Practitioners who use informatics tools should be clinically qualified and adequately trained in using the software products.
3. The tools themselves should be carefully evaluated and validated.
4. Health informatics tools and applications should be evaluated not only in terms of performance, including efficacy, but also in terms of their influences on institutions, institutional cultures, and workplace social forces.
5. Ethical obligations should extend to system developers, maintainers, and supervisors as well as to clinician users.
6. Education programs and security measures should be considered essential for protecting confidentiality and privacy while improving appropriate access to personal patient information.

Table 10.2. Consortium recommendations for monitoring and regulating clinical software systems.[a]

Variable	Regulatory class			
	A	B	C	D
Supervision by FDA	Exempt from regulation	Excluded from regulation	Simple registration and postmarket surveillance required	Premarket approval and postmarket surveillance required
Role of software oversight committee	Optional	Mandatory	Mandatory	Mandatory
Software risk category	Monitor locally	Monitor locally instead of monitoring by FDA	Monitor locally and report problems to FDA as appropriate	Assure adequate local monitoring without replicating FDA activity
1. Informational or generic systems[b]	All software in category	—	—	—
2. Patient-specific systems that provide low-risk assistance with clinical problems[c]	—	All software in category	—	—
3. Patient-specific systems that provide intermediate-risk support on clinical problems[d]	—	Locally developed or locally modified systems	Commercially developed systems that are not modified locally	—
4. High-risk, patient-specific systems[e]	—	Locally developed, noncommercial systems	—	Commercial systems

[a] FDA = Food and Drug Administration.

[b] Includes systems that provide factual content or simple, generic advice (such as "give flu vaccine to eligible patients in midautumn") and generic programs, such as spreadsheets and databases.

[c] Systems that give simple advice (such as suggesting alternative diagnoses or therapies without stating preferences), and give ample opportunity for users to ignore or override suggestions.

[d] Systems that have higher clinical risk (such as those that generate diagnoses or therapies ranked by score) but allow users to ignore or override suggestions easily; net risk is therefore intermediate.

[e] Systems that have great clinical risk and give users little or no opportunity to intervene (such as a closed-loop system that automatically regulates ventilator settings). (*Source*: Miller R.A., Gardner R.M. (1997). Summary recommendations for responsible monitoring and regulation of clinical software systems. *Annals of Internal Medicine*, 127(9):842.)

7. Adequate oversight should be maintained to optimize ethical use of electronic patient information for scientific and institutional research.

New sciences and technologies always raise interesting and important ethical issues. Much the same is true for legal issues, although in the absence of precedent or legislation any legal analysis will remain vague. Similarly important challenges confront people who are trying to determine the appropriate role for government in regulating health care software. The lack of clear public policy for such software underscores the importance of ethical insight and education as the exciting new tools of health informatics become more common.

Suggested Readings

Goodman K.W. (Ed.) (1998). *Ethics, Computing, and Medicine: Informatics and the Transformation of Health Care*. Cambridge: Cambridge University Press.
This volume—the first devoted to the intersection of ethics and informatics—contains chapters on informatics and human values, responsibility for computer-based decisions, evaluation of medical information systems, confidentiality and privacy, decision support, outcomes research and prognostic scoring systems, and meta-analysis.

Miller R.A. (1990). Why the standard view is standard: People, not machines, understand patients' problems. *Journal of Medicine and Philosophy*, 15:581–591.
This contribution lays out the standard view of health informatics. This view holds, in part, that because only humans have the diverse skills necessary to practice medicine or nursing, machine intelligence should never override human clinicians.

Miller R.A., Schaffner K.F., Meisel, A. (1985). Ethical and legal issues related to the use of computer programs in clinical medicine. *Annals of Internal Medicine*, 102:529–536.
This article constitutes a major early effort to identify and address ethical issues in informatics. By emphasizing the questions of appropriate use, confidentiality, and validation, among others, it sets the stage for all subsequent work.

National Research Council (1997). *For the Record: Protecting Electronic Health Information*. Washington, D.C.: National Academy Press.
A major policy report, this document outlines leading challenges for privacy and confidentiality in medical information systems and makes several important recommendations for institutions and policymakers.

Questions for Discussion

1. What is meant by the standard view of appropriate use of medical information systems? Identify three key criteria for determining whether a particular use or user is appropriate.
2. Can quality standards for system developers and maintainers simultaneously safeguard against error and abuse and stimulate scientific progress? Explain your answers. Why is there an ethical obligation to adhere to a standard of care?

3. Identify (a) two major threats to patient confidentiality, and (b) policies or strategies that you propose for protecting confidentiality against these threats.

4. Many prognoses by humans are subjective and are based on faulty memory or incomplete knowledge of previous cases. What are the two drawbacks to using objective prognostic scoring systems to determine whether to allocate care to individual patients?

5. People who are educated about their illnesses tend to understand and to follow instructions, to ask insightful questions, and so on. How can the World Wide Web improve patient education? How, on the other hand, might Web access hurt traditional physician–patient and nurse–patient relationships?

11
Evaluation and Technology Assessment

CHARLES P. FRIEDMAN, JEREMY C. WYATT, AND DOUGLAS K. OWENS

After reading this chapter, you should know the answers to these questions:

- Why are empirical studies based on the methods of evaluation and technology assessment important to the successful implementation of information resources to improve health care?
- What challenges make studies in informatics difficult to carry out? How are these challenges addressed in practice?
- Why can all evaluations be classified as empirical studies?
- What are the major assumptions underlying objectivist and subjectivist approaches to evaluation? What are the advantages and disadvantages of each?
- What are the factors that distinguish the three stages of technology assessment?
- How does one distinguish measurement and demonstration aspects of objectivist studies, and why are both aspects necessary?
- What steps are typically undertaken in a measurement study? What designs are typically used in demonstration studies?
- What is the difference between cost-effectiveness and cost-benefit analyses? How can investigators address issues of cost effectiveness and cost benefit of medical information resources?
- What steps are followed in a subjectivist study? What techniques are employed by subjectivist investigators to ensure rigor and credibility of their findings?
- Why is communication between investigators and clients central to the success of any evaluation?

11.1   Introduction and Definitions of Terms

This chapter is about the formal study of medical information resources—computer systems that support health care, education, research, and biomedical research—to address questions of importance to developers, users, and other people. We explore the methods of performing such studies, which are essential to the field of informatics but are often challenging to carry out successfully. Fortunately, every study is not designed from a blank tablet. To guide us, there exist two closely related and highly overlapping bodies of methodological knowledge: evaluation and technology assessment. These methodological fields, which have largely developed over the past four decades, are together the subject of this chapter.[1]

---

[1]This chapter is heavily drawn from the textbook on evaluation by co-authors Friedman and Wyatt (2006); refer to that text for further details.

11.1.1   Evaluation and Technology Assessment

Most people understand the term evaluation to mean a measurement or description of an organized, purposeful activity. Evaluations are usually conducted to answer questions or to help make decisions. Whether we are choosing a holiday destination or a word processor, we evaluate what the options are and how well they fit key objectives or personal preferences. The forms of the evaluation differ widely, according to what is being evaluated and how important the decision is. Thus, in the case of holiday destinations, we may ask our friend which Hawaiian island she prefers and may browse color brochures from the travel agent; for a word processor, we may gather technical details, such as the time to open and spell check a 1,000-word document or the compatibility with our printer. Thus, the term **evaluation** describes a wide range of data-collection activities, designed to answer questions ranging from the casual, "What does my friend think of Maui?" to the more focused, "Is word processor A faster than word processor B on my personal computer?"

In medical informatics, we study the collection, processing, and communication of health care information and build **information resources**—usually consisting of computer hardware or software—to facilitate these activities. Such information resources include systems to collect, store, and retrieve data about specific patients (e.g., clinical workstations and databases) and systems to assemble, store, and reason about medical knowledge (e.g., medical knowledge–acquisition tools, knowledge bases, decision-support systems, and intelligent tutoring systems). Thus, there is a wide range of medical information resources to evaluate.

Further complicating the picture, each information resource has many different aspects that can be evaluated. The technically minded might focus on inherent characteristics, asking such questions as, "Is the code compliant with current software engineering standards and practices?" or "Is the data structure the optimal choice for this type of application?" Clinicians, however, might ask more pragmatic questions such as, "Is the knowledge in this system completely up-to-date?" or "How long must we wait until the decision-support system produces its recommendations?" People who have a broader perspective might wish to understand the influence of these resources on users or patients, asking questions such as, "How well does this database support a clinical audit?" or "What effects will this decision-support system have on clinical practice, working relationships, and patients?" Thus, evaluation methods in medical informatics must address a wide range of issues, from technical characteristics of specific systems to systems' effects on people and organizations.

Technology assessment is a field of study closely aligned with evaluation (Garber and Owens, 1994). The Institute of Medicine (1985, p. 2) defines technology assessment as "any process of examining and reporting properties of a medical technology used in health care, such as safety, efficacy, feasibility, and indication for use, cost, and cost effectiveness, as well as social, economic, and ethical consequences, whether intended or unintended."

But what is a medical technology? **Medical technology** usually is defined broadly and consists of the "techniques, drugs, equipments, and procedures used by health care professionals in delivering medical care to individuals, and the systems within which such care is delivered" (Institute of Medicine, 1985, pp. 1–2). Medical information resources clearly fit within this definition. Technology assessment is relevant to informatics because many of the techniques from this field are applicable to the study of information resources.

We shall not dwell here on the differences between evaluation and technology assessment. Such differences are ones of emphasis and focus. Individuals who do evaluation and technology assessment are interested in much the same issues and use similar methods.

11.1.2   Reasons for Performing Studies

Like all complex and time-consuming activities, evaluation and technology assessment can serve multiple purposes. There are five major reasons why we study clinical information resources (Wyatt and Spiegelhalter, 1990):

- *Promotional*: If we are to encourage the use of information resources in medicine, we must be able to reassure physicians that these systems are safe and that they benefit both patients and institutions through improved cost effectiveness.
- *Scholarly*: One of the main activities in medical informatics is developing clinical information resources using computer-based tools. To obtain a deeper understanding of the links between the structure, function, and effects of these information resources on clinical decisions and actions requires careful evaluation. The knowledge we gain from such studies will help to build the foundations of medical informatics as a discipline (Heathfield and Wyatt, 1995).
- *Pragmatic*: Without evaluating their systems, developers will never know which techniques or methods are more effective or why certain approaches failed. Equally, other developers will not be able to learn from previous mistakes and may reinvent a square wheel.
- *Ethical*: Clinical professionals are under an obligation to practice within an ethical framework. For example, before using an information resource, health care providers must ensure that it is safe. Equally, those responsible for commissioning the purchase of a hospital-wide clinical information system costing several million dollars must be able to justify this in preference to other information resources or the many other health care innovations that compete for the same budget.
- *Medicolegal*: To reduce the risk of liability, developers of an information resource should obtain accurate information to allow them to assure users that the resource is safe and effective. Users need evaluation results to enable them to exercise their professional judgment before using systems so that the law will regard these users as "learned intermediaries." An information resource that treats users merely as automata, without allowing them to exercise their skills and judgment, risks being judged by the strict laws of product liability instead of by the more lenient principles applied to provision of professional services (Brahams and Wyatt, 1989) (also see Chapter 10).

The motivation for every study is one or more of these factors. Awareness of the major reason for conducting an evaluation will often help the investigators to frame the questions to be addressed and to avoid disappointment.

11.1.3   The Stakeholders in Evaluation Studies and Their Roles

Figure 11.1 shows the actors who pay for (solid arrows) and regulate (shaded arrows) the health care process. Each of them may be affected by a medical information resource, and each may have a unique view of what constitutes benefit. More specifically, in a typical clinical information resource project, the key stakeholders are the developers, the users, the patients whose management may be affected, and the people responsible for purchasing and maintaining the system. Each may have different questions to be answered (Figure 11.2).

Whenever we design evaluation or technology assessment studies, it is important to consider the perspectives of all stakeholders in the information resource. Because studies are often designed to answer specific questions, any one study is unlikely to satisfy all of the questions that concern stakeholders. Sometimes, due to the intricacy of health care systems and processes, it can be a challenge for an evaluator to identify all the relevant stakeholders and to distinguish those whose questions must be satisfied from those whose satisfaction is optional.

11.2   The Challenges of Study Design and Conduct

The work of evaluation and technology assessment in informatics lies at the intersection of three areas, each notorious for its complexity: (1) medicine and health care delivery,

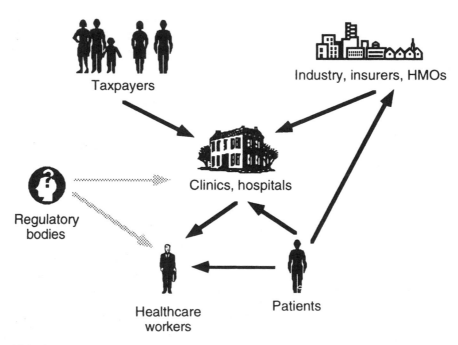

Figure 11.1. Some of the actors involved in health care delivery, administration, policy making, and regulation, each of whom may have a stake in an evaluation study. (*Source*: Friedman and Wyatt, 1997a.)

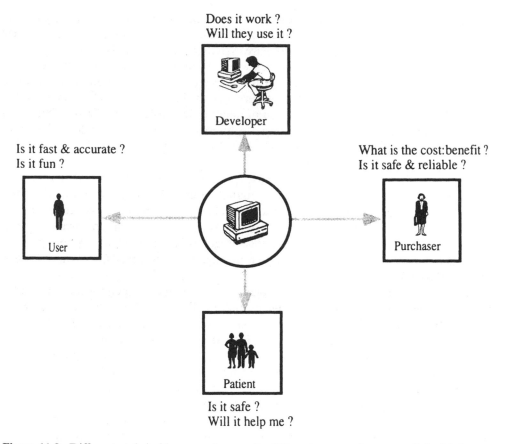

Figure 11.2. Different stakeholders may have quite different perspectives on a clinical information resource and questions that they wish to be answered by an evaluation study. (*Source*: Friedman and Wyatt, 1997a.)

(2) computer-based information systems, and (3) the general methodology of study conduct itself. Because of the complexity of each area, any work that combines them necessarily poses serious challenges.

11.2.1 The Complexity of Medicine and Health Care Delivery

Donabedian (1966) informs us that any health care innovation may influence three aspects of the health care system. The first is the health care system's **structure**, including the space it takes up; the equipment available; the financial resources required; and the number, skills, and interrelationships of the staff. The second is the **processes** that take place during health care activity, such as the number and appropriateness of diagnoses, and the investigations and therapies administered. The third is the health care **outcomes** for both individual patients and the community, such as quality of life, complications of procedures, and length of survival. Thus, when we study the influence of an information resource on a health care system, we may see effects on any of these three aspects. An information resource may lead to an improvement in one area (e.g., patient outcomes) but to deterioration in another (e.g., the costs of running the service).

Also, it is well known that the roles of nursing and clinical personnel are well defined and hierarchical in comparison to those in many other professions. Thus information resources designed for one specific group of professionals, such as a residents' information system designed for one hospital (Young, 1980), may be of little benefit to other groups.

Because health care is a safety-critical area, with more limited budgets and a less tangible currency than, for example, retail or manufacturing, rigorous proof of safety and effectiveness is required in evaluation studies of clinical information resources. Complex regulations apply to people who develop or market clinical therapies or investigational technology. It is not yet clear whether these regulations apply to all computer-based information resources or to only those that manage patients directly, without a human intermediary (Brannigan, 1991).

Medicine is well known to be a complex domain. Students spend a minimum of 7 years gaining qualifications. A single internal-medicine textbook contains approximately 600,000 facts (Wyatt, 1991b); practicing experts have as many as 2 to 5 million facts at their fingertips (Pauker et al., 1976). Also, medical knowledge itself (Wyatt, 1991b), and methods of health care delivery, change rapidly so that the goalposts for a medical information resource may move during the course of an evaluation study.

Patients often suffer from multiple diseases, which may evolve over time at differing rates and may be subject to a number of interventions and other influences over the course of the study period, confounding the effects of changes in information management. There is even variation in how doctors interpret patient data (e.g., prostate-specific antigen results) across medical centers. Thus, simply because an information resource is safe and effective when used in one center on patients who have a given diagnosis, we are not entitled to prejudge the results of using it in another center or with patients who have a different disease profile.

The causal links between introducing an information resource and achieving improvements in patient outcome are long and complex compared with those for direct patient care interventions such as medications. In addition, the functioning and influence of an information resource may depend critically on input from health care workers or patients. It is thus unrealistic to look for quantifiable changes in patient outcomes after the introduction of many information resources until we have documented changes in the structure or processes of health care delivery.

The processes of medical decision making are complex and have been studied extensively (Elstein et al., 1978; Patel. et. al, 2001). Clinicians make many kinds of decisions—including diagnosis, monitoring, therapy, and prognosis—using incomplete and fuzzy data, some of which are appreciated intuitively and are not recorded in the clinical notes. If an information resource generates more effective management of both patient data and medical knowledge, it may intervene in the process of medical decision making in a number of ways, making difficult the determination of which component of the resource is responsible for observed changes.

There is a general lack of gold standards in medicine. Thus, for example, diagnoses are rarely known with 100 percent certainty, because it is unethical to do all possible tests on every patient, (to follow up patients without good cause), because tests and ability to interpret them are imperfect, and because the human body is simply too complex. When a clinician attempts to establish a diagnosis or the cause of death, even if it is possible to perform a postmortem examination, correlating the patients' symptoms or clinical findings before death with the observed changes may prove impossible. Determining the correct management for a patient is even more complicated, because there is wide variation in **consensus opinions** (Leitch, 1989), as reflected in wide variations in clinical practice even in neighboring areas.

Doctors practice under strict legal and ethical obligations to give their patients the best care that is available, to do patients no harm, to keep patients informed about the risks of all procedures and therapies, and to maintain confidentiality. These obligations may well impinge on the design of evaluation studies. For example, because health care workers have imperfect memories and patients take holidays and participate in the unpredictable activities of real life, it is impossible to impose strict discipline in data recording, and study data are often incomplete. Similarly, before a randomized controlled trial can be undertaken, health care workers and patients are entitled to a full explanation of the possible benefits and disadvantages of being allocated to the control and intervention groups before giving their consent.

11.2.2   The Complexity of Computer-Based Information Resources

From the perspective of a computer scientist, the goal of evaluating a computer-based information resource might be to predict that resource's function and effects from a knowledge of its structure. Although software engineering and formal methods for specifying, coding, and evaluating computer programs have become more sophisticated, even systems of modest complexity challenge these techniques. To formally verify a program rigorously (to obtain proof that it performs all and only those functions specified), we must invest effort that increases exponentially with the program's size—the problem is "**NP hard**." Put simply, to test a program rigorously requires the application of every combination of possible input data in all possible orders. Thus, it entails at least n factorial experiments, where n is the number of input data items. The size of n factorial increases exponentially with small increases in n, so the task rapidly becomes unfeasible. In some technology-led projects, the goals of the new information resources are not defined precisely. Developers may be attracted by technology and may produce applications without first demonstrating the existence of a clinical problem that the application is designed to meet (Heathfield and Wyatt, 1993). An example was a conference entitled "Medicine Meets Virtual Reality: Discovering Applications for 3D Multimedia." The lack of a clear need for an information resource makes it hard to evaluate the ability of the information resource to alleviate a clinical problem. Although one can still evaluate the structure and function of the system in isolation, it will be hard to interpret the results of such an evaluation in clinical terms.

Some computer-based systems are able to adapt themselves to their users or to data already acquired, or they may be deliberately tailored to a given institution; it may then be difficult to compare the results of one evaluation with a study of the same information resource conducted at a different time or in another location. Also, the notoriously rapid evolution of computer hardware and software means that the time course of an evaluation study may be greater than the lifetime of the information resource itself.

Medical information resources often contain several distinct components, including the interface, database, reasoning and maintenance programs, patient data, static medical knowledge, and dynamic inferences about the patient, the user, and the current activity of the user. Such information resources may perform a wide range of functions for users. Thus, if evaluators are to answer questions such as, "What part of the information resource is responsible for the observed effect?" or "Why did the information resource fail?" they must be familiar with each component of the information resource, know its functions, and understand potential interactions (Wyatt, 1989, 1991a).

11.2.3   The Complexity of Study Methods

Studies do not focus solely on the structure and function of an information resource, they also address the resource's effects on the care providers who are customarily its users and on patient outcomes. To understand users' actions, investigators must confront the gulf between peoples' private opinions, public statements, and actual behavior. Humans vary widely in their responses to stimuli, both from minute to minute and from one to another, making the results of measurements subject to random and systematic errors. Thus, studies of medical information resources require analytical tools from the behavioral and social sciences, statistics, and other fields.

Studies require test material, such as clinical cases, and information resource users, such as physicians or nurses. Both are often in shorter supply than the study design requires; the availability of patients also is usually overestimated, sometimes many times over. In addition, it may be unclear what kind of cases or users should be recruited for a study. Often, study designers are faced with a trade-off between selecting cases, users, and study settings with high fidelity to real life and selecting those who will help to achieve adequate experimental control. Finally, one of the more important determinants of the results of an evaluation study is the manner in which case data are abstracted and presented to users. For example, we would expect differing results in a study of an information resource's accuracy depending on whether the test data were abstracted by the developers or by the intended users.

There are many reasons for performing studies, ranging from assessing a student's work to formulating health policy to understanding a specific technical advance. Such reasons will in turn determine the kinds of questions that will be asked about the information resource. To help those who are trying to determine the broad goals of an evaluation study, in Table 11.1 we list some of the many questions that can arise about information resources and about their influence on users, patients, and the health care system.

Table 11.1. Possible questions that may arise during the study of a medical information resource.

About the resource itself	About the resource's impact
Is there a clinical need for it?	Do people use it?
Does it work?	Do people like it?
Is it reliable?	Does it improve users' efficiency?
Is it accurate?	Does it influence the collection of data?
Is it fast enough?	Does it influence users' decisions?
Is data entry reliable?	For how long do the observed effects last?
Are people likely to use it?	Does it influence users' knowledge or skills?
Which parts cause the effects?	Does it help patients?
How can it be maintained?	Does it change consumption of resources?
How can it be improved?	What might ensue from widespread use?

(*Source*: Friedman and Wyatt, 1997a.)

11.3   The Full Range of What Can Be Studied

When evaluating a medical information resource, there are five major aspects of interest: (1) the clinical need the resource is intended to address, (2) the process used to develop the resource, (3) the resource's intrinsic structure, (4) the functions that the resource carries out, and (5) the resource's effects on users, patients, and other aspects of the clinical environment. In a theoretically complete evaluation, separate studies of a particular resource might address each aspect. In the real world, however, it is difficult to be comprehensive. Over the course of its development and deployment, a resource may be studied many times with the studies in their totality touching on many or most of these aspects, but few resources will be studied completely and many will, inevitably, be studied only minimally.

The evaluation focus changes as we study the different aspects:

1. *The need for the resource*: Evaluators study the clinical status quo absent the resource. They determine the nature of the problems that the resource is intended to address and the frequency with which these problems arise.
2. *The development process*: Evaluators study the skills of the development team and the methodologies employed to understand whether the design is likely to be sound.
3. *The resource's intrinsic structure*: Evaluators study specifications, flowcharts, program codes, and other representations of the resource that they can inspect without running the program.
4. *The resource's functions*: Evaluators study how the resource performs when it is used.
5. *The resource's effects*: Evaluators study not the resource itself but rather its influence on users, patients, and health care organizations.

Several factors characterize an evaluation study:

- *The focus of study*: The focus can be the status quo before introduction of the information resource, the design process adopted, the resource's structure or function, the resource users' simulated decisions or real decisions, or the clinical actions and patient outcomes once the resource is made available in the workplace.

- *Study setting*: Studies of the design process, the resource's structure, and the resource's functions can be conducted outside the active clinical environment, in a laboratory setting, which is easier logistically and may allow greater control over the evaluation process. Studies to elucidate the need for a resource and studies of the resource's effects on users both usually take place in clinical settings. The effects of a resource on patients and health care organizations can take place in only a true clinical setting where the resource is available for use at the time and place where patient-management decisions are made.
- *Clinical data employed*: For many studies, the resource will actually be run. That will require clinical data, which can be simulated data, data abstracted from real patients' records, or actual patient data. Clearly, the kind of data employed in a study has serious implications for the study results and the conclusions that can be drawn.
- *User of the resource*: Most information resources function in interaction with one or more users. In any particular study, the users of the resource can be members of the development team or the evaluation team, or other individuals not representative of those people who will interact with the resource after it is deployed; or the users in a study could be representative of the end users for whose use the resource is ultimately designed. Again, the selection of resource users can affect study results profoundly.
- *The decisions affected by use of the resource*: Many information resources, by providing information or advice to clinicians, seek to influence the decisions made by these clinicians. As a study moves from the laboratory to the clinical setting, the information provided by the resource potentially has greater implications for the decisions being made. Depending on a study's design and purposes, only simulated decisions may be affected (clinicians are asked what they would do, but no action is taken), or real decisions involved in the care of actual patients may be affected.

Table 11.2 lists nine broad types of studies of clinical information resources that can be conducted: the focus of each type, the setting in which it occurs, the kind of clinical data employed as input to the resource, the person who uses the resource during the study, and the kind of clinical decisions affected by the resource during the study. For example, a laboratory-user impact study would be conducted outside the active clinical environment based on simulated or abstracted clinical data. Although it would involve individuals representative of the end-user population, the study would yield primary results derived from simulated clinical decisions, so the clinical care of patients would not be affected. Read across each row of the table to obtain a feel for the contrasts among these study types.

11.4   Approaches to Study Design

Having established a large number of reasons why it can be difficult to study medical information resources, we now introduce the methods that have been developed to address these challenges. We begin by describing a generic structure that all studies share. Then we introduce, in turn, more specific methods of evaluation and the closely related methods of technology assessment.

Tables 11.2 Generic types of evaluation studies of clinical information resources.

Study type	Study setting	Version of the Resource	Sampled users	Sampled tasks	What is observed
1. Needs Assessment	Field	None, or pre-existing resource to be replaced	Anticipated resource users	Actual tasks	User skills, knowledge, decisions or actions; care processes, costs, team function or organization; patient outcomes
2. Design Validation	Development lab	None	None	None	Quality of design method or team
3. Structure Validation	Lab	Prototype or released version	None	None	Quality of resource structure, components, architecture
4. Usability Test	Lab	Prototype or released version	Proxy, real users	Simulated, abstracted	Speed of use, user comments, completion of sample tasks
5. Laboratory Function Study	Lab	Prototype or released version	Proxy, real users	Simulated, abstracted	Speed & quality of data collected or displayed; accuracy of advice given
6. Field Function Study	Field	Prototype or released version	Proxy, real users	Real	Speed & quality of data collected or displayed; accuracy of advice given
7. Lab User Effect Study	Lab	Prototype or released version	Real users	Abstracted, real	Impact on user knowledge, simulated / pretend decisions or actions
8. Field User Effect Study	Field	Released version	Real users	Real	Extent and nature of resource use. Impact on user knowledge, real decisions, real actions
9. Problem Impact Study	Field	Released version	Real users	Real	Care processes, costs, team function, cost effectiveness

11.4.1   The Anatomy of All Studies

The structural elements that all studies share are illustrated in Figure 11.3. Evaluations are guided by someone's or some group's need to know. No matter who that someone is—the development team, the funding agency, or other individuals and groups—the evaluation must begin with a process of negotiation to identify the questions that will be a starting point for the study. The outcomes of these negotiations are an understanding of how the evaluation is to be conducted, usually stated in a written contract or agreement, and an initial expression of the questions the evaluation seeks to answer. The next element of the study is investigation: the collection of data to address these questions and, depending on the approach selected, possibly other questions that arise during the study. The mechanisms are numerous, ranging from the performance of the resource on a series of benchmark tasks to observations of users working with the resource.

The next element is a mechanism for reporting the information back to the individuals who need to know it. The format of the report must be in line with the stipulations of the contract; the content of the report follows from the questions asked and the data collected. The report is most often a written document, but it does not have to be—the purposes of some evaluations are well served by oral reports or by live demonstrations. We emphasize that it is the evaluator's obligation to establish a process through which the results of her study are communicated, thus creating the potential for the study's findings to be put to constructive use. No investigator can guarantee a constructive outcome for a study, but there is much they can do to increase the likelihood of a salutary result. Also note that a salutary result of a study is not necessarily one that casts the resource under study in a positive light. A salutary result is one where the stakeholders learn important information from the study findings.

11.4.2   Philosophical Bases of Approaches to Evaluation

Several authors have developed classifications, or **typologies**, of evaluation methods or approaches. Among the best is that developed in 1980 by Ernest House. A major

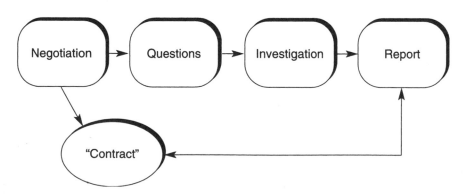

Figure 11.3. Anatomy of all evaluation studies. (*Source*: Friedman and Wyatt, 1997a.)

advantage of House's typology is that each approach is linked elegantly to an underlying philosophical model, as detailed in his book. This classification divides current practice into eight discrete approaches, four of which may be viewed as **objectivist** and four of which may be viewed as **subjectivist**. This distinction is very important. Note that these approaches are not entitled objective and subjective, because those words carry strong and fundamentally misleading connotations: of scientific precision in the former case and of imprecise intellectual voyeurism in the latter.

The objectivist approaches derive from a **logical–positivist** philosophical orientation—the same orientation that underlies the classic experimental sciences. The major premises underlying the objectivist approaches are as follows:

- In general, attributes of interest are properties of the resource under study. More specifically, this position suggests that the merit and worth of an information resource— the attributes of most interest in evaluation—can in principle be measured with all observations yielding the same result. It also assumes that an investigator can measure these attributes without affecting how the resource under study functions or is used.
- Rational persons can and should agree on what attributes of a resource are important to measure and what results of these measurements would be identified as a most desirable, correct, or positive outcome. In medical informatics, making this assertion is tantamount to stating that a gold standard of resource performance can always be identified and that all rational individuals can be brought to consensus on what this gold standard is.
- Because numerical measurement allows precise statistical analysis of performance over time or performance in comparison with some alternative, numerical measurement is prima facie superior to a verbal description. Verbal, descriptive data (generally known as qualitative data) are useful in only preliminary studies to identify hypotheses for subsequent, precise analysis using quantitative methods.
- Falsification: while it is possible to disprove a well-formulated scientific hypothesis, it is never possible to fully prove one; thus science proceeds by successive disproof of previously plausible hypotheses.
- Through these kinds of comparisons, it is possible to demonstrate to a reasonable degree that a resource is or is not superior to what it replaced or to a competing resource.

Contrast these assumptions with a set of assumptions that derives from an **intuitionist–pluralist** philosophical position that spawns a set of subjectivist approaches to evaluation:

- What is observed about a resource depends in fundamental ways on the observer. Different observers of the same phenomenon might legitimately come to different conclusions. Both can be objective in their appraisals even if they do not agree; it is not necessary that one is right and the other wrong.
- Merit and worth must be explored in context. The value of a resource emerges through study of the resource as it functions in a particular patient care or educational environment.

- Individuals and groups can legitimately hold different perspectives on what constitutes the most desirable outcome of introducing a resource into an environment. There is no reason to expect them to agree, and it may be counterproductive to try to lead them to consensus. An important aspect of an evaluation would be to document the ways in which they disagree.
- Verbal description can be highly illuminating. Qualitative data are valuable, in and of themselves, and can lead to conclusions as convincing as those drawn from quantitative data. The value of qualitative data, therefore, goes far beyond that of identifying issues for later "precise" exploration using quantitative methods.
- Evaluation should be viewed as an exercise in argument, rather than as a demonstration, because any study appears equivocal when subjected to serious scrutiny.

The approaches to evaluation that derive from this subjectivist philosophical perspective may seem strange, imprecise, and unscientific when considered for the first time. This perception stems in large part from the widespread acceptance of the objectivist worldview in biomedicine. The importance and utility of subjectivist approaches in evaluation is, however, emerging. Within medical informatics, there is growing support for such approaches (Rothschild et al., 1990; Forsythe and Buchanan, 1992; Ash et al., 2003; Anderson et al., 1995). As stated earlier, the evaluation mindset includes methodological eclecticism. It is important for people trained in classic experimental methods at least to understand, and possibly even to embrace, the subjectivist worldview if they are to conduct fully informative evaluation studies.

11.4.3   Multiple Approaches to Evaluation

House (1980) classifies evaluation into eight approaches. Although most evaluation studies conducted in the real world can be unambiguously tied to one of these approaches, the categories are not mutually exclusive. Some studies exhibit properties of several approaches and are thus not cleanly classified. The first four approaches derive from the objectivist position; the second four are subjectivist.

Comparison Based

The **comparison-based approach** employs experiments and quasi-experiments. The information resource under study is compared with a control condition, a placebo, or a contrasting resource. The comparison is based on a relatively small number of **outcome variables** that are assessed in all groups; randomization, controls, and statistical inference are used to argue that the information resource was the cause of any differences observed. Examples of comparison-based studies include McDonald's work on physician reminders (McDonald et al., 1984a) and the studies from Stanford on rule-based systems (Yu et al., 1979a; Hickam et al., 1985a). The 98 controlled trials of medical decision-support systems reviewed by Hunt and co-workers (1998) fall under the comparison-based approach. The Turing test (Turing, 1950) can be seen as a specific model for a comparison-based evaluation.

Objectives Based

The **objectives-based approach** seeks to determine whether a resource meets its designer's objectives. Ideally, such objectives are stated in great detail, so there is little ambiguity in developing procedures to measure their degree of attainment. These studies are comparative only in the sense that the observed performance of the resource is viewed in relation to stated objectives. The concern is whether the resource is performing up to expectations; it is not whether the resource is outperforming what it replaced. The objectives that are the benchmarks for these studies are typically stated at an early stage of resource development. Although clearly suited to laboratory testing of a new resource, this approach can also be applied to testing of an installed resource. Consider the example of a resource to provide advice to emergency-room physicians (Wyatt, 1989). The designers might set as an objective that the system's advice be available within 15 minutes of the time the patient is first seen. An evaluation study that measured the time for this advice to be delivered, and compared that time with this objective, would be objectives based.

Decision Facilitation

In the **decision facilitation approach**, evaluation seeks to resolve issues important to developers and administrators so that these individuals can make decisions about the future of the resource. The questions that are posed are those that the decision makers state, although the people conducting the evaluation may help the decision makers to frame these questions to be amenable to study. The data-collection methods follow from the questions posed. These studies tend to be formative in focus. The results of studies conducted at the early stages of resource development are used to chart the course of further development, which in turn generates new questions for further study. A systematic study of alternative formats for computer-generated advisories, conducted while the resource to generate the advisories is still under development, is a good example of this approach (de Bliek et al., 1988).

Goal Free

In the three approaches described, the evaluation is guided by a set of goals for the information resource or by specific questions that the developers either state or play a profound role in shaping. Any such study will be polarized by these manifest goals and may be more sensitive to anticipated than to unanticipated effects. In the **goal-free approach**, the people conducting the evaluation are purposefully blinded to the intended effects of an information resource and pursue whatever evidence they can gather to enable them to identify all the effects of the resource, intended or not (Scriven, 1973). This approach is rarely applied in practice, but it is useful to individuals designing evaluations to remind them of the many effects an information resource can engender.

Quasi-Legal

The **quasi-legal approach** establishes a mock trial, or other formal adversary proceeding, to judge a resource. Proponents and opponents of the resource offer testimony and may be examined and cross-examined in a manner resembling standard courtroom procedure. A jury that is witness to the proceedings can then, on the basis of this testimony, make a decision about the merit of the resource. As in a debate, the issue can be decided by the persuasive power of rhetoric as well as by the persuasive power of what is portrayed as fact. There are few examples of this technique formally applied to medical informatics, but the technique has been applied to facilitate difficult decisions in other medical areas such as treatment of sickle cell disease (Smith, 1992).

Art Criticism

The **art criticism approach** relies on methods of art criticism and the principle of connoisseurship (Eisner, 1991). Under this approach, an experienced and respected critic, who may or may not be trained in the domain of the resource but who has a great deal of experience with resources of this generic type, works with the resource. The critic then writes a review highlighting the benefits and shortcomings of the resource. Clearly, the art criticism approach cannot be definitive if the critic is not an expert in the subject domain of a medical informatics resource, because the critic will be unable to judge the clinical or scientific accuracy of the resource's knowledge base or of the advice that it provides. Nonetheless, the thoughtful and articulate comments of an experienced reviewer can help other people to appreciate important features of a resource. Software reviews are examples of this approach in common practice.

Professional Review

The **professional-review approach** is well known in the form of **site visits**. This approach employs panels of experienced peers who spend several days in the environment where the resource is installed. Site visits are often guided by a set of guidelines specific to the type of project under study but sufficiently generic to accord the reviewers a great deal of control over the conduct of any particular visit. The reviewers are generally free to speak with whomever they wish and to ask these individuals whatever they consider important to know. They may also request documents for review. Over the course of a site visit, unanticipated issues may emerge. The site visitors typically explore both the anticipated issues and the questions articulated in the guidelines and those that emerge during the site visit itself. The result is a report usually drafted on site or very soon after the visit is completed.

Responsive–Illuminative

The **responsive–illuminative approach** seeks to represent the viewpoints of both users of the resource and people who are an otherwise significant part of the clinical environment where the resource operates (Hamilton et al., 1977). The goal is understanding or illumination rather than judgment. The methods used derive largely from ethnography. The investigators immerse themselves in the environment where the resource is operational. The designs of these studies are not rigidly predetermined. They develop dynamically as the investigators' experience accumulates. The study team begins with a minimal set of orienting questions; the deeper questions that receive thoroughgoing study evolve over time. Many examples of studies using this approach can be found in the literature of medical informatics (Fafchamps et al., 1991; Forsythe, 1992; Ash et. al., 2003).

Note that the study types described in Table 11.2 relate to the purposes, foci, settings, and logistics of evaluation studies. The evaluation approaches introduced in this section address a complementary issue, What methods will be used to identify specific questions and to collect data as part of the actual conduct of these studies? Although it is perhaps extreme to state that every evaluation approach can apply to every type of study, there is certainly potential to use both objectivist and subjectivist approaches throughout Table 11.2. At the two extremes, for example, both need-validation studies and clinical-effects studies provide opportunities for application of subjectivist as well as objectivist approaches.

11.4.4   Stages of Technology Assessment

Yet another way to categorize studies is according to the three stages of technology assessment (Fuchs and Garber, 1990; Garber and Owens, 1994). The first stage emphasizes **technical characteristics**, such as the response time of an information system to a query or the resolution of an imaging system. The second stage emphasizes the **efficacy** or effectiveness of a device, information system, or diagnostic or therapeutic strategy (Fuchs and Garber, 1990). Clinical trials of information systems usually fit this category, as do randomized trials of clinical interventions. The trials often use **process measures**, such as the degree of physician compliance with computer-generated reminders or the change in laboratory parameters in response to treatment rather than the endpoints that matter to patients: mortality, morbidity, and cost. Studies that determine the sensitivity and specificity of diagnostic tests are another example of second-stage assessments (see Chapter 3).

Third-stage assessments directly evaluate effectiveness via health and economic **outcomes**; therefore, these evaluations are the most comprehensive technology assessments (Fuchs and Garber, 1990). A third-stage evaluation of a computer-based reminder system for breast cancer screening would examine changes in mortality or morbidity from breast cancer rather than physician compliance with guidelines. Typically, a third-stage evaluation also would evaluate the costs of such a system. When outcomes are infrequent or occur after a long delay (such as the occurrence of breast cancer), third-stage evaluations may be substantially more difficult to perform than are second-stage evaluations; thus, third-stage assessments are uncommon in medical informatics (see Garg et al., 1998). Third-stage evaluations also may consider the importance of patients' preferences in assessing the outcomes of an intervention (Nease and Owens, 1994; Owens, 1998a).

We now examine the types of studies that investigators may initiate for each of the stages of technology assessment.

Stage I Assessments: Technical Characteristics

The choice of what to evaluate during a first-stage technology assessment depends on the purpose of the evaluation (Friedman and Wyatt, 1997b). Possibilities include the evaluation of the design and development process of a clinical information resource or of the structure of the resource (the hardware, input and output devices, user interface, internal data, knowledge structures, processor, algorithms, or inference methods). An assessment of the design and development process could evaluate the software engineering of the resource. Such an evaluation might be important to assess how the resource could be integrated with other systems or platforms. The rationale for studying the structure of the resource is the assumption that, if the resource contains appropriately designed components linked together in a suitable architecture, the system is more likely to function correctly.

Stage II Assessments: Clinical Efficacy

Second-stage assessments move beyond evaluation of operating parameters to an evaluation of the function of the information resource. These evaluations are increasingly common. Recent systematic reviews report over 100 clinical trials of information resources (Balas et al., 1996; Shea et al., 1996; Hunt et al., 1998). Examples of second-stage evaluations include studies of computer-assisted drug dosing; preventive care reminder systems; and computer-aided quality assurance programs for active medical problems. The majority of these second-stage evaluations assess the effect of information resources on the process of care. Did the clinician prescribe the right drug dose? Did the patient receive an influenza vaccine? In situations in which a process measure correlates closely with health outcome (e.g., use of thrombolytic therapy for patients who have heart attacks correlates closely with decreased mortality rates), use of the process measure will not adversely affect validity and will increase the feasibility of the study (Mant and Hicks, 1995). The link from many interventions to the intended health and economic outcomes is not, however, well defined; in these circumstances, a second-stage technology assessment may not be sufficient to justify implementation of a system, particularly if the system is costly.

Stage III Assessments: Comprehensive Clinical Effectiveness, Economic, and Social Outcomes

Rising health care costs have forced policymakers, clinicians, and developers to assess whether health interventions provide sufficient value for the required economic investment. Thus, a demonstration of efficacy is often not sufficient. Proponents of a technology must also establish its cost effectiveness (see Section 11.5.5 for a more detailed explanation of cost-effectiveness studies). The third stage of technology assessment encompasses these more sophisticated assessments. The hallmark of these evaluations is a comprehensive assessment of health and economic outcomes. Studies that evaluate comprehensive outcomes will be more useful than studies that evaluate narrowly defined outcomes. Thus, a study that evaluates the cost effectiveness of an information resource in terms of dollars per quality-adjusted life year (QALY) saved (see Chapter 3) would enable clinicians and policymakers to compare the cost effectiveness of an information resource to a wide variety of other interventions. In contrast, a study that evaluates an information resource in terms of dollars per case of cancer prevented would provide a useful comparison only for other interventions that prevent cancer.

The choice of outcome measures for a third-stage assessment depends on the purpose of the study and on the cost and feasibility of measuring the outcome. Common choices include the number of lives saved, life-years saved, quality-adjusted life years saved, cancers prevented, and cases of disease averted. For example, a third-stage evaluation of a computer-generated protocol for treatment of hypertension could measure changes in blood pressure of patients whose care was governed by the protocol. The evaluation could also assess the costs of implementing the protocol and subsequently the cost effectiveness of the implementation of the computer-generated protocol. An evaluation of computer-based guidelines for care of people who have human immunodeficiency virus (HIV) evaluated the effect of the guideline on the rate of hospitalization for opportunistic infection (Safran et al., 1995). The study found that, under the guidelines, providers responded more rapidly to changes in patient status (such as abnormal laboratory tests), but this prompt action did not change the rate of hospitalization. This study highlights the difficulty of demonstrating that a beneficial change in the process of care has led to improved health outcomes. In fact, few studies have demonstrated that information resources improve health outcomes (Garg et al., 1998). The studies may not show benefit because of inadequate sample sizes, use of outcome measures that are difficult to assess, inadequate follow-up, other weaknesses in study design, or interventions that do not work (Rotman et al., 1996).

In summary, the requirements of a technology assessment have expanded to include comprehensive health, economic, and social outcomes. Third-stage technology assessment is a particular challenge in medical informatics. Although the use of process measures will be appropriate for third-stage assessment when evidence from systematic reviews shows that process measures correlate very well with patient outcomes, until that time investigators will need to plan studies that explicitly incorporate comprehensive health and economic outcomes.

11.5   Conduct of Objectivist Studies

In this section, we focus on the comparison-based approach, which is the most widely used objectivist approach and which also is the basis of most work in technology assessment.

11.5.1   Structure and Terminology of Comparative Studies

In a comparative study, the investigator typically creates a contrasting set of conditions to compare the effects of one with those of another. Usually, the goal is to attribute cause and effect or to answer scientific questions raised by other kinds of studies. After identifying a sample of participants for the study, the researcher assigns each participant, often randomly, to one or a set of conditions. Some variable of interest is measured for each participant. The aggregated values of this variable are compared across the conditions. To understand the many issues that affect design of comparative studies, we must develop a precise terminology.

The participants in a study are the entities about which data are collected. A specific study will employ one sample of participants, although this sample might be subdivided if, for example, participants are assigned to conditions in a comparative design. It is key to emphasize that participants are often people—either care providers or recipients—but also may be information resources, groups of people, or organizations. In informatics, medical care is conducted in hierarchical settings with naturally occurring groups (a "doctor's patients"; the "care providers in a ward team"), so we often face the challenging question of exactly who the subjects are.

Variables are specific characteristics of the participants that either are measured purposefully by the investigator or are self-evident properties of the participants that do not require measurement. In the simplest study, there may be only one variable, for example, the time required for a user of an information system to complete a particular task.

Some variables take on a continuous range of values. Others have a discrete set of levels corresponding to each of the measured values that that variable can have. For example, in a hospital setting, physician members of a ward team can be classified as residents, fellows, or attendings. In this case, the variable "physician's level of qualification" has three levels.

The **dependent variables** form a subset of the variables in the study that captures the outcomes of interest to the investigator. For this reason, dependent variables are also called **outcome variables**. A study may have one or more dependent variables. In a typical study, the dependent variable will be computed, for each subject, as an average over a number of tasks. For example, clinicians' diagnostic performance may be measured over a set of cases, or "tasks", that provide a range of diagnostic challenges. (In studies in which computers or people solve problems or work through clinical cases, we use the term "task" generically to refer to those problems or cases. Designing or choosing tasks can be the most challenging aspect of an evaluation.)

The **independent variables** are included in a study to explain the measured values of the dependent variables. For example, whether a computer system is available, or not, to support certain clinical tasks could be the major independent variable in a study designed to evaluate that system. A purely descriptive study has no independent variables; comparative studies can have one or many independent variables.

Measurement challenges almost always arise in the assessment of the outcome or dependent variable for a study. Often, for example, the dependent variable is some type of performance measure that invokes concerns about reliability (precision) and validity (accuracy) of measurement. Depending on the study, the independent variables may also raise measurement challenges. When the independent variable is gender, for example, the measurement problems are relatively straightforward. If the independent variable is an attitude, level of experience, or extent of resource use, however, profound measurement challenges can arise.

11.5.2   *Issues of Measurement*

Measurement is the process of assigning a value corresponding to the presence, absence, or degree of a specific attribute in a specific object, as illustrated in Figure 11.4. Measurement usually results in either (1) the assignment of a numerical score representing the extent to which the attribute of interest is present in the object, or (2) the assignment of an object to a specific category. Taking the temperature (attribute) of a patient (object) is an example of the process of measurement.[2]

From the premises underlying objectivist studies (see Section 11.4.2), it follows that proper execution of such studies requires careful and specific attention to methods of measurement. It can never be assumed, particularly in informatics, that attributes of interest are measured without error. Accurate and precise measurement must not be an afterthought. Measurement is of particular importance in medical informatics because, as a relatively young field, informatics does not have a well-established tradition of "variables worth measuring" or proven instruments for measuring them. By and large, people planning studies are faced first with the task of deciding what to measure and then with that of developing their own measurement methods. For most researchers, these tasks prove to be harder and more time consuming than initially anticipated. In some cases, informatics investigators can adapt the measures used by other investigators, but often they need to apply their measures to a different setting where prior experience may not apply.

We can underscore the importance of measurement by establishing a formal distinction between studies undertaken to develop methods for making measurements, which

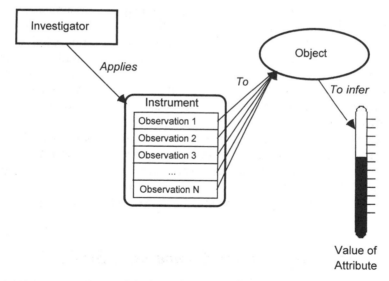

Figure 11.4. The process of measurement. (*Source*: Friedman and Wyatt, 1997a.)

---

[2]When we speak specifically of measurement, it is customary to use the term "object" to refer to the entity on which measurements are made.

we call measurement studies, and the subsequent use of these methods to address questions of direct importance in informatics, which we call demonstration studies. **Measurement studies** seek to determine how accurately an attribute of interest can be measured in a population of objects. In an ideal objectivist measurement, all observers will agree on the result of the measurement. Any disagreement is therefore due to error, which should be minimized. The more agreement among observers or across observations, the better the measurement. Measurement procedures developed and validated through measurement studies provide researchers with what they need to conduct **demonstration studies** that directly address questions of substantive and practical concern. Once we know how accurately we can measure an attribute using a particular procedure, we can employ the measured values of this attribute as a variable in a demonstration study to draw inferences about the performance, perceptions, or effects of an information resource. For example, once a measurement study has explored how accurately the speed of an information resource can be measured, a related demonstration study would explore whether a particular resource has sufficient speed—speed being measured using methods developed in the measurement study—to meet the needs of busy clinicians.

A detailed discussion of measurement issues is beyond the scope of this chapter. The bottom line is that investigators should know that their measurement methods will be adequate before they collect data for their studies. It is necessary to perform a measurement study, involving data collection on a small scale, to establish the adequacy of all measurement procedures if the measures to be used do not have an established track record. Even if the measurement procedures of interest do have a track record in a particular health care environment and with a specific mix of cases and care providers, they may not perform equally well in a different environment, so measurement studies may still be necessary. Researchers should always ask themselves, "How good are my measures in this particular setting?" whenever they are planning a study, before they proceed to the demonstration phase. The importance of measurement studies for informatics was explained in 1990 by Michaelis and co-workers. A more recent study (Friedman et al., 2003) has demonstrated that studies of clinical information systems have not systematically addressed the adequacy of the methods used to measure the specific outcomes reported in these studies.

Whenever possible, investigators planning studies should employ established measurement methods, with a "track record", rather than developing their own. While there exist relatively few compendia and measurement instruments specifically for informatics, web-based resource listing over 50 instruments asscoiated with the development, usability, and impact of information systems at http://www.isworld.org/ surveyinstruments/surveyinstruments.htm.

11.5.3   Control Strategies in Comparative Studies

One of the most challenging questions in comparative study design is how to obtain control. We need a way to monitor all the other changes taking place that are not attributable to the information resource. In clinical medicine, it is occasionally possible to predict patient outcomes with good accuracy from a small set of initial clinical findings—for example, the survival of patients in intensive care (Knaus et al., 1991). In these unusual circumstances, where we have a mechanism to tell us what would have happened to patients if we had not intervened, we can compare what actually happens with what is predicted to draw tentative conclusions about the benefit of the information resource. Such accurate predictive models are, however, extremely unusual in medicine (Wyatt and Altman, 1995). Instead, we use various types of controls: subjects who complete tasks that are not affected by the intervention of interest.

In the following sections we review a series of control strategies. We employ as a running example a reminder system that prompts doctors to order prophylactic antibiotics for orthopedic patients to prevent postoperative infections. In this example, the intervention is the installation and commissioning of the reminder system; the subjects are the physicians; and the tasks are the patients cared for by the physicians. The dependent variables derive from the outcome measurements made and would include physicians' ordering of antibiotics and the rate of postoperative infections averaged across the patients cared for by each physician.

Descriptive (Uncontrolled) Studies

In the simplest possible design, an uncontrolled or **descriptive study**, we install the reminder system, allow a suitable period for training, and then make our measurements. There is no independent variable. Suppose that we discover that the overall postoperative infection rate is 5 percent and that physicians order prophylactic antibiotics in 60 percent of orthopedic cases. Although we have two measured dependent variables, it is hard to interpret these figures without any comparison—it is possible that there has been no change due to the system.

Historically Controlled Experiments

As a first improvement to a descriptive study, let us consider a **historically controlled experiment**, sometimes called a **before–after study**. The investigator makes **baseline** measurements of antibiotic ordering and postoperative infection rates before the information resource is installed, and then makes the same measurements after the information resource is in routine use. The independent variable is time and has two levels: before and after resource installation. Let us say that, at baseline, the postoperative infection rates were 10 percent and doctors ordered prophylactic antibiotics in only 40 percent of cases; the postintervention figures are the same as before (see Table 11.3).

The evaluators may claim that the halving of the infection rate can be safely ascribed to the information resource, especially because it was accompanied by a 20 percent improvement in doctors' antibiotic prescribing. Many other factors might, however, have changed in the interim to cause these results, especially if there was a long interval between the baseline and postintervention measurements. New staff could have taken over, the case mix of patients could have altered, new prophylactic antibiotics may have been introduced, or clinical audit meetings may have highlighted the infection problem and thus caused greater clinical awareness. Simply assuming that the reminder system alone caused the reduction in infection rates is naive. Other factors, known or unknown,

Table 11.3. Hypothetical results of historically controlled study of an antibiotic reminder system.

	Antibiotic prescribing rate	Postoperative infection rate
Baseline results (before installation)	40%	10%
Postinstallation results	60%	5%

(*Source*: Friedman and Wyatt, 1997a.)

could have changed meanwhile, making untenable the simple assumption that our intervention is responsible for all of the observed effects.

An improvement on this design is to add either internal or external controls—preferably both. The internal control should be a measure likely to be affected by any nonspecific changes happening in the local environment, but unaffected by the intervention. The external control can be exactly the same measure as in the target environment, but in a similar external setting, e.g., another hospital. If the measure of interest changes while there is no change in either internal or external controls, a skeptic needs to be quite resourceful to claim that the system is not responsible (Wyatt & Wyatt, 2003).

Simultaneous Nonrandomized Controls

To address some of the problems with historical controls, we might use **simultaneous controls**, which requires us to make our outcome measurements in doctors and patients who are not influenced by the prophylactic antibiotic reminder system but who are subject to the other changes taking place in the environment. Taking measurements both before and during the intervention strengthens the design, because it gives an estimate of the changes due to the nonspecific factors taking place during the study period.

This study design would be a parallel group comparative study with simultaneous controls. Table 11.4 gives hypothetical results of such a study, focusing on postoperative infection rates as a single outcome measure or dependent variable. The independent variables are time and group, both of which have two levels of intervention and control. There is the same improvement in the group where reminders were available, but no improvement—indeed a slight deterioration—where no reminders were available. This design provides suggestive evidence of an improvement that is most likely to be due to the reminder system. This inference is stronger if the same doctors worked in the same wards during the period the system was introduced, and if similar kinds of patients, subject to the same nonspecific influences, were being operated on during the whole time period.

Table 11.4. Hypothetical results of simultaneous controlled study of antibiotic reminder system.

	Postoperative infection rates	
	Reminder group	Control group
Baseline results	10%	10%
Postintervention results	5%	11%

(*Source*: Friedman and Wyatt, 1997a.)

Even though the controls in this example are simultaneous, skeptics may still refute our argument by claiming that there is some systematic, unknown difference between the clinicians or patients in the two groups. For example, if the two groups comprised the patients and clinicians in two adjacent wards, the difference in the infection rates could be attributable to systematic or chance differences between the wards. Perhaps hospital-staffing levels improved in some wards but not in others, or there was cross infection by a multiple-resistant organism only among the patients in the control ward. To overcome such criticisms, we could expand the study to include all wards in the hospital—or even other hospitals—but that would clearly take considerable resources. We could try to measure everything that happens to every patient in both wards and to build complete psychological profiles of all staff to rule out systematic differences. We would still, however, be vulnerable to the accusation that some variable that we did not measure—did not even know about—explains the difference between the two wards. A better strategy is to ensure that the controls really are comparable by randomizing them.

Simultaneous Randomized Controls

The crucial problem in the previous example is that, although the controls were simultaneous, there may have been systematic, unmeasured differences between them and the subjects receiving the intervention. A simple and effective way of removing systematic differences, whether due to known or unknown factors, is to randomize the assignment of subjects to control or intervention groups. Thus, we could randomly allocate one-half of the doctors on both wards to receive the antibiotic reminders and the remaining doctors to work normally. We would then measure and compare postoperative infection rates in patients managed by doctors in the reminder and control groups. Provided that the doctors never look after one another's patients, any difference that is statistically "significant" (conventionally, for which the p value is less than 0.05) can be attributed reliably to the reminders. The only way other differences could have emerged is by chance.

Table 11.5 shows the hypothetical results of such a study. The baseline infection rates in the patients managed by the two groups of doctors are similar, as we would expect, because the patients were allocated to the groups by chance. There is a greater reduction in infection rates in patients of reminder physicians compared with those of control physicians. Because random assignment means that there was no systematic difference in patient characteristics between groups, the only systematic difference between the two groups of patients is receipt of reminders by their doctors.

Table 11.5. Hypothetical results of a simultaneous randomized controlled study of antibiotic reminder system.

	Postoperative infection rates	
	Reminder physicians	Control physicians
Baseline results	11%	10%
Postinstallation results	6%	8%

(*Source*: Friedman and Wyatt, 1997a.)

Provided that the sample size is large enough for these results to be statistically significant, we might begin to conclude with some confidence that providing doctors with reminders caused the reduction in infection rates. One lingering question is why there was also a small reduction, from baseline to installation, in infection rates in control cases, even though the control group should have received no reminders.

11.5.4   *Threats to Inference and Validity*

We all want our studies to be valid. There are two aspects to this: internal and external validity. If a study has **internal validity**, we can be confident in the conclusions drawn from the specific circumstances of the experiment—the population of subjects studied, the measurements made, and the interventions provided. Are we justified in concluding that the differences observed are due to the attributed causes? Even if all threats to internal validity are overcome to our satisfaction, we would also like our study to have **external validity**, such that the conclusions can be generalized from the specific setting, subjects, and intervention studied to the broader range of settings that other people will encounter. Thus, even if we demonstrate convincingly that our antibiotic reminder system reduces postoperative infection rates in our own hospital, this finding is of little interest to other clinicians unless we can convince them that the results can be generalized safely to other reminder systems or to the same system in other hospitals.

When we conduct a comparative study, there are four possible outcomes. We illustrate them in the context of a study that explores the effectiveness of an information resource and that uses an appropriate comparative design as follows:

1. The information resource was truly effective, and our study shows that it was.
2. The information resource was truly ineffective, and our study shows that it was.
3. The information resource was truly effective, but for some reason our study mistakenly failed to show that it was.
4. The information resource was truly ineffective, but for some reason our study mistakenly suggested that it was effective.

Outcomes 1 and 2 are salutary from a methodological viewpoint, the results of the study mirror reality. Outcome 3 is a false-negative result, or **type II error**. In the language of inferential statistics, we mistakenly accept the **null hypothesis**. Type II errors can arise because the size of the information resource's effect on the measure of interest is small and too few subjects have been included for the study to detect it (Freiman et al., 1978). Alternatively, we may have failed to measure the outcome variable on which the example resource is having an effect. In outcome 4, we have concluded that the resource is valuable when it is not; we have a false-positive result or **type I error**. We have mistakenly rejected the null hypothesis. A risk of a type I error is built into every study. When we accept, for example, the conventional value of $p < 0.05$ as a criterion for statistical significance, we are consciously accepting a 5 percent risk of making a type I error as a consequence of using randomization as a mechanism of experimental control. If we feel uncomfortable with this 5 percent risk of a false-positive result or type I error, we can reduce it by reducing the threshold for statistical significance to 0.01, which carries only a 1 percent chance of a type I error.

The more important threats to internal validity of studies are the following:

- **Assessment bias**: It is important to ensure that all persons involved in making measurements do not allow their own feelings and beliefs about an information resource—positive or negative—to bias the results. Consider a study in which the same clinicians who are users of an antibiotic reminder system also collect the clinical data used for determining whether the advice generated by the system is correct, such as the incidence of significant wound or chest infections. If they had some prejudice against the reminder system and wished to undermine it, they might massage the clinical infection data to prove themselves right and the reminder system wrong in certain patients. Thus, they might record that a patient was suffering from a nonexistent postoperative cough with productive sputum to justify an antibiotic prescription that the reminder system had not advised.

- **Allocation bias**: Early studies of information resources often take place in the environment in which the resources were developed and often arouse strong (positive or negative) feelings among study subjects. In a study where patients are randomized and the subjects have strong beliefs about the information resource, two biases may arise. Investigators may cheat the randomization method and systematically allocate easier (or more difficult) cases to the information resource group (allocation bias), or they may avoid recruiting a particularly easy (or difficult) case to the study if they know in advance that the next patient will be allocated to the control group recruitment bias (Schulz et al., 1995).

- The **Hawthorne effect**: The Hawthorne effect is the tendency for humans to improve their performance if they know it is being studied. Psychologists measured the effect of ambient lighting on workers' productivity at the Hawthorne factory in Chicago (Roethligsburger and Dickson, 1939). Productivity increased as the room illumination level was raised, but productivity increased again when the illumination level was accidentally reduced. The study itself, rather than changes in illumination, caused the increases. During a study of a medical information resource, the attention of the investigators can lead to an improvement in the performance of all subjects in all study groups, intervention and control, due to the Hawthorne effect.

- The **checklist effect**: The checklist effect is the improvement observed in decision making due to more complete and better-structured data collection when paper-based or computer-based forms are used to collect patient data. The effect of forms on decision making can equal that of computer-generated advice (Adams et al., 1986), so it must either be controlled for or quantified. To control for the checklist effect, investigators should collect the same data in the same way in the control and information resource groups, even though the information resource's output is available only in the latter group (see for e.g., Wyatt, 1989).

- The **placebo effect**: In some drug trials, simply giving patients an inactive tablet or other placebo can cause a measurable improvement in some clinical variables such as well-being, sleep pattern, and exercise tolerance, because patients feel good about receiving attention and potentially useful medication. This placebo effect may be more powerful than the drug effect itself and may obscure a complete absence of pharmaceutical benefit. In a study of a medical information resource, if some patients watch their doctors consult an impressive workstation while others have no such experience, this experience could unbalance the groups and overestimate the value of the information resource. Alternatively, some patients might believe that a care provider who needs a computer workstation is less competent than one who can manage without. Several studies have, however, shown that patients show more confidence in clinicians who use technology than in those who get by without it.

These and a number of other biases that may apply in certain kinds of studies are more fully discussed in Chapter 7 of Friedman and Wyatt (2006).

11.5.5   Cost-Effectiveness and Cost-Benefit Studies

The purpose of cost-effectiveness and cost-benefit analyses is to assess quantitatively the benefits obtained from a health intervention relative to the costs of the intervention. In short, cost-effectiveness and cost-benefit analyses provide a mechanism to assess the relative value of different interventions in producing health benefits, such as longer life or greater quality of life. Our description of these analyses is brief; for further details, see Gold (1996), Weinstein and Fineberg (1980), and Sox et al. (1988). In a **cost-effectiveness analysis**, the analyst expresses the health benefits in units of health outcomes (e.g., lives saved) and the costs in dollars. The analysts can choose the health outcomes that they believe as appropriate for the purpose of the analysis, such as life years saved, quality-adjusted life years saved, or cases of disease prevented. Usually the analyst seeks to compare the cost and health effects of one treatment relative to the costs and health effects of another treatment. In such a situation, the appropriate estimate of the relative value of the interventions is the **incremental cost-effectiveness ratio**. To calculate the incremental cost-effectiveness ratio for intervention "b" relative to intervention "a", we divide the difference in the costs with the two interventions by the difference in health benefits. For example, for interventions whose benefits are measured as increases in life expectancy (LE), we calculate the incremental cost-effectiveness ratio for intervention "b" relative to intervention "a" as

$$(C_b - C_a)/(LE_b - LE_a)$$

where C_b is the cost of intervention "b", C_a is the cost of intervention "a", LE_b is the life expectancy with intervention "b", and LE_a is life expectancy with intervention "a."

In contrast to cost-effectiveness analyses, a **cost-benefit analysis** values all benefits and costs in dollars. Thus, if a health intervention averts a death, the analyst must express the value of that averted death in dollars. The goal of such an analysis is to determine whether the benefit (expressed in dollars) is larger than the cost (expressed in dollars).

To perform a cost-effectiveness analysis, the analyst must perform the following steps (Office of Technology Assessment, 1980; Gold et al., 1996): (1) define the problem, including identification of the objective and perspective of the analysis, and the alternative interventions under consideration; (2) identify and analyze the benefits; (3) identify and analyze the costs; (4) perform discounting; (5) analyze uncertainties; (6) address ethical questions; and (7) interpret the results. We shall illustrate these concepts with the example that we used in Section 11.5.3 of a computer-based reminder system that prompts physicians to order prophylactic antibiotics before orthopedic surgery.

The first step of a cost-effectiveness analysis is to define the problem clearly. Failure to define the problem carefully can lead to many difficulties. One approach to defining the problem is to determine the decision context. What decision does the analyst, or the consumer of the analysis, need to make? Is the decision whether to implement a computer-based antibiotic reminder system or a manual system? Or, is the decision which computer-based antibiotic reminder system to implement? Or, do the decision makers seek to know whether to implement a computer-based system or to hire a nurse practitioner to check the antibiotic orders? Answers to these questions will enable the analyst to frame the analysis appropriately.

To ensure that the cost-effectiveness ratio that the analyst calculates will be helpful for the decision makers, the analyst should also identify the objective of the study. Is the objective to reduce hospital costs or all costs? A program that reduced hospital costs could do so by shifting certain costs to the outpatient setting. Is that a concern? The analyst should also determine the perspective of the analysis, because the perspective determines whose costs and whose benefits belong in the analysis. For example, if the perspective is that of the hospital, outpatient costs may not matter. If the perspective of the analysis is societal, however, as is typically true, the analyst should include outpatient costs. Finally, the analyst should identify the alternatives that the decision makers will (or should) consider. Rather than install an expensive hospital information system, perhaps the hospital should sign a contract with another hospital to perform all orthopedic surgeries. If the analyst has evaluated the decision context carefully, the important alternatives should be clear.

The next step in a cost-effectiveness analysis is to identify and analyze the health outcomes and costs of the alternative interventions. How should the analyst evaluate the cost effectiveness of the antibiotic reminder system? First, the analyst should decide how to measure the health benefit of the system, and then could quantify the health benefit by assessing the number of postoperative infections before and after implementation of the computer-based system. The units of the cost-effectiveness ratio would therefore be dollars expended per postoperative infection prevented. Such a ratio may be helpful to decision makers, but the decision makers could compare the cost effectiveness of the system only with other interventions that prevent postoperative infections; for example, they could not compare the cost effectiveness of the system with that of a computer-based reminder system for breast cancer screening. To remedy this problem, the analyst could choose a more comprehensive measure of health outcome, such as quality-adjusted life years (see Chapter 3). The analysts would then estimate the number of quality-adjusted life years saved for each postoperative infection prevented. Decision modeling provides one approach to make such estimates (see Chapter 3). Thus, use of quality-adjusted life years would enable policymakers to evaluate the cost effectiveness of the antibiotic reminder system relative to other interventions, but would impose an additional analytic burden on the analyst.

To evaluate the incremental cost effectiveness of the reminder system, the analysts must also estimate the costs with the old system and the costs with the computer-based system. The literature often refers to *direct costs* and *indirect costs*, but these terms are not used consistently. We shall follow the definitions and conventions of Gold and co-workers (1996) and refer to costs as either direct costs or productivity costs. With this approach, certain costs that we classify as direct costs formerly were considered as indirect costs. The **direct costs** include the value of all the goods, services, and other resources that are required to produce an intervention, including resources consumed because of future consequences (intended or unintended) of the intervention (Gold et al., 1996). Direct costs include changes in the use of health care resources, of non-health care resources, of informal caregiver time, and of patient time. The direct health care costs include the costs of drugs, tests, procedures, supplies, health care personnel, and facilities. For the antibiotic reminder system, the direct health care costs include the costs of installation, maintenance, personnel, supplies, drugs (antibiotics), and the future cost savings that may result from a reduction in postoperative infection, among others. Direct nonhealth care costs include other services required for the delivery of an intervention, such as patients' transportation costs associated with medical care. If family members provide ancillary care, the value of their time is also a cost of the intervention. The time a patient must spend to receive the intervention is also a cost. Because implementation of an antibiotic reminder system would not change these costs, the analyst does not need to include them in an analysis. **Productivity costs** are those costs that accrue because of changes in productivity due to illness or death; they could be relevant to the analysis of the antibiotic reminder system if prevention of postoperative infection changed substantially the time away from work for patients in whom infection was prevented (for further discussion, see Gold et al., 1996).

To complete the analysis, the analyst should discount health and economic outcomes, address uncertainty and ethical considerations, and interpret the results. **Discounting** enables the analyst to account for time preference in the analysis: Expenditures and health benefits that occur in the future have less value than do those expenditures or benefits that occur immediately. The analyst performs discounting by calculating the net present value of health outcomes and costs; this calculation reduces the influence of future health and economic outcomes relative to those that occur in the present (for further explanations, see Gold et al., 1996). Both health and economic outcomes should be discounted (Gold et al., 1996). Sensitivity analyses (described in Chapter 3) provide a mechanism for assessing the importance of uncertainty. Ethical concerns include how to ensure equity in policy alternatives, how to value outcomes, and how to choose a cost-effectiveness threshold (also see Chapter 10). The **cost-effectiveness threshold** (e.g., $50,000 per quality-adjusted life year saved) reflects the value judgment of the decision makers about the maximum value of a year of life saved. Although currently there is not a consensus on the appropriate threshold, many interventions that are used widely cost[3] less than $50,000 to $60,000 per quality-adjusted life year gained (Owens, 1998b). Interpretation of the results should incorporate statements both about the influence of uncertainty on the estimated cost-effectiveness ratio and about ethical concerns.

Cost-effectiveness and cost-benefit analyses provide tools for helping policymakers and clinicians to understand the relationship between the health outcomes and costs of

---

[3] See http://www.nice.org.uk

alternative health interventions, including information resources. We emphasize that they provide information about one important aspect of an intervention, or information system, but are insufficient alone for decision making. Other social, ethical, and political factors will be important for most decisions. Evaluation of comprehensive information systems poses formidable challenges because the benefits of such systems may be diffuse, varied, and difficult to quantify. Nonetheless, like other health care interventions and innovations, information resources must provide sufficient benefit to justify their expense.

11.6   Conduct of Subjectivist Studies

The objectivist approaches to evaluation, described in the previous section, are useful for addressing some, but not all, of the interesting and important questions that challenge investigators in medical informatics. The subjectivist approaches described here address the problem of evaluation from a different set of premises. They use different but equally rigorous methods.

11.6.1   The Rationale for Subjectivist Studies

Subjectivist methods enable us to address the deeper questions that arise in informatics: the detailed "whys" and "according to whoms" in addition to the aggregate "whethers" and "whats." As defined earlier, the responsive–illuminative approach, within the subjectivist family of approaches, seeks to represent the viewpoints of people who are users of the resource or are otherwise significant participants in the clinical environment where the resource operates. The goal is illumination rather than judgment. The investigators seek to build an argument that promotes deeper understanding of the information resource or environment of which it is a part. The methods used derive largely from **ethnography**. The investigators immerse themselves physically in the environment where the information resource is or will be operational, and they collect data primarily through observations, interviews, and reviews of documents. The designs—the data-collection plans—of these studies are not rigidly predetermined and do not unfold in a fixed sequence. They develop dynamically and nonlinearly as the investigators' experience accumulates.

Although subjectivist approaches may run counter to common ideas of how we ought to conduct empirical investigations, these methods and their conceptual underpinnings are not altogether foreign to the worlds of information and computer science. The pluralistic, nonlinear thinking that underlies subjectivist investigation shares many features with modern conceptualizations of the information-resource design process. For example, Winograd and Flores (1987, p. 170) argued as follows:

> In designing computer-based devices, we are not in the position of creating a formal "system" that covers the functioning of the organization and the people within it. When this is attempted, the resulting system (and the space of potential action for people within it) is inflexible and unable to cope with new breakdowns or potentials. Instead we design additions and changes to the network of equipment (some of it computer based) within which people

work. The computer is like a tool, in that it is brought up for use by people engaged in some domain of action. The use of the tool shapes the potential for what those actions are and how they are conducted. Its power does not lie in having a single purpose ... but in its connection to the larger network of communication (electronic, telephone, paper-based) in which organizations operate.

Another connection is to the methodology of **formal systems analysis**, which is generally accepted as an essential component of information resource development. Systems analysis uses many methods that resemble closely the subjectivist methods for evaluation that we introduce here. People recognize that systems analysis requires a process of information gathering, heavily reliant on interviews with people who use the existing system in various ways. Information gathering for systems analysis is typically portrayed as a cyclic, iterative process rather than as a linear process (Davis, 1994). In the literature of systems analysis, we find admonitions, analogous to those made by proponents of subjectivist evaluation, that an overly structured approach can misportray the capabilities of workers in the system's environment, misportray the role of informal communication in the work accomplished, underestimate the prevalence of exceptions, and fail to account for political forces within every organization that shape much of what actually happens (Bansler and Bødker, 1993). Within the field of systems analysis, then, there has developed an appreciation of some of the shortcomings of objectivist methods and of the potential value of subjectivist methods (Zachary et al., 1984).

11.6.2   A Rigorous, but Different, Methodology

The subjectivist approaches to evaluation, like their objectivist counterparts, are empirical methods. Although it is easy to focus only on their differences, these two broad classes of evaluation approaches share many features. In all empirical studies, for example, evidence is collected with great care; the investigators are always aware of what they are doing and why. The evidence is then compiled, interpreted, and ultimately reported. Investigators keep records of their procedures, and these records are open to audit by the investigators themselves or by individuals outside the study team. The principal investigator or evaluation-team leader is under an almost sacred scientific obligation to report their methods. Failure to do so will invalidate a study. Both classes of approaches also share a dependence on theories that guide investigators to explanations of the observed phenomena, as well as to a dependence on the pertinent empirical literature such as published studies that address similar phenomena or similar settings. In both approaches, there are rules of good practice that are generally accepted; it is therefore possible to distinguish a good study from a bad one.

There are, however, fundamental differences between objectivist and subjectivist approaches. First, subjectivist studies are **emergent** in design. Objectivist studies typically begin with a set of hypotheses or specific questions, and with a plan for addressing each member of this set. The investigator assumes that, barring major unforeseen developments, the plan will be followed exactly. Deviation, in fact, might introduce bias. The investigator who sees negative results emerging from the exploration of a particular question or use of a particular measurement instrument might change strategies in hope of obtaining more positive findings. In contrast, subjectivist studies typically begin with general **orienting issues** that stimulate the early stages of investigation. Through these initial investigations, the important questions for further study emerge. The subjectivist investigator is willing, at virtually any point, to adjust future aspects of the study in light of the most recent information obtained. Subjectivist investigators tend to be **incrementalists**; they change their plans from day-to-day and have a high tolerance for ambiguity and uncertainty. In this respect, they are much like good software developers. Also like software developers, subjectivist investigators must develop the ability to recognize when a project is finished, when further benefit can be obtained only at too great a cost in time, money, or work.

A second feature of subjectivist studies is a **naturalistic** orientation, a reluctance to manipulate the setting of the study, which in most cases is the environment in to which the information resource is introduced. They do not alter the environment to study it. Control groups, placebos, purposeful altering of information resources to create contrasting interventions, and other techniques that are central to the construction of objectivist studies typically are not used. Subjectivist studies will, however, employ quantitative data for descriptive purposes and may offer quantitative comparisons when the research setting offers a "natural experiment" where such comparisons can be made without deliberate intervention. For example, when physicians and nurses both use a clinical system to enter orders, their experiences with the system offer a natural basis for comparison. Subjectivist researchers are opportunists where pertinent information is concerned; they will use what they see as the best information available to illuminate a question under investigation.

A third important distinguishing feature of subjectivist studies is that their end product is a report written in narrative prose. These reports may be lengthy and may require significant time investment from the reader; no technical understanding of quantitative research methodology or statistics is required to comprehend them. Results of subjectivist studies are therefore accessible—and may even be entertaining—to a broad community in a way that results of objectivist studies are not. Objectivist study reports often can be results of inferential statistical analyses that most readers will not find easy to read and will typically not understand. Reports of subjectivist studies seek to engage their audience.

11.6.3 Natural History of a Subjectivist Study

As a first step in describing the methodology of subjectivist evaluation, Figure 11.5 illustrates the stages or natural history of a study. These stages constitute a general sequence, but, as we mentioned, the subjectivist investigator must always be prepared to revise his thinking and possibly return to earlier stages in light of new evidence. Backtracking is a legitimate step in this model.

1. *Negotiation of the ground rules of the study*: In any empirical research, and particularly in evaluation studies, it is important to negotiate an understanding between the study team and the people commissioning the study. This understanding should embrace the general aims of the study; the kinds of methods to be used; the access to various sources of information, including health care providers, patients, and various

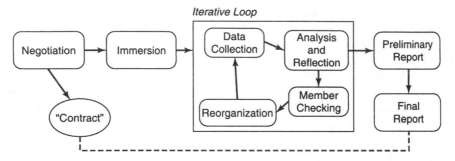

Figure 11.5. Natural history of subjectivist studies. (*Source*: Friedman and Wyatt, 1997a.)

documents; and the format for interim and final reports. The aims of the study may be formulated in a set of initial **orienting questions**. Ideally, this understanding will be expressed in a **memorandum of understanding**, analogous to a contract.

2. *Immersion into the environment*: At this stage, the investigators begin spending time in the work environment. Their activities range from formal introductions to informal conversations, or to silent presence at meetings and other events. Investigators use the generic term **field** to refer to the setting, which may be multiple physical locations, where the work under study is carried out. Trust and openness between the investigators and the people in the field are essential elements of subjectivist studies to ensure full and candid exchange of information.

   Even as immersion is taking place, the investigator is already collecting data to sharpen the initial questions or issues guiding the study. Early discussions with people in the field, and other activities primarily targeted toward immersion, inevitably begin to shape the investigators' views. Almost from the outset, the investigator is typically addressing several aspects of the study simultaneously.

3. *Iterative loop*: At this point, the procedural structure of the study becomes akin to an iterative loop, as the investigator engages in cycles of data collection, analysis and reflection, member checking, and reorganization. Data collection involves interview, observation, document analysis, and other methods. Data are collected on planned occasions, as well as serendipitously or spontaneously. The data are recorded carefully and are interpreted in the context of what is already known. Analysis and reflection entail the contemplation of the new findings during each cycle of the loop. **Member checking** is the sharing of the investigator's emerging thoughts and beliefs with the participants themselves. Reorganization results in a revised agenda for data collection in the next cycle of the loop.

   Although each cycle within the iterative loop is depicted as linear, this representation is misleading. Net progress through the loop is clockwise, as shown in Figure 11.5, but backward steps are natural and inevitable. They are not reflective of mistakes or errors. An investigator may, after conducting a series of interviews and studying what participants have said, decide to speak again with one or two participants to clarify their positions on a particular issue.

4. *Preliminary report*: The first draft of the final report should itself be viewed as a research instrument. By sharing this report with a variety of individuals, the investigator obtains a major check on the validity of the findings. Typically, reactions to the preliminary report will generate useful clarifications and a general sharpening of the study findings. Because the report usually is a narrative, it is vitally important that it be well written in language understandable by all intended audiences. Circulation of the report in draft can ensure that the final document communicates as intended. Use of anonymous quotations from interviews and documents makes a report highly vivid and meaningful to readers.

5. *Final report*: The final report, once completed, should be distributed as negotiated in the original memorandum of understanding. Distribution is often accompanied by "meet the investigator" sessions that allow interested persons to ask the author of the report to expand or explain what has been written.

11.6.4 *Data-Collection and Data-Analysis Methods*

What data-collection strategies are in the subjectivist researcher's black bag? There are several, and they are typically used in combination. We shall discuss each one, assuming a typical setting for a subjectivist study in medical informatics, the introduction of an information resource into patient care activities in a hospital.

Observation

The investigators typically immerse themselves into the setting under study in one of two ways. The investigator may act purely as a detached observer, becoming a trusted and unobtrusive feature of the environment but not a participant in the day-to-day work and thus reliant on multiple "informants" as sources of information. True to the naturalistic feature of this kind of study, great care is taken to diminish the possibility that the presence of the observer will skew the work activities that occur or that the observer will be rejected outright by the ward team. An alternative approach is participant observation, where the investigator becomes a member of the work team. Participant observation is more difficult to engineer; it may require the investigator to have specialized training in the study domain. It is time consuming but can give the investigator a more vivid impression of life in the work environment. During both kinds of observation, data accrue continuously. These data are qualitative and may be of several varieties: statements by health care providers and patients, gestures and other nonverbal expressions of these same individuals, and characteristics of the physical setting that seem to affect the delivery of health care.

Interviews

Subjectivist studies rely heavily on interviews. Formal interviews are occasions where both the investigator and interviewee are aware that the answers to questions are being recorded (on paper or tape) for direct contribution to the evaluation study. Formal interviews vary in their degree of structure. At one extreme is the **unstructured interview**, where there are no predetermined questions. Between the extremes is the **semistructured interview**, where the investigator specifies in advance a set of topics that he would like to address but is flexible as to the order in which these topics are addressed, and is open to discussion of topics not on the prespecified list. At the other extreme is the **structured interview**, with a schedule of questions that are always presented in the same words and in the same order. In general, the unstructured and semistructured interviews are preferred in subjectivist research. Informal interviews—spontaneous discussions between the investigators and members of a ward team that occur during routine observation— are also part of the data collection process. Informal interviews are invariably considered a source of important data.

Document and Artifact Analysis

Every project produces a trail of papers and other artifacts. These include patient charts, the various versions of a computer program and its documentation, memoranda prepared by the project team, perhaps a cartoon hung on the office door by a ward clerk. Unlike the day-to-day events of patient care, these artifacts do not change once created or introduced. They can be examined retrospectively and referred to repeatedly, as necessary, over the course of a study. Also included under this heading are **unobtrusive measures**, which are the records accrued as part of the routine use of the information resource. They include, for example, user trace files of an information resource. Data from these measures are often quantifiable.

Anything Else that Seems Useful

Subjectivist investigators are supreme opportunists. As questions of importance to a study emerge, the investigators will collect any information that they perceive as bearing on these questions. This data collection could include clinical chart reviews, questionnaires, tests, simulated patients, and other methods more commonly associated with the objectivist approaches.

Analysis of Subjectivist Data

There are many procedures for analysis of qualitative data. The important point is that the analysis is conducted systematically. In general terms, the investigator looks for themes or trends emerging from several different sources. He collates individual statements and observations by theme, as well as by source. Some investigators transfer these observations to file cards so they can be sorted and resorted in a variety of ways. Others use software especially designed to facilitate analysis of qualitative data (Fielding and Lee, 1991). Because they allow electronic recording of the data will the investigator is "in the field", palm-tops and other hand-held devices are changing the way subjectivist research is carried out.

The subjectivist analysis process is fluid, with analytic goals shifting as the study matures. At an early stage, the goal is primarily to focus the questions that themselves will be the targets of further data elicitation. At the later stages of study, the primary goal is to collate data that address these questions. Conclusions derive credibility from a process of "triangulation", which is the degree to which information from different independent sources generate the same theme or point to the same conclusion. Subjectivist analysis also employs a strategy known as "member checking" whereby investigators take preliminary conclusions back to the persons in the setting under study, asking if these conclusions make sense, and if not, why not. In subjectivist investigation, unlike objectivist studies, the agenda is never completely closed. The investigator is constantly on the alert for new information that can require a significant reorganization of the findings and conclusions that have been drawn to date.

11.7   Conclusions: The Mindset of Evaluation and Technology Assessment

The previous sections probably make evaluation and technology assessment look difficult. If scholars of the field disagree in fundamental ways about how these studies should be done, how can relative novices proceed at all, much less with confidence? To address this dilemma, we conclude this chapter by offering a mindset for evaluation, a general orientation that anyone conducting an evaluation might constructively bring to their work. The components of this mindset apply, to varying degrees, across all study types and approaches.

- *Tailor the study to the problem and key stakeholder questions*: Every study is made to order. Evaluation and technology assessment differ from mainstream views of research in that a study derives importance from the needs of clients rather than from the unanswered questions of an academic discipline. If an evaluation contributes new knowledge of general importance to an academic discipline, that is a serendipitous by-product.
- *Collect data that will be useful to make decisions*: There is no theoretical limit to the questions that can be asked and, consequently, to the data that can be collected in a study. What is done is determined by the decisions that need ultimately to be made and the information seen as useful to inform these decisions.
- *Look for intended and unintended effects*: Whenever a new information resource is introduced into an environment, there can be many consequences, only some of which relate to the stated purpose of the resource. In a complete evaluation, it is important to look for and document effects that were anticipated as well as those that were not, and to continue the study long enough to allow these effects to manifest themselves.
- *Study the resource while it is under development and after it is installed*: In general, the kinds of decisions evaluation can facilitate are of two types. **Formative decisions** are made as a result of studies undertaken while a resource is under development. They affect the resource before it can go online. **Summative decisions** are made after a resource is installed in its envisioned environment and deal explicitly with how effectively the resource performs in that environment. Often, it will take many years for an installed resource to stabilize within an environment. Before summative studies are conducted, it may be necessary for this amount of time to pass.
- *Study the resource in the laboratory and in the field*: Completely different questions arise when an information resource is still in the laboratory and when it is in the field.

In vitro studies, conducted in the developer's laboratory, and *in vivo* studies, conducted in an ongoing clinical or educational environment, are both important aspects of evaluation.

- *Go beyond the developer's point of view*: The developers of an information resource usually are empathic only up to a point and are often not predisposed to be detached and objective about the resource's performance and utility. People doing evaluation often see it as part of their job to get close to the end user and to portray the resource as the user sees it.
- *Take the environment into account*: Anyone who conducts an evaluation study must be, in part, an ecologist. The function of an information resource must be viewed as an interaction among the resource itself, a set of users of the resource, and the social, organizational, and cultural context that largely determines how work is carried out in that environment. Whether a new resource functions effectively is determined as much by its goodness of fit with its environment as by its compliance with the resource designers' operational specifications as measured in the laboratory.
- *Let the key issues emerge over time*: Evaluation studies are dynamic. The design for a study, as it might be stated in a project proposal, is often just a starting point. Rarely are the important questions known, with total precision or confidence, at the outset of a study. In the real world, evaluation designs, even those employing objectivist approaches, must have some leeway to evolve as the important issues come into focus.
- *Be methodologically catholic and eclectic*: It is best to derive overall approaches, study designs, and data collection methods from the questions to be explored rather than to bring predetermined methods or instruments to a study. Certain questions are better answered with qualitative data collected through open-ended interviews and observation. Others are better answered with quantitative data collected via structured questionnaires, patient chart audits, and logs of user behavior.

Finally, remember that the perfect study has never been performed and probably never will be. This chapter has introduced various approaches to study design and execution that can minimize bias and maximize credibility, but the findings of every study can be questioned. It is sufficient for a study to be guiding, clarifying, or illuminating.

Suggested Readings

Anderson J.G., Aydin C.E., Jay S.J. (Eds.) (1994). *Evaluating Health Care Information Systems: Methods and Applications*. Thousand Oaks, CA: Sage Publications.
This is an excellent edited volume that covers a wide range of methodological and substantive issues in evaluation, including both objectivist and subjectivist approaches. Although not formally constructed as a textbook, it is written at a basic level for individuals more familiar with medical informatics than study methodology.

Ash, J.S., Gorman, P.N., Lavelle, M., Payne, T.H., Massaro, T.A., Frantz, G.L., Lyman JA. (2003). A cross-site qualitative study of physician order entry. *Journal of the American Medical Informatics Association,* 10(2),188–200.

Cohen P.R. (1995). *Empirical Methods for Artificial Intelligence*. Cambridge, MA: MIT Press.
This is a nicely written, detailed book that is focused on evaluation of artificial intelligence applications, not necessarily those operating in medical domains. It emphasizes objectivist methods and could serve as a basic statistics course for computer science students.

Friedman C.P., Wyatt J.C. (2006). *Evaluation Methods in Biomedical Informatics*. New York: Springer-Verlag.
This is the book on which the current chapter is based. It offers expanded discussion of almost all issues and concepts raised in the current chapter.

Jain R. (1991). *The Art of Computer Systems Performance Analysis: Techniques for Experimental Design, Measurement, Simulation, and Modeling*. New York: John Wiley & Sons.
This work offers a technical discussion of a range of objectivist methods used to study computer systems. The scope is broader than Cohen's book (1995) described earlier. It contains many case studies and examples and assumes knowledge of basic statistics.

Lincoln Y.S., Guba E.G. (1985). *Naturalistic Inquiry*. Beverly Hills, CA: Sage Publications.
This is a classic book on subjectivist methods. The work is very rigorous but also very easy to read. Because it does not focus on medical domains or information systems, readers must make their own extrapolations.

Rossi P.H., Freeman H.E. (1989). *Evaluation: A Systematic Approach* (4th ed.). Newbury Park, CA: Sage Publications.
This is a valuable textbook on evaluation, emphasizing objectivist methods, and is very well written. Like the book of Lincoln and Guba (1985), described earlier, it is generic in scope, and the reader must relate the content to medical informatics. There are several excellent chapters addressing pragmatic issues of evaluation. These nicely complement the chapters on statistics and formal study designs.

Questions for Discussion

1. Choose any alternative area of biomedicine (e.g., drug trials) as a point of comparison, and list at least four factors that make studies in medical informatics more difficult to conduct successfully than in that area. Given these difficulties, discuss whether it is worthwhile to conduct empirical studies in medical informatics or whether we should use intuition or the marketplace as the primary indicators of the value of an information resource.

2. Assume that you run a philanthropic organization that supports medical informatics. In investing the scarce resources of your organization, you have to choose between funding a new system or resource development, or funding empirical studies of resources already developed. What would you choose? How would you justify your decision?

3. To what extent is it possible to be certain how effective a medical informatics resource really is? What are the most important criteria of effectiveness?

4. Do you believe that independent, unbiased observers of the same behavior or outcome should agree on the quality of that outcome?

5. Many of the evaluation approaches assert that a single unbiased observer is a legitimate source of information in an evaluation, even if that observer's data or judgments are

unsubstantiated by other people. Give examples drawn from our society where we vest important decisions in a single experienced and presumed impartial individual.

6. Do you agree with the statement that all evaluations appear equivocal when subjected to serious scrutiny? Explain your answer.

7. Associate each of the following hypothetical studies with a particular approach to evaluation:[4]

   a. A comparison of different user interfaces for a computer-based medical-record system, conducted while the system is under development.

   b. A site visit by the U.S. National Library of Medicine's Biomedical Library Review Committee to the submitters of a competing renewal of a research grant.

   c. A noted consultant on user interface design being invited to spend a day at an academic department to offer suggestions regarding the prototype of a new system.

   d. Patient chart reviews conducted before and after the introduction of an information resource, without the reviewer being told anything about the nature of the information resource or even that the intervention is the information resource.

   e. Videotapes of attending rounds on a service where a knowledge resource has been implemented and periodic interviews with members of the ward team.

   f. Determination of whether a new version of a resource executes a standard set of performance tests at the speed the designers projected.

   g. Patients being randomly assigned such that their medical records are maintained either by a new computer system or by standard procedures, and then an investigator seeking to determine whether the new system affects clinical protocol recruitment and compliance.

   h. A mock debate at a research-group retreat.

8. For each of the following hypothetical evaluation scenarios, list which of the nine types of studies in Table 11.2 they include. Some scenarios may include more than one type of study.[5]

   a. An order-communication system is implemented in a small hospital. Changes in laboratory workload are assessed.

   b. A study team performs a thorough analysis of the information required by psychiatrists to whom patients are referred by community social workers.

   c. A medical-informatics expert is asked for opinion about a doctoral student's project. The expert requests copies of the student's programming code and documentation for review.

   d. A new intensive care unit system is implemented alongside manual paper charting for one month. Then, the qualities of the computer-based data and of the data recorded on the paper charts are compared. A panel of intensive care physicians is asked to identify episodes of hypotension from each dataset, independently.

---

[4] Answers: (a) decision facilitation; (b) professional review; (c) art criticism; (d) goal free; (e) responsive–illuminative; (f) objectives based; (g) comparison based; (h) quasi-legal.

[5] Answers: (a) field user effect; (b) needs assessment; (c) structure validation; (d) field function; (e) needs assessment and design validation; (f) laboratory function; (g) laboratory user effect and laboratory function; (h) problem impact.

e. A medical-informatics professor is invited to join the steering group for a clinical-workstation project in a local hospital. The only documentation available for the professor to critique at the first meeting is a statement of the project goals, a description of the planned development method, and the advertisements and job descriptions for team members.

f. Developers invite clinicians to test a prototype of a computer-aided learning system as part of a workshop on user-centered design.

g. A program is built that generates a predicted 24-hour blood glucose profile using seven clinical parameters. Another program uses this profile and other patient data to advise on insulin dosages. Diabetologists are asked to prescribe insulin for the patient given the 24-hour profile alone and then again after seeing the computer-generated advice. They are also asked their opinion of the advice.

h. A program to generate drug-interaction alerts is installed in a geriatric clinic that already has a computer-based medical record system. Rates of clinically significant drug interactions are compared before and after installation of the alerting resource.

Unit II
Biomedical Informatics Applications

12
Electronic Health Record Systems

PAUL C. TANG AND CLEMENT J. MCDONALD

After reading this chapter, you should know the answers to these questions:

- What is the definition of an electronic health record (EHR)?
- How does an EHR differ from the paper record?
- What are the functional components of an EHR?
- What are the benefits of an EHR?
- What are the impediments to development and use of an EHR?

12.1 What Is An Electronic Health Record?

The preceding chapters introduced the conceptual basis for the field of biomedical informatics, including the use of patient data in clinical practice and research. We now focus attention on the **patient record**, commonly referred to as the patient's **chart** or **medical record**. The patient record is an amalgam of all the data acquired and created during a patient's course through the health care system. The use of medical data was covered extensively in Chapter 2. We also discussed the limitations of the paper record in serving the many users of patient information. In this chapter, we examine the definition and use of computer-based patient record systems, discuss their potential benefits and costs, and describe the remaining challenges to address in their dissemination.

12.1.1 Purpose of a Patient Record

Stanley Reiser (1991) wrote that the purpose of a patient record is "to recall observations, to inform others, to instruct students, to gain knowledge, to monitor performance, and to justify interventions." The many uses described in this statement, although diverse, have a single goal—to further the application of health sciences in ways that improve the well-being of patients, including the conduct of research and public health activities that address population health. Yet, observational studies of physicians' use of the paper-based record find that logistical, organizational, and other practical limitations reduce the effectiveness of traditional records for storing and organizing an ever-increasing number of diverse data. An electronic health record (EHR) is designed to overcome many of these limitations, as well as to provide additional benefits that cannot be attained by a static view of events.

An electronic health record (EHR) is a repository of electronically maintained information about an individual's lifetime health status and health care, stored such that it can serve the multiple legitimate users of the record. Traditionally, the patient record was a record of care provided when a patient is ill. Managed care (discussed in Chapter 23) encourages health care providers to focus on the continuum of health and health care from wellness to illness and recovery. Consequently, the record must integrate elements regarding a patient's health and illness acquired by multiple providers across diverse settings. In addition, the data should be stored such that different views of those data can be presented to serve the many uses described in Chapter 2.

A **electronic health record (EHR) system** adds information management tools to provide clinical reminders and alerts, linkages with knowledge sources for health care decision support, and analysis of aggregate data both for care management and for research. To use a paper-based patient record, the reader must manipulate data either mentally or on paper to glean important clinical information. In contrast, an EHR system provides computer-based tools to help the reader organize, interpret, and react to data. Examples of tools provided in current EHR systems are discussed in Section 12.3.

A number of large institutions have installed EHRs and described their many different approaches and the lessons learned (Pryor et al., 1983; Giuse and Mickish, 1996; Halamka et al., 1998; Hripcsak et al., 1999; McDonald et al., 1999; Slack and Bleich, 1999; Teich et al., 1999; Yamazaki and Satomura, 2000; Cheung et al., 2001; Duncan et al., 2001; Brown et al., 2003).

12.1.2   Ways in Which an Electronic Health Record Differs from a Paper-Based Record

In contrast to a traditional patient record, whose functionality is tethered by the static nature of paper—a single copy of the data stored in a single format for data entry and retrieval—an EHR is flexible and adaptable. Data may be entered in a format that simplifies the input process (which includes electronic interfaces to other computers where patient data are stored) and displayed in different formats suitable for their interpretation. Further, the EHR can integrate multimedia information such as radiology images and echocardiographic video loops that were never part of the traditional medical record. Data can be used to guide care for a single patient or in aggregate form to help administrators develop policies for a population. Hence, when considering the functions of an EHR, we do not confine discussion to the uses of a single, serial recording of provider–patient encounters. An EHR system extends the usefulness of patient data by applying information-management tools to the data.

Inaccessibility is a common drawback of paper records. In large organizations, the traditional record may be unavailable to others for days while the clinician finishes documentation of an encounter. For example, paper records are often sequestered in a medical records department until the discharge summary is completed and every document is signed. During this time, special permission and extra effort are required to locate and retrieve the record. Individual physicians often borrow records for their convenience, with the same effect. With computer-stored records, all authorized personnel can access patient data immediately as the need arises. Remote access to EHRs also is possible.

When the data are stored on a secure network, authorized clinicians with a need to know can access them from the office, home, or emergency room, to make timely informed decisions. At the same time that EHR systems make data more available to authorized users for legitimate uses, they also provide the tools needed to control and track access to patient records to enforce the privacy policies required by the Health Insurance Portability and Accountability Act (HIPAA; see Chapter 10).

Documentation in an EHR can be more legible because it is recorded as printed text rather than as handwriting, and it is better organized because structure is imposed on input. The computer can even improve completeness and quality by automatically applying validity and required field checks on data as they are entered. For example, numerical results can be checked against reference ranges. Typographical errors can be detected via spell checkers and restricted input menus. Moreover, an interactive system can prompt the user for additional information. In this case, the data repository not only stores data but also enhances their completeness.

Data entered into a computer can be reused. For example, a physician could cut and paste parts of their visit note into a letter to a referring physician and into an admission note. Reusability of data is one way that an EHR increases the provider's efficiency. Data entered as part of the patient care process can also be reused in reports that support patient safety, quality improvement, and regulatory or accreditation requirements.

The degree to which a particular EHR demonstrates these benefits depends on several factors:

1. *Comprehensiveness of information.* Does the EHR contain information about health as well as illness? Does it include information from all clinicians who participated in a patient's care? Does it cover all settings in which care was delivered (e.g., office practice, hospital)? Does it include the full spectrum of clinical data, including clinicians' notes, laboratory test results, medication details, and so on?
2. *Duration of use and retention of data.* A record that has accumulated patient data over 5 years will be more valuable than one that contains only the last month's worth of records.
3. *Degree of structure of data.* Medical data that are stored simply as narrative text entries will be more legible and accessible than similar entries in a paper medical record. Uncoded information, however, is not standardized (see Chapter 7), and inconsistent use of medical terminology limits the ability to search for data, but as anyone who has used an Internet search tool knows, clever use of synonyms and statistics improves the hit rates. Use of a controlled, predefined vocabulary (see Chapter 7) facilitates computer-supported decision making and clinical research, but at the cost of "coding" time to the provider who is entering such data.
4. *Ubiquity of access.* A system that is accessible from a few sites will be less valuable than one accessible from any computer by an authorized user (see Chapter 5).

A computer-stored medical record system has disadvantages. It requires a larger initial investment than its paper counterpart due to hardware, software, training, and support costs. The human and organizational factors often dominate the technical challenges. Physicians and other key personnel will have to take time from their work to learn how to use the system and to redesign their work flow to use the system efficiently.

Another risk associated with computer-based systems is the potential for subtle as well as catastrophic failures. If the computer system fails, stored information may be unavailable for an indeterminate time. Paper records fail one chart at a time. On the other hand, if the average paper chart is unavailable up to 10 percent of the time, that would be equivalent to a 10 percent downtime for the average patient. Furthermore, modern computers with fully redundant components, *swappable memory* and computers and disk units and *mirrored servers*, have very high reliability. Yet, nothing provides complete protection; so contingency plans must be developed for handling brief or longer computer outages Physicians record large amounts of clinical information in their history, physical examination, and progress notes. Capture of this information directly from the physician is a major goal of medical informatics because it provides the most timely, accurate, and useful content. However, the goal is elusive. The time cost of physician input can be high, so the physician input may be infeasible in some settings. Although new input devices are introduced or improved each year (e.g., pen-based entry, speech input), none of these have become time-competitive with dictation or handwriting. The wireless personal digital assistants (PDAs) and slate computers improve accessibility compared with fixed workstations, but battery life and physical attributes still limit their widespread applicability.

Some institutions are scanning selected parts of the patient chart (including the physicians' notes) into the computer (Teich, 1997). Scanning and storing chart notes into an EHR does solve the availability problems of the paper chart, and the solution can be applied to any kind of document. Indeed, many hospitals now scan in the entire paper chart at discharge for easy retrieval. However, a typical scanned page occupies 50 to 80 kilobytes, so high-speed communication links are required for quick display. Further no option exists for searching or analyzing the content of a scanned document without an abstraction step.

Although it takes time to learn how to use the system and to change workflows, there is mounting recognition that an EHR system is required to support the care process, as well as the regulatory and business side of health care. One of the largest health maintenance organizations (HMOs) recently committed $1.8 billion to implementing an EHR throughout its health system.

12.2   Historical Perspective

The historical development of the medical record parallels the development of science in clinical care. The development of automated systems for dealing with health care data parallels the need for data to comply with reimbursement requirements. Early health care systems focused on inpatient-charge capture to meet billing requirements in a fee-for-service environment. Contemporary systems need to capture clinical information in a managed care environment focusing on clinical outcomes in ambulatory care.

12.2.1   Early Hospital Focus

The Flexner report on medical education was the first formal statement made about the function and contents of the medical record (Flexner, 1910). Mayo clinic had begun to record the diagnoses for every admitted patient 3 years earlier (Melton, 1996). In advocating a scientific approach to medical education, the Flexner report also encouraged physicians to keep a patient-oriented medical record. The contents of medical records in hospitals became the object of scrutiny in the 1940s, when hospital-accrediting bodies began to insist on the availability of accurate, well-organized medical records as a condition for accreditation. Since then, these organizations also have required that hospitals abstract certain information from the medical record and submit that information to national data centers. Such discharge abstracts contain (1) demographic information, (2) admission and discharge diagnoses, (3) length of stay, and (4) major procedures performed. The national centers produce statistical summaries of these case abstracts; an individual hospital can then compare its own statistical profile with that of similar institutions.

In the late 1960s, computer-based hospital information systems (HISs) began to emerge (see also Chapter 13). These systems were intended primarily for communication. They collected orders from nursing stations, routed the orders to various parts of the hospital, and identified all chargeable services. They also gave clinicians electronic access to results of laboratory tests and other diagnostic procedures. Although they contained some clinical information (e.g., test results, drug orders), their major purpose was to capture charges rather than to assist with clinical care. Many of the early HISs stored and presented much of their information as text, which is difficult to analyze. Moreover, these early systems rarely retained the content for long after a patient's discharge.

The introduction of the **problem-oriented medical record (POMR)** by Lawrence Weed (1969) influenced medical thinking about both manual and automated medical records. Weed was among the first to recognize the importance of an internal structure of a medical record, whether stored on paper or in a computer. He suggested that the primary organization of the medical record should be by the medical problem; all diagnostic and therapeutic plans should be linked to a specific problem.

Morris Collen (1972) was an early pioneer in the use of hospital-based systems to store and present laboratory test results as part of preventive care. He also wrote an extensive history of the field (Collen, 1995). Use of computers to screen for early warning signs of illness was a basic tenet of HMOs. Other early university hospital-based systems provided feedback to physicians that affected clinical decisions and ultimately patient outcomes. The HELP system (Pryor, 1988) at LDS Hospital, the CCC system at Beth Israel Deaconess Medical Center (Slack and Bleich, 1999), and the Regenstrief System (Tierney et al., 1993; McDonald et al., 1999) at Wishard Memorial Hospital continue to add more clinical data and decision-support functionality.

12.2.2 Influence of Managed Care and the Integrated Delivery System

Until recently, the ambulatory care record has received less attention from the commercial vendors than the hospital record because of differences in financing and regulatory requirements. The status of ambulatory care records was reviewed in a 1982 report (Kuhn et al., 1984). Under the influence of managed care (described in detail in Chapter 13), the reimbursement model has shifted from a **fee-for-service model** (payers pay providers for all services the provider deemed necessary) toward a payment scheme where providers are paid a **fixed fee** for a specific service (payers pay a fixed amount for services approved by the payer). Information management tools that facilitate effective management of patients outside of the hospital setting help providers manage patients' disease more cost-effectively. The emphasis on ambulatory care brought new attention to the ambulatory care record.

Thirty years ago, a single family physician provided almost all of an individual's medical care. Today, however, responsibility for ambulatory care is shifting to teams of health care professionals in outpatient clinics and HMOs (see Chapter 13). Ambulatory care records may contain lengthy notes written by many different health care providers, large numbers of laboratory test results, and a diverse set of other data elements, such as X-ray examination and pathology reports and hospital discharge summaries. Accordingly, the need for information tools in ambulatory practice has increased. COSTAR (Barnett, 1984), the Regenstrief Medical Record System (RMRS) (McDonald et al., 1975), STOR (Whiting-O'Keefe et al., 1985), and TMR (Stead and Hammond, 1988) are among the early systems that focused on ambulatory care. Costar and RMRS are still in use today.

12.3   Functional Components of an Electronic Health Record System

As we explained in Section 12.1.2, an EHR is not simply an electronic version of the paper record. When the record is part of a comprehensive EHR system, there are linkages and tools available to facilitate communication and decision making. In Sections 12.3.1 to 12.3.5, we summarize components of a comprehensive EHR system and illustrate functionality with examples from systems currently in use. The five functional components are:]

- Integrated view of patient data
- Clinical decision support
- Clinician order entry
- Access to knowledge resources
- Integrated communication and reporting support

12.3.1   Integrated View of Patient Data

Clearly, providing integrated access to all patient data is the primary purpose of an EHR. Although this task may seem relatively simple, acquisition and organization of these data are major challenges because of the complexity and diversity of the data— ranging from simple numbers to graphs to images to motion images—and the large number and organizationally distributed sources of patient data such as clinical laboratories, radiology departments, free-standing magnetic resonance imaging (MRI) centers, community pharmacies, home health agencies. Furthermore, no unique national patient identifier exists in the United States for linking patient data obtained from many sites (patient indexes to link disparate patient identifiers are discussed in Chapter 10). The fact that different patient data source systems use different identifiers, data content terminologies, and data formats creates substantial work. Administrators of each EHR system must revise the message formats and map coding systems from the source system to the format and codes that are acceptable to their EHR system. Today most clinical data sources can deliver the clinical content as **health level 7 (HL7)** messages, but senders deviate from the standard and use local codes as identifiers for clinical observations and orders in these messages. So, some small amount of message tweaking and a large amount of code mapping is usually required. Interface engines facilitate the management and tweaking of the messages (see Chapter 7); Figure 12.1 shows an example of architecture to integrate data from multiple source systems. The database interface depicted not only provides message-handling capability but can also automatically translate codes from the source system to the preferred codes of the receiving EHR. However, human labor is needed to define the mappings that drive this automatic translation. The **interface engine** provides a technical and translation buffer between systems manufactured by different vendors. In this way, organizations can mix different vendors' products and still achieve the goal of integrated access to patient data for the clinician.

The idiosyncratic, local terminologies used to identify clinical variables and their values in many source systems represent major barriers to integration of medical record data by EHRs. Code systems such as LOINC (McDonald et al., 2003) and SNOMED (Wang et al., 2002), which have been adopted by the U.S. federal government

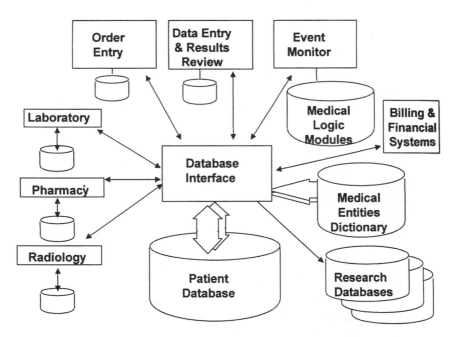

Figure 12.1. A block diagram of multiple-source-data systems that contribute patient data ultimately reside in a CPR. The database interface, commonly called an interface engine, may perform a number of functions. It may simply be a router of information to the central database. Alternatively, it may provide more intelligent filtering, translating, and alerting functions. as it dose at Columbia presbyterian Medical Center. (Source: Courtesy of Columbia Presbyterian Medical Center, New York.)

agencies for their health-related data and are discussed in Chapter 10, help overcome these barriers.

Clinicians need more than just integrated access to patient data; they also need various **views** of these data (e.g., in chronologic order by report date) so providers can easily find the newest individual results, in a flowsheet format to highlight changes over time across multiple variables, and in focused views tailored to specialties and settings An example of such a snapshot for general medicine in an outpatient setting visit is shown in Figure 12.2. This summary view of patient data shows the active patient problems, active medications, medication allergies, health maintenance reminders, and other relevant summary information. Such a view presents a current summary of patient context that is updated automatically at every encounter; such updating is not possible in a paper record.

Web browsers for finding and viewing information on the Internet (see Chapters 13 and 24) also provide health care workers with tools to view patient data from remote systems. Advanced security features (e.g., Secure Socket Layer (SSL)) are required to ensure the confidentiality of patient data transmitted over the public Internet. Figure 12.3a shows an integrated view of a flowsheet of the radiology impressions with the rows representing all kinds of radiology examinations and the columns representing Web dates. Clicking on the radiology image icon ⊠ brings up the radiology images, e.g., the quarter resolution PA and lateral chest X-ray views in Figure 12.3b. An analogous

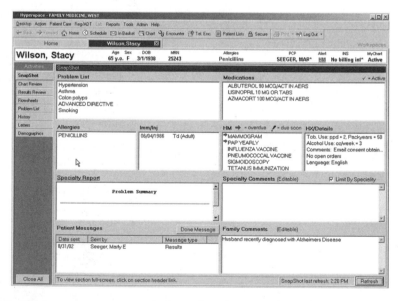

Figure 12.2. Quick access to summary information about a patient. The patient's active medical problems, current medications, and drug allergies are among the core data that physicians must keep in mind when making any decision on patient care. This one-page screen provides an instant display of these core clinical data elements as well as reminders about required preventive care. (*Source:* Courtesy of Epic Systems, Madison, WI.)

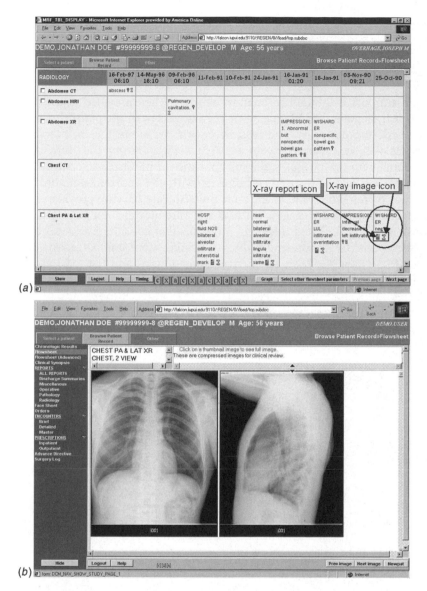

Figure 12.3. Web resources. (*a*) Web-browser flowsheet of radiology reports. The rows all report one kind of study, the columns one date. Each cell shows the impression part of the radiology report as a quick summary of the content of that report. The cells include two icons. Clicking on the report icon provides the full radiology report. Clicking on the radiology image icon ☒ provides the images. (*b*) Shows the chest X-ray images on radiology images obtained by clicking on the "bone" icon. What shows by default is a quarter-sized view of both the PA and lateral chest view X-ray. By clicking on various options, users can obtain up to the full (2,000 × 2,300) resolution, and window and level the images over the 12 bits of a radiographic image, using a control provided by Medical Informatics Engineering (MIE), Fort Wayne Indiana. (*Source*: Courtesy of Regenstrief Institute, Indianapolis, IN.)

process applies to EKG measurements where clicking on the EKG icon for a particular result brings up the full EKG tracing in Portable Document Format (PDF) form.

12.3.2   Clinical Decision Support

Decision support is thought to be most effective when provided at the point of care, while the physician is formulating his or her assessment of the patient's condition and is making ordering decisions. The most successful decision-support intervention makes complying with the suggested action easy (e.g., simply hitting the "Enter key" or clicking "Accept" with the mouse), while still allowing the physician to control the final decision. Providing access to a brief rationale with the recommendation may increase acceptance of reminders and at the same time educate the care provider.

Figure 12.4 shows the suggestions of a software module in a large HIS. The patient diagnosis uses sophisticated treatment protocols that consider a wide spectrum of clinical information to recommend antibiotic choice, dose, and duration of treatment. Clinicians can view the basis for the recommendations and the logic used. A notable part of this program is its solicitation of feedback when the clinician decides not to follow the recommendations. This feedback is used to improve the clinical protocol and the software program. Providing online advice on antimicrobial selection has resulted in

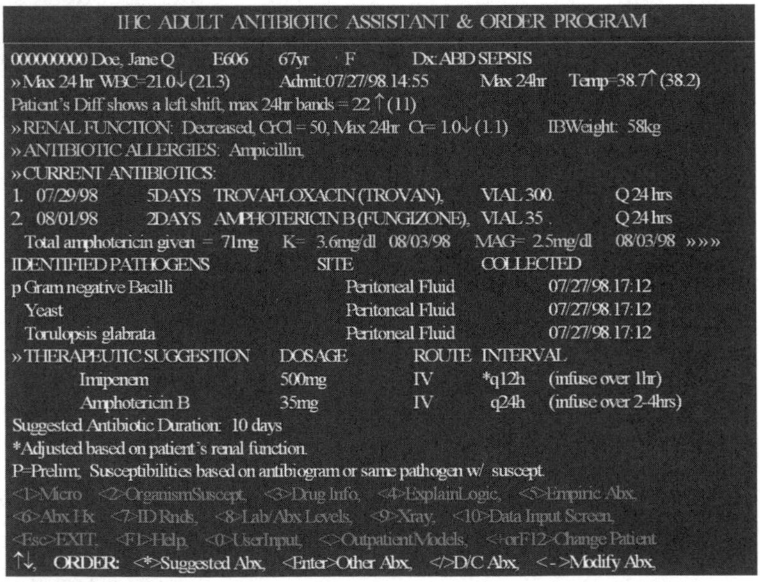

Figure 12.4. Example of the main screen from the Intermountain Health Care Antibiotic Assistant program. The program displays evidence of an infection-relevant patient data (e.g., kidney function, temperature), and recommendations for antibiotics based on the culture results. (*Source*: Courtesy of R. Scott Evans, Stanley L. Pestotnik, David C. Classen, and John P. Burke, LDS Hospital, Salt Lake City, UT.)

significantly improved clinical and financial outcomes for patients whose infectious diseases were managed through the use of the program.

Reminders and alerts can be raised during outpatient encounters as well. Indeed the outpatient setting is where the most formal reminder studies have been performed (Garg et al., 2005). Figure 12.5 shows how alerts and reminders are included on a preprinted encounter form for use during an outpatient visit. The system searches for applicable decision-support rules and prints relevant reminders on the encounter form during batch printing the night before the scheduled visit. Figure 12.6 shows computer-based suggestions regarding health maintenance topics from the Veterans Administration EHRS. These suggestions were derived from rules that examine the patient's problems

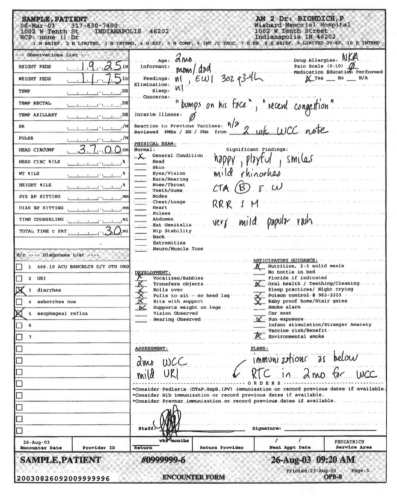

Figure 12.5. Pediatric encounter form. The questions on these forms vary by age. Reminders for routine immunizations appear at the bottom. (*Source*: Courtesy of Regenstrief Institute, Indianapolis, IN.)

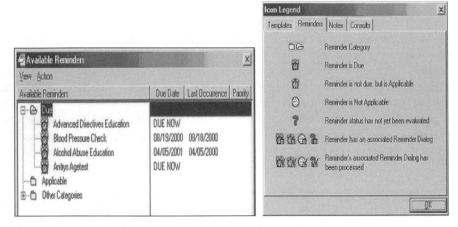

Figure 12.6. A powerful feature of electronic medical records is their use of protocols or algorithms to review the patient's electronic data and provide alerts and reminders about any unmet goals of those protocols to clinical decision makers. The first figure shows adult advisories for preventive services produced by the Veterans Administration computer-based patient record system (CPRS)—released as VISTA open source system (web reference accessed sep 17, 2005 http://www.vistasoftware.org/). Clinical users may optionally complete any "due" reminders, browse applicable reminders, or review completed reminders. The second screen defines the meaning of the icons from that same system functionality. (*Source*: Courtesy of Veterans Administration, 2003, Salt Lake City, UT.)

and medications and the timing of laboratory test orders. Even for hospitalized patients, reminders about preventive health procedures can improve compliance. In one study, there was a 50-fold increase in influenza immunization orders among eligible patients (Dexter et al., 2001).

12.3.3 Clinician Order Entry

If the ultimate goal of an EHR system is to help clinicians make informed decisions, then the system should present relevant information at the time of order entry. Several systems have the capability of providing decision support during the order-entry process (Dexter et al., 2001; Steen, 1996; Evans et al., 1999; Sanders and Miller, 2001; Kuperman et al., 2003). For example, a clinical team in the medical intensive care unit (ICU) at Vanderbilt University Hospital can use an electronic chart rack to view active orders and enter new orders. The WIZ Order screen integrates information about a patient's active orders, clinical alerts based on current data from the electronic patient record, and abstracts of relevant articles from the literature. Clinical alerts attached to a laboratory test result can also include suggestions for appropriate actions (Geissbuhler and Miller, 1996). Figure 12.7 shows computer suggestions for dosing and follow-up of intravenous heparin orders at Vanderbilt. Physician order-entry systems can warn the physician about allergies and drug interactions before they complete a medication order as exemplified by the screen from Partner's outpatient medical record shown in Figure 12.8.

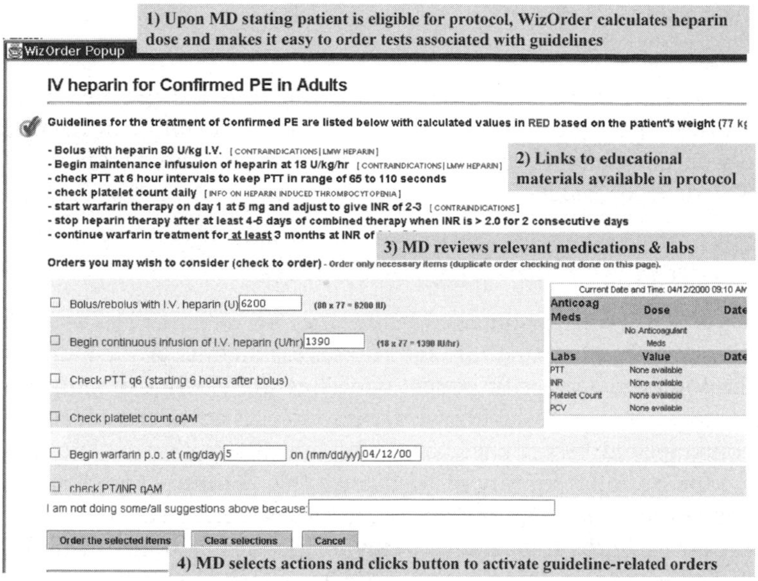

Figure 12.7. An example of computer-assisted decision support. At the top left, this screen specifies the actions required for intravenous (IV) heparin drip and provides access to text knowledge about them, and alternatives. To the right, the screen displays computer-relevant laboratory and medication information, and at the bottom, patient-specific protocol-based values for the bolus and infusion rate. The provider can complete the order (with a single click) or can modify the order as needed. (*Source*: Courtesy of Vanderbilt University, Nashville, TN.)

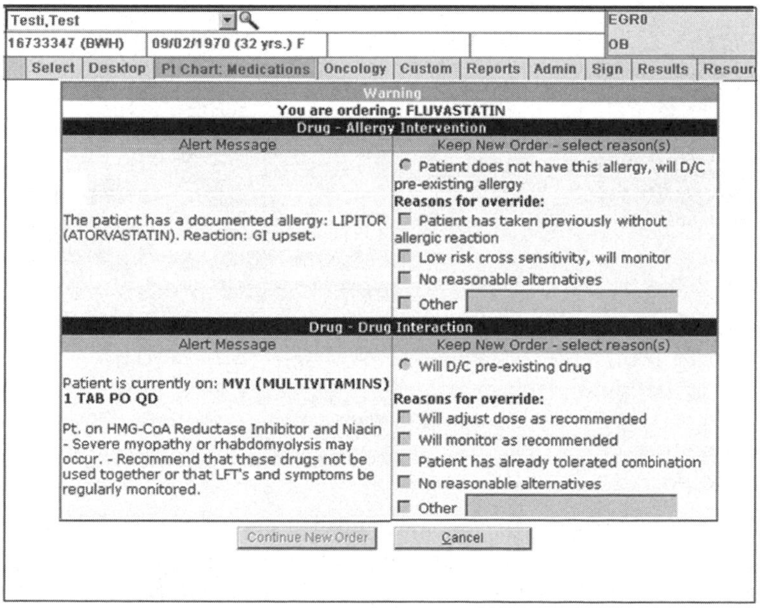

Figure 12.8. Drug-alert display screen from Partners outpatient medical record application (Longitudinal Medical Record, LMR). The screen shows a drug-allergy alert and a drug–drug interaction alert in response to a proposed prescription for fluvastatin. (*Source*: Courtesy of Partners Health Care System, Chestnut Hill, MA.)

Once a physician order-entry system is adopted into the practice culture, simply changing the default drug or dosing based on the latest scientific evidence can significantly change the physician's ordering behavior. Clinical quality and financial costs can be changed virtually overnight.

12.3.4 Access to Knowledge Resources

Most queries of knowledge resources, whether they are satisfied by consulting another human colleague or by searching through reference materials or the literature, are conducted in the context of a specific patient (Covell et al., 1985). Consequently, the most effective time to provide access to knowledge resources is at the time decisions or orders are being contemplated by the clinician. Today a rich selection of knowledge sources ranging from the National Library of Medicine's free literature search site, PubMed to full-text resources such as OVID and online references such as Up-To-Date are available for perusal. Consequently, it is relatively easy for physicians to get medical knowledge while reviewing results or writing notes or orders online. However, active presentation of literature relevant to a particular clinical situation, such as an "Infobutton" would increase the chance that the knowledge will influence clinicians' decisions (Cimino et al., 2003) (Figure 12.9).

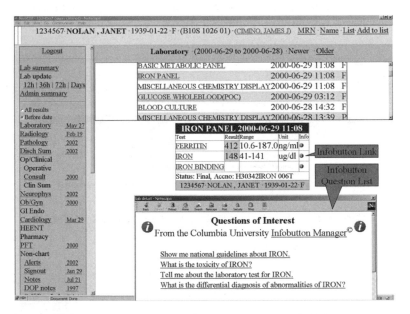

Figure 12.9. A Computer-based patient record (CPR) linked to knowledge resources so that context-specific information can be displayed at the time of clinical decision making. This figure shows the use of Columbia University's info buttons – during results review. Clicking on the info button adjacent to the Iron result generates a window (below) with a menu of questions. When the user clicks on one of the questions—he/she gets the answers. (*Source*: Courtesy of Columbia Presbyterian Medical Center, New York.)

12.3.5   *Integrated Communication and Reporting Support*

As the care function becomes increasingly distributed among multidisciplinary health care professionals, the effectiveness and efficiency of communication among the team members affect the overall coordination and timeliness of care provided. Most messages are associated with a specific patient. Thus, communication tools should be integrated with the EHR system such that messages (including system messages or laboratory test results) are electronically attached to a patient's record, i.e., the patient's record should be available at the touch of a button. Geographic separation of team members creates the demand for networked communication that reaches all sites where providers make decisions on patient care. These sites include the providers' offices, the hospital, the emergency room, and the home. Connectivity to the patient's home will provide an important vehicle for monitoring health (e.g., home blood-glucose monitoring, health status indicators) and for enabling routine communication. Communication also can be "pushed" to the user via e-mail and or pager services (Major et al., 2002; Poon et al., 2002) or "pulled" by providers at their routine interactions with the computer. Figure 12.10 shows a screen that can be viewed after the immediate notification via pager about a critically low serum potassium level in a patient taking digitalis.

An EHR system can also help with routine patient handoffs, where the responsibility for care is transferred from one clinician to another. Typically, a brief verbal or written exchange helps the covering clinician understand the patient's problems, as is important for making decisions when the primary clinician is unavailable. An example of a screen

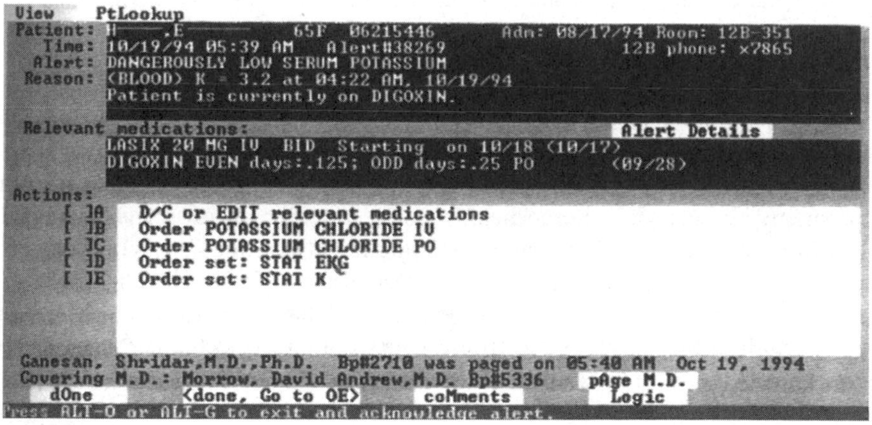

Figure 12.10. When such a laboratory test is completed, the computer identifies critically abnormal results of special importance then sends a message to the ordering physician's pager announcing the result. The physician can find details on a nearby computer screen (shown in figure) that displays the relevant facts, and suggests remedial actions, such as an order for potassium replacement. The example in the figure is based on a rule that checks for serum potassium concentrations of less than 3.3 mEq/L when a patient is also taking dioxin. (*Source*: Courtesy of Brigham and Women's Hospital, Boston, MA.)

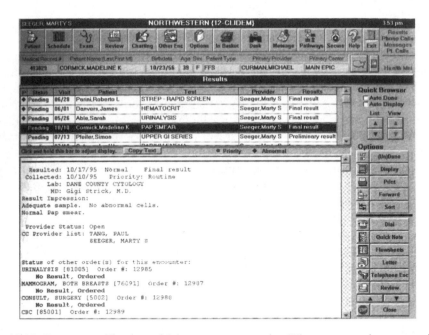

Figure 12.11. Prompt notification of laboratory test results. When a messaging system is integrated with the CPR system, test results can be directed to the provider's in-basket as soon as they are available. By clicking on the Review button at the lower right corner, the clinician can retrieve the patient's CPR instantly and with it any relevant information that he/she reviewed before acting on the most recent result or message. Telephone messages and other patient-related information can be handled in the same manner. (*Source*: Courtesy of Epic Systems, Madison, WI.)

that contains instructions from the primary physician, as well as system-provided information (e.g., recent laboratory test results), is shown in Figure 12.11.

Although a patient encounter is usually defined by a face-to-face visit (e.g., outpatient visit, inpatient bedside visit, home health visit), provider decision making occurs in response to other events such as patient telephone calls about new symptoms or prescription renewal requests and the arrival of test results. Ideally, the clinician or a key office staff should be notified of these events and have the EHR tools needed to respond, including the patient's electronic chart content, mechanisms for electronic renewal authorizations, templates for producing reports to patients about normal test results, and back-to-work forms as shown in Figure 12.11. In addition, when the physician asks the patient to schedule a diagnostic test such as a mammogram, an EHR system can keep track of the time since the order was written and can notify the physician that a test result has not appeared in a specified time. This tracking function prevents diagnostic plans from falling through the cracks.

EHRs are usually bounded by the institution in which they reside. The National Health Information Infrastrucuture (NHII) (NCVHS, 2001) reaches beyond the single institution with an infrastructure that would permit an authorized provider caring for

Mr. Jones to automatically obtain relevant medical data about that patient from other organizations within their community, e.g., from the hospital across town. Examples of such community-based "EHRs" are operating in Indianapolis (McDonald et al., 2005) and Santa Barbara to serve emergency, and other urgent, care needs. The Boston NEHEN Collaborative has created an analogous community-wide system for managing eligibility, preauthorization, and claim status information (www.nehen.net/technology.htm) (NEHEN, 2003).

Communication tools that support timely and efficient communication between patients and the health care team can enhance coordination of care and more effective disease management. eHealth applications can provide patients with secure access to their EHR and provide integrated communication tools to ask medical questions or perform other clinical (e.g., renew a prescription) or administrative tasks (e.g., schedule an appointment) conveniently online (Tang, 2003).

In addition to supporting communication among health care professionals and patients, community-based EHRs can facilitate the efficient creation and transmission of reports that support patient safety, quality improvement, public health, research, and other health care operations. (NCVHS, 2001) The creation of aggregate reports from such data, however, requires standardization as described in Chapter 10.

12.4   Fundamental Issues for Computer-Based Patient Record Systems

All medical record systems must serve the same functions, whether they be automated or manual. From a user's perspective, the two approaches differ fundamentally in the way data are entered into and information is extracted from the record. In this section, we explore the issues and alternatives related to data entry and then describe the options for displaying and retrieving information from an EHR.

12.4.1   Data Capture

Data entry of information into the EHR remains a formidable challenge, because it requires significant time and effort on the part of its users. There are two general methods of **data capture** in EHRs: electronic interfaces from systems, such as laboratory systems that are already fully automated and manual data entry, when no such electronic source exists. A third method, scanning paper reports, is available, but unless OCR methods are used the resulting format is not searchable or understandable to the computer.

Electronic Interfaces

The preferred method of capturing EHR data is to implement an electronic interface between the EHR and existing electronic data sources (e.g., laboratory systems, electronic instruments, registration systems, scheduling systems).

Though interfaces can require real effort as described under Section 12.3.1, they provide near-instant availability of the clinical data and avoid the labor costs and potential errors of manual transcription. Generally, the information technology department will invest resources needed to develop these electronic interfaces when the volume of data makes it worth the initial investment. This typically occurs when the organization that owns the EHR system also owns or is tightly affiliated with the owner of the source system. Efforts to capture data from systems outside the organizational boundary can be more difficult. Solutions require personal negotiations with sites that frequently provide care to a practice's patients and place extra work on the part of the practice.

The above discussion focuses on data produced by the home organization and/or produced by an outside organization in response to an order from the home organization. But even when all of the patient data produced, or ordered, by the home organization are captured, important clinical information produced by other organizations will not be included. For example, if the organization is a hospital system, it would not automatically capture pediatric immunizations. That information would be scattered across the pediatric and public health offices around town. So, the hospital would have to develop special procedures to collect immunization records if they wanted to help to improve immunization rates for children cared for in their clinics The trend toward larger, more integrated, and more self-contained health care systems and community-based health information infrastructures described by the NHII report will tend to reduce such problems of data capture. Nevertheless, the standards required to move data faithfully and automatically from source systems to EHRs within a health care delivery system remain a significant challenge (see Chapters 7 and 13).

Data Entry

The data-entry step is burdensome because of the personnel time required. People must interpret or translate the data, as well as enter them into the computer. Data may be entered in free-text form, in coded form, or in a form that combines both **free text** and **codes**. Trade-offs between the use of codes and narrative text exist.

The major advantages of coding are that data are classified and standardized, thus facilitating selective retrieval of patient data for clinical research, quality improvement, and administration. Coding lets the computer "understand" the data and thereby process them more intelligently. Immediate coding by physicians yields codes that the EHR can use to guide physicians' decisions. If selection methods are carefully designed, physician coding can be more accurate than coding by other personnel. The major disadvantage of coding is the human time it takes to translate the source text into valid codes. There also is the potential for coding errors, which, in contrast to errors in free-text entry, are difficult to detect, because coded information lacks the internal redundancy of text. For example, a transposition error causing a substitution of code 392 for 329 may not be detected unless the computer displays the associated text and the data-entry operator notices the error. Natural-language processing offers hope for automatic encoding of narrative text (Hripcsak et al., 2004).

In Chapter 7, we described alternative schemes for classifying diagnoses and medical procedures. Various computer sources of coded data, including laboratory systems, pharmacy systems, and electrocardiogram (ECG) carts, exist in health care settings.

Data from these systems can flow automatically to the EHR through message standards such as HL7 (described in Chapter 7). Here, the challenge is the variety of local coding systems. The solution is to use standard coding systems—such as LOINC for identification of laboratory tests and clinical measurements (McDonald et al., 2003), and Rx.Norm NDFRT (Nelson et al., 2002; RxNorm Overview, A guide to RxNorm. Accessed Sep 17, 2005 http://www.nlm.nih.gov/research/nmls/rxnorm_overview.htm/) or one of the commercial drug database codes for the identification of drug products, and SNOMED for diagnosis and findings (see Chapter 7).

Physician-Entered Data

Physician-gathered patient information requires special comment because it presents the most difficult challenge to developers and operators of EHR systems. Physicians' notes can be entered via one of three general mechanisms: transcription of dictated or written notes, entry of data recorded on structured encounter forms, or direct data entry by physicians (direct entry may include use of electronic templates or macros). Dictation and **transcription** is a common option for data entry of textual information into EHRs because it is widely and comfortably used by physicians. This method is especially attractive when the practice has already invested in dictation services, because then the cost of keying already has been absorbed. If physicians dictate their reports using standard formats (e.g., present illness, past history, physical examinations, and treatment plan), then the transcriptionist maintains this structure in the transcribed document. Voice recognition software offers a very attractive option for "dictating" without the cost or delay of transcription. The technology is improving as hardware processing speeds increase. However, even with accuracy rates of 95 to 98 percent, finding and correcting the few errors takes time and inhibits the use of this technology.

Although dictation is a preferred means of note writing, in many settings, physicians are recognizing the benefits of direct data entry because it eliminates the turnaround time required for the dictation to be transcribed and for someone to review, correct, sign, and file the transcribed document. All these steps leave room for errors and delays in completing the record. The lack of encoding further reduces the benefits of using an EHR. The problem with direct physician entry of their notes via templates and typing is cost of physician time.

The second data-entry method is to have physicians use a **structured encounter form** from which their notes are transcribed and possibly scanned in which case some of the content can be automatically encoded via an optical character reader (OCR) and/or mark-sense reading while some is stored as scanned image as is done at Regenstrief (Downs et al., 2005) and Mayo (Hagen et al., 1998). The handwritten numbers on the left side and the computer-printed numbers at the bottom left of Figure 12.5 are read by OCR techniques.

The third alternative is the **direct entry** of data, by a care provider, via a computer. This alternative has the advantage that the computer can immediately check the entry for consistency with previously stored information and can generate reminders about further questions that should be asked based on the information just entered.

Physician orders are specially important for the medical record because they specify what is to be done for the patient. Because of the many potential advantages for care quality and efficiency, organizations are being encouraged to move to direct computerized physician order entry (CPOE). CPOE can be facilitated by custom menus that contain standing orders for specific problems (e.g., postoperative orders for patients who undergo coronary artery bypass operations). Menus must be carefully structured. They must not contain lists that are too long, require scrolling, or impose a rigid hierarchy (Kuhn et al., 1984). Direct entry of the patient's history, physical findings, and progress notes has been challenging because of the extra time it takes the physician to enter such information into the computer compared with scribbling a note. Yet some physicians do enter all of their notes into the computer in some EHRs, while transcribed dictation remains an important source of physcians' notes in many EHR implementations.

Data Validation

Because of the chance of transcription errors occurring when clinical information is entered into the computer, EHR systems must apply **validity checks** scrupulously. A number of different kinds of checks apply to clinical data (Schwartz et al., 1985). **Range checks** can detect or prevent entry of values that are out of range (e.g., a serum potassium level of 50.0 mEq/L—the normal range for healthy individuals is 3.5 to 5.0 mEq/L). **Pattern checks** can verify that the entered data have a required pattern (e.g., the three digits, hyphen, and four digits of a local telephone number). **Computed checks** can verify that values have the correct mathematical relationship (e.g., white blood cell differential counts, reported as percentages, must sum to 100). **Consistency checks** can detect errors by comparing entered data (e.g., the recording of cancer of the prostate as the diagnosis for a female patient). **Delta checks** warn of large and unlikely differences between the values of a new result and of the previous observations (e.g., a recorded weight that changes by 100 pounds in 2 weeks). **Spelling checks** verify the spelling of individual words. No such syntactic checks can catch all errors.

12.4.2   Data Display

Once stored in the computer, data can be presented in numerous formats for different purposes without further entry work. In addition, computer-stored records can be produced in novel formats that are unavailable in manual systems. We discuss a few helpful formats.

Flowsheets of Patient Data

A **flowsheet** is similar to a spreadsheet; it organizes patient data according to the time that they were generated, thus emphasizing changes over time. Figure 12.12 shows the popular pocket rounds report that provides laboratory and nursing measurements as a very compact flowsheet that fits in a white coat pocket (McDonald et al., 1992). A flowsheet used to monitor patients who have hypertension (high blood pressure) might contain values for weight, blood pressure, heart rate, and doses of medications that control hypertension. Other pertinent information could be added, such as results of laboratory tests that monitor complications associated with hypertension, or complications of

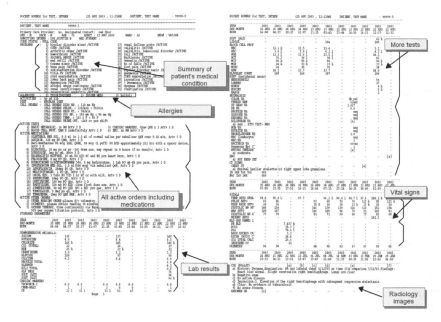

Figure 12.12. The very popular Pocket rounds report – so called because it fits in the clinician's white coat pocket when folded in half. The report is a very dense (16 lines per inch 2 characters per inch) printed in landscape mode on one 8 1/2 × 11 inch page) summary of the patient's medical state, and includes the all active orders (including medications), recent laboratory results, vital signs and the summary impressions of radiology, endoscopy, and cardiology reports (*Source*: Courtesy of Regenstrief Institute, Indianapolis, IN.)

medications used to control hypertension. Flowsheets are potentially problem-, patient-, or specialty-specific. The time granularity may change from one setting to another. For example, when a patient is in the ICU, minute-to-minute changes in the patient's clinical state may be of interest. On the other hand, an outpatient physician is more likely to want to know how that patient's data have changed over weeks or months. For convenience of human review, the temporal granularity should be appropriate to the intensity of care. Thus, of the hundreds of blood pressure measurements taken every 20 minutes in an ICU not all are of interest to the physician taking care of the same patient later in the clinic after the patient's condition has stabilized.

Summaries and Abstracts

EHRs can highlight important components (e.g., active allergies, active problems, active treatments, and recent observations) in a clinical summary (Tang et al., 1999). In the future, we can expect more sophisticated summarizing strategies, such as automated detection of adverse events (Bates, 2003) or automated time-series events (e.g., cancer chemotherapy cycles). We may also see reports that distinguish abnormal changes that have been treated from those that have not and displays that dynamically organize the supporting evidence for existing problems (Tang, 1994a). Ultimately, computers should be able to produce concise and flowing summary reports that are like an experienced physician's hospital discharge summary.

Dynamic Displays

Anyone who has reviewed a patient's chart knows how hard it can be to find a particular piece of information. From 10 percent (Fries, 1974) to 81 percent (Tang et al., 1994b) of the time, physicians do not find patient information that has been previously recorded and belongs in the medical record. Furthermore, the questions clinicians routinely ask are often the ones that are difficult to answer from perusal of a paper-based record. Common questions include whether a specific test has ever been performed, what kinds of medications have been tried in the past, and how the patient has responded to particular treatments (e.g., a class of medications) in the past. Physicians constantly ask these questions as they flip back and forth in the chart searching for the facts to support or refute one in a series of evolving hypotheses. Search tools help the physician to locate relevant data, and specialized presentation formats (e.g., flowsheets or graphics) make it easier for them to glean information from the data. Special displays can identify problem-specific parameters to help the physician retrieve relevant information, and a graphical presentation can help the physician to assimilate the information quickly and to draw conclusions (Fafchamps et al., 1991; Tang et al., 1994a; Starren and Johnson, 2000).

12.4.3   Query and Surveillance Systems

The **query** and **surveillance** capabilities of computer-stored records have no counterpart in manual systems. Medical personnel, quality and patient safety professionals, and administrators can use these capabilities to analyze patient outcomes and practice patterns. Public health professionals can use the reporting functions of computer-stored records for surveillance, looking for emergence of new diseases or other health threats that warrant medical attention.

Although these functions are different, their internal logic is similar. In both, the central procedure is to examine a patient's medical record and, if the record meets prespecified criteria, to generate an appropriate output. Queries generally address a large subset, or all, of a patient population; the output is a tabular report of selected raw data on all the patient records retrieved or a statistical summary of the values contained in the records. Surveillance generally addresses only those patients under active care; its output is an **alert** or **reminder message** (McDonald, 1976). Query and surveillance systems can be used for clinical care, clinical research, retrospective studies, and administration.

Clinical Care

Computer reminders have increased substantially physicians' use of preventive care for eligible patients. Surveillance systems can identify patients who are due for periodic screening examinations such as immunizations, mammograms, and cervical Pap tests and can remind physicians to perform these procedures during the next visit. For example, physicians given computer reminders quadrupled the use of certain vaccines in eligible patients compared with those who did not receive reminders (McDonald et al., 1984a; McPhee et al., 1991; Hunt, 1998; Teich, 2000). Query systems are particularly useful for conducting ad hoc searches such as those required to identify and notify patients who have been receiving a recalled drug. Such systems can also facilitate quality management and patient safety activities. They can identify candidate patients for concurrent review and can gather many of the data required to complete such audits.

Clinical Research

Query systems can be used to identify patients who meet eligibility requirements for prospective clinical trials. For example, an investigator could identify all patients seen in a medical clinic who have a specific diagnosis and meet eligibility requirements while not having any exclusionary conditions. Surveillance facilities can support the execution of a study by tracking patients through their visits and by following the steps of a clinical trial as described in the study protocol to ensure that treatments are given and measurements obtained when required (Tierney and McDonald, 1991). Some existing systems use reminder logic to request the provider's permission to invite a patient into an ongoing study. The entry of back pain as the visit diagnosis, for example, could trigger a request about an ongoing trial of physical therapy for back pain. If the physician agrees, the computer sends an electronic page to the nurse recruiter for that study so that he/she can get to the clinic to invite the patient into the study.

Retrospective Studies

Randomized **prospective studies** are the gold standard for clinical investigations, but **retrospective studies** of existing data have contributed much to medical progress. Retrospective studies can obtain answers at a small fraction of the time and cost of comparable prospective studies.

EHR systems can provide many of the data required for a retrospective study. They can, for example, identify study cases and comparable control cases, and they can perform the statistical analyses needed to compare the two groups (McDonald et al., 2005; Bleich et al., 1989; Safran, 1991; Mahon et al., 2000).

Computer-stored records do not eliminate all the work required to complete an epidemiologic study; chart reviews and patient interviews may still be necessary if some patient information is recorded as narrative text. The more information that can be retrieved from the computer record, however, the less frequently and less intensively such time-consuming tasks must be conducted. Computer-stored records are likely to be most complete and accurate with respect to drugs administered, laboratory test results, and visit diagnoses, especially if the first two types of data are entered directly from automated laboratory and pharmacy systems. Consequently, computer-stored records are most likely to contribute to research on a physician's practice patterns, on the efficacy of tests and treatments, and on the toxicity of drugs.

Administration

In the past, administrators had to rely on data from billing systems to understand practice patterns and resource utilization. However, claims data are notoriously unreliable for understanding clinical practice because the source data are often entered by nonclinical personnel not directly involved with the care decisions. Medical query systems can provide information about the relationships among diagnoses, indices of severity of illness, and resource consumption. Thus, query systems are important tools for administrators who wish to make informed decisions in the increasingly cost-sensitive world of health care.

12.5   Challenges Ahead

Although many commercial products are labeled as EHR systems, they do not all satisfy the criteria that we defined at the beginning of this chapter. Even beyond matters of definition, however, it is important to recognize that the concept of an EHR is neither unified nor static. As the capability of technology evolves, the function of the EHR will expand. A review of current products would be obsolete by the time that it was published. We have included examples from various systems in this chapter, both developed by their users and commercially available, to illustrate a portion of the functionality of EHR systems currently in use.

The future of EHR systems depends on both technical and nontechnical considerations. Hardware technology will continue to advance, with processing power doubling every 2 years according to Moore's law. Software will improve with more powerful applications, better user interfaces, and more integrated decision support. Perhaps the greater need for leadership and action will be in the social and organizational foundations that must be laid if EHRs are to serve as the information infrastructure for health care. We touch briefly on these challenges in this final section.

12.5.1   Users' Information Needs

We discussed the importance of clinicians directly using the EHR system to achieve maximum benefit from computer-supported decision making. On the one hand, organizations that require providers to enter all of their order, notes, and data directly into the EHR will gain the most efficiency and care quality. But it will be the physicians who will bear the time costs of entering this information and face disruptions to their routines. So, some balance between the organization' and providers' interests must be struck, and this balance is easiest to reach when the physicians are part of the organization's leadership.

Developers of EHR systems must thoroughly understand clinicians' information needs and workflows in the various settings where health care is delivered. The most successful systems have been developed either by clinicians or through close collaborations with practicing clinicians.

Studies of clinicians' information needs reveal that common questions that physicians ask concerning patient information (e.g., Is there evidence to support a specific patient diagnosis? Has a patient ever had a specific test? Has there been any follow up because of a particular laboratory test result?) are difficult to answer from the perusal of the paper-based chart (Tang et al., 1994b). Regrettably, most clinical systems in use now cannot answer many of the common questions that clinicians ask. Developers of EHR systems must have a thorough grasp of users' needs and workflows if they are to produce systems that help health care providers use these tools efficiently to deliver care effectively.

12.5.2   User Interfaces

An intuitive and efficient user interface is an important part of the system. Designers must understand the cognitive aspects of the human and computer interaction if they are to build interfaces that are easy-to-learn and easy-to-use. Improving human–computer interfaces will require changes not only in how the system behaves but also in how humans interact with the system. What information the provider needs and what tasks the provider performs should influence what and how information is presented. Development of human-interface technology that matches the data-processing power of computers with the cognitive capability of humans to formulate insightful questions and to interpret data is still a rate-limiting step (Tang and Patel, 1993). User interface requirements of clinicians entering patient data are different from the user interfaces developed for clerks entering patient charges. Among the most potent functions of EHRs is CPOE. To facilitate use by busy health care professionals, health care applications developers must focus on clinicians' unique information needs.

12.5.3   Standards

We alluded to the importance of standards earlier in this chapter, when we discussed the architectural requirements of integrating data from multiple sources. Standards were discussed in Chapter 7. Here, we stress the critical importance of national standards in the development, implementation, and use of EHR systems (McDonald et al., 1997b). Health information should follow patients as they interact with different providers in different care settings. Uniform standards are essential for systems to interoperate and exchange data in meaningful ways. Having standards reduces development costs, increases integration, and facilitates the collection of meaningful aggregate data for quality improvement and health policy development. The HIPAA legislation has mandated standards for administrative messages, privacy, security, and clinical data. Regulations based on this legislation have been promulgated for the first three of these categories. These can be obtained at http://www.cms.hhs.gov/hipaa/hipaa2/regulations/default.asp. A Consolidated Health Informatics (CHI) group within the U.S. federal government is selecting standards that will be required for transmission of clinical data within federal agencies. They have selected HL7 Version. 2.4 as the primary message standard, DICOM for radiology images, LOINC for laboratory test observations. They are working on a host of additional selections to cover units of measures, test answers, medication identifier codes, general clinical terminology (likely SNOMED), and more (see Chapter 7). The interested reader can follow their progress at the Web site http://www.hhs.gov/healthit/chi.html. A public-private consortium, connecting for Health, is also making recommendations that have influenced CHI. Standards for clinical data transmission will not be mandated in the United States but they will be encouraged and incented. Those who wish to implement EHRs should promote and adopt clinical information standards.

12.5.4   Legal and Social Issues

In addition to legislation on standards, federal laws and policies regarding other aspects of the use of EHR systems must be established before widespread adoption will occur. HIPAA has also established key regulations to protect the confidentiality of individually identifiable health information and the security of computer systems that store and transmit patient information (see http://cms.hhs.gov/hipaa). With appropriate laws and policies computer-stored data can be more secure and confidential than those data maintained in paper-based records (Barrows and Clayton, 1996).

12.5.5   Costs and Benefits

The Institute of Medicine declared the EHR an essential infrastructure for the delivery of health care (Institute of Medicine Committee on Improving the Patient Record, 1997) and the protection of patient safety (IOM, 2001). Like any infrastructure project, the benefits specifically attributable to infrastructure are difficult to establish; an infrastructure plays an enabling role in all projects that take advantage of it. Part of the difficulty in comparing costs and benefits of an EHR is our inability to measure accurately the actual costs and opportunity costs of using paper-based records. Many randomized controlled clinical studies have shown that computer-based decision-support systems that are integrated in an EHR reduce costs and improve quality compared with usual care supported with a paper medical record (Tierney et al., 1993; Bates et al., 1997, 2003; Classen et al., 1997). It is difficult, however, to determine the scalability and longevity of such benefits.

Because of the significant resources needed and the significant broad-based potential benefits, the decision to implement an EHR system is a strategic one. Hence, the evaluation of the costs and benefits must consider the effects on the organization's strategic goals, as well as the objectives for individual health care. Recently, the federal government and professional organizations have both expressed interest in the **Open Source** options for EHR software (McDonald et al., 2003).

12.5.6   Leadership

Leaders from all segments of the health care industry must work together to articulate the needs, to define the standards, to fund the development, to implement the social change, and to write the laws to accelerate the development and routine use of EHR systems in health care. Because of the prominent role of the federal government in health care—as a payer, provider, policymaker, and regulator—federal leadership to create incentives for developing and adopting standards and for promoting the implementation and use of EHRs is crucial. Technological change will continue to occur at a rapid pace, driven by consumer demand for entertainment, games, and business tools. Nurturing the use of information technology in health care requires leaders who promote the use of EHR systems and work to overcome the obstacles that impede widespread use of computers for the benefit of health care.

Suggested Readings

Barnett G.O. (1984). The application of computer-based medical-record systems in ambulatory practice. *New England Journal of Medicine*, 310(25):1643–1650.
This seminal article compares the characteristics of manual and automated ambulatory patient record systems, discusses implementation issues, and predicts future developments in technology.

Collen M.F. (1995). *A history of medical informatics in the United States, 1950–1990*. Indianapolis: American Medical Informatics Association, Hartman Publishing.
This rich history of medical informatics from the late 1960s to the late 1980s includes an extremely detailed set of references.

Institute of Medicine Committee on Improving the Patient Record (1997). *The Computer-Based Patient-Record: An Essential Technology for Health Care* (2nd ed). Washington, D.C.: National Academy Press.
This landmark study by the Institute of Medicine defines the EHR, describes the users and uses of the medical record, examines technologies employed in EHRs, and recommends actions to accelerate the development and routine use of EHRs in the United States. The second edition adds commentaries on the status of EHRs in the United States and Europe 5 years after the release of the original report.

McDonald C.J. (Ed.) (1988). Computer-stored medical record systems. *MD Computing*, 5(5):1–62.
This issue of *MD Computing* contains invited papers on the STOR, HELP, RMRS, and TMR systems. The objective of the issue is to describe the design goals, functions, and internal structure of these established, large-scale EHR systems.

McDonald C.J., Tierney W.M. (1986). The medical gopher: A microcomputer system to help find, organize and decide about patient data. *Western Journal of Medicine*, 145(6):823–829.
McDonald and Tierney describe research conducted at the Regenstrief Institute for Health Care in developing a PC-based medical workstation that can help physicians to organize, review, and record medical information.

Osheroff J. (Ed.) (1995). *Computers in Clinical Practices. Managing Patients, Information, and Communication*. Philadelphia: American College of Physicians.
This text looks at the practical use of computers in the office practice with a special emphasis on medical records.

Pryor T.A., Gardner R.M., Clayton P.D., Warner H.R. (1983). The HELP system. *Journal of Medical Systems*, 7(2):87–102.
This article summarizes the HELP system's objectives and describes HELP's use in clinical decision making.

Van Bemmel J.H., Musen, M.A. (1997). *Handbook of Medical Informatics*. Heidelberg: Bohn Stafleu Van Loghum, Houten.

This book provides a comprehensive survey of work being performed to develop information technology for the clinical workplace.

Weed L.L. (1969). *Medical Records, Medical Evaluation and Patient Care: The Problem-Oriented Record as a Basic Tool*. Chicago: Year Book Medical Publishers.
In this classic book, Weed presents his plan for collecting and structuring patient data to produce a problem-oriented medical record.

Questions for Discussion

1. What is the definition of an EHR? Define an EHR system. What are five advantages of a EHR over a paper-based record? What are three limitations of an EHR?
2. What are the five functional components of an EHR? Think of the information systems used in health care institutions in which you work or that you have seen. Which of the components that you named do those systems have? Which are missing? How do the missing elements limit the value to the clinicians or patients?
3. Discuss three ways in which a computer system could facilitate information transfer between hospitals and ambulatory care facilities, thus enhancing continuity of care for previously hospitalized patients who have been discharged and are now being followed up by their primary physicians.
4. How does the health care financing environment affect the use, costs, and benefits of an EHR system? How has the financing environment affected the functionality of information systems? How has it affected the user population?
5. Would a computer scan of a paper-based record be an EHR? What are two advantages and two limitations of this approach?
6. Among the key issues for designing an EHR system are what information should be captured and how it should be entered into the system.
    a. Physicians may enter data directly or may record data on a paper worksheet (encounter form) for later transcription by a data-entry worker. What are two advantages and two disadvantages of each method?
    b. Discuss the relative advantages and disadvantages of entry of free text instead of entry of fully coded information. Describe an intermediate or compromise method.
7. Identify four locations where clinicians need access to the information contained in an EHR. What are the major costs or risks of providing access from each of these locations?
8. What are three important reasons to have physicians enter orders directly into an EHR system? What are three challenges in implementing such a system?
9. Consider the task of creating a summary report for clinical data collected over time and stored in an EHR system. Clinical laboratories traditionally provide summary test results in flowsheet format, thus highlighting clinically important changes over time. A medical record system that contains information for patients who have chronic diseases must present serial clinical observations, history information, and medications, as well as laboratory test results. Suggest a suitable format for presenting the information collected during a series of ambulatory-care patient visits.

10. The public demands that the confidentiality of patient data must be maintained in any patient record system. Describe three protections and auditing methods that can be applied to paper-based systems. Describe three technical and three nontechnical measures you would like to see applied to ensure the confidentiality of patient data in an EHR. How do the risks of privacy breaches differ for the two systems?

13
Management of Information in Healthcare Organizations

LYNN HAROLD VOGEL AND LESLIE E. PERREAULT

After reading this chapter, you should know the answers to these questions:

- What are the primary information requirements of healthcare organizations?
- What are the clinical, financial, and administrative functions provided by a healthcare information system (HCIS), and what are the potential benefits of implementing such a system?
- How have changes in healthcare delivery models changed the scope and capabilities of HCISs over time?
- How do differences among business strategies and organizational structures influence information systems choices?
- What are the major challenges to implementing and managing HCISs?
- How are ongoing healthcare reforms, technological advances, and changing social norms likely to affect HCIS requirements in the future?

13.1   Overview

Healthcare organizations (HCOs), like all business entities, are information-intensive enterprises. Healthcare personnel require sufficient data and information management tools to make appropriate decisions, both while caring for patients and while managing and running the enterprise, to document and communicate plans and activities, and to meet the requirements of regulatory and accrediting organizations. Clinicians assess patient status, plan patient care, administer appropriate treatments, and educate patients and families regarding clinical management of various conditions. Primary-care physicians and care managers assess the health status of new members of a health plan. Medical directors evaluate the clinical outcomes, quality, and cost of health services provided. Administrators determine appropriate staffing levels, manage inventories of drugs and supplies, and negotiate payment contracts for services. Governing boards make decisions about investing in new business lines, partnering with other organizations, and eliminating underutilized services. Collectively, healthcare professionals comprise a heterogeneous group with diverse objectives and information requirements.

The purpose of a **healthcare information system** (HCIS) is to manage the information that health professionals need to perform their jobs effectively and efficiently. HCISs facilitate communication, integrate information, and coordinate action among multiple healthcare professionals. In addition, they assist in the organization and storage of information, and they support certain record-keeping and reporting functions. Many of the clinical information functions of an HCIS were detailed in our discussion of the computer-based patient record (CPR) in Chapter 12; systems to support nurses and other care providers are discussed in Chapter 16. An HCIS also supports the financial and administrative functions of a health organization and associated operating units, including the operations of ancillary and other clinical-support departments. The evolving complexities of HCOs place great demands on an HCIS. The HCIS must organize, manage, and integrate large numbers of clinical and financial data collected by diverse users in a variety of settings and must provide healthcare workers (and, increasingly, patients) with timely access to complete, accurate, and up-to-date information presented in a useful format.

13.1.1   Evolution from Automation of Specific Functions, to Departmental, to Hospital-wide and then Healthcare System Information Systems

Chapter 23 details the economic and regulatory factors, and the resultant healthcare reforms, that have altered the delivery-of-care model in the United States. These changes radically transformed the structure, strategic goals, and operational processes of healthcare organizations through a gradual shifting of financial risk from third party payers (such as Blue Cross and Blue Shield, Medicare and Medicaid programs in the 1960s and 1970s, and then managed care companies in the 1980s) to the hospitals themselves. This shifting of risk also brought about a rapid consolidation of healthcare providers into **integrated delivery networks** (IDNs) in the 1990s. More recently, we have seen a retreat from the most restrictive models of managed care toward greater consumer choice, a slowing of mergers and acquisitions activities, several high profile IDN failures (Shortell et al., 2000, Weil, 2001, Kastor, 2001), and major new regulatory requirements aimed at improved efficiency and greater patient privacy and safety. All these changes have had tremendous implications for information systems.

The evolution of HCISs has paralleled the organizational evolution of the healthcare industry itself. The earliest HCISs were largely focused on the automation of specific functions within hospitals including, initially, patient registration and billing. The justification for these systems was relatively straightforward since large mainframe computers were easily capable of performing the largely clerical tasks associated with tracking patients and sending out bills. In the 1960s and 1970s, additional functions were added to the financial systems as hospitals realized the benefits of installing computer systems to support ancillary departments such as radiology, the pharmacy, and the laboratories. Collectively these disparate functional systems have become known as **hospital information systems** (HISs), even though in most cases they remain quite separate not only in function but in terms of computer hardware, operating systems, and even programming languages. The lack of connectivity among these various systems created significant obstacles to keeping track of where patients were located in a hospital, and more importantly, what kinds of care were being provided and the clinical results of that care. It was not uncommon for care givers to have to log on to several different computer systems just to learn the status of specific clinical results. By the late 1980s, **clinical information**

system (CIS) components of HISs offered clinically oriented capabilities, such as order writing and results communications. During the same period, **ambulatory medical record systems** (AMRSs) and **practice management systems** (PMSs) were being developed to support large outpatient clinics and physician offices, respectively. These systems performed functions analogous to those of hospital systems, but were generally less complex, reflecting the lower volume and complexity of patient care delivered in outpatient settings. Typically, these various systems were implemented within organizational boundaries, with no integration between hospital and ambulatory settings.

The presence of so many different, functionally specific information systems is one of the unique attributes of HCOs. These systems were often developed in isolation from one another as vendors focused on developing as much highly specialized functionality as possible—in effect, striving for a "best of breed" designation in the marketplace for their particular type of system. The isolation of these systems, even within a single organizational structure, was overcome in part by the development of interfaces between the various systems. Initially these interfaces focused on delivering patient demographic information from registration systems to the ancillary systems and data on specific clinical events (e.g., laboratory tests, radiology exams, medications ordered) from the ancillary systems to the billing system. However, as more information systems were added to the HCIS environment, the challenge of moving data from one system to another became overwhelming. In response, two unique developments occurred: 1) the development of the **interface engine**; and 2) the creation of HL7, a process for standardizing the content of the data messages that were being sent from one information system to another.

The challenge of sharing data among many different information systems was daunting. As we noted earlier, the various components of the HCIS were in most cases developed by different vendors, using different hardware (e.g., DEC, IBM), operating systems (e.g., PICK, Altos, DOS, VMS, and IBM's OS on mainframes) and programming languages (e.g., BASIC, PL1, COBOL, and even assembler). Sharing data among two different systems typically requires a two-way interface—one to send data from A to B, the other to send data back or acknowledge receipt from B back to A. Adding a third system didn't require simply one additional interface because the new system would in many cases have to be interfaced to both of the original systems, resulting in the possibility of six interfaces. Introducing a fourth system into the HCIS environment could create the need for two-way interfaces to each of the original three systems, for a total of twelve. With the prospect of interfaces increasing exponentially with the addition of each new system (represented by the formula, $n=n(n-1)$) where n represents the number of systems, it was clear that a new solution was needed to address the complexity and cost of interfacing. In response, a new industry niche was born in the late 1980s which focused on creating a new software application the purpose of which was to manage the interfacing challenges among disparate systems in the HCIS environment. Instead of each system having to interface to every other system, the interface engine served as the central connecting point for all interfaces. Each system had only to connect to the interface engine; the engine then managed the sending of data to any other system that needed it. The initial **interface engine** concept, which originated in healthcare, has given rise to a whole series of strategies for managing multiple systems called Enterprise Application

Integration. Many of the vendors who got their start in healthcare interfacing have found new markets in the financial services as well as other industries.

The creation of HL7 (see Chapter 7) was yet another response to the challenge of moving data among disparate systems in healthcare. HL7 is a healthcare-based initiative, also started in the late 1980s, to develop standards for the sharing of data among the many individual systems that comprise an HCIS. The basic idea was to create a virtually integrated HCIS through the use of messaging standards so that data could be moved in standard formats within the HCIS environment. Most of the departmental systems that were introduced at this time were the products of companies focused on specific niche markets, including laboratories, pharmacies and radiology departments. Consequently there was strong support for both the interface engine and the HL7 efforts as mechanisms to permit smaller vendors to compete successfully in the marketplace. In recent years, many of these pioneering vendors have been purchased and their products included as components of larger product families. In spite of this consolidation, strong demand for HL7 and interface engines has continued because, even within larger product families, there is still a need to move data as seamlessly as possible from one functional application to another.

The decade of the 1990s was marked by a large number of mergers and affiliations among previously independent and often competing organizations designed to drive excess capacity from the system (e.g., an oversupply of hospital beds) and to secure regional market share. First, hospitals and medical centers began to build satellite ambulatory-care clinics and to reach out to community physician practices in an attempt to feed patient referrals to their specialty services and to fill their increasingly vacant inpatient beds. Later, facing competition with vertically integrated for-profit healthcare chains and with other integrating organizations, hospitals started at first affiliating and then more tightly banding into the regional aggregates of healthcare service providers called Integrated Delivery Networks (IDNs) (See Figure. 13.1).

By 2000, IDNs were prominent in every healthcare market in the United States and in several cases, spanned large geographic regions or multiple states. Each IDN typically consisted of multiple acute-care facilities, satellite ambulatory health centers, and owned or managed physicians' practice groups. In addition, larger IDNs might have skilled nursing homes, hospices, home-care agencies, and for-profit subcorporations to deliver support services back to the healthcare providers, including regional laboratories, separate organizations for purchasing and distributing drugs and medical supplies, and remote billing services. A major goal of such IDNs was to reduce their costs (both internally and from suppliers), as well as to retain or increase revenues by improving their negotiating strength with third party payers. Because they controlled a significant regional market share and were positioned to provide and manage comprehensive health services, IDNs expected to negotiate favorable purchasing contracts with suppliers and very competitive service contracts with payers or directly with large employers. Some IDNs went further and affiliated with a regional health maintenance organization (HMO) or developed their own health-plan organizations to act as their own insurance carriers. The largest of the IDNs had pooled annual revenues of billions of dollars, had staffs comprising or contracting with thousands of physicians and nurses, and managed contracts to provide comprehensive care for more than one million patients.

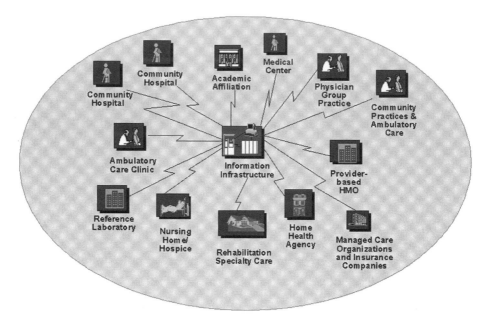

Figure 13.1. Major organizational components of an integrated delivery network (IDN). A typical IDN includes multiple acute-care facilities, ambulatory-care clinics, and owned or managed physicians' practices that jointly operate to provide comprehensive health services. In addition, an IDN may own or affiliate with other healthcare facilities, for-profit subcorporations, and managed care or health plan organizations. HMO = Health Maintenance Organization.

A second goal of IDNs was to cut costs by achieving economies of scale; for example, by consolidating administrative and financial functions and combining clinical services. Such IDNs were challenged to coordinate patient care and manage business operations throughout an extensive network of community and regional resources. As a result, HCISs were developed to share information and coordinate activities not only within, but among multiple hospitals, ambulatory care sites, physicians' practice groups, and other affiliated organizations.

Although IDNs are still a prominent feature in most healthcare markets, recent years have seen a decrease in the rate of market consolidation and some highly visible IDN failures. While the most successful of IDNs have achieved a measure of structural and operational integration, gains from the integration of clinical activities and from the consolidation of information systems has been much more difficult (See Figure 13.2). Many IDNs have scaled back their original goals for combining clinical activities and are in the process of shedding home care services, physician practices, health plans and managed care entities. It appears that the expertise gained from managing an inpatient-driven organization (e.g., a hospital) does not translate easily to the successful management of other organizational activities, nor in some cases, even to other hospitals. To date, none have gained the degree of cost savings and efficiencies they had originally

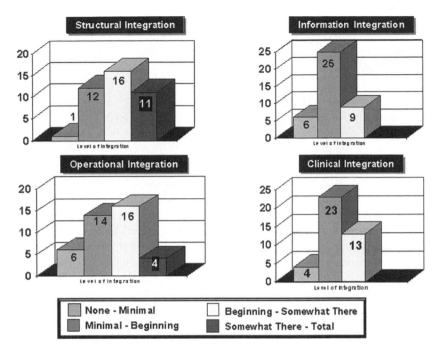

Figure 13.2. Relative progress in structural, operational, clinical, and information integration among 40 IDNs from a 1996 survey of organizational members of the Center for Clinical Integration. Clinical integration and information systems typically lag behind structural and operational integration in emerging IDNs. (*Source:* Copyright First Consulting Group. Reprinted with permission.)

projected. The immense up-front costs of implementing the required HCISs have contributed to the limited success, and sometimes to the demise, of IDNs. Regardless of organizational structure, all healthcare organizations are striving toward greater information access and integration, including improved information linkages with physicians and patients. The "typical" HCO is a melding of diverse organizations, and the associated information systems infrastructure is still far from integrated; rather, it is an amalgam of heterogeneous systems, processes, and data stores.

13.1.2 Information Requirements

From a clinical perspective, the most important function of an HCIS is to present patient-specific data to care givers so that they can easily interpret the data and use it in decision-making and to support the necessary communication among the many healthcare workers who cooperate in providing health services to patients. From an administrative perspective, the most pressing information needs are those related to the daily operation and management of the organization—bills must be generated accurately and rapidly, employees and vendors must be paid, supplies must be ordered, and so on. In addition, administrators need information to make short-term and long-term planning decisions. We can classify an HCO's operational information needs into four broad categories of support: daily operations, planning, communication, and documentation and reporting.

- *Operational requirements.* Healthcare workers—both care givers and administrators—require detailed and up-to-date factual information to perform the daily tasks that keep a hospital, clinic, or physician practice running—the bread-and-butter tasks of the institution. Here are examples of queries for operational information: Where is patient John Smith? What drugs is he receiving? What tests are scheduled for Mr. Smith after his discharge? Who will pay his bill? Is the staffing skill mix sufficient to handle the current volume and special needs of patients in Care Center 3 West? What are the names and telephone numbers of patients who have appointments for tomorrow and need to be called for a reminder? What authorization is needed to perform an ultrasound procedure on Jane Blue under the terms of her health insurance coverage? An HCIS can support these operational requirements for information by organizing data for prompt and easy access. Because the HCO may have developed product-line specialization within a particular facility (e.g., a diagnostic imaging center or women's health center), however, answering even a simple request may require accessing information stored in different systems at many different facilities.
- *Planning requirements.* Health professionals also require information to make short-term and long-term decisions about patient care and organizational management. The importance of appropriate clinical decision-making is obvious—we devoted all of Chapter 3 to explaining methods to help clinicians select diagnostic tests, interpret test results, and choose treatments for their patients. The decisions made by administrators and managers are no less important in their choices concerning the acquisition and use of healthcare resources. In fact, clinicians and administrators alike must choose wisely in their use of resources to provide high-quality care and excellent service at a competitive price. An HCIS should help healthcare personnel to answer queries such as these: What are the organization's clinical guidelines for managing the care of patients with this condition? Have similar patients experienced better clinical outcomes with medical treatment or with surgical intervention? What are the financial and medical implications of closing the maternity service? If we added six care managers to the outpatient-clinic staff, can we improve patient outcomes and reduce emergency admissions? Will the proposed contract to provide health services to Medicaid patients be profitable given the current cost structure and current utilization patterns? Often, the data necessary for planning are generated by many sources. An HCIS can help planners by aggregating, analyzing, and summarizing the information relevant to decision-making.
- *Communication requirements.* It should be clear that communication and coordination of patient care and operations across multiple personnel, multiple business units, and far-flung geography is not possible without investment in an underlying technology infrastructure. For example, the routing of paper medical records, a cumbersome process even within a single hospital, is an impossibility for a regional network of providers trying to act in coordination. Similarly, it is neither timely nor cost effective to copy and distribute hard copy documents to all participants in a regionally dis-

tributed organizational structure. An HCO's technology infrastructure can enable information exchange via web-based access to shared databases and documents, electronic mail, standard document-management systems, and on-line calendaring systems, as well as providing and controlling HCIS access for authorized users at the place and time that information is required.

- *Documentation and reporting requirements.* The need to maintain records for future reference or analysis and reporting makes up the fourth category of informational requirements. Some requirements are internally imposed. For example, a complete record of each patient's health status and treatment history is necessary to ensure continuity of care across multiple providers and over time. External requirements create a large demand for data collection and record keeping in HCOs. As discussed in Chapter 2, the medical record is a legal document. If necessary, the courts can refer to the record to determine whether a patient received proper care. Insurance companies require itemized billing statements, and medical records substantiate the clinical justification of services provided and the charges submitted to them. The Joint Commission for Accreditation of Healthcare Organizations (JCAHO) has specific requirements concerning the content and quality of medical records, as well as requirements for organization-wide information-management processes. Furthermore, to qualify for participation in the Medicare and Medicaid programs, JCAHO requires that hospitals follow accepted procedures for auditing the medical staff and monitoring the quality of patient care, and they must be able to show that they meet the safety requirements for infectious disease management, buildings, and equipment. Employer and consumer groups are also joining the list of external monitors. In response to the Institute of Medicine's 1999 report, "To Err is Human", which documented the large number of preventable medication errors in hospitals, a consortium of large employers and other healthcare purchasers formed The Leapfrog Group, which now exerts pressure on hospitals to participate in their patient safety surveys and implement their recommended safety practices. Survey results are publicly reported and used by purchasers in contract discussions.

13.1.3   Integration Requirements

If an HCO is to manage patient care effectively, to project a focused market identity, and to control its operating costs, it must perform in a unified and consistent manner. For these reasons, information technologies to support data and process integration are recognized as critical to an HCO's operations. From an organizational perspective, information should be available when and where it is needed; users must have an integrated view, regardless of system or geographic boundaries; data must have a consistent interpretation; and adequate security must be in place to ensure access only by authorized personnel and only for appropriate uses.

Data Integration

In hospitals, clinical and administrative personnel have traditionally had distinct areas of responsibility and performed many of their functions separately. Thus, it is not surprising that administrative and clinical data were often managed separately—administrative data in business offices and clinical data in medical-records departments. When computers were used at all, the hospital's information processing was often performed on separate computers with separate databases, thus minimizing conflicts about priorities in services and investment. As we have seen earlier in this chapter, information systems to support hospital functions and ambulatory care historically have, with a few notable exceptions (Bleich et al., 1985), developed independently. Many organizations have rich databases for inpatient data but maintain less information for outpatients—often only billing data such as diagnosis and procedure codes, and charges for services provided. Even today, relatively little clinical data is available in electronic format for most ambulatory-care clinics and physician offices in the United States, although this disparity is beginning to diminish as IDNs and larger physician group practices make investments in information systems. In contrast, some countries in Western Europe (e.g., the Netherlands, Norway, and Great Britain) have implemented electronic patient records in most primary-care offices.

The lack of integration of data from diverse sources creates a host of problems. If clinical and administrative data are stored on separate systems, then data needed by both must either be entered directly into both systems or be copied from one system to the other. In addition to the expense of redundant data entry and data maintenance incurred by this approach, the consistency of information tends to be poor because data may be updated in one place and not in the other, or information may be copied incorrectly. In the extreme example, the same data may be referred to differently in different settings. Within the hospital setting, many of these issues have been addressed through the development of automated interfaces to transfer demographic data, orders, results, and charges between clinical systems and billing systems. Even with an interface engine managing data among disparate systems, however, an organization still must solve the thorny issues of synchronization of data and comparability of similar data types.

With the development of IDNs and other complex HCOs, the sharing of data elements among operating units becomes more critical and more problematic. Data integration issues are further compounded in IDNs by the acquisition of previously independent organizations that have clinical and administrative information systems incompatible with those of the rest of the IDN. It is still not unusual to encounter minimal automated information exchange among settings in an IDN. Patients register and reregister at the physician's office, diagnostic imaging center, ambulatory surgery facility, and acute-care hospital—and sometimes face multiple registrations even within a single facility. Each facility keeps its own clinical records, and *shadow files* include copies of critical information such as operative reports and hospital discharge summaries. Inconsistencies in the databases can result in inappropriate patient management and inappropriate resource allocation. For example, medications that are first given to a patient while she is a hospital inpatient may inadvertently be discontinued when she is transported to a rehabilitation hospital or nursing home. Also, information about a patient's known allergies and medication history may be unavailable to physicians treating an unconscious patient in an emergency department.

The objectives of coordinated, high-quality, and cost-effective health care cannot be completely satisfied if an organization's multiple computer systems operate in isolation.

Unfortunately, free-standing systems within HCOs are still common, and there are still few examples of organizations investing heavily in implementing new common systems in all their facilities or in integrating existing systems to allow data sharing. In Section 13.4, we discuss architectural components and strategies for data integration.

Process Integration

To be effective, information systems must mesh smoothly with operational workflow and human organizational systems. Such process integration poses a significant challenge for HCOs. Today's healthcare-delivery models represent a radical departure from more traditional models of care delivery. They demand, for example, changes in the responsibilities and work patterns of physicians, nurses, and other care providers; the development of entirely new job categories (such as care managers who coordinate a patient's care across facilities and between encounters); and the more active participation of patients in personal health management (Table 13.1). Process integration in IDNs is further complicated in that component entities of an IDN typically have evolved substantially different operational policies and procedures, which reflect each component organization's history and leadership. The most progressive IDNs are developing new enterprise-wide processes for providing easy and uniform access to health services, for deploying consistent clinical guidelines, and for coordinating and managing patient care across multiple care settings throughout the IDN (Drazen & Metzger, 1999). Integrated information technologies are essential to supporting such enterprise-wide processes. Thus, mechanisms for information management aimed at integrating operations across entities must address not only the migration from legacy systems but also the migration from legacy work processes to new, consistent policies and processes across entities.

Table 13.1. The changing healthcare environment and its implications for an IDN's core competencies.

Characteristic	Old care model	New care model
Goal of care	Manage sickness	Manage wellness
Center of delivery system	Hospital	Primary-care providers/ambulatory settings
Focus of care	Episodic acute and chronic care	Population health, primary and preventive care
Driver of care decisions	Specialists	Primary-care providers/patients
Metric of system success	Number of admissions	Number of enrollees
Performance optimization	Optimize individual provider performance	Optimize system-wide performance
Utilization controls	Externally controlled	Internally controlled
Quality measures	Defined as inputs to system	Defined as patient outcomes and satisfaction
Physician role	Autonomous and independent	Member of care team; user of system-wide guidelines of care
Patient role	Passive receiver of care	Active partner in care

Source: Copyright First Consulting Group. Reprinted with Permission.

The introduction of new information systems almost always changes the workplace. In fact research has shown that in most cases the real value from an investment in information systems comes only when underlying work processes are changed to take advantage of the new information technology (Vogel, 2003). At times, these changes can be fundamental. The implementation of a new system offers an opportunity to rethink and redefine existing work processes to take advantage of the new information-management capabilities, thereby reducing costs, increasing productivity, or improving service levels. For example, providing electronic access to information that was previously accessible only on paper can shorten the overall time required to complete a multistep activity by enabling conversion of serial processes (completed by multiple workers using the same record sequentially) to concurrent processes (completed by the workers accessing an electronic record simultaneously). More fundamental business transformation is also possible with new technologies; for example, direct entry of medication orders by physicians, linked with a decision-support system, allows immediate checking for proper dosing and potential drug interactions, and the ability to recommend less expensive drug substitutes.

Few healthcare organizations today have the time or resources to develop entirely new information systems and redesigned processes; therefore, most opt to purchase existing software products or to partner with commercial systems vendors in codevelopment projects. Although these commercial systems allow some degree of custom tailoring, they also reflect an underlying model of work processes that may have evolved through development in other healthcare organizations with different underlying operational policies and procedures. Most clinical sites must adapt their own work processes to those embodied in the systems they are installing. (For example, some commercial systems require care providers to discontinue and then reenter all orders when a patient is admitted to the hospital after being monitored in the emergency department.) Furthermore, once the systems are installed and once workflow has been adapted to them, they become part of the organization's culture—and any subsequent change to the new system may be arduous because of these workflow considerations. Thus, decision-makers should take great care when selecting and tailoring a new system to support and enhance desired work processes. Such organizational workflow adaptation represents a significant challenge to the HCO and its systems planners. Too often organizations are unable to realize the full potential return on their information-technology investments; inappropriate management practices and suboptimal workflow absorb much of the potential gains.

To meet the continually evolving requirements of today's healthcare environment, HCOs must change—and they must change quickly. Although an HCO's business plans and information-systems strategies may be reasonable and necessary, changing ingrained organizational behavior can be many times more complex than changing the underlying information systems. Successful process integration requires not only successful deployment of the technology but also sustained commitment of resources; dedicated leadership with the willingness to make difficult, sometimes unpopular decisions; education; and new performance incentives to overcome cultural inertia and politics.

13.1.4   Security and Confidentiality Requirements

As we discussed in Chapter 10, the protection of health information from unwanted or inappropriate use is governed not only by the trust of patients in their health providers but also by law. In accordance with the Health Insurance Portability and Accountability Act (HIPAA) of 1996 (Chapter 10), the Secretary of Health and Human Services recommended that "Congress enact national standards that provide fundamental privacy rights for patients and define responsibilities for those who serve them." These laws now mandate standardized data transactions for sending data to payer organizations, the development and adherence to formal policies for securing and maintaining access to patient data, and under privacy provisions, prohibit disclosure of patient-identifiable information by most providers and health plans, except as authorized by the patient or explicitly permitted by legislation. HIPAA also provides consumers with significant new rights to be informed about how and by whom their health information will be used, and to inspect and sometimes amend their health information. Stiff criminal penalties including fines and possible imprisonment are associated with noncompliance or the knowing misuse of patient-identifiable information. HIPAA security measures, the means by which HCOs implement the privacy rules, are less specifically identified. They recommend a set of administrative procedures, physical safeguards, and technical security mechanisms for data and networks (see Table 13.2), but not the particular technologies or implementation methods.

Computer systems can be designed to provide security, but only people can promote the trust necessary to protect the confidentiality of patients' clinical information. To achieve the goal of delivering coordinated and cost-effective care, clinicians need to access information on specific patients from many different locations. Unfortunately, it is difficult to predict in advance which clinicians will need access to which patient data. Therefore, an HCO must strike a balance between restricting information access and ensuring the accountability of the users of patient information. To build trust with its patients and meet HIPAA requirements, an HCO should adopt a three-pronged approach to securing information. First, the HCO needs to designate a security officer and develop a uniform security and confidentiality policy, including specification of sanctions, and to enforce this policy rigorously. Second, the HCO needs to train employees so they understand the appropriate uses of patient-identifiable information and the consequences of violations. Third, the HCO must use electronic tools such as access controls and information audit trails not only to discourage misuse of information, but also to teach employees and patients that people who access confidential information can be tracked and will be held accountable.

13.1.5   The Benefits of Healthcare Information Systems

In a 1966 study of three New York hospitals, researchers found that information handling to satisfy requirements such as those discussed in Section 13.1.2 accounted for approximately 25 percent of the hospital's total operating costs (Jydstrup & Gross, 1966). On average, workers in administrative departments spent about three-fourths of

Table 13.2 HIPAA security standards and implementation specifications.

Area of Focus	Standards	Required Components	Addressable Components
Administrative Safeguards	Security Management Process	• Risk Analysis • Risk Management • Sanction Policy • Information System Activity Review	
	Assigned Security Responsibility	• Assigned Responsibility for Security	
	Workforce Security		• Authorization and/or Supervision • Workforce Clearance Procedure • Termination Procedures
	Information Access Management	• Isolating Healthcare Clearinghouse Function	• Access Authorization • Access Establishment and Modification
	Security Awareness and Training		• Security Reminders • Protection from Malicious Software • Log-in Monitoring • Password Management
	Security Incident Procedures	• Response and Reporting	
	Contingency Plan	• Data Backup Plan • Disaster Recovery Plan • Emergency Mode Operation Plan	• Testing and Revision Procedure • Applications and Data Criticality Analysis
	Evaluation	• Evaluation Process	
	Business Associate Contracts and Other Arrangement	• Written Contract or Other Arrangement	
Physical Safeguards	Facility Access Controls		• Contingency Operations • Facility Security Plan • Access Control and Validation Procedures • Maintenance Records
	Workstation Use	• Controls on Workstation Use	
	Workstation Security	• Control of Workstation Security	
	Device and Media Controls	• Secure Disposal of Media • Secure Media Re-use	• Accountability • Data Backup and Storage
Technical Safeguards	Access Control	• Unique User Identification • Emergency Access Procedure	• Automatic Logoff • Encryption and Decryption
	Audit Controls	• Audit trails	
	Integrity		• Mechanism to Authenticate Electronic Protected Health Information
	Person or Entity Authentication	• Person or Entity Authentication	
	Transmission Security		• Integrity Controls • Encryption

Source: Federal Register Vol 68, No 34, February 20, 2003/Rules and Regulations

their time handling information; workers in nursing units spent about one-fourth of their time on these tasks. Almost forty years later, the basic conclusions of the study hold true: information management in healthcare organizations is still a costly activity. The collection, storage, retrieval, analysis, and dissemination of the clinical and administrative information necessary to support the organization's daily operations, to meet external and internal requirements for documentation, and to support short-term and strategic planning remain important and time-consuming aspects of the jobs of healthcare workers.

Today, the justifications for implementing HCISs include cost reduction, productivity enhancement, and quality and service improvement, as well as regulatory compliance and strategic considerations related to competitive advantage:

- *Cost reduction*. Much of the initial impetus for implementing HCISs was their potential to reduce the costs of information management in hospitals and other facilities. HCOs continue to make tactical investments in information systems to streamline administrative processes and departmental workflow. Primary benefits that may offset some information-systems costs include reductions in labor requirements, reduced waste (e.g., dated surgical supplies that are ordered but unused or food trays that are delivered to the wrong destination and therefore are wasted), and more efficient management of supplies and other inventories. Large savings can be gained through efficient scheduling of expensive resources such as operating suites and imaging equipment. In addition, HCISs can help to eliminate inadvertent ordering of duplicate tests and procedures. Once significant patient data are available online, information systems can reduce the costs of storing, retrieving, and transporting charts in the medical-records department.
- *Productivity Enhancements*. A second area of benefit from an HCIS comes in the form of improved productivity of clinicians and other staff. With continuing (and at times increasing) constraints on reimbursements, HCOs are continually faced with the challenge of "doing more with less". Providing information systems support to staff can in many cases enable them to manage a larger variety of tasks and data than would otherwise be possible using strictly manual processes. Interestingly, in some cases hospital investments in an HCIS support the productivity improvement of staff who are not employed by the hospital, namely the physicians, and can even extend to payers by lowering their costs.
- *Quality and service improvement*. As HCISs broadened in scope to encompass support for clinical processes, the ability to improve the quality of care became an additional benefit. Qualitative benefits of HCISs include improved accuracy and completeness of documentation, reductions in the time clinicians spend documenting (and associated increases in time spent with patients), fewer drug errors and quicker response to adverse events, and improved provider-to-provider communication. Through telemedicine and remote linkages (see Chapter 14), HCOs are able to expand their geographical reach and improve delivery of specialist care to rural and outlying areas. As described in Chapter 20, the use of clinical decision-support systems in conjunction with an HCIS or CPR can produce impressive benefits, improving the quality of care while reducing costs. (Bates et al., 1997; Classen et al., 1997; Teich et al., 1996; Tierney et al., 1993; Bates & Gawande, 2003).

- *Competitive advantage.* Information technologies must be deployed appropriately and effectively; however, with respect to HCISs, the question is no longer whether to invest, but rather how much and what to buy. Although some organizations still attempt to cost justify all information-systems investments, many HCOs have recognized information technology as an investment that is necessary for survival: without an enabling technology infrastructure, an organization cannot meet its needs for integrated operations and coordinated patient care. Some HCOs are considering upgrades to their security infrastructures in light of return on security investment (ROSI)—the benefits of avoiding security breaches. Access to clinical information is necessary not only to carry out patient management, but also to attract and retain the loyalty of physicians who care for (and thus control much of the HCO's access to) the patients. The long-term benefits of clinical systems include the ability to influence clinical practices by reducing large unnecessary variations in medical practices, to improve patient outcomes, and to reduce costs—although these costs might be more broadly economic and societal than related to specific reductions for the hospital itself (Leatherman, et. al., 2003). Physicians ultimately control the great majority of the resource-utilization decisions in health care through their choices in prescribing drugs, ordering diagnostic tests, and referring patients for specialty care. Thus, providing physicians with access to information on "best practices" based on the latest available clinical evidence, as well as giving them other clinical and financial data to make appropriate decisions, is an essential HCIS capability. Other examples of competitive advantages are the ability to satisfy external organizations (such as Leapfrog's recommendation to implement computer-based physician order entry), and to identify patients for enrollment in research trials.
- *Regulatory compliance.* Increasingly, regulators are including information systems solutions in their requirements. For example, the Food and Drug Administration now mandates the use of barcodes on all drugs. Similarly, HIPAA rules specify the required content and format for certain electronic data transactions for those HCOs that exchange data electronically.

13.1.6   *Managing Information Systems in a Changing Healthcare Environment*

Despite the importance of integrated information systems, implementation of HCISs has proved to be a daunting task, often requiring a multiyear capital investment of tens of millions of dollars and forcing fundamental changes in the types and ways that health professionals perform their jobs. To achieve the potential benefits, health organizations must plan carefully and invest wisely. The grand challenge for an HCO is to design and implement an HCIS that is sufficiently flexible and adaptable to meet the changing needs of the organization. Given the rapidly changing environment and the multiyear effort involved, people must be careful to avoid implementing a system that is obsolete functionally or technologically before it becomes operational. Success in implementing an HCIS entails consistent and courageous handling of numerous technical, organizational, and political challenges.

Changing Technologies

As we discussed in Chapter 5, past decades have seen dramatic changes in computing and networking technologies. These advances are important in that they allow quicker and easier information access, less expensive computational power, greater flexibility, and other performance advantages. A major challenge for many HCOs is how to decide whether to retain their "best of breed" strategy, with its requirement either to upgrade individual systems and interfaces to newer products or to migrate from their patchwork of legacy systems to a more integrated systems environment. Such migration requires integration and selective replacement of diverse systems that are often implemented with closed or nonstandard technologies and medical vocabularies. Unfortunately the trade off between migrating "best of breed" or implementing more integrated systems is that vendors offering more integrated approaches seldom match the functionality of the best of breed environment. Furthermore, the end point is not fixed—HCOs must move aggressively to implement new systems, while progress continues in development of standards (see Chapter 7), functional enhancements, regulatory requirements, distributed database architecture, and Internet/Intranet tools. In a sense, it is the information content of the systems that is much more important than the underlying technology—as long as the data are accessible, the choice of specific technology is less critical.

Changing Culture

In the current healthcare environment, physicians are confronted with significant obstacles to the practice of medicine as they have historically viewed it. With a seventy-five year history of entrepreneurial practice, physicians face significant adjustments as they are confronted by pressures to practice in accordance with institutional standards aimed at reducing variation in care, and to focus on the costs of care even when those costs are borne either by hospitals or by third party payers. They are expected to assume responsibility not simply for healing the sick, but for the wellness of people who come to them not as patients but as members of health plans and health maintenance organizations. In addition, they must often work as members of collaborative patient-care teams. The average patient length of stay in a hospital is decreasing; concomitantly, the complexity of the care provided after discharge is increasing. The time allotted for an individual patient visit in the ambulatory setting is decreasing as individual clinicians face economic incentives to increase the number of patients for whom they care each day. Some HCOs are now instituting pay-for performance incentives to reward desired work practices. At the same time, it is well known that the amount of knowledge about disease diagnosis and treatment increases exponentially each year, with whole new areas of medicine being added from major breakthroughs in areas such as genomic and imaging research. To cope with the increasing workload, greater complexity of care, extraordinary amounts of new medical knowledge, new skills requirements, and the wider availability of medical knowledge to consumers through the Internet, both clinicians and health executives must become effective information managers, and the supporting information systems must meet their workflow and information requirements. As the healthcare culture and the roles of clinicians and health executives continue to change, HCOs must constantly reevaluate the role of information technology to ensure that the implemented systems continue to match user requirements.

Changing Process

Developing a new vision of how health care will be delivered and managed, designing processes and implementing supporting information systems are all critical to the success of evolving HCOs. Changes in process affect the jobs that people do, the skills required to do those jobs, and the fundamental ways in which they relate to one another. For example, models of cross-continuum care management encourage interdisciplinary care teams that work in symphony to promote health as well as treat illness. Although information systems are not the foremost consideration for people who are redesigning process, a poor information-systems implementation can institutionalize bad processes.

Organizations must and will undertake various process redesign initiatives—and these initiatives can lead to fundamental transformations of the enterprise. Indeed, work process redesign is essential if information systems are to become truly valuable to HCOs. Too often, however, the lack of a clear understanding of existing organizational dynamics leads to a misalignment of incentives—a significant barrier to change—or to the assumption that simply installing a new computer system will be sufficient to generate value. Moreover, organizations, as collections of individuals, have natural fears about and reluctance to change. Even under the best circumstances, there are limits to the amount of change that any organization can absorb. The magnitude of work required to plan and manage organizational change is often underestimated or ignored. It is the handling of people and process issues that has emerged as one of the most critical success factors for HCOs as they implement new work methods and new and upgraded information systems.

Management and Governance

Figure 13.3 illustrates the information-technology environment of an HCO composed of two hospitals, an owned physician practice, affiliated nursing homes and hospice, and several for-profit service organizations. Even this relatively simple environment presents significant challenges for the management and governance of information systems. For example, to what extent will the information management function be controlled centrally versus decentralized to the individual operating units and departments? How should limited resources be allocated between new investment in strategic projects (such as office-based data access for physicians) and the often critical operational needs of individual entities (e.g., replacement of an obsolete laboratory information system)? Academic medical centers with distinct research and educational needs raise additional issues for managing information across operationally independent and politically powerful constituencies.

Trade-offs between functional and integration requirements, and associated contention between users and information-systems departments, will tend to diminish over time with the development and widespread adoption of technology standards and

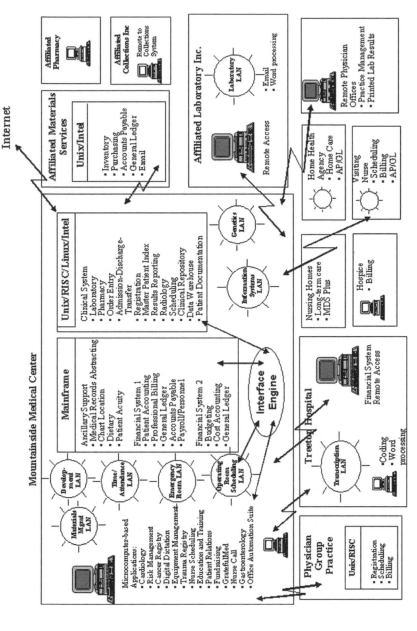

Figure 13.3. An information-systems environment for a small healthcare organization (HCO). Even this relatively simple HCO has a complex mix of information systems that poses integration and information-management challenges for the organization. MDS = minimum data set; LAN = local area network; AP = accounts payable; GL = general ledger.

common clinical-data models and vocabulary. On the other hand, an organization's information-systems "wants" and "needs" will always outstrip its ability to deliver these services. Political battles will persist, as HCOs and their component operating units wrestle with the age-old issues of how to distribute scarce resources among competing, similarly worthy projects.

A formal governance structure with representation from all major constituents provides a critical forum for direction setting, prioritization, and resource allocation across an HCO. Leadership by respected clinical peers has proved a critical success factor for CIS planning, implementation, and acceptance. In addition, development of a strategic information-management plan, accompanied by an Information Systems Advisory or Steering Committee composed of the leaders of the various constituencies within the HCO, can be a valuable exercise if the process engages the organization's clinical, financial, and administrative leadership and results in their gaining not only a clear understanding of the highest-priority information technology investments but a sense of accountability and ownership over the HCIS and its applications. Because of the dynamic nature of both healthcare business strategies and the supporting technologies, many HCOs have seen the timeframes of their strategic information-management plans shrink from five years to three, and then be changed yet again through annual updates.

13.2   Functions and Components of a Healthcare Information System

A carefully designed computer-based system can increase the effectiveness and productivity of health professionals, improve the quality and reduce the costs of health services, and improve levels of service and of patient satisfaction. As described in Section 13.1, the HCIS supports a variety of functions, including the delivery and management of patient care and the administration of the health organization. From a functional perspective, an HCIS typically consists of components that support five distinct purposes: (1) patient management and billing, (2) departmental management, (3) care delivery and clinical documentation, (4) clinical decision support, (5) financial and resource management.

13.2.1   Patient Management and Billing

Systems that support patient management functions perform the basic centralized functions of HCO operations related to patients, such as identification, registration, scheduling, admission, discharge, transfer among locations, and billing. Within hospitals, maintenance of the hospital census and a patient billing system were the first tasks to be automated—largely because a patient's location determined not only the daily room/bed charges (since an ICU bed was more expensive than a regular medical/surgical bed) but where medications were to be delivered, where clinical results were to be posted, etc. Today, virtually all hospitals and ambulatory centers and many physician offices use a computer-based **master patient index** (MPI) to store patient-identification information, basic demographic data that are acquired during the patient-registration process, and simple encounter-level information such as dates and locations where services were provided. The MPI can also be integrated within the registration module of an ambulatory care or physician-practice system or even elevated to an **enterprise master patient index** (EMPI) across several facilities. Within the hospital setting, the census is maintained by the **admission–discharge–transfer** (ADT) module, which updates the census whenever a patient is admitted to the hospital, discharged from the hospital, or transferred to a new bed.

Registration and census data serve as a reference base for the financial programs that perform billing functions. When an HCIS is extended to other patient-care settings— e.g., to the laboratory, pharmacy, and other ancillary departments—patient-management systems provide a common reference base for use by these systems as well. Without access to the centralized database of patient financial, demographic, registration and location data, these subsystems would have to maintain duplicate patient records. In addition, the transmission of registration data can trigger other activities, such as automatic retrieval of medical records from archival storage for patients scheduled to be seen in the clinic or notification of hospital housekeeping when a bed becomes free. The billing function in these systems serves as a collection point for all of the chargeable patient activity that occurs in a facility, including room/bed charges, ancillary service charges, and supplies used during a patient's stay.

Scheduling in a healthcare organization is complicated because patient load and resource utilization can vary by day, week, or season or even through the course of a single day simply due to chance or to patterns of patient and physician behavior. Effective resource management requires that the appropriate resources be on hand to meet such fluctuations in demand. At the same time, resources cannot remain unnecessarily idle since that results in an inefficient use of resources. The most sophisticated scheduling systems have been developed for the operating rooms and radiology departments, where scheduling constraints include matching up the patient not only with the providers but also with special equipment, support staff, and technicians. **Patient-tracking** applications monitor patient movement in multistep processes; for example, they monitor and manage patient wait times in the emergency department.

Within a multi-facility HCO, the basic tasks of patient management are compounded by the need to manage patient care across multiple settings, some of which may be supported by independent information systems. Is the Patricia C. Brown who was admitted last month to Mountainside Hospital the same Patsy Brown who is registering for her appointment at the Seaview Clinic? Integrated delivery networks ensure unique patient identification either through conversion to common registration systems or, more frequently, through implementation of an enterprise EMPI (see Section 13.4) that links patient identifiers and data from multiple registration systems.

13.2.2   Departmental Management

Ancillary departmental systems support the information needs of individual clinical departments within an HCO. From a systems perspective, those areas most commonly automated are the laboratory, pharmacy, radiology, blood-bank, and medical-records departments. Such systems serve a dual purpose within an HCO. First, ancillary systems perform many dedicated tasks required for departmental operations. Such tasks include generating specimen-collection lists and capturing results from automated laboratory instruments in the clinical laboratory, printing medication labels and managing inventory in the pharmacy, and scheduling examinations and supporting the transcription of image interpretations in the radiology department. In addition, information technology coupled with robotics can have a dramatic impact on the operation of an HCO's ancillary departments, particularly in pharmacies (to sort and fill medication carts) and in clinical laboratories (where in some cases the only remaining manual task is the collection of the specimen and its transport to the laboratory's robotic system). Second, the ancillary systems contribute major data components to online patient records, including laboratory-test results and pathology reports, medication profiles, digital images (see Chapter 18), records of blood orders and usage, and various transcribed reports including history and physical examinations, operative, and radiology reports. HCOs that consolidate ancillary functions outside hospitals to gain economies of scale—for example, creating outpatient diagnostic imaging centers and reference laboratories—increase the complexity of integrated patient management, financial, and billing processes.

13.2.3   Care Delivery and Clinical Documentation

Computer-based patient record systems (CPRs) that support care delivery and clinical documentation are discussed at length in Chapter 12. Although comprehensive CPRs are the ultimate goal of most HCOs, many organizations today are still building more basic clinical-management capabilities. Automated **order entry** and **results reporting** are two important functions provided by the clinical components of an HCIS. Health professionals can use the HCIS to communicate with ancillary departments electronically, eliminating the easily misplaced paper slips or the transcription errors often associated with translating hand-written notes into typed requisitions, thus minimizing delays in conveying orders. The information then is available online, where it is accessible to health professionals who wish to review a patient's medication profile or previous laboratory-test results. Ancillary departmental data represent an important subset of a patient's clinical record. A comprehensive clinical record, however, also includes various data that clinicians have collected by questioning and observing the patient. In the hospital, an HCIS can help health personnel perform an initial assessment when a patient is admitted to a unit, maintain patient-specific care plans, chart vital signs, maintain medication-administration records, record diagnostic and therapeutic information, document patient and family teaching, and plan for discharge (also see Chapter 16). Many organizations have developed diagnosis-specific **clinical pathways** that identify clinical goals, interventions, and expected outcomes by time period; using the clinical pathway, case managers or care providers can document actual versus expected outcomes and are alerted to intervene when a significant unexpected event occurs. More hospitals are now implementing systems to support what are called "closed loop medication systems" in which every task from the initial order for medication to its administration to the patient is recorded in the HCIS—one outcome of increased attention to patient safety issues.

With the shift toward delivering more care in outpatient settings, clinical systems are becoming more common in ambulatory clinics and physician practices. Numerous vendors have introduced **personal digital assistants** (PDAs) with software designed specifically for physicians in ambulatory settings, so that they can access appropriate information even as they move from exam room to exam room. Such systems allow clinicians to record problems and diagnoses, symptoms and physical examinations, medical and social history, review of systems, functional status, active and past prescriptions, access to therapeutic and medication guidelines, etc. The most successful of such systems, integrated with a practice management system, provide additional support for physician workflow and typical clinic functions, such as by documenting telephone follow-up calls or printing prescriptions. In addition, specialized clinical information systems have been developed to meet the specific requirements of intensive-care units (see Chapter 17), long-term care facilities, home-health organizations, and specialized departments such as cardiology and oncology.

13.2.4   Clinical Decision Support

Clinical decision-support systems directly assist clinical personnel in data interpretation and decision-making. Once the basic clinical components of an HCIS are well developed, clinical decision-support systems can use the information stored there to monitor patients and issue alerts, to make diagnostic suggestions, to provide limited therapeutic advice, and to provide information on medication costs. These capabilities are particularly useful when they are integrated with other information-management functions. For example, a useful adjunct to **computer-based physician order-entry** (CPOE) is a decision-support program that alerts physicians to patient food or drug allergies; helps physicians to calculate patient-specific drug-dosing regimens; performs advanced order logic, such as recommending an order for prophylactic antibiotics before certain surgical procedures; automatically discontinues drugs when appropriate or prompts the physician to reorder them; suggests more cost-effective drugs with the same therapeutic effect; or activates and displays applicable clinical-practice guidelines (see Chapter 12). Clinical-event monitors integrated with results-reporting applications can alert clinicians to abnormal results and drug interactions by electronic mail or page. In the outpatient setting, these event monitors may produce reminders to provide preventive services such as screening mammograms and routine immunizations. The same event monitors might trigger access to the HCO's approved formulary, displaying information that includes costs, indications, contraindications, approved clinical guidelines, and relevant online medical literature (Perreault & Metzger, 1999; Teich et al., 1997; Kaushal et. al., 2003).

13.2.5   Financial and Resource Management

Financial and administrative systems assist with the traditional business functions of an HCO, including management of the payroll, human resources, general ledger, accounts payable, and materials purchasing and inventory. Most of these data-processing tasks are well structured, and have been historically labor intensive and repetitious—ideal opportunities for substitution with computers. Furthermore, with the exception of patient-billing functions, the basic financial tasks of an HCO do not differ substantially from those of organizations in other industries. Not surprisingly, financial and administrative applications have typically been among the first systems to be standardized and centralized in IDNs.

Conceptually, the tasks of creating a patient bill and tracking payments are straightforward, and financial transactions such as claims submission and electronic funds transfer have been standardized to allow **electronic data interchange** (EDI) among providers and payers. In operation, however, patient accounting requirements are complicated by the myriad reimbursement requirements of government and third-party payers. These requirements vary substantially by payer, by insurance plan, by type of facility where service was provided, and often by state. As the burden of financial risk for care has shifted from third party payers to providers (through per diem or diagnosis-based reimbursements), these systems have become even more criticial to the operation of a successful HCO. As another example, the growth of managed care (see Chapter 23), has added even more complexity, necessitating processes and information systems to check a patient's health-plan enrollment and eligibility for services, to manage referrals and preauthorization for care, to price claims based on negotiated contracts, and to create documentation required to substantiate the services provided.

As HCOs go "at risk" for delivery of health services by negotiating per diem, diagnosis-based, and capitated payments (to provide comprehensive care for a specified patient population at a preset cost), their incentives focus not only on reducing the cost per unit service but also on maintaining the health of members while using health resources effectively and efficiently. Similarly, the HCO's scope of concern broadens from a relatively small population of sick patients to a much larger population of plan members, most of whom are still well.

Provider-profiling systems support utilization management by tracking each provider's resource utilization (costs of drugs prescribed, diagnostic tests and procedures ordered, and so on) compared with severity-adjusted outcomes of that provider's patients such as their rate of hospital readmission and mortality by diagnosis. Such systems are also being used by government bodies and consumer advocate organizations to publicize their findings, often through the Internet. **Contract-management systems** have capabilities for estimating the costs and payments associated with potential managed care contracts and comparing actual with expected payments based on the contracts' terms. More advanced managed-care information systems handle **patient triage** and **medical management** functions, helping the HCOs to direct patients to appropriate health services and to proactively manage the care of chronically ill and high-risk patients. Health plans, and IDNs that incorporate a health plan, also must support payer and insurance functions such as claims administration, premium billing, marketing, and member services.

13.3   Historical Evolution of Healthcare Information Systems

Technological advances and changes in the information and organizational requirements of HCOs have driven the transformation of underlying system architecture, hardware, software, and functionality of HCISs over time. The tradeoff between richness of function and ease of integration is another important factor that accounts for choices in systems design. In this section, we outline the evolution of HCISs from the earliest mainframe-based systems to the networked and Internet-accessible systems of today.

13.3.1 Central and Mainframe-based Systems

The earliest HCISs (typically found in hospitals) were designed according to the philosophy that a single comprehensive or **central system** could best meet an HCO's information needs. Advocates of the centralized approach emphasized the importance of first identifying all the hospital's information needs and then designing a single, unified framework to meet these needs. As we have seen, patient management and billing functions were the initial focus of such efforts. One natural product of this design goal was the development of systems in which a single, large computer performed all information processing and managed all the data files using application-independent file-management programs. Users obtained information via general-purpose video-display terminals (VDTs).

One of the first clinically-oriented HCISs was the Technicon Medical Information System (TMIS; the precursor of Eclipsys Corporation's TDS 7000). System development began in 1965 as a collaborative project between Lockheed and El Camino Hospital, a community hospital in Mountain View, California. By 1987, the system had been installed in more than 85 institutions by Technicon Data Systems (TDS), which purchased the system from Lockheed in 1971. TDS was one of the earliest examples of what we could expect from a large, centrally operated, clinically focused HCIS. Depending on the size of the central machine, the TDS center could support from several hundred to a few thousand hospital beds. Because of this high capacity, one computer installation could serve multiple hospitals in an area. The hospitals were connected via high-speed dedicated telephone lines to the central computer. Within a hospital, a switching station connected the telephone lines to an onsite network that led to stations on all the patient-care units. Each unit had at least one VDT and one printer with which users could access, display, and print information. Because the TDS system was designed for use by both nurses and physicians it was one of the first systems to support both nursing clinical documentation and physician order entry. Forty years later, the TDS system, with its forty column screens and display using only capital letters, is still in use in some hospitals—a testament both to its enduring usefulness and to its roots in the programming tools of the 1960s.

The Center for Clinical Computing (CCC) system, developed by Howard Bleich and Warner Slack as a centralized clinical computing system, was first deployed in 1978 at the Beth Israel Medical Center in Boston (now part of the Beth Israel Deaconess Medical Center and the CareGroup IDN). Still in operation through ongoing development, this system is designed around a single common registry of patients, with tight integration of all its departmental systems. It was remarkable in the breadth of its functionality to support physicians and the intensity of its use by clinicians. For example, the system records over 70,000 lookups of patient data per week by clinicians. It was the first system to offer hospital-wide electronic mail, as well as end-user access to Medline via PaperChase. In addition, CCC was among the first to employ audit trails on who was looking at patient data, a feature now common in most clinical systems (and a HIPAA requirement). In ambulatory clinics, an electronic patient record including support for problem lists, clinic notes, prescription writing, and other functions is used by over 1,000 clinicians in more than 30 primary-care and specialty areas (Safran et al., 1991). On the other hand, the system provided only limited support for order entry, alerts, and reminders. The CCC also has a MUMPS database that functions as a clinical-data repository and an online data warehouse, called ClinQuery (Safran et al., 1989). With records from more than 300,000 consecutive hospitalizations since 1983, the database contains complete data on all test results and medications, as well as ICD-9 and SNOMED diagnosis codes. The CCC was transferred to the Brigham and Women's Hospital in 1983 and was subsequently developed separately as the Brigham Integrated Computer System (BICS), a distributed client–server system. The Eclipsys Corporation later licensed the BICS internal processing logic, which is still found in current product offerings.

Central systems integrated and communicated information well because they provided users with a single data store and a general method to access information simply and rapidly. On the other hand, the biggest limitation of central systems was their inability to accommodate the diverse needs of individual application areas. There is a tradeoff between the uniformity (and relative simplicity) of a general system and the nonuniformity and greater power of custom-designed systems that solve specific problems. Generality—a characteristic that enhances communication and data integration in a homogeneous environment—can be a drawback in an HCO because of the complexity and heterogeneity of the information-management tasks. In general, central systems have proved too unwieldy and inflexible to support current HCO requirements, except in smaller facililties.

13.3.2 *Departmental Systems*

By the 1970s, departmental systems began to emerge. Decreases in the price of hardware and improvements in software made it feasible for individual departments within a hospital to own and operate their own computers. In a **departmental system**, one or a few machines are dedicated to processing specific functional tasks within the organization. Distinct software application modules carry out specific tasks, and a common framework, which is specified initially, defines the interfaces that will allow data to be shared among the modules. Laboratory systems with their support of specific laboratory areas (e.g., hematology, chemistry) are examples of this type of system.

The most ambitious project based on the departmental approach was the Distributed Hospital Computer Program (DHCP) for the Veterans Administration (VA) hospitals. The system had a common database and a database system (Fileman), which was written to be both hardware- and operating-system-independent. A small number of support centers in the VA developed the software modules in cooperation with user groups. The CORE—the first set of applications to be developed and installed—consisted of modules for patient registration, ADT, outpatient scheduling, laboratory, outpatient pharmacy, and inpatient pharmacy. Modules to support other clinical departments (such as radiology, dietetics, surgery, nursing, and mental health) and administrative functions (such as financial and procurement applications) were developed subsequently. By 1985, the VA had installed DHCP in more than one-half of its approximately 300 hospitals and clinics. The software was in the public domain and was also used in private hospitals and other government facilities (Kolodner and Douglas, 1997). Interestingly, one of the reasons for the success of the VA system was its ability to focus on the clinical environment. Given the nature of government reimbursement for the care of veterans, there was no need to develop or integrate a billing function into the DHCP system.

The departmental approach solved many of the problems of central systems. Although individual departmental systems are constrained to function with predefined interfaces, they do not have to conform to the general standards of the overall system, so they can be designed to accommodate the special needs of specific areas. For example, the processing capabilities and file structures suitable for managing the data acquired from a patient-monitoring system in the intensive-care unit (analog and digital signals acquired in real time) differ from the features that are appropriate for a system that reports radiology results (text storage and text processing). Furthermore, modification of departmental systems, although laborious with any approach, is simpler because of the smaller scope of the system. As long as the interfaces are undisturbed, subsystems can be modified or replaced without the remainder of the HCIS being disrupted. The price for this greater flexibility is increased difficulty in integrating data and communicating among modules. In reality, installing a subsystem never is as easy as simply plugging in the connections.

By the 1980s, HCISs based on network-communications technology were being developed. As **distributed systems**, connected through electronic networks, these HCIS consisted of a federation of independent systems that had been tailored for specific application areas. The computers operated autonomously and shared data (and sometimes programs and other resources, such as printers) by exchanging information over a local area network (LAN; see Chapter 5) using a standard protocol such as HL7 for communication and in many cases utilizing the interface engine strategy we discussed earlier in Section 13.1.1.

Researchers at the University of California, San Francisco (UCSF) Hospital successfully implemented one of the first LANs to support communication among several of the hospital's standalone systems in the early 1980s. Using technology developed at the Johns Hopkins University, they connected minicomputers serving patient registration, medical records, radiology, the clinical laboratory, and the outpatient pharmacy. In the historical sense, each of the four computers was incompatible with the other three: the computers were made by different manufacturers and ran different operating systems (McDonald et al., 1984a).

The University of Michigan Hospital in Ann Arbor later adopted a hybrid strategy to meet its information needs. The hospital emphasized the central model of architecture and operated a mainframe computer to perform core HCIS functions. In 1986, however, it installed a LAN to allow communication among all its internal clinical laboratories and to allow physicians to obtain laboratory-test results directly from the laboratory information system. At the time of installation, more than 95 percent of all the peripheral devices in the laboratories were connected to the network rather than hardwired to the laboratory computer. A second clinical host computer, which supported the radiology information system, was later added to the LAN, allowing physicians to access radiology reports directly. Although the mainframe HCIS initially was not connected to the LAN, the hospital later adopted the strategy of installing universal workstations that could access both the mainframe computer and the clinical hosts via the LAN (Friedman & Dieterle, 1987).

The advantage of a distributed system is that individual departments have a great deal of flexibility in choosing hardware and software that optimally suits their needs. Even smaller ancillary departments such as Respiratory Therapy, which previously could not justify a major computer acquisition, could now purchase microcomputers and participate in the HCIS. Healthcare providers in nursing units or at the bedside, physicians in their offices or homes, and managers in the administrative offices can access and analyze data locally using microcomputers. On the downside, the distribution of information processing and responsibility for data among diverse systems makes the tasks of data integration, communication, and security difficult. Development of industry-wide standard network and interface protocols such as HL7 have eased the technical problems of electronic communication considerably. Still, there are problems to overcome in managing and controlling access to a patient database that is fragmented over multiple computers, each with its own file structure and method of file management. Furthermore, when no global structure is imposed on an HCIS, individual departments and entities may encode data values in ways that are incompatible with the definitions chosen by other areas of the organization. The promise of sharing among independent departments, entities, and even independent institutions increases the importance of defining clinical data standards (see Chapter 7). Some HCOs pursue a "best of breed" strategy in which they choose the best system, regardless of vendor and technology, then work to integrate that system into their overall HCIS. Some HCOs modify this strategy by choosing suites of related applications (e.g., selecting all ancillary systems from a single vendor) thereby reducing the overall number of vendors they work with and, in theory, reducing the costs and difficulty of integration.

Today, the distributed architecture for information systems is the norm, and all viable large commercial systems support a distributed model. PC-based **universal workstations** are the norm as well; however, separate access to independent ancillary systems has been largely eliminated by interfaces that join such systems to a core clinical system or through the use of a centralized clinical data repository that receives clinical data from each ancillary system. For example, whereas staff working in the laboratory access the laboratory system directly, clinicians view consolidated clinical results (laboratory, radiology, and so on) stored in the HCIS database by accessing the HCIS clinical applications. The ability to access patient databases (by clinicians), shared documents (by employees), and basic information about facilities, departments, and staff (by the public) is also becoming common.

13.3.3   Integrated Systems from Single Vendors

Today, many smaller HCOs opt for implementation of turnkey systems, which are in effect departmental functions integrated into application suites, developed by a single systems vendor. These systems offer a relatively inexpensive means to achieve reasonable function and integration, but allow minimal customization to meet institution-specific workflows and requirements. In addition, they may not be as "feature rich" as systems designed for specific departmental functions. Numerous debates have been held at national conferences regarding the desirability of an integrated system versus "best of breed" approaches in which the various systems have to be interfaced in order to function in effect as a "virtual" HCIS. In the late 1990s, several large IDNs developed their IT strategies based on the use of integrated systems from vendors historically focused on smaller hospitals. This has provided greater credibility to these vendors and at the same time challenged the long held assumption that the greater functionality of best of breed strategies, with their inherently greater cost and interface requirements, is the only viable strategy for large IDNs.

13.4 Architecture for a Changing Environment

As the complexity of the healthcare business continues to increase, HCOs and IDNs present new challenges to information systems planners. As we described in Section 13.1, most IDNs have developed through the merger or acquisition of independent organizations. Thus, the information systems environment of a new or evolving IDN usually is a jumble of disparate legacy systems, technologies, and architectures. In such an environment, how can an IDN's information systems planners design systems and processes to support new business strategies (such as a diabetes management program or a central call center) and provide integrated information access throughout the IDN, while maintaining uninterrupted operational support for the IDN's existing business units? Most importantly, how can such integration challenges be met within the constraints of reimbursement levels that seem to decline almost annually?

Sometimes, an IDN will selectively replace specific systems to fit its new organizational structure and strategies (e.g., consolidation of the finance and human resources departments and migration to common corporate general ledger, accounts payable, payroll, and human resources systems for all business entities). As always, resources (both money and staff) are limited; and often it is simply not feasible for an IDN to replace all legacy systems with new common systems. Therefore, more creativity is required to develop an architecture that can support the emerging IDN and flexibly grow with it as business conditions (and associated information requirements) change.

The particular legacy systems environment and business strategy in both large HCOs and IDNs present unique information requirements; therefore a single architecture is unlikely to suffice for all. Nonetheless, a few lessons can be learned from past implementations. First, a strategy for data preservation must be developed by providing access to data and implementing an approach for standardizing the meaning of those data. Second, to the extent possible, IDNs and HCOs should separate three conceptual layers—data management, applications and business logic, and user interface—to allow greater flexibility (See Figure. 13.4).

The first layer of architecture is the **data layer**. Data—the facts of process that are collected as part of the health enterprise—are of central importance. One fundamental

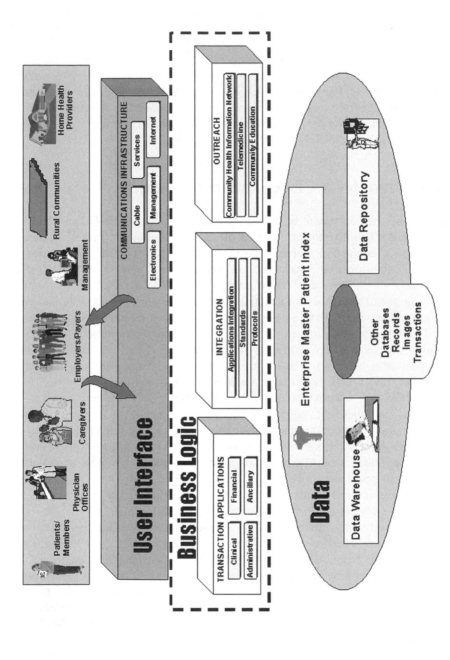

Figure 13.4. Three conceptual layers of an IDN's architectural model illustrate separation of data, business logic, and user interface which allows system developers to modify applications and interfaces over time to meet changing needs while preserving the HCO's long-term data asset.

mistake that a healthcare organization can make is to fail to provide access to its data. Organizations that choose information systems based on the functionality available to meet short-term needs may find that these needs are no longer as important as the HCO or IDN continues to evolve. For this reason, a long-term data strategy needs to be a separate component of the information-management plan. This plan must include access to data for applications and a method to ensure that demographic, clinical, and financial data collected across business units are consistent and comparable. Security and confidentiality safeguards (see Section 13.1.4) should also be part of the data strategy.

With respect to clinical data, HCOs and IDNs need data for both real-time operations and retrospective data analysis. These needs generate different requirements for data management. In the first case, detailed data need to be stored and optimized for retrieval for the individual patient. In the second case, the data need to be optimized for aggregation across a population of patients. Although the terms are sometimes used interchangeably, the distinction should be made between a **clinical data repository** (CDR), which serves the needs of patient care and day-to-day operations, and a **data warehouse**, which serves longer term business and clinical needs such as contract management and outcomes evaluation. Both the CDR and data warehouse should be purchased or developed for their ability to model, store, and retrieve efficiently the organization's data. Quite often, vendors of a CDR or warehouse include programs to view and manipulate these data. Conceptually, this packaging makes sense.

The second component of a clinical data strategy is an ability to keep patient information comparable. At the simplest level one needs to identify the patient. When a health organization consisted of only one hospital and one major information system, the authority over patient identification was relatively simple and usually resided in the HCIS's admitting or registration module (see Section 13.2.1). As HCOs evolve into IDNs, there is no one authority that can identify the patient or resolve a conflicting identification. Thus, as we noted earlier, a new architectural component, the **enterprise master patient index** (EMPI), has arisen as the **name authority**. In its simplest form, the EMPI is an index of patient names and identification numbers used by all information systems in the IDN that store a patient registry. Using this type of EMPI requires considerable manual intervention to ensure data synchrony, but it does enable an IDN to uniquely identify its patients and link their data. Alternatively, an EMPI can be configured as the name authority for all systems that hold patient information even within a single HCO. Then all systems must interact with the EMPI in order to get a patient-identification number assigned. This type of EMPI requires that all other systems disable their ability to assign identification numbers and use the external—and unique—EMPI-generated identification numbers.

Uniquely identifying patients within the HCO and the IDN is just a necessary first step in ensuring data comparability and consistency. Healthcare providers also may want to know which of their patients are allergic to penicillin, which patients should be targeted for new cardiac-disease prevention services, or which patients are likely to need home services when they are discharged from the hospital or emergency room. To store and evaluate the data that could be used to make such determinations, a consistent approach must be developed for naming data elements and defining their values. Some institutions, such as Columbia Presbyterian Medical Center (CPMC) in New York City, have developed their own internal vocabulary standards, or **terminology authority**. CPMC separates the storage and retrieval of data from the meaning of the terms in the database using a medical entities dictionary (MED) that defines valid database terms and synonyms for use by its clinical applications. An alternative approach is to develop a set of **terminology services**. These services fall into three categories: (1) linking or normalizing the data contained within the HCO's or IDN's legacy databases before these data are copied to a CDR; (2) reregistering all terms used by new applications and linking them to external authoritative vocabulary terms, such as those contained within the Unified Medical Language System's Metathesaurus (see Chapter 7); and (3) providing real-time help in selecting the appropriate term to describe a clinical situation.

The second layer of architecture is the **business-logic layer**. As we discussed in Section 13.1.6, once a system has been installed, its users will usually resist change. The reason for this inertia is not just that there is a steep learning curve for a new system but also that historical systems embody institutional workflow. Separating the workflow or business logic from the database will enable more natural migrations of systems as the HCO or IDN evolves. Organizations should not, however, assume that old workflow is correct or should necessarily be embodied in new information systems. The point here is that a modern architecture that separates the workflow from the data allows prior data to be carried forward as the systems migrate. This also enables organizations to change workflow as new features and functions become available in newer products or product releases.

The third layer, the **user-interface layer**, is the one most subject to frequent change. The cost of desktop devices and support represents a significant portion of HCO and IDN information systems budgets—often as much as one-third of the total budget. For example, an IDN that supports 10,000 workstations will incur ongoing costs for hardware and software alone of $10 million per year, assuming a $3,000 unit cost and a 3-year life span per workstation. Thin client and browser-based technologies, which minimize processing at the workstation level, can substantially reduce this cost by allowing simpler maintenance and support as well as decreased cost per device.

Future network and computer system architecture will likely increasingly rely on the tools and technological developments driven by the ubiquity of the Internet. PDAs, cell phones, pagers and other devices continue to shrink in size while increasing in functionality. However, often due to size limitations (and specifically the limits of keyboards and display screens available on PDAs), these systems are currently better suited for one-way retrieval and presentation of information and do not adequately support clinicians' requirements for data input. But even with shrinking size, these devices are still suitable for accessing electronic schedule and contact lists and have (modified) handwriting recognition capabilities, and support other productivity tools which have become popular. Voice-entry devices have found some utility where noncontinuous speech is supported by good screen design (see Chapter 5). The introduction of computer tablets with handwriting recognition show promise for use in specialized clinical applications. Most probably, clinician end users will require a variety of devices—some that are application specific and some that vary with personal preference. The important design consideration is that, if possible, the design of the display and the nature of the input devices should not be so tied to the application that change and modification are difficult.

13.5 Forces That Will Shape the Future of Healthcare Information Systems

As we have discussed throughout this chapter, the changing landscape of the healthcare industry and the strategic and operational requirements of HCOs and IDNs have accelerated the acquisition and implementation of HCISs. Although there are many obstacles to implementation and acceptance of smoothly functioning, fully integrated HCISs, few people today would debate the critical role that information technology plays in an HCO's success or in an IDN's efforts at clinical and operational integration.

We have emphasized the dynamic nature of today's healthcare environment and the associated implications for HCISs. The information architecture described in Section 13.4 can help to carry HCOs and IDNs through this dynamic time, but a host of new requirements loom that will challenge today's available solutions. We anticipate additional requirements associated with the changing organizational landscape, technological advances, and broader societal changes.

13.5.1 Changing Organizational Landscape

Although the concepts underlying HCOs and IDNs are no longer new, the underlying organizational forms and business strategies of these complex organizations continue to evolve. The success of individual HCOs varies widely. Some, serving target patient populations such as those with heart disease or cancer or age-defined groups such as children, appear to be relatively more successful that those attempting to serve patients across a wide range of illnesses or those attempting to combine diverse missions of clinical care, teaching and research. IDNs, on the other hand, have by and large failed to achieve the operational improvements and cost reductions they were designed to deliver. It is possible that we will witness the emergence of entirely new forms of HCOs and IDNs, and in fact we have already witnessed the reversal in some areas of the trend toward consolidation. Key to understanding the magnitude of the information systems challenge for IDNs in particular is recognizing the extraordinary pace of change—IDNs reorganize, merge, uncouple, acquire, sell off, and strategically align services and organizational units in a matter of weeks. On the other hand, today's state-of-the-art systems (computer systems and people processes) may require months or years to build and refine.

All too frequently, business deals are cut with insufficient regard to the cost and time required to create the supporting information infrastructure. For IDNs even in the best of circumstances, the cultural and organizational challenges of linking diverse users and care-delivery settings will tax their ability to change their information systems environments quickly enough. These issues will increase in acuity as operational budgets continue to shrink—today's IDNs are spending significant portions of their capital budgets on information-systems investments. In turn, these new investments translate into increased annual operating costs (costs of regular system upgrades, maintenance, user support, and staffing). Still most healthcare organizations devote at most 3 to 4 percent of their total revenues to their information systems operating budgets; in other information-intensive industries, the percentage of operating budgets devoted to information technology investment can be 3 to 4 times higher.

13.5.2 Technological Changes Affecting Healthcare Organizations

Although future changes in technology are hard to predict (e.g., we have heard for over two decades that voice-entry systems are 5 years away from practical use!), the best clues to the future may be found in our recent past. First, the emergence of the powerful microprocessor and the cost performance of storage media will continue to be a dominant factor in future health-systems design. These technologies ensure that sufficient processing and storage will be available for almost any healthcare application that currently can be imagined. Second, the ever expanding availability of Internet access as well as the trend in the communications industry to integrate voice, video, and data will ensure that HCOs and IDNs will have broadband capacity not only within their traditional domain but also to an extended enterprise that may include even patients' homes, schools, and workplaces. Third, the design of modern software based on the replicability of code and code standards such as XML, should eventually yield more flexible information technology systems.

If security and confidentiality concerns can be resolved, the emergence of a networked society will profoundly change our thinking about the nature of healthcare delivery. Health services are still primarily delivered locally—we seldom leave our local communities to receive health care except under the most dire of circumstances. In the future, providers and even patients will have access to healthcare experts that are dispersed over state, national, and even international boundaries. Distributed healthcare capabilities will enable the implementation of collaborative models that could include virtual house calls and routine remote monitoring via telemedical linkages (see Chapter 14).

13.5.3 Societal Change

At the beginning of the twenty-first century, clinicians find themselves spending less time with each patient and spending more time with administrative and regulatory concerns. This decrease in clinician–patient contact has contributed to declining patient and provider satisfaction with care-delivery systems. At the same time, empowered health consumers interested in self-help and unconventional approaches have access to more health information than ever before. These factors are changing the interplay among physicians, care teams, patients, and external (regulatory and financial) forces. The changing model of care, coupled with changing economic incentives, places a greater focus on wellness and preventative and lifelong care. Although we might agree that aligning economic incentives with wellness is a good thing, this alignment also implies a shift in responsibility.

Like the healthcare environment, the technology context of our lives is also changing. The Internet has already dramatically changed our approaches to information access and system design in the workplace. Concurrent with the development of new standards of information display and exchange is a push led by the entertainment industry (and others) to deliver broadband multimedia into our homes. Such connectivity will catalyze changing care models more than any other factor we can imagine by bringing fast, interactive, and multimedia capabilities to the household level. Finally, vast amounts of information can now be stored efficiently on movable media. If past performance predicts future availability, we can assume almost unlimited and inexpensive storage of consumer-oriented health information, including, for example, video segments that show the appearance and sounds of normal and abnormal conditions or demonstrate common procedures for home care and health maintenance.

With societal factors pushing our HCOs and IDNs to change, and the likely availability of extensive computing and communication capacity in the homes, in the work place, and in the schools, health organizations and health providers are increasingly challenged to rethink the basic operating assumptions about how to deliver care. The traditional approach has been facility and physician centric—patients usually come to the hospital or to the physician at a time convenient for the hospital or the physician. The HCO and IDN of the twenty-first century may be truly a healthcare delivery system without walls, where routine health management is conducted in nontraditional settings, such as homes and workplaces, using the power of telemedicine and consumer informatics.

Suggested Readings

Drazen E., Metzger J. (1999). Strategies for Integrated Health Care. San Francisco: Jossey-Bass Publishers.
This book reviews descriptive research covering the organizational and information systems aspects of new healthcare delivery strategies being pursued by pioneering IDNs. Prominent in the book are discussions of new models for providing access to health services, for delivering coordinated services across distributed care settings, and for integrating physician and IDN patient care activities.

Gross M.S., Lohman P. (1997). The technology and tactics of physician integration. Journal of the Healthcare Information and Management Systems Society, 11(2):23–41.
This article discusses physician integration, which is the process of aligning the activities and incentives of individual and groups of physicians with the other components of an IDN. The article examines alternative IDN models, common problems associated with physicians' changing roles, and the influence of physician culture on these problems. The article recommends integration tactics and discusses how management style and information technology can address the goals of the IDN and the interests of its physicians.

Lorenzi N. M., Riley R.T., Blyth A.J., Southon G., Dixon, B.J. (1997). Antecedents of the people and organizational aspects of medical informatics: review of the literature. Journal of the American Medical Informatics Association, 4(2):79–93.
This article reviews the contributions of behavioral science and organizational management disciplines and their implications for processes for creating future direction, managing complex change processes, involving individuals and groups in implementation projects, and managing the altered organization.

Overhage J. M. (1998). Proceedings of the Fourth Annual Nicholas E. Davies CPR Recognition Symposium. July 9–10. Renaissance Mayflower Hotel, Washington, D.C. Computer-based Patient Record Institute, Schaumburg, IL
This conference proceedings includes detailed and organized summaries of the management, function, technology, and effects of provider information systems for the 1998 Davies award-winning organizations. These organizations have demonstrated an ability to integrate data from multiple sources, provide decision support, and be used by caregivers as the primary source of information in patient care. The 1998 winners were Northwestern Memorial Hospital (Chicago) and Kaiser-Permanente Northwest (Portland, OR). Prior years' proceedings summarize the systems of Intermountain Health Care, Columbia Presbyterian Medical Center (New York City), Department of Veterans Affairs (1995); Brigham and Women's Hospital (1996); Kaiser-Permanente of Ohio, North Mississippi Health Services, and the Regenstrief Institute for Health Care (1997). The winning HCISs represent both inhouse-developed and commercial systems.

Questions for Discussion

1. Briefly explain the differences among an HCO's operational, planning, communications, and documentary requirements for information. Give two examples in each category. Choose one of these categories, and discuss similarities and differences in the environments of a tertiary-care medical center, a community-based ambulatory-care clinic, and a specialty-care physician's office. Describe the implied differences in these units' information requirements.
2. Describe three situations in which the separation of clinical and administrative information could lead to inadequate patient care, loss of revenue, or inappropriate administrative decisions. Identify and discuss the challenges and limitations of two methods for improving data integration.
3. Describe three situations in which lack of integration of information systems with clinicians' workflow can lead to inadequate patient care, reduced physician productivity, or poor patient satisfaction with an HCO's services. Identify and discuss the challenges and limitations of two methods for improving process integration.
4. Describe the trade-off between functionality and integration. Discuss three strategies currently used by HCOs to minimize this tradeoff.
5. Assume that you are the chief information officer of a multi-facility HCO. You have just been charged with planning a new HCIS to support a large tertiary care medical center, two smaller community hospitals, a nursing home, and a 40-physician group practice. Each organization currently operates its own set of integrated and stand-alone technologies and applications. What technical and organizational factors must you consider? What are the three largest challenges you will face over the next 24 months?
6. How do you think the implementation of HCISs will affect the quality of relationships between patients and providers? Discuss at least three potential positive and three potential negative effects. What steps would you take to maximize the positive value of these systems?

14
Consumer Health Informatics and Telehealth

PATRICIA FLATLEY BRENNAN AND JUSTIN B. STARREN

After reading this chapter you should know the answers to these questions:

- What factors contribute to the increasing pressure for lay people to actively participate in health care?
- How does direct access to health information technologies assist patients in participating in their own health care?
- Critically appraise the informatics requirements for successful telehealth.
- How can lay people determine the value of a telehealth innovation such as a health-related Web site or an on-line disease management service?

14.1   Introduction

Complexity and collaboration characterize health care in the early 21st century. Complexity arises from increasing sophistication in the understanding of health and disease, wherein etiological models must take into account both molecular processes and physical environments. Collaboration reflects not only inter-professional collaboration, but also a realization that successful attainment of optimal well-being and effective management of disease processes necessitate active engagement of clinicians, lay persons, concerned family members, and society as a whole. This chapter introduces the concepts of **telemedicine**, **telehealth**, and **consumer health informatics** (CHI) and illustrates how maturing computer networks like the Internet make possible the collaborations necessary to achieve the full benefits of our growing understanding of health promotion, disease management and disability prevention. Consider the following situation:

> Jeffery is an 18-year old high school senior, who is newly diagnosed with Type I diabetes following an acute hyperglycemic episode which required hospitalization. After four days he is medically stable and ready for discharge. He is able to measure his blood glucose and can safely administer the appropriate dose of insulin. The nurse notes that Jeffery sometimes has trouble calibrating the insulin dose to the blood glucose reading. She also notes that his father is short and impatient with Jeffery, expressing many concerns that Jeffery "may not be able to handle such a complex medical problem on his own".

14.1.1   Telemedicine, Telehealth and Reducing the Distance Between the Consumer and the Healthcare System?

Warner Slack calls the patient "the most underused resource in the health care delivery system." Telehealth and telemedicine approaches have the ability to bring professionals and patients closer together, and CHI innovations insure that the patient has access to the information resources necessary for them to participate fully in the health care process.

Historically, health care has usually involved travel. Either the health care provider traveled to visit the patient, or more recently, the patient traveled to visit the provider. Diabetic patients, like Jeffery, typically meet with their physician every two to six months to review data and plan therapy changes. Travel has costs, both directly, in terms of gasoline or transportation tickets, and indirectly, in terms of travel time, delayed treatment, and lost productivity. In fact, travel has accounted for a significant proportion of the total cost of healthcare. (Starr, 1983) Because of this, both patients and providers have been quick to recognize that rapid electronic communications have the potential to improve care by reducing the costs and delays associated with travel. This has involved both access to information resources, as well as direct communication among various participants, including patients, family members, primary care providers and specialists.

As is the case with informatics, the formal definitions of telemedicine and telehealth tend to be very broad. One widely circulated definition is:

> Telemedicine involves the use of modern information technology, especially two-way inter-active audio/video communications, computers and telemetry to deliver health services to remote patients and to facilitate information exchange between primary care physicians and specialists at some distance from each other. (Bashshur, *et al.*, 1997).

It is clear from the definition above that there is considerable overlap between telemedicine and biomedical informatics. In fact, one will frequently find papers on telemedicine systems presented at biomedical informatics conferences and presentations on informatics at telemedicine meetings. The major distinction is one of emphasis. Telemedicine emphasizes the distance, especially the provision of care to remote or isolated patients and communities. In contrast, biomedical informatics emphasizes methods for handling the information, irrespective of the distance between patient and provider. A question that frequently arises in any discussion of this topic is the distinction between telemedicine and telehealth. Although not formalized, a frequent distinction between the two terms is that telemedicine is an older and a narrower term, connoting communication between two persons. Telemedicine is often associated with video-conferencing between patients and providers. In contrast, telehealth is a newer and broader term that has been used to include both traditional telemedicine as well as interactions with automated systems or information resources. Because of its broader scope, we are using the term telehealth in this chapter. Another topic of discussion is whether consumer-health informatics (CHI) is a sub-domain of telehealth or whether they are two separate domains. This question lacks a simple answer. As can be seen in Figure 14.1, both CHI and telehealth are ways to bridge the distance between patients

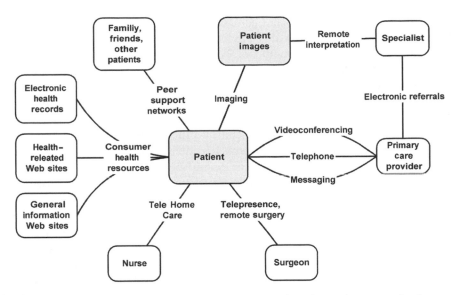

Figure 14.1. Connections. The figure shows different ways that electronic communications can be used to link patients with various health resources. Only connections directly involving the patient are shown (e.g., use of the EHR by the clinician is not shown). Some of the resources, such as Web sites or telehome care, can be accessed from the patient's home. Other resources, such as remote surgery or imaging, would require the patient to go to a telehealth-equipped clinical facility.

and necessary health resources. Those resources could involve interaction with specific persons, such as physicians, nurses or other patients. They could also involve interactions with computerized information, such as Web sites, or with expert knowledge, such as the remote interpretation of a images. Collectively, CHI and telehealth transport healthcare knowledge and expertise to where they are needed, and are ways to involve the patient as an active partner in care. In spite of their similarities, CHI and telehealth come from very different historical foundations. Telehealth derived from traditional patient care, while CHI derived from the self-help movements of the 1970's. (See Section 14.2) Largely owing to this historical separation, practitioners and researchers in the two fields tend to come from different backgrounds. For these reasons, we are presenting CHI and telehealth as two distinct, but closely related domains with central ties to biomedical informatics.

14.1.2 Consumerism, Self-Help, and Consumer Health Informatics

Contemporary consumers experience greater demands to participate in their own care than have patients at any time since the emergence of modern health care. Patient participation takes many forms: shared decision-making, self-care, and collaborative practices. In essence, it reflects a shift from the patient as the silent recipient of ministrations from a wise, beneficent clinician to an active collaborator whose values, preferences, and lifestyle not only alter predisposition to certain illnesses but also shape the characteristics of desirable treatments. The legacy of the self-help movement of the 1970s and the **consumerism** of the 1980s is growth in the importance of the patient as a full participant in health care. Patients participate by self-monitoring, by evaluating and choosing therapeutic strategies from a set of acceptable alternatives, by implementing the therapies, and by evaluating the effects. Recent social and clinical changes in the manner in which care is provided shift clinical-practice activities that were once the purview of licensed professionals to patients and their family caregivers. The failure of 50 years of bioscience research to produce definitive clinical remedies for more than a handful of disease states requires that medical science be tempered with patient preferences (e.g., between surgical and radiation therapies). Furthermore, there is growing belief that behavioral interventions and alternative therapies hold great promise as adjuncts, or even replacements, for traditional medical therapies. These trends contribute to a contemporary healthcare environment that is more diffuse and involves more people than ever before. The home and the community are fast becoming the most common sites where health care is provided. Information technologies necessary to support patients and their family caregivers must not only migrate from the inpatient institution to the community but also be populated with information resources that help to guide patients in complex healthcare decision-making, to communicate with health professionals and to access the clinical records and health science knowledge necessary to help them comprehend their health states and participate in appropriate treatments.

The role of the consumer as a full partner in health promotion and disease management has never been more necessary than now. In the distributed-managed-care models of health care, consumers serve as their own case managers, brokering care from generalists, specialists, and ancillary groups. Rarely do consumers receive all of their needed clinical services from a single provider. Informatics tools, such as the **electronic health record**, provide an integrated record and communication service. Consumers require access to this record so that they can contribute timely observations, monitor their own progress toward health, and comprehend the plethora of clinical interventions available to them.

The development of inexpensive, reliable computers and telecommunications technology enables healthcare providers, payers, patients, and the general public to access health information and healthcare resources directly from their homes and from public gathering places, such as libraries, schools, and workplaces. Through computer networks, telephone messaging services, and other initiatives, clinicians have a unique opportunity to reach patients and clients with health-promotion, disease-prevention, and illness-management clinical interventions. Telecommunications-based health services also pose unique challenges to modify existing clinical interventions and to devise new ones to take appropriate advantage of the electronic environment.

14.2 Historical Perspectives

The use of communication technology to convey health-related information at a distance is nothing new. The earliest known example may be the use of so-called "leper bells" carried by individuals during Roman times. Sailing ships would fly a yellow flag to indicate a ship was under quarantine and awaiting clearance by a doctor, or a yellow and black "plague flag" to indicate that infected individuals were on board. By some accounts, when Alexander Graham Bell said "Mr. Watson. Come here. I need you" in 1876, it was because he had spilled acid on his hand and needed medical assistance. In 1879, only three years later, the first description of telephone use for clinical diagnosis appeared in a medical journal. (Practice by Telephone, 1879)

14.2.1   Early Experiences

One of the earliest and most long-lived telchealth projects is the Australian Royal Flying Doctor Service (RFDS), founded in 1928. In addition to providing air ambulance services, the RFDS provides telehealth consultations. These consultations first used Morse Code, and later voice, radio communications to the remote sheep stations in the Australian outback. Lay people played a significant role here, clearly communicating their concerns and clinical findings to the RFDS and carefully carrying out instructions while awaiting, if necessary, the arrival of the physician. The RFDS is most famous for its standardized medical chest, introduced in 1942. The chest contains diagnostic charts and medications, identified only by number. This allowed the consulting clinician to localize symptoms by number and then prescribe care, such as "take one number five and two number fours." Modern telehealth can be traced to 1948 when the first transmission of a radiograph over a phone line was reported. Video-based telehealth can be traced to 1955 when the Nebraska Psychiatric Institute began experimenting with a closed-circuit video network on its campus. In 1964 this was extended to a remote state mental health facility to support education and **teleconsultation**. In 1967, Massachusetts General Hospital (MGH) was linked to Logan International Airport via a microwave video link. In 1971 the National Library of Medicine began the Alaska Satellite Biomedical Demonstration project linking 26 remote Alaskan villages utilizing NASA satellites.

The period from the mid 1970's to the late 1980's was a time of much experimentation, but few fundamental changes in telehealth. A variety of pilot projects demonstrated the feasibility and utility of video-based telehealth. The military funded a number of research projects aimed at developing tools for providing telehealth care on the battlefield. The early 1990's saw several important advances. Military applications developed during the previous decades began to be deployed. Military **teleradiology** was first deployed in 1991 during Operation Desert Storm. Telehealth in military field hospitals was first deployed in 1993 in Bosnia. Several states, including Georgia, Kansas, North Carolina and Iowa implemented statewide telehealth networks. Some of these were pure video networks, based on broadcast television technology. Others were built using evolving Internet technology. During this same period, *correctional telehealth* became much more common. For example, in 1992 East Carolina University contracted with the largest maximum-security prison in North Carolina to provide telehealth consultation. Telehealth projects in the early 1990s continued to be plagued by two problems that had hampered telehealth since its inception: high cost and poor image quality. Both hardware and high-bandwidth connections were prohibitively expensive. A single telehealth station typically cost over \$50,000 and connectivity could cost thousands of dollars per month. Most programs were dependent on external grant funding for survival. Even with this, image resolution was frequently poor and motion artifacts were severe. The Internet revolution of the late 1990s drove fundamental change in telehealth. Advances in computing power both improved image quality and reduced hardware costs to the point that, by 2000, comparable systems cost less than a tenth of what they had a decade earlier. Improvements in **image compression** made it possible to transmit low-resolution, full-motion video over standard telephone lines, enabling the growth of *telehome care*. With the increasing popularity of the World Wide Web, high-bandwidth connections became both more available and less expensive. Many telehealth applications that had relied on expensive, dedicated, point-to-point connections were converted to utilize commodity Internet connections. The availability of affordable hardware and connectivity also made access to health-related electronic resources from the home, school or work place possible and fueled the growth of CHI.

14.2.2   *Engaging Consumers in Health Care*

Patients, family members and the general public have long-played an active role in health care, and have actively sought information from health professionals and government agencies. During the early 20th century, the US Federal Children's Bureau served as a major source of health information for the public. Mothers could write to this federal agency, asking questions about normal child development, nutrition, and disease management. Written materials, such as letters and pamphlets served as the primary mechanism for delivering information that supported lay people in their handling of health challenges. Broadcast and reproduction media, including television, videotapes and audiotapes, were quickly harnessed by health professionals as a means for presenting complex information and health care instructions to people in their homes.

Computers and telecommunications have been used since the early 1940's for patient assessment, patient education, and clinical information sharing. Morris Collen and colleagues at Kaiser Permanente created a health appraisal system that prompted for patient data and returned a systematic risk appraisal. Slack and colleagues at the University of Wisconsin used a **mainframe computer** system as a health assessment tool. Patients sat at a **cathode ray tube** (CRT) terminal and responded to text questions, receiving a printed summary of their health appraisal at the end of the session. At MGH in the late 1950's, computer-driven telephone systems were used to conduct home-based follow-up with post-surgery cardiac patients, calling them daily to obtain pulse readings.

In the 1980's clinicians and health educators capitalized on the increasingly common personal computers as vehicles for health education. Initially, computers were used primarily for **computer-assisted learning** programs, providing general coaching regarding topics such as nutrition and home care of the elderly. The Body Awareness Resource Network (BARN), developed in the 1980's by Gustafson and colleagues at the University of Wisconsin, engaged adolescents in game-type interaction to help them learn about growth and development, develop healthy attitudes towards avoidance of risky behaviors, and rehearse strategies for negotiating the complex interpersonal world of adolescents. Later developments in the 1980's and 1990's moved beyond computer aided learning to values clarification and risk appraisal exercises, thus capitalizing on the computational power as well as the visual display capabilities of the computer.

Social trends, coupled with the introduction of **managed care** and the rapid growth of computer tools, networks, and multimedia, led to both an explosion of need for health-care information by the lay public and a dramatic rise in the use of information technology to meet that need. Lay persons need information about health promotion, illness prevention, and disease management. Special computer programs, health-focused CD-ROMs, and health-related, Internet-based World Wide Web sites all provide information likely to be useful to the lay public in participating in health care. Browsers linked to the World Wide Web allow consumers to access their health records and communicate with health care providers in a secure fashion. Labeled consumer-health informatics (CHI), these applications of medical informatics technologies to health care focuses on the patient as the primary user.

14.3   Bridging Distance with Informatics: Real-world Systems

There are many ways to categorize CHI and telehealth resources, including classifications based on participants, bandwidth, information transmitted, medical specialty, immediacy, health care condition, and financial reimbursement. The categorization in Table 14.1 is based loosely on bandwidth and overall complexity. This categorization was chosen because each category presents different challenges for informatics researchers and practitioners.

A second categorization of telehealth systems that overlaps the previous one is the separation into *synchronous* (or *real-time*) and *asynchronous* (or *store-and-forward*

Table 14.1. Categories of telehealth and consumer health informatics.

Telehealth category	Bandwidth	Applications
Information Resources	Low to moderate	Web-based information resources, patient access to electronic medical records
Messaging	Low	E-mail, chat groups, consumer health networks, personal clinical electronic communications (PCEC)
Telephone	Low	Scheduling, triage
Remote monitoring	Low to moderate	Remote monitoring of pacemakers, diabetes, asthma, hypertension, CHF.
Remote interpretation	Moderate	PACS, remote interpretation of radiographic studies and other images, such as dermatologic and retinal photographs.
Videoconferencing	Low to high	Wide range of applications, from low-bandwidth telehome care over telephone lines, to high-bandwidth telementoring and telepsychiatry
Telepresence	High	Remote Surgery, telerobotics

CHF = Congestive Heart Failure.

systems). Video conferencing is the archetypal synchronous telehealth application. Synchronous telehealth encounters are analogous to conventional office visits. Telephony, chat-groups, and **telepresence** are also examples of synchronous telehealth. A major challenge in all synchronous telehealth is scheduling. All participants must be at the necessary equipment at the same time. Store-and-forward, as the name implies, involves the preparation of a dataset at one site that is sent asynchronously to a remote recipient. Remote interpretation, especially teleradiology, is the archetypal example of store-and-forward telehealth. Images are obtained at one site and then sent, sometimes over very low bandwidth connections, to another site where the domain expert interprets them. Other examples of store-and-forward include access to Web sites, e-mail and text messaging. Some store-and-forward systems support the creation of multimedia "cases" that contain multiple clinical data types, including text, scanned images, wave forms and videos.

14.3.1   Direct Access to Health Information Resources by Consumers

> A classmate tells Jeffery – "it's too bad you have diabetes – you can't have sex – all guys with diabetes are impotent sooner or later". Later that night, Jeffery goes on the Internet and tries to find out if his friend's dire warning is true.

Patients like Jeffery need quick, private access to accurate information that can calm fears and ensure direct access to currently accepted treatment for their illness. Existing healthcare delivery systems are woefully inadequate in providing such information to their patients. At best, a busy clinician may be able to take a few minutes to explain terms and likely consequences and perhaps to provide the patient with additional brochures and printed information. Computer technology can supplement clinicians' teaching with more detailed information that can be referenced repeatedly by a patient in the privacy of his home.

Consumer health informatics resources provide substantive and procedural knowledge about health problems and promising interventions (Table 14.2). Information resources developed for consumers vary in content and sophistication. Some of these resources are little more than digitized brochures, presenting in an electronic form exactly what can be found in available printed materials. Others include interactive or multimedia presentations of information about specific conditions and appropriate actions to prevent, cure, or ameliorate the problem. Multimedia presentations capitalize on the features of computer systems to enrich the presentation of health-related materials with pictures, short movies, and drawings.

Consumer health informatics resources provide patients with condition-specific and disease-specific information about the problems they face. Some resources explain the etiology and natural history of disease in terms comprehensible to lay people. Other resources provide procedural information, explain diagnostic procedures or services, detail expected treatment activities, and provide any relevant warnings and precautions. The presentation of CHI is heavily influenced by the perspective of the system developer. Medically oriented clinical resources demonstrate an emphasis on locally accepted

Table 14.2. Selected consumer health Web sites on the Internet.

Federal resources
 The U.S. Department of Health and Human Services primary consumer health information resource:
  http://www.healthfinder.gov/
 The National Library of Medicine's Consumer Resources
  General Information http://www.nlm.nih.gov/medlineplus/
  Clinical Trials Update www.clinicaltrials.gov
  Genetics Health Information http://ghr.nlm.nih.gov/
 Agency for Health Care Policy and Research Consumer Health Guides http://www.ahcpr.gov/consumer/

National resources
 Statement of the Institute of Medicine on the Electronic Health Record
  http://www.nap.edu/books/NI000427/html/
 ebMD Health Resources (Commercial) http://www.webmd.com/

Regional resources
 Healthy Wisconsin http://www.healthywisconsin.org/
 Mayo Clinic's Health References: http://www.MayoClinic.com/

Condition or disease-specific information on the Web
 Nutrition Navigator http://navigator.tufts.edu/
 Foot Care http://www.nia.nih.gov/health/agepages/footcare.htm
 Diabetes http://ndep.nih.gov/get-info/info-control.htm

Evaluating health information on the Web:
 Information Quality Tool (Mitertek, Inc) – an interactive tool for consumers
  http://hitiweb.mitretek.org/iq/
 Guidelines from the University of British Columbia
  http://www.library.ubc.ca/home/evaluating/Easyprint.html

Quality assurance indicators for health-related Web sites
 URAC, also known as the American Accreditation HealthCare Commission *http://www.urac.org/*
 Health on the Net Foundation: http://www.hon.ch/

medical practice. Community health-oriented resources are more likely to include information relevant to living in the community with a specific disease or condition.

Consumer health informatics resources originate from two major perspectives: professional and self-help. **Professional-developed CHI resources** are those developed by healthcare clinicians and their organizations. Healthcare organizations—such as HMOs, managed-care companies, and group practices—develop information resources as a service to the patient populations that they treat. These resources tend to complement and extend the clinical services offered by the professional group and may be based on a desire to ensure adherence with accepted therapies or to triage and manage access to care for common health problems. Examples include Kaiser Permanente Health Facts, a program designed to help Kaiser members answer questions about common health problems, and the Mayo Health Advisor, a commercially available CD-ROM that any interested person can purchase and use to help manage his health at home. Examples of other commercially available programs that have a professional orientation include Health Wise and Health Desk. Figure 14.2 shows an example of professional-developed CHI resources accessible via the Internet.

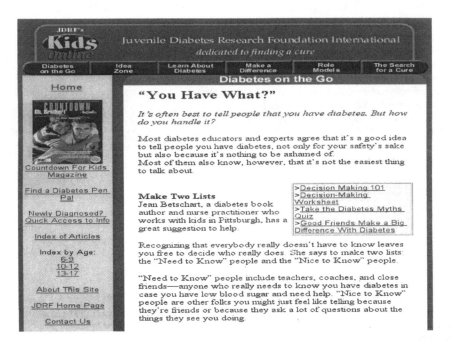

Figure 14.2. Consumer Health Web site designed for use by children. Note the casual language style, the mix of information and skill building, and the colors and graphics. (© 2003 JDRF)

Consumer health informatics resources developed from a self-help perspective complement and augment those provided by the formal healthcare delivery system. A self-help perspective is generally more inclusive than a professional perspective. The information may address daily living concerns and lifestyle issues along with, or in place of, content deemed credible by established medical authorities.

Many CHI resources represent a combination of professional and self-help perspectives. Web-based resources, such as those provided by the Fred Hutchinson Cancer Research Center, provide pointers to other Web sites that represent professional or self-help perspectives. Commercial vendors, such as HealthGate Data Corporation, provide access via a Web site to professional-developed and self-help–oriented CHI resources for a subscription or transaction-based fee.

As the electronic health record (EHR) (Chapter 12) gains acceptance, its relevance to individual patients also grows. Many hospitals and clinics have begun providing direct patient access to the clinical record, allowing individuals to electronically access sections of their records to recall salient instructions or obtain results of tests. Figure 14.3 shows the PatCIS system developed at Columbia University.(Cimino *et al.*, 1998) Critical aspects of security, privacy and accurate identification of patients must be addressed, as well as compliance with government regulations (See Chapter 5.) Additionally, designers must take special care to insure that the language used in presenting personal health data enhances the patient's understanding of his or her health concerns. Many of these

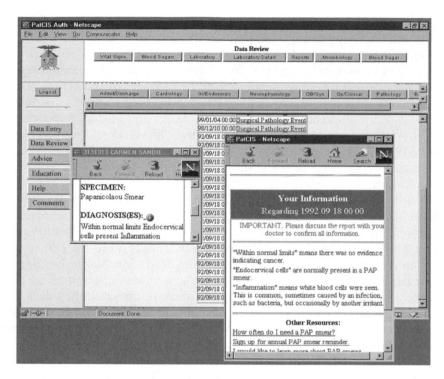

Figure 14.3. PatCIS screen. The Patient Clinical Information System (PatCIS) allows patients to enter and review data in the Central Data Repository at Columbia University/New York Presbyterian Hospital. In this screen the patient has selected to review a Pap smear result. Definitions of commonly misinterpreted words are automatically generated, along with links to related information. (*Source*: Cimino et al., 2003.)

portals also provide secure messaging systems, allowing patients to communicate concerns about their clinical record to their health care providers.

14.3.2 Consumer Health Networks and Health-Related Messaging

Recognizing the concerns expressed in her latest coaching session with Jeffery, the Diabetes Educator believes that giving Jeffery a greater sense of control in his life management may help reduce the fears he currently has. She provides him with a network-equipped PalmPilot that he can use to record his exercise and eating patterns, schedule alarms to remind him to complete blood glucose testing, store the current sliding-scale insulin management plan, and automatically send reports to his care providers for evaluation. After the first two weeks, Jeffery reports that he likes the device, as it helps him remember when to do the testing. He also adds that he's figured out how to instant-message (IM) with friends using the Palm, and how to download games. The Diabetes Educator sighs, and considers ways to use the Palm to engage Jeffery in more learning and self-management.

Computer networks not only provide patients with access to information; they provide the additional opportunity for individuals to connect with other people who share similar concerns and with their healthcare providers. Network-based consumer-health services include both specialty and public access networks. Examples of two specialty systems that have been heavily researched are the ComputerLink (Brennan, 1998), a specialized computer network service for homebound patients and their caregivers, and the Comprehensive Health Evaluation and Social Support System (CHESS), which targets the needs of people living with AIDS and women diagnosed with breast cancer (Gustafson et al., 2002). Public access systems include the health-related Usenet discussion groups and the health forums available on CompuServe and America Online.

Network-based CHI resources generally provide both static information about health problems and management and specialized health-communications utilities. Some professional-developed CHI resources not only provide information to members of a health plan but also facilitate communication between the patient and the health plan. The Kaiser model allows patients who determine that the health problem they face requires a visit to a clinician to cease the information-resource portion and to activate a communication module that links them to the scheduling desk of their local health clinic, where they can request an appointment to see a clinician. Information resources that reside on the Web generally provide a question-answering service—a utility where interested persons can leave a question to be answered by a professional. Still others support direct electronic mail between patients and clinicians. Some offer discussion groups and chat rooms, where people interested in a specific disease or condition can post and read messages. These discussion areas function as electronic support groups and demonstrate many of the same features found in face-to-face support groups. Professionals participate in these discussions, providing advice or counsel.

Patient-to-patient communication services are generally the most actively used aspects, with a ratio of 10 contacts with a communication service for each access to an information service. These communication services offer great opportunity for health professionals to clarify information, to guide people in wellness behavior, and to recommend specific activities for managing existing health conditions.

Timely access to staged, tailored informational services may have the greatest positive health benefit (Bass et al., 1998; Brennan et al, 2001). For some users, even infrequent access to information resources has led to improved health outcomes. Because of their convenience and accessibility, it is possible that the network-based services offer timely, private access to information when needed by the individual. It is also possible that the network access, supporting both communication and information access, permits lay people to obtain factual knowledge in the context of peer support.

> Two weeks later Jeffery's physician notes a slight but persistent rise in his blood glucose readings. He sends Jeffery a message on the Palm to schedule an appointment and review the medication administration strategy. Later realizing that Jeffery regularly tests his blood but doesn't always record the insulin dosing, the physician and nurse set up a plan for Jeffery to message them at each dose administration point. They use this messaging to provide reassurance, encouragement and to insure that the medication is actually being taken.

Text messaging is emerging as a popular mode of communication between patients and providers. It began with patients sending conventional e-mails to physician. The popularity of this grew so rapidly that national guidelines were developed.(Kane & Sands, 1998) However, e-mail has a number of disadvantages for health related messaging: delivery is not guaranteed; security is problematic; e-mail is transient (there was no automatic logging or audit trail); and the messages are completely unstructured. To address these limitations, a variety of Web-based messaging solutions, called Personal Clinical Electronic Communications, have been developed (Sarkar & Starren, 2002). The Medem system, developed in conjunction with eight medical societies, has emerged as the most popular such system. In these systems, patients and providers log onto a secure Web site to send or view messages. Rather than completely unstructured messages, the Web-based systems typically used structured forms and limit messages to specific categories, such as medication refill, appointment request, or second-opinion consultation. Because the messages never leave the Web site, many of the problems associated with conventional e-mail are avoided. Some of these systems are also being interfaced directly to EHRs to facilitate prescription renewals and reporting of test results to patients.

14.3.3   The Forgotten Telephone

Until recently, the telephone was the forgotten component in teleheath. The field of telemedicine and telehealth focused on video and largely ignored the audio-only telehealth. Few studies were done and few articles written. This is paradoxical given that up to 25% of all primary care encounters occur via the telephone. These include triage, case management, results review, consultation, medication adjustment and logistical issues, like scheduling. In part, this can be traced to the fact that telephone consultations are not reimbursed by most insurance carriers. More recently, increased interest in cost control through case management has driven renewed interest in use of audio-only communication between patients and providers. Multiple articles have appeared on the value of telephone follow-up for chronic conditions. Several managed care companies have set up large telephone triage centers. The National Health Service in the UK is investing £90 million per year in NHS Direct, a nation wide telephone information and triage system. With some insurance providers reimbursing for e-mails and text messaging, providers are asking why not reimburse for telephone calls also.

14.3.4   Remote Monitoring

Remote monitoring is a subset of telehealth focusing on the capture of clinically relevant data in the patients' homes or other locations outside of conventional hospitals, clinics or healthcare provider offices, and the subsequent transmission of the data to central locations for review. The conceptual model underlying nearly all remote monitoring is that clinically significant changes in patient condition occur between regularly scheduled visits and that these changes can be detected by measuring physiologic parameters. The care model presumes that, if these changes are detected and treated sooner, the overall condition of the patient will be improved. An important distinction between remote monitoring and many conventional forms of telemedicine is that remote monitoring focuses on management, rather than on diagnosis. Typically, remote monitoring involves patients who have already been diagnosed with a chronic disease or condition. Remote monitoring is used to track parameters that guide management. Any measurable parameter is a candidate for remote monitoring. The collected data may include continuous data streams or discrete measurements. The collection of discrete measurements is the most common approach. Another important feature of most remote monitoring is that the measurement of the parameter and the transmission of the data are typically separate events. The measurement devices have a memory that can store multiple measurements. The patient will send the data to the caregiver in one of two ways. For many studies, the patient will log onto a server at the central site (either over the Web or by direct dial-up) and then type in the data. Alternately, the patient may connect the measurement device to a personal computer or specialized modem and transfer the readings electronically. A major advantage of direct electronic transfer is that it eliminates problems stemming from manual entry, including falsification, number preference and transcription errors.

Virtually any condition that is evaluated by measuring a physiologic parameter is a candidate for remote monitoring. (See Chapter 17 for more on patient monitoring systems.) The parameter most measured in the remote setting is blood glucose for monitoring diabetes. A wide variety of research projects and commercial systems have been developed to monitor patients with diabetes. Patients with asthma can be monitored with peak-flow or full-loop **spirometers**. Hypertensives can be monitored with automated blood pressure cuffs. Patients with congestive heart failure (CHF) are monitored by measuring daily weights to detect fluid gain. Remote monitoring of pacemaker function has been available for a number of years and has recently been approved for reimbursement. Home coagulation meters have been developed that allows the monitoring of patients on chronic anticoagulation therapy. Several factors limit the widespread use of remote monitoring. First is the question of efficacy. While these systems have proven acceptable to patients and beneficial in small studies, few large-scale controlled trials have been done. Second is the basic question of who will review the data. Research studies have utilized specially trained nurses at centralized offices but it is not clear that this will scale up. Third is money—for most conditions, remote monitoring is still not a reimbursed activity.

14.3.4   Remote Interpretation

Remote interpretation is a category of store-and-forward telehealth that involves the capture of images, or other data, at one site and transmission to another site for interpretation. This may include radiographs (teleradiology), photographs (teledermatology, teleophthalmology, telepathology), or wave forms, such as ECGs (telecardiology). By far, teleradiology is the largest category of remote interpretation, and probably the largest category of telehealth. Teleradiololgy and telepathology represent the most mature clinical domains in telehealth. With the deployment of **picture archiving and communications systems** (PACS) that capture, store, transmit and displays digital radiology images, the line between teleradiology and conventional radiology is blurring.

(Radiology image management is discussed in more detail in Chapter 18.) One factor leading to the more rapid adoption of teleradiology and telepathology is the relationship between these specialists and the patients. In both cases, the specialist rarely interacts directly with the patient. The professional role is often limited to the interpretation of images. To the patient, there is little difference between a radiologist in the next building and one in the next state. The most important factor driving the growth of teleradiology is that it is reimbursable. Because image interpretation does not involve direct patient contact, few payers make any distinction about where the interpretation occurred.

Another area of remote interpretation that is growing rapidly is teleophthalmology, particularly for diabetic retinopathy screening. Systems have been developed that allow nurses in primary care offices to obtain high quality digital retinal photographs. These images are sent to regional centers for interpretation. If diabetic retinopathy is suspected, the patient is referred for a full ophthalmologic examination.

The store-and-forward modalities have benefited most from the development of the commodity Internet and the increasing availability of affordable high bandwidth connections. The shared commodity Internet provides relatively high bandwidth, but the available bandwidth is continuously varying. This makes it much better suited to the transfer of files rather than for streaming data, like video connections. Although the image files are often tens or hundreds of megabytes, the files are typically transferred to the interpretation site and cached there for later interpretation.

14.3.5   Video-based Telehealth

To many people telehealth *is* videoconferencing. Whenever the words "telehealth" or "telemedicine" are mentioned, most people have a mental image of a patient talking to a doctor over some type of synchronous video connection. Indeed, most early telehealth research did focus on synchronous video connections. For many of the early studies, the goal was to provide access to specialists in remote or rural areas. Nearly all of the early systems utilized a hub-and-spoke topology where one hub, usually an academic medical center, was connected to many spokes, usually rural clinics. Many of the early telehealth consults involved the patient and the primary care provider at one site conferring with a specialist at another site. Most of the state-wide telehealth networks operated on this model. This was so engrained in the telehealth culture, that the first legislation allowing Medicare reimbursement of telehealth consults required a "presenter" at the remote site. This requirement for a "presenter" exacerbated the scheduling problem. Because synchronous video telehealth often uses specialized videoconferencing rooms, the televists need to be scheduled at a specific time. Getting the patient and both clinicians (expert and presenter) at the right places at the right time has forced many telehealth programs to hire a full-time scheduler. The scheduling problem, combined with the advent of more user-friendly equipment, ultimately led Medicare to drop the presenter requirement. Even so, scheduling is often the single biggest obstacle to greater use of synchronous video consultations. A second obstacle has been the availability of relevant clinical information. Because of the inability to interface between various EHRs, it was not unusual for staff to print out results from the EHR at one site and then to fax those to the other site prior to a synchronous video consultation.

Unlike store-and-forward telehealth, synchronous video requires a stable data stream. Although video connection can use conventional phone lines, diagnostic quality video typically requires at least 128Kbs and more commonly 384Kbs (see Chapter 5). In order to guarantee stable data rates, synchronous video still relies heavily on dedicated circuits, either **Integrated Service Digital Network** (ISDN) connections or leased lines. Within single organizations, **Internet Protocol** (IP) based video conferencing is being used with increasing frequency. Synchronous video telehealth has been used in almost every conceivable situation. In addition to traditional consultations, the systems have been used to transmit grand rounds and other educational presentations. Video cameras have been placed in operation rooms in hub sites to transmit surgeries for educational purposes. Video cameras were placed in emergency departments and operating rooms of spoke sites to allow experts to "telementor" less experienced physicians in the remote location. Video cameras have been placed in ambulances to provide remote triage.

In contrast to the wide variety of research and demonstration projects, few applications of synchronous video have been sustainable. Most programs begun with grant funding ended soon after the grant funding ended. This is in spite of the fact that Medicare has begun reimbursing for synchronous video under limited circumstances. Three categories of synchronous video telehealth stand in marked contrast to the general trend: *telepsychiatry*, *correctional telehealth* and *home telehealth*.

Telepsychiatry

In many ways, psychiatry is the ideal clinical domain for synchronous video consultation. Diagnosis is based primarily on observing and talking to the patient. The interactive nature of the dialog means that store-and-forward video is rarely adequate. Physical examination is relatively unimportant, so that the lack of physical contact is not limiting. There are very few diagnostic studies or procedures, so that interfacing to other clinical systems is less important. In addition, state offices of mental health deliver a significant fraction of psychiatric services, minimizing reimbursement issues. This is illustrated by two projects. In 1995, the South Carolina Department of Mental Health established a telepsychiatry network to allow a single clinician to provide psychiatric services to deaf patients throughout the state (Afrin & Critchfield, 1997). The system allowed clinicians, who had previously driven all over the state, to spend more time in patient care and less time traveling. The system was so successful that it was expanded to multiple providers and roughly 20 sites. The second example comes from the New York State Psychiatric Institute (NYSPI), which is responsible for providing expert consultation to mental health facilities and prisons throughout the state. As in South Carolina, travel time was a significant factor in providing this service. To address the problem, the NYSPI created a videoconference network among the various state mental health centers. The system allows specialists at NYSPI in New York City to provide consultations in a timelier manner, improving care and increasing satisfaction at the remote sites.

Correctional Telehealth

Prisons tend to be located far from major metropolitan centers. Consequently, they are also located far from the specialists in major medical centers. Transporting prisoners to medical centers is an expensive proposition, typically requiring two officers and a vehicle. Depending on the prisoner and the distance, costs for a single transfer range from hundreds to thousands of dollars. Because of the high cost of transportation, correctional telehealth was economically viable even before the advent of newer low cost systems. Correctional telehealth also improves patient satisfaction. A fact surprising to many is that inmates typically do not want to leave a correctional institution to seek medical care. Many dislike the stigma of being paraded through a medical facility in prison garb. In addition, the social structure of prisons is such that any prisoner who leaves for more than a day risks losing privileges and social standing. Correctional telehealth follows the conventional model of providing specialist consultation to supplement to on-site primary care physicians. This has become increasingly important with the rising prevalence of AIDS in the prison population.

Home Telehealth

> After Jeffrey misses two scheduled visits, the Diabetes Educator calls see what is the matter. Jeffery explains that it is a three hour drive from his home to the diabetes center and that his father had trouble taking time off from work to drive Jeffery. The Diabetes Educator notes that Jeffery lives in a rural area and is eligible to receive educational services via teleheath. She signs Jeffery up to receive a Home Telehealth Unit and schedules delivery. After the unit arrives, Jeffery rarely misses a video education session. At one visit, Jeffery complains that is father is always "on his case" about his injections. She schedules the next video visit during an evening when Jeffery's father can attend. She also schedules Jeffery to have a video visit with the dietitian.

Somewhat paradoxically, one of the most active areas of telehealth growth is at the lowest end of the bandwidth spectrum—telehealth activities into patients' homes. In response to this, the American Telemedicine Association released new guidelines for Home Telehealth in 2002. Synchronous video is provided over so-called plain old telephone service (POTS) connections. In the late 1990s, many believed that home broadband access would soon become ubiquitous and a number of vendors abandoned POTS-based systems in favor or IP-based video solutions. The broadband revolution was slower than expected, especially in rural and economically depressed areas most in need of home telehealth services. A few research projects paid to have broadband or ISDN installed in patients' homes. Most vendors have returned to POTS-based solutions and a number of new products have appeared in the past three years. In addition to video, the devices typically have data ports for connection of various peripheral devices, such as a digital stethoscope, glucose meter, blood pressure meter, or spirometer. Although the video quality would not be adequate for many diagnostic purposes, it is adequate for the management of existing conditions. Figure 14.4B and 14.4C shows actual POTS video quality. Home telehealth can be divided into two major categories. The first category, often called *telehome care*, is the telehealth equivalent of home

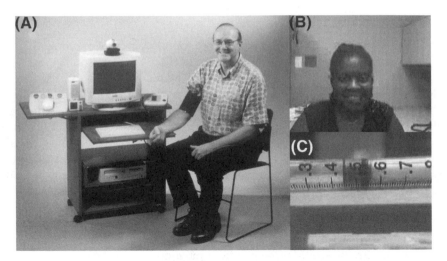

Figure 14.4. Plain old telephone service (POTS)–based home telehealth. Panel (A) shows the IDEATel Home Telemedicine Unit. Panel (B) shows a typical full-motion video image transmitted over POTS. Because of frame-to-frame compression, images of nonmoving objects can be of even higher quality. Many home telehealth systems are also equipped with close-up lenses to allow providers to monitor medications or wounds. Panel (C) shows a close-up video image of a syringe indicating that the patient has drawn up 44 units of insulin. The small markings are roughly 0.6 mm apart. (*Source*: Starren, 2003.)

nursing care. It involves frequent video visits between nurses and, often homebound, patients. With the advent of prospective payment for home nursing care, telehome care is viewed as a way for home care agencies to provide care at reduced costs. As with home nursing care, telehome care tends to have a finite duration, often focused on recovery from a specific disease or incident. Several studies have shown that telehome care can be especially valuable in the management of patients recently discharged from the hospital and can significantly reduce readmission rates.

The second category of home telehealth centers on the management of chronic diseases. Compared with telehome care, this type of home telehealth frequently involves a longer duration of care and less frequent interactions. Video interactions tend to focus on patient education, more than on evaluation of acute conditions. The largest such project to date is the Informatics for Diabetes Education and Telemedicine (IDEATel) project.(Starren *et al.*, 2002) Started in February 2000, the IDEATel project is a 4-year, $28 million demonstration project funded by the Center for Medicare and Medicaid Services (CMS, formerly the Health Care Financing Administration, or HCFA) involving 1665 diabetic Medicare patients in urban and rural New York State. In this randomized clinical trial, half of the patients received Home Telemedicine Units (HTU) (Figure 14.4), and half continued to receive standard care. At peak, 636 patients were actively using the HTU's. In addition to providing 2-way POTS-based video, the HTU allows patients to interact in multiple ways with their online charts. When patients measure blood pressure or fingerstick glucose with devices connected directly to the

HTU, the results are automatically encrypted and transmitted over the Internet into the Columbia Web-based Clinical Information System (WebCIS) at New York Presbyterian Hospital (NYPH) and to diabetes-specific case management software. Nurse case managers monitor patients by viewing the uploaded results, participating in bulletin board discussions, videoconferencing, and answering e-mailed questions daily. The case manager receives an alert when a patient's transmitted values exceed set thresholds. An important distinction between telehome care and disease management telehealth is that interaction in the former are initiated and managed by the nurse. Measurements, such as blood pressure, are typically collected during the video visit and uploaded as part of the video connection. For disease management, the HTU also needs to support remote monitoring, patient-initiated data uploads and, possibly, Web-based access to educational or disease management resources.

A project that reversed the conventional notion of home telehealth was the Baby CareLink project.(Gray *et al.*, 2000) This project focused on very low birth weight infants who typically spend months in neonatal intensive care units (NICU). The project used high-speed (ISDN) video connections to connect from the NICU into the parents' home. This allowed parents who could not visit the NICU regularly to maintain daily contact with their infants. The video connection was supplemented by communication and educational material on a project Web site.

14.3.6   *Telepresence*

Telepresence involves systems that allow clinicians to not only view remote situations, but also to act on them. The archetypal telepresence application is *telesurgery*. Although largely still experimental, a trans-Atlantic gall bladder operation was demonstrated in 2001. The military has funded considerable research in this area in the hope that surgical capabilities could be extended to the battlefield. Telepresence requires high bandwidth, low latency connections. Optimal telesurgery requires not only teleoperation of robotic surgical instruments, but also accurate force feedback. Such haptic feedback requires extremely low network latencies. Accurate millisecond **force feedback** has been historically limited to distances under 100 miles. The endoscopic gall bladder surgery mentioned above is an exception to this general principle because that specific procedure relied almost exclusively on visual information. It used a dedicated and custom configured 10Mb/s fiberoptic network with a 155 millisecond latency. Providing tactile feedback over large distances actually requires providing the surgeon with simulated feedback while awaiting transmission of the actual feedback data. Such simulation requires massive computing power and is an area of active research. Telesurgery also require extremely high reliability connections. Loss of a connection is an annoyance during a consultation; it can be fatal during a surgical procedure.

A novel form of telepresence gives clinicians the ability to not only to see, but also to walk around. A system called the Companion combined conventional video telehealth system with a remote controlled robot. (Figure 14.5). The system is geared toward nursing home and other long-term facilities. It allows clinicians to literally make remote video rounds. A frequent problem with telehealth systems is having the equipment where it is needed. With this system, the telehealth equipment is literally able take itself

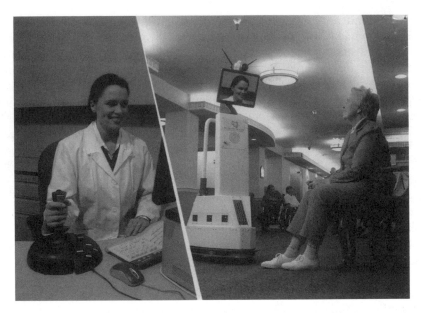

Figure 14.5. "Companion" telehealth robot. The remote clinician (left) is able to control the robot using a joystick. (*Source*: InTouch Health.)

to wherever it is needed. It is too early to tell whether this model of telepresence will be come widely adopted, but, like many earlier innovative systems, it raises many interesting questions.

14.4   Challenges and Future Directions

As CHI and telehealth evolve from being research novelties, to being the way health care is delivered, many challenges must be overcome. Some of these challenges arise because the one patient, one doctor model no longer applies. Basic questions of identity and trust become paramount. At the same time, the shifting focus from treating illness to managing health and wellness requires that clinicians know not only the history of the individuals they treat but also information about the social and environmental context within which those individuals reside. In the diabetes example, knowledge of the family history of risk factors diseases in an area and the appropriate diagnostic and interventional protocols aid the clinical staff in providing timely and appropriate treatment.

14.4.1   Quality of Information and Content Credentialing

The amount of information available to consumers is growing rapidly. This volume of information can be overwhelming. Therefore, consumers may need help in sifting through the mass of available resources. Furthermore, the quality of such information varies widely not only in terms of the extent to which it is accepted by the formal medical industry but also in its basic clinical or scientific accuracy. Therefore, a key issue in CHI lies in determining the quality and relevance of health information found on CD-ROMs or Web sites. **Credentialing** or certification by recognized bodies, such as respected healthcare providers or clinical professional associations, represents one approach to ensuring the quality of health information available to consumers. This approach bases its quality ratings on reviews and evaluations conducted by established knowledgeable sources. It has the advantage of delivering an imprimatur to a CD-ROM or Web site, which informs the user that the information presented meets a standard of quality. Credentialing is most useful when the credential itself is accompanied by a statement indicating the perspectives and biases of those granting it. Information presented by alternative therapies and other non-clinical groups is no less susceptible to bias than is information presented by professional sources.

Inherent in the credentialing approach are three disadvantages. First, the challenge to ensure that every information element—every link in a decision program or pathway in a Web site—is tested and evaluated fully exceeds the resources available to do so (see Chapter 20). In many cases, the credentialing approach rests on certification of the group or individuals providing the information rather than approval of the content itself. Second, the credentialing approach leaves control of the authority for healthcare information in the hands of traditional care providers, reflecting both the expertise and the biases of established medical sources. Third, credentialing alone is inherently contradictory to healthcare consumerism, which empowers the consumer to make choices consistent with her own worldview. A source's credential is just an additional piece of information that may be considered in making personal health decisions.

An approach to evaluating the quality and relevance of CHI resources that is consistent with a philosophy of patient participation is based on teaching patients and lay people how to evaluate CHI resources. Consumers with sufficient literacy and evaluation skills can locate CHI resources and determine these resources' relevance to their individual health concerns. Consumers can use six criteria to evaluate the quality and relevance of CHI resources to their situations (Table 14.3). Applying the criteria listed in Table 14.3 to the samples presented in Figures 14.2 and 14.3 illustrates the strengths and weaknesses of the various presentations.

14.4.2   Challenges to Using the Internet for Consumer Health and Telehealth Applications

Because of the public, shared nature of the Internet, its resources are widely accessible by citizens and healthcare organizations. This public nature also presents challenges to the security of data transmitted along the Internet. The openness of the Internet leaves the transmitted data vulnerable to interception and inappropriate access. In spite of significant improvements in the security of Web browsing several areas, including protection against viruses, authentication of individuals and the security of email, remain problematic.

Ensuring every citizen access to the Internet represents a second important challenge to the ability to use it for public health and consumer health purposes. Access

Table 14.3. Sample criteria for evaluating consumer health information resources on the Web.

Criteria for Evaluating Internet Health Information

- **Credibility:** includes the source, currency, relevance/utility, and editorial review process for the information.
- **Content:** must be accurate and complete, and an appropriate disclaimer provided.
- **Disclosure:** includes informing the user of the purpose of the site, as well as any profiling or collection of information associated with using the site.
- **Links:** evaluated according to selection, architecture, content, and back linkages.
- **Design:** encompasses accessibility, logical organization (navigability), and internal search capability.
- **Interactivity:** includes feedback mechanisms, means for exchange of information among users, and tailoring of information to individual needs.
- **Caveats:** clarification of whether site function is to market products and services or is a primary information content provider.

(*Source:* Criteria for Assessing the Quality of Health Information on the Internet Policy Paper. http://hitiweb.mitretek.org/docs/criteria.html [Accessed August 8, 2003].)

to the Internet presently requires computer equipment that may be out of reach for persons with marginal income levels. Majority-language literacy and the physical capability to type and read present additional requirements for effective use of the Internet. Preventing unequal access to healthcare resources delivered via the Internet will require that healthcare agencies work with other social service and educational groups to make available the technology necessary to capitalize on this electronic environment for health care.

As health care becomes increasingly reliant on internet-based telecommunications technology, the industry faces challenges in insuring the quality and integrity of many devices and network pathways. These challenges differ from previous medical device concerns, because the diversity and reliability of household equipment is under the control of the household, not the health care providers. There is an increased interdependency between the providers of health services, those who manage telecommunication infrastructure and the manufacturers of commercial electronics. Insuring effective use of telehealth for home and community based care requires that clinical services be supported by appropriate technical resources.

14.4.3   Licensure and Economics in Telehealth

Licensure is frequently cited as the single biggest problem facing telemedicine (meaning direct patient-provider interactions over telehealth). This is because medical licensure in the United States is state-based, while telemedicine frequently crosses state or national boundaries. The debate revolves around the questions of whether the patient "travels" through the wire to the clinician, or the clinician "travels" through the wire to the patient. Several states have passed legislation regulating the manner in which clinicians may deliver care remotely or across state lines. Some states have enacted "full licensure models" that require practitioners to hold a full, unrestricted license in each state where a patient resides. Many of these laws have been enacted specifically to restrict the out-of-state practice of telemedicine. To limit Web-based prescribing and other types of asynchronous interactions, several states have enacted or are considering regulations that would require a face-to-face encounter *before* any electronically delivered care would be allowed. In contrast, some states are adopting regulations to facilitate telehealth by exempting out-of-state physicians from in-state licensure requirements provided that electronic care is provided on an irregular or episodic basis. Still other models would include states agreeing to either a mutual exchange of privileges, or some type of "registration" system whereby clinicians from out of state would register their intent to practice via electronic medium.

At the same time, national organizations representing a variety of health care professions (including nurses, physicians and physical therapists) have proposed a variety of approaches to these issues. While the existing system is built around individual state licensure, groups that favor telemedicine have proposed various interstate or national licensure schemes. The Federated State Board of Medical Examiners has proposed that physicians holding a full, unrestricted license in any state should be able to obtain a limited telemedicine consultation license using a streamlined application process. The American Medical Association is fighting to maintain the current state-based licensure model while encouraging some reciprocity. The American Telemedicine Association supports the position that—since patients are "transported" via telemedicine to the clinician—the practitioner need only be licensed in his or her home state. The National Council of State Boards of Nursing has promoted an Interstate Nurse Licensure Compact whereby licensed nurses in a given state are granted multi-state licensure privileges and are authorized to practice in any other state that has adopted the compact. As of 2002, 19 states had enacted the compact.

The second factor limiting the growth of telehealth is reimbursement. Prior to the mid-1990s there was virtually no reimbursement for telehealth outside of teleradiology. At present Medicare routinely reimburses for synchronous video only for rural patients. Nineteen states provide coverage for synchronous video for Medicaid recipients. Five states also mandate payments by private insurers. A few insurers have begun experimenting with reimbursement for electronic messaging and online consultation, although this has been limited to specific pilot projects. Although teleradiology is often reimbursed, payments for other types of store-and-forward telehealth or remote monitoring remain rare. Few groups have even considered reimbursement for telehealth services that do not involve patient-provider interaction. An expert system could provide triage services; tailored on-line educational material, or customized dosage calculations. Such systems are expensive to build and maintain, but only services provided directly by humans are currently reimbursed by insurance. Determining whether, and how much, to pay for automatically delivered telehealth services will likely be a topic of debate for years to come.

14.4.4 Roles of Health Professionals in Consumer-Health Informatics

Healthcare professionals play three key roles in CHI. First, professionals serve as sources for content. Working in conjunction with software designers, clinicians provide relevant information on the nature and course of illnesses and expected treatment. To be most effective as content experts, clinicians should consider not only the physiological causes of disease but also the social and environmental causes and consequences of illnesses. Second, professionals provide important guidance in moderating public electronic discussion groups and responding to patients' electronic messages. This responsibility challenges clinicians to modify existing interventions to ensure proper interpretation and clear communication when interacting with patients electronically. Third, clinicians become information brokers and interpreters for patients, directing patients to relevant resources and using time in the clinical encounter to discuss observations, to help interpret the meaning and relevance of particular information, and to aid patients to translate information into behavioral changes in their lives.

14.4.5   Future Directions

Through the Internet and private intranets, a wealth of public health information and provider-oriented information resources are available to clinicians in practice. Workstations connected to secure or public networks facilitate access to public-health information that can help clinicians to diagnose disease and to plan treatment. The primary challenge of the future will be how to best match human professional resources with technology and patient self-management in a way that achieves optimal health outcomes.

From the provider perspective, clinicians now encounter patients who come to the appointment prepared with citations from Medline or comments pulled down from an electronic chat group. Working with enlightened patients demands new skills for clinicians and changes the nature of the clinical encounter. Time must be allotted to discuss the information that patients have read, to help patients interpret the relevance of the information to their own situations, and to refer patients to appropriate resources. Clinicians are challenged to become information brokers and to devise new ways to ensure that patients are prepared to participate in the clinical interaction.

Traditional medical care uses a workflow model based on synchronous interactions between clinicians and individual patients. The workflow model is also a sequential one in that the clinician may deal with multiple clinical problems or data trends but only within the context of treating a single patient at a time. Medical records, both paper and electronic, as well as billing and administrative systems all rely on this sequential paradigm, in which the fundamental unit is the "visit." Advances in telehealth are disrupting this paradigm. Devices have been developed that allow remote electronic monitoring of diabetes, hypertension, asthma, congestive heart failure (CHF), and chronic anticoagulation. As a result, clinicians will soon be inundated by hundreds of electronic results and messages every day. The clinician will no longer function in an assembly-line fashion, but will become more like a dispatcher or air-traffic controller, electronically monitoring many processes simultaneously. Clinicians will no longer ask simply, "How is Mrs. X today?" They will also ask the computer "Among my 2000 patients, which ones need my attention today?" Neither clinicians, nor EHRs, are prepared for this change.

Technology alone will not determine the extent to which these changes occur. A major social change is needed on the part of both clinicians and patients if they are to become full partners in health care. Patients have been socialized to assume a passive, dependent role in health care, presenting themselves for diagnosis and treatment with little planning. At the same time, clinicians have enjoyed the privilege of control, holding fast to the possession of expert knowledge and therefore direction to patients. In addition, not all clinicians and patients now or ever will have computers. Furthermore, there will always be many situations where use of technology is not feasible or is inappropriate due to the patient's physical or mental health status, level of literacy, comfort with technology, or access to information resources.

Contemporary pressures to share decision-making with patients and to assume a longitudinal perspective to health problems necessitate that we involve patients early and continuously in their own care. Further development of consumer-health technologies will allow patients to have access to the knowledge that they need for care and the analytical tools necessary to ensure that they know their own minds. Technology also will increasingly support the clinician in integrating patient preferences, scientific knowledge, and practical realities of care into efficient treatment plans. The availability of new and integrated public-health technologies will ensure the expansion of reference from the individual in the clinic, to her home, community, and life.

Perhaps the greatest long-term effect of the information/communications revolution will be the breaking down of role, geographic, and social barriers. Medicine is already benefiting greatly from this effect. Traditional "doctors and nurses" are collaborating with public health professionals; the sick and the well can easily access information that only 5 years ago was unavailable to the lay public (or did not exist at all); everyone with computer access can potentially communicate with experts around the world. We now have the tools to develop new healthcare models, wherein clinicians, community leaders, families, and friends collaborate to prevent illness, promote health, care for the sick, and develop and administer new therapies. This vision is no longer a pipe dream: We can do it today. The challenge will be to facilitate productive collaborations between patients, their caregivers, biomedical scientists, and information technology experts.

Suggested Readings

Brennan P. F. (1996). The future of clinical communication in an electronic environment. Holistic Nursing Practice, 11(1):97–104.
Dyadic interaction forms the core of the clinician–patient relationship. Modifications in familiar skills are needed to form those relationships in a healthcare environment that increasingly relies on technology to maintain contact with patients.

Gray, J. E., Safran, C., Davis, R. B., Pompilio-Weitzner, G., Stewart, J. E., Zaccagnini, L., & Pursley, D. (2000). Baby CareLink: using the internet and telemedicine to improve care for high-risk infants. *Pediatrics* **106**, 1318-1324.
Families of very-low-birthweight babies use interactive television and the world-wide-web to monitor the babies' progess while in hospital and to receive professional coaching and support once the babies return home.

Eysenbach G. Powell J. Kuss O. Sa ER. Empirical studies assessing the quality of health information for consumers on the world wide web: a systematic review. [Review] [122 refs] [Journal Article. Review. Review, Academic] *JAMA. 287(20):2691-700, 2002 May 22-29*
Appraising quality of health information on the web from the perspective of health professionals provides criteria that are also useful to lay people.

Bashshur, R.L., Mandil, S.H., Shannon, G.W. (eds). State-of-the-art telemedicine/telehealth symposium: An international perspective. (2002) Telemedicine Journal and e-Health. 8(1) (entire issue).
This special issue provides an excellent overview of many telehealth applications as diverse field.

Starren, J., Hripcsak, G., Sengupta, S., Abbruscato, C.R., Knudson, P., Weinstock, R.S. and Shea, S. (2002) Columbia University's Informatics for Diabetes Education and Telemedicine (IDEATel) project: Technical implementation. J Am Med Inform Assoc 9:25-36.
Providing telehealth care to over 600 patients spread across an entire state requires new thinking about the technology, systems and processes.

Questions for Discussion

1. Telehealth has evolved from systems designed primarily to support consultations between clinicians to systems that provide direct patient care. This has required changes in hardware, user interfaces, software, and processes. Discuss some of the changes that must be made when a system designed for use by health care professionals is modified to be used directly by patients.
2. Some people involved in CHI advocate that any publicly accessible health information be credentialed (reviewed and certified as accurate) by a professional body. Other people argue that credentialing is antithetical to the consumerist perspective. Assume and defend one of these perspectives.
3. Using CHI and telehealth systems, patients can now have interaction with a large number of health care providers, organizations and resources. As a result, coordination of care becomes increasingly difficult. Two solutions have been proposed. One is to develop better ways to transfer patient-related information among existing EHRs. The other is to give the give the patient control of the health record, either by giving them a smart card or placing the records on a central web site controlled by the patient. Assume and defend one of these perspectives.

15
Public Health Informatics and the Health Information Infrastructure

WILLIAM A. YASNOFF, PATRICK W. O'CARROLL, AND ANDREW FRIEDE

After reading this chapter you should know the answers to these questions:

- What are the three core functions of public health, and how do they help shape the different foci of public health and medicine?
- What are the current and potential effects of a) the genomics revolution; and b) 9/11 on public health informatics?
- What were the political, organizational, epidemiological, and technical issues that influenced the development of immunization registries? How do registries promote public health, and how can this model be expanded to other domains (be specific about those domains)? How might it fail in others? Why?
- What is the vision and purpose of the National Health Information Infrastructure? What kinds of impacts will it have, and in what time periods? Why don't we have one already? What are the political and technical barriers to its implementation? What are the characteristics of any evaluation process that would be used to judge demonstration projects?

15.1 Introduction

Biomedical informatics includes a wide range of disciplines that span information from the molecular to the population level. This chapter is primarily focused on the population level, which includes informatics applied to public health and to the entire health care system (**health information infrastructure**). Population-level informatics has its own special problems, issues, and considerations. Creating information systems at the population level has always been very difficult because of the large number of data elements and individuals that must be included, as well as the need to address data and information issues that affect health in the aggregate (e.g., environmental determinants of health). With faster and cheaper hardware and radically improved software tools, it has become financially and technically feasible to create information systems that will provide the information about individuals and populations necessary for optimized decision-making in medical care and public health. However, much work remains to fully achieve this goal.

This chapter deals with public health informatics primarily as it relates to the medical care of populations. However, it should be emphasized that the domain of public health informatics is not limited to the medical care environment. For example, information technology is being applied to automatically detect threats to health from the food supply, water systems, and even driving conditions (such as obstacles on the roadway beyond the reach of visible headlight beams), and to assist in man-made or natural disaster management. Monitoring the environment for health risks due to biological, chemical, and radiation exposures (natural and made-made) is of increasing concern to protecting the public's health. For example, systems are now being developed and deployed to rapidly detect airborne bioterror agents. Although they do not directly relate to medical care, these applications designed to protect human health should properly be considered within the domain of public health informatics.

15.2   Public Health Informatics

Public health informatics has been defined as the systematic application of information and computer science and technology to public health practice, research, and learning (Friede et al., 1995; Yasnoff et al., 2000). Public health informatics is distinguished by its focus on populations (versus the individual), its orientation to prevention (rather than diagnosis and treatment), and its governmental context, because public health nearly always involves government agencies. It is a large and complex area that is the focus of another entire textbook in this series (O'Carroll et al., 2003).

The differences between public health informatics and other informatics specialty areas relate to the contrast between public health and medical care itself (Friede & O'Carroll, 1998; Yasnoff et al., 2000). Public health focuses on the health of the community, as opposed to that of the individual patient. In the medical care system, individuals with specific diseases or conditions are the primary concern. In public health, issues related to the community as the patient may require "treatment" such as disclosure of the disease status of an individual to prevent further spread of illness or even quarantining some individuals to protect others. Environmental factors, especially ones that that affect the health of populations over the long term (e.g. air quality), are also a special focus of the public health domain. Public health places a large emphasis on the prevention of disease and injury versus intervention after the problem has already occurred. To the extent that traditional medical care involves prevention, its focus is primarily on delivery of preventive services to individual patients.

Public health actions are not limited to the clinical encounter. In public health, the nature of a given intervention is not predetermined by professional discipline, but rather by the cost, expediency, and social acceptability of intervening at any potentially effective point in the series of events leading to disease, injury, or disability. Public health interventions have included (for example) wastewater treatment and solid waste disposal systems, housing and building codes, fluoridation of municipal water supplies, removal of lead from gasoline, and smoke alarms. Contrast this with the modern healthcare system, which generally accomplishes its mission through medical and surgical encounters.

Public health also generally operates directly or indirectly through government agencies that must be responsive to legislative, regulatory, and policy directives, carefully balance competing priorities, and openly disclose their activities. In addition, certain public health actions involve authority for specific (sometimes coercive) measures to protect the community in an emergency. Examples include closing a contaminated pond or a restaurant that fails inspection.

15.2.1   What Is Public Health?

Public health itself is a complex and varied discipline, encompassing a wide variety of specialty areas. The broad scope and diversity of activities makes it difficult to readily and concisely define and explain public health. One useful conceptualization defines public health in terms of its three core functions of assessment, policy development, and assurance (Institute of Medicine (IOM), 1988). Assessment involves monitoring and tracking the health status of populations including identifying and controlling disease outbreaks and epidemics. By relating health status to a variety of demographic, geographic, environmental, and other factors, it is possible to develop and test hypotheses about the etiology, transmission, and risk factors that contribute to health problems.

Policy development is the second core function of public health. It utilizes the results of assessment activities and etiologic research in concert with local values and culture (as reflected via citizen input) to recommend interventions and public policies that improve health status. For example, the relationship between fatalities in automobile accidents and ejection of passengers from vehicles led to recommendations, and eventually laws, mandating seat belt use. Although, at present, there is intense interest in the promise of enhanced public health surveillance using information technology to provide near-real-time access to clinical data stores, it is in the area of policy development that information technology may have its greatest impact.

Because public health is primarily a governmental activity, it depends upon and is informed by the consent of those governed. Policy development in public health is (or should be) based on science, but it is also derived from the values, beliefs, and opinions of the society it serves. Today, e-mail, Web sites, on-line discussion groups, and instant messaging are the most heavily used Internet applications. In comparison, only a minuscule fraction of the populace ever concerns itself with surveillance data. Public health officials who wish to promote certain health behaviors, or to promulgate regulations concerning, say, fluoridated water or bicycle helmets, would do well to tap into the online marketplace of ideas—both to understand the opinions and beliefs of their citizenry, and to (hopefully) influence them.

The third core function of public health is assurance, which refers to the duty of public health agencies to assure their constituents that services necessary to achieve agreed upon goals are provided. Note that the services in question (including medical care) might be provided directly by the public health agency or by encouraging or requiring (through regulation) other public or private entities to provide the services. For example, in some communities, local public health agencies provide a great deal of direct clinical care. In Multnomah County, Oregon, for example, the local public health agency currently provides health care services in seven primary care clinics, three county jails, thirteen schools, four community sites and in people's homes. In other communities (e.g., Pierce County, Washington), local public health agencies have sought to minimize or eliminate direct clinical care services, instead working with and relying on community partners to provide such care. Though there is great variation across juris-dictions, the fundamental assurance function is unchanged: to assure that all members of the community have adequate access to needed services. The assurance function is not limited to access to clinical care. Rather, it refers to assurance of the conditions that allow people to be healthy and free from avoidable threats to health—which includes access to clean water, a safe food supply, well-lighted streets, responsive and effective public safety entities, and so forth.

This "core functions" framework has proven to be highly useful in clarifying the fun-damental, over-arching responsibilities of public health. But if the core functions describe what public health is *for*, a more detailed and grounded delineation was needed to describe what public health agencies *do*. To meet this need, a set of ten essential pub-lic health services (Table 15.1) was developed through national and state level delibera-tions of public health providers and consumers (Department of Health and Human Services (DHHS), 1994). It is through these ten services that public health carries out its mission to assure the conditions in which people can be healthy.

The core function of assessment, and several of the essential public health services rely heavily on public health **surveillance**, one of the oldest systematic activities of the public health sector. Surveillance in the public health context refers to the ongoing col-lection, analysis, interpretation, and dissemination of data on health conditions (e.g., breast cancer) and threats to health (e.g., smoking prevalence). Surveillance data repre-sent one of the fundamental means by which priorities for public health action are set. Surveillance data are useful not only in the short term (e.g., in surveillance for acute infectious diseases such as influenza, measles, and HIV/AIDS), but also in the longer term, e.g., in determining leading causes of premature death, injury, or disability. In either case, what distinguishes surveillance is that the data are collected for the purposes of action—either to guide a public health response (e.g., an outbreak investigation, or mitigation of a threat to a food or water source) or to help direct public health policy. A recent example of the latter is the surveillance data showing the dramatic rise in obe-sity in the United States. A tremendous amount of energy and public focus has been brought to bear on this problem—including a major DHHS program, the *Healthier US* initiative—driven largely by compelling surveillance data.

Table 15.1. Ten essential services of public health (DHHS, 1994).

1. Monitor the health status of individuals in the community to identify community health problems
2. Diagnose and investigate community health problems and community health hazards
3. Inform, educate, and empower the community with respect to health issues
4. Mobilize community partnerships in identifying and solving community health problems
5. Develop policies and plans that support individual and community efforts to improve health
6. Enforce laws and rules that protect the public health and ensure safety in accordance with those laws and rules
7. Link individuals who have a need for community and personal health services to appropriate commu-nity and private providers
8. Ensure a competent workforce for the provision of essential public health services
9. Research new insights and innovate solutions to community health problems
10. Evaluate the effectiveness, accessibility, and quality of personal and population-based health services in a community

15.2.2   *Information Systems in Public Health*

The fundamental science of public health is **epidemiology**, which is the study of the prevalence and determinants of disability and disease in *populations*. Hence, most public health information systems have focused on information about aggregate populations. Almost all medical information systems focus almost exclusively on identifying information about *individuals*. For example, almost any clinical laboratory system can quickly find Jane Smith's culture results. What public health practitioners want to know is the time trend of antibiotic resistance for the *population* that the clinic serves, or the trend for the population that the clinic actually covers.

Most health care professionals are surprised to learn that there is no uniform national routine reporting – never mind information system – for most diseases, disabilities, risk factors, or prevention activities in the United States. In contrast, France, Great Britain, Denmark, Norway and Sweden have comprehensive systems in selected areas, such as occupational injuries, infectious diseases, and cancer; no country, however, has complete reporting for every problem. In fact, it is only births, deaths, and – to a lesser extent – fetal deaths that are uniformly and relatively completely reported in the United States by the National Vital Statistics System, operated by the states and the Centers for Disease Control and Prevention (CDC). If you have an angioplasty and survive, nobody at the state or federal level necessarily knows.

Public health information systems have been designed with special features. For example, they are optimized for retrieval from very large (multi-million) record databases, and to be able to quickly cross-tabulate, study secular trends, and look for patterns. The use of personal identifiers in these systems is very limited, and their use is generally restricted to linking data from different sources (e.g., data from a state laboratory and a disease surveillance form). A few examples of these kinds of population-focused systems include CDC systems such as the HIV/AIDS reporting system, which collects millions of observations concerning people infected with the Human Immunodeficiency Virus (HIV) and those diagnosed with Acquired Immunodeficiency Syndrome (AIDS) and is used to conduct dozens of studies (and which does not collect personal identifiers; individuals are tracked by pseudo-identifiers); the National Notifiable Disease Surveillance System, which state epidemiologists use to report some 60 diseases (the exact number varies as conditions wax and wane) every week to the CDC (and which makes up the center tables in the Morbidity and Mortality Weekly Report [MMWR]). The CDC WONDER system (Friede et al., 1996), which contains tens of millions of observations drawn from some 30 databases, explicitly blanks cells with fewer than three to five observations (depending on the dataset), specifically to prevent individuals with unusual characteristics from being identified.

If there is no national individual reporting, how are estimates obtained for, say, the trends in teenage smoking or in the incidence of breast cancer? How are epidemics found? Data from periodic surveys and special studies, surveillance systems, and disease registries are handled by numerous stand-alone information systems. These systems – usually managed by state health departments and federal health agencies (largely the CDC) or their agents – provide periodic estimates of the incidence and prevalence of diseases and of certain risk factors (for example, smoking and obesity); however, because the data are from population samples, it is usually impossible to obtain estimates at a level of geographic detail finer than a region or state. Moreover, many of the behavioral indices are patient self-reported (although extensive validation studies have shown that they are good for trends and sometimes are more reliable than are data obtained from clinical systems). In the case of special surveys, such as CDC's National Health and Nutrition Examination Survey (NHANES), there is primary data entry into a CDC system. The data are complete, but the survey costs many millions of dollars, is done only every few years, and it takes years for the data to be made available.

There are also disease registries that track – often completely – the incidence of certain conditions, especially cancers, birth defects, and conditions associated with environmental contamination. They tend to focus on one topic or to cover certain diseases for specific time periods. The CDC maintains dozens of surveillance systems that attempt to track completely the incidence of many conditions, including lead poisoning, injuries and deaths in the workplace, and birth defects. (Some of these systems use samples or cover only certain states or cities). As discussed above, there is also a list of about 60 notifiable diseases (revised every year) that the state epidemiologists and the CDC have determined are of national significance and warrant routine, complete reporting; however, it is up to providers to report the data, and reporting is still often done by telephone or mail, so the data are incomplete. Finally, some states do collect hospital discharge summaries, but now that more care is being delivered in the ambulatory setting, these data capture only a small fraction of medical care. They are also notoriously difficult to access.

What all these systems have in common is that they rely on special data collection. It is rare that they are seamlessly linked to ongoing clinical information systems. Even clinical data such as hospital infections is reentered. Why? All these systems grew up at the same time that information systems were being put in hospitals and clinics. Hence, there is duplicate data entry, which can result in the data being shallow, delayed, and subject to input error and recall bias. Furthermore, the systems themselves are often unpopular with state agencies and health care providers precisely because they require duplicate data entry (a child with lead poisoning and salmonella needs to be entered in two different CDC systems). The National Electronic Disease Surveillance System (NEDSS) is a major CDC initiative that addresses this issue by promoting the use of data and information system standards to advance the development of efficient, integrated, and interoperable surveillance systems at federal, state and local levels (see www.cdc.gov/nedss). This activity is designed to facilitate the electronic transfer of appropriate information from clinical information systems in the health care industry to public health departments, reduce provider burden in the provision of information, and enhance both the timeliness and quality of information provided.

Now that historical and epidemiological forces are making the world smaller and causing lines between medicine and public health to blur, systems will need to be multifunctional, and clinical and public health systems will, of necessity, coalesce. What is needed are systems that can tell us about individuals *and* the world in which those individuals live. To fill that need, public health and clinical informaticians will need to work closely together to build the tools to study and control new and emerging threats such as bioterror, HIV/AIDS, SARS and its congeners, and the environmental effects of the shrinking ozone layer and greenhouse gases. It can be done. For example, in the late 1990's, Columbia Presbyterian Medical Center and the New York City Department of Health collaborated on the development of a tuberculosis registry for northern Manhattan, and the Emory University System of Health Care and the Georgia Department of Public Health built a similar system for tuberculosis monitoring and treatment in Atlanta. It is not by chance that these two cities each developed tuberculosis systems; rather, tuberculosis is a perfect example of what was once a public health problem (that affected primarily the poor and underserved) coming into the mainstream population as a result of an emerging infectious disease (AIDS), immigration, increased international travel, multidrug resistance, and our growing prison population. Hence, the changing ecology of disease, coupled with revolutionary changes in how health care is managed and paid for, will necessitate information systems that serve both individual medical and public health needs.

15.3   Immunization Registries: A Public Health Informatics Example

Immunization registries are confidential, population based, computerized information systems that contain data about children and vaccinations (National Vaccine Advisory Committee, 1999). They represent a good example for illustrating the principles of public health informatics. In addition to their orientation to prevention, they can only function properly through continuing interaction with the health care system. They also must exist in a governmental context because there is little incentive (and significant organizational barriers) for the private sector to maintain such registries. Although immunization registries are among the largest and most complex public health information systems, the successful implementations show conclusively that it is possible to overcome the challenging informatics problems they present.

15.3.1   History and Background of Immunization Registries

Childhood immunizations have been among the most successful public health interventions, resulting in the near elimination of nine vaccine preventable diseases that historically extracted a major toll in terms of both morbidity and mortality (IOM, 2000a). The need for immunization registries stems from the challenge of assuring complete immunization protection for the approximately 11,000 children born each day in the United States in the context of three complicating factors: the scattering of immunization records among multiple providers; an immunization schedule that has become increasingly complex as the number of vaccines has grown; and the conundrum that the very success of mass immunization has reduced the incidence of disease, lulling parents and providers into a sense of complacency.

The 1989-91 U.S. measles outbreak, which resulted in 55,000 cases and 123 preventable deaths (Atkinson et al., 1992), helped stimulate the public health community to expand the limited earlier efforts to develop immunization registries. Because CDC was proscribed by Congress from creating a single national immunization registry (due to privacy concerns), the Robert Wood Johnson Foundation, in cooperation with several other private foundations, established the All Kids Count (AKC) program that awarded funds to 24 states and communities in 1992 to assist in the development of immunization registries. AKC funded the best projects through a competitive process, recruited a talented staff to provide technical assistance, and made deliberate efforts to ensure sharing of the lessons learned, such as regular, highly interactive meetings of the grantees. Subsequent funding of 13 states by CDC and the Woodruff Foundation via the Information Network for Public Health Officials (INPHO) project (Baker et al., 1995) was greatly augmented by a presidential commitment to immunization registries announced in 1997 (White House, 1997). This resulted in every state's involvement in registry development.

Immunization registries must be able to exchange information to ensure that children who relocate receive needed immunizations. To accomplish this, standards were needed to prevent the development of multiple, incompatible immunization transmission formats. Beginning in 1995, CDC worked closely with the Health Level 7 standards development organization (see Chapter 7) to define HL7 messages and an implementation guide for immunization record transactions. The initial data standard was approved by HL7 in 1997 and an updated implementation guide was developed in 1999. CDC continues its efforts to encourage the standards-based exchange of immunization records among registries.

As more experience accumulated, AKC and CDC collaborated to develop an immunization registry development guide (CDC, 1997) that captured the hard-won lessons developed by dozens of projects over many years. By 2000, a consensus on the 12 needed functions of immunization registries had emerged (Table 15.2), codifying years of experience in refining system requirements. CDC also established a measurement system for tracking progress that periodically assesses the percentage of immunization registries that have operationalized each of the 12 functions (Figure 15.1). Further formalizing the public policy commitment to the development of immunization

Table 15.2. Twelve functional standards for immunization registries (CDC, 2002).

1. Electronically store data regarding all National Vaccine Advisory Committee-approved core data elements
2. Establish a registry record within 6 weeks of birth for each child born in the catchment area
3. Enable access to vaccine information from the registry at the time of the encounter
4. Receive and process vaccine information within 1 month of vaccine administration
5. Protect the confidentiality of medical information
6. Protect the security of medical information
7. Exchange vaccination records by using Health Level 7 standards
8. Automatically determine the immunization(s) needed when a person is seen by the health care provider for a scheduled vaccination
9. Automatically identify persons due or late for vaccinations to enable the production of reminder and recall notices
10. Automatically produce vaccine coverage reports by providers, age groups, and geographic areas
11. Produce authorized immunization records
12. Promote accuracy and completeness of registry data

Figure 15.1. Measurement system for tracking progress of immunization registries.

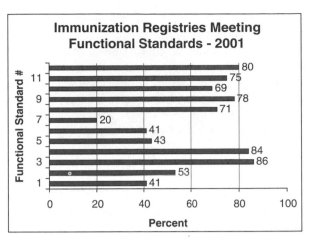

registries, the national Healthy People 2010 objectives include the goal of having 95% of all U.S. children covered by fully functioning immunization registries (DHHS, 2000).

15.3.2 Key Informatics Issues in Immunization Registries

The development and implementation of immunization registries presents challenging informatics issues in at least four areas: 1) interdisciplinary communication; 2) organizational and collaborative issues; 3) funding and sustainability; and 4) system design. While the specific manifestations of these issues are unique to immunization registries, these four areas represent the typical domains that must be addressed and overcome in public health informatics projects.

15.3.2.1 Interdisciplinary Communications

Interdisciplinary communications is a key challenge in any biomedical informatics project—it is certainly not specific to public health informatics. To be useful, a public health information system must accurately represent and enable the complex concepts and processes that underlie the specific business functions required. Information systems represent a highly abstract and complex set of data, processes, and interactions. This complexity needs to be discussed, specified, and understood in detail by a variety of personnel with little or no expertise in the terminology and concepts of information technology. Therefore, successful immunization registry implementation requires clear communication among public health specialists, immunization specialists, providers, IT specialists, and related disciplines, an effort complicated by the lack of a shared vocabulary and differences in the usage of common terms from the various domains.

Added to these potential communication problems are the anxieties and concerns inherent in the development of any new information system. Change is an inevitable part of such a project—and change is uncomfortable for everyone involved. Furthermore, information is power—and power shifts are unavoidable with the implementation of information systems. In this context, tensions and anxieties can further degrade communications.

To deal with the communications challenges, particularly between IT and public health specialists, it is essential to identify an interlocutor who has familiarity with both information technology and public health. The interlocutor should spend sufficient time in the user environment to develop a deep understanding of the information processing context of both the current and proposed systems. It is also important for individuals from all the disciplines related to the project to have representation in the decision-making processes.

15.3.2.2   Organizational and Collaborative Issues

The organizational and collaborative issues involved in developing immunization registries are daunting because of the large number and wide variety of partners. Both public and private sector providers and other organizations are likely participants. For the providers, particularly in the private sector, immunization is just one of many concerns. However, it is essential to mobilize private providers to submit immunization information to the registry. In addition to communicating regularly to this group about the goals, plans, and progress of the registry, an invaluable tool to enlist their participation is a technical solution that minimizes their time and expense for registry data entry, while maximizing the benefit in terms of improved information about their patients. It is critical to recognize the constraints of the private provider environment, where income is generated mostly from "piecework" and time is the most precious resource.

Governance issues are also critical to success. All the key stakeholders need to be represented in the decision-making processes, guided by a mutually acceptable governance mechanism. Large information system projects involving multiple partners — such as immunization registries — often require multiple committees to ensure that all parties have a voice in the development process. In particular, all decisions that materially affect a stakeholder should be made in a setting that includes their representation.

Legislative and regulatory issues must be considered in an informatics context because they impact the likelihood of success of projects. With respect to immunization registries, the specific issues of confidentiality, data submission, and liability are critical. The specific policies with respect to confidentiality must be defined to allow access to those who need it while denying access to others. Regulatory or legislative efforts in this domain must also operate within the context of the federal Health Insurance Portability and Accountability Act (HIPAA) that sets national minimum privacy requirements for personal health information. Some jurisdictions have enacted regulations requiring providers to submit immunization data to the registry. The effectiveness of such actions on the cooperation of providers must be carefully evaluated. Liability of the participating providers and of the registry operation itself may also require legislative and/or regulatory clarification.

15.3.2.3   Funding and Sustainability

Funding and sustainability are continuing challenges for all immunization registries. In particular, without assurances of ongoing operational funding, it will be difficult to secure the commitments needed for the development work. Naturally, an important tool for securing funding is development of a business case that shows the anticipated costs and benefits of the registry. While a substantial amount of information now exists about costs and benefits of immunization registries (Horne et al., 2000), many of the registries that are currently operational had to develop their business cases prior to the availability of good quantitative data. Specific benefits associated with registries include preventing duplicative immunizations, eliminating the necessity to review the vaccination records for school and day care entry, and efficiencies in provider offices from the immediate availability of complete immunization history information and patient-specific vaccine schedule recommendations. The careful assessment of costs and benefits of specific immunization registry functions may also be helpful in prioritizing system requirements. As with all information systems, it is important to distinguish "needs" (those things people will pay for) from "wants" (those things people would like to have but are not willing to spend money on) (Rubin, 2003). Information system "needs" are typically supported by a strong business case, whereas "wants" often are not.

15.3.2.4   System Design

System design is also an important factor in the success of immunization registries. Difficult design issues include data acquisition, database organization, identification and matching of children, generating immunization recommendations, and access to data, particularly for providers. Acquiring immunization data is perhaps the most challenging system design issue. Within the context of busy pediatric practices (where the majority of childhood immunizations are given), the data acquisition strategy must of necessity be extremely efficient. Ideally, information about immunizations would be extracted from existing electronic medical records or from streams of electronic billing data; either strategy should result in no additional work for participating providers. Unfortunately neither of these options is typically available. Electronic medical records are currently implemented only in roughly 10-15% of physician practices. While the use of billing records is appealing, it is often difficult to get such records on a timely basis without impinging on their primary function—namely, to generate revenue for the practice. Also, data quality, particularly with respect to duplicate records, is often a problem with billing information. A variety of approaches have been used to address this issue, including various forms of direct data entry as well as the use of bar codes (Yasnoff, 2003).

Database design also must be carefully considered. Once the desired functions of an immunization registry are known, the database design must allow efficient implementation of these capabilities. The operational needs for data access and data entry, as well as producing individual assessments of immunization status, often require different approaches to design compared to requirements for population-based immunization assessment, management of vaccine inventory, and generating recall and reminder notices. One particularly important database design decision for immunization registries is whether to represent immunization information by vaccine or by antigen. Vaccine-based representations map each available preparation, including those with multiple antigens, into its own specific data element. Antigen-based representations translate multi-component vaccines into their individual antigens prior to storage. In some cases, it may be desirable to represent the immunization information both ways. Specific consideration of required response times for specific queries must also be factored into key design decisions.

Identification and matching of individuals within immunization registries is another critical issue. Because it is relatively common for a child to receive immunizations from multiple providers, any system must be able to match information from multiple sources to complete an immunization record. In the absence of a national unique patient identifier, most immunization registries will assign an arbitrary number to each child. Of course, provisions must be made for the situation where this identification number is lost or unavailable. This requires a matching algorithm, which utilizes multiple items of demographic information to assess the probability that two records are really data from the same person. Development of such algorithms and optimization of their parameters has been the subject of active investigation in the context of immunization registries, particularly with respect to deduplication (Miller et al., 2001).

Another critical design issue is generating vaccine recommendations from a child's prior immunization history, based on guidance from the CDC's Advisory Committee on Immunization Practices (ACIP). As more childhood vaccines have become available, both individually and in various combinations, the immunization schedule has become increasingly complex, especially if any delays occur in receiving doses, a child has a contraindication, or local issues require special consideration. The language used in the written guidelines is sometimes incomplete, not covering every potential situation. In addition, there is often some ambiguity with respect to definitions, e.g., for ages and intervals, making implementation of decision support systems problematic. Considering that the recommendations are updated relatively frequently, sometimes several times each year, maintaining software that produces accurate immunization recommendations is a continuing challenge. Accordingly, the implementation, testing, and maintenance of decision support systems to produce vaccine recommendations has been the subject of extensive study (Yasnoff & Miller, 2003).

Finally, easy access to the information in an immunization registry is essential. While this may initially seem to be a relatively simple problem, it is complicated by private providers' lack of high-speed connectivity. Even if a provider office has the capability for Internet access, for example, it may not be immediately available at all times, particularly in the examination room. Immunization registries have developed alternative data access methods such as fax-back and telephone query to address this problem. Since the primary benefit of the registry to providers is manifest in rapid access to the data, this issue must be addressed. Ready access to immunization registry information is a powerful incentive to providers for entering the data from their practice.

15.4   Health Information Infrastructure

In the United States, the first major report calling for a Health Information Infrastructure was issued by the Institute of Medicine of the National Academy of Sciences in 1991 (IOM, 1991). This report, "The Computer-Based Patient Record," was the first in a series of national expert panel reports recommending transformation of the health care system from reliance on paper to electronic information management. In response to the IOM report, the Computer-based Patient Record Institute (CPRI), a private not-for-profit corporation, was formed for the purpose of facilitating the transition to computer-based records. A number of community health information networks (CHINs) were established around the country in an effort to coalesce the multiple community stakeholders in common efforts towards electronic information exchange. The Institute of Medicine updated its original report in 1997 (IOM, 1997), again emphasizing the urgency to apply information technology to the information intensive field of health care.

However, most of the community health information networks were not successful. Perhaps the primary reason for this was that the standards and technology were not yet ready for cost-effective community-based electronic health information exchange. Another problem was the focus on availability of aggregated health information for secondary users (e.g., policy development), rather than individual information for the direct provision of patient care. Also, there was neither a sense of extreme urgency nor were there substantial funds available to pursue these endeavors. However, at least one community, Indianapolis, continued to move forward throughout this period and has now emerged as an a national example of the application of information technology to health care both in individual health care settings and throughout the community.

The year 2000 brought widespread attention to this issue with the IOM report "To Err is Human" (IOM, 2000b). In this landmark study, the IOM documented the accumulating evidence of the high error rate in the medical care system, including an estimated 44,000 to 98,000 preventable deaths each year in hospitals alone. This report has proven to be a milestone in terms of public awareness of the consequences of paper-based information management in health care. Along with the follow-up report, "Crossing the Quality Chasm" (IOM, 2001), the systematic inability of the health care system to operate at high degree of reliability has been thoroughly elucidated. The report clearly placed the blame on the system, not the dedicated health care professionals who work in an environment without effective tools to promote quality and minimize errors.

Several additional national expert panel reports have emphasized the IOM findings. In 2001, the President's Information Technology Advisory Committee (PITAC) issued a report entitled "Transforming Health Care Through Information Technology" (PITAC, 2001). That same year, the Computer Science and Telecommunications Board of the National Research Council (NRC) released "Networking Health: Prescriptions for the Internet" (NRC, 2001) which emphasized the potential for using the Internet to improve electronic exchange of health care information. Finally, the National Committee on Vital and Health Statistics (NCVHS) outlined the vision and strategy for building a National Health Information Infrastructure (NHII) in its report, "Information for Health" (NCVHS, 2001). NCVHS, a statutory advisory body to DHHS, indicated that federal government leadership was needed to facilitate further development of an NHII.

On top of this of bevy of national expert panel reports, there has been continuing attention in both scientific and lay publications to cost, quality, and error issues in the health care system. The anthrax attacks of late 2001 further sensitized the nation to the need for greatly improved disease detection and emergency medical response capabilities. What has followed has been the largest-ever investment in public health information infrastructure in the history of the United States. Some local areas, such as Indianapolis and Pittsburgh, have begun to actively utilize electronic information from the health care system for early detection of bioterrorism and other disease outbreaks. In 2003, separate large national conferences were devoted to both the CDC's Public Health Information Network (PHIN) (CDC, 2003) and the DHHS NHII initiative (DHHS, 2003 Yasnoff et al., 2004).

While the discussion here has focused on the development of NHII in the United States, many other countries are involved in similar activities and in fact have progressed further along this road. Canada, Australia, and a number of European nations have devoted considerable time and resources to their own national health information infrastructures. The United Kingdom, for example, has announced its intention to allocate several billion pounds over the next few years to substantially upgrade its health information system capabilities. It should be noted, however, that all of these nations have centralized, government-controlled health care systems. This organizational difference from the multifaceted, mainly private health care system in the U.S. results in a somewhat different set of issues and problems. Hopefully, the lessons learned from health information infrastructure development activities across the globe can be effectively shared to ease the difficulties of everyone who is working toward these important goals.

15.4.1   Vision and Benefits of NHII

The vision of the National Health Information Infrastructure is anytime, anywhere health care information at the point of care. The intent to is to create a distributed system, not a centralized national database. Patient information would be collected and stored at each care site. When a patient presented for care, the various existing electronic records would be located, collected, integrated, and immediately delivered to allow the provider to have complete and current information upon which to base clinical decisions. In addition, clinical decision support (see Chapter 20) would be integrated with information delivery. In this way, clinicians could receive reminders of the most recent clinical guidelines and research results during the patient care process, thereby avoiding the need for superhuman memory capabilities to assure the effective practice of medicine.

The potential benefits of NHII are both numerous and substantial. Perhaps most important are error reduction and improved quality of care. Numerous studies have shown that the complexity of present-day medical care results in very frequent errors of both omission and commission. This problem was clearly articulated at the 2001 meeting of the Institute of Medicine: "Current practice depends upon the clinical decision making capacity and reliability of autonomous individual practitioners, for classes of problems that routinely exceed the bounds of unaided human cognition" (Masys, 2001). Electronic health information systems can contribute significantly to improving this problem by reminding practitioners about recommended actions at the point of care. This can include both notifications of actions that may have been missed, as well as warnings about planned treatments or procedures that may be harmful or unnecessary. Literally dozens of research studies have shown that such reminders improve safety and reduce costs (Kass, 2001; Bates, 2000). In one such study (Bates et al., 1998), medication errors were reduced by 55%.

A more recent study by the Rand Corporation showed that only 55 % of U.S. adults were receiving recommended care (McGlynn et al., 2003). The same techniques used to reduce medical errors with electronic health information systems also contribute substantially to ensuring that recommended care is provided. This is becoming increasingly important as the population ages and the prevalence of chronic disease increases.

Guidelines and reminders also can improve the effectiveness of dissemination of new research results. At present, widespread application of a new research in the clinical setting takes an average of 17 years (Balas & Boren, 2000). Patient-specific reminders delivered at the point of care highlighting important new research results could substantially increase the adoption rate.

Another important contribution of NHII to the research domain is improving the efficiency of clinical trials. At present, most clinical trials require creation of a unique information infrastructure to insure protocol compliance and collect essential research data. With NHII, where every practitioner would have access to a fully functional electronic health record, clinical trials could routinely be implemented through the dissemination of guidelines that specify the research protocol. Data collection would occur automatically in the course of administering the protocol, reducing time and costs. In addition, there would be substantial value in analyzing deidentified aggregate data from routine patient care to assess the outcomes of various treatments, and monitor the health of the population.

Another critical function for NHII is early detection of patterns of disease, particularly early detection of possible bioterrorism. Our current system of disease surveillance, which depends on alert clinicians diagnosing and reporting unusual conditions, is both slow and potentially unreliable. Most disease reporting still occurs using the Postal Service, and the information is relayed from local to state to national public health authorities. Even when fax or phone is employed, the system still depends on the ability of clinicians to accurately recognize rare and unusual diseases. Even assuming such capabilities, individual clinicians cannot discern patterns of disease beyond their sphere of practice. These problems are illustrated by the seven unreported cases of cutaneous anthrax in the New York City area two weeks before the so-called "index" case in Florida in the Fall of 2001 (Lipton & Johnson, 2001). Since all the patients were seen by different clinicians, the pattern could not have been evident to any of them even if the diagnosis had immediately been made in every case. Wagner et al have elucidated nine categories of requirements for surveillance systems for potential bioterrorism outbreaks—several categories must have immediate electronic reporting to insure early detection (Wagner et al., 2003).

NHII would allow immediate electronic reporting of both relevant clinical events and laboratory results to public health. Not only would this be an invaluable aid in early detection of bioterrorism, it would also serve to improve the detection of the much more frequent naturally occurring disease outbreaks. In fact, early results from a number of electronic reporting demonstration projects show that disease outbreaks can routinely be detected sooner than was ever possible using the current system (Overhage et al., 2001). While early detection has been shown to be a key factor in reducing morbidity and mortality from bioterrorism (Kaufmann et al., 1997), it will also be extremely helpful in reducing the negative consequences from other disease outbreaks. This aspect of NHII is discussed in more detail in section 15.5.

Finally, NHII can substantially reduce health-care costs. The inefficiencies and duplication in our present paper-based health care system are enormous. Recent study showed that the anticipated nationwide savings from implementing advanced computerized provider order entry (CPOE) systems in the outpatient environment would be $44 billion per year (Johnston et al., 2003), while a related study (Walker et al., 2004) estimated $78 billion more is savings from health information exchange (for a total of $112 billion per year). Substantial additional savings are possible in the inpatient setting—numerous hospitals have reported large net savings from implementation of electronic health records. Another example, electronic prescribing, would not only reduce medication errors from transcription, but also drastically decrease the administrative costs of transferring prescription information from provider offices to pharmacies. A more recent analysis concluded that the total efficiency and patient safety savings from NHII would be in range of $142-371 billion each year (Hillestad et al., 2005). While detailed studies of the potential savings from comprehensive implementation of NHII, including both electronic health records and effective exchange of health information, are still ongoing, it is clear that the cost reductions will amount to hundreds of billions of dollars each year. It is important to note that much of the savings depends not just on the widespread implementation of electronic health records, but the effective interchange of this information to insure that the complete medical record for every patient is immediately available in every care setting.

15.4.2   Barriers and Challenges to NHII

There are a number of significant barriers and challenges to the development of NHII. Perhaps the most important of these relates to protecting the confidentiality of electronic medical records. The public correctly perceives that all efforts to make medical records more accessible for appropriate and authorized purposes simultaneously carry the risk of increased availability for unscrupulous use. While the implementation of the HIPAA privacy and security rules (see Chapter 10) has established nationwide policies for access to medical information, maintaining public confidence requires mechanisms that affirmatively prevent privacy and confidentiality breaches before they occur. Development, testing, and implementation of such procedures must be an integral part of any NHII strategy.

Another important barrier to NHII is the misalignment of financial incentives in the health care system. Although the benefits of NHII are substantial, they do not accrue equally across all segments of the system. In particular, the benefits are typically not proportional to the required investments for a number of specific stakeholder groups. Perhaps most problematic is the situation for individual and small group health care providers, who are being asked to make substantial allocations of resources to electronic health record systems that mostly benefit others. Mechanisms must be found to assure the equitable distribution of NHII benefits in proportion to investments made. While this issue is the subject of continuing study, early results indicate that most of the NHII financial benefit accrues to payers of care. Therefore, programs and policies must be established to transfer appropriate savings back to those parties who have expended funds to produce them.

One consequence of the misaligned financial incentives is that the return on investment for health information technology needed for NHII is relatively uncertain. While a number of health care institutions, particularly large hospitals, have reported substantial cost improvements from electronic medical record systems, the direct financial benefits are by no means a forgone conclusion, especially for smaller organizations. The existing reimbursement system in the United States does not provide ready access to the substantial capital required by many institutions. For health care organizations operating on extremely thin margins, or even in the red, investments in information technology are impractical regardless of the potential return.

In addition, certain legal and regulatory barriers prevent the transfer of funds from those who benefit from health information technology to those who need to invest but have neither the means nor the incentive of substantial returns. Laws and regulations designed to prevent fraud and abuse, payments for referrals, and private distribution of disguised "profits" from nonprofit organizations are among those needing review. It is important that mechanisms be found to enable appropriate redistribution of savings generated from health information technology without creating loopholes that would allow abusive practices.

Another key barrier to NHII is that many of the benefits relate to exchanges of information between multiple health care organizations. The lack of interoperable electronic medical record systems that provide for easy transfer of records from one place to another is a substantial obstacle to achieving the advantages of NHII. Also, there is a "first mover disadvantage" in such exchange systems. The largest value is generated when all health care organizations in a community participate electronic information exchange. Therefore, if only a few organizations begin the effort, their costs may not be offset by the benefits.

15.4.3   *Approaches to Accelerating HII Progress*

A number of steps are currently under way to accelerate the progress towards NHII in the United States. These include establishing standards, fostering collaboration, funding demonstration projects in communities that include careful evaluation, and establishing consensus measures of progress.

15.4.3.1   Establishing Standards

Establishing electronic health record standards that would promote interoperability is the most widely recognized need in health information technology at the present time. Within institutions that have implemented specific departmental applications, extensive time and energy is spent developing and maintaining interfaces among the various systems. Although much progress has been made in this area by organizations such as Health Level 7, even electronic transactions of specific health care data (such as laboratory results) are often problematic due to differing interpretations of the implementation of existing standards.

Recently, the U.S. government has made substantial progress in this area. NCVHS, the official advisory body on these matters to DHHS, has been studying the issues of both message and content standards for patient medical record information for several years (NCVHS, 2000). The Consolidated Healthcare Informatics (CHI) initiative recommended five key standards (HL7 version 2.x, LOINC, DICOM, IEEE 1073, and NCPDP SCRIPT) that were adopted for government-wide use in early 2003, followed by 15 more that were added in 2004.

In July, 2003, the Federal government licensed the comprehensive medical vocabulary known as SNOMED (Systematized NOmenclature of MEDicine; see Chapter 7), making it available to all U.S. users at no charge. This represents a major step forward in the deployment of vocabulary standards for health information systems. Unlike message format standards, such as HL7, vocabulary standards are complex and expensive to develop and maintain and therefore require ongoing financial support. Deriving the needed funding from end users creates a financial obstacle to deployment of the standard. Removing this key barrier to adoption should promote much more widespread use over the next few years.

Another important project now under way is the joint effort of the Institute of Medicine and HL7 to develop a detailed functional definition of the electronic health record (EHR). These functional standards will provide a benchmark for comparison of existing and future EHR systems, and also may be utilized as criteria for possible financial incentives that could be provided to individuals and organizations that implement such systems. The elucidation of a consensus functional definition of the EHR also should help prepare the way for its widespread implementation by engaging all the stakeholders in an extended discussion of its desired capabilities.

This functional standardization of the EHR is expected to be followed by the development of a formal Interchange Format Standard (IFS) to be added to HL7 version 3. This standard would enable full interoperability of EHR systems through the implementation of an import and export capability to and from the IFS. While it is possible at the present time to exchange complete electronic health records with existing standards, is both difficult and inconvenient. The IFS will greatly simplify the process, making it easy to accomplish the commonly needed operation of transferring an entire electronic medical record from one facility to another.

Another key standard that is needed involves the representation of guideline recommendations. While the standard known as Arden Syntax (HL7, 2003; see Chapter 7) partially addresses this need, many real-world medical care guidelines are too complex to be represented easily in this format. At the present time, the considerable effort required to translate written guidelines and protocols into computer executable form must be repeated at every health care organization wishing to incorporate them in their EHR. Development of an effective guideline interchange standard would allow medical knowledge to be encoded once and then distributed widely, greatly increasing the efficiency of the process (Peleg at al., 2003).

15.4.3.2   Promoting Collaboration

Collaboration is another important strategy in promoting NHII. To enable the massive changes needed to transform the health care system from its current paper-based operation to the widespread utilization of electronic health information systems, the support of a very large number of organizations and individuals with highly varied agendas is required. Gathering and focusing this support requires extensive cooperative efforts and specific mechanisms for insuring that everyone's issues and concerns are expressed, appreciated, and incorporated into the ongoing efforts. This process is greatly aided by a widespread recognition of the serious problems that exist today in the U.S. healthcare system. A number of private collaboration efforts have been established such as the e-Health Initiative and the National Alliance for Health Information Technology (NAHIT). In the public sector, National Health Information Infrastructure (NHII) has become a focus of activity at DHHS. As part of this effort, the first ever national stakeholders meeting for NHII was convened in mid-2003 to develop a consensus national agenda for moving forward (Yasnoff et al., 2004).

These multiple efforts are having the collective effect of both catalyzing and promoting organizational commitment to NHII. For example, many of the key stakeholders are now forming high-level committees to specifically address NHII issues. For some of these organizations, this represents the first formal recognition that this transformational process is underway and will have a major impact on their activities. It is essential to include all stakeholders in this process. In addition to the traditional groups such as providers, payers, hospitals, health plans, health IT vendors, and health informatics professionals, representatives of groups such as consumers (e.g., AARP) and the pharmaceutical industry must be brought into the process.

15.4.3.3   Demonstration Projects

The most concrete and visible strategy for promoting NHII is the encouragement of demonstration projects in communities, including the provision of seed funding. By establishing clear examples of the benefits and advantages of comprehensive health information systems in communities, additional support for widespread implementation can be garnered at the same time that concerns of wary citizens and skeptical policymakers are addressed.

There are several important reasons for selecting a community-based strategy for NHII implementation. First and foremost, the existing models of health information infrastructures (e.g., Indianapolis and Spokane, WA) are based in local communities. This provides proof that it is possible to develop comprehensive electronic health care information exchange systems in these environments. In contrast, there is little or no evidence that such systems can be directly developed on a larger scale. Furthermore, increasing the size of informatics projects disproportionately increases their complexity and risk of failure. Therefore, keeping projects as small as possible is always a good strategy. Since NHII can be created by effectively connecting communities that have developed local health information infrastructures (LHIIs), it is not necessary to invoke a direct national approach to achieve the desired end result. A good analogy is the telephone network, which is composed of a large number of local exchanges that are then connected to each other to form community and then national and international networks.

Another important element in the community approach is the need for trust to overcome confidentiality concerns. Medical information is extremely sensitive and its exchange requires a high degree of confidence in everyone involved in the process. The level of trust needed seems most likely to be a product of personal relationships developed over time in a local community and motivated by a common desire to improve health care for everyone located in that area. While the technical implementation of information exchange is non-trivial, it pales in comparison to the challenges of establishing the underlying legal agreements and policy changes that must precede it. For example, when Indianapolis implemented sharing of patient information in hospital emergency rooms throughout the area, as many as 20 institutional lawyers needed to agree on the same contractual language (Overhage, 2002).

The community approach also benefits from the fact that the vast majority of health care is delivered locally. While people do travel extensively, occasionally requiring medical care while away from home, and there are few out-of-town consultations for difficult and unusual medical problems, for the most part people receive their health care in the community in which they reside. The local nature of medical care results in a natural interest of community members in maintaining and improving the quality and efficiency of their local health care system. For the same reasons, it is difficult to motivate interest in improving health care beyond the community level.

Focusing NHII efforts on one community at a time also keeps the implementation problem more reasonable in its scope. It is much more feasible to enable health information interchange among a few dozen hospitals and a few hundred or even a few thousand providers than to consider such a task for a large region or the whole country. This also allows for customized approaches sensitive to the specific needs of each local community. The problems and issues of medical care in a densely populated urban area are clearly vastly different than in a rural environment. Similarly, other demographic and organizational differences as well as the presence of specific highly specialized medical care institutions make each community's health care system unique. A local approach to HII development allows all these complex and varied factors to be considered and addressed, and respects the reality of the American political landscape, which gives high priority to local controls.

The community-based approach to HII development also benefits from the establishment of national standards. The same standards that allow effective interchange of information between communities nationwide can also greatly facilitate establishing effective communication of medical information within a community. In fact, by encouraging (and even requiring) communities to utilize national standards in building their own LHIIs, the later interconnection of those systems to provide nationwide access to medical care information becomes a much simpler and easier process.

Demonstration projects also are needed to develop and verify a replicable strategy for LHII development. While there are a small number of existing examples of LHII systems, no organization or group has yet demonstrated the ability to reliably and successfully establish such systems in multiple communities. From the efforts of demonstration projects in numerous communities, it should be possible to define a set of strategies that can be applied repeatedly across the nation.

Seed funding is essential in the development of LHII systems. While health care in United States is a huge industry, spending approximately $1.5 trillion each year and representing 14% of the GDP, shifting any of the existing funds into substantial IT investments is problematic. The beneficiaries of all the existing expenditures seem very likely to strongly oppose any such efforts. On the other hand, once initial investments begin to generate the expected substantial savings, it should be possible to develop mechanisms to channel those savings into expanding and enhancing LHII systems. Careful monitoring of the costs and benefits of local health information interchange systems will be needed to verify the practicality of this approach to funding and sustaining these projects.

Finally, it is important to assess and understand the technical challenges and solutions applied to LHII demonstration projects. While technical obstacles are usually not serious in terms of impeding progress, understanding and disseminating the most effective solutions can result in smoother implementation as experience is gained throughout the nation.

15.4.3.4   Measures to Evaluate Progress

The last element in the strategy for promoting a complex and lengthy project such as NHII is careful measurement of progress. The measures used to gauge progress define the end state and therefore must be chosen with care. Measures may also be viewed as the initial surrogate for detailed requirements. Progress measures should have certain key features. First, they should be sufficiently sensitive so that their values change at a reasonable rate (a measure that only changes value after five years will not be particularly helpful). Second, the measures must be comprehensive enough to reflect activities that impact most of the stakeholders and activities needing change. This ensures that efforts in every area will be reflected in improved measures. Third, the measures must be meaningful to policymakers. Fourth, periodic determinations of the current values of the measures should be easy so that the measurement process does not detract from the actual work. Finally, the totality of the measures must reflect the desired end state so that when the goals for all the measures are attained, the project is complete.

A number of different types or dimensions of measures for NHII progress are possible. Aggregate measures assess NHII progress over the entire nation. Examples include the percentage of the population covered by an LHII and the percentage of health care personnel whose training occurs in institutions that utilize electronic health record systems.

Another type of measure is based on the setting of care. Progress in implementation of electronic health record systems in the inpatient, outpatient, long-term care, home, and community environments could clearly be part of an NHII measurement program. Yet another dimension is health care functions performed using information systems support, including, for example, registration systems, decision support, CPOE, and community health information exchange.

It is also important to assess progress with respect to the semantic encoding of electronic health records. Clearly, there is a progression from the electronic exchange of images of documents, where the content is only readable by the end user viewing the image, to fully encoded electronic health records where all the information is indexed and accessible in machine-readable form using standards. Finally, progress can also be benchmarked based on usage of electronic health record systems by health care professionals. The transition from paper records to available electronic records to fully used electronic records is an important signal with respect to the success of NHII activities.

15.5   Example: NHII and Homeland Security

To illustrate some of the informatics challenges inherent in NHII, the example of its application to homeland security will be used. Bioterrorism preparedness in particular is now a key national priority, especially following the anthrax attacks that occurred in the Fall of 2001. Early detection of bioterrorism is critical to minimize morbidity and mortality. This is because, unlike other terrorist attacks, bioterrorism is usually silent at first. Its consequences are usually the first evidence that an attack has occurred. Traditional public health surveillance depends on alert clinicians reporting unusual diseases and conditions. However, it is difficult for clinicians to detect rare and unusual diseases since they are neither familiar with their manifestations nor suspicious of the possibility of an attack. Also, it is often difficult to differentiate potential bioterrorism from more common and benign manifestations of illness.

This is clearly illustrated by the seven cases of cutaneous anthrax that occurred in the New York City area two weeks prior to the "index " case in Florida the Fall of 2001 (Lipton & Johnson, 2001). All these cases presented to different clinicians, none of whom recognized the diagnosis of anthrax with sufficient confidence to notify any public health authority. Furthermore, such a pattern involving similar cases presenting to multiple clinicians could not possibly be detected by any of them. It seems likely that had all seven of these patients utilized the same provider, the immediately evident pattern of unusual signs and symptoms alone would have been sufficient to result in an immediate notification of public health authorities even in the absence of any diagnosis.

Traditional public health surveillance also has significant delays. Much routine reporting is still done via postcard and fax to the local health department, and further delays occur before information is collated, analyzed, and reported to state and finally to federal authorities.

There is also an obvious need for a carefully coordinated response after a bioterrorism event is detected. Health officials, in collaboration with other emergency response agencies, must carefully assess and manage health care assets and ensure rapid deployment of backup resources. Also, the substantial increase in workload created from such an incident must be distributed effectively among available hospitals, clinics, and laboratories, often including facilities outside the affected area.

15.5.1   Vision for HII in Homeland Security

The vision for the application of NHII to homeland security involves both early detection of bioterrorism and the response to such an event. Clinical information relevant to public health would be reported electronically in near real-time. This would include clinical lab results, emergency room chief complaints, relevant syndromes (e.g., flu-like illness), and unusual signs, symptoms, or diagnoses. By generating these electronic reports automatically from electronic health record systems, the administrative reporting burden currently placed on clinicians would be eliminated. In addition, the specific diseases and conditions reported could be dynamically adjusted in response to an actual incident or even information related to specific threats. This latter capability would be extremely helpful in carefully tracking the development of an event from its early stages.

NHII could also provide much more effective medical care resource management in response to events. This could include automatic reporting of all available resources so they could be allocated rapidly and efficiently, immediate operational visibility of all health care assets, and effective balancing of the tremendous surge in demand for medical care services. This would also greatly improve decision making about deployment of backup resources.

Using NHII for these bioterrorism preparedness functions avoids developing a separate, very expensive infrastructure dedicated to these rare events. As previously stated, the benefits of NHII are substantial and fully justify its creation even without these bioterrorism preparedness capabilities, which would be an added bonus. Furthermore, the same infrastructure that serves as an early detection system for bioterrorism also will allow earlier and more sensitive detection of routine naturally occurring disease outbreaks (which are much more common) as well as better management of health care resources in other disaster situations.

15.5.2   Informatics Challenges of HII in Homeland Security

The application of NHII to homeland security involves a number of difficult informatics challenges. First, this activity requires participation from a very wide range of both public and private organizations. This includes all levels of government and organizations that have not had significant prior interactions with the health care system such as agriculture, police, fire, and animal health. Needless to say, these organizations have divergent objectives and cultures that do not necessarily mesh easily. Health and law enforcement in particular have a significantly different view of a bioterrorism incident. For example, an item that is considered a "specimen" in the health care system may be regarded as "evidence" by law enforcement.

Naturally, this wide variety of organizations has incompatible information systems, since for the most part they were designed and deployed without consideration for the issues raised by bioterrorism. Not only do they have discordant design objectives, but they lack standardized terminology and messages to facilitate electronic information exchange. Furthermore, there are serious policy conflicts among these various organizations, for example, with respect to access to information. In the health care system, access to information is generally regarded as desirable, whereas in law enforcement it must be carefully protected to maintain the integrity of criminal investigations.

Complicating these organizational, cultural, and information systems issues, bioterrorism preparedness has an ambiguous governance structure. Many agencies and organizations have legitimate and overlapping authority and responsibility, so there is often no single clear path to resolve conflicting issues. Therefore, a high degree of collaboration and collegiality is required, with extensive pre-event planning so that roles and responsibilities are clarified prior to any emergency.

Within this complex environment, there is also a need for new types of systems with functions that have never before been performed. Bioterrorism preparedness results in new requirements for early disease detection and coordination of the health care system. Precisely because these requirements are new, there are few (if any) existing systems that have similar functions. Therefore careful consideration to design requirements of bioterrorism preparedness systems is essential to ensure success.

Most importantly, there is an urgent need for interdisciplinary communication among an even larger number of specialty areas than is typically the case with health information systems. All participants must recognize that each domain has its own specific terminology and operational approaches. As previously mentioned in the public health informatics example, the interlocutor function is vital. Since it is highly unlikely that any single person will be able to span all or even most of the varied disciplinary areas, everyone on the team must make a special effort to learn the vocabulary used by others.

As a result of these extensive and difficult informatics challenges, there are few operational information systems supporting bioterrorism preparedness. It is interesting to note that all the existing systems developed to date are local. This is most likely a consequence of the same issues previously delineated in the discussion of the advantages of community-based strategies for NHII development.

One such system performs automated electronic lab reporting in Indianapolis (Overhage et al., 2001). The development of this system was led by the same active informatics group that developed the LHII in the same area. Nevertheless, it took several years of persistent and difficult efforts to overcome the technical, organizational, and legal issues involved. For example, even though all laboratories submitted data in "standard" HL7 format, it turned out that many of them were interpreting the standard in such a way that the electronic transactions could not be effectively processed by the recipient system. To address this problem, extensive reworking of the software that generated these transactions was required for many of the participating laboratories.

Another example of a bioterrorism preparedness system involves emergency room chief complaint reporting in Pittsburgh (Tsui et al., 2003). This is a collaborative effort of multiple institutions with existing electronic medical record systems. It has also been led by an active informatics group that has worked long and hard to overcome technical, organizational, and legal challenges. It provides a near real-time "dashboard" for showing the incidence rates of specific types of syndromes, such as gastrointestinal and respiratory. This information is very useful for monitoring the patterns of diseases presenting to the area's emergency departments.

Note that both of these systems were built upon extensive prior work done by existing informatics groups. They also took advantage of existing local health information infrastructures that provided either available or least accessible electronic data streams. In spite of these advantages, it is clear from these and other efforts that the challenges in building bioterrorism preparedness systems are immense. However, having an existing health information infrastructure appears to be a key prerequisite. Such an infrastructure implies the existence of a capable informatics group and available electronic health data in the community.

15.6   Conclusions and Future Challenges

Public health informatics may be viewed as the application of biomedical informatics to populations. In a sense, it is the ultimate evolution of biomedical informatics, which has traditionally focused on applications related to individual patients. Public health informatics highlights the potential of the health informatics disciplines as a group to integrate information from the molecular to the population level.

Public health informatics and the development of health information infrastructures are closely related. Public health informatics deals with public health applications, whereas health information infrastructures are population-level applications primarily focused on medical care. While the information from these two areas overlaps, the orientation of both is the community rather than the individual. Public health and health care have not traditionally interacted as closely as they should. In a larger sense, both really focus on the health of communities—public health does this directly, while the medical care system does it one patient at a time. However, it is now clear that medical care must also focus on the community to integrate the effective delivery of services across all care settings for all individuals.

The informatics challenges inherent in both public health informatics and the development of health information infrastructures are immense. They include the challenge of large numbers of different types of organizations including government at all levels. This results in cultural, strategic, and personnel challenges. The legal issues involved in interinstitutional information systems, especially with regard to information sharing, can be daunting. Finally, communications challenges are particularly difficult because of the large number of areas of expertise represented, including those that go beyond the health care domain (e.g., law enforcement). To deal with these communication issues, the interlocutor function is particularly critical.

However, the effort required to address the challenges of public health informatics and health information infrastructures is worthwhile because the potential benefits are so substantial. Effective information systems in these domains can help to assure effective prevention, high-quality care, and minimization of medical errors. In addition to the resultant decreases in both morbidity and mortality, these systems also have the potential to save hundreds of billions of dollars in both direct and indirect costs.

It has been previously noted that one of the key differences between public health informatics and other informatics disciplines is that it includes interventions beyond the medical care system, and is not limited to medical and surgical treatments (Yasnoff et al., 2000). So despite the focus of most current public health informatics activities on population-based extensions of the medical care system (leading to the orientation of this chapter), applications beyond this scope are both possible and desirable. Indeed, the phenomenal contributions to health made by the hygienic movement of the 19th and early 20th centuries suggest the power of large-scale environmental, legislative, and social changes to promote human health (Rosen, 1993). Public health informatics must explore these dimensions as energetically as those associated with prevention and clinical care at the individual level.

The effective application of informatics to populations through its use in both public health and the development of health information infrastructures is a key challenge of the 21st century. It is a challenge we must accept, understand, and overcome if we want to create an efficient and effective health care system as well as truly healthy communities for all.

Suggested Readings

Centers for Disease Control and Prevention (1997). Community Immunization Registries Manual. Available at http://www.cdc.gov/nip/registry/cir-manual.htm. While some of the particulars are a little dated, this accessible document shows how public health professionals approach informatics problems.

Hellestad R, Bigelow J, Bower A, Girosi F, Meili R, Scoville R, Taylor R 2005: Can Electronic Medical Record Systems Transform   Health Care? Potential Health Benefits, Savings, and Costs *Health Affairs* 2005; 24:1103–1117.

Yasnoff WA,Humphreys BL, Overhage JM, Detmer DE, Brenman PF, Morris RW, Middleton B, Bates DW, Fanning JP: A Consensus Action Agenda for Achieving the National Health Information Infrastructure. J Am Med Informatics Assoc 11(4)-332-338. Summarizes the results of a recent conference; presents a broad overview and many forward-looking perspectives.

Friede A, Blum HL, McDonald M (1995). Public health informatics: how information-age technology can strengthen public health. *Annu Rev Public Health* 16:239-52. The seminal article on public health informatics.

Koo D, O'Carroll PW, LaVenture M (2001). Public health 101 for informaticians. *Journal of the American Medical Informatics Association* 8(6):585-97. An accessible document that introduces public health thinking.

O'Carroll PW, Yasnoff WA, Ward ME, Ripp LH, Martin EL (eds.) (2003): *Public Health Informatics and Information Systems*. New York: Springer-Verlag. A new and comprehensive textbook.

Walker J, Pan E, Johnston D, Adler-Milstein J, Bates DW, Middleton B. (2004). *The Value of Healthcare information Exchange and Interoperability*. Boston, MA: Center for Information Technology Leadership.

Yasnoff WA, Humphreys BL, Overhage JM, Detmer DE, Brennan PF, Morris RW, Middlleton B, Bates DW, Fanning JP (2004): A Consensus Action Agenda for Achieving the National Health Information Infrastructure. *J Am Med Informatics Assoc* 11(4):332–338, 2004. Summarizes the results of a recent conference; presents a broad overview and many forward-working perspectives.

Yasnoff WA, O'Carroll PW, Koo D, Linkins RW, Kilbourne EM (2000). Public Health Informatics: Improving and transforming public health in the information age. *Journal of Public Health Management & Practice* 6(6):67-75. A concise yet comprehensive introduction to the field.

Questions for further study:

1. What are the current and potential effects of a) the genomics revolution; and b) 9/11 on public health informatics?
2. How can the successful model of immunization registries be used in other domains of public health (be specific about those domains)? How might it fail in others? Why?
3. Fourteen percent of the US GDP is spent on medical care (including public health). How could public health informatics help use those monies more efficiently? Or lower the figure absolutely?
4. Compare and contrast the database desiderata for clinical versus public health information systems. Explain it from non-technical and technical perspectives.
5. Make the case for and against investing billions in an NHII.
6. What organizational options would you consider if you were beginning the development of a local health information infrastructure? What are the pros and cons of each? How would you proceed with making a decision about which one to use?
7. If public health informatics (PHI) involves the application of information technology in any manner that improves or promotes human health, does this necessarily involve a human "user" that interacts with the PHI application? For example, could the information technology underlying anti-lock braking systems be considered a public health informatics application?

16
Patient-Care Systems

JUDY G. OZBOLT AND SUZANNE BAKKEN

After reading this chapter, you should know the answers to these questions:

- What are the four major information-management issues in patient care?
- How have patient-care systems evolved during the past four decades?
- How have patient-care systems influenced the process and outcomes of patient care?
- Why are patient-care systems essential to the computer-based patient record?
- How can they be differentiated from the computer-based patient record itself?

16.1 Information Management in Patient Care

Patient care is the focus of many clinical disciplines—medicine, nursing, pharmacy, nutrition, therapies such as respiratory, physical, and occupational, and others. Although the work of the various disciplines sometimes overlaps, each has its own primary focus, emphasis, and methods of care delivery. Each discipline's work is complex in itself, and collaboration among disciplines adds another level of complexity. In all disciplines, the quality of clinical decisions depends in part on the quality of information available to the decision-maker. The systems that manage information for patient care are therefore a critical tool. Their fitness for the job varies, and the systems enhance or detract from patient care accordingly. This chapter describes information-management issues in patient care, the evolution of patient care systems in relation to these issues, and current research. It will also show how patient care systems provide the infrastructure that determines the quality and functions of the computer-based patient record.

16.1.1 Concepts of Patient Care

Patient care is an interdisciplinary process centered on the care recipient in the context of the family, significant others, and community. Typically, patient care includes the services of physicians, nurses, and members of other health disciplines according to patient needs: physical, occupational, and respiratory therapists; nutritionists; psychologists; social workers; and many others. Each of these disciplines brings specialized perspectives and expertise. Specific cognitive processes and therapeutic techniques vary by discipline, but all disciplines share certain commonalities in the provision of care.

In its simplest terms, the process of care begins with collecting data and assessing the patient's current status in comparison to criteria or expectations of normality. Through

564

cognitive processes specific to the discipline, diagnostic labels are applied, therapeutic goals are identified with timelines for evaluation, and therapeutic interventions are selected and implemented. At specified intervals, the patient is reassessed, the effectiveness of care is evaluated, and therapeutic goals and interventions are continued or adjusted as needed. If the reassessment shows that the patient no longer needs care, services are terminated. This process was illustrated for nursing in 1975 (Goodwin & Edwards, 1975) and was updated and made more general in 1984 (Ozbolt et al., 1985). The flowchart reproduced in Figure 16.1 could apply equally well to other patient-care disciplines.

Although this linear flowchart helps to explain some aspects of the process of care, it is, like the solar-system model of the atom, a gross simplification. Frequently, for example, in the process of collecting data for an initial patient assessment, the nurse may recognize (diagnose) that the patient is anxious about her health condition. Simultaneously with continuing the data collection, the nurse sets a therapeutic goal that the patient's anxiety will be reduced to a level that increases the patient's comfort and ability to participate in care. The nurse selects and implements therapeutic actions of modulating the tone of voice, limiting environmental stimuli, maintaining eye contact, using gentle touch, asking about the patient's concerns, and providing information. All the while, the nurse observes the effects on the patient's anxiety and adjusts his behavior accordingly. Thus, the complete care process can occur in a microcosm while one step of the care process—data collection—is underway. This simultaneous, nonlinear quality of patient care poses challenges to informatics in the support of patient care and the capture of clinical data.

Each caregiver's simultaneous attention to multiple aspects of the patient is not the only complicating factor. Just as atoms become molecules by sharing electrons, the care provided by each discipline becomes part of a complex molecule of **interdisciplinary care**. Caregivers and developers of informatics applications to support care must recognize that true interdisciplinary care is as different from the separate contributions of the various disciplines as an organic molecule is from the elements that go into it. The contributions of the various disciplines are not merely additive; as a force acting on the patient, the work of each discipline is transformed by its interaction with the other disciplines in the larger unity of patient care.

For example, a 75-year-old woman with rheumatoid arthritis, high blood pressure, and urinary incontinence might receive care from a physician, a home-care nurse, a nutritionist, a physical therapist, and an occupational therapist. From a simplistic, additive perspective, each discipline could be said to perform the following functions:

1. Physician: diagnose diseases, prescribe appropriate medications, authorize other care services
2. Nurse: assess patient's understanding of her condition and treatment and her self-care abilities and practices; teach and counsel as needed; help patient to perform exercises at home; report findings to physician and other caregivers
3. Nutritionist: assess patient's nutritional status and eating patterns; prescribe and teach appropriate diet to control blood pressure and build physical strength
4. Physical therapist: prescribe and teach appropriate exercises to improve strength and flexibility and to enhance cardiovascular health, within limitations of arthritis

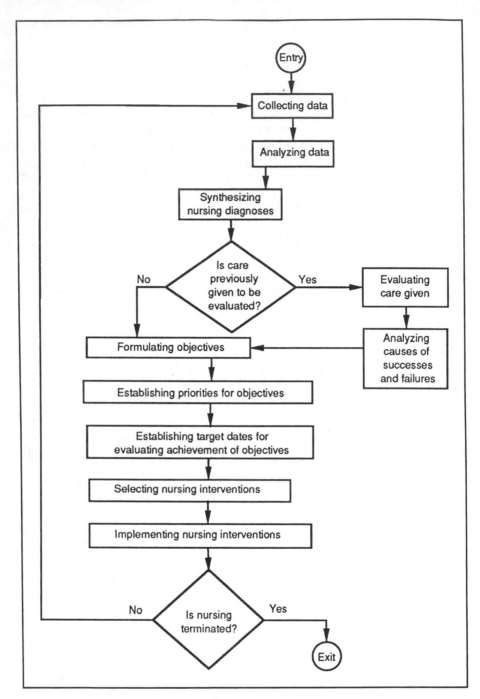

Figure 16.1. The provision of nursing care is an iterative process that consists of steps to collect and analyze data, to plan and implement interventions, and to evaluate the results of interventions. (*Source:* Adapted with permission from Ozbolt J.G., et al. [1985]. A proposed expert system for nursing practice. *Journal of Medical Systems,* 9:57–68.

5. Occupational therapist: assess abilities and limitations for performing activities of daily living; prescribe exercises to improve strength and flexibility of hands and arms; teach adaptive techniques and provide assistive devices as needed

In a collaborative, interdisciplinary practice, the nurse might discover that the patient was not taking walks each day as prescribed because her urinary incontinence was exacerbated by the diuretic prescribed to treat hypertension, and the patient was embarrassed to go out. The nurse would report this to the physician and the other caregivers so that they could understand why the patient was not carrying out the prescribed regime. The physician might then change the strategy for treating hypertension while initiating treatment for urinary incontinence. The nurse would help the patient to understand the interaction of the various treatment regimes, would provide practical advice and assistance in dealing with incontinence, and would help the patient to find personally acceptable ways to follow the prescribed treatments. The nutritionist might work with the patient on the timing of meals and fluid intake so that the patient could exercise and sleep with less risk of urinary incontinence. The physical and the occupational therapists would adjust their recommendations to accommodate the patient's personal needs and preferences while moving toward the therapeutic goals. Finally, the patient, rather than being assailed with sometimes conflicting demands of multiple caregivers, would be supported by an ensemble of services. Such collaboration, however, requires exquisite communication and feedback. The potential for information systems to support or sabotage this kind of care is obvious.

Although the care of individual patients is thus complex, it is far from being the totality of patient care. Because patients receive services from multiple caregivers, someone must coordinate those services. Coordination includes seeing that patients receive all the services they need in logical sequence without scheduling conflicts and ensuring that each caregiver communicates as needed with the others. Sometimes, a **case manager** is designated to do this coordination. In other situations, a physician or a nurse assumes the role by default. Sometimes, coordination is left to chance, and both the processes and the outcomes of care are put at risk. In recognition of this, the IOM recently designated coordination of care as one of 14 priorities for national action to transform health care quality (Institute of Medicine, 2002).

Delivering and managing the interdisciplinary care of each patient would seem to be sufficiently challenging, but patient care has yet another level of complexity. Each caregiver is usually responsible for the care of multiple patients. In planning and executing the work of caregiving, each professional must consider the competing demands of all the patients for whom she is responsible, as well as the exigencies of all the other professionals involved in each patient's care. Thus, the nurse on a post-operative unit must plan for scheduled treatments for each of her patients to occur near the optimal time for that patient. She must take into account that several patients may require treatments at nearly the same time and that some of them may be receiving other services, such as X-ray or physician's visits, at the time when it might be most convenient for the nurse to administer the treatment. When unexpected needs arise, as they often do—an emergency, an unscheduled patient, observations that could signal an incipient complication—the nurse must set priorities, organize, and delegate to be sure that at least the critical needs are met. Similarly, the physician must balance the needs of various patients who may be widely dispersed throughout an institution. Decision-support systems have the potential to provide important assistance for both clinical and organizational decisions.

Finally, caregivers not only deliver services to patients, with all the planning, documenting, collaborating, referring, and consulting attendant on direct care; they are also responsible for **indirect-care** activities, such as teaching and supervising students, attending staff meetings, participating in continuing education, and serving on committees. Each caregiver's plan of work must allow for both the direct-care and the indirect-care activities. Because the caregivers work in concert, these plans must be coordinated.

In summary, patient care is an extremely complex undertaking with multiple levels. Each caregiver's contributions to the care of every patient must take into account the ensemble of contributions of all caregivers and the interactions among them, all coordinated to optimize effectiveness and efficiency. Moreover, these considerations are multiplied by the number of patients for whom each caregiver is responsible. Patient care is further complicated by the indirect-care activities that caregivers must intersperse among the direct-care responsibilities and coordinate with other caregivers. It is little wonder that managing, processing, and communicating data, information, and knowledge are integral and critical to every aspect of patient care.

16.1.2   *Information to Support Patient Care*

As complex as patient care is, the essential information for direct patient care is defined in the answers to the following questions:

- Who is involved in the care of the patient?
- What information does each professional require to make decisions?
- From where, when, and in what form does the information come?
- What information does each professional generate? Where, when, and in what form is it needed?

The framework described by Zielstorff and others (1993) provides a useful heuristic for understanding the varied types of information required to answer each of these questions. As listed in Table 16.1, this framework delineates three information categories: (1) patient-specific data, which are those data about a particular patient acquired from a variety of data sources; (2) agency-specific data, which are those data relevant to the specific organization under whose auspices the health-care is provided; and (3) domain information and knowledge, which is specific to the health-care disciplines.

The framework further identifies four types of information processes that information systems may apply to each of the three information categories. **Data acquisition** entails the methods by which data become available to the information system. It may include data entry by the care provider or acquisition from a medical device or from another computer-based system. **Data storage** includes the methods, programs, and structures used to organize data for subsequent use. Examples of standardized coding and classification systems useful in representing patient care concepts are listed in Table 16.2. This topic is discussed in greater detail in Chapters 2, 7, and 12. **Data**

Table 16.1. Framework for design characteristics of a patient-care information system with examples of patient-specific data, agency-specific data, and domain information and knowledge for patient care.

Types of data	System processes			
	Acquiring	Storing	Transforming	Presenting
Domain-specific	Downloading relevant scientific or clinical literature or practice guidelines	Maintaining information in electronic journals or files, searchable by key words	Linking related literature or published findings; updating guidelines based on research	Displaying relevant literature or guidelines in response to queries
Agency-specific	Scanning, downloading, or keying in agency policies and procedures; keying in personnel, financial, and administrative records	Maintaining information in electronic directories, files and databases	Editing and updating information; linking related information in response to queries; analyzing information	Displaying on request continuously current policies and procedures shoring relevant policies and procedures in response to queries; generating management reports
Patient-specific	Point-of-care entry of data about patient assessment, diagnoses, treatments planned and delivered, therapeutic goals patient outcomes	Moving patient data into a current electronic record or an aggregate data repository	Combining relevant data on a single patient into a cue for action in a decision-support system; performing statistical analyses on data from many patients	Displaying reminders, alerts probable diagnoses, or suggested treatments; displaying vital signs graphically; displaying statistical results

Source. Framework adapted with permission from *Next Generation Nursing Information Systems*, 1993, American Nurses Association, Washington, DC.

Table 16.2. Examples of standardized coding and classification systems with utility for patient care.

System	Problems	Interventions	Goals/Outcomes
International Classification of Diseases	x		
NANDA Taxonomy 1	x		
Current Procedural Terminology		x	
Nursing Interventions Classification		x	
Nursing Outcomes Classification			x
Omaha System	x	x	x
Home Health Care Classification	x	x	x
SNOMED Clinical Terms	x	x	x
Patient Care Data Set	x	x	x

transformation or **processing** comprises the methods by which stored data or information are acted on according to the needs of the end user—for example, calculation of a pressure ulcer risk-assessment score at admission or calculation of critically ill patients' acute physiology and chronic health evaluation (APACHE) scores. Figure 16.2 illustrates the transformation (abstraction, summarization, aggregation) of patient-specific data for multiple uses. **Presentation** encompasses the forms in which information is delivered to the end user after processing.

Transformed patient-specific data can be presented in a variety of ways. Numeric data may be best presented in chart or graph form to allow the user to examine trends,

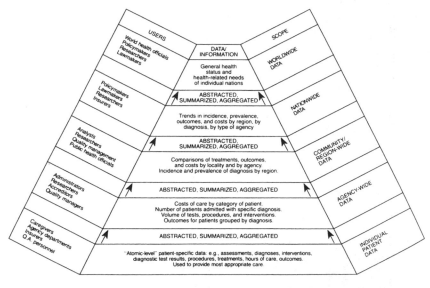

Figure 16.2. Examples of uses for atomic-level patient data collected once but used many times. (Source: Reprinted with permission from R. D. Zielstorff, C. I. Hudgings, S. J. Grobe, and The National Commission on Nursing Implementation Project Task Force on Nursing Information Systems. Next-Generation Nursing Information Systems, © 1993 American Nurses Publishing, American Nurses Foundation/American Nurses Association, Washington, DC.)

whereas the compilation of potential diagnoses generated from patient-assessment data lends itself to an alphanumeric-list format. Different types of agency-specific data lend themselves to a variety of presentation formats. Common among all, however, is the need for presentation at the point of patient care; for example, the integration of up-to-the-minute patient-specific data with agency-specific guidelines or parameters can produce alerts, reminders, or other types of notifications for immediate action. See Chapter 17, on patient-monitoring systems, for an overview of this topic. Presentation of domain information and knowledge related to patient care is most frequently accomplished through interaction with databases and knowledge bases, such as Medline or Micromedex (see Chapter19). Another approach is the Infobutton at New York Presbyterian Hospital. Through the Infobutton Manager, data about the patient, the provider, and the area in the clinical information system is taken into account so that context-specific knowledge is presented at the point of care (Cimino et al., 2002).

To support patient care, information systems must be geared to the needs of all the professionals involved in care. The systems should acquire, store, process, and present each type of information (patient-, agency-, and domain-specific) where, when, and how each function is needed by each professional. These systems not only support each professional's care of individual patients but also, through appropriate use of patient-specific information (care requirements), agency-specific information (caregivers and their responsibilities and agency policies and procedures), and domain information (guidelines), such systems can greatly aid the coordination of interdisciplinary services for individual patients and the planning and scheduling of each caregiver's work activities. Patient acuity is taken into account in scheduling nursing personnel, but most often is entered into a separate system rather than derived directly from care requirements. Integrated systems—still an ideal today—would enhance our understanding of each patient's situation and needs, improve decision-making, facilitate communications, aid coordination, and use clinical data to provide feedback for improving clinical processes.

Clearly, when patient-care information systems fulfill their potential, they will not merely replace oral and paper-based methods of recording and communicating. They will not only support but also transform patient care. How far have we come toward the ideal? What must we do to continue our progress?

16.2   Historical Evolution of Patient-Care Systems

The genesis of patient care systems occurred in the mid-1960s. One of the first and most successful systems was the Technicon Medical Information System (TMIS), begun in 1965 as a collaborative project between Lockheed and El Camino Hospital in Mountain View, California (see Chapter 13). Designed to simplify documentation through the use of standard order sets and care plans, TMIS defined the state of the art when it was developed. Four decades later, versions of TMIS are still widely used, but the technology has moved on. The hierarchical, menu-driven arrangement of information in TMIS required users to page through many screens to enter or retrieve data and precluded aggregation of data across patients for statistical analysis. Today's users have a different view of what can be done with data, and they demand systems that support those uses.

Part of what changed users' expectations for patient care systems has been the development and evolution of systems that support clinical decision making. The HELP system (see Chapters 12, 13, and 17) at LDS Hospital in Salt Lake City, Utah, initially provided decision support to physicians during the process of care (in addition to managing and storing data). HELP subsequently became able to support nursing care decisions and to aggregate data for research, leading to improved patient care. Other systems that provide decision support for physician order-entry, such as those developed at Partners Health Care in Boston and at Vanderbilt University Medical Center in Nashville, Tennessee, have been translated into commercial systems. By demonstrating that these systems can improve patient outcomes while containing costs, developers and vendors raise expectations in the marketplace. Still other systems, such as the order-entry system developed at Vanderbilt, are beginning to explore the effects of feedback about care effectiveness on the processes and outcomes of care.

Today, many commercially available information systems for patient care incorporate decision support, integration of information from multiple sources, care planning and documentation, organization of the clinician's workflow, and support for care management. Both vendors of information systems and researchers in health-care enterprises are working to advance these features in systems that use the latest technologies for navigating and linking information. Although knowledge-based systems have been in existence since the early years of biomedical informatics, we are seeing the infancy of systems that aggregate and analyze clinical data to produce new knowledge and apply it in practice. As clinical knowledge and workflow, rather than financial models, become the basis for system design, emerging generations of patient care systems appear poised to fulfill the promises of clinical informatics.

16.2.1 Societal Influences

The historical evolution of information systems that support patient care is not solely a reflection of the available technologies. Societal forces—including delivery-system structure, practice model, payer model, and quality focus—have influenced the design and implementation of patient-care systems (Table 16.3).

Delivery-System Structure

Authors have noted the significant influence of the organization and its people on the success or failure of informatics innovations (Ash, 1997; Kaplan, 1997; Lorenzi et al., 1997; Southon et al., 1997). As delivery systems shifted from the predominant single-institution structure of the 1970s to the **integrated delivery networks** of the 1990s to the complex linkages of the 21st Century, the information needs changed, and the challenges of meeting those information needs increased in complexity. See Chapters 13, 14, and 15 for discussions of managing clinical information in integrated delivery systems, in consumer-provider partnerships in care, and in the public health information infrastructure.

Table 16.3. Societal forces that have influenced the design and implementation of patient care systems.

	1970s	1980s	1990s
Delivery-system structure	Single institution	Single organization	Integrated delivery systems
Professional-practice model	Team nursing	Primary nursing	Patient-focused care
	Single or small group physician practice	Group models for physicians	Interdisciplinary care
			Case management
			Variety of constellations of physician group practice models
Payer model	Fee for service	Fee for service	Capitation
		Prospective payment, diagnosis-related groups (DRGs)	Managed Care
Quality focus	Professional Standards Review Organizations (PSROs)	Continuous quality improvement	Risk-adjusted outcomes
		Joint Commission on Accreditation of Health Care Organization (JCAHO)'s Agenda for Change	Benchmarking
	Retrospective chart review		Practice guidelines
			Critical paths/care maps
	Joint Commission on Accreditation of Hospitals' Peer Evaluation Program		Health Employer Data and Information set (HEDIS)
	Quality of Patient Care System (QUALPACS)		

Professional Practice Models

Professional practice models have also evolved for nurses and physicians. In the 1970s, team nursing was the typical practice model for the hospital, and the nursing care plan—a document for communicating the plan of care among nursing team members—was most frequently the initial computer-based application designed for use by nurses. The 1990s were characterized by a shift to interdisciplinary-care approaches necessitating computer-based applications such as critical paths to support case management of aggregates of patients, usually with a common medical diagnosis, across the **continuum of care**. The 21ˢᵗ Century sees advanced practice nurses increasingly taking on functions previously provided by physicians while maintaining a nursing perspective on collaborative, interdisciplinary care. These changes broaden and diversify the demands for decision support, feedback about clinical effectiveness, and quality improvement as a team effort.

Physician practice models have shifted from single physician or small group offices to complex constellations of provider organizations. The structure of the model (e.g., staff model health-maintenance organization, captive-group model health-maintenance organization, or independent-practice association; see Chapter 23) determines the types of relationships among the physicians and the organizations. These include issues—such as location of medical records, control of practice patterns of the physicians, and data-reporting requirements—that have significant implications for the design and implementation of patient-care systems. In addition, the interdisciplinary and distributed care approaches of the 1990s and the 2000s have given impetus to system-design strategies, such as the creation of a single patient problem list, around which the patient-care record is organized, in place of a separate list for each provider group (e.g., nurses, physicians, respiratory therapists).

Payer Models

Changes in payer models have been a significant driving force for information-system implementation in many organizations. With the shift from fee for service to prospective payment in the 1980s, and then toward capitation in the 1990s, information about costs and quality of care has become an essential commodity for rational decision-making in the increasingly competitive healthcare marketplace. Because private, third-party payers often adopt federal standards for reporting and regulation, health care providers and institutions have struggled in the early 2000s to keep up with the movement toward data and information system standards accelerated by the Health Insurance Portability and Accountability Act (HIPAA) and the initiatives to develop a National Health Information Infrastructure. See Chapter 23 for a thorough discussion of the effects of healthcare financing on health-care information systems.

Quality Focus

Demands for information about quality of care have also influenced the design and implementation of patient-care systems. The quality-assurance techniques of the 1970s were primarily based on retrospective chart audit. In the 1980s, continuous-quality-improvement techniques became the modus operandi of most healthcare organizations. The quality-management techniques of the 1990s were much more focused on concurrently influencing the care delivered than on retrospectively evaluating its quality. In the 21st Century, patient-care systems-based approaches—such as critical paths, practice guidelines, alerts, and reminders—are an essential component of **quality management**. In addition, institutions must have the capacity to capture data for benchmarking purposes and to report process and outcomes data to regulatory and accreditation bodies, as well as to any voluntary reporting programs (e.g., Maryland Hospital Indicator Program) to which they belong. Increasingly, concurrent feedback about the effectiveness of care guides clinical decisions in real time.

16.2.2   Patient-Care Systems

The design and implementation of **patient-care systems**, for the most part, occurred separately for hospital and ambulatory-care settings. Early patient-care systems in the hospital settings included the University of Missouri-Columbia System (Lindberg, 1965), the Problem-Oriented Medical Information System (PROMIS) (Weed, 1975), the Tri-

Service Medical Information System (TRIMUS) (Bickel, 1979), the Health Evaluation Logical Processing (HELP) System (Kuperman et al., 1991), and the Decentralized Hospital Computer Program (DHCP) (Ivers & Timson, 1985). The Computer-Stored Ambulatory Record (COSTAR), the Regenstrief Medical Record System (McDonald, 1976), and The Medical Record (TMR) were among the earliest ambulatory care systems. For a comprehensive review, see Collen (1995).

According to Collen (1995), the most commonly used patient-care systems in hospitals of the 1980s were those that supported nursing care planning and documentation. Systems to support capture of physicians' orders, communications with the pharmacy, and reporting of laboratory results were also widely used. Some systems merged physician orders with the nursing care plan to provide a more comprehensive view of care to be given. This merging, such as allowing physicians and nurses to view information in the part of the record designated for each other's discipline, was a step toward integration of information. It was still, however, a long way from support for truly collaborative interdisciplinary practice.

Early ambulatory-care systems most often included paper-based, patient encounter forms that were either computer-scannable mark-sense format or were subsequently entered into the computer by clerical personnel. Current desktop, laptop, or hand-held systems use keyboard, mouse, or pen-based entry of structured information, with free text kept to a minimum. These systems also provide for retrieval of reports and past records. Some systems provide decision support or alerts to remind clinicians about needed care, such as immunizations or screening examinations, and to avoid contraindicated orders for medications or unnecessary laboratory analyses. Depending on network capabilities, systems may facilitate communications among the professionals and settings involved in the patient's care. Voice-recognition technology is advancing and is beginning to permit direct dictation into the record. Although this mode of data entry has the advantages of ease and familiarity to clinicians, free text in the record inhibits search, retrieval, and analysis of data. Before dictated notes can become as useful as structured data, the entry systems will have to become able to recognize the meanings of words and their context and to store the data in databases. Although this level of intelligent processing of natural language remains in the future (See Chapter 8), systems to support ambulatory care have clearly made great strides. The best provide good support for traditional medical care. Support for comprehensive, collaborative care that gives as much attention to health promotion as to treatment of disease presents a challenge not only to the developers of information systems but also to practitioners and healthcare administrators who must explicate the nature of this practice and the conditions under which agencies will provide it.

Patient-care information systems in use today represent a broad range in the evolution of the field. Versions of some of the earliest systems are still in use. These systems were generally designed to speed documentation and to increase legibility and availability of the records of patients currently receiving care. Most lack the capacity to aggregate data across patients, to query the data about subsets of patients, or to use data collected for clinical purposes to meet informational needs of administrators or researchers. These shortcomings seem glaring today, but they were not apparent when the very idea of using computers to store and communicate patient information required a leap of the imagination.

More recently developed systems attempt with varying success to respond to the edict "collect once, use many times." Selected items of data from patient records are abstracted manually or electronically to aggregate databases where they can be analyzed for administrative reports, for quality improvement, for clinical or health-services research, and for required patient safety and public health reporting. See Chapter 15 for a full discussion of public health informatics.

Some recently developed systems offer some degree of coordination of the information and services of the various clinical disciplines into integrated records and plans. Data collected by one caregiver can appear, possibly in a modified representation, in the "view" of the patient record designed for another discipline. When care-planning information has been entered by multiple caregivers, it can be viewed as the care plan to be executed by a discipline, by an individual, or by the interdisciplinary team. Some patient-care systems offer the option to organize care temporally into **clinical pathways** and to have variances from the anticipated activities, sequence, or timing reported automatically. Others offer a patient "view" so that individuals can view and contribute to their own records records (Pyper et al, 2002; Cimino, Patel, Kushniruk, 2002).

Doolan et al. (2003) studied information system functionality for clinical care in five sites that had won the Computer-based Patient Record Institute Davies' Award:

- LDS Hospital, Salt Lake City (LDSH) in 1995
- Brigham and Women's Hospital, Boston (BWH) in 1996
- Wishard Memorial Hospital, Indianapolis (WMH) in 1997
- Queen's Medical Center, Honolulu (QMC) in 1999
- Veteran's Affairs Purget Sound Healthcare System, Seattle and Tacoma (VAPS) in 2000

All sites had broadscale computer-based results reporting and order entry for medications and other therapeutics. As compared to many other organizations, the patient care systems these sites also had some functionality related to documentation of clinical notes (See Table 16.4). It is noteworthy that even in these sites that are widely recognized for their advanced clinical information systems, clinicians' progress notes are not completely computer-based.

Computerized Notes

The publication of the Institute of Medicine's reports *To Err is Human* (2000) and *Crossing the Quality Chasm* (2001) resulted in increasing demands from health care providers for information systems that reduce errors in patient care. Information system vendors are responding by developing such systems themselves and by purchasing the rights to patient care systems developed in academic medical centers that have demonstrated reductions in errors and gains in quality of care and cost control. "**Closed loop**" medication systems use technologies such as bar codes and decision support to guard against errors throughout the process of prescribing, dispensing, administering, and

Table 16.4. Computerized Notes*

	LDSH	WMH	BWH	QMC†	VAPS
Inpatient	Physicians: admission, allergies, medications, procedures, discharge summary. Nurses: initial assessment, progress, vital signs, handover, medication administration record. Therapists: all notes	Physicians: problem list, allergies, medications, admission note, progress (60% house staff, 100% attending physicians), procedures (50%), discharge summary. Nurses: initial assessment (70%), vital signs. Therapists: most notes	Physicians: problem list, allergies, medications, some progress in the form of a handover summary, procedure notes, discharge summary	Physicians: problem list, allergies, medications, history, procedures. Nurses: initial assessment, vital signs (general wards), operative notes, medication administration record	Physicians: problem list (85%), allergies, medications, admission, progress, procedures, discharge summary. Nurses: initial assessment, progress notes, vital signs (50%), operative notes, medication administration record (80%), discharge summary. Therapists: all notes
Ambulatory	Physicians: problem list, allergies, medications, history and physical findings, procedures. Nurses: vital signs	Physicians: problem list, allergies, medications, history and physical findings (50%), vital signs, procedures (70%). Nurses: vital signs	Physicians: problem list, allergies, medications, history and physical findings. Nurses: vital signs	Physicians: problem list, allergies, medications, history and physical findings, procedures. Nurses: initial assessment, vital signs	Physicians: problem list (85%), allergies, medications, history and physical findings, procedures. Nurses: initial assessment (80%), vital signs (90%). Therapists: all notes
Emergency department	Physicians: allergies, medications, discharge summary. Nurses: initial assessment, progress, vital signs, transfer, medication administration record, discharge summary	Physicians: problem list, allergies, medications (discharge only), discharge summary	Physicians: allergies, medications, summary note by attending physician on all patients	Physicians: summary note by attending physician on all patients. Nurses: initial assessment, discharge summary	Physicians: problem list (85%), allergies, medications (67%), history and physical findings, progress, discharge summary. Nurses: initial assessment, vital signs (10%)

*Indicates 100% of listed function unless otherwise statement.

†At QMC internal hospital ambulatory clinics and 11 out of 237 affiliated physician clinics using computerized notes.

Reprinted with permission. Doolan, DF, Bates, DW, & James, BC (2003). Journal of the American Medical Informatics Association, 10(1), p. 99.

recording. In other contexts, decision support systems offer "best practice" guidelines, protocols, and order sets as a starting point for planning individualized patient care; provide alerts and reminders; use knowledge bases and patient data bases to assess orders for potential contraindications; and offer point-and-click access to knowledge summaries and full-text publications. See Chapter 20 for more information about these systems.

Many healthcare agencies have substantial investment in legacy systems and cannot simply switch to more modern technology. Finding ways to phase the transition from older systems to newer and more functional ones is a major challenge to health informatics. To make the transition from a patchwork of systems with self-contained functions to truly integrated systems with the capacity to meet emerging information needs is even more challenging (see Chapter 13). Approaches to making this transition are described in the Proceedings of the 1996 IAIMS Symposium (IAIMS, 1996) and in the Journal of the American Medical Informatics Association (Stead et al., 1996).

The cornerstone of good patient-care systems is the ability to capture clinical data in the process of care, to store the data, to aggregate them, to analyze them, and to produce reports that not only describe care but also yield knowledge of quality, effectiveness, and costs that can be the basis of improved clinical processes. The key to performing these operations is data standards (see Chapters 2, 7, 12, 13, and 15). It is vital that the data standards support the care delivery and evaluation processes of the variety of healthcare professionals who participate in patient care. In this regard, the nursing profession has made substantial efforts in the creation of standardized nursing languages. More recently through the development of SNOMED CT (see Chapter 7 for more details), data reflective of the care provided others such as dentists, podiatrists, nutritionists, and physical therapists have augmented the standardized terms typically used by physicians and nurses.

If patient-care systems are to be effective in supporting better care, healthcare professionals must possess the informatics competencies to use the systems. Consequently, many are integrating informatics competencies into health science education (See Chapter 21). For example at the Columbia University School of Nursing, basic and advanced practice nursing students document their clinical encounters using personal digital assistants and receive educational content designed to meet professional standards for informatics competencies for beginning and experienced nurses, respectively (Bakken et al, 2003).

To what degree do patient-care disciplines need to prepare their practitioners for roles as informatics specialists? To the degree that members of the discipline use information in ways unique to the discipline, the field needs members prepared to translate the needs of clinicians to those who develop, implement, and make decisions about information systems. If the information needs are different from those of other disciplines, some practitioners should be prepared as system developers.

16.3   Current Research

Friedman (1995) proposed a typology of the science in medical informatics. The four categories build from fundamental conceptualization to evaluation as follows:

- Formulating models for acquisition, representation, processing, display, or transmission of biomedical information or knowledge
- Developing innovative computer-based systems, using these models, that deliver information or knowledge to healthcare providers
- Installing such systems and then making them work reliably in functioning healthcare environments
- Studying the effects of these systems on the reasoning and behavior of health-care providers, as well as on the organization and delivery of health care

Following are examples of recent research on patient-care systems in each category.

16.3.1   Formulation of Models

In recent years standards development organizations (SDOs) and professional groups alike have focused on the formulation of models that describe the patient care process and the formal structures that support management and documentation of patient care. The efforts of SDOs are summarized in Chapter 7. As a complement to SDO efforts, the Nursing Terminology Summit is an informal, interdisciplinary professional collaboratory whose participants develop and evaluate formal models such as reference information models, reference terminology models, and clinical document and EHR architectures from the perspective of nursing practice. Since the first Summit Conference in 1999, the participants' efforts have resulted in a number of significant achievements. These include among others: 1) agreement to collaborate to develop terminology models of diagnoses and interventions; 2) contribution to the development of a proposal to the International Standards Organization (ISO) from the Nursing Informatics Special Interest Group of the International Medical Informatics Association (IMIA) and the International Council of Nurses (ICN) to develop terminology models for nursing and to integrate those models with comprehensive models for health terminologies; 3) testing of the LOINC semantic structure for ability to represent standardized nursing assessments and subsequent integration of selected nursing content into LOINC; and 4) recommendations for extension to HL7 RIM in order to represent educational interventions (Ozbolt, 2000; Hardiker, Hoy, & Casey, 2000; Bakken, Cimino, Haskell, Kukafka, Matsumoto, Chan, & Huff, 2000).

16.3.2   Development of Innovative Systems

New systems to support patient care often take advantage of information entered in one context for use in other contexts. For example, the Brigham Integrated Computing System (BICS), a PC-based client–server HIS developed at Brigham and Women's Hospital in Boston, used information from the order entry, scheduling, and other systems to prepare drafts of the physician's discharge orders and the nurse's discharge abstract, thus minimizing the information to be entered manually. The professionals reviewed the drafts and edited as needed (O'Connell et al., 1996). The BICS system's success in this and other functions led to its acquisition for commercial deployment.

The principle of entering information once for multiple uses also drove development of the low-cost bedside workstations for intensive-care units at the University Hospital of Giessen, Germany (Michel et al., 1996). The client–server architecture combined local data-processing capabilities with a central relational patient database, permitting, for example, clinical nursing data to be used in calculating workload. These workstations also combined data from many sources, including medical devices, to support the integrated care of physicians, nurses, and other caregivers.

Even as systems such as these begin to fulfill some of the promises of informatics to support patient care, research and development continue to address the demands that the complexities of patient care place on information systems. Hoy and Hyslop (1995) reported a series of projects directed toward the development of a person-based health record. They found problems with traditional approaches to automating paper-based care-planning systems that resulted in loss of data detail, inability to use data for multiple purposes, and limitations in the capacity to aggregate and query patient data. Hoy and Hyslop (1995) recommended:

- Making the structure of the clinical record (including the care plan) more flexible and extensible to allow summarized higher-level data, with lower-level details where appropriate
- Simplifying the elements of that structure to make data entry and retrieval easier and more effective

Hoy and Hyslop (1995) built a prototype system to demonstrate their recommendations. Like other investigators, they concluded that "the issues of language and structures must be dealt with before the integration of person-based systems can be realized." As noted in Chapter 7, significant headway has been made in this regard during the last 5 years.

At Vanderbilt University Medical Center, patient-care systems have evolved since the mid-1990s to support patient safety and quality of care in a variety of ways. Clinical teams, assisted by specially trained clinical librarians, develop evidence-based order sets as templates for interdisciplinary care. These order sets are instantiated in Vanderbilt's order-entry system, where they serve as the starting point for planning and documenting each patient's care. When a patient is admitted to the hospital, a decision-support tool helps the physician to identify the appropriate evidence-based order set and then to edit the template to produce an individualized plan of care. In this way, the most current clinical knowledge provides the basis for each patient's care. Ozdas et al (2006) demonstrated that use of the evidence-based order set increased physician compliance with quality indicators for treating acute myocardial infarction. Other research opportunities are to explore the impact (positive or negative) of deviations from the template order sets in the context of different patient characteristics and comorbidities, thereby refining the evidence base and adding to clinical knowledge. Patient care systems like this make it possible to learn from data collected in the course of patient care about the effectiveness and safety of specific care practices and to integrate that emerging knowledge in continual quality improvement (Ozbolt, 2001, 2003).

16.3.3   Implementation of Systems

Higgins and associates (see Rotman et al., 1996) described the lessons learned from a failed implementation of a computer-based physician workstation that had been designed to facilitate and improve ordering of medications. Those lessons are not identical to, but are consistent with, the recommendations of Leiner and Haux (1996) in their protocol for systematic planning and execution of projects to develop and implement patient-care systems. As these experiences demonstrate, the implementation of patient-care systems is far more complex than the replacement of one technology with another. Such systems transform work and organizational relationships. If the implementation is to succeed, attention must be given to these transformations and to the disruptions that they entail. Southon and colleagues (1997) provided an excellent case study of the role of organizational factors in the failed implementation of a patient-care system that had been successful in another site. To realize the promise of informatics for health and clinical management, people who develop and promote the use of applications must anticipate, evaluate, and accommodate the full range of consequences. In early 2003, these issues came to the attention of the public-at-large when a large academic medical center decided to temporarily halt implementation of its CPOE system due to mixed acceptance by the physician staff (Chin, 2003). A case series study by Doolan, Bates, and James (2003) identified five key factors associated with successful implementation: 1) having organizational leadership, commitment, and vision; 2) improving clinical processes and patient care; 3) involving clinicians in the design and modification of the system; 4) maintaining or improving clinical productivity; and 5) building momentum and support amongst clinicians.

16.3.4   Study of the Effects of Systems

Many studies of the effects of patient care systems have looked at impact on process of care. A frequent expectation of systems to support nursing care planning and documentation is that they will decrease the time required for documentation, improve the quality and relevance of data in the record, and increase the proportion of nursing time spent in direct patient care. Pabst and colleagues (1996) found that an automated system designed to replace just 40 percent of manual documentation decreased the time required for documentation by one third, or by 20 minutes per shift. Nurses using the system spent more time in direct patient care and were more likely than were nurses using only manual documentation to complete documentation during their shifts rather than staying over into the next shift. Quality of documentation was not affected. Oniki et al. (2003) demonstrated a significant decrease in charting deficiencies in the ICU following computer-based reminders. Adderley and associates (1997) described the benefits of a phased implementation of a paperless record as related to accessibility of the record. Verbal orders were eliminated, and progress notes were more likely to be entered. Communications among caregivers were enhanced. Prospective, rather than retrospective, reviews of clinical data provided concurrent assessment of patient progress, care planning, medication use, and ancillary services. Annual cost avoidance from using the electronic patient record was estimated at more than $300,000. Lusignan et al. (2003) showed that feedback improved the quality of computer-based records in primary care in aspects such as linking prescriptions to diagnosis.

While improvements in processes of care are important, many patient care systems are designed with improving patient safety and outcomes in mind. Ruland (2002) reported that a handheld support system for preference-based care planning (CHOICE) not only improved the consistency of nursing care with patient preferences, but also increased patient achievement related to functional status. Bates et al. (2003) conducted a systematic review of information technologies for detecting adverse events and concluded that tools such as event monitoring and natural language processing can inexpensively detect adverse events such as adverse drug events and nosocomial infections. Wilson et al. (1997) demonstrated that the use of a shared computer-based medication record by pharmacy and nursing led to a statistically significant decrease in medication occurrences. .Chapters 12, 17, and 20 provide additional details about the effects of particular types of systems used in patient care.

Improving the methods of evaluating information resources was the driving force behind the Institute of Medicine's 1996 report on telemedicine (Field, 1996). Finding assessments of technical performance insufficient, the report recommended that evaluations focus on effects on patient welfare and on the processes and costs of care in comparison to those of reasonable alternatives. Members of the committee who developed the report noted that telemedicine may be considered a subset of medical informatics and that the methods of research and evaluation applicable to telemedicine are like those applicable to other patient-care systems (also see Chapter 14).

16.4   Outlook for the Future

Patient-care systems are changing in two ways. First, legacy systems designed primarily for charge capture and other administrative functions are being replaced by systems designed to support and improve clinical practice, as well as to send clinical data to the various locations where these data are needed for practice, management, and research. Second, systems designed to support each discipline separately are yielding to those based on integrated, interdisciplinary concepts of care. Research is continuing to develop structured clinical languages, standards, and data models; to develop innovative systems; to determine more effective and efficient ways to implement systems; and to investigate the effects of changing information resources on the processes of care and the functioning of the organization.

This environment is a fertile one for the development and growth of patient-care systems. In the first decade of the 21st Century, systems that will perform all the desired functions at a high level remain just out of reach. Many factors—evolution of technology, development of standards, and societal demands among them—are converging to stimulate rapid progress. Real-world systems are extending their mastery over more and more of the functions needed to support patient care: intelligent support for clinical decisions; better organization and communication; feedback on clinical effectiveness; linked databases for research; and administrative analyses based on pertinent clinical data. Such tools will make available to clinicians, managers, and policy-makers the data, information, and knowledge required for sound decisions and effective action. By complementing and extending cognitive processes, patient-care systems become an integral and essential technology for patient care.

Suggested Readings

Doolan, DF, Bates, DW, & James, BC (2003). The use of computers for clinical care: A case series of advanced U.S. sites. Journal of the American Medical Informatics Association, 10(1), 94-107.
This article describes the clinical information systems in 5 U.S. hospitals that have won the Davies Award for outstanding systems. The article describes similarities and differences in the systems and experiences at these sites and identifies factors important to successful implementation.

Ruland, CM (2002). Handheld technology to improve patient care. Journal of the American Medical Informatics Association, 9(2), 192-200.
This research study evaluates the effectiveness of a handheld application to elicit patients' preferences for functional performance. Use of the application improved the frequency with which patients' preferences were respected.

Ida M. Androwich, Carol J. Bickford, Patricia S. Button, Kathleen M. Hunter, Judy Murphy, and Joyce Sensmeier (2002) Clinical Information Systems: A Framework for Reaching the Vision. Washington, DC: ANA Publishing.
This concise synthesis of healthcare informatics articulates an organizing framework for clinical information systems from a professional nursing perspective, and addresses how to best design, develop, and implement them.

Questions for Discussion

1. What is the utility of a linear model of patient care as the basis for a decision-support system? What are two primary limitations? Discuss two challenges that a nonlinear model poses for representing and supporting the care process in an information system?
2. Compare and contrast "segregated" versus "integrated" models of interdisciplinary patient care. What are the advantages and disadvantages of each model as a mode of care delivery? As the basis for developing information systems to plan, document, and support patient care?
3. Imagine a patient-care information system that assists in planning the care of each patient independently of all the other patients in a service center or patient-care unit. What are three advantages to the developer in choosing such an information architecture? What would be the likely result in the real world of practice? Does it make a difference whether the practice setting is hospital, ambulatory care, or home care? What would be the simplest information architecture that would be sufficiently complex to handle real-world demands? Explain.
4. Zielstorff et al. (1993) proposed that data routinely recorded during the process of patient care could be abstracted, aggregated, and analyzed for management reports,

policy decisions, and knowledge development. What are three advantages of using patient care data in this way? What are three significant limitations?

5. A number of patient-care information systems designed in the 1970s are still in use. How do the practice models, payer models, and quality focus of today differ from those of the past? What differences do these changes require in information systems? What are two advantages and two disadvantages of "retrofitting" these changes on older systems versus designing new systems "from scratch"?

6. What are three advantages and three disadvantages of free text (including oral narrative entered by dictation) versus structured data for recording observations, assessments, goals, and plans? What is the impact of using free text on the ability to retrieve and aggregate data? Should developmental efforts focus on interpreting natural language or on creating data standards? Explain your position.

7. What are four major purposes of patient care information systems? What criteria should be used to evaluate them? What methods of evaluation could be used to assess the system with respect to these criteria?

17
Patient-Monitoring Systems

REED M. GARDNER AND M. MICHAEL SHABOT

After reading this chapter,[1] you should know the answers to these questions:

- What is patient monitoring, and why is it done?
- What are the primary applications of computerized patient-monitoring systems in the intensive-care unit?
- How do computer-based patient monitors aid health professionals in collecting, analyzing, and displaying data?
- What are the advantages of using microprocessors in bedside monitors?
- What are the important issues for collecting high-quality data either automatically or manually in the intensive-care unit?
- Why is integration of data from many sources in the hospital necessary if a computer is to assist in critical-care-management decisions?

17.1 What Is Patient Monitoring?

Continuous measurement of patient parameters such as heart rate and rhythm, respiratory rate, blood pressure, blood-oxygen saturation, and many other parameters have become a common feature of the care of critically ill patients. When accurate and immediate decision-making is crucial for effective patient care, electronic monitors frequently are used to collect and display physiological data. Increasingly, such data are collected using non-invasive sensors from less seriously ill patients in a hospital's medical-surgical units, labor and delivery suites, nursing homes, or patients' own homes to detect unexpected life-threatening conditions or to record routine but required data efficiently.

We usually think of a **patient monitor** as something that watches for—and warns against—serious or life-threatening events in patients, critically ill or otherwise. **Patient monitoring** can be rigorously defined as "repeated or continuous observations or measurements of the patient, his or her physiological function, and the function of life support equipment, for the purpose of guiding management decisions, including when to make therapeutic interventions, and assessment of those interventions" (Hudson, 1985, p. 630). A patient monitor may not only alert caregivers to potentially life-threatening

---

[1]Portions of this chapter are based on Shabot M.M., Gardner R.M. (Eds.) (1994). Decision Support Systems in Critical Care, Boston, Springer-Verlag; and Gardner R.M., Sittig D.F., Clemmer T.P. (1995). Computers in the ICU: A Match Meant to Be! In Ayers S.M., et al. (Eds.), Textbook of Critical Care (3rd ed., p. 1757). Philadelphia, W.B. Saunders.

events; many also provide physiologic input data used to control directly connected life-support devices.

In this chapter, we discuss the use of computers to assist caregivers in the collection, display, storage, and decision-making, including interpretation of clinical data, making therapeutic recommendations, and alarming and alerting. In the past, most clinical data were in the form of heart and respiratory rates, blood pressures, and flows, but today they include integrating data from bedside instruments which measure blood gases, chemistry, and hematology as well as integrating data from many sources outside the intensive-care unit (ICU). Although we deal primarily with patients who are in ICUs, the general principles and techniques are also applicable to other hospitalized patients. For example, patient monitoring may be performed for diagnostic purposes in the emergency room or for therapeutic purposes in the operating room. Techniques that just a few years ago were used only in the ICU are now routinely used on general hospital units and in some situations by patients at home.

17.1.1   A Case Report

We will use a case report to provide a perspective on the problems faced by the health-care team caring for a critically ill patient: A young man is injured in an automobile accident. He has multiple chest and head injuries. His condition is stabilized at the accident scene by skilled paramedics using a microcomputer-based **electrocardiogram** (ECG) monitor, and he is quickly transported to a trauma center. Once in the trauma center, the young man is connected via sensors to computer-based monitors that determine his heart rate and rhythm and his blood pressure. Because of the head injury, the patient has difficulty breathing, so he is connected to a microprocessor-controlled ventilator. Later, he is transferred to the ICU. A fiberoptic pressure-monitoring sensor is inserted through a bolt drilled through his skull to continuously measure intracranial pressure with another computer-controlled monitor. Clinical chemistry and blood-gas tests are performed in two minutes at the bedside with a microcartridge inserted into the physiologic monitor, and the results are transmitted to the laboratory computer system and the ICU system using a Health Level 7 (HL7) interface over a standard Ethernet network. With intensive treatment, the patient survives the initial threats to his life and now begins the long recovery process.

Unfortunately, a few days later, he is beset with a problem common to multiple trauma victims—he has a major *nosocomial* (hospital-acquired) *infection* and develops **sepsis, adult respiratory distress syndrome** (ARDS), and multiple organ failure. As a result, even more monitoring sensors are needed to acquire data and to assist with the patient's treatment; the quantity of information required to care for the patient has increased dramatically.

The ICU computer system provides suggestions about how to care for the specific problems, provides visual alerts for life-threatening situations, and organizes and reports the mass of data so that caregivers can make prompt and reliable treatment decisions. The patient's physicians are automatically alerted to critical laboratory and blood gas results as well as to complex physiological conditions by detailed alphanumeric pager messages. His ARDS is managed with the assistance of a computer-monitored and controlled protocol. Figure 17.1 shows a nurse at the patient's bedside surrounded by a **bedside monitor**, **infusion pumps** and a **microprocessor** controlled **ventilator**. Figure 17.2 shows an example of a computer-generated ICU report produced by the HELP system (HELP is discussed in Chapter 13). This report summarizes 24 hours of patient data and is used by physicians to review a patient's status during daily rounds (daily visits by physicians to their hospitalized patients).

17.1.2 *Patient Monitoring in Intensive-Care Units*

There are at least five categories of patients who need physiological monitoring:

1. Patients with unstable physiological regulatory systems; for example, a patient whose respiratory system is suppressed by a drug overdose or anesthesia
2. Patients with a suspected life-threatening condition; for example, a patient who has findings indicating an acute myocardial infarction (heart attack)
3. Patients at high risk of developing a life-threatening condition; for example, patients immediately after open-heart surgery or a premature infant whose heart and lungs are not fully developed
4. Patients in a critical physiological state; for example, patients with multiple trauma or septic shock.
5. Mother and baby during the labor and delivery process.

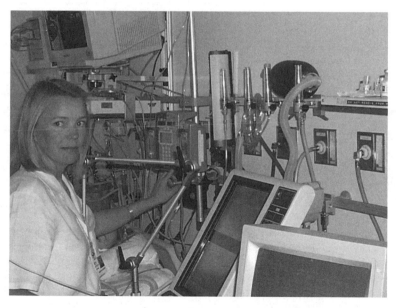

Figure 17.1. A nurse at a patient's ICU bedside. Above the nurse's head is the bedside monitor which measurse and displays key physiological data, above her left hand is an IV pump connected to a Medical Information Bus (MIB), to her right are two screens of a patient ventilator and to the far right is a bedside computer terminal used for data entry and data review. (*Source:* Courtesy of Dr. Reed M. Gardner)

```
                        L D S   H O S P I T A L   I C U   R O U N D S   R E P O R T
                                       DATA WITHIN LAST 24 HOURS

NAME:        , STEVEN                NO.    10072      ROOM: E609                      DATE: JAN 29 14:17
DR. STINSON, JAMES B.          SEX: M   AGE:  43   HEIGHT: 178  WEIGHT:  75.40   BSA: 1.93   BEE: 1697  MOF:  0
ADMT DIAGNOSIS: FEVER UNK ORIGN, S/P KIDNEY TR   ADMIT DATE: 14 DEC 88
_____
CARDIOVASCULAR:  0                                               EXAM: _____
    -- NO CARDIAC OUTPUT DATA AVAILABLE
                SP   DP   MP   HR  | LACT       CPK        CPK-MB     LDH-1      LDH-2
    LAST VALUES 121   68   89  113 |
    MAXIMUM     194   97  126  124 |  (    )    (    )    (    )    (    )    (    )
    MINIMUM     101   58   72   83 *
_____
RESPIRATORY:   0
            pH   PCO2  HCO3   BE    HB   CO/MT   PO2  SO2  O2CT  %O2  AVO2  VO2   C.O.   A-a  QS/QT PK/ PL/PP  MR/SR
29 06:21 A 7.43  27.3  18.0  -4.5  10.0   2/ 1   80   94  13.2   30                      66        0/ 0/ 5  17/ 0
         SAMPLE # 74, TEMP 38.4, BREATHING STATUS : ASSIST/CONTROL
         NORMAL ARTERIAL ACID-BASE CHEMISTRY
         SEVERELY REDUCED O2 CONTENT (13.2) DUE TO ANEMIA (LOW HB)

         ------- machine settings ------- | ---------------------------- patient values ----------------------------
         VENT  MODE   VR   Vt   O2%    PF   IP    MAP   PK  PL  PP  m-Vt  c-Vt  s-Vt   MR   SR   TR   m-VE  s-VE  t-VE  Cth   Pc
29 14:15 B-I   A/C   16  700   30     50        32  26   5  866   731        29        21.2                    34.8
29 06:05 B-I   A/C   16  700   30     50        22  20   5  830   745        19        14.2                    49.7
29 14:15  5/14:16   INTERFACE: TRACH TUBE;  ALARMS CHECKED; POSITION: SUPINE;  THERAPIST: DAVIS, TERIANNE, CRTT
29 06:05 10/06:08   INTERFACE: TRACH TUBE;  ALARMS CHECKED; POSITION: SEMI-FOWLER;  PATIENT CONDITION: CALM;  SUCTIONED, 3 CC,
         HEMOPTIC;  THERAPIST: TARR, TED, RRT

   DATE   TIME    HR   VR    VT   VC    VE   MIP  MEP  MVV  PK FLOW THERAPIST                EXAM: _____
01/29/89 07:15  109   20   600       12.0  -60              DAVIS, TERIANNE                       _____
_____
NEURO AND PSYCH:   0
     GLASCOW  6 (08:00)  VERBAL _____  EYELIDS _____  MOTOR _____  PUPILS _____  SENSORY _____

     DTR _____    BABIN. _____   ICP _____    PSYCH _____
_____
COAGULATION:  0
     PT:   14.2   (05:15   )  PTT:    50 (05:15   )  PLATELETS:   89 (05:15   )  FIBRINOGEN:   0(00:00) EXAM:_____
     FSP-CON:   0 (00:00  )  FSP-PT:   0 (00:00   )  3P:         (00:00   )                                 _____
_____
RENAL, FLUIDS, LYTES:   0
   IN   3430 CRYST  1025  COLLOID  1035  BLOOD      NG/PO  1340 | NA       (    ) K       (    ) CL     (    )
   OUT  2689 URINE   800  NGOUT     500  DRAINS  25 OTHER  1364 | CO2 21.0 (05:15) BUN  51 (05:15) CRE  4.2 (05:15)
   NET   741 WT    75.40  WT-CHG         S.G.     1.015        | AGAP  16.7         UOSM           UNA      CRCL
_____
METABOLIC --- NUTRITION:   0
   KCAL    2630  GLU  138   (05:15)  ALB   2.9 (05:15) | CA   7.7 (05:15) FE    .0 (00:00) TIBC    0 (00:00)
   KCAL/N2  891  UUN   .0 (00:00)  N-BAL   .0         | PO4  1.9 (05:15) MG   1.9 (05:15) CHOL  228 (05:15)
_____
GI, LIVER, AND PANCREAS:   0                                                                  EXAM:
   HCT    29.4 (05:15)  TOTAL BILI   23.1 (05:15)  SGOT   73 (05:15)  ALKPO4  957 (05:15)  GGT    768 (05:15) _____
   GUAIAC      (    )   DIRECT BILI  17.4 (05:15)  SGPT   99 (05:15)  LDH     237 (05:15)  AMYLASE  0 (00:00) _____
_____
INFECTION:   0
   WBC  5.2(05:15 )  TEMP  40.3 (28/06:00)  DIFF  26 B, 70P,  3L,  1M,  E (05:15) GRAM STAIN: SPUTUM _____  OTHER _____
_____
SKIN AND EXTREMITIES:
   PULSES _____   RASH _____   DECUBITI _____
_____
TUBES:
   VEN _____    ART _____   SG _____   NG _____   FOLEY _____   ET _____   TRACH _____   DRAIN_____

   CHEST _____   RECTAL _____   JEJUNAL _____   DIALYSIS _____   OTHER _____
_____
MEDICATIONS:

MORPHINE, INJ                          MGM  IV     20   AMPHOJEL, LIQUID                        ML   NG       30
MEPERIDINE (DEMEROL), INJ              MGM  IV    150   DIPHENHYDRAMINE (BENADRYL), INJ         MGM  IV      100
PHENYTOIN (DILANTIN), SUSPENSION       MGM  NG    300   HYDROCORTISONE NA SUCCINATE (SOLU-CORTEF)MGM, IV     200
MIDAZOLAM (VERSED), INJ                MGM  IV      5   AMIN-AID FULL STRENGTH, LIQUID          ML   NG D    1380
AMPHOTERICIN B, INJ                    MGM  IV     40   TAP WATER, LIQUID                       ML   NG       60
CEFTAZIDIME (FORTAZ), INJ              MGM  IV   1000   MAGNESIUM SULFATE 50%, INJ              GM   IV        2
SUCRALFATE (CARAFATE), TAB             MGM  NG   4000   POTASSIUM CHLORIDE, INJ                 MEQ  IV       20
FAMOTIDINE (PEPCID), INJ               MGM  IV     40   NOVOLIN REGULAR, INJ                    UNITS IV      58
                                                                                               #087 · pgl
```

Figure 17.2. Rounds report used at LDS Hospital in Salt Lake City for evaluation of patients each day during teaching and decision-making rounds. The report abstracts data from diverse locations and sources and organizes them to reflect the physiological systems of interest. Listed at the top of the report is patient-identification and patient-characterization information. Next is information about the cardiovascular system; data for other systems follow. (*Source:* Courtesy of LDS Hospital.)

Care of the critically ill patient requires prompt and accurate decisions so that life-protecting and life-saving therapy can be appropriately applied. Because of these requirements, ICUs have become widely established in hospitals. Such units use computers almost universally for the following purposes:

- To acquire physiological data frequently or continuously, such as blood pressure readings
- To communicate information from data-producing systems to remote locations (e.g., laboratory and radiology departments)
- To store, organize, and report data
- To integrate and correlate data from multiple sources
- To provide clinical alerts and advisories based on multiple sources of data
- To function as a decision-making tool that health professionals may use in planning the care of critically ill patients
- To measure the severity of illness for patient classification purposes
- To analyze the outcomes of ICU care in terms of clinical effectiveness and cost effectiveness

17.2 Historical Perspective

The earliest foundations for acquiring physiological data date to the end of the Renaissance period.[2] In 1625, Santorio, who lived in Venice at the time, published his methods for measuring body temperature with the spirit thermometer and for timing the pulse (heart) rate with a pendulum. The principles for both devices had been established by Galileo, a close friend. Galileo worked out the uniform periodicity of the pendulum by timing the period of the swinging chandelier in the Cathedral of Pisa, using his own pulse rate as a timer. The results of this early biomedical-engineering collaboration, however, were ignored. The first scientific report of the pulse rate did not appear until Sir John Floyer published "Pulse-Watch" in 1707. The first published course of fever for a patient was plotted by Ludwig Taube in 1852. With subsequent improvements in the clock and the thermometer, the temperature, pulse rate, and respiratory rate became the standard **vital signs**.

In 1896, Scipione Riva-Rocci introduced the sphygmomanometer (blood pressure cuff), which permitted the fourth vital sign, arterial blood pressure, to be measured. A Russian physician, Nikolai Korotkoff, applied Riva-Rocci's cuff with a stethoscope developed by the French physician Rene Laennec to allow the auscultatory measurement[3] of both systolic and diastolic arterial pressure. Harvey Cushing, a preeminent U.S. neurosurgeon of the early 1900s, predicted the need for and later insisted on routine arterial blood pressure monitoring in the operating room. Cushing also raised two questions familiar even at the turn of the century: (1) Are we collecting too much data?

---

[2] This section has been adapted, with permission, from Glaeser D.H., Thomas L.J. Jr. (1975). Computer monitoring in patient care. Annual Review of Biophysics and Bioengineering, 4:449–476, copyright Annual Reviews, Inc.

[3] In medicine, auscultation is the process of listening to the sounds made by structures within the body, such as by the heart or by the blood moving within the vessels.

(2) Are the instruments used in clinical medicine too accurate? Would not approximated values be just as good? Cushing answered his own questions by stating that vital-sign measurements should be made routinely and that accuracy was important (Cushing, 1903).

Since the 1920s, the four vital signs—temperature, respiratory rate, heart rate, and arterial blood pressures—have been recorded in all patient charts. In 1903, Willem Einthoven devised the string galvanometer for measuring the electrocardiogram (ECG), for which he was awarded the 1924 Nobel Prize in physiology. The ECG has become an important adjunct to the clinician's inventory of tests for both acutely and chronically ill patients. Continuous measurement of physiological variables has become a routine part of the monitoring of critically ill patients.

At the same time that advances in monitoring were made, major changes in the therapy of life-threatening disorders were also occurring. Prompt quantitative evaluation of measured physiological and biochemical variables became essential in the decision-making process as physicians applied new therapeutic interventions. For example, it is now possible—and in many cases essential—to use ventilators when a patient cannot breathe independently, cardiopulmonary bypass equipment when a patient undergoes open-heart surgery, hemodialysis when a patient's kidneys fail, and intravenous (IV) nutritional and electrolyte (e.g., potassium and sodium) support when a patient is unable to eat or drink.

17.2.1   Development of Intensive-Care Units

To meet the increasing demands for more acute and intensive care required by patients with complex disorders, new organizational units—the ICUs—were established in hospitals beginning in the 1950s. The earliest units were simply postoperative recovery rooms used for prolonged stays after open-heart surgery. Intensive-care units proliferated rapidly during the late 1960s and 1970s. The types of units include burn, coronary, general surgery, open-heart surgery, pediatric, neonatal, respiratory, and multipurpose medical-surgical units. Today there are an estimated 75,000 adult, pediatric, and neonatal intensive care beds in the United States.

The development of **transducers** and electronic instrumentation during World War II dramatically increased the number of physiological variables that could be monitored. Analog-computer technology was widely available, as were oscilloscopes, electronic devices used to depict changes in electrical potential on a cathode-ray tube (CRT) screen. These devices were soon used in specialized cardiac-catheterization[4] laboratories, and they rapidly found their way to the bedside.

Treatment for serious cardiac arrhythmias (rhythm disturbances) and cardiac arrest (abrupt cessation of heartbeat)—major causes of death after myocardial infarctions—became possible. As a result, there was a need to monitor the ECGs of patients who had suffered heart attacks so that these episodes could be noticed and

---

[4]A procedure whereby a tube (catheter) is passed into the heart through an artery or vein, allowing the cardiologist to measure pressure within the heart's chambers, to obtain blood samples, to inject contrast dye for radiological procedures, and so

treated immediately. In 1963, Day reported that treatment of postmyocardial-infarction patients in a coronary-care unit reduced mortality by 60 percent. As a consequence, coronary-care units—with ECG monitors—proliferated. The addition of online blood-pressure monitoring quickly followed. **Pressure transducers**, already used in the cardiac-catheterization laboratory, were easily adapted to the monitors in the ICU.

With the advent of more automated instruments, the ICU nurse could spend less time manually measuring the traditional vital signs and more time observing and caring for the critically ill patient. Simultaneously, a new trend emerged; some nurses moved away from the bedside to a central console where they could monitor the ECG and other vital-sign reports from many patients. Maloney (1968) pointed out that this was an inappropriate use of technology when it deprived the patient of adequate personal attention at the bedside. He also suggested that having the nurse record vital signs every few hours was "only to assure regular nurse–patient contact" (Maloney, 1968, p. 606).

As monitoring capabilities expanded, physicians and nurses soon were confronted with a bewildering number of instruments; they were threatened by **data overload**. Several investigators suggested that the digital computer might be helpful in solving the problems associated with data collection, review, and reporting.

17.2.2   Development of Computer-Based Monitoring

Teams from several cities in the United States introduced computers for physiological monitoring into the ICU, beginning with Shubin and Weil (1966) in Los Angeles and then Warner and colleagues (1968) in Salt Lake City. These investigators had several motives: (1) to increase the availability and accuracy of data, (2) to compute derived variables that could not be measured directly, (3) to increase patient-care efficacy, (4) to allow display of the time trend of patient data, and (5) to assist in computer-aided decision-making. Each of these teams developed its application on a mainframe computer system, which required a large computer room and special staff to keep the system operational 24 hours per day. The computers used by these developers cost over $200,000 each in 1965 dollars! Other researchers were attacking more specific challenges in patient monitoring. For example, Cox and associates (1972) in St. Louis developed algorithms to analyze the ECG for heart rhythm disturbances in real-time. The arrhythmia-monitoring system, which was installed in the coronary-care unit of Barnes Hospital in 1969, ran on a relatively inexpensive microcomputer.

As we described in Chapter 5, the advent of integrated circuits and other advances allowed computing power per dollar to increase dramatically. As hardware became smaller, more reliable, and less expensive, and as better software tools were developed, simple analog processing gave way to digital signal processing. Monitoring applications developed by the pioneers using large central computers now became possible using dedicated microprocessor-based machines at the bedside.

The early bedside monitors were built around "bouncing-ball" or conventional oscilloscopes and analog-computer technology. As computer technology has advanced, the definition of **computer-based monitoring** has changed. The early developers spent a major part of their time deriving data from analog physiological signals. Soon the data-storage and decision-making capabilities of the computer monitoring systems came under the investigator's scrutiny. Therefore, what was considered computer-based patient monitoring in the late 1960s and early 1970s is now entirely built into bedside monitors and is considered simply a "bedside monitor." Systems with database functions, report-generation systems, and some decision-making capabilities are usually called **computer-based patient monitors**.

17.3   Data Acquisition and Signal Processing

The use of microcomputers in bedside monitors has revolutionized the acquisition, display, and processing of physiological data. There are virtually no bedside monitors or ventilators marketed today that do not use at least one microcomputer. Figure 17.3 shows a block diagram of a bedside monitor. Physiological signals such as the ECG are derived from sensors that convert biological signals (such as pressure, flow, or mechanical movement) into electrical signals. In modern computerized monitors, these signals are digitized as close to the patient as possible.

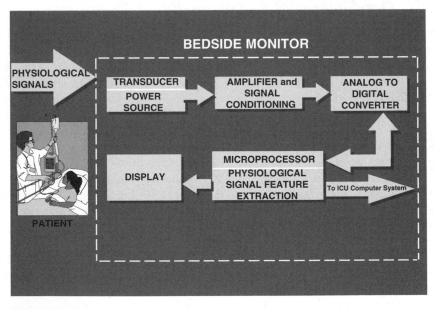

Figure 17.3. Block diagram of a modern Bedside Monitor. Physiological signals from the patient are acquired by transducers. These transducers convert the appropriate physiological signal into an electrical signal that is then amplified and conditioned (usually an analog filter of some sort) and then present the signal to an Analog to Digitial converter (ADC) . The ADC sends the data to a microprocessor based signal processor which extracts features such as heart rate and blood pressure. After processing, the physiological signals are displayed on a display device and usually sent to a centralized ICU display system and frequently to a electronic patient record.

Some biological signals are already in electrical form, such as the currents that traverse the heart and are recorded as the ECG. The ECG voltage signal derived from the electrodes at the body surface is small—only a few millivolts in amplitude. The patient is electrically isolated from the bedside monitor, and the analog ECG signal is amplified to a level sufficient for conversion to digital data using an analog-to-digital converter (ADC). Digital data then can be processed and the results displayed (Weinfurt, 1990, p. 130) (Figure 17.4).

As discussed in Chapter 5, the sampling rate is an important factor that affects the correspondence between an analog signal and that signal's digital representation. Figure 17.5 shows an ECG that has been sampled at four different rates. At a rate of 500 measurements per second (Figure 17.5a), the digitized representation of the ECG looks like an analog recording of the ECG. All the features of the ECG, including the shape of the P wave (atrial depolarization), the amplitude of the QRS complex (ventricular depolarization), and the shape of the T wave (ventricular recovery), are reproduced faithfully. When the sampling rate is decreased to 100 measurements per second, however, the amplitude and shape of the QRS complex begin to be distorted. When only 50 observations per second are recorded, the QRS complex is grossly distorted, and the other features also begin to distort. At a recording rate of only 25 measurements per second, gross signal distortion occurs, and even estimating heart rate by measuring intervals from R to R is problematic.

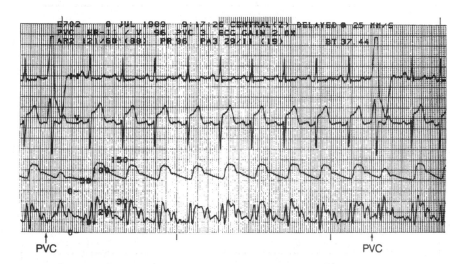

Figure 17.4. Electrocardiogram (first and second traces), arterial pressure (third trace), and pulmonary-artery pressure (fourth trace) recorded from a patient's bedside. Annotated on the recording are the bed number (E702), date (8 Jul 1989), and time (9:17:25). Also noted are a regular rhythm, a heart rate from the ECG (V) of 96 beats per minute, a systolic arterial pressure of 121, a diastolic pressure of 60, a mean pressure of 88 mm Hg, and a heart rate from pressure (PR) of 96. The patient is having premature ventricular contractions (PVCs) at a rate of three per minute; two PVCs can be seen in this tracing (at the beginning and near the end). The pulmonary-artery pressure is 29/11, with a mean of 19 mm Hg, and the blood temperature is 37.44°C. The self-contained monitoring system has determined the values and generated the calibrated graphical plot.

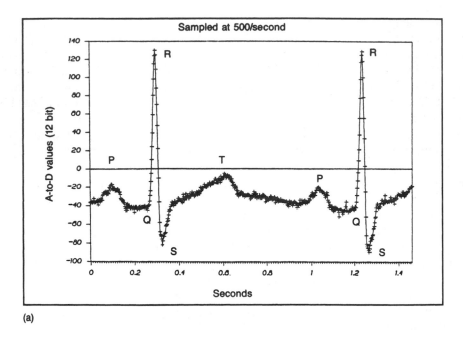

(a)

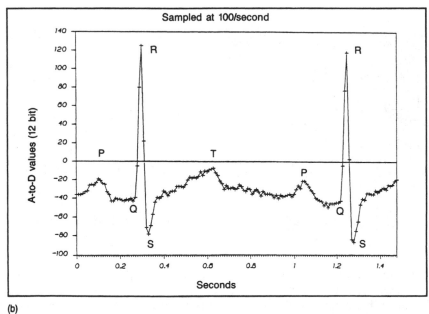

(b)

Figure 17.5. The sampling rate of the analog-to-digital converter determines the quality of the ECG. All four panels show the same ECG, sampled at different rates. Note the degradation of the quality of the signal as one proceeds from a to d. The ECG is sampled at 500 (a), 100 (b), 50 (c), and 25 (d) measurements per second.

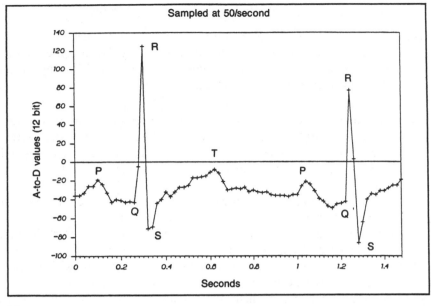

(c)

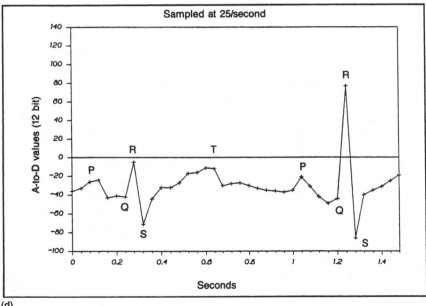

(d)

Figure 17.5. (*Continued*)

17.3.1   Advantages of Built-In Microcomputers

Today, bedside monitors contain multiple microcomputers, with much more computing power and memory than was available in the systems used by the computer monitoring pioneers. Bedside monitors with built-in microcomputers have the following advantages over their analog predecessors (Weinfurt, 1990):

* The digital computer's ability to store patient waveform information such as the ECG permits sophisticated **pattern recognition** and physiological signal **feature extraction**. Modern microcomputer-based bedside monitors use multiple ECG channels and pattern recognition schemes to identify abnormal waveform patterns and then to classify ECG arrhythmias.
* Signal quality from multiple ECG leads can now be monitored and interference noise minimized. For example, the computer can watch for degradation of ECG skin–electrode contact resistance. If the contact is poor, the monitor can alert the nurse to change the specified problematic electrode.
* Physiological signals can be acquired more efficiently by converting them to digital form early in the processing cycle. The waveform processing (e.g., calibration and filtering, as described in Chapter 5) then can be done in the microcomputer. The same process simplifies the nurse's task of setting up and operating the bedside monitor by eliminating the manual calibration step.
* Transmission of digitized physiological waveform signals is easier and more reliable. Digital transmission of data is inherently noise-free. As a result, newer monitoring systems allow health-care professionals to review a patient's waveform displays and derived parameters, such as heart rate and blood pressure, at the bedside, at a central station in the ICU, or at home via modem on a laptop computer. Figure 17.6 is a closeup of the signals and values from a typical bedside patient monitor.
* Selected data can be retained easily if they are digitized. For example, ECG strips of interesting physiological sequences, such as periods of arrhythmias (Figure 17.7), can be stored in the bedside monitor for later review. Today's monitors typically store all of the waveform data from multiple leads of ECG and blood pressure transducers for at least 24 hours and sometimes for even longer.
* Measured variables, such as heart rate and blood pressure, can be graphed over prolonged periods to aid with detection of life-threatening trends.
* Alarms from bedside monitors are now much "smarter"and raise fewer false alarms. In the past, analog alarm systems used only high–low threshold limits and were susceptible to **signal artifacts** (Gardner, 1997). Now, computer-based bedside monitors often can distinguish between artifacts and real alarm situations by using the information derived from one signal to verify that from another and can confidently alert physicians and nurses to real alarms. For example, heart rate can be derived from either the ECG or the arterial blood pressure. If both signals indicate dangerous tachycardia (fast heart rate), the system sounds an alarm. If the two signals do not agree, the monitor can notify the health-care professional about a potential instrumentation or medical problem. The procedure is not unlike that performed by a human verifying possible problems by using redundant information from simpler bedside monitor alarms. Despite these

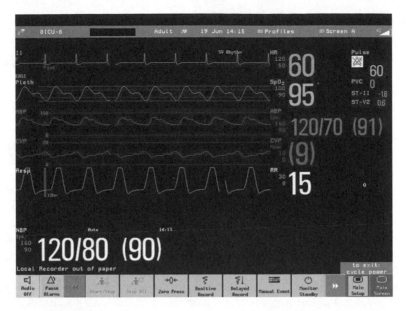

Figure 17.6. Close-up display of the screen of a modern bedside monitor showing physiological waveforms and numerical values derived from processing the diaplayed physiological data.

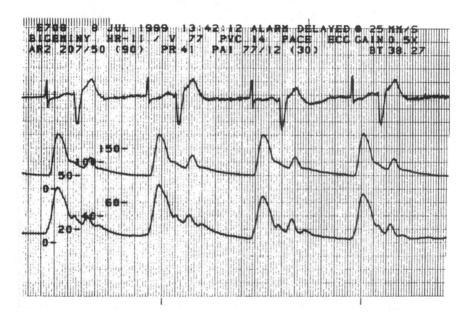

Figure 17.7. A strip showing a patient's ECG (upper trace) and arterial (middle trace) and pulmonary-artery (lower trace) pressure waveforms. The patient has a potentially life-threatening arrhythmia in which heart beats occur in pairs—a pattern called bigeminy. Note that, for two extra beats on the ECG pattern, the resulting pressure waveform pulsation is unusually small, indicating that the heart has not pumped much blood for that extra beat. The patient's heart rate, as determined from the ECG, is 77 beats per minute, whereas that determined from blood pressure is only 41 beats per minute. The heart is effectively beating at a very slow rate of 41 beats per minute.

advancements in bedside monitors, however, false alarms are still very prevalent (Tsien & Fackler, 1997, Koski et al 1995, Goldstein B 2003).

• Systems can be upgraded easily. Only the software programs in read-only memory (ROM) need to be changed; older analog systems required hardware replacement.

17.3.2   *Arrhythmia Monitoring—Signal Acquisition and Processing*

Although general-purpose computer-based physiological monitoring systems are now being more widely adopted, computer-based ECG arrhythmia-monitoring systems were accepted quickly (Weinfurt, 1990). Electrocardiographic arrhythmia analysis is one of the most sophisticated and difficult of the bedside monitoring tasks. Conventional arrhythmia monitoring, which depends on people observing displayed signals, is expensive, unreliable, tedious, and stressful to the observers. One early approach to overcoming these limitations was to purchase an arrhythmia-monitoring system operating on a time-shared central computer. Such minicomputer-based systems usually monitored 8 to 17 patients and cost at least $50,000.

The newest bedside monitors, in contrast, have built-in arrhythmia-monitoring systems. These computers generally use a 32-bit architecture, waveform templates, and real-time feature extraction in which the computer measures such features as the R-R interval and QRS complex width; and template correlation, in which incoming waveforms are compared point by point with already classified waveforms (Weinfurt, 1990). Figure 17.8 shows the output from a commercial bedside monitor. Using signals from four ECG leads the computer has correctly classified a rhythm abnormality—in this

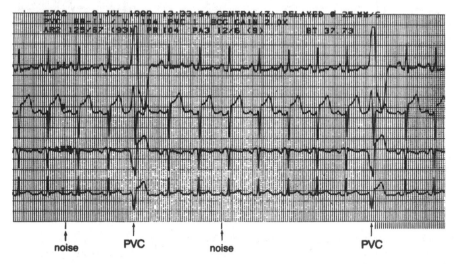

Figure 17.8. Two time-trend plots of systolic, mean, and diastolic pressure: a, 8 hours; b, 24 hours. Indicated across the bottom are the time of day at each of the tick marks. These plots show relatively stable blood-pressure trends over the 24-hour period.

case, a premature ventricular contraction (PVC). The bedside monitor also retains an ECG tracing record in its memory so that at a later time a health professional can review the information.

Wave Form Classification

Computer algorithms for processing ECG rhythms take sampled data, such as those shown in Figure 17.5, and extract features, such as the amplitude and duration of the QRS complex (Weinfurt, 1990). In most schemes, each time the QRS detector is tripped, it signals a beat classification subprogram, which receives four channels of ECG data at the same time. Such a beat-classification scheme compares the waveform of each incoming beat with that of one or more clinically relevant waveform classes already established for the patient. If the new waveform matches any of those already classified, the "template" of that waveform class is updated to reflect any minor evolutionary changes in the shape. Most beat-classification schemes have the capacity to store up to 30 templates. The performance of these multilead monitors has been dramatic; however, such arrhythmia monitors are still not perfect.

Detecting and identifying pacemaker signals poses special problems for digital computer-based monitoring systems. Pacemaker signals do not reliably traverse the analog acquisition circuitry, and the pacemaker "spikes" are very narrow such that they can occur between data samples and be missed entirely. As a result, special analog "injection" methods are used to enhance the pacemaker "spike" so that it can be more easily detected (Weinfurt, 1990).

Full-Disclosure and Multilead ECG Monitoring

Contemporary **central monitors** combine the advantages of digital waveform analysis as described above with high-capacity disk drives to store one or more days worth of continuous waveform data, including ECG. Some of these monitors can support recording full disclosure or synthesis of the entire 12-lead ECG on a second by second basis. Figure 17.9 shows a run of ventricular tachycardia in a portion of a 24-hour **full disclosure** ECG display. Figure 17.10 shows a bedside physiologic monitor displaying a Web page view of a full 12-lead ECG with computerized interpretations.

ST segment analysis of the ECG has also become very important because ST segment displacement is indicative of ischemic episodes of the heart muscle. Changes in open-heart procedure and administration of thrombolytic therapy are predicated on ST segment analysis. Multilead monitors now offer the opportunity to monitor ST segment changes.

17.3.3   Bedside Point of Care Laboratory Testing

Over the past decade, laboratory chemical, hematologic, and blood gas testing processes have progressed from "wet" methods in which specific liquid reagents were mixed with blood or serum to perform analyses to a more or less "dry" phase in which analyses are performed by bringing a blood sample in contact with a reagent pack. Additional development has miniaturized both the blood-analysis cartridge and the blood-analysis

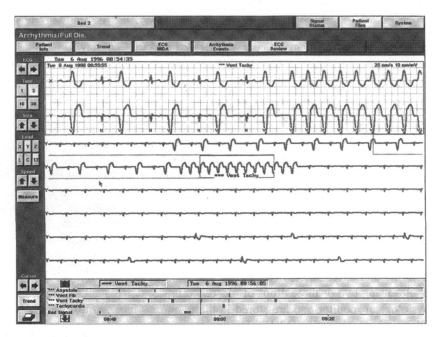

Figure 17.9. "Full disclosure" ECG display. This system stores continuous waveforms for 48 hours along with arrhythmia information. Waveforms may be displayed in a highly compressed format similar to Holter displays. (*Source:* Courtesy of Philips Medical Systems.)

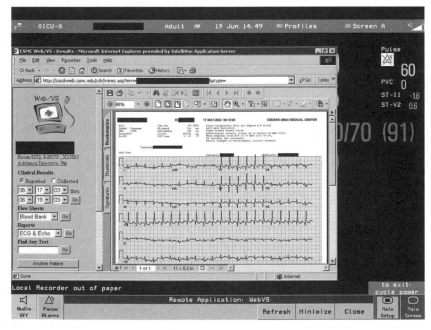

Figure 17.10. Web view of a "Full disclosure" 12-lead ECG with computerized ECG interpretations viewed on a bedside physiologic monitor. (*Source:* Courtesy of Dr. M. Michael Shabot)

machine to the point that the entire analysis system consists of a small plug-in module to a bedside physiological monitor (Figure 17.11).

Many laboratory tests, including pH, Po2, Pco2, Hco3, electrolytes, glucose, ionized calcium, other chemistries, hemoglobin, and hematocrit, can be performed in 2 minutes using two or three drops of blood. Results are displayed on the bedside physiological monitor and are stored in the monitor's database for comparison with previous results (Figure 17.12). These laboratory results obtained at the bedside are also automatically transmitted through the monitoring network and hospital's backbone network to the laboratory computer system, and other systems as required, so that the results can be integrated into the patient's long-term records.

17.3.4 Commercial Development of Computer-Based Monitoring and Intensive-Care-Unit Information Systems

The development of central stations and integrated arrhythmia systems based on standard microcomputer-based server hardware and software platforms has led to wide-scale distribution in the clinical environment. These systems possess database and analysis functions previously reserved for larger systems, and well over 2000 such systems are in use in ICUs worldwide.

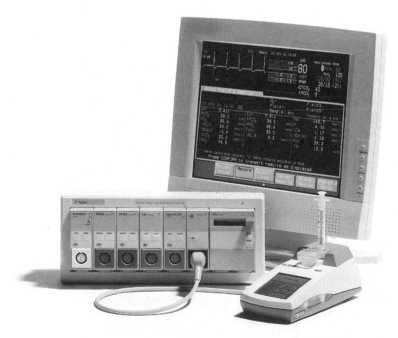

Figure 17.11. Blood analysis point of care device and a bedside physiological monitor. (*Source:* Courtesy of Philips Medical Systems.)

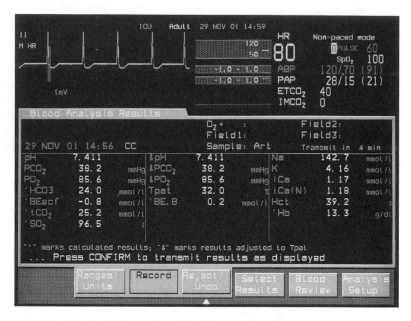

Figure 17.12. Philips Medical Systems IntelliVue Monitoring System physiological monitor display of bedside blood gas test results. Previous measurements are stored in the monitor and displayed with the current results. (*Source:* Courtesy of Philips Medical Systems.)

In recent years, the bedside monitor has become a focal point for data entry and presentation. In fact, most bedside monitoring systems sold today can also acquire and display data from clinical laboratories, bedside laboratory devices such as blood chemistry machines, and a host of other devices such as ventilators. Unfortunately each of these monitors has its own proprietary communications protocol and data acquisition scheme. As a result, the user community is faced with bedside monitors that function like "mini" patient-data-management systems. Furthermore, the desire to capture and manage all clinical data for patients in a critical care setting (not just patient monitoring data) has resulted in development of specialized ICU information systems (see Section 17.4). It is common for hospitals to acquire computer-based bedside monitors, which must be interfaced to an ICU information system, which in turn may be interfaced with a hospital's clinical information system. Several large, capable, and reputable manufacturers have supplied over 350 computer-based ICU information systems worldwide. Three of the major companies involved in the development of such computer-based charting and monitoring systems are Philips Medical Systems with its CareVue system (Shabot, 1997b), GE Medical Systems formerly Marqueette Electronics with its Centricity Clinical Information system, and Eclipsys (formerly EMTEK) with its Continuum 2000 computerized charting application (Brimm, 1987; Cooke & Barie, 1998).

During the time that commercially available physiological monitoring systems were being developed, imaging systems – **x-ray**, **computed tomagraphy** (CT) and **magnetic resonance imaging** (MRI) were also undergoing major developments and transformations (See Chapter 18). Medical imaging plays a major role in the diagnosis and treatment of the critically ill. With most medical images now available in digital format it is now convenient for care providers to have fast and convenient access to medical images via the web. Figure 17.13 shows an abdominal CT scan from a patient at Cedars-Sinai Medical Center's ICU.

17.4   Information Management in the Intensive-care Unit

One of the goals of bedside patient monitoring is to detect life-threatening events promptly so that they can be treated before they cause irreversible organ damage or death. Care of the critically ill patient requires considerable skill and necessitates prompt, accurate treatment decisions. Healthcare professionals collect numerous data through frequent observations and testing, and more data are recorded by continuous-monitoring equipment. Physicians generally prescribe complicated therapy for such patients. As a result, enormous numbers of clinical data accumulate (Buchman, 1995; Kahn, 1994; Sailors & East, 1997; Shabot, 1995;Morris 2003). Professionals can miss

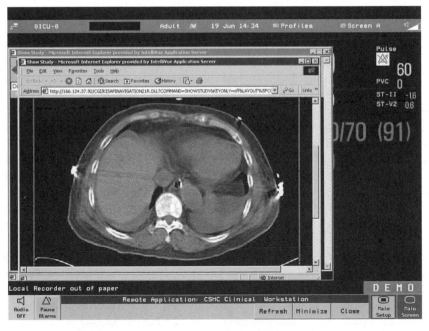

Figure 17.13. Abdominal CT image shown on a bedside physiologic monitor at Cedars-Sinai Medical Center (*Source:* Courtesy of Dr. M. Michael Shabot.)

important events and trends if the accumulated data are not presented in a compact, well-organized form. In addition, the problems of managing these patients have been made even more challenging by economic pressures to reduce the cost of diagnostic and therapeutic interventions.

Continuity of care is especially important for critically ill patients. Such patients are generally served by teams of physicians, nurses, and therapists. Data often are transferred from one individual to another (e.g., the laboratory technician calls a unit clerk who reports the information to a nurse who in turn passes it on to the physician who makes a decision). Each step in this transmission process is subject to delay and error. The medical record is the principal instrument for ensuring the continuity of care for patients.

17.4.1   Computer-Based Charting

As discussed in Chapters 2 and 12, the traditional medical record has several limitations. The problems of poor or inflexible organization, illegibility, and lack of physical availability are especially pertinent to the medical records of critically ill patients due to the large number of data collected and the short time allowed for many treatment decisions.

The importance of having a unified medical record was demonstrated by a study conducted at LDS Hospital in the mid-1980s (Bradshaw et al., 1984). Investigators kept detailed records of the data used by physicians to make treatment decisions in a shock–trauma ICU (Figure 17.14). The investigators were surprised to find that laboratory and blood-gas data were used most frequently (42 percent total), given that physiological bedside monitors are always present in the ICU. Clinicians' observations (21 percent) and drug and fluid-balance data (22 percent) also were used frequently. The bedside physiological monitor accounted for only 13 percent of the data used in making therapeutic decisions. These findings clearly indicate that data from several sources, not just from the traditional physiological monitoring devices, must be communicated to and integrated into a unified medical record to permit effective decision-making and treatment in the ICU. More recent studies by investigators at Stanford University and Cedars-Sinai Medical Center further support the need for integrated records and methods to assist in the "communal reasoning" required by the ICU team (Reddy, 2002).

To be effective, computer charting in the ICU must support multiple types of data collection. As Figure 17.14 shows, a large percentage of the data collected comes from what are typically manual tasks, such as administering a medication or auscultating breath or heart sounds. Furthermore, many instruments that present data in electronic form require their data to be observed by a person and entered into the patient chart. Thus, computer charting systems must be able to collect a wide variety of data from automated and remote sites, as well as from health-care providers at the bedside. Dictated and transcribed reports (e.g., history, physical, and X-ray reports) still represent a large and important source of computer readable but uncoded information for the clinical staff in an ICU. Unfortunately, most computer-charting systems have dealt with a limited set of the data that need to be charted (usually only the bedside monitoring data).

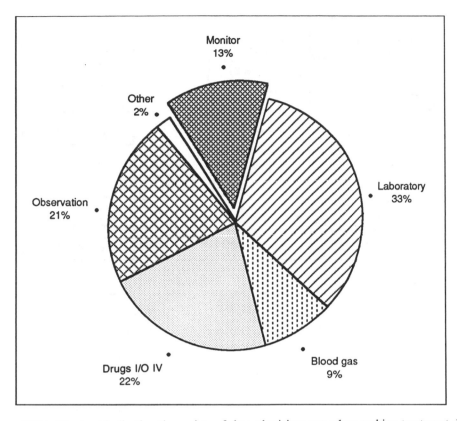

Figure 17.14. Pie chart indicating the variety of data physicians use when making treatment decisions in a shock–trauma intensive care unit. I/O5input–output; IV5intravenous.

Figure 17.15 illustrates the complexity of ICU charting. Modern computerized ICU flowsheet and medication administration record (MAR) displays are shown in Figures 17.16 and 17.17. The chart must document the actions taken by the medical staff to meet both medical and legal requirements (items 1 and 2 in Figure 17.15).

In addition, many of the data logged in the chart are used for management and billing purposes (items 3 and 4 in Figure 17.15). Many computer systems have ignored these requirements and thus have unwittingly forced the clinical staff to chart the same information in more than one place. Efficient management in hospitals is required, especially given the implementation of managed care strategies (see Chapter 23). Hospitals now have strong incentives to know the cost of procedures and to control these costs. As a result, it is necessary to know how sick the patient is, which in turn allows administrators to project nurse staffing needs and to account for the care of a patient by degree of illness. Communications (item 5 in Figure 17.15) to other departments within the hospital is mandatory. Access from office or home to clinical and administrative

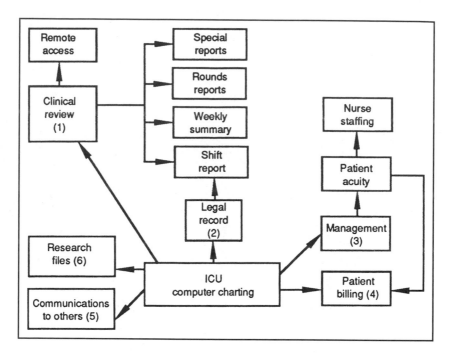

Figure 17.15. Block diagram showing the six major areas in which healthcare professionals interact with computer-based ICU charting to make patient care more effective and efficient. See text for explanations of functions. (*Source:* Reprinted with permission from Gardner R.M., Sittig D.F, Budd, M.C. [1989]. Computers in the intensive care unit: match or mismatch? In Shoemaker W.C., et al. (Eds.), *Textbook of Critical Care* (2nd ed, (p. 249). Philadelphia: W.B. Saunders.

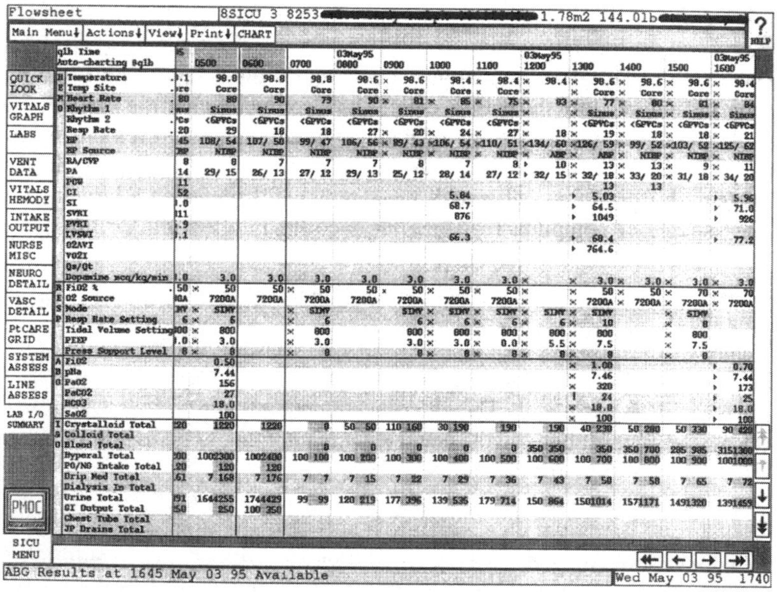

Figure 17.16. CareVue QuickLook Summary Display. The Quicklook display contains a summary of important data from different parts of the flowsheet. The content and appearance of the QuickLook display can be configured for each clinical area. (*Source:* M. Michael Shabot.)

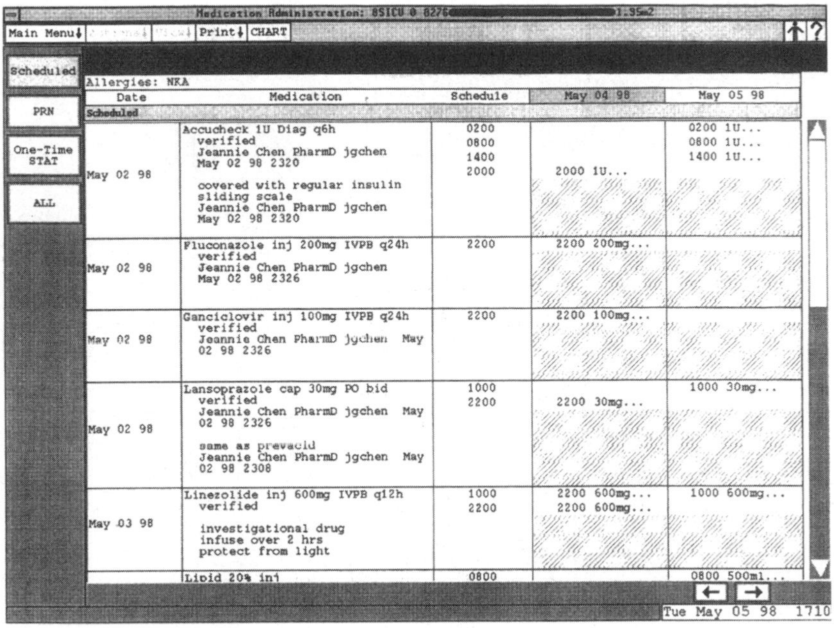

Figure 17.17. CareVue medication administration record (MAR) display. All medications are charted dose by dose in this system. (*Source:* M. Michael Shabot.)

information is a great convenience to physicians. Such communication is easier with a computer-based record. Because the computer-based ICU record is stored in the system, it is readily available for research purposes (item 6 in Figure 17.15). Anyone who has tried to retrieve data from manual patient charts for research purposes will recognize the value of the computer's capability.

To meet the clinical management needs required by critically ill patients as well as to provide an adequate legal record, most patient data-management systems generate a variety of reports. At the LDS Hospital, in addition to the rounds report shown in Figure 17.2, there are a variety of other reports. Figure 17.18 show a nursing shift report. The 12-hour report documents the physiological data and summarizes the laboratory data in its upper section. In the lower section, it displays a record of each drug given and each IV fluid administered. It lists the nurses who care for the patient; the nurses place their initials next to their names to indicate that they have verified the data. Total fluid-intake data are derived from the IV data, and fluid-output data are summarized as well. This allows a calculation of the net intake–output balance for the shift.

For the patient who is in the ICU for several days, a broader view of the course of the recovery process is essential. Thus, the system at LDS Hospital prepares weekly reports that summarize the data for each of the past seven 24-hour periods (Figure 17.19). The data already are stored in the computer, so no additional data entry is required to generate the report. A program abstracts and formats the data.

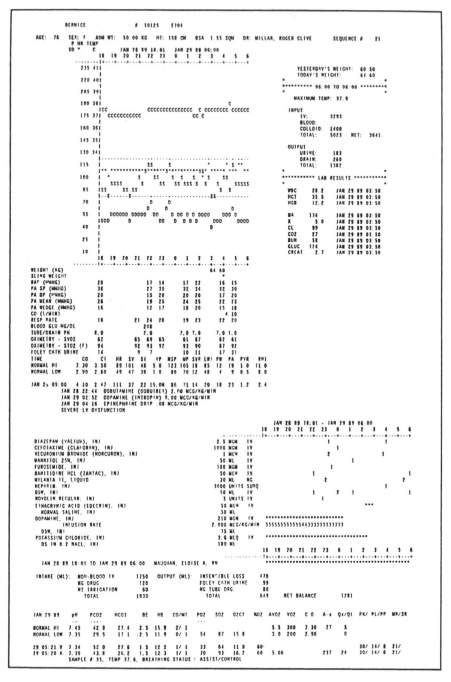

Figure 17.18. Shift report for 12-hour ICU nursing shift at LDS Hospital. (*Source:* Courtesy of LDS Hospital.)

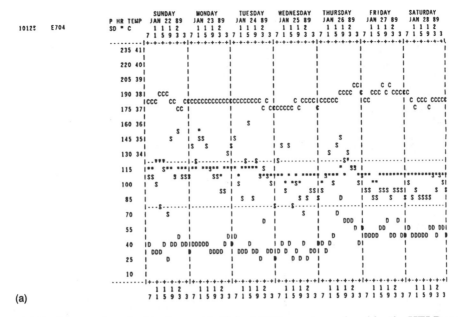

(a)

Figure 17.19. Two portions (a, b) of a weekly (7-day) ICU report, produced by the HELP system at LDS Hospital. The report provides a daily weight, fluid-balance, drug, and physiological-data summary for an individual patient. (*Source:* HELP System, LDS Hospital.)

Figure 17.20 shows a blood-gas report indicating the acid–base status of the patient's blood, as well as the blood's oxygen-carrying capacity. Note that, in addition to the numerical parameters for the blood, the patient's breathing status is indicated. Based on all these clinical data, the computer provides an interpretation. For life-threatening situations, the computer prompts the staff to take the necessary action

17.4.2   Calculation of Derived Variables

Increased sophistication of hemodynamic, renal, and pulmonary monitoring resulted in the need to calculate **derived parameters**; for the first time, ICU staff had to crunch numbers. At first, pocket calculators were used, with each step performed by a careful nurse. Then programmable calculators took over this task, making the computation simpler, faster, and more accurate (Shabot, 1982; Shabot et al., 1977). Soon these devices were replaced by portable computers. Some of these systems also provided graphical plots and interpretations.

17.4.3   Decision-Making Assistance

One mark of a good physician is having the ability to make sound clinical judgments. Medical decision-making traditionally has been considered an intuitive, as well as a scientific, process. More recently, however, formal methods for decision-making have

			JAN 22	JAN 23	JAN 24	JAN 25	JAN 26	JAN 27	JAN 28
MORPHINE, INJ	MGM	IV	37.0	21.0	2.0			7.0	6.0
ACETAMINOPHEN, SUPP	MGM	RECT					1300	650	
DIAZEPAM (VALIUM), INJ	MGM	IV						10.0	5.0
CEFOTAXIME (CLAFORAN), INJ	MGM	IV							1000
GENTAMICIN, INJ	MGM	IV						60.0	60.0
CEFUROXIME (ZINACEF), INJ	MGM	IV	3000	3000	3000	3000	3000	3000	
DOBUTAMINE (DOBUTREX), INJ	MGM	IV	732	582	792	810	270	87	222
EPINEPHRINE DRIP, INJ	MGM	IV	22.20	11.46	3.96	0.00			1.53
VECURONIUM BROMIDE (NORCURON), INJ	MGM	IV	39	26	18	13	10	3	7
DOPAMINE, INJ	MGM	IV	648	492	420	396	522	864	738
METOLAZONE (ZAROXOLYN), TAB	MGM	NG					5.00		
NITROPRUSSIDE (NIPRIDE), INJ	MGM	IV	0						
AMRINONE (INOCOR), INJ	MGM	IV	0						
FUROSEMIDE, INJ	MGM	IV	80	80	80	80	120	80	280
MANNITOL 25%, INJ	ML	IV							50
ETHACRYNIC ACID (EDECRIN), INJ	MGM	IV							50
ACETAZOLAMIDE (DIAMOX), INJ	MGM	IV			250	250		250	
RANITIDINE HCL (ZANTAC), INJ	MGM	IV	150	100	150	150	150	150	150
MYLANTA II, LIQUID	ML	NG		60	30	120	90	60	180
MYLANTA, LIQUID	ML	NG			30	60			
HEPARIN, INJ	UNITS	SUBQ						3000	6000
HEPARIN FLUSH, INJ	UNITS	IV	400	300		300	500	200	100
ARTIFICAL TEARS (LACRIL), SOLUTION	GTTS	OPTH	6	4					
PLASMANATE 5%, INJ	ML	IV						250	1400
PACKED RBC	ML	IV					500		
ALBUMIN 25%, INJ	ML	IV	100	50	50	150			
PLATELETS (RANDOM DONOR)	ML	IV	400		150				
AMINOSYN 8.5%, INJ	ML	IV	311	621	472	529	608	1079	617
POTASSIUM	MEQ	IV	25.2	50.3	38.2	59.7	73.0	131.0	94.9
CALCIUM	MEQ	IV	3.1	6.2	4.7	5.3	5.7	9.9	5.8
MAGNESIUM	MEQ	IV	14.9	35.0	28.3	31.7	12.7	17.3	9.9
ZINC	MGM	IV	3.4	6.8	5.2	5.8	6.7	11.9	6.4
COPPER	MGM	IV	0.7	1.4	1.0	1.2	1.3	2.4	1.3
MANGANESE	MGM	IV	0.3	0.6	0.5	0.5	0.6	1.1	0.6
CHROMIUM	MCG	IV	6.8	13.7	10.4	11.6	13.4	23.7	12.7
CHLORIDE	MEQ	IV	20.8	41.6	31.6	35.4	35.0	50.6	47.5
ACETATE	MEQ	IV	24.9	49.7	37.8	42.3	41.5	69.7	52.2
PHOSPHATE	MEQ	IV	14.9	29.8	22.7	25.4	65.8	138.5	45.5
SULFATE	MEQ	IV	9.9	25.1	20.8	23.3	10.1	17.3	7.6
GLUCONATE	MEQ	IV	3.1	6.2	4.7	5.3	5.7	9.9	5.8
FAT EMULSION 10% (LIPOSYN), INJ	ML	IV							500
NORMAL SALINE, INJ	ML	IV	6	2		2	154	10	40
FAT EMULSION 20% (LIPOSYN), INJ	ML	IV	200	200	200	200	200	66	134
POTASSIUM CHLORIDE, INJ	MEQ	IV	67.9	78.0	183.7	51.9	51.6	104.3	17.6
D5W, INJ	ML	IV	410	215	25	150	5	10	
HETASTARCH (HESPAN), INJ	ML	IV					250	0	
MAGNESIUM SULFATE 50%, INJ	GM	IV	2.00						
NOVOLIN REGULAR, INJ	UNITS	IV	18	15					3

		JAN 22	JAN 23	JAN 24	JAN 25	JAN 26	JAN 27	JAN 28
INTAKE (ML):	BLOOD	400		150		500		
	COLLOID	100	50	50	150		250	1400
	NON-BLOOD IV	2783	3046	2707	2395	2254	3145	3293
	NG DRUG		60	60	180	90	60	180
	TOTAL	3313	3216	2967	2815	2874	3485	5023
OUTPUT (ML):	INSENSIBLE LOSS	937	946	943	873	1016	1077	939
	FOLEY CATH URINE	360	740	210	902	2950	895	183
	NG TUBE DRG.	50	200	80	125	40	75	260
	WATERSEAL DRG, 1	180	50					
	TOTAL	3918	3936	4023	2512	5226	2470	1382
NET BALANCE (ML):		-605	-720	-1056	303	-2352	1015	3641
WEIGHT (KG)		61.2	61.4	60.8	62.2	60.4	60.5	64.6
NUTRITIONAL:	NP ENERGY KCAL (IV)	1468	2143	1784	1803	1953	2813	2395
	TOTAL ENERGY KCAL (IV)	1573	2354	1944	1982	2160	3181	2605
	PROTEIN GM	26	53	40	45	52	92	52
	FAT GM	40	40	40	40	40	13	77
	CHO GM	315	513	407	413	456	789	464
	NP ENERGY/N2 KCAL/GM	367	238	254	257	244	200	266
	N2 IN GM	4	9	7	7	8	14	9

BERNICE   # 10125   E704

TIME OUT: JAN 29 89 13:53   PROCESS TIME: 00:18
(END)

Figure 17.19. (*Continued*)

been applied to medical problem-solving (see Chapter 3), and computer-assisted medical decision-making has gained wider acceptance (see the discussions of decision-support systems in Chapter 20). We now have the opportunity to use the computer to assist staff in the complex task of medical decision-making in the ICU. For example, the

L D S   H O S P I T A L   B L O O D   G A S   R E P O R T

```
        STEVEN                    NO.  10072    DR. STINSON, JAMES B.        RM E609
                      SEX: M  AGE: 43

  JAN 05 89    pH    PCO2   HCO3    BE    HB   CO/MT   PO2   SO2   O2CT   %O2  AVO2  VO2   C.O.   A-a  Qs/Qt  PK/ PL/PP  MR/S
  NORMAL HI   7.45  40.6   25.9   2.5  17.7   2/ 1                            5.5  300  7.30    22    5
  NORMAL LOW  7.35  27.2   15.7  -2.5  13.7   0/ 1    64    91   18.5         3.0  200  2.90           0

  05 04:36 V  7.43  34.5   22.7  -.4  11.5   2/ 1    42    76   12.3   40                                   30/ 28/ 5  20/
  05 04:35 A  7.48  29.3   21.7       11.6   2/ 1   128    96   15.9   40   3.43               75   12     30/ 28/ 5  20/
              SAMPLE # 37, TEMP 37.3, BREATHING STATUS : ASSIST/CONTROL
              MILD ACID-BASE DISORDER
              MODERATELY REDUCED O2 CONTENT
              SUPRA-NORMAL PO2
              PULSE OXIMETER SO2  96.0

  04 04:20 V  7.45  36.1   24.9   1.9  10.2   2/ 1    37    72   10.4   40                                   26/ 20/ 5  21/
  04 04:19 A  7.49  31.6   24.0   2.0  10.2   2/ 1    90    95   13.7   40   3.36  353  10.50  111   48     26/ 20/ 5  21/
              SAMPLE # 36, TEMP 37.5, BREATHING STATUS : ASSIST/CONTROL
              MILD ACID-BASE DISORDER
              SEVERELY REDUCED O2 CONTENT (13.7) DUE TO ANEMIA (LOW HB)
              PULSE OXIMETER SO2  93.0

  03 06:05 A  7.44  35.8   24.1   1.0  11.7   2/ 1    91    95   15.7   40                      105          26/ 22/ 5  23/
              SAMPLE # 35, TEMP 37.0, BREATHING STATUS : ASSIST/CONTROL
              NORMAL ARTERIAL ACID-BASE CHEMISTRY
              MODERATELY REDUCED O2 CONTENT
              PULSE OXIMETER SO2  93.0

  02 04:16 V  7.46  37.4   26.4   3.4   9.1   1/ 1    35    71    9.1   40                                   32/ 25/10  20/
  02 04:15 A  7.51  32.4   25.8   3.9   9.5   2/ 1    91    95   12.8   40   3.29  237  7.20  109   17     32/ 25/10  20/
              SAMPLE # 34, TEMP 37.1, BREATHING STATUS : ASSIST/CONTROL
              MODERATE METABOLIC ALKALOSIS
              SEVERELY REDUCED O2 CONTENT (12.8) DUE TO ANEMIA (LOW HB)
              PULSE OXIMETER SO2  95.0

  01 10:53 A  7.47  37.0   26.8   4.0  11.1   1/ 1    77    94   14.7   60                      238          36/ 27/10  20/
              SAMPLE # 33, TEMP 37.7, BREATHING STATUS : ASSIST/CONTROL
              MILD ACID-BASE DISORDER
              MODERATELY REDUCED O2 CONTENT
              PULSE OXIMETER SO2  93.0

  01 03:59 V  7.41  46.2   29.0   4.5  10.0   1/ 1    42    73   10.2   80                                    /  /12  20/
  01 03:58 A  7.46  39.2   27.7   4.5   9.9   1/ 1   146    97   13.7   80   3.64  331  9.10  287   23       /  /12  20/
              SAMPLE # 32, TEMP 38.4, BREATHING STATUS : ASSIST/CONTROL
              MILD ACID-BASE DISORDER
              SEVERELY REDUCED O2 CONTENT (13.7) DUE TO ANEMIA (LOW HB)
              SUPRA-NORMAL PO2

  01 00:39 A  7.44  42.2   28.4   4.7  10.0   1/ 1   104    95   13.5   90                      386          /  /10  20/
              SAMPLE # 31, TEMP 38.9, BREATHING STATUS : ASSIST/CONTROL
              MILD ACID-BASE DISORDER
              SEVERELY REDUCED O2 CONTENT (13.5) DUE TO ANEMIA (LOW HB)
              PULSE OXIMETER SO2  91.0

  31 23:35 A  7.42  42.4   27.2   3.2  10.1   1/ 1    63    87   12.3   65                      276          /  / 5  20/
              SAMPLE # 30, TEMP 39.0, BREATHING STATUS : ASSIST/CONTROL
              MILD ACID-BASE DISORDER
              MODERATE HYPOXEMIA
              SEVERELY REDUCED O2 CONTENT (12.3) DUE TO ANEMIA (LOW HB)
              PULSE OXIMETER SO2  83.0

  31 16:00 A  7.49  34.4   26.1   3.8   9.7   1/ 1    87    95   13.1   40                      111          /  / 5  21/
              SAMPLE # 29, TEMP 37.8, BREATHING STATUS : ASSIST/CONTROL
              MILD ACID-BASE DISORDER
              SEVERELY REDUCED O2 CONTENT (13.1) DUE TO ANEMIA (LOW HB)
```

```
  PRELIMINARY INTERPRETATION -- BASED ONLY ON BLOOD GAS DATA.  ***(FINAL DIAGNOSIS REQUIRES CLINICAL CORRELATION)***
  KEY: CO=CARBOXY HB, MT=MET HB, O2CT=O2 CONTENT, AVO2=ART VENOUS CONTENT DIFFERENCE (CALCULATED WITH AVERAGE OF A &V HB VALU
  VO2=OXYGEN CONSUMPTION, C.O.=CARDIAC OUTPUT, A-a=ALVEOLAR arterial O2 DIFFERENCE, Qs/Qt=SHUNT, PK=PEAK, PL=PLATEAU, PP=PEE
  MR=MACHINE RATE, SR=SPONTANEOUS RATE.         *** SPECIMEN IDENTIFICATION: BLOOD (A=ARTERIAL, V=VENOUS, C=CAPILLARY, W=WEDG
                                               FLUIDS (P=PLEURAL, J=JOINT, B=ABDOMINAL, S=ABSCESS); E=EXPIRED AIR;
                                               ECCo2R (I=INFLOW, M=MIDFLOW, O=OUTFLOW)
```

`KEEP FULL PAGE FOR RECORDS`
`(END)`

Figure 17.20. Blood-gas report showing the patient's predicted values, as well as the measured values. The computer provides a decision-making interpretation and alerting facility. Note that this report summarizes, in reverse chronological order, the patient's blood-gas status over the course of 8 days. (*Source:* Courtesy of LDS Hospital.)

HELP computer system at the LDS Hospital in Salt Lake City has been used effectively to assist in ICU antibiotic use decision-making (Evans et al., 1998; Garibaldi, 1998). The so called "antibiotic assistant" provides recommendations as to the specific antibiotic recommended for a specific patient and further recommends the dose to be given and the mode of delivery (for example IV) also based on the patient's size and renal function (Figure 17.21). The system collects and integrates data for the ICU patient from a wide variety of sources. The data are processed automatically by the HELP decision-making system to determine whether the new information, by itself or in combination with other data in the patient record (such as a laboratory result or a previously generated decision), leads to a new medical decision. These computer-generated medical decisions are based on predefined criteria stored in the system's knowledge base.

The HELP decision-making system has been used in the following areas:

- Interpretation of data; for example, interpretation of breathing status based on blood-gas reports and hemodynamic parameters
- Alerts; for example, notification that a drug is contraindicated at the time the drug is being ordered

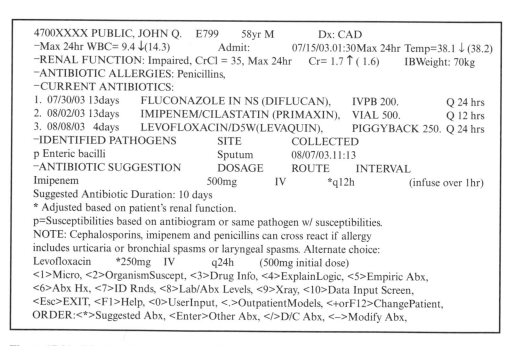

Figure 17.21. Display of a screen from the Antibiotic Assistant at LDS Hospital. Screen shows important patient information such as maximum temperature, microbiology data and then makes recommendations for medicatiion with its dose, route of administration and recommended duration (*Source:* Courtesy of Dr. R. Scott Evans at LDS Hospital).

- Diagnoses; for example, detection of hospital-acquired infections
- Treatment suggestions; for example, suggestions about the most effective antibiotics to order

The ICU component of HELP is one of the most mature of the system's clinical applications. The basic requirements for data acquisition, decision support, and information reporting are similar for patients in the ICU and on the general patient-care units of the LDS Hospital. The number of variables and the volume of observations that must be integrated, however, are much greater for patients in the ICU.

At Cedars-Sinai Medical Center, all laboratory and flowsheet data are continuously analyzed for critical laboratory results and adverse combinations of clinical (nonlaboratory) events. When such events are detected, they are transmitted to the responsible physician via an encrypted alphanumeric pager. Figure 17.22 shows a low Serum Potassium laboratory alert (K$^+$ 2.8), and Figure 17.23 warns of a critical Penicillan allergy sent by an encrypted transmission to a BlackBerry$^{™}$ device.

17.4.4 Response by Nurses and Physicians

Currently, bedside terminals are functioning in all ICUs at LDS Hospital, and nurses use a computer-based system to create nursing care plans and to chart ICU data. The goals of automation were (1) to facilitate the acquisition of clinical data, (2) to improve

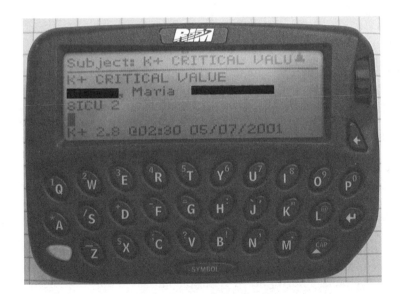

Figure 17.22. A Blackberry$^{™}$ alphanumeric pager displays a real-time alert message for a serum potassium level of 2.8 mg/dl. All laboratory data coming into CareVue is transferred to another computer system where it is run through a rules engine, which generates the pager alert messages at Cedars-Siani Medical Center (*Source:* Courtesy of Dr. M. Michael Shabot).

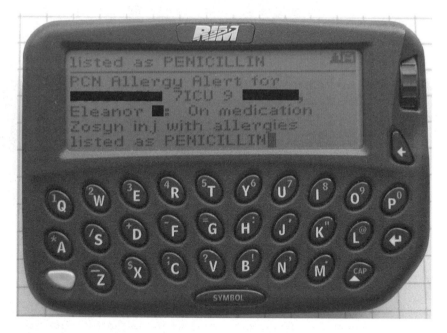

Figure 17.23. A Blackberry™ alphanumeric pager displays an alert for a potentially serious drug allergy at Cedars-Siani Medical Center (*Source:* Courtesy of Dr. M. Michael Shabot).

the content and legibility of medical documentation, and (3) to increase the efficiency of the charting process so that nurses could devote more time to direct patient care. Studies have shown wide acceptance by nurses and physicians of the HELP system and its decision-support capabilities (Gardner & Lundsgaarde, 1994). Also, the content and quality of nursing charts has improved markedly (Bradshaw et al., 1988). To date, however, the studies have not shown improvements in the efficiency of information management by ICU nurses (time savings) that could be credited to use of the system.

The lack of demonstrable time savings may be due to several factors. First, the new system affected only selected aspects of the nursing process. For example, physiological and laboratory data were already acquired automatically, so the effects of these computer-based systems were not included in the analyses. Second, the computer-based charting system is not yet comprehensive; nurses still hand write some data in the patient chart. Third, nurses do not always take advantage of the capabilities of the charting system. For example, they sometimes reenter vital signs that have already been stored in the computer. Fourth, the intervals of time saved may have been too small to be measured using the work-sampling methods employed in the studies. Fifth, these small savings in time are easily absorbed into other activities. Despite the lack of widespread improvement in efficiency, the clinical staff at LDS Hospital are enthusiastic about using computers (Gardner & Lundsgaarde, 1994).

At Cedars-Sinai Medical Center, a national healthcare consulting firm was employed in 1989 to measure time savings associated with the computerized system in the surgical ICUs compared with the standard paper charting system in noncomputerized ICUs. The consultants drew their conclusions from observations of caregiver activities in both kinds of ICUs, as well as from detailed interviews. They concluded that the system saved about 20 percent of the nurses time spent in charting, about 25 percent of surgical residents' time reviewing data, and about 33 percent of attending surgeons' time reviewing data (Dorenfest and Associates, 1989, Chicago, IL, unpublished report). In addition a "vision" of what technology can do for nursing has recently been presented by Dr. Shabot (Shabot 2003).

17.5   Current Issues in Patient Monitoring

As more health services are shifted to outpatient settings, the acuity of hospitalized patients continues to increase; thus, the future of computer-based ICU monitoring systems is bright. Developments in bedside monitors have accelerated because of the availability of more powerful and affordable microcomputers. Nonetheless, some important areas of research in patient monitoring have not yet been addressed effectively.

17.5.1   Data Quality and Data Validation

There are still major problems with acquiring ICU data either automatically or manually (Gardner, 1997, p. 126). A system must provide feedback at various levels to verify correct operation, to carry out quality control, and to present intermediate and final results. As discussed earlier, some **cross validation** between signals is possible, but this process is performed by very few of the bedside monitors in use today. An ICU study of early, standalone pulse oximetry monitors revealed that up to 46.5 percent of low saturation alarms were neither observed nor responded to by any caregiver in large part due to constant false alarms associated with such devices (Bentt et al., 1990). Some newer patient-monitoring devices, such as integrated pulse oximeters and direct pressure measuring systems, have built in noise-rejection algorithms to improve the quality of the data presented (Gardner et al., 1986). Data validation, however, is one area of patient monitoring that still offers much opportunity for technological development and improvement (Dalto et al., 1997; Strong et al., 1997; Young et al., 1997). Figure 17.24 illustrates a problem with manual charting of data from bedside devices. During an implementation of IV pumps with the **Medical Information Bus** (MIB) at one our our hospitals, we had nurses chart "manually" and also logged IV drip rate changes with the MIB. Shown in Figure 17.24 are the "time delays" between the time an IV drip rate was "changed" and when the data were logged into the electronic medical record. Note that only about 1/3 of the drip rate changes were logged within 10 minutes of the change. Also note it took over 190 minutes to have 90% of the rate changes charted. Then, even at 300 minutes only 95% of the changes were charted. Physicians and nurses will recognize such a charting practices as waiting until the "end of shift" to log ALL the results. Such a manual charting process not only makes it impossible to follow what is going on

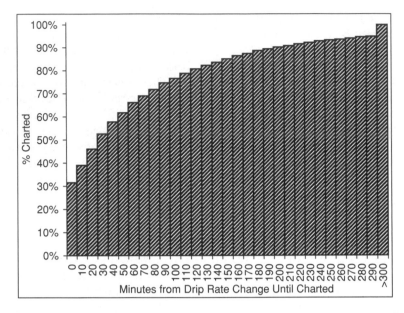

Figure 17.24. IV Charting comparison – Delay time between when an IV drip rate actually occurred and it was manually charted by a nurse in the ICU. Horizonatl axis is the time in minutes and the vertical axis is the cumulate percentage of values that are recorded within each of the 10 minute time slots. For example in the first 10 minutes about 33% of drip rates would have been entered into a bedside manual charting system.

with the patient – for example, if a **vasoactive drug** caused the blood pressure to stabilize, but can also lead to major treatment errors. Suprisingly, these same types of delays were seen with simple IV fluid infusions such as normal saline, but were also seen with important, short vasoactive medication agents.

17.5.2 *Continuous Versus Intermittent Monitoring*

One of the persistent questions facing people who monitor patients is: Should I measure a parameter continuously, or is intermittent sampling enough? A related question is: How often do I make the measurement? These questions have no simple answer. If we are measuring the ECG and want to display it continuously, we must sample the signal at a rate of at least twice the rate of the maximum frequency of interest in the signal (the Nyquist frequency; see Chapter 5). Thus, for an ECG, the sampling rate should be at least 200 measurements per second.

To perform intermittent monitoring—periodic measurement of blood pH, for example—the overriding concerns in determining sampling rate are how rapidly the parameter can change, and how long before a dangerous change will result in irreversible damage. Sudden heart stoppage or severe dysrhythmias are the most frequent causes of sudden death. Therefore, heart-rate and rhythm monitors must function continuously and should sound alarms within 15 to 20 seconds after detecting a problem. Other physiological parameters are not as labile and can be monitored less frequently. For the most part, medical measurements are made intermittently, and even continuously measured parameters are displayed at intervals. For example, heart rate can change with each beat (by 0.35 to 1 second). To provide data that a human can interpret, however, a bedside monitor usually updates its display every 3 seconds.

17.5.3   Data Recording: Frequency and Quantity

In the past, because analog and early digital bedside monitors and central stations could not store continuous waveforms from all patients, it was acceptable for nurses to archive periodic strip chart recordings ("snapshots") in the patient's ICU chart. Most ICUs have policies and procedures for pasting waveform recordings during the nursing shift and for critical events. The newer central stations, however, record digitized waveforms to hard disk on a continuous basis, and theoretically these data could be archived with the patient's electronic chart or printed out for a paper chart. But must second-by-second waveform data be archived permanently? Will it improve the quality of patient care? Or will it simply increase the cost of care in the form of increased magnetic or optical storage media, paper usage, and material for lawyers to haggle over for years to come?

There is a worrisome precedent with fetal monitoring recordings (See Figure 17.25): When it became possible to make a continuous record—first on paper and more recently in electronic form — it became mandatory for hospitals to do so. The fate of continuous recordings of routine ICU waveforms remains to be decided.

17.5.4   Invasive Versus Noninvasive Monitoring

Physiological and biochemical parameters commonly used in monitoring can be measured by instruments and devices that are either invasive (require breaking the skin or entering the body) or noninvasive. After several decades of development of **invasive techniques**, the recent trend has been to design **noninvasive methods**. Much of the

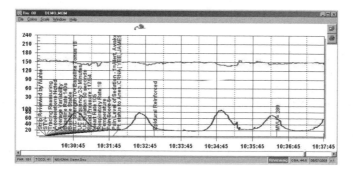

Figure 17.25. Stork-bytes. (*Source:* Courtesy of LDS Hospital.)

development of noninvasive technology can be attributed to the availability of microcomputers and solid-state sensors.

The development of inexpensive light-emitting diodes (LED), small solid-state light detectors, and new computer methods made possible, for example, the development of the *pulse oximeter*, an exciting example of noninvasive monitoring technology. When alternately red and then infrared light is shined from the LEDs through a finger or an ear, the device can detect the pulsations of blood and determine arterial oxygen saturation and heart rate (Severinghaus & Astrup, 1986). Pulse oximetry is one of the most significant technological advances ever made in monitoring. The technology is quite reliable, yet inexpensive, and, because it is noninvasive, it does not subject the patient to the costs and risks of invasive techniques (e.g., infection and blood loss). Recently several manufacturers have produced "next-generation oximeters" (Health Devices 2003). These newer pulse oximeters use advanced signal-processing algorithms that allow the devices to eliminate motion artifact and detect poor perfusion. As a consequence of these improvements, the quality of the derived signals and the number of false alarms have been dramatically reduced.

17.5.5   *Integration of Patient-Monitoring Devices*

Most bedside patient-support devices, such as IV pumps, ventilators, and physiological monitors, are microcomputer based. Each has its own display and, because each comes from a different manufacturer, each is designed as a standalone unit. As a result, it is common for a nurse or therapist to read a computer display from one of these devices and then to enter the data through a workstation into a different computer. The need to integrate the outputs of the myriad devices in the ICU is apparent. The absence of standards for medical-device communications has stymied the acceptance and success of automated clinical data management systems. Due to the large number and variety of medical devices available and to the peculiar data formats, it is impractical to interface the growing number of bedside devices to computers by building special software and hardware interfaces. For these reasons, an Institute of Electrical and Electronic Engineers (IEEE) **Medical Information Bus (MIB)** standards committee 1073 was established (Dalto et al., 1997; Kennelly & Gardner, 1997; Shabot, 1989; Wittenber & Shabot, 1990; Young et al., 1997). Automated data capture from bedside medical devices is now possible using the IEEE 1073 communications standards.[5] With these standards in place, it is possible for vendors and hospitals to implement "plug and play" interfaces to a wide variety of bedside medical devices such as bedside monitors, IV pumps, and ventilators.

Work at LDS Hospital (Gardner et al., 1992) and many other medical centers using the MIB has demonstrated that the use of a common bus system facilitates timely and accurate data acquisition from bedside devices such as pulse oximeters, ventilators, infusion pumps, pH meters, and mixed venous oxygen saturation monitoring systems. As a result of the standardization of MIB, it is much easier to establish communications with these devices in the ICU (Figure 17.26). The larger information challenges in the ICU

---

[5]http://ieee.1073org.

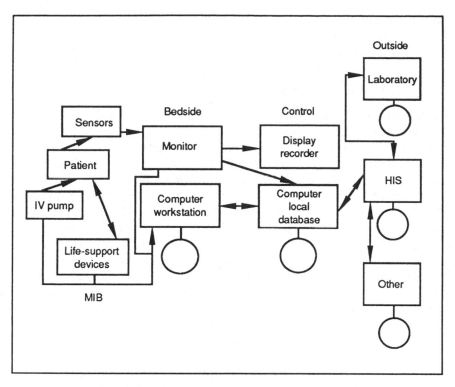

Figure 17.26. Block diagram of a distributed-database ICU system with networking. The database has been distributed to improve response time and reliability; the communications network has been implemented to enhance the integration function needed to care for the critically ill patient. MIB5medical information bus; HIS5hospital information system; IV5intravenous.

now include integration of patient-monitoring data and observations charted by clinicians within ICU management systems and subsequent integration of the critical-care records with the overall computerized patient record (Chapter 12).

17.5.6   Closed-Loop Therapy

The natural outcome from the remarkable developments noted above would seem to be **closed-loop control** of physiological processes. It can be argued that pacemakers and implantable defibrillators are such devices. In the ICU, however, precisely controlled intravenous pumps are available for drug infusions, and there is no shortage of digitized physiological signals available at the bedside and on the monitoring network. Despite Sheppard (Sheppard 1968) and colleagues' pioneering work in automated blood infusion therapy after open-heart surgery 35 years ago, however, very few examples exist of successful similar work. Although a closed-loop nitroprusside pump was marketed briefly a few years ago, no commercial products are available at this time. The major impediments include the difficulty of creating closed-loop systems with tolerance for the kind of artifacts and measurement errors seen in ICU patients and the difficult medicolegal environment in many industrialized countries.

17.5.7   Treatment Protocols

As in other areas of medical practice, there is considerable interest in developing standard treatment protocols to improve the consistency, quality, and cost effectiveness of critical-care settings. Two different examples will demonstrate the value of treatment protocols in the ICU. The first is an expert system for management of mechanical ventilation, and the second is a computer-assisted management program for antibiotics. Researchers at LDS Hospital initially implemented a program to manage the therapy of patients who have Adult Respiratory Distress Syncrome (ARDS) and who were enrolled in a controlled clinical trial (Sittig, 1987). More recently a broader set of protocols has been developed (East et al., 1992). These computerized protocols were developed to standardize therapy, ensure uniformity of care, provide equal intensity and frequency of monitoring, improve the consistency of decision-making strategies, and achieve common therapeutic goals. The HELP system automatically generates therapeutic instructions regarding ventilator management to healthcare providers based on data input by the laboratory and by physicians, nurses, and respiratory therapists. The system has been used successfully to manage complex patient trials with great success (Henderson et al., 1991, Morris 2001, Morris 2003).

In contrast, the **antibiotic-assistant program** developed by Evans and colleagues (1998) (also at LDS Hospital) acquires data from the rich coded database of the HELP system and provides "consultation" to physicians ordering antibiotics for patients who have or who are suspected of having an infection. The program is designed to fit into the work flow pattern of practitioners. It provides physicians with the latest pertinent information about individual patients. The computer provides decision support to suggest the appropriate antibiotic for the patient or even to indicate the lack of a need for such a medication. The program uses the patient's admission diagnosis, white-blood cell count, temperature, surgical-procedure data, chest radiograph interpretation (free text), and information from the pathology and microbiology laboratories to make its recommendations. The knowledge base used to drive the clinical recommendations was created from analysis of historical "antibiograms" and the knowledge of clinical and infectious disease experts. Physicians have been enthusiastic users of the system because it provides the relevant data in about 5 seconds, whereas it may take 15 minutes or more to acquire the same data from patient records. In addition, the system was shown to improve the quality of patient care and reduce costs (Evans et al., 1998).

17.5.8   Demonstrating the Efficacy of Care in the Intensive-Care Unit

Intensive-care-unit care is expensive. Given the current pressures to control healthcare spending (see Chapter 23), there is growing concern about the cost effectiveness of such care. In a 1984 study prepared for the Office of Technology Assessment, one researcher estimated that 15 to 20 percent of the nation's hospital budget, or almost 1 percent of the gross national product, was spent for ICU care (Berenson, 1984). Unfortunately, the problems of assessing the benefit of each element in the ICU are many; to date, no definitive studies have been performed. It is difficult to identify and isolate all the factors in the ICU setting that affect patient recovery and outcome. To this end, a Coalition of Critical Care Excellence of the Society of Critical Care Medicine recently reviewed the issues related to developing evidence about the safety and effectiveness of critical care monitoring devices and related interventions (Bone, 1995). Furthermore, the ethical implications of withholding potentially beneficial care from patients in the control group of a randomized clinical trial make such studies almost impossible to perform. As discussed in Section 17.4.3 and 17.5.7, a computer-assisted program for management of antibiotics at LDS Hospital was found to improve the quality of patient care while reducing associated costs (Evans et al., 1998). Recently work by Clemmer and colleagues has shown important improvements in quality of care and outcomes using collaborative methods supported by computer technology. (Clemmer 1999). Also, work by Adhikari and Lapinsky gives an outline of technology assessment techniques (Adhikari 2003). Further, several intensivists have projected the current and future value of critical care computing (Seiver 2000, Seiver 2003, McIntosh 2002, Varon 2002).

At Cedar-Sinai Medical Center, physiological data, ICU utilization data, and measurable outcomes for specific subsets of ICU patients have been analyzed to determine which patients require care or observation that can only be performed in an ICU. Using these results, the medical center has developed guidelines and pathways for use of the ICU by similar patients. These guidelines have been approved by the various divisions of surgery. Intensive-care unit pathways, including guidelines for nonadmission to the ICU in some cases, are in place for elective craniotomy, thoracotomy, carotid endarterectomy, infrainguinal arterial surgery, ovarian cancer surgery, kidney transplantation, and liver transplantation. Use of these pathways and guidelines has reduced the average ICU cost of caring for these groups of patients, with no adverse changes in outcome (Amir et al., 1997; Chandra et al., 1995; Cunneen et al., 1998; McGrath et al., 1996; Shabot, 1997a). Figure 17.27 shows part of the pathway for infrainguinal arterial surgery, and Figure 17.28 shows the pop-up guideline for ICU admission for these patients.

17.5.9   Responsible Use of Medical Software

Use of medical software has become ubiquitous, especially in the ICU. There is a growing literature documenting how computerized systems improve health-care delivery (Garibaldi, 1998). There are also concerns, however, about patient safety that must still be addressed. The Food and Drug Administration (FDA) has called for discussions about further regulating of such software (Miller & Gardner, 1997a). The American Medical Informatics Association and others have made recommendations about how such software should be monitored and evaluated (Miller & Gardner, 1997b). See Chapter 10 for a discussion of legal issues in healthcare informatics and Chapter 11 for a detailed discussion of software evaluation.

Pathway		Apr 01 96	Apr 02 96	Apr 03 96	
1	1 INFRAINGUINL BYPASS GRAFT	Pathway Day 1	Pathway Day 2	Pathway Day 3 (Floor Care)	▲
2	2 LEVEL OF CARE (B1)	1. Operating Room	1. SICU		
3		2. Recovery Room	2. Floor Care		
4		3. G2 - GUIDELINE FOR TRANSFER TO ICU VS. FLOOR CARE			
5	3 DIAGNOSTIC TESTS/PROCS (B1)		CBC + Chem I		
6			PT		
			PTT		
7	4 MEDICATIONS (B1)	Ancef q8h	Ancef q8h		
8		Heparin Drip	Heparin Drip		
		Pain Management (PCA)	Pain Management (PCA)		
LAB I/O SUMMARY	5 TREATMENTS (B1)	Intravenous line	D/C IV		
10		O2 PRN	D/C O2		
		Pulse Oximeter	D/C Pulse Oximeter		
11	6 ACTIVITY (B1)	Bedrest	OOB to chair		
12		Leg elevated	PT eval		
SICU MENU	7 NUTRITION (B1)	NPO	1. Start Clears	▼	

Figure 17.27. Cedars-Sinai Medical Center pathway for managing infrainguinal bypass graft patient. Note the embedded guideline for ICU versus floor care after the Recovery Room (Pathway Day 1). (*Source:* Courtesy of Cedars-Sinai Medical Center.)

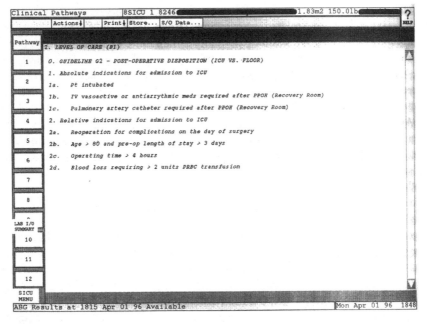

Clinical Pathways   8SICU 1 8246   1.83m2 150.0lb   ? HELP

Actions↓   Print↓ Store... S/O Data...

Pathway | 2. LEVEL OF CARE (B1)

1 ▲
2
3
4
5
6
7
8
LAB I/O SUMMARY
10
11
12
SICU MENU

0. GUIDELINE G2 - POST-OPERATIVE DISPOSITION (ICU VS. FLOOR)

1. Absolute indications for admission to ICU

1a.   Pt intubated

1b.   IV vasoactive or antiarrythmic meds required after PPOH (Recovery Room)

1c.   Pulmonary artery catheter required after PPOH (Recovery Room)

2. Relative indications for admission to ICU

2a.   Reoperation for complications on the day of surgery

2b.   Age > 80 and pre-op length of stay > 3 days

2c.   Operating time > 4 hours

2d.   Blood loss requiring > 2 units PRBC transfusion

ABG Results at 1815 Apr 01 96 Available   Mon Apr 01 96 1848

Figure 17.28. Pop-up guideline for admission to ICU versus floor care after infrainguinal bypass graft. The evidence-based criteria were derived from the actual ICU courses of hundreds of patients undergoing this operation at Cedars-Sinai Medical Center. (*Source:* Courtesy of Cedars-Sinai Medical Center.)

17.5.10   Integration of Bioinformatics and Genomics with Critical Care

Critically ill patients are monitored extensively and intensively with methods discussed in this Chapter. However, up to now the goal of monitoring has been to measure the degree of injury and to prevent further injury, rather than to measure "repair." In the future we may be able to monitor the progress of "repair" by using genomic and proteomic markers (Hopf 2003). These types of monitors would enable clinicians to control the healing environment using these biomarkers. For example, diagnosis of infection in the critically ill patient requires that cultures of pathogens be made. Culturing and subsequent determination of the sensitivity of an appropriate antibiotic can take days. With the ability to detect bacterial DNA we should be able to detect and identify the active bacteria using genetic markers. These new techniques will require the use of computierized patient records and tools developed by our Bioinformatics colleagues.

17.5.11   Consensus Conference on Critical-Care Medicine

A global perspective on what should be done to improve critical-care patient-data management can be gained from a 1983 consensus conference organized by the National Institutes of Health (Ayers, 1983). Although formulated in the mid-1980s, the conclusions of this conference concerning areas of improvement in treatment of critically ill patients remain pertinent today. Many of these problems are amenable to computer assistance. Technical difficulties, errors in data interpretation, and increasing interventions caused by continuous monitoring are potential nosocomial hazards for ICU patients. Based on the findings of the original conference, we identify eight areas in which computers can assist in the practice of critical-care medicine.

1. All ICUs should be capable of arrhythmia monitoring. Bedside physiological monitors with microcomputers now provide excellent arrhythmia monitoring.
2. Invasive monitoring should be performed safely. Computer-based charting of invasive events such as the insertion of an arterial catheter, analyzed in combination with data from the microbiology laboratory, can help to avoid infection (a major complication of invasive monitoring).
3. Generated data should be correct. The computer can check data as they are entered to verify that they are reasonable. In addition, data communications and calculation errors can be reduced or eliminated by letting the computer do the work.
4. Derived data should be interpreted properly. The computer can assist in the integration of data from multiple sources. In addition, the computer can derive parameters and also can provide prompt, accurate, and consistent interpretations and alerts.
5. Therapy should be employed safely. The computer can assist physicians by suggesting therapy, calculating appropriate drug doses, and flagging combinations of interacting drugs.
6. Access to laboratory data should be rapid and comprehensive. Computer networking provides quick access to all laboratory data and can even interpret the results and provide alerts.

7. Enteral (tube-feeding) and parenteral (IV) nutritional-support services should be available. There are interactive computer programs that help physicians to prescribe care by assisting with the complex task of determining the appropriate volume and content of nutritional supplements.
8. Titrated[6] therapeutic interventions with infusion pumps should be available. In theory, closed-loop systems for controlling the administration of fluids and intravenous drugs could facilitate patient care. In reality, however, work to date in this area has proved unsuccessful.

The availability of microcomputers has greatly enhanced the ability to generate and process the physiological data used in patient monitoring. The use of computers in the ICU is still an area of growth, however. Although advances in signal processing and ICU information systems have been significant, many challenges remain in the exploration of ways with which the computer can be used effectively to integrate, display results, evaluate, and simplify the complex data used in caring for critically ill patients.

Suggested Readings

Gardner R.M., Sittig D.F., Clemmer T.P. (1995). Computers in the intensive care unit: a match meant to be! In W.C. Shoemaker et al. (Eds.), Textbook of Critical Care (3rd ed., pp. 1757–1770). Philadelphia: W.B. Saunders.
This chapter summarizes the current status of medical practice in the ICU. Other chapters in the handbook will be of interest to the medical computer scientist who is exploring the use of computers in critical-care settings.

Ginzton L.E., Laks M.M. (1984). Computer aided ECG interpretation. M.D. Computing, 1:36.
This article summarizes the development of computer-based ECG interpretation systems, discusses the advantages and disadvantages of such systems, and describes the process by which a typical system obtains and processes ECG data.

Strong D.M., Lee Y.W., Wang R.T. (1997). 10 potholes in the road to information quality. IEEE Computer, 31:38–46.
This article provides an entertaining and thoughtful presentation of the problems we all face as we acquire data. Its use of a general strategy to discuss data-quality problems and relate them to the medical field is refreshing.

Morris AH. Rational use of computerized protocols in the intensive care unit. Crit Care 2001 Oct;5(5):249-254.
Excess information in complex ICU environments exceeds human decisiion-making limits. This article outlines the strategies needed to use computerized protocols in a busy clinical critical care unit. The author bases his recommendations on decades of experience.

---

[6]Determination of the concentration of a dissolved substance. Titration is a method for adjusting the concentration of a drug to achieve a desired effect—for example, adjusting nitroprusside infusion to control blood pressure.

Questions for Discussion

1. Describe how the integration of information from multiple bedside monitors, the pharmacy, and the clinical laboratory can help to improve the sensitivity and specificity of the alarm systems used in the ICU.
2. What factors must you consider when deciding when and how often a physiological, biochemical, or observational variable should be measured and stored in a computer's database?
3. You have been asked to design part of an electronic exercise bicycle. Sensors in the hand grips of the bicycle will be used to pick up transmitted electrical signals reflecting the rider's heart activity. Your system then will display the rider's heart rate numerically in a liquid crystal display (LCD).
   a. Describe the steps your system must take in converting the heart's electrical signals (essentially a single ECG lead) into the heart rate displayed on the LCD.
   b. Describe how computerized data acquisition can be more efficient and accurate than manual methods of data acquisition.

18
Imaging Systems in Radiology

ROBERT A. GREENES AND JAMES F. BRINKLEY

18.1 Introduction

In chapter 9 we introduce the concept of **digital images** as a fundamental datatype that, because of its ubiquity, must be considered in many applications. We define biomedical **imaging informatics** as the study of methods for generating, manipulating, managing, and integrating images in many biomedical applications. We describe many of the methods for generating and manipulating images, particularly as applied to the brain, and discuss the relationship of these methods to structural informatics.

In this chapter we continue the study of imaging informatics by describing methods for managing and integrating images, focusing on how images are acquired from imaging equipment, stored, transmitted, and presented for interpretation. We also focus on how these processes and the image information are integrated with other clinical information and used in the health care enterprise, so as to have a maximal impact on patient care.

We discuss these issues in the context of Radiology, since imaging is the primary focus of that field[1]. Yet imaging is an important part of many other fields as well, including Pathology, Dermatology, Ophthalmology, Gastroenterology, Cardiology, Surgery (for minimally invasive procedures especially) and Obstetrics, which often do their own imaging procedures; most other fields that use imaging rely on Radiology and Pathology for their imaging needs.

The distribution of imaging responsibility has given rise to the need of many departments to address issues of image acquisition, storage, transmission, and interpretation. As these modalities have gradually become largely digital in format, the development of electronic systems to support these tasks has been needed.

We begin by describing some of the roles of imaging in all of biomedicine, then concentrate on their management and integration in radiology systems, bringing in illustrative examples from other disciplines where appropriate. We further focus primarily on the needs of the medical center-based Radiology department. Many Radiology departments are becoming highly distributed enterprises, with acquisition sites in intensive care unit areas, regular patient floors, emergency departments, vascular services,

---

[1]The name Radiology is itself a misnomer, since the field is involved in using ultrasound, magnetic resonance, optical, thermal, and other non-radiation imaging modalities when appropriate. Radiology departments in some institutions are thus referred to alternatively as Departments of Medical Imaging.

626

screening centers, ambulatory clinics, and in affiliated community-based practice settings. Interpretation of images may be in those locations when dedicated onsite radiologists are needed, but increasingly, due to high-speed network availability, interpretation can be done at central sites, or according to different methods of organization, since image acquisition and interpretation can be effectively decoupled. Independent imaging centers in a community face some of the same issues and opportunities, although to a lesser degree, so we focus primarily on the distributed medical center-based Radiology department in this chapter.

18.2   Basic Concepts and Issues

18.2.1   Roles for Imaging in Biomedicine

Imaging is a central part of the healthcare process for diagnosis, treatment planning, image-guided treatment, assessment of response to treatment, and estimation of prognosis. In addition, it plays important roles in medical communication and education, as well as in research.

18.2.1.1   Detection and diagnosis

Among the primary uses of images are for detection of medical abnormalities and for diagnostic purposes. Detection focuses on identifying the presence of an abnormality, but in the case in which the findings are not sufficiently specific to be characteristic of a particular disease, other methods must be used for actual diagnosis. This is the case, for example, for mammograms, which are often used for screening for breast cancer; once a suspicious abnormality is detected, usually a biopsy procedure is required for diagnosis. In other circumstances, the image finding is adequate to diagnose the abnormality, for example, the finding of focal stenosis or obstruction of a coronary artery during angiography is diagnostic in itself, and some tumors, congenital abnormalities, or other diseases have highly characteristic appearances. More often there is a continuum between detection and diagnosis, with a test able to not only detect but narrow the range of possibilities.

Diagnosis and detection can be done with a wide variety of imaging procedures. Images produced by visible light, as in ophthalmology, for example, can be used for retinal photography; in dermatology, to view skin lesions; and in pathology, for gross specimen viewing and for light microscopy. The visible-light spectrum is also responsible for producing images seen endoscopically, rendered typically as video images or sequences. Sound energy, in the form of echoes from internal structures, is used to form images in ultrasound, a modality used primarily in cardiac, abdominal, pelvic, breast, and obstetrical imaging, as well as in imaging of small parts, such as the thyroid and testes. In addition, **Doppler shifts** of sound frequency are used to evaluate blood flow in many organs and in major vessels. X-ray energy produces radiographic and **computed-tomography** (CT) images of most parts of the body: The differential absorption of X-rays by various tissues produces the varying densities that enable the images to characterize normal and abnormal structures. Isotope emissions of radioactive particles are used to produce nuclear-medicine images, which result from the differential concentration of radioactively tagged molecules in various tissues. **Magnetic-resonance imaging** (MRI) depicts energy fluctuations of certain atomic nuclei—primarily of hydrogen—when they are aligned in a magnetic field and then perturbed by an orthogonal radiofrequency pulse. Parameters such as proton density, rate at which the nuclei return to alignment, and rate of loss of phase coherence after the pulse can be measured in various combinations, depending on equipment configurations and pulse sequences. These quantities differ in various tissues due to differential concentrations of hydrogen atoms, thus enabling MRI to distinguish among them.

18.2.1.2   Assessment and Planning

In addition to being used for detection and diagnosis, imaging is often used to assess a patient's health status in terms of progression of a disease process (such as determination of tumor stage), response to treatment, and estimation of prognosis. We can analyze cardiac status by assessing the heart's size and motion echographically. Similarly, we can use ultrasound to assess fetal size and growth, as well as development. Computed tomography is used frequently to determine approaches for surgery or for radiation therapy. In the latter case, precise calculations of radiation-beam configuration can be determined to maximize dose to the tumor while minimizing absorption of radiation by surrounding tissues. This calculation is often performed by simulating alternative radiation-beam configurations. For surgical planning, three-dimensional volumes of CT or MRI data can be constructed and presented for viewing from different perspectives to facilitate determination of the most appropriate surgical approach.

18.2.1.3   Guidance of Procedures

Images can provide real-time guidance when virtual-reality methods are used to superimpose a surgeon's visual perspective on the appropriate image view in the projection that demonstrates the abnormality. With endoscopic and minimally invasive surgery, this kind of imaging can provide a localizing context for visualizing and orientating the endoscopic findings, and can enable monitoring of results of interventions such as focused ultrasound, cryosurgery, or thermal ablation.

Such minimally invasive surgery can be conducted at a distance (see Chapter 14), although practical to do so only in limited settings. Because the abnormality is viewed through a video monitor that displays the endoscopic field, the view can be physically remote, a technique called telepresence. Similarly, the manipulation of the endoscope itself can be controlled by a robotic device that reproduces the hand movements of a remote operator, along with **haptic feedback** reproducing the sensations of tissue textures, margins, and resistance, a technique called **telerobotics**.

18.2.1.4   Communication

Medical decision-making, including diagnosis and treatment planning, is often aided by allowing clinicians to visualize images concurrently with textual reports and discussions of interpretations. Thus, we consider imaging to be an important adjunct to communication and images to be a desirable component of a multimedia electronic medical record. Communicating digital images is essential to enable remote viewing, interpretation, and consultation, as in techniques such as **teleradiology, telepathology**, and **teledermatology**, collectively referred to as **telemedicine** (see Chapter 14).

18.2.1.5   Education and Training

Images, both still and in motion form, are an essential part of medical education and training, because so much of medical diagnosis and treatment depends on imaging and on the skills needed to interpret such images (see Chapter 21). Case libraries, tutorials, atlases, three-dimensional models, quiz libraries, and other resources using images can provide this kind of educational support.

Taking a history, performing a physical examination, and conducting medical procedures also demand appropriate visualization and observation skills. Training in these skills can be augmented by viewing images and video sequences, as well as through practice in simulated situations. An example of the latter is an approach to training individuals in endoscopy techniques by using a mannequin and video images in conjunction with tactile and visual feedback that correlate with the manipulations being carried out. An often-overlooked aspect of education that is aided by access to appropriate images is the provision of instructions and educational materials to patients—about their diseases, about procedures to be carried out, about follow-up care, and about healthy lifestyles.

18.2.1.6   Research

Imaging is, of course, also intimately involved in many aspects of research. An example is structural modeling of DNA and proteins, including their three-dimensional configurations (see Chapter 22). Another is the images obtained in molecular or cellular biology to follow the distributions of fluorescent or radioactively tagged molecules. The quantitative study of **morphometrics**, or growth and development, depends on the use of imaging methods. **Functional mapping**—for example, of the human brain—relates specific sites on images to particular functions.

18.2.2   The Radiologic Process and Its Interaction

As noted in the introduction, we concentrate in this chapter on the subset of imaging that falls under the purview of **Radiology**. Radiology departments are engaged in all aspects of the healthcare process, from detection and diagnosis to treatment, follow-up and prognosis assessment, and they illustrate well the many issues involved in acquiring and managing images, interpreting them, and communicating those interpretations. Space does not permit us to discuss the other disciplines that utilize imaging, but the processes involved and issues faced, which we discuss in the context of radiology, pertain to the other disciplines also. Occasionally, we intersperse examples from other areas, where we wish to emphasize a particular point, and imaging for educational purposes is discussed at length in Chapter 21.

The primary function of a Radiology department is the acquisition and analysis of medical images. Through imaging, healthcare personnel obtain information that can help them to establish diagnoses, to plan or administer therapy, and to follow the courses of diseases or therapies.

Diagnostic studies in the Radiology department are provided at the request of referring clinicians, who then use the information for decision-making. The Radiology department produces the images, and the radiologist provides the primary analysis and interpretation of the radiologic findings. Thus, radiologists play a direct role in clinical problem-solving and in diagnostic-work-up planning. **Interventional radiology** and image-guided surgery (if done by the radiologist) are activities in which the radiologist plays a primary role in treatment.

The radiologic process (Greenes, 1989) is characterized by seven kinds of tasks, each of which involves information exchange and which can be augmented and enhanced by information technology, as illustrated in Figure 18.1. The first five tasks occur in sequence, whereas the final two are ongoing and support the other five.

1. The process begins with an evaluation by a clinician of a clinical problem and determination of the need for an imaging procedure.
2. The procedure is requested and scheduled, the indication for the procedure is stated, and relevant clinical history is made available.
3. The imaging procedure is carried out, and images are acquired. The procedure may be tailored for particular clinical questions or patient status considerations.
4. The radiologist reviews the images in terms of the clinical history and questions to be answered and may manipulate the images. This task actually involves two interrelated subtasks: (a) perception of the relevant findings and (b) interpretation of those findings in terms of clinical meaning and significance.
5. The radiologist creates a report and may otherwise also directly communicate the results to the referring clinician, as well as making suggestions for further evaluation as needed. The process may then be repeated if a subsequent procedure is considered to be helpful.
6. Quality control and monitoring are carried out, with the aim of improving the foregoing processes. Factors such as patient waiting times, workloads, numbers of exposures obtained per procedure, quality of images, radiation dose, yields of procedures, and incidence of complications are measured and adjusted.
7. Continuing education and training are carried out through a variety of methods, including access to atlases, review materials, teaching-file cases, and feedback of subsequently confirmed diagnoses to interpreting radiologists.

All these tasks are now, in a growing number of departments, computer-assisted, and most of them involve images in some way. In fact, radiology is one branch of medicine in which even the basic data can be produced by computers and stored directly in computer memory. Radiology has also contributed strongly to advances in computer-aided instruction (see Chapter 21), in technology assessment (see Chapter 11), and in clinical decision support (see Chapter 20).

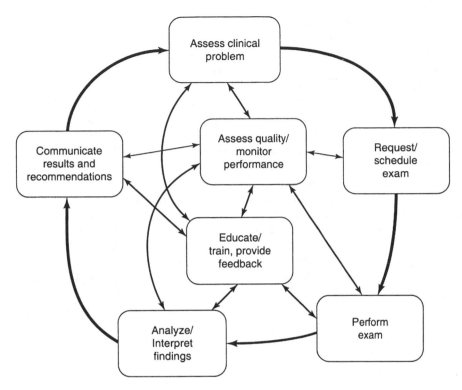

Figure 18.1. The radiologic process. The typical flow of activity begins when a clinician assesses a clinical problem and determines that an imaging procedure would be useful (top-most box). Subsequently, four classes of activities (moving clockwise around the circle) ensue, ending with a report to the clinician of the interpretation and possible recommendations for additional studies. The process may continue iteratively as needed. All these activities involve interaction between the clinical and imaging departments (e.g., performance of a particular imaging examination may require tailoring or special views, depending on the clinical question), and all depend on information exchange and information-technology support. The two classes of activity at the center of the diagram are not part of the workflow for individual procedures but are essential to maintaining quality and supporting the professional growth and development of participants; thus, ideally, they need to interact with all of the department-level workflow activities in the outer circle.

18.2.3   *Image Management and Display*

One of the major burdens implied by the radiologic process is the storage and retrieval of the images relating to specific examinations, which are required for interpretation by radiologists, for review by referring physicians, for consultation, for treatment planning, for education, and for research. As healthcare delivery networks disperse geographically, the need for remote access to images increases. These factors create a strong push toward digital capture, storage, transmission, interpretation, and review of images.

Although imaging modalities increasingly generate their images in digital form, many medical imaging studies were until recently primarily or secondarily recorded and stored on film. Even images produced by CT and MRI scans, which are inherently digital, had been often transferred to film after the technologist optimized them for viewing. Radiologists then placed the filmed images on illuminated light boxes, where the films could be analyzed in comparison to previous and related studies. For certain procedures—for example, ultrasound and fluoroscopic studies—the images would be recorded on videotape or videodisk rather than on film.

Before widespread digital imaging, and in those institutions still film-based, the management procedures have been typically as follows: Radiology personnel prepare a film folder for each examination (or type of examination), label it with patient-identification information, and file it with the patient's master film jacket in the film library. The staff must locate and retrieve the master jacket each time that the images are needed for review or for comparison with previous studies. If a clinician wishes to take a film out of the department, the staff must make a duplicate film or transact a loan.

Film storage requires a large amount of space. Typically, departments have the capacity to store films for only those patients whose studies were completed within the past 6 to 12 months. Older studies, usually retained for at least 7 years, are stored in a basement or warehouse (possibly off-site). Film is also expensive; radiology departments typically sell film from outdated examinations for recycling of silver content.

Digital acquisition of images has enabled dramatic reduction of the physical space requirements, material cost, and manual labor of traditional film-handling tasks through on-line digital archiving, rapid retrieval of images via querying of image databases, and high-speed transmission of images over communications networks. Researchers and industry have worked to develop systems that have such capabilities—**picture-archiving and communication systems** (PACS) (Fig. 18.2) (Dwyer, 1996; Bauman, 1996; Honeyman, 2003; Napoli, 2003; Huang, 2003). Many complex problems had to be solved for PACS to be practical, including development of technology for high-resolution acquisition, high capacity storage, and high-speed networking; standardization of image-transmission and storage formats; development of storage-management schemes for enormous volumes of data; and design of workstations, or display consoles, that are as convenient and acceptable to radiologists for the interpretation of digital images as are the illuminated light boxes used for film-based interpretation. Soft copy interpretation—that is, by the radiologist viewing digital images of a study at a workstation—is done in the growing number of departments that have become filmless, and increasingly for interpretation of remotely acquired studies in the practice of teleradiology. Dissemination of images along with reports for viewing by referring physicians throughout a healthcare enterprise, has been made possible by advances in image compression and in internet-based web technology.

18.2.3.1   Image Acquisition

The primary requirement for PACS is that it must obtain images in digital form (Horii, 1996). As discussed in Section 18.2, most imaging modalities—even those traditionally done on film—are now capable of producing direct digital output, yet replacement of

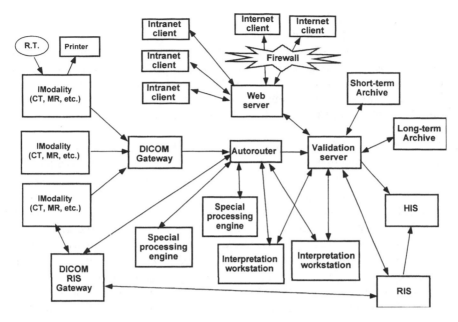

Figure 18.2. Architecture of a typical picture-archiving and communication system (PACS). Images are acquired by facilities specific to the various imaging modalities (such as computed radiography, CT, MRI, angiography, ultrasound, or nuclear medicine), and the facilities are operated largely by radiology (or imaging) technologists (denoted R.T.). Local printing of images on film or paper may be performed. Image procedures are scheduled through a radiology information system (RIS), and patient-identification and schedule information is transmitted to the modality workstation through a DICOM RIS gateway. Remote imaging centers operate in the same way.

The images produced are transmitted through a DICOM gateway to a server (autorouter), which is responsible for sending the images where they are needed and for managing workflow. The autorouter validates the linkage of images to the appropriate study (by interaction with a validation server) and distributes them according to rules (e.g., MRIs and CTs are sent to workstation x for interpretation).

Images can be viewed on interpretation workstations, both special purpose and generic, and manipulated by imaging professionals who use built-in workstation tools and invoke special processing functions through servers (e.g., for three-dimensional rendering, registration, and fusion of data from images obtained by two different modalities, for feature extraction, or for computer-aided detection).

Multiple images from a particular examination need to be associated, and both prior and other associated studies and reports may need to be available. This linkage is accomplished by the validation server, which is able to query for and retrieve information from the RIS or hospital information system (HIS), as well as from the PACS archives. The validation server is responsible for coordinating the association of image and nonimage information. Referring physicians may access images at internal and Internet based workstations, typically through a Web interface. Access from a browser through a Web server permits the user to obtain study information, including reports and images, through the validation server, which interacts with the PACS archive and with the HIS and RIS. (*Source:* Adapted from Brigham and Women's Hospital Department of Radiology internal document by William B Hanlon.)

all imaging equipment with digital units is expensive and has proceeded gradually as old equipment has needed to be updated or as departments have expanded.

In departments in which traditional imaging devices are still being used for some modalities, the only option for achieving a full PACS is digital scanning of film. Such scanning has been rarely done, however, because it requires considerable manual handling, for transport and manipulation of examination folders and films, for operating the scanner, and for recording of the patient and examination identification information.

In a growing number of departments of radiology, particularly those in academic medical centers, all imaging is digital with the exception of mammography. Digital mammography is still in use in only a small number of departments, since its assessment as a replacement for film mammography for breast cancer screening is, as of this writing, yet undergoing a large scale clinical trial known as DMIST. The DMIST trial is sponsored by the National Cancer Institute and conducted under the auspices of the American College of Radiology Imaging Network (ACRIN), a consortium of radiology departments and imaging centers (Hillman, 2002). Digital mammography has special problems, not only in terms of acquisition, because of the extremely high resolution requirements for detection of subtle abnormalities, but also because of issues of storage, and display for interpretation. The issues are discussed further in section 18.2.3.5.

18.2.3.2   Storage Requirements

On-line digital archiving of image data for a busy radiology department requires vast amounts of storage. Image modalities differ substantially in their storage requirements, depending on the contrast and spatial resolution needed, the number of images or the size of the data sets, whether raw or processed data are stored, and whether data-compression techniques are used.

Table 18.1 indicates typical raw-data storage requirements (that is, with no preprocessing or postprocessing and no compression) for examinations of a variety of image types. A CT image, for example, consists of a 512×512 array of pixels. If the full dynamic range of CT numbers is saved, each pixel is represented by 12 bits. Once the radiologist or technologist has determined the optimal brightness and contrast settings for displaying the region of interest, however, perhaps only 8 bits per pixel need to be saved. A typical CT examination still consists of 40 to 80 cross-sectional slices. Additional slices are required if both precontrast and postcontrast images, or other special slices, are desired. Assuming that a CT examination consists of 60 images and that the full dynamic range is retained for each, then $60 \times 512 \times 512 \times 12$ bits, or approximately 180 million bits, must be saved. Because 12 bits of data typically are stored as 2 bytes, this storage requirement corresponds to 30 million bytes. CT scanning is becoming increasingly higher in resolution, with slice thickness decreasing, and thus with many more slices obtained to cover a given field, such as a patient's chest. Storage requirements of course increase correspondingly.

A single-view chest X-ray (or CR) image consists of $2,048 \times 2,560 \times 12$ bits of data; therefore, a typical two-image (front and side views) examination contains about 120 million bits. A real-time ultrasound examination generates video images at 30 frames

Table 18.1. Comparative imaging parameters for alternative imaging modalities.

	CR	MRI	CT	US	NM
Pixels per image	2048×2560	256×256	512×512	512×512	128×128
Bits per pixel	12	10	12	8	8
Typical no. of mages per study	2	100	60	30 (plus dynamic series)	30
Bytes per study*	20M	12M	30M	7.5M (for static images only)	0.5M
Contrast resolution	low	high	high	low	low
Spatial resolution	high	Low	mod	mod	low
Temporal resolution	low	low	mod	high	high
Radiation	mod	none	mod	none	mod
Portability	some	no	no	no	yes
Physiologic function	no	yes	no	no	yes
Cost	mod	high	high	low	mod

CR = computed radiography, MRI = magnetic resonance imaging, CT = computed tomography, US = ultrasound, NM = nuclear medicine.
*Assume 2 bytes needed per pixel for images with pixel depth of 10 or 12 bits.

per second. Of these, a radiologist usually selects 30 to 40 frames for later analysis. Occasionally, dynamic sequences, such as those portraying a cardiac arrhythmia, are retained at the full rate of 30 images per second. Resolution per image is 512×512 pixels; about 8 bits per pixel are required to store the acoustical signal once the image has been postprocessed for optimal viewing. Nuclear-medicine images have lower resolution—typically, $128 \times 128 \times 8$, or about 130,000 bits of data per image are sufficient. Magnetic resonance imaging has intermediate resolution but uses multiple images similar to CT except that data are available for a volume of the body rather than for single slices, and data on several parameters at each voxel are potentially useful.

Considering that a typical radiology department performs 250 examinations per day, and nominally assuming 10 megabytes per study, then, in an average day, approximately 2.5 gigabytes of data must be transmitted from the image-acquisition nodes to the image archive. Assuming 250 working days per year (ignoring weekends for simplicity), we estimate that the storage requirements per year for examination image data are on the order of 625 gigabytes. These requirements are only increasing, however, due to the aforementioned trend to higher resolution cross-sectional imaging, as well as to the increasing proportion of imaging studies that involve such technologies.

In addition to the on-line maintenance of active images, an image archiving system must provide for the storage of older image data. Because of the large storage requirements, practical systems will use some form of hierarchical storage management, whereby the most current images are easily and rapidly accessible, and images that are less likely to be retrieved are stored in a less costly, less accessible form.

Magnetic disks and optical disks are the most practical media for on-line storage of image data. Magnetic disks currently available can store over 80 gigabytes for half-height drives. Cost per megabyte continues to drop dramatically. Optical write-once compact disks (CDs) are still only 650 megabytes, but 4.6 gigabyte (or greater) digital video (DVD) drives are available in writable form. Magneto-optical (MO) disks are 5.2

gigabyte or greater. Magneto-optical media are expensive and have slow read and write times. Jukeboxes are available, however, in 150-, 500-, and 1,000-platter sizes. For archiving, dense media (such as tape) are still needed, so most departments must maintain an unattractive three-tiered storage scheme, using magnetic disks for active data, optical or MO disks for intermediate storage, and tape, optical disks, or laser cards for inactive storage.

An alternate strategy uses large magnetic disks of 500 gigabytes (0.5 terabytes) or more, sufficient to store approximately 1 year's image data in a typical department; and a digital-tape library functioning for long-term storage, with radiology information systems (RISs) scheduling and pre-fetching to retrieve older examinations for comparison before they are needed (see Section 18.2.3.2).

Data compression and prior selection or preprocessing of image data can reduce storage requirements considerably. Compression may be lossless or lossy (Dwyer, 1996; Woods, 1991). **Lossless compression** uses simple run-length encoding (RLE) or variations on other sequence coding schemes such as Huffman encoding, which assigns the shortest codes to most frequently occurring values. Maximum compression ratios achievable with lossless methods are on the order of 2:1 or 3:1.

Lossy compression uses methods to filter the image's frequency spectrum and to encode data selectively at various frequencies more compactly and to eliminate other frequencies, which primarily contain noise. A widely used method developed by the Joint Photographic Experts Group is JPEG compression, which codes images for hue and saturation (or color and intensity). Because the eye is less sensitive to variations in hue than it is to variations in intensity, the hue values can be stored with lower resolution. Compression ratios as high as 20:1 can be obtained with JPEG compression, but with variable quality. The latest version, JPEG 2000, includes the option for progressive JPEG, allowing lower resolution images to be transmitted initially, and the image gradually enhanced with more detail, based on transmission speed. An extension of JPEG 2000 allows for encoding of 12-bit gray-scale image data, as needed in medical images, rather than just 8-bit data per color, as in standard JPEG. The 12-bit extended capabilities, while defined, are not widely supported with available tools, however. Fractal compression is another method that has been explored.

Wavelet compression is now widely accepted as a superior method for image compression (Vetterli & Kovarevic, 1995). Wavelets are basis functions for representing discrete data or continuous functions; they operate more locally than the **Fourier transform**. They have compact support: There is no truncation error when finite signals, such as those for radiological images, are processed. Wavelet basis functions are orthonormal, meaning that the terms in a wavelet series are nonredundant. Wavelet series provide multiresolution representations for data, organizing them into a hierarchy according to spatial frequency and spatial position. Wavelet compression may eventually become the standard method adopted by JPEG, in future releases, but standardization of wavelet methods is not as far along currently as is JPEG.

Wavelet compression at ratios as high as 80:1 for plain films such as mammograms have being evaluated, and found to be satisfactory, although ratios of more than 60:1 are rarely used. Wavelet compression may actually *enhance* image appearance by preferentially eliminating nonstructural noise, such as artifacts. Lower compression ratios are achievable for other modalities, depending on how much redundant information is present; for example, 20:1 to 30:1 is possible for chest X-ray images. CT scans are less compressible, with ratios on the order of 6:1.

Another consideration in storage relates to speed of access. Storage on a local workstation provides fastest access from the point of view of responsiveness to user manipulations; storage on a server may be sufficient if the network speeds are sufficiently high. Images stored on a local workstation must be transmitted there in advance—for example, at off-peak network-traffic times. An examination may have multiple images, and the same image may need to be processed, enhanced, or viewed in multiple different ways (see Section 18.2.2.6), all of which require storage. After she completes the interpretation, the radiologist may indicate that only a few of the images contain clinically important information. It then may be practical to archive the other images on optical disk or on another slower access medium. After the examination is complete and has been reviewed by all relevant clinical practitioners, it can also be archived *in toto*. As a consequence, however, when a practitioner wants to compare an older study with a current study—for example, to evaluate progression of disease—the archived images must be retrieved from the slower access medium. Thus, hierarchies of storage and algorithms for deciding where to place image data based on patterns of expected use and network traffic are required for smooth functioning of a PACS.

18.2.3.3   Image Transmission

The integration of distributed viewing stations, on-line image databases, image-management systems, and broadband local-area networks (LANs) and wide-area networks (WANs) allows imaging data to be shared among health professionals at remote viewing sites. Furthermore, the data can be viewed at multiple locations simultaneously. Thus, health personnel throughout an institution or extended health-care enterprise can have timely and convenient access to medical images.

The principal media for image transmission and networking are broadband **coaxial cable** and **fiberoptic cable** (see Chapter 5). Coaxial cable, used in the cable-television industry, supports a variety of network topologies. Coaxial networks are relatively inexpensive, and they are reliable, although they are susceptible to electrical and radiofrequency interference. Fiberoptic networks offer a high degree of reliability without interference problems, but they are somewhat more limited with respect to the topologies that they can support and the ease with which connections can be added. Slow-speed connections using modems have maximum transmission rates of 56 kilobits per second (Kbps). Wide-area optical-network backbones can now transmit data at 2.4 gigabits per second (Gbps). Many options are available between these extremes, depending on cost limitations and distance requirements, and a network can be configured to combine different components via gateways. The network configuration and the capacity of each part must be planned in relation to considerations such as patterns of expected use and cost. Particular *network topologies* and protocols available for both LAN and WAN connectivity, and their influence on transmission speeds, are discussed in Chapter 5. Because of the large sizes of image files, image transmission times can vary from hours to seconds, depending on choice of network method and degree of compression.

18.2.3.4   Standardization of Formats

TCP/IP (see Chapters 5 and 7) is the dominant low-level protocol used in medical imaging. Transmission of data about a medical imaging procedure, however, including patient, examination, and image data, require higher level messaging formats. Layered protocols are organized to build such messages. The seven-layer Open Standards Interconnect (OSI) protocol of the International Standards Organization (ISO) is a conceptual model that provides for application, presentation, session, transport, network, data link, and physical layers (see Chapter 5). In practice, higher-level protocols at the application or presentation level tend to combine several of the layers of the OSI/ISO model.

For PACS to succeed, developers have needed to agree on a vendor-neutral format for patient demographic and clinical data, examination-specific data, and image-specific data to be stored, as well as on protocols for network communication of these data. The format, developed as an outgrowth of work by the American College of Radiology (ACR) and the National Equipment Manufacturers Association (NEMA), and known as Digital Imaging and Communications in Medicine (**DICOM**), has been adopted to a large extent worldwide for both radiological and other medical images (also see Chapter 7).

In DICOM, the higher-level transmission protocol is loosely based on the OSI/ISO reference model but embraces traditional computer networks for the transport layer and below. DICOM is intended to ensure that a wide variety of equipment (acquisition devices, archive nodes, interpretation consoles, review workstations, servers doing special processing, and so on) can be interfaced with the network and that the data can be recognized and interpreted correctly by all the nodes on the network.

In contrast to the original ACR-NEMA standards, which dealt with only point-to-point transmission protocols, DICOM adopts an object-oriented model and consists of definitions of information objects, service classes (functions performed on or with objects), and network protocols. DICOM 3.0 is a complex multipart standard consisting of 13 parts, specifications for which are available by purchase from the NEMA website (NEMA, 2004). The most current summary is available only on the Radiology Society of North America (RSNA) website (RSNA, 2004). The parts include object definitions, service-class specifications, data structures and encoding, data dictionary, network protocols, and media-storage and file-format specifications.

18.2.3.5   Display Capabilities

A major task of PACS researchers is to develop workstations on which users can view and interpret digital images. The design of image-viewing consoles that are suitable for interpretation of examinations by radiologists poses a host of technical and human engineering problems: Consoles must match the low cost, convenience, and flexibility of illuminated light boxes that radiologists use for interpreting film-based images.

Radiologists usually interpret an examination by comparing multiple images from both the current examination and previous or correlative studies. Flexibility is crucial as radiologists organize and reorganize the images to display temporal sequence, to reflect anatomic organization, and to compare *preintervention* versus *postintervention* (e.g., images obtained before and after injection of a contrast medium). Furthermore, when radiologists analyze an image, their attention shifts rapidly between overview or general pattern-recognition modes of viewing and detailed inspection of specific areas. The ability to reshuffle images, to shift attention, to zoom in on a specific area, and to step back again to get an overview are all essential to the interpretive and analytic processes. These effects are easy to achieve with film, but are difficult to replicate on a viewing console (Figure. 18.3).

Mammography presents especially difficult challenges for soft-copy interpretation. As we indicated in section 18.2.3.1, mammography requires extremely high resolution for microcalcification detection. Further, user interface requirements are demanding for optimal interpretation of microcalcifications, nodules, and regions of asymmetry. In conventional film-screen mammography, typically four film images are obtained (views of each breast in two orthogonal planes), which are used to localize potential abnormalities within a breast, and for comparing one side vs. the other in both planes. If available, four images from the most recent prior study are also compared, for determining whether any change has occurred. These can be arranged readily on a fluorescent light box, but manipulation of eight high-resolution images on one or two display screens to facilitate the same kind of evaluations is a challenge. A countervailing advantage for digital mammography is the ability to preprocess images with computer-aided detection (CAD) algorithms for highlighting potential nodules and microcalcifications.

Because of the above challenges, a multi-site national clinical trial (DMIST: the Digital Mammography Imaging Screening Trial) is currently underway, as noted in Section 18.2.3.1, for comparing conventional vs. digital mammography, conducted by ACRIN and sponsored by the National Cancer Institute.

Experience with CT underscores the challenges of designing viewing consoles for image interpretation. Computed tomography is the quintessential digital imaging modality. Furthermore, viewing consoles are available to and operated by radiologists. Nonetheless, interpretation of CT scans still until recently was done on film. The viewing console associated with a CT scanner for many years had limited flexibility, permitting the technologist to retrieve single images (slices) one at a time, to manipulate the image's gray scale for detailed inspection, and to perform some analysis. Typically, however, it did not allow the operator to view all the images of a study concurrently, to rearrange them, or to zoom in rapidly on particular images for detailed inspection. For these reasons, the CT console was used only to determine whether patients had been positioned properly, to monitor the progress of studies, and to optimize the display before images were photographed onto sheets of film. Radiologists then did the interpretations from the film or from satellite workstations.

Interpretation consoles or workstations have advanced considerably, and now support general image-manipulation operations (such as gray scale manipulation, histogram equalization, edge enhancement, image subtraction, and on-line measurement), and other operations that radiologists need to perform while analyzing images. Significant issues that have been dealt with have concerned size and number of display

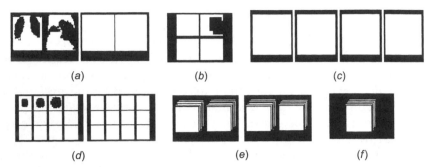

Figure 18.3. Workstation-display alternatives for multi-image data. Because most imaging studies involve more than one image per study, and because comparison with prior studies is frequently needed, a single monitor is almost never sufficient for viewing an entire study in full resolution.

Considering only gray scale modalities, most examinations produce images of more than 8 bits of data per pixel (more than 256 gray levels). Monitors are constrained to 8-bit pixel depth; however, brightness and contrast adjustment (window and level manipulation) are almost always needed so that the viewer can adapt the display to the particular kind of image and type of tissue or process being visualized. Horizontal and vertical dimensions of an image need to be considered, a task that involves many factors, including pixel dot resolution (how close pixels are to one another), physical size of monitor, typical viewing distance of user, and desired physical size of the image.

Examples *a–c* are three alternative views of chest X-rays (posteroanterior and lateral views of the current study compared with same two views of a previous study—four images in all). On either a 1,000 or 2,000 pixel-wide monitor, the images could be positioned in landscape mode (*a* and *b*) or in portrait mode (*c*). Whether or not reduced in size, areas of an image or an entire image can be zoomed to higher magnification as depicted by the inset in (*b*).

For studies with large numbers of images, such as CT and MRI studies, rather than proliferating monitors to view an entire study and comparisons, it is often preferable to link the current and previous study such that the viewer can compare similar portions of both studies—for example, by anatomic region, cross-sectional orientation, or window/level setting, as shown in *d*, where the entire study is not visible. The user can scroll through a study on each monitor independently, on both monitors as single continuous series, or simultaneously through subsets of images on both monitors (they are linked).

Alternatively, cross-sectional images can be viewed as linked volumes of stacked images, which are scrolled through, one slice at a time, either automatically (movie mode) or manually (*e*). Example (*f*) shows another way to view large numbers of slices that represent a volume: by reconstructing them as three-dimensional volumes.

Other factors to be determined in workstation design include luminance, orientation (landscape versus portrait), and nondisplay qualities such as kinds of controls (e.g., zoom, pan, measurement, enhancement), cost, quality of graphical user interface, and general ease of use, including degree to which functions are integrated into and facilitate workflow.

monitors to be used, resolution of the monitors, and design of the user interface to provide convenient and natural access to needed functionality (Lou,1996).

The display of three-dimensional imaging data places even greater demands on consoles to calculate and redisplay oblique slices and rotated views rapidly (Vannier, 1996).

Another mode that is frequently used is to view a sequence of slices as an animated image as the user scrolls through the volume either up or down, in a particular plane, or doing the same thing in an automated "movie" mode. This is especially needed as the resolution and number of images per study continue to increase, as discussed earlier, for many cross-sectional imaging examinations. In addition, some interpretation requires image-specific processing capabilities; for example, a program may use mathematical models to calculate cardiac volume or fetal weight (Greenes, 1982).

Special capabilities can be incorporated in the design of viewing consoles, e.g., for MRI data manipulation because of the specialized nature of an MRI database. MRI data are inherently three dimensional. Each point typically is associated with multiple data values, the interpretations of which are also dependent on a variety of data acquisition and examination parameters. The design of practical image-interpretation workstations thus requires considerable human engineering and experimentation.

For distribution of images to referring clinicians, to enable them to review examinations that already have been preprocessed and interpreted, lower resolution may be acceptable, as well as less processing and data-transmission volume and smaller local memory. Workstations for review and consultation, however, must be easily accessible and thus must be conveniently distributed throughout an institution, or throughout an extended integrated delivery network. Access via the World Wide Web provides a means for meeting this need, coupled with image compression methods.

18.2.3.6   Cost

Image management and PACS development were initially conceived as having significant benefits for radiology departments in terms of reductions in film-library space and personnel time, as well as immediacy of access to images. Direct acquisition of high-quality digital images took longer than anticipated for some modalities—notably plain-film radiography and, still in transition, mammography. Secondary digitization by scanning from film is not cost-effective. As a result, some parts of radiology departments (such as the CT, MRI, ultrasound, and nuclear medicine sections, in which images are intrinsically digital) were more amenable to PACS than other parts, giving rise to mini-PACS systems.

It is now recognized that much of the benefit of PACS accrues from the provision of image results to clinicians in a timely fashion to facilitate clinical management, the ability to conduct distant consultations, and the performance of teleradiology services (Goldberg, 1996; Brown, 2004). The push in those directions shifted the emphasis in development and cost justification. As a result, implementation of full-department PACS has often been an evolutionary process in an institution or integrated delivery system, concurrent with the evolution of the entire healthcare enterprise to a multimedia-capable environment suitable for image distribution. Interest has also grown in distributing nonradiology image-based examination results (e.g., cardiology, pathology) as well (Siegel, 1997; Kalinski, 2002). Costs for the network infrastructure and for image acquisition, storage, and review can be shared by the entire healthcare system rather than falling exclusively to radiology departments.

18.2.4   Integration with Other Healthcare Information

Health-care images are useful only to the extent that they are accessible to applications that make use of them. For clinical practice, images must be integrated with the data about them, including data indicating the examinations through which they were obtained and the patients to whom they relate. Radiological images and the associated data need to be available to interpreting radiologists as well as to clinicians. They need to be reviewed for diagnosis, treatment planning, and procedure guidance. Practitioners may need to consult about the images perhaps via a network. Images may also need to be shown to patients, with whom the findings are discussed.

Medical images arising from procedures carried out by specialists other than radiologists pose many of the same challenges. As healthcare practice becomes increasingly distributed, the needs for image distribution and access become more varied, and timeliness of availability of the image, the associated report, and other relevant clinical information is key. In addition, uses of images in medical education and training, and in research, create further needs for image distribution and access. In this section, we discuss a variety of aspects of this challenge and approaches to fostering image integration.

Healthcare information systems require both vertical and horizontal integration (Greenes, 1996). Specialized functionality—such as for image manipulation or interpretation, for education, or for decision support—as well as more comprehensive capabilities embodied in HISs have tended to develop in relative isolation over many years or even decades. As a result, the software architectures of systems that implement these capabilities often are incompatible and frequently are inflexible with respect to ease of integration with one another. Newer systems approaches that rely on open architectures and standard interfaces and data models facilitate such integration (Deibel, 1996; Wong, 2003; Chu 2000) but often cannot simply replace existing legacy systems; instead, evolutionary strategies must be developed (also see Chapter 13). This often involves development of Web-based front ends to specialized databases and services. The longevity of older legacy back-end services is thereby increased, and the back-end services can be upgraded or replaced without major redesign of the front-end client interface.

18.2.4.1   Radiology Information Systems

The workings of a radiology department illustrate the many tasks in producing and managing clinical images. Management of work flow in a radiology department is a complex activity that involves not only maintenance of the film library and digital archive but also scheduling of examinations, registration of patients, performance of examinations, review and analysis of studies by radiologists, creation of interpretations, transcription of dictated reports (or generation of structured reports directly by radiologists), distribution of radiology reports to referring physicians, and billing for services. In addition, department managers must collect and analyze process-control and financial data to prepare budgets, to make appropriate informed decisions regarding staffing levels and the purchase of additional equipment, and to identify problems, such as overly large numbers of retakes of images, too many portable or urgent examination requests, excessive patient waiting times, poor image quality, and unacceptable delays in report transcription or signatures. Inventory control, quality assurance, radiation-exposure monitoring, and preventive-maintenance scheduling are other important managerial functions.

As noted in previous chapters, many information-intensive tasks yield readily to automation; computer-based **Radiology Information Systems** (RISs) have been developed to handle almost the entire spectrum of information-management tasks in the radiology department. RISs have been implemented either as standalone systems or as components of HISs. In either case, an RIS must be integrated with other information systems within an institution to allow reconciliation of patient data, to support examination scheduling and results reporting, and to facilitate patient billing.

Picture-archiving and communication system (PACS) image-management functions must be integrated with RISs and HISs. Because an RIS (or, in some cases, an HIS) keeps track of examinations and associates them with patients, and a PACS keeps track of images and associates them with examinations, the task is to provide coordination between the examination data on the two systems. Several different implementation approaches are possible. For example, the RIS (or HIS) can be augmented such that examination records indicate the presence of associated images. The path to the images can be stored directly with the examination record on the RIS (or HIS), or the examination data can be duplicated on the PACS, where pointers to the images for each examination are maintained. Alternatively, the PACS can be augmented with patient-lookup and examination-lookup capabilities and the databases from an RIS or HIS duplicated on it. Whenever a user application submits a query about images, the query is sent to a PACS server; queries about other clinical information are sent to the RIS or HIS. Again, a Web-based front end could integrate with appropriate back-end services of HIS, RIS, and PACS to eliminate such duplication. Such new architectures are beginning to be developed, but the transition from legacy systems with limited integration via the Web is only slowly occurring.

18.2.4.2 Reporting Methodology

We consider the tasks of producing and distributing radiology reports separately because they pose unique challenges. Traditionally, most reporting of image interpretations has been done by means of dictation by the radiologist, with transcription by typists and editing and approval by the radiologist. In recent years, digital dictation systems have enabled retrieval of voice reports by referring physicians or even voice-report automatic distribution.

Considerable work has gone into voice-recognition systems; the user's voice may trigger canned phrases or complete prestructured templates, or it may add free-text comments. Until recently, these systems have been cumbersome to use and did not have great success. The biggest impediment has been the poor ability to handle continuous speech—a hurdle that systems have begun to overcome. Even with the best systems, if there is a non-negligible error rate, the radiologist must view the text and correct the errors, causing a slowdown of the reporting process and thus reducing acceptability.

A compromise that is used as a transition to full voice recognition operation is to use voice recognition to create a draft report which a transcriptionist/editor reads along with the voice dictation, and corrects as needed. This reduces typing effort and thus improves turnaround time for the same size transcription staff. It does little to reduce report turnaround delays, however, since the biggest component of turnaround time is typically the time between completion of transcription and report editing/signing by the radiologist.

Reporting of interpretations using structured methods that encode findings in databases is desirable to facilitate retrieval for research studies. It also avoids the need for transcription and subsequent editing/signing. Structured reporting using computer interaction has been explored for many years. The idea here is that radiologists could compose reports by concatenating prestored phrases, augmenting the phrases by limited free-text keyboard or voice entry. They could use templates, for certain classes of examinations, that mimic typical report formats, which can then be tailored, or they could simply compose reports de novo through phrase selection from hierarchical or alphabetic menus. This approach has been used successfully in certain areas—for example, in obstetrical ultrasound (Greenes, 1982), where the entry of data on fetal size can be augmented by automatic calculation of fetal gestational age, weight, and percentile; in ultrasound generally, where findings can be initially entered by technologists, for radiological review (Bell, 1994); and in mammography, where the range of abnormalities is fairly limited and where a standardized vocabulary exists (BI-RADS, a mammography vocabulary standard developed by the American College of Radiology) (D'Orsi, 1997; Liberman, 2002).

18.2.4.3   Enterprise Integration

Beyond the integration of the HIS, RIS, and PACS, further challenges are posed by geographically distributed integrated delivery networks (IDNs) that have formed to deliver health care in a region more efficiently and effectively and to support the complete needs of patients in the networks. In an IDN environment, clinical data and images typically are obtained from multiple sources (hospitals, offices, imaging centers) and distributed for interpretation (to the imaging specialist) and for review (to the requesting clinician and other specialists). Multiway consultations can be carried out, with all parties concurrently or asynchronously viewing and perhaps annotating the images. Images from different sources may need to be fused or used in image-guided treatment.

Beyond the tasks of reconciling patient identification and of providing a consistent user interface to a virtual or real clinical repository (discussed in Chapter 13), IDNs must provide an information-technology infrastructure that supports multimedia-capable high-speed network connectivity among all participants to achieve enterprise-wide integration of images. The infrastructure must also provide the necessary servers for managing the imaging and clinical-data repositories and must ensure that these servers are readily available and able to handle the loads required. Client workstations must have the necessary hardware and software configurations to run the applications; in a distributed network with 10,000 or more workstations, as is not atypical, workstation management may require central resources for automatically checking client workstations and remotely installing software updates.

The multiple sources of image data and the diverse uses of data for clinical practice, education, and research all require an infrastructure that facilitates flexible integration of distributed software components, as opposed to design of comprehensive integrated, monolithic software. As demands become more complex, applications at a user work-station are increasingly functioning as the locus for integration of specialized services that are obtained over the network and for control of the **presentation layer**, or user interface. **Middleware** components are being developed that support access, processing, analysis, and composition of lower-level resources available through basic services, such as access to image data or clinical data (Fig. 18.4). The software architecture in some of these approaches permits middleware components to run either on workstations or on servers (with workstations in this case functioning as "thin clients"), thus enabling adaptation to workstation capacity, network speeds, traffic loads, and other factors that can affect performance.

18.3   Historical Development

18.3.1   The Evolution of Image Management in Picture-Archiving and Communication Systems

Over the past 20 years, many researchers have worked to develop PACS implementations. Based on the experience of early projects in the 1980s, it became clear that researchers had to devote considerable work to building an infrastructure that would support (1) image acquisition from the various modalities; (2) storage of image data to accommodate both clinical use (short term) and archiving (long term); (3) transmission of image data within a LAN among the PACS acquisition, storage, and display nodes; (4) workstation display for interpretation and review; (5) integration with RISs and hospital information systems (HISs); and (6) generation of hard copy film recordings (Dwyer, 1996). Teleradiology uses WANs, but otherwise requires much of the same infrastructure.

Some early projects focused on one or two aspects of the overall PACS problem, whereas others attempted to incorporate all aspects of a PACS. A problem faced by early researchers was the rapid evolution of network, storage, and workstation technology, causing obsolescence of the initial systems. At the University of Kansas, Templeton and colleagues (Templeton,1984) developed one of the earliest prototype systems to study the image-management requirements of a PACS-supported radiology department, investigating a hierarchical storage strategy and developing projections about network capacity and archival storage requirements. Blaine and colleagues (Blaine, 1983) at the Mallinckrodt Institute of Radiology in St. Louis developed a **PACS workbench**: a set of tools to study PACS design and to conduct experiments related to image acquisition, transmission, archiving, and viewing. Another prototype system developed by Arenson and colleagues (Arenson, 1988) at the Hospital of the University of Pennsylvania was designed to provide a comprehensive image database that could be used for image review and consultation, with an initial focus on the intensive-care unit. A fiberoptic network, in a star configuration, linked digital image-acquisition devices, image-archiving nodes, and image-review stations, with the central node of the

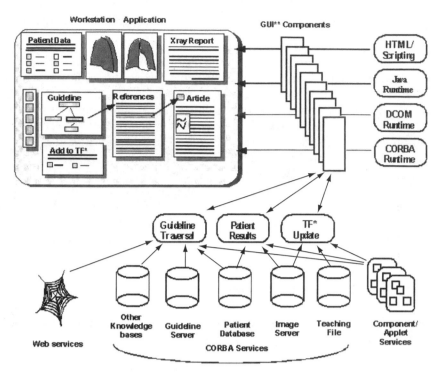

Figure 18.4. New architectures for imaging workstation applications. Workstations for both imaging specialists and clinicians should be able to bring together data, images, and knowledge resources of a variety of types, as required for a particular application. Consider a radiologist interpreting an examination, needing to retrieve the examination-request data, the images, and other relevant data about the patient and then creating a report (possibly through a voice-recognition interface). The radiologist may wish to review current guidelines for the clinical situation, including retrieval of pertinent references, before making a recommendation for further workup, to include in the report. Also, because the case had unusual findings, the radiologist may select relevant images for addition to a departmental teaching file, enter a brief description, and select diagnostic code terms.

The workstation must be able to assemble information from the HIS, the RIS, the PACS, a guideline library, and other knowledge bases and Web resources and to update the teaching file (TF). All of these resources may exist on separate hardware platforms, independent systems both old and new, and incompatible formats. A wide variety of capabilities must be integrated into the application, so complexity is managed by an approach in which each resource type responds to requests for services in a standard manner. That is, interfaces allow resources to be considered externally as well-defined components, independent of how they are implemented internally. They represent the message in a syntax and semantics understood by both sender and receiver and use a standard invocation and transport method. Evolving standards for messages include HL 7 for clinical data and DICOM for image data. Active X/DCOM, CORBA, HTML, and Java provide alternative standards for invocation and transport of the messages. Note that the workstation does not need to perform all the work of integration. Components can be developed to do many of these tasks—an approach that is particularly desirable if there is likely to be a need to reuse that component in another application. As such *middleware* components proliferate, they can carry out increasingly sophisticated tasks, including invocation of other middle components. Components may have client-side graphical-user-interface (GUI) responsibilities as well for visual display and interaction with the user.

network—the image manager—connected to the department's RIS. Nondigital images were scanned manually.

Progress since those early systems has been substantial on several fronts. Acquisition initially required hand-crafting of interfaces to proprietary imaging hardware. Gradually, DICOM was adopted as the format for transmission of image, examination, and patient data from acquisition devices to storage devices. Storage of the huge volumes of data required for a typical radiology department's images was initially hampered by the cost and capacity limitations of disk storage systems. We have seen a marked expansion in disk capacities, dramatic decreases in costs, and the advent of read–write optical disks and jukebox units that provide multiple terabytes of storage. Hierarchical storage-management schemes schedule migration of image files from high-speed storage to slower media based on predictions of decreased likelihood of future access. Compression methods, such as the use of wavelet-transform encoding, can also greatly reduce storage requirements.

Workstation display also has greatly improved, with screens and image memory enabling 2,000 × 2,500 pixel resolution becoming relatively inexpensive. Workstation random-access memory (RAM) and video graphic board memory have increased, thus enabling local storage of image files at full resolution, with rapid selective display of reduced-size images, regions of interest, zoomed portions of images, and alterations in brightness or contrast characteristics. Luminance of a video monitor is one of the key factors enabling sufficient gray-scale range to be visualized; high-luminance monitors have been available for a number of years.

Workstation software enabling management of the images on the screen, in terms of placement, size, and sort sequence, as well as access to image-manipulation tools, has become progressively more user friendly, with brightness and contrast control, zoom, pan, various image enhancement methods, measurement, annotation, and methods of image processing (Lou, 1996). Higher end workstations permit three-dimensional reconstruction of images, rotations, exposure of arbitrary planes, and selective removal of specific anatomic structures that are identified by their imaging characteristics (Vannier, 1996); these machines are used increasingly in surgical planning and image-guided therapy. For some image enhancement and for three-dimensional modeling, the computations involved are often performed by a networked server rather than at the workstation directly.

Network technology for the earliest systems was limited to slow-speed Ethernet. Fiber Distributed Data Interface (FDDI), asynchronous transfer mode (ATM), and fast Ethernet have all become widely available, and gateways among them have been developed for both LAN and WAN applications. Linkage of PACS with RISs and with HISs now has been accomplished in a number of ways by various commercial implementations. Such connection facilitates definitive patient identification, attachment of demographics, and association of radiology examination and report data with the relevant images, as discussed in Section 18.2.4.

As noted earlier, the initial PACS implementations were designed to support the all-digital, filmless radiology department. Although this goal has been achieved in a growing number of sites, the emphasis has now included image distribution and access to facilitate enterprise-wide communication and rapid image and result review.

18.3.2   Integration of Images with Radiology Information Systems

Information management for procedures associated with clinical-imaging activities had its origins in RISs. Over the years, similar information systems have been developed to handle the procedure flow in pathology, as well as in other departments that deal with images. In some cases, these services have been incorporated in the functionality of HISs; in other cases, they have been developed as separate systems that operate independently and have limited interface to an HIS. Gradually, as integrated delivery networks have forced the development of more highly modular and comprehensive software architectures, and as demands for both image and information access have spread enterprise-wide, a new level of integration has been developed between legacy systems and newer systems.

18.3.2.1   Computer-Based Information Management Systems

The first applications of computers to radiology information management were developed in the late 1960s. At that time, a study at the Massachusetts General Hospital (MGH) identified two major bottlenecks in the hospital's radiology department: (1) patient-examination scheduling and (2) film-library management. The researchers designed and implemented a system to automate these two functions (Bauman, 1975a,b). The examination-scheduling system checked for conflicting or duplicate examinations, assigned patients to examination rooms, and assisted in the registration of essential patient data. It produced flashcards to identify patients' imaging studies, generated requests for patients' master folders in the film library, and automatically produced daily worklists for each examination area. The film-library management system demonstrated one of the first medical uses of bar-code readers and labels; bar-code labels identified and tracked film jackets. In addition, the system maintained a database of film-library loan transactions.

The system was a precursor of today's RISs and evolved to include a variety of other functions. Particularly important was on-line transcription of radiology reports, including the capability for on-line editing and approval of reports by radiologists. Another feature, incorporated into the MGH system in the late 1970's by Greenes and colleagues (1978), was a link to a computer-based surgical-pathology accessioning system. Radiologists had automated access to confirmed pathologic diagnoses and thus could receive automated feedback on their interpretations (Greenes, 1978). Links to other hospital systems were later incorporated.

With the development of new imaging techniques, the volume of and demand for radiologic studies grew, stressing existing manual systems for image and information handling. At the same time, radiology departments faced increasing pressures to control costs and to manage resources efficiently. Computer-based RISs rapidly became necessary to schedule equipment and examination rooms for maximum usage, to assist in film-library management, to track the locations of films, and to collect and analyze the data necessary for evaluation and planning decisions. A number of RISs currently exist. Some are one-of-a-kind systems that have been developed within a particular institution; others are available commercially.

Until the mid-1980s, one of the most comprehensive RISs in operation was that developed by Arenson and his associates at the Hospital of the University of Pennsylvania (HUP) (see Arenson, 1984). It was based on the MGH system but was expanded to support a wide range of department functions, including scheduling, patient tracking, film-library management, billing, and management reporting. Although the system provided essentially all of the functionality outlined, it was not commercially available. Under Arenson's leadership, however, a group of university-based radiology departments formed the Radiology Information Systems Consortium (RISC) in the early 1980s, which developed a comprehensive specification for an RIS, based in large part on the HUP experience (Arenson, 1982). Digital Equipment Corporation (DEC) was the vendor chosen to work with RISC to implement the system, known as DECRad. Since that time the product changed hands and is now marketed and supported by IDX Corporation under the name IDXRad. Several other RISs are on the market, although IDXRad is the most widely installed.

18.3.2.2   Report Generation

Also in the late 1960s, several groups explored methods to allow radiologists to enter reports directly into computer-based systems rather than dictating reports for later transcription. The most elaborate was a system developed by Margulies and later enhanced by Wheeler at Johns Hopkins University Hospital (Margulies, 1972). Researchers created a set of large, graphically oriented displays on film. The displays could be selected randomly and back-projected onto a touch-sensitive screen. Radiologists were able to compose narrative reports by touching appropriate areas of the screen to select words, phrases, and even pictures. Branching from one display to another was controlled by the choices selected by the radiologist. SIREP, a commercial version of this system, marketed by Siemens, had limited acceptance; other companies explored reimplementations.

Bauman and colleagues at MGH also experimented with using branching hierarchical menus of displays as a means for entry of radiologic reports but abandoned this project because the approach did not seem to fit well with the radiologists' desire for freedom of expression when creating reports (Bauman, 1972). A similar menu-driven system, called CLIP, was developed by Leeming, Simon, and Bleich at Beth Israel Hospital in Boston (see Leeming, 1982). Radiologists chose from lists of statements by indicating the alphanumeric code for the desired phrase and then modified the selected statements by inserting appropriate adjectives and adverbs. A report-generation system developed in the late 1960s by Lehr and colleagues at the University of Missouri at Columbia allowed radiologists to compose reports by concatenating symbols that represented sentences or phrases. They could append free text to the report by typing it into the terminal. This system later added patient-registration, scheduling, and film-tracking capabilities, to become a full-function RIS known as MARS (Lehr, 1973). Subsequently, specialized systems—such as for obstetrical ultrasonography (Greenes, 1982) and for ultrasonography generally (Bell, 1994)—have been successful in limited areas, but structured reporting has not progressed significantly, even with the improved graphical user interfaces now available. To create a standardized way of formatting report documents, whether fully structured or not, and to be able to link annotations and comments to images, the DICOM standard includes a section for Structured Reporting (Bidgood, 1998; Hussein, 2004).

In the 1980s, developers explored combining voice input with selection from screen-based menus (Robbins, 1988). Several such commercial systems were introduced, but success was limited because of the need for use of disconnected speech (e.g., enunciation of single words), persistent error rates of 2 to 5 percent, and awkward user interfaces. Recent improvements in the recognition of continuous speech have now made such systems easier to use and substantially reduced error rates, as a result of which new product offerings with such capabilities are increasingly available.

18.4   Current Status

18.4.1   Image Management

Digital methods for image acquisition, transmission, storage, and interpretation for most imaging modalities are gradually appearing. The full integration of these capabilities is still realized in relatively few sites, but is growing rapidly. It is still much more prevalent in Radiology departments, but is beginning to make inroads in the other image-intensive specialties. In addition, the motivations for accomplishing such integration have shifted due to increased focus on enterprise-wide perspectives.

18.4.1.1   Picture Archiving and Communication Systems

The completely filmless radiology department is still limited by the fact that film mammography has not yet been supplanted by digital modalities to a significant extent. As noted in Section 18.2.3.1, mammography has the highest resolution demands (50 micron), and digital mammography has only recently become available commercially and is still being evaluated vs. conventional film-screen mammography in a large national clinical trial, although preliminary assessments are encouraging. Devices providing digital capture of other traditional plain film studies (e.g., examinations of the chest, bone, and abdomen) are widely available, and units are being acquired by radiology departments as new needs arise or as older film-based units are replaced.

Soft copy radiology interpretation at workstations has largely overcome early technical difficulties and user resistance. Interpretation of examinations is now more smoothly coupled with access to clinical information including old reports. Dictation systems are now integrated with interpretation workstations, enabling a toggle button for a case on a workstation to automatically transmit the user, patient, and case identification header information to the dictation station and prepare the latter for accepting a dictation.

A popular misconception is that barriers to soft copy interpretation are removed by higher resolution display screens. If a 20-inch diagonal monitor can display 1,000 × 1,000 pixels, the question is whether it is inherently inferior to a 2,000 × 2,000 monitor or a 4,000 × 4,000 monitor, with a screen of the same 20-inch physical size. Clearly, each pixel in the 1,000 × 1,000 monitor is four times the area of an individual pixel on a 2,000 × 2,000 monitor and 16 times the area of a pixel on a 4,000 × 4,000 monitor. If individual pixels are sufficiently close together on a $1,000 \times 1,000$ monitor so that the eye cannot resolve them at normal viewing distance (as is the case), however, then the additional resolution of the $2,000^2$ or $4,000^2$ monitors will not improve perceived image quality.

Displaying a $4,000 \times 4,000$ image on a $1,000 \times 1,000$ monitor requires that each displayed pixel (of a $1,000 \times 1,000$ reduced image) summarizes the value in a corresponding 4×4 pixel area of the original image occupying the same physical size on the screen. How the value of that pixel is computed is the key determinant of image quality on the reduced image. Subsampling (e.g., every fourth pixel), or averaging, does not work well. A function that computes the brightness level that the eye would detect in that 4×4 area on a higher resolution monitor is the optimal way to determine the value of the single pixel on the lower resolution monitor. In fact, for certain classes of abnormalities (e.g., calcifications or masses on a mammogram) that are indicated by brighter areas, simply displaying the maximum pixel value in the 4×4 region is a satisfactory substitute. The question of optimal resolution for interpretation of most studies has not yet been satisfactorily answered. A few projects have assessed the adequacy of soft copy interpretation, but convincing receiver operating characteristic (ROC) studies (see Chapter 11) have generally not been done, except for specific kinds of abnormalities (e.g., a pneumothorax or interstitial disease on a chest X-ray image).

18.4.1.2 Teleradiology

Although some limitations remain, workstation and network capacity for interpretation, acquisition and transmission of radiological examinations over a distance has rapidly grown, and Web clients with Java-based wavelet decompression enable high resolution viewing of original image detail (subject to degree of compression). It is now common for radiology departments to enable their radiologists to provide coverage from home, especially for interpretations of CT and MRI examinations obtained during nights or weekends and review of interpretations made by radiology residents before finalization of reports. Teleradiology—the provision of remote interpretations—is increasing as a mode of delivery of radiology services. Typically, a radiology center will offer these services to facilities that are generally understaffed or that seek coverage for specialized areas of interpretation. In the United States, expansion of teleradiology is still limited by the requirement that interpreting radiologists be licensed in the state in which the images are acquired.

Current work emphasizes enterprise-wide image distribution and access not only for radiology but also for other kinds of procedures—a major departure from the functionality of most clinical information systems, which have not traditionally been multimedia-capable. In addition to supporting the need for remote interpretation by imaging specialists, electronic distribution and access meet strong demands for review and consultation among clinicians, for surgical planning, and for teaching. To implement these capabilities, as well as to provide a variety of other functions for education and decision support, enterprises have developed intranet and Internet technologies, typically using the Web. Client-based viewing applications are often augmented by Java to provide needed user-interface features for image manipulation. At the back end of the systems is generally an image repository of images stored in a DICOM-compatible format, and often compressed by wavelet methods. Patient-identification information permits linkage to an RIS or HIS, associating images with specific examinations and to reports (Khorasani, 1998). A number of commercial enterprise-wide distribution software applications are available now.

18.4.1.3   Indexing and Image Retrieval

In a typical PACS system, images are archived on a file server. Identification data, usually obtained from the DICOM header, are stored in an associated relational database. Specific images are retrieved based on information that was entered in the database at the same time that the images were acquired, either directly or via linkage to an RIS. For routine radiology this information is usually sufficient, because current and previous images are retrieved mostly by patient identifier and imaging modality.

For research or education, however, it is often desirable to retrieve images that "look like this one"—for example, to show other examples of a particular disease process or to perform a retrospective research study. The standard approach to this task, for educational and research databases, is to index images manually according to keywords. The DICOM standard has provisions to include these keywords (Bidgood, 1997), and controlled vocabularies, such as the *Systematized Nomenclature of Medicine* (SNOMED) (Wang 2002), *Neuro-names* (Bowden, 1995), and the *Digital Anatomist Foundational Model* (Rosse, 1997) (all of which are part of the National Library of Medicine's **Unified Medical Language System** [UMLS] [Lindberg, 1993]), provide many of the needed source keywords (see Chapter 7).

In most routine cases, however, the relevant keywords will not have been entered, because it was not known ahead of time what the query would be. What is needed is content-based image retrieval, which allows the computer to index the images based on their content (Tagare, 1997).

As described in Chapter 9, image understanding is not likely to be available in the near future. Simpler methods have, however, been applied successfully in certain image domains. For example, color images can be indexed according to their relative percentages of red, green, and blue (Flickner, 1995). Asking for images with large amounts of blue from a collection of natural scenes will retrieve images showing a large amount of sea or sky. Of course most medical images are gray scale, so a color-based approach will not work. An alternative developed at Yale, called qualitative arrangement (Tagare, 1995), looks at the relative relationships of regions in the image, without trying to identify them, and retrieves images that have similar relationships. When applied to cardiac MRI images, this approach was able to retrieve images acquired in the same plane of section. See [Muller, 2004] for a review of content-based image retrieval. Sinha and colleagues [Sinha, 2002] address a number of approaches and challenges in image description and integration with clinical environments.

Although much more research is required before these kinds of techniques become widely used, the availability of digital images, PACS, and powerful display workstations provide a good foundation on which to implement them.

18.4.2   Integration in Radiology Information Systems

The Radiology department provides examples of some of the most dramatic health-care computing applications to date. The use of computers in radiology has produced fundamental advances in image generation and image analysis, in addition to facilitating the communication and management of images and radiologic information. Radiology information systems (or incorporation of RIS functionality with HISs) are now widespread. Structured reporting using mouse and keyboard interaction has seen a few success stories but is not being widely adopted. Primary attention currently is focused on voice dictation systems which incorporate continuous-speech recognizers.

Infrastructure is gradually shifting to a client–server, distributed-computing model, using the Internet, World Wide Web, Java for enhanced presentation layer, and standards-based APIs for invoking remote distributed networked services. Progress is relatively slow because of the investment in legacy systems, the size and diversity of IDNs, and the difficulty of creating the hardware and communications infrastructure necessary for integrating all the elements and connecting the various users.

18.4.2.1   PACS, HIS, and RIS Integration

The evolution of radiology at the Brigham and Women's Hospital is probably representative of that at many institutions. The Brigham is part of an IDN, the Partners HealthCare System, serving eastern Massachusetts. The Brigham has a large and successful HIS, known as BICS, and an IDXRad RIS. A homegrown PACS was developed for acquisition and archiving of the digital modalities, later replaced by a commercial system from General Electric Corp. The HIS and RIS are interlinked for transfer of patient demographic, billing, and report information, and the RIS and PACS are interlinked to enable the RIS to keep track of images on the PACS associated with particular examinations (Hanlon, 1996). Ultrasound reports are generated by separate reporting modules (Bell, 1994) and are integrated into the RIS through an HL7 interface (see Chapter 6). Other semi-independent reporting modules can be linked to the RIS in similar fashion. Voice-recognition systems for reporting have been introduced. Mostly, these are used to provide draft reports to transcription editors who revise them as necessary.

A major focus of PACS development at the Brigham has been distributing images to referring physicians and making them available in the homes of staff radiologists who are on call to residents and fellows. A commercial Web interface to the RIS and PACS enables examinations to be retrieved based on a variety of search criteria (such as patient name or medical-record number, examination type, date, location, interpreting radiologist). The reports can be reviewed and the images accessed if available. These files can be sent in different formats and image sizes, and gray scale can be modified. Images also can be selected by radiologists for storage as teaching-file cases. The system is now a combined home-grown and commercial effort.

18.4.2.2   DICOM and HL7

Integration among PACS, RIS, and HIS has been aided by the evolution of two standards, DICOM and HL7. DICOM, as discussed in Section 18.2.3.4, is a standard format for transmitting image information, including patient, exam, and study series information. It has been important in making it possible for different imaging modality devices and consoles to transmit images to common PACS archives, and enabling the images to be manipulated on common interpretation workstations, while maintaining the association between images and the series and exams of which they are part, for specific patients. Patient demographic and exam ordering information, result reporting, and billing, on the other hand, have been the province of messaging standards developed by HL7. Thus RISs and PACS must communicate using both DICOM and HL7 standards, in order to fully integrate the above information. The HL7 and DICOM standards development communities, in fact, participate jointly in an Image Management Special Interest Group of HL7, to resolve areas of interface and overlap. A particular area of overlap that is the subject of continuing discussion is the Structured Reporting part of DICOM, since this overlaps with the foci of the Compound Document Architecture Technical Committee and Template Special Interest Group of HL7 {HL7, 2004).

18.4.2.3   IHE

Specification of a standard and ensuring that it works in practice are two different tasks. Because of the variety of parameters that can be specified, for example, in an HL7 message, it is not guaranteed, just because two systems use HL7, that their messages can be exchanged and fully understood. To address this issue, the Radiology Society of North America (RSNA) and the Health Information Management Systems Society (HIMSS) developed a joint initiative termed "Integrating the Healthcare Enterprise" (IHE) (Channin 2002) aimed at promoting true operational integration. This was begun in 1998, and consisted of annual successively more elaborate suites of communication capabilities that were demonstrated by vendors at the meetings of the two organizations. The goal was to be able to satisfy the requirements of a variety of clinical and management scenarios by operating environments in which applications or components from various vendors worked together through DICOM and HL7 communication.

A set of precisely detailed specifications have been developed by the IHE committee each year, and a suite of tools to validate conformance with those specifications has been implemented. Those vendors that have been able to satisfy conformance have participated in the IHE demonstration. The first year focused on ordering of a radiologic procedure, communication of the order information to the imaging modality, and transmission of the completed examination with images to the viewing station, and included various settings in which updating of patient demographic or examination information needed to occur. In subsequent years the demonstration has involved more activities involving scheduling, reporting, enterprise-wide distribution of images and reports, and extension beyond radiology. IHE was not intended to develop standards but rather to support and encourage adoption of those already developed, to select from those standards, particular subsets that could be implemented and shown to work, and to inform the standards development organizations where deficiencies were found in the specifications. The 2004 IHE demonstration was held in conjunction with HL7's exhibit at the HIMSS meeting, a testimony to how effective the IHE process has been as a market force to encourage vendors to focus on interoperability.

18.4.3   Other Examples of Image-Based Systems

As noted earlier, there are many other examples of image-based system, not only in clinical departments such as pathology, surgery, cardiology and obstetrics, but also in basic science and education. Educational applications are described in chapter 21. In this section we describe a few other examples out of the many that could be mentioned.

18.4.3.1   Surgical Planning and Image-Guided Therapy

A major revolution has occurred in the use of volumetric image data as an aid to surgery (Dohi, 2002). Images can be modeled and reconstructed in a variety of projections, with certain layers removed and others enhanced or colored to enable abnormalities to be visualized clearly in context. The projections can be conformed to the exact perspective of a surgeon looking at an operating field by reconciling position on a head-mounted display with exact coordinates of the patient and superimposed on the operative field. Pioneering work at the Brigham and Women's Hospital (Jolesz, 1997) has integrated surgery and imaging more closely through use of an open MRI magnet that enables interventional procedures to be carried out directly while the patient is being imaged.

Through similar approaches, minimally invasive techniques like focused ultrasound, cryosurgery, and thermal ablation can be monitored in real time through tissue changes on MRI scans. (Dohi 2002).

18.4.3.2   Brain Map Information Systems

Most of this chapter describes clinical uses of images generated in the radiology department. However, there are many research uses as well. For example, chapter 9 describes methods for acquiring, processing and visualizing 3-D structural and functional brain images, most or all of which are acquired in the radiology department. Like clinical images, these images, and the results of processing applied to them, must be managed and integrated in information systems if they are to be optimally useful for neuroscience research. Thus, there are a growing number of examples of image-based information systems for brain mapping that have been funded by the Human Brain Project and other efforts.

As one example, chapter 9, section 9.5, describes a visualization-based approach for mapping the location of cortical language sites onto the surface of the brain, and for relating these sites to other measures of language activation, such as those obtained from functional MRI. As part of this project we [JB] have developed a web-based distributed information system for managing and visualizing images, derived 3-D models and maps, and other experimental data required by this approach (Figure 9.9). Images and 3-D models are stored on a fileserver. Metadata describing the location of these images and models, as well as non-image based experimental data, are stored in a relational database. A software toolkit called the Web Interfacing Repository Manager (WIRM) (Jakobovits, 2001) maintains consistency between these two sources of data, and generates a web interface that allows users to upload images and other data, and to browse existing data. A separate visualization server, when invoked with a patient identifier, consults the database to find the appropriate image and 3-D model files, loads these files, renders the resulting 3-D scene, and returns the rendering to the web client as a 2-D snapshot. The user can then manipulate the resulting scene with the mouse, which causes the server to re-render the scene with the new parameters. The advantage of the visualization server is that remote users do not need expensive or complex hardware and software to interact with the scenes. The overall system is an example of a multi-media Experiment Management System (Jakobovits, 2002) of the type that will assume increasing importance as researchers need to manage, visualize and share large amounts of complex image-based data.

18.5   Future Directions for Imaging Systems

It should be clear from this chapter's discussion that computers are an essential tool in radiology, as well as in other imaging-oriented specialties. As processing power and storage have become less expensive, newer, computationally intensive capabilities have been widely adopted. To date, this trend shows no signs of slowing.

The overall trend with respect to image generation is ever-increasing numbers of imaging modalities; almost every modality provides unique information, so most of them will remain available. For each modality, the trend is toward higher spatial, contrast, and temporal resolution, up to the physical limits. In addition, all modalities will continue the trend toward three-dimensional or four-dimensional data. New methods will continue to be found to image physiological function and genetic and molecular expression, and modalities will be combined to maximize the information content.

Widespread access to images and reports will be demanded throughout health-care delivery networks, as well as across wider geographic areas for teleradiology services. Methodology for meeting this demand probably will continue to build on the World Wide Web, augmented by Java for support of image-manipulation user interfaces. At the back end, systems will use distributed servers not only for storage and for connection to the patient's electronic medical record but also for various kinds of image manipulation. These systems will use the DICOM standard for format of image messages and HL7 for clinical-data exchange and will invoke functionality on the various servers through standardized distributed object management protocols.

Image retrieval for research and educational purposes will become much easier due to widespread use of controlled vocabularies such as SNOMED, and the metathesaurus of the UMLS to link to other appropriate vocabularies, and to continued progress in content-based retrieval. Much of this progress will depend on research in image-manipulation techniques.

Images will be delivered via high-speed networks to increasingly powerful workstations equipped with commercially available software packages for image manipulation and visualization. These software packages will take advantage of advances that are now only at the research stage. Sophisticated user interfaces will be combined with high-level anatomical knowledge, often in the form of shape-based deformable models, to allow rapid creation of instantiations of the models to fit the image data for the given patient. Such three-dimensional instantiated models will provide a framework not only for visualizing and manipulating the three-dimensional anatomy and pathology of individual patients but also for superimposing nonimage information in a structure-based visual medical record.

Soft copy interpretation of radiology images will become ubiquitous as user interfaces are improved and radiologists become more comfortable with the process. For reporting, continuous-speech recognition offers the best hope for an acceptable automated method of capturing radiologist interpretations. Use of voice recognition for free text and for selecting phrases for structured reports will provide the best combination of methods, ultimately replacing dictation and transcription.

Enterprise integration will continue to occur in stages. As digital images replace analog images in the Radiology department, PACS will increasingly assume the functions of the film library. Databases of medical images, available for clinical and research purposes, will be indexed for retrieval by image, by case, by diagnosis, or by feature. The integration of RIS and PACS will then allow coordination of all the major activities of the Radiology department, from examination scheduling and patient registration; to image acquisition, storage, and retrieval; to report generation and distribution.

The Radiology department systems in turn will be increasingly integrated with the enterprise health-information system of the IDN. Thus, healthcare personnel throughout an enterprise will have on-line access to the images, in addition to radiologists' reports. At the same time, linkages between the RIS and patients' computer-based medical records will allow radiologists to access the clinical data that they need to interpret images and to obtain feedback on their work. Other imaging-based specialties will also be integrated increasingly into the enterprise network for distribution of their images and for teleconsulting.

We will see significant growth in image-guided surgery and advances in image-guided minimally invasive therapy as imaging is integrated in real time with the treatment process. Telesurgery will be feasible: Video images are currently used by endoscopists to guide their maneuvers, and techniques are improving to provide tactile feedback sensations to users as resistance is encountered by remote probes. Combining these haptic techniques with the ability to visualize the anatomic context through real-time MR imaging of the body part could permit an expert interventionalist to conduct an endoscopic procedure entirely remotely, with only a lesser-trained individual on site to perform preprocedure and postprocedure tasks and to deal with problems, should they occur.

As we have described throughout this chapter, many parts of this future scenario already are operational or are well underway at different institutions. Key determinants of the pace of evolution of radiology-imaging systems include the adoption of software architectures that provide a distributed component infrastructure; the cost of computer processors, storage, displays, network servers, and other hardware; and continued advances in user interfaces and software functionality.

Suggested Readings

Bauman R.A., Gell G., Dwyer S.J. 3rd. (1996). Large picture archiving and communication systems of the world, Part 2. Journal of Digital Imaging, 9(4):172-177.
This comprehensive survey describes the state of the art, in 1996, of operational PACS implementations.

D'Orsi C.J., Kopans D.B. (1997). Mammography interpretation: the BI-RADS method. American Family Physician, 55(5):1548-1550, 1997.
This article describes the use of the BI-RADS structured data encoding scheme, which was developed by the American College of Radiology for generating mammographic reports.

Dohi, T.; Kikinis, R. (Eds.) (2002). Medical Image Computing and Computer-Assisted Intervention -MICCAI 2002 ċ 5th International Conference, Tokyo, Japan, September 25-28, 2002, Proceedings, Part I ISBN 3-540-44224-3, EUR 80.-* Part II ISBN 3-540-44225-1, EUR 72.-*
The two volumes of this book constitute the refereed proceedings of the 5th International Conference on Medical Image Computing and Computer-Assisted Intervention, MICCAI 2002, held in Tokyo, Japan, in September 2002. The 184 revised full papers offer main topical sections on medical robotics and endoscopic devices; validation; brain tumor, cortex, vascular, and imaging and analysis; segmentation; cardiac applications; computer-assisted diagnosis; tubular structures; interventions; simulation; modelling; statistical shape modelling; image registration; visualization; and novel imaging techniques.

Greenes R.A., Bauman R.A. (Eds.) (1996). Imaging and information management: computer systems for a changing health care environment. Radiology Clinics of North America, 34(3):463-697.
This issue is an update of a 1986 survey on the use of computers in radiology, with more emphasis on image management and applications. Sections include image acquisition, PACS, networks, workstation design, three-dimensional imaging, image processing for diagnosis, reporting, decision aids, educational uses, telemedicine, and technology assessment.

Jolesz F.A. (1997). 1996 RSNA Eugene P. Pendergrass New Horizons Lecture.
Image-guided procedures and the operating room of the future. Radiology, 204(3), 601-612.
This article, by a leader in MRI-guided surgical planning and interventional procedures, describes major uses of imaging in treatment.

Siegel E.L., Protopapas Z., Reiner B.I., Pomerantz S.M. (1997). Patterns of utilization of computer workstations in a filmless environment and implications for current and future picture archiving and communication systems. Journal of Digital Imaging, 10(3 Suppl 1):41-43.
This article describes one of the first and most comprehensive implementations of an all-digital, filmless radiology department, at the Baltimore Veterans Administration Medical Center.

Questions for Discussion

1. Describe the various factors that a planner must consider when estimating the storage requirements for image data in an all-digital radiology department. What are the major factors that reduce the volume of data that are maintained in on-line storage?
2. Refer to Table 18.1. How many bytes are needed to store a digitized chest X-ray image? How many bytes are needed to store a 15-image CT study? If you have a communication line that transmits 56,000 bits per second, how long will it take to transmit each of these images to the display workstations within the hospital? What are the implications of your answer for widespread transmission of image data?
3. What are the economic and technologic factors that determine how quickly hospitals and clinics can adopt all-digital radiology departments?
4. What are the ways in which radiology reports of examination interpretations can be generated, and what are the advantages and disadvantages of each approach, in terms of ease and efficiency of report creation, timeliness of availability of report to clinicians, usefulness for retrieval of cases for research and education?

19
Information Retrieval and Digital Libraries

WILLIAM HERSH, P. ZOË STAVRI, AND WILLIAM M. DETMER

After reading this chapter, you should know the answers to these questions:

- What types of online content are available and useful to health care practitioners, researchers, and consumers?
- What are the major components of the information retrieval process?
- How do techniques differ for indexing various types of knowledge-based biomedical information?
- What are the major approaches to retrieval of knowledge-based biomedical information?
- How effectively do searchers utilize information retrieval systems?
- What are the important research directions in information retrieval?
- What are the major challenges to making digital libraries effective for health and biomedical users?

Information retrieval (IR) is the field concerned with the acquisition, organization, and searching of knowledge-based information (Hersh, 2003). Although biomedical informatics has traditionally concentrated on the retrieval of text from the biomedical literature, the domain over which IR can be effectively applied has broadened considerably with the advent of multimedia publishing and vast storehouses of chemical structures, cartographic materials, gene and protein sequences, video clippings, and a wide range of other digital media of relevance to biomedical education, research, and patient care. With the proliferation of IR systems and online content, the notion of the library has changed substantially, and new **digital libraries** have emerged (Humphreys, 2000).

19.1 Evolution of Biomedical Information Retrieval

As with many chapters in this volume, this area has changed substantially over the three editions of this book. In the first edition, this chapter was titled "Bibliographic-Retrieval Systems," reflecting the type of knowledge that was accessible at the time. In this edition, we add "Digital Libraries" to the chapter name, reflecting that the entire biomedical library and beyond is now part of online knowledge that is available.

Although this chapter focuses on the use of computers to facilitate IR, methods for finding and retrieving information from medical sources have been in existence for over a century. In 1879 Dr. John Shaw Billings created ***Index Medicus*** to help medical professionals find relevant journal articles (DeBakey, 1991). Journal articles were indexed by author name(s) and subject heading(s) and then aggregated in bound volumes. A scientist or practitioner seeking an article on a topic could manually search the index for the single best-matching subject heading and then be directed to citations of published articles.

The printed *Index Medicus* served as the main biomedical IR source until 1966, when the National Library of Medicine (NLM) unveiled an electronic version, the **Medical Literature Analysis and Retrieval System (MEDLARS)** (Miles, 1982). Because computing power and disk storage were very limited, MEDLARS and its follow-on **MEDLARS Online (MEDLINE)**, stored only limited information for each article, such as author name(s), article title, journal source, and publication date. In addition, the NLM assigned to each article a number of terms from its **Medical Subject Heading (MeSH)** thesaurus (see Chapter 7). Searching was done in batch mode, with users having to mail a paper search form to the NLM and receiving results back a few weeks later. Only librarians who had completed a specialized course were allowed to submit searches.

As computing power grew and disk storage became more plentiful in the 1980s, full-text databases began to emerge. These new databases allowed searching of the entire text of medical documents. Although lacking graphics, images, and tables from the original source, these databases made it possible to retrieve the full text of important documents quickly and in remote locations. Likewise, with the growth of time-sharing networks, end users were now allowed to search the databases directly, though at a substantial cost.

In the early 1990s, the pace of change in the IR field quickened. The advent of the **World Wide Web (WWW or Web)** and the exponentially increasing power of computers and networks brought a world where vast quantities of medical information from multiple sources with various media extensions were now available over the global Internet (Berners-Lee et al., 1994). In the late 1990s, the NLM made all of its databases available to the entire world for free. Also during this time, the notion of digital libraries developed, with the recognition that the entire array of knowledge-based information could be accessed using this technology (Borgman, 1999).

Now in the early twenty-first century, use of IR systems and digital libraries has become mainstream. Estimates vary, but among individuals who use the Internet in the United States, over 40 percent have used it to search for personal health information (Baker et al., 2003). Among physicians, over 90 percent use the Internet, with those spending more time in clinical care using it more frequently (Taylor and Leitman, 2001). Furthermore, access to systems has gone beyond the traditional personal computer and extended to new devices, such as **personal digital assistants (PDAs)**.

19.2   Knowledge-Based Information in Health and Biomedicine

IR systems and digital libraries store and disseminate knowledge-based information. What exactly does that mean? Although there are many ways to classify biomedical information and the informatics applications that use them, in this chapter we will broadly divide them into two categories. **Patient-specific information** applies to individual patients. Its purpose is to tell health care providers, administrators, and researchers about the health and disease of a patient. This information comprises the patient's medical record. The second category of biomedical information is **knowledge-based information**. This is information that has been derived and organized from observational or experimental research. In the case of clinical research, this information provides clinicians, administrators, and researchers with knowledge derived from experiments and observations, which can then be applied to individual patients. This information is most commonly provided in books and journals but can take a wide variety of other forms, including clinical practice guidelines, consumer health literature, Web sites, and so forth.

Knowledge-based information can be subdivided into two categories. **Primary knowledge–based information** (also called primary literature) is original research that appears in journals, books, reports, and other sources. This type of information reports the initial discovery of health knowledge, usually with either original data or reanalysis of data (e.g., meta-analyses). **Secondary knowledge–based information** consists of the writing that reviews, condenses, and/or synthesizes the primary literature. The most common examples of this type of literature are books, monographs, and review articles in journals and other publications. Secondary literature also includes opinion-based writing such as editorials and position or policy papers. It also encompasses clinical practice guidelines, systematic reviews, and health information on Web pages. In addition, it includes the plethora of pocket-sized manuals that are a staple for practitioners in many professional fields. As will be seen later, secondary literature is the most common type of literature used by physicians. Finally, secondary literature also includes the growing quality of patient/consumer-oriented health information that is increasingly available via the Web.

Libraries have been the historical place where knowledge-based information has been stored. Libraries actually perform a variety of functions, including the following:

- Acquisition and maintenance of collections.
- Cataloging and classification of items in collections to make them more accessible to users.
- Serving as a place where individuals can go to seek information with assistance, including information on computers.
- Providing work or studying space (particularly in universities).

Digital libraries provide some of the same services, but their focus tends to be on the digital aspects of content.

19.2.1 Information Needs and Seeking

Different users of knowledge-based information have differing needs based on the nature of what they need the information for and what resources are available. The information needs and information seeking of physicians have been most extensively studied. Gorman (1995) has defined four states of **information need** in the clinical context:

- Unrecognized need—clinician unaware of information need or knowledge deficit.
- Recognized need—clinician aware of need but may or may not pursue it.
- Pursued need—information seeking occurs but may or may not be successful.
- Satisfied need—information seeking successful.

There is a great deal of evidence that these information needs are not being met and that IR applications may help. Among the reasons that physicians do not adhere to the most up-to-date clinical practices is that they often do not recognize that their knowledge is incomplete. While this is not the only reason for such practices, the evidence is compelling. For example, physicians continue to prescribe antibiotics inappropriately (Gonzales et al., 2001), not adhere to established guidelines (Knight et al., 2000), and vary widely in how they provide care (Weiner et al., 1995).

When physicians recognize an information need, they are likely to pursue only a minority of unanswered questions. A variety of studies have demonstrated that physicians in practice have unmet information on the order of two questions for every three patients seen and only pursue answers for about 30 percent of these questions (Covell et al., 1985; Gorman and Helfand, 1995; Ely et al., 1999). When answers to questions are actually pursued, these studies showed that the most frequent source for answers to questions was colleagues, followed by paper-based textbooks. Usage of computers to answer these questions is relatively low, even in more recent studies of physician information seeking (Arroll et al., 2002). Therefore it is not surprising that barriers to satisfying information needs remain (Ely et al., 2002). One possible approach to lowering the barrier to knowledge-based information is to link it more directly with the context of the patient in the **electronic health record** (EHR). Cimino (1996) has pioneered much work in EHR and continues to carry out research into the best ways to make it useful to clinicians. Another promising approach is to deliver information to the point of need via handheld and wireless devices.

A small but growing amount of research has looked at the information needs and seeking of consumers and patients. This group includes not only patients but also people looking for wellness information (Stavri, 2001) who often have to contend with the affective nature of their information needs and information source preferences (Brennan and Strombom, 1998). Patients have become "coproducers" of their own health care (Bopp, 2000), and Web-enabled patients have impacted the patient–physician relationship (Anderson et al., 2003). The Pew Internet & American Life Project continues to do extensive research into the characteristics of users of the Internet for health information and the cultural and literacy barriers they encounter (Lenhart et al., 2003).

19.2.2   Changes in Publishing

The Internet and the Web have had a profound impact in the publishing of knowledge-based information. The technical impediments to electronic publishing of journals have largely been solved. Most scientific journals are published electronically in some form already. Journals that do not publish electronically likely could do so easily, since most of the publishing process has already been converted to the electronic mode. A modern

Internet connection is sufficient to deliver most of the content of journals. Indeed, a near-turnkey solution is already offered through Highwire Press (www.highwire.org), a spin-off from Stanford University, which has an infrastructure that supports the tasks of journal publishing, from content preparation to searching and archiving.

There is great enthusiasm for electronic availability of journals, as evidenced by the growing number of titles to which libraries provide access. When available in electronic form, journal content is easier and more convenient to access. Furthermore, since most scientists have the desire for widespread dissemination of their work, they have incentive for their papers to be available electronically. Not only is there the increased convenience of redistributing reprints, but Lawrence (2001) has found that papers (at least from computer science) freely available on the Web have a higher likelihood of being cited by other papers than those that are not. As citations are important to authors for academic promotion and grant funding, authors have incentive to maximize the accessibility of their published work.

The technical challenges to electronic scholarly publication have been replaced by economic and political ones (Hersh and Rindfleisch, 2000; Anonymous, 2001c). Printing and mailing, tasks no longer needed in electronic publishing, comprised a significant part of the "added value" from publishers of journals. There is still however value added by publishers, such as hiring and managing editorial staff to produce the journals, and managing the peer review process. Even if publishing companies as they are known were to vanish, there would still be some cost to the production of journals. Thus, while the cost of producing journals electronically is likely to be less, it is not zero, and even if journal content is distributed "free," someone has to pay the production costs. The economic issue in electronic publishing, then, is who is going to pay for the production of journals. This introduces some political issues as well. One of them centers around the concern that much research is publicly funded through grants from federal agencies such as the National Institutes of Health (NIH) and the National Science Foundation (NSF). In the current system, especially in the biomedical sciences (and to a lesser extent in other sciences), researchers turn over the copyright of their publications to journal publishers. The political concern is that the public funds the research and the universities carry it out, but individuals and libraries then must buy it back from the publishers to whom they willingly cede the copyright. This problem is exacerbated by the general decline in funding for libraries that has occurred over the last couple of decades (Boyd and Herkovic, 1999; Meek, 2001).

Some proposed models of "open access" scholarly publishing keep the archive of science freely available. Harnad (1998) proposes that authors and their institutions pay the cost of production of manuscripts up front after they are accepted through a peer review process. He suggests this cost could even be included in the budgets of grant proposals submitted for funding agencies. After the paper is published, the manuscript would be freely available on the Web. The collection of journals published by **Biomed Central** (**BMC**, www.biomedcentral.com) adhere to a variant of this model.

Another model that has emerged is **PubMed Central** (**PMC**, pubmedcentral.gov). Proposed by former NIH director Harold Varmus, PMC began as an initiative called "E-Biomed" (Varmus, 1999). Modified extensively since its original proposal, PMC provides free access to published literature that allows publishers to maintain copyright as well as optionally keep the papers on their own servers. A lag time of up to 6 months is allowed so that journals can reap the revenue that comes with initial publication. The newer approach to PMC has been accepted by many leading journals, with nearly 200 journals contributing to it. Varmus himself is now leading the Public Library of Science (www.plos.org), another open-access, Web-based journal for publication of scientific research.

19.2.3   Quality of Information

The growth of the Internet and the Web has led to another concern, which is the quality of information available. A large fraction of Web-based health information is aimed at nonprofessional audiences. Many laud this development as empowering those most directly affected by health care—those who consume it (Eysenbach et al., 1999). Others express concern about patients misunderstanding or being purposely misled by incorrect or inappropriately interpreted information (Jadad, 1999). Some clinicians also lament the time required to go through stacks of printouts patients bring to the office. The Web is inherently democratic, allowing virtually anyone to post information. This is no doubt an asset in a democratic society like the United States. However, it is potentially at odds with the operation of a professional field, particularly one like health care, where practitioners are ethically bound and legally required to adhere to the highest standard of care. Thus, a major concern with health information on the Web is the presence of inaccurate or out-of-date information. A recent systematic review of studies assessing the quality of health information found that 55 of 79 studies came to the conclusion that quality of information was a problem (Eysenbach et al., 2002).

Another concern about health information on the Web for consumers is **readability**. It has been found that most patients (Williams et al., 1996) and parents of child patients (Murphy, 1994) read at an average of a fifth- to sixth-grade level. Reading ability also declines with age (Gazmararian et al., 1999). Berland et al. (2001) determined that no health-related site they evaluated had readability below the tenth-grade level, while over half were written at a college level and 11 percent at a graduate school level.

Eysenbach and Diepgen (1998) note that the problem of poor-quality and hard-to-read information on the Web is exacerbated by a **context deficit** that makes poor-quality information more difficult to distinguish. These authors note that there are fewer clear "markers" of the type of document (e.g., professional textbook vs. patient handout) and that the reader of a specific page may not be aware of the "context" of a Web site that includes disclaimers, warnings, and so forth. Furthermore, information may be correct in one context but incorrect in another, and this difference may not be detectable on a random page within a Web site (e.g., the differences in treatment in children vs. adults or across different ethnic groups).

The impact of this poor-quality information is unclear. A recent systematic review of whether harm has resulted from information obtained on the Internet found 15 case reports (Crocco et al., 2002). The review noted that larger studies of whether Internet information has caused general harm to patients have not been done. A dissenting view has been provided by Ferguson (2002), who argues that patients and consumers actually are savvy enough to understand the limits of quality of information on the Web and that they should be trusted to discern quality using their own abilities to consult different sources of information and communicate with health care practitioners and others who share their condition(s). Indeed, the ideal situation may be a partnership among patients and their health care practitioners, as it has been shown that patients desire that their practitioners be the primary source of recommendations for online information (Tang et al., 1997).

This lack of quality information has led a number of individuals and organizations to develop guidelines for assessing the *quality of health information*. These guidelines usually have explicit criteria for a Web page that a reader can apply to determine whether a potential source of information has attributes consistent with high quality. One of the earliest and most widely quoted set of criteria was published in *JAMA* (Silberg et al., 1997). These criteria stated that Web pages should contain the name, affiliation, and credentials of the author; references to the claims made; explicit listing of any perceived or real conflict of interest; and date of most recent update.

Another early set of criteria was the **Health on the Net (HON)** codes (www.hon.ch), a set of voluntary codes of conduct for health-related Web sites. Sites that adhere to the HON codes can display the HON logo. Another approach to insuring Web site quality may be accreditation by a third party. The American Accreditation HealthCare Commission (called URAC) recently announced a process for such accreditation (www.accreditation.urac.org). The URAC standards manual provides 53 standards to support accreditation. The URAC standards cover six general issues: health content editorial process, disclosure of financial relationships, linking to other Web sites, privacy and security, consumer complaint mechanisms, and internal processes required to maintain quality over time. To receive accreditation, sites have to meet the requirements listed in the standards manual. Thirteen commercial Web sites were in the first group awarded accreditation (Fox, 2001).

19.2.4   *Evidence-Based Medicine*

The growing quantity of clinical information available in IR systems and digital libraries requires new approaches to select that which is best to use for clinical decisions. The philosophy guiding this approach is **evidence-based medicine (EBM)**, which can be viewed a set of tools to inform clinical decision making. It allows clinical experience ("art") to be integrated with best clinical science (Haynes et al., 2002). Also, EBM makes the medical literature more clinically applicable and relevant. In addition, it requires the user to be facile with computers and IR systems. There are many well-known books and Web resources for EBM. The original textbook by Sackett et al. (2000) is now in a second edition. A series of articles published in *JAMA* is now available in a handbook (Guyatt and Rennie, 2001) and reference book format (Guyatt et al., 2001).

The process of EBM involves three general steps:

• Phrasing a clinical question that is pertinent and answerable.
• Identifying evidence (studies in articles) that address the question.
• Critically appraising the evidence to determine whether it applies to the patient.

The phrasing of the clinical question is an often-overlooked portion of the EBM process. There are two general types of clinical question: background questions and foreground questions (Sackett et al., 2000). **Background questions** ask for general knowledge about a disorder, whereas **foreground questions** ask for knowledge about managing patients with a disorder. Background questions are generally best answered with textbooks and classical review articles, whereas foreground questions are answered using EBM techniques. There are four major foreground question categories:

- Therapy (or intervention)—benefit of treatment or prevention.
- Diagnosis—test diagnosing disease.
- Harm—detrimental health effects of a disease, environmental exposure (natural or man-made), or medical intervention.
- Prognosis—outcome of disease course.

Identifying evidence involves selecting the best evidence for a given type of question. EBM proponents advocate, for example, that randomized controlled trials or a meta-analysis that combines multiple trials are the best evidence for health care interventions. Likewise, diagnostic test accuracy is best assessed with comparison to a known gold standard in an appropriate spectrum of patients to whom the test will be applied (see Chapter 3). Questions of harm can be answered by randomized controlled trials when it is not unethical to do so; otherwise they are best answered with observational case control or cohort studies. There are checklists of attributes for these different types of studies that allow their critical appraisal and applicability to a given patient in the EBM resources described above.

The original approach to EBM, called "first-generation" EBM by Hersh (1999), focused on finding original studies in the primary literature and applying critical appraisal. As already discussed, accessing the primary literature is challenging and time-consuming for clinicians for a variety of reasons. This has led to what Hersh (1999) calls "next-generation" EBM and focuses on the use of "synthesized" resources, where the literature searching, critical appraisal, and extraction of statistics operations are performed ahead of time. This approach puts EBM resources in the context of more usable information resources as advocated in systematic reviews (Mulrow et al., 1997), the **InfoMastery** concept of Shaughnessy et al. (1994) and Chueh and Barnett's **"just-in-time" information model** (Chueh and Barnett, 1997). Haynes (2001) has developed the "4S" model of the hierarchy of EBM resources: the original studies themselves, syntheses of those studies in systematic review, synopses of those syntheses in digestible form for clinicians, and systems that incorporate the knowledge of those studies for clinician decision support (see Chapter 20).

19.2.5   *Content of Knowledge-Based Information Resources*

The previous sections of this chapter have described some of the issues and concerns surrounding the production and use of knowledge-based information in biomedicine. It is useful to classify the information to gain a better understanding of its structure and function. In this section, we classify content into bibliographic, full-text, database/collection, and aggregated categories.

Bibliographic Content

The first category consists of **bibliographic content**. It includes what was for decades the mainstay of IR systems: **literature reference databases**. Also called **bibliographic databases**, this content consists of citations or pointers to the medical literature (i.e., journal articles). The best-known and most widely used biomedical bibliographic database is **MEDLINE**, which contains bibliographic references to all of the biomedical articles, editorials, and letters to the editors in approximately 4,500 scientific journals. The journals are chosen for inclusion by an advisory committee of subject experts convened by NIH. At present, about 500,000 references are added to MEDLINE yearly. It now contains over 12 million references.

The current MEDLINE record contains up to 49 fields. A clinician may be interested in just a handful of these fields, such as the title, abstract, and indexing terms. But other fields contain specific information that may be of great importance to a smaller audience. For example, a genome researcher might be highly interested in the *Supplementary Information* (SI) field to link to genomic databases. Even the clinician may, however, derive benefit from some of the other fields. For example, the *Publication Type* (PT) field can help in the application of EBM, such as when one is searching for a practice guideline or a randomized controlled trial. The NLM also partitions MEDLINE into subsets for users wishing to search on a focused portion of the database, such as *AIDS* or *Complementary and Alternative Medicine*. MEDLINE is accessible by many means and available without charge via the **PubMed** system (pubmed.gov), produced by the **National Center for Biotechnology Information** (**NCBI**, www.ncbi.nlm.nih.gov) of the NLM, which provides access to other databases as well.

A number of other Web sites provide MEDLINE for free. Some information vendors, such as Ovid Technologies (www.ovid.com) and Aries Systems (www.ariessys.com), license the content and provide value-added services that can be accessed for a fee by individuals and institutions.

MEDLINE is only one of many databases produced by the NLM (Anonymous, 2000c). Other more specialized databases are also available, covering topics from AIDS to space medicine and toxicology. There are several non-NLM bibliographic databases that tend to be more focused on subjects or resource types. The major non-NLM database for the nursing field is the **Cumulative Index to Nursing and Allied Health Literature** (**CINAHL**, CINAHL Information Systems, www.cinahl.com), which covers nursing and allied health literature, including physical therapy, occupational therapy, laboratory technology, health education, physician assistants, and medical records.

Another well-known series of large databases is part of **Excerpta Medica** (Elsevier Science Publishers, www.excerptamedica.com). **EMBASE**, the electronic version of *Excerpta Medica*, is referred to by some as the "European MEDLINE" (www.embase.com). It contains over 8 million records dating back to 1974. EMBASE covers many of the same medical journals as MEDLINE but with a more international focus, including more non-English-language journals. These journals are often important for those carrying out meta-analyses and systematic reviews, which need access to all the studies done across the world.

A second, more modern type of bibliographic content is the **Web catalog**. There are increasing numbers of such catalogs, which consist of Web pages containing mainly links to other Web pages and sites. It should be noted that there is a blurry distinction between Web catalogs and aggregations (the fourth category). In general, the former contain only links to other pages and sites, while the latter include actual content that is highly integrated with other resources. Some well-known Web catalogs include:

- *HealthWeb* (healthweb.org)—topics maintained by a consortium of 12 midwestern universities (Redman et al., 1997).
- *HealthFinder* (healthfinder.gov)—consumer-oriented health information maintained by the Office of Disease Prevention and Health Promotion of the U.S. Department of Health and Human Services.
- *OMNI* (Organising Medical Networked Information, omni.ac.uk)—a UK-based Web catalog (Norman, 1996) that includes a recent subset devoted to nursing, midwifery, and allied health professions (NMAP, nmap.ac.uk).
- *HON Select* (www.hon.ch/HONselect)—a European catalog of quality-filtered, clinician-oriented Web content from the HON foundation.

There are a number of large general Web catalogs that are not limited to health topics. Two examples are Yahoo (www.yahoo.com) and Open Directory (dmoz.org), both of which have significant health components.

The final type of bibliographic content is the **specialized registry**. This resource is very close to a literature reference database except that it indexes more diverse content than scientific literature. One specialized registry of great importance for health care is the **National Guidelines Clearinghouse (NGC**, www.guideline.gov). Produced by the Agency for Healthcare Research and Quality (AHRQ), it contains exhaustive information about clinical practice guidelines. Some of the guidelines produced are freely available, published electronically and/or on paper. Others are proprietary, in which case a link is provided to a location at which the guideline can be ordered or purchased. The overall goal of the NGC is to make evidence-based clinical practice guidelines and related abstract, summary, and comparison materials widely available to health care and other professionals.

Full-text Content

The second type of content is **full-text content**. A large component of this content consists of the online versions of books and periodicals. As already noted, a wide variety of the traditional paper-based medical literature, from textbooks to journals, is now available electronically. The electronic versions may be enhanced by measures ranging from the provision of supplemental data in a journal article to linkages and multimedia content in a textbook. The final component of this category is the Web site. Admittedly, the diversity of information on Web sites is enormous, and sites may include every other type of content described in this chapter. However, in the context of this category, "Web site" refers to the vast number of static and dynamic Web pages at a discrete Web location.

Electronic publication of journals allows additional features not possible in the print world. Journal editors often clash with authors over the length of published papers (editors want them short for readability whereas authors want them long to be able to present all ideas and results). To address this situation, the *British Medical Journal* (BMJ) has initiated an **electronic-long, paper-short (ELPS)** system that provides on the Web site supplemental material that did not appear in the print version of the journal. Journal Web sites can provide additional description of experiments, results, images, and even raw data. A journal Web site also allows more dialog about articles than could be published in a "Letters to the Editor" section of a print journal. Electronic publication allows true bibliographic linkages, both to other full-text articles and to the MEDLINE record.

The Web also allows linkage directly from bibliographic databases to full text. PubMed maintains a field for the Web address of the full-text paper. This linkage is active when the PubMed record is displayed, but users may be met by a password screen if the article is not available for free. There is often an option to enter a credit card number to gain access, but the typical price for electronic access ($10 to $15 per article at the time of this writing) is an impediment to many. Other publishers, such as Ovid and MDConsult (www.mdconsult.com), provide access within their own password-protected interfaces to articles from journals that they have licensed for use in their systems.

The most common secondary literature source is traditional textbooks, an increasing number of which are available in computer form. A common approach with textbooks is bundling them, sometimes with linkages across the bundled texts. An early bundler of textbooks was Stat!-Ref (Teton Data Systems, www.statref.com) that, like many, began as a CD-ROM product and then moved to the Web. Stat!-Ref offers over 30 textbooks. Another product that implemented linking early was Harrison's Online (McGraw-Hill, www.harrisonsonline.com), which contains the full text of *Harrison's Principles of Internal Medicine* and the drug reference *Gold Standard Pharmacology*. Another textbook collection of growing stature is the NCBI Bookshelf, which contains many volumes on biomedical research topics (http://www.ncbi.nlm.nih.gov/entrez/query.fcgi?db=Books).

Electronic textbooks offer additional features beyond text from the print version. While many print textbooks do feature high-quality images, electronic versions offer the ability to have more pictures and illustrations. They also have the ability to use sound and video, although few do at this time. As with full-text journals, electronic textbooks can link to other resources, including journal references and the full articles. Many Web-based textbook sites also provide access to continuing education self-assessment questions and medical news. Finally, electronic textbooks let authors and publishers provide more frequent updates of the information than is allowed by the usual cycle of print editions, where new versions come out only every 2 to 5 years.

As noted above, Web sites are another form of full-text information. Probably the most effective provider of Web-based health information is the U.S. government. The bibliographic databases of the NLM, the National Cancer Institute (NCI), AHRQ, and others have already been described. These agencies have also been innovative in providing comprehensive full-text information for health care providers and consumers as well. Some of these will be described later as aggregations, since they provide many different types of resources. A large number of private consumer health Web sites have emerged in recent years. Of course, they include more than just collections of text; they also include interaction with experts, online stores, and catalogs of links to other sites. There are also Web sites that provide information geared toward health care providers, typically overviews of diseases, their diagnosis, and treatment; medical news and other resources for providers are often offered as well.

Databases/Collections

The third category consists of databases and other specific collections of information. These resources are usually not stored as freestanding Web pages but instead are often housed in **database management systems**. This content can be further subcategorized into discrete information types:

1. **Image databases**—collections of images from radiology, pathology, and other areas.
2. **Genomics databases**—information from gene sequencing, protein characterization, and other genomic research.
3. **Citation databases**—bibliographic linkages of scientific literature.
4. **EBM databases**—highly structured collections of clinical evidence.
5. **Other databases**—miscellaneous other collections.

A great number of image databases are available on the Web. One collection of note is the **Visible Human Project** of the NLM, which consists of three-dimensional representations of normal male and female bodies (Spitzer et al., 1996). This resource is built from cross-sectional slices of cadavers, with sections of 1 mm in the male and 0.3 mm in the female. Also available from each cadaver are transverse computerized tomography (CT) and magnetic resonance (MR) images. In addition to the images themselves, a variety of searching and browsing interfaces have been created which can be accessed via the project Web site (www.nlm.nih.gov/research/visible/visible_human.html).

Many genomics databases are available across the Web. The first issue each year of the journal *Nucleic Acids Research* catalogs and describes these databases (Baxevanis, 2003). The most important of these databases are available from NCBI. All their databases are linked among themselves, along with PubMed and OMIM, and are searchable via the **Entrez** system (www.ncbi.nlm.nih.gov/Entrez). More details on the specific content of genomics databases is provided in Chapter 22.

Citation databases provide linkages to articles that cite others across the scientific literature. The best-known citation databases are the *Science Citation Index* (SCI, ISI Thompson) and *Social Science Citation Index* (SSCI, ISI Thompson). A recent development is the Web of Science, a Web-based interface to these databases. Another system for citation indexing is the Research Index (formerly called CiteSeer, citeseer.nj.nec.com) (Lawrence et al., 1999). This index uses a process called *autonomous citation indexing* that adds citations into its database by automatically processing of papers from the Web. It also attempts to identify the context of citations, showing words that are similar across citations such that the commonality of citing papers can be observed.

EBM databases are devoted to providing synopses of evidence-based information in forms easily accessible by clinicians. Some examples of these databases include:

- *The Cochrane Database of Systematic Reviews*—one of the original collections of systemtatic reviews (www.cochrane.org).
- *Clinical Evidence*—an "evidence formulary" (www.clinicalevidence.com).
- *Up-to-Date*—content centered around clinical questions (www.uptodate.com).
- *InfoPOEMS*—"patient-oriented evidence that matters" (www.infopoems.com).
- *Physicians' Information and Education Resource* (PIER)—"practice guidance statements" for which every test and treatment has associated ratings of the evidence to support them (pier.acponline.org).

There are a variety of other databases/collections that do not fit into the above category, such as the ClinicalTrials.gov database that contains details of ongoing clinical trials sponsored by the NIH.

Aggregations

The final category consists of **aggregations** of content from the first three categories. The distinction between this category and some of the highly linked types of content described above is admittedly blurry, but aggregations typically have a wide variety of different types of information serving the diverse needs of users. Aggregated content has been developed for all types of users from consumers to clinicians to scientists.

Probably the largest aggregated consumer information resource is **Medline Plus** (medlineplus.gov) from the NLM (Miller et al., 2000). Medline Plus includes all of the types of content previously described, aggregated for easy access to a given topic. At the top level, Medline Plus contains health topics, drug information, medical dictionaries, directories, and other resources. Medline Plus currently contains over 700 health topics. The initial selection of topics is based on analysis of those used by consumers to search for health information on the NLM Web site (Miller et al., 2000). Each topic contains links to health information from the NIH and other sources deemed credible by its selectors. There are also links to current health news (updated daily), a medical encyclopedia, drug references, and directories, along with a preformed PubMed search, related to the topic. Figure 19.1 interface has changed-see following shows the top of the Medline Plus page for *cholesterol*.

Aggregations of content have also been developed for clinicians. **Merck Medicus** (www.merckmedicus.com), developed by the well-known publisher and pharmaceutical house, is available for free to all licensed U.S. physicians, and includes such well-known resources as Harrison's Online, MDConsult, and DXplain. Another aggregated resource for clinicians that combines several applications is **MedWeaver** (Unbound Medicine, www.unboundmedicine.com) (Detmer et al., 1997). MedWeaver combines three applications:

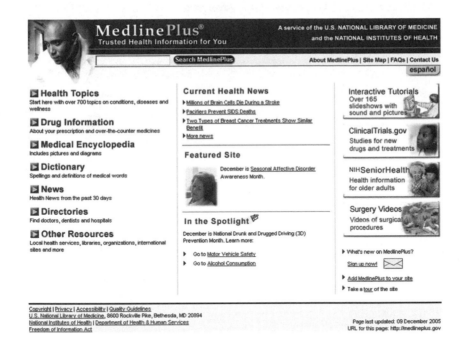

Figure 19.1. A screen display of MEDLINEplus. (Courtesy of NLM.)

1. MEDLINE
2. **DXplain**—a diagnostic decision support that maintains profiles of findings for over 2,000 diseases and generates differential diagnoses when cases of findings are entered (Barnett et al., 1987)
3. A Web catalog

Figure 19.2 shows MedWeaver links elicited by a case of a middle-aged man with *chest pain* and *shortness of breath*. A differential diagnosis is generated, with links to the DXplain disease profile, MEDLINE, and entries in a Web catalog. The *Explain* option lists the diagnostic reasoning of DXplain.

Another well-known group of aggregations of content for biomedical researchers is the **model organism databases**. These databases bring together bibliographic databases, full text, and databases of sequences, structure, and function for organisms whose genomic data have been highly characterized, such as the mouse, fruit fly, and Saccharomyces yeast (Bahls et al., 2003). More detail is provided in Chapter 22.

19.3   Information Retrieval

Now that we have a general understanding of the types, production, and use of knowledge-based biomedical information, we can focus on IR systems. A model for the IR

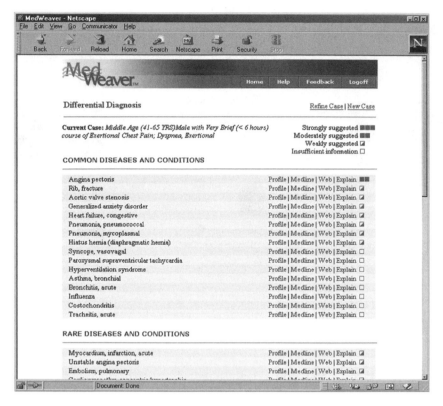

Figure 19.2. A screen display of MedWeaver. (Courtesy of Unbound Medicine.)

system and the user interacting with it is shown in Figure 19.3 (Hersh, 2003). Based on our previous discussion, we know that the ultimate goal of the user is to access content, which may be in the form of a digital library. For that content to be accessible, it must be described with **metadata**.

The major intellectual processes of IR are **indexing** and **retrieval**. These will be described next, followed by discussion on the **evaluation** of IR systems and research directions.

19.3.1 Indexing

Most modern commercial content is indexed in two ways:

1. **Manual indexing**—where human indexers, usually using standardized terminology, assign indexing terms and attributes to documents, often following a specific protocol.
2. **Automated indexing**—where computers make the indexing assignments, usually limited to breaking out each word in the document (or part of the document) as an indexing term.

Figure 19.3. A graphic representation of the information retrieval (IR) process. (Courtesy of Springer-Verlag.)

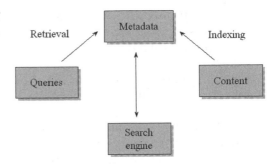

Manual indexing is done most commonly with bibliographic databases. In this age of proliferating electronic content, such as online textbooks, practice guidelines, and multimedia collections, manual indexing has become either too expensive or outright unfeasible for the quantity and diversity of material now available. Thus there are increasing numbers of databases that are indexed only by automated means.

Controlled Terminologies

Before discussing specific terminologies, it is useful to define some terms, since different writers attach different definitions to the various components of thesauri. A **concept** is an idea or object that occurs in the world, such as the condition under which human blood pressure is elevated. A **term** is the actual string of one or more words that represent a concept, such as *Hypertension* or *High Blood Pressure*. One of these string forms is the preferred or **canonical form**, such as *Hypertension* in the present example. When one or more terms can represent a concept, the different terms are called **synonyms**.

A **controlled terminology** usually contains a list of terms that are the canonical representations of the concepts. They are also called **thesauri** and contain relationships between terms, which typically fall into three categories:

1. *Hierarchical*—terms that are broader or narrower. The hierarchical organization not only provides an overview of the structure of a thesaurus but also can be used to enhance searching (e.g., MeSH tree explosions described in Chapter 7).
2. *Synonymous*—terms that are synonyms, allowing the indexer or searcher to express a concept in different words.
3. *Related*—terms that are not synonymous or hierarchical but are somehow otherwise related. These usually remind the searcher of different but related terms that may enhance a search.

The MeSH terminology is used to manually index most of the databases produced by the NLM (Coletti and Bleich, 2001). The latest version contains nearly 23,000 *subject headings* (the word MeSH uses for the canonical representation of its concepts). It also contains over 100,000 supplementary concept records in a separate chemical thesaurus. In addition, MeSH contains the three types of relationships described in the previous paragraph:

1. Hierarchical—MeSH is organized hierarchically into 15 **trees**, such as Diseases, Organisms, and Chemicals and Drugs.
2. Synonymous—MeSH contains a vast number of **entry terms**, which are synonyms of the headings.
3. Related—terms that may be useful for searchers to add to their searches when appropriate are suggested for many headings.

The MeSH terminology files, their associated data, and their supporting documentation are available on the NLM's MeSH Web site (www.nlm.nih.gov/mesh/). There is also a **browser** that facilitates exploration of the terminology (www.nlm.nih.gov/mesh/MBrowser.html).

There are features of MeSH designed to assist indexers in making documents more retrievable (Anonymous, 2000b). One of these is **subheadings**, which are qualifiers of subject headings that narrow the focus of a term. In *Hypertension*, for example, the focus of an article may be on the diagnosis, epidemiology, or treatment of the condition. Another feature of MeSH that helps retrieval is **check tags**. These are MeSH terms that represent certain facets of medical studies, such as age, gender, human or nonhuman, and type of grant support. Related to check tags are the geographical locations in the Z tree. Indexers must also include these, like check tags, since the location of a study (e.g., *Oregon*) must be indicated. Another feature gaining increasing importance for EBM and other purposes is the **publication type**, which describes the type of publication or the type of study. A searcher who wants a review of a topic may choose the publication type *Review* or *Review Literature*. Or, to find studies that provide the best evidence for a therapy, the publication type *Meta-Analysis*, *Randomized Controlled Trial*, or *Controlled Clinical Trial* would be used.

MeSH is not the only thesaurus used for indexing biomedical documents. A number of other thesauri are used to index non-NLM databases. CINAHL, for example, uses the **CINAHL Subject Headings**, which are based on MeSH but have additional domain-specific terms added (Brenner and McKinin, 1989). EMBASE has a terminology called **EMTREE**, which has many features similar to those of MeSH (www.elsevier.nl/home-page/sah/spd/site/locate_embase.html).

One problem with controlled terminologies, not limited to IR systems, is their proliferation. As already described in Chapter 7, there is great need for linkage across these different terminologies. This was the primary motivation for the **Unified Medical Language System (UMLS) Project**, which was undertaken in the 1980s to address this problem (Humphreys et al., 1998). There are three components of the **UMLS Knowledge Sources**: the **Metathesaurus**, the **UMLS Semantic Network**, and the **Specialist Lexicon**. The Metathesaurus component of the UMLS links parts or all of over 100 terminologies.

In the Metathesaurus, all terms that are conceptually the same are linked together as a **concept**. Each concept may have one or more **terms**, each of which represents an expression of the concept from a source terminology that is not just a simple lexical variant (i.e., differs only in word ending or order). Each term may consist of one or more **strings**, which represent all the lexical variants that are represented for that term in the source terminologies. One of each term's strings is designated as the preferred form, and the preferred string of the preferred term is known as the **canonical form** of the concept. There are rules of precedence for determining the canonical form, the main one being that the MeSH heading is used if one of the source terminologies for the concept is MeSH. Each Metathesaurus concept has a single *concept unique identifier* (*CUI*). Each term has one *term unique identifier* (*LUI*), all of which are linked to the one (or more) CUIs with which they are associated. Likewise, each string has one *string unique identifier* (*SUI*), which likewise are linked to the LUIs in which they occur.

Figure 19.4 depicts the English-language concepts, terms, and strings for the concept *atrial fibrillation*. The canonical form of the concept and one of its terms is *atrial fibrillation*. Within both terms are several strings, which vary in word order and case. The Metathesaurus contains a wealth of additional information. In addition to the synonym relationships between concepts, terms, and strings described earlier, there are also nonsynonym relationships between concepts. There are a great many attributes for the concepts, terms, and strings, such as definitions, lexical types, and occurrence in various data sources. Also provided with the Metathesaurus is a word index that connects each word to all the strings it occurs in, along with its concept, term, and string identifiers.

Manual Indexing

Manual indexing of bibliographic content is the most common and developed use of indexing. Bibliographic manual indexing is usually done by means of a controlled terminology of terms and attributes. Most databases utilizing human indexing usually have a detailed protocol for assignment of indexing terms from the thesaurus. The MEDLINE database is no exception. The principles of MEDLINE indexing were laid

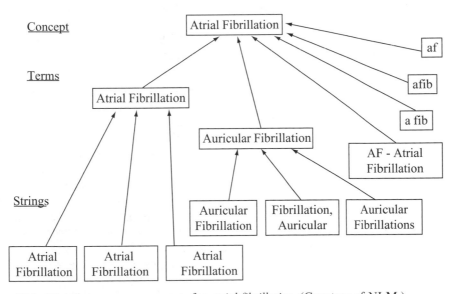

Figure 19.4. Metathesaurus components for *atrial fibrillation*. (Courtesy of NLM.)

out in the two-volume *MEDLARS Indexing Manual* (Charen, 1976, 1983). Subsequent modifications have occurred with changes to MEDLINE, other databases, and MeSH over the years (Anonymous, 2000a). The major concepts of the article, usually from two to five headings, are designed as *main headings*, and designated in the MEDLINE record by an asterisk. The indexer is also required to assign appropriate subheadings. Finally, the indexer must also assign check tags, geographical locations, and publication types.

Few full-text resources are manually indexed. One type of indexing that commonly takes place with full-text resources, especially in the print world, is that performed for the index at the back of the book. However, this information is rarely used in IR systems; instead, most online textbooks rely on automated indexing (see below). One exception to this is MDConsult (www.mdconsult.com), which uses back-of-book indexes to point to specific sections in its online books.

Manual indexing of Web content is challenging. With several billion pages of content, manual indexing of more than a fraction of it is not feasible. On the other hand, the lack of a coherent index makes searching much more difficult, especially when specific resource types are being sought. A simple form of manual indexing of the Web takes place in the development of the Web catalogs and aggregations as described above. These catalogs contain not only explicit indexing about subjects and other attributes, but also implicit indexing about the quality of a given resource by the decision of whether to include it in the catalog.

Two major approaches to manual indexing have emerged on the Web, which are often complementary. The first approach, that of applying metadata to Web pages and sites, is exemplified by the **Dublin Core Metadata Initiative (DCMI**, www.dublincore.org). The second approach, to build directories of content, was popularized initially by the Yahoo search engine (www.yahoo.com). A more open approach to building directories has been the Open Directory Project (dmoz.org), which carries on the structuring of the directory and entry of content by volunteers across the world.

One of the first frameworks for metadata on the Web was the DCMI (Weibel, 1996). The goal of the DCMI has been to develop a set of standard data elements that creators of Web resources can use to apply metadata to their content. The specification has defined 15 elements, as shown in Table 19.1 (Anonymous, 1999). The DCMI was recently approved as a standard by the **National Information Standards Organization (NISO)** with the designation Z39.85 (Anonymous, 2001b).

There have been several medical adaptations of the DCMI. Malet et al. (1999) proposed the Medical Core Metadata (MCM) project, which would extend the DCMI to allow more health-specific tagging in fields such as *Subject* (i.e., using MeSH terms) and *Type* (using a controlled set of names to describe resource type). Another project applying the DCMI to health care resources is the Catalogue et Index des Sites Médicaux Francophones (CISMeF) (Darmoni et al., 2000). A catalog of French-language health resources on the Web, CISMeF has used DCMI to catalog over 13,000 Web pages, including information resources (e.g., practice guidelines, consensus development conferences), organizations (e.g., hospitals, medical schools, pharmaceutical companies), and databases. The *Subject* field uses the French translation of MeSH (http://dicdoc.kb.inserm.fr:2010/basismesh/mesh.html) but also

Table 19.1. Elements of Dublin Core metadata.

Dublin Core element	Definition
DC.title	The name given to the resource
DC.creator	The person or organization primarily responsible for creating the intellectual content of the resource
DC.subject	The topic of the resource
DC.description	A textual description of the content of the resource
DC.publisher	The entity responsible for making the resource available in its present form
DC.date	A date associated with the creation or availability of the resource
DC.contributor	A person or organization not specified in a creator element who has made a significant intellectual contribution to the resource but whose contribution is secondary to any person or organization specified in a creator element
DC.type	The category of the resource
DC.format	The data format of the resource, used to identify the software and possibly hardware that might be needed to display or operate the resource
DC.identifier	A string or number used to uniquely identify the resource
DC.source	Information about a second resource from which the present resource is derived
DC.language	The language of the intellectual content of the resource
DC.relation	An identifier of a second resource and its relationship to the present resource
DC.coverage	The spatial or temporal characteristics of the intellectual content of the resource
DC.rights	A rights management statement, an identifier that links to a rights management statement, or an identifier that links to a service providing information about rights management for the resource

(*Source*: Anonymous, 1999.)

includes the English translations. For *Type*, a list of common Web resources has been enumerated.

While Dublin Core Metadata was originally envisioned to be included in **Hypertext Markup Language (HTML)** Web pages, it became apparent that many non-HTML resources exist on the Web and that there are reasons to store metadata external to Web pages. For example, authors of Web pages might not be the best people to index pages or other entities might wish to add value by their own indexing of content. An emerging standard for cataloging metadata is the **Resource Description Framework (RDF)** (Miller, 1998). A framework for describing and interchanging metadata, RDF is usually expressed in **Extensible Markup Language (XML)**, a standard for data interchange on the Web. Key features of XML are its ability to express complex data, its readability, and the growing array of tools to parse and extract data from encoded documents. Increasingly, XML is being used to interchange data between databases and has been designated the preferred interchange format in the **Clinical Document Architecture** of the **Health Level 7 (HL7**, www.hl7.org) standard (Dolin et al., 2001). RDF also forms the basis of what some call the future of the Web as a repository not only of content but also of knowledge, which is also referred to as the **Semantic Web** (Lassila et al., 2001). Dublin Core Metadata (or any type of metadata) can be represented in RDF (Beckett et al., 2000).

Another approach to manually indexing content on the Web has been to create directories of content. The first major effort to create these was the Yahoo! search engine, which created a subject hierarchy and assigned Web sites to elements within it (www.yahoo.com). When concern began to emerge that the Yahoo directory was proprietary and not necessarily representative of the Web community at large (Caruso, 2000), an alternative movement sprung up: the Open Directory Project.

Manual indexing has a number of limitations, the most significant of which is inconsistency. Funk and Reid (1983) evaluated indexing inconsistency in MEDLINE by identifying 760 articles that had been indexed twice by the NLM. The most consistent indexing occurred with check tags and central concept headings, which were only indexed with a consistency of 61 to 75 percent. The least consistent indexing occurred with subheadings, especially those assigned to non-central-concept headings, which had a consistency of less than 35 percent. Manual indexing also takes time. While it may be feasible with the large resources the NLM has to index MEDLINE, it is probably impossible with the growing amount of content on Web sites and in other full-text resources. Indeed, the NLM has recognized the challenge of continuing to have to index the growing body of biomedical literature and is investigating automated and semiautomated means of doing so (Aronson et al., 2000).

Automated Indexing

In automated indexing, the work is done by a computer. Although the mechanical running of the automated indexing process lacks cognitive input, considerable intellectual effort may have gone into development of the system for doing it, so this form of indexing still qualifies as an intellectual process. In this section, we will focus on the automated indexing used in operational IR systems, namely the indexing of documents by the words they contain.

We tend not to think of extracting all the words in a document as "indexing," but from the standpoint of an IR system, words are descriptors of documents, just like human-assigned indexing terms. Most retrieval systems actually use a hybrid of human and word indexing, in that the human-assigned indexing terms become part of the document, which can then be searched by using the whole controlled term or individual words within it. As will be seen in the next chapter, most MEDLINE implementations have always allowed the combination of searching on human indexing terms and on words in the title and abstract of the reference. With the development of full-text resources in the 1980s and 1990s, systems that allowed only word indexing began to emerge. This trend increased with the advent of the Web.

Word indexing is typically done by taking all consecutive **alphanumeric** sequences between **white space** (which consists of spaces, punctuation, carriage returns, and other nonalphanumeric characters). Systems must take particular care to apply the same process to documents and the user's query, especially with characters such as hyphens and apostrophes. Many systems go beyond simple identification of words and attempt to assign weights to words that represent their importance in the document (Salton, 1991).

Many systems using word indexing employ processes to remove common words or conflate words to common forms. The former consists of filtering to remove **stop words**, which are common words that always occur with high frequency and are usually of little value in searching. The stop word list, also called a **negative dictionary**, varies in size from the seven words of the original MEDLARS stop list (*and, an, by, from, of, the, with*) to the list of 250 to 500 words more typically used. Examples of the latter are the 250-word list of van Rijsbergen (1979), the 471-word list of Fox (1992), and the PubMed stop list (Anonymous, 2001d). Conflation of words to common forms is done via **stemming**, the purpose of which is to ensure words with plurals and common suffixes (e.g., *-ed, -ing, -er, -al*) are always indexed by their stem form (Frakes, 1992). For example, the words *cough, coughs,* and *coughing* are all indexed via their stem *cough*. Both stop word remove and stemming reduce the size of indexing files and lead to more efficient query processing.

A commonly used approach for **term weighting** is **TF*IDF weighting**, which combines the **inverse document frequency (IDF)** and **term frequency (TF)**. The IDF is the logarithm of the ratio of the total number of documents to the number of documents in which the term occurs. It is assigned once for each term in the database, and it correlates inversely with the frequency of the term in the entire database. The usual formula used is:

$$\text{IDF(term)} = \log \frac{\text{number of documents in database}}{\text{number of documents with term}} + 1 \qquad (19.1)$$

The TF is a measure of the frequency with which a term occurs in a given document and is assigned to each term in each document, with the usual formula:

$$\text{TF(term,document)} = \text{frequency of term in document} \qquad (19.2)$$

In TF*IDF weighting, the two terms are combined to form the indexing weight, WEIGHT:

$$\text{WEIGHT(term,document)} = \text{TF(term,document)}^*\text{IDF(term)} \qquad (19.3)$$

Another automated indexing approach generating increased interest is the use of **link-based** methods, fueled no doubt by the success of the **Google** (www.google.com) search engine. This approach gives weight to pages based on how often they are cited by other pages. The **PageRank (PR) algorithm** is mathematically complex, but can be viewed as giving more weight to a Web page based on the number of other pages that link to it (Brin and Page, 1998). Thus, the home page of the NLM or a major medical journal is likely to have a very high PR, whereas a more obscure page will have a lower PR.

Word indexing has a number of limitations, including:

- **Synonymy**—different words may have the same meaning, such as *high* and *elevated*. This problem may extend to the level of phrases with no words in common, such as the synonyms *hypertension* and *high blood pressure*.
- **Polysemy**—the same word may have different meanings or senses. For example, the word *lead* can refer to an element or to a part of an electrocardiogram machine.
- **Content**—words in a document may not reflect its focus. For example, an article describing *hypertension* may make mention in passing to other concepts, such as *congestive heart failure* (CHF) that are not the focus of the article.

- **Context**—words take on meaning based on other words around them. For example, the relatively common words *high, blood,* and *pressure*, take on added meaning when occurring together in the phrase *high blood pressure*.
- **Morphology**—words can have suffixes that do not change the underlying meaning, such as indicators of plurals, various participles, adjectival forms of nouns, and nominalized forms of adjectives.

Granularity—queries and documents may describe concepts at different levels of a hierarchy. For example, a user might query for *antibiotics* in the treatment of a specific infection, but the documents might describe specific antibiotics themselves, such as *penicillin*.

19.3.2 Retrieval

There are two broad approaches to retrieval. **Exact-match searching** allows the user precise control over the items retrieved. **Partial-match searching**, on the other hand, recognizes the inexact nature of both indexing and retrieval, and instead attempts to return the user content ranked by how close it comes to the user's query. After general explanations of these approaches, we will describe actual systems that access the different types of biomedical content.

Exact-Match Retrieval

In exact-match searching, the IR system gives the user all documents that exactly match the criteria specified in the search statement(s). Since the **Boolean operators** AND, OR, and NOT are usually required to create a manageable set of documents, this type of searching is often called **Boolean searching**. Furthermore, since the user typically builds sets of documents that are manipulated with the Boolean operators, this approach is also called **set-based searching**. Most of the early operational IR systems in the 1950s through 1970s used the exact-match approach, even though Salton was developing the partial-match approach in research systems during that time (Salton and Lesk, 1965). In modern times, exact-match searching tends to be associated with retrieval from bibliographic databases, while the partial-match approach tends to be used with full-text searching.

Typically the first step in exact-match retrieval is to select terms to build sets. Other attributes, such as the author name, publication type, or gene identifier (in the secondary source identifier field of MEDLINE), may be selected to build sets as well. Once the search term(s) and attribute(s) have been selected, they are combined with the Boolean operators. The Boolean AND operator is typically used to narrow a retrieval set to contain only documents with two or more concepts. The Boolean OR operator is usually used when there is more than one way to express a concept. The Boolean NOT operator is often employed as a subtraction operator that must be applied to another set. Some systems more accurately call this the ANDNOT operator.

Some systems allow terms in searches to be expanded by using the *wild-card character*, which adds all words to the search that begin with the letters up until the wild-card character. This approach is also called *truncation*. Unfortunately, there is no standard approach to using wild-card characters, so syntax for them varies from system to system. PubMed, for example, allows a single asterisk at the end of a word to signify a wild-card character. Thus the query word *can** will lead to the words *cancer* and *Candida*, among others, being added to the search. The AltaVista search engine (www.altavista.com) takes a different approach. The asterisk can be used as a wild-card character within or at the end of a word but only after its first three letters. For example, *col*r* will retrieve documents containing *color*, *colour*, and *colder*.

Partial-Match Retrieval

Although **partial-match searching** was conceptualized very early, it did not see widespread use in IR systems until the advent of Web search engines in the 1990s. This is most likely because exact-match searching tends to be preferred by "power users" whereas partial-match searching is preferred by novice searchers. Whereas exact-match searching requires an understanding of Boolean operators and (often) the underlying structure of databases (e.g., the many fields in MEDLINE), partial-match searching allows a user to simply enter a few terms and start retrieving documents.

The development of partial-match searching is usually attributed to Salton (1991), who pioneered the approach in the 1960s. Although partial-match searching does not exclude the use of nonterm attributes of documents, and for that matter does not even exclude the use of Boolean operators (e.g., Salton et al., 1983), the most common use of this type of searching is with a query of a small number of words, also known as a **natural language query**. Because Salton's approach was based on vector mathematics, it is also referred to as the **vector-space model** of IR. In the partial-match approach, documents are typically ranked by their closeness of fit to the query. That is, documents containing more query terms will likely be ranked higher, since those with more query terms will in general be more likely to be relevant to the user. As a result this process is called **relevance ranking**. The entire approach has also been called **lexical–statistical retrieval**.

The most common approach to document ranking in partial-match searching is to give each a score based on the sum of the weights of terms common to the document and query. Terms in documents typically derive their weight from the TF*IDF calculation described above. Terms in queries are typically given a weight of one if the term is present and zero if it is absent. The following formula can then be used to calculate the document weight across all query terms:

$$\text{Document weight} = \sum_{\text{all query terms}} \text{Weight of term in query} * \text{Weight of term in document} \quad (4)$$

This may be thought of as a giant OR of all query terms, with sorting of the matching documents by weight. The usual approach is for the system to then perform the same stop word removal and stemming of the query that was done in the indexing process. (The equivalent stemming operations must be performed on documents and queries so that complementary word stems will match.)

Retrieval Systems

This section describes searching systems used to retrieve content from the four categories previously described in Section 19.2.6.

As noted above, PubMed is the system at NLM that searches MEDLINE and other bibliographic databases. Although presenting the user with a simple text box, PubMed does a great deal of processing of the user's input to identify MeSH terms, author names, common phrases, and journal names (Anonymous, 2001d). In this automatic term mapping, the system attempts to map user input, in succession, to MeSH terms, journals names, common phrases, and authors. Remaining text that PubMed cannot map is searched as text words (i.e., words that occur in any of the MEDLINE fields).

PubMed allows the use of wild-card characters. It also allows phrase searching whereby two or more words can be enclosed in quotation marks to indicate they must occur adjacent to each other. If the specified phrase is in PubMed's phrase index, then it will be searched as a phrase. Otherwise the individual words will be searched. PubMed allows specification of other indexing attributes via the PubMed "Limits" screen (see Figure 19.5). These include publication types, subsets, age ranges, and publication date ranges.

As in most bibliographic systems, users search PubMed by building search sets and then combining them with Boolean operators to tailor the search. Consider a user searching for studies assessing the reduction of mortality in patients with CHF through the use of medications from the *angiotensin-converting* (*ACE*) *inhibitor* class of drugs. A simple approach to such a search might be to combine the terms *ACE Inhibitors* and *CHF* with an AND. The easiest way to do this is to enter the search string *ace inhibitors AND CHF*. (The operator *AND* must be capitalized because PubMed treats the lower-

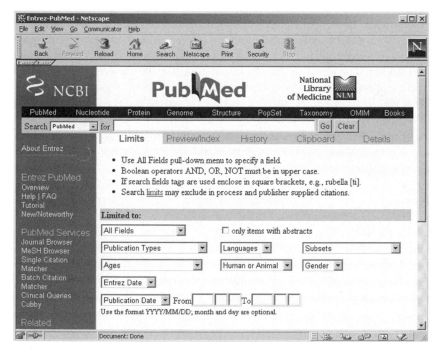

Figure 19.5. PubMed limits. (Courtesy of NLM.)

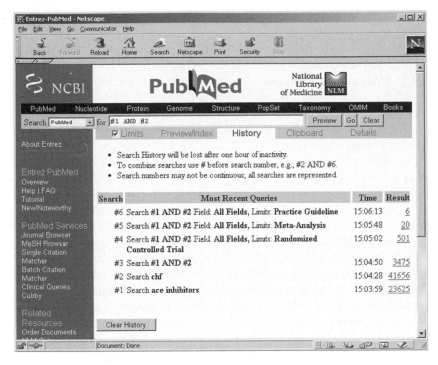

Figure 19.6. PubMed history screen. (Courtesy of NLM.)

case "and" as a text word, since some MeSH terms, such as *Bites and Strings*, have the word "and" in them.) Figure 19.6 shows the PubMed History screen such a searcher might develop. This searcher has limited the output (using the screen in Figure 19.5) with various publication types known to contain the best evidence for this question.

PubMed has another approach to finding the best evidence that is simpler though not as flexible. PubMed allows the user to enter *clinical queries*, where the subject terms are limited by search statements designed to retrieve the best evidence based on principles of EBM. There are two different approaches. The first uses strategies for retrieving the best evidence for the four major types of clinical questions. These strategies arise from research assessing the ability of MEDLINE search statements to identify the best studies for therapy, diagnosis, harm, and prognosis (Haynes et al., 1994). The second approach to retrieving the best evidence aims to retrieve evidence-based resources that are syntheses and synopses, in particular meta-analyses, systematic reviews, and practice guidelines. The strategy derives in part from research by Boynton et al. (1998). When the clinical queries interface is used, the search statement is processed by the usual automatic term mapping and the resulting output is limited (via AND) with the appropriate statement.

There are other ways to access MEDLINE without charge on the Web. WebMEDLINE (www.medweaver.com/webmedline/new.html) provides a simpler user interface to PubMed. Searches created by using its interface are sent to PubMed, with results redisplayed in another simple view. Another site that puts a different interface in front of PubMed is Infotrieve (www.infotrieve.com). BioMedNet (www.biomednet.com), owned by Reed-Elsevier, provides free MEDLINE to those who register on the site. Access to full-text and other resources linked from MEDLINE is provided at a cost. Medscape (www.medscape.com) provides access to MEDLINE through a licensed version of the Knowledge Finder system. Studies in the past have shown considerable variation in the search results of different systems searching the same underlying MEDLINE database (Haynes et al., 1985; Haynes et al., 1994). There is no reason to believe the same situation does not still exist.

As noted already, a great number of biomedical journals use the Highwire system for online access to their full text. The Highwire system provides a retrieval interface that searches over the complete online contents for a given journal. Users can search for authors, words limited to the title and abstract, words in the entire article, and within a date range. The interface also allows searching by citation by entering volume number and page as well as searching over the entire collection of journals that use Highwire. Users can browse through specific issues as well as collected resources.

Once an article has been found, a wealth of additional features are available (see Figure 19.7). First, the article is presented both in HTML and **Portable Document Format (PDF)** form, with the latter providing a more readable and printable version. Links are also provided to related articles from the journal as well as the PubMed reference and its related articles. Also linked are all articles in the journal that cited this one, and the site can be configured to set up a notification e-mail when new articles cite the item selected. Finally, the Highwire software provides for "Rapid Responses," which are online letters to the editor. The online format allows a much larger number of responses than could be printed in the paper version of the journal.

A good example of the functionality used for retrieval from a database/collection can be seen with the ClinicalTrials.Gov database of clinical trials. At the home page, the user can enter a natural language search or use a "Focused Search" that provides an interface to search by disease, location, treatment, sponsor, and so forth. The natural language search results page provides an option of "Query Details" that:

- Attempts to refine the query by mapping words into terms from the various fields, e.g., disease, location, and treatment into "Query Suggestions" that the user can perform by clicking on the appropriate link.
- Provides links to "Possibly Relevant MEDLINEplus Topics" from disease words and terms it can map from the query.
- Lists individual words and phrases it has mapped and the count of the number of matches in the database.

As an example, if the user enters the query *heart attack beta blockers portland*, the "Query Details" will map the phrase *heart attack* to *myocardial infarction*, recognize the phrase *beta blocker*, and look for clinical trials in Portland (Oregon or Maine!).

The MEDLINEplus system of aggregated consumer health resources provides a simple text box but also features a more advanced interface that allows exact versus approximate (using stemming) match of words as well as the requirement for matching all

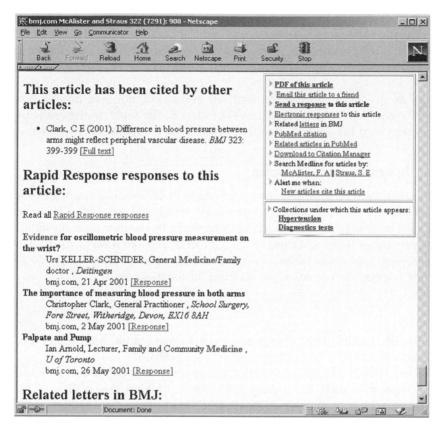

Figure 19.7. Highwire options for a retrieved article. (Courtesy of BMJ)

words (AND) or just some (OR). The user can also look up terms in a medical dictionary to check their spelling and have the search run against the entire site or just for
information in certain areas.

19.3.3   *Evaluation*

There has been a great deal of research over the years devoted to evaluation of IR systems. As with many areas of research, there is controversy as to which approaches to
evaluation best provide results that can assess searching in the systems they are using.
Many frameworks have been developed to put the results in context. One of those
frameworks organized evaluation around six questions that someone advocating the use
of IR systems might ask (Hersh and Hickam, 1998):

1. Was the system used?
2. For what was the system used?

3. Were the users satisfied?
4. How well did they use the system?
5. What factors were associated with successful or unsuccessful use of the system?
6. Did the system have an impact?

A simpler means for organizing the results of evaluation, however, groups approaches and studies into those which are *system-oriented*, i.e., the focus of the evaluation is on the IR system, and those which are *user-oriented*, i.e., the focus is on the user.

19.3.3.1   System-Oriented Evaluation

There are many ways to evaluate the performance of IR systems, the most widely used of which are the relevance-based measures of **recall** and **precision**. These measures quantify the number of relevant documents retrieved by the user from the database and in his or her search. They make use of the number of *relevant documents* (Rel), *retrieved documents* (Ret), and *retrieved documents that are also relevant* (Retrel). Recall is the proportion of relevant documents retrieved from the database:

$$\text{Recall} = \frac{\text{Retrel}}{\text{Rel}} \tag{19.5}$$

In other words, recall answers the question, for a given search, what fraction of all the relevant documents have been obtained from the database?

One problem with Equation (19.5) is that the denominator implies that the total number of relevant documents for a query is known. For all but the smallest of databases, however, it is unlikely, perhaps even impossible, for one to succeed in identifying all relevant documents in a database. Thus most studies use the measure of **relative recall**, where the denominator is redefined to represent the number of relevant documents identified by multiple searches on the query topic.

Precision is the proportion of relevant documents retrieved in the search:

$$\text{Precision} = \frac{\text{Retrel}}{\text{Ret}} \tag{19.6}$$

This measure answers the question, for a search, what fraction of the retrieved documents are relevant?

One problem that arises when one is comparing systems that use ranking versus those that do not is that nonranking systems, typically using Boolean searching, tend to retrieve a fixed set of documents and as a result have fixed points of recall and precision. Systems with relevance ranking, on the other hand, have different values of recall and precision depending on the size of the retrieval set the system (or the user) has chosen to show. For this reason, many evaluators of systems featuring relevance ranking will create a recall precision table (or graph) that identifies precision at various levels of recall. The "standard" approach to this was defined by Salton (1983), who pioneered both relevance ranking and this method of evaluating such systems.

To generate a recall-precision table for a single query, one first must determine the intervals of recall that will be used. A typical approach is to use intervals of 0.1 (or 10 percent), with a total of 11 intervals from a recall of 0.0 to 1.0. The table is built by determining the highest level of overall precision at any point in the output for a given interval of recall. Thus, for the recall interval 0.0, one would use the highest level of precision at which the recall is anywhere greater than or equal to zero and less than 0.1. An approach that has been used more frequently in recent times has been the **mean average precision (MAP)**, which is similar to precision at points of recall but does not use fixed recall intervals or interpolation (Voorhees, 1998). Instead, precision is measured at every point at which a relevant document is obtained, and the MAP measure is found by averaging these points for the whole query.

No overview of IR evaluation can ignore the **Text REtrieval Conference (TREC,** trec.nist.gov) organized by the U.S. **National Institute for Standards and Technology (NIST,** www.nist.gov) (Voorhees and Harman, 2000). Started in 1992, TREC has provided a testbed for evaluation and a forum for presentation of results. TREC is organized as an annual event at which the tasks are specified and queries and documents are provided to participants. Participating groups submit "runs" of their systems to NIST, which calculates the appropriate performance measure, usually recall and precision. TREC is organized into tracks geared to specific interests. Voorhees recently grouped the tracks into general IR tasks (Voorhees and Harman, 2001):

- Static text—ad hoc
- Streamed text—routing, filtering
- Human in the loop—interactive
- Beyond English (cross-lingual)—Spanish, Chinese, and others
- Beyond text—optical character recognition (OCR), speech, video
- Web searching—very large corpus, Web
- Answers, not documents—question-Answering

Relevance-based measures have their limitations. While no one denies that users want systems to retrieve relevant articles, it is not clear that the quantity of relevant documents retrieved is the complete measure of how well a system performs (Swanson, 1988; Harter, 1992). Hersh (1994) has noted that clinical users are unlikely to be concerned about these measures when they simply seek an answer to a clinical question and are able to do so no matter how many other relevant documents they miss (lowering recall) or how many nonrelevant ones they retrieve (lowering precision).

What alternatives to relevance-based measures can be used for determining performance of individual searches? Harter admits that if measures using a more situational view of relevance cannot be developed for assessing user interaction, then recall and precision may be the only alternatives. Thus Egan et al. (1989) evaluated the effectiveness of Superbook by assessing how well users could find and apply specific information in this manner. Mynatt et al. (1992) used a similar approach in comparing paper and electronic versions of an online encyclopedia, while Wildemuth et al. (1995) assessed the ability of students to answer testlike questions by using a medical curricular database. Hersh et al. have adapted these methods to searching for answers to medical questions in an electronic textbook (Hersh et al., 1994) and MEDLINE (Hersh et al., 1996). The Interactive Track at the TREC has also demonstrated the feasibility of this approach (Hersh, 2001).

19.3.3.2 User-Oriented Evaluation

A number of user-oriented evaluations have been performed over the years looking at users of biomedical information. Most of these studies have focused on clinicians.

One of the original studies measuring searching performance in clinical settings was performed by Haynes et al. (1990). This study also compared the capabilities of librarian and clinician searchers. In this study, 78 searches were randomly chosen for replication by both a clinician experienced in searching and a medical librarian. During this study, each original ("novice") user had been required to enter a brief statement of information need before entering the search program. This statement was given to the experienced clinician and librarian for searching on MEDLINE. All the retrievals for each search were given to a subject domain expert, blinded with respect to which searcher retrieved which reference. Recall and precision were calculated for each query and averaged. The results (Table 19.2) showed that the experienced clinicians and librarians achieved comparable recall, although the librarians had statistically significant precision. The novice clinician searchers had lower recall and precision than either of the other groups. This study also assessed user satisfaction of the novice searchers, who despite their recall and precision results said that they were satisfied with their search outcomes. The investigators did not assess whether the novices obtained enough relevant articles to answer their questions, or whether they would have found additional value with the ones that were missed.

A follow-up study yielded some additional insights about the searchers (McKibbon et al., 1990). As was noted, different searchers tended to use different strategies on a given topic. The different approaches replicated a finding known from other searching studies in the past, namely, the lack of overlap across searchers of overall retrieved citations as well as relevant ones. Thus, even though the novice searchers had lower recall, they did obtain a great many relevant citations not retrieved by the two expert searchers. Furthermore, fewer than 4 percent of all the relevant citations were retrieved by all three searchers. Despite the widely divergent search strategies and retrieval sets, overall recall and precision were quite similar among the three classes of users.

Recognizing the limitations of recall and precision for evaluating clinical users of IR systems, Hersh and coworkers have carried out a number of studies assessing the ability of systems to help students and clinicians answer clinical questions. The rationale for these studies is that the usual goal of using an IR system is to find an answer to a question. While the user must obviously find relevant documents to answer that question, the quantity of such documents is less important than whether the question is success-

Table 19.2. Recall and precision of MEDLINE searchers.

Users	Results (percent)	
	Recall	Precision
Novice clinicians	27	38
Experienced clinicians	48	49
Medical librarians	49	58

(*Source*: Haynes et al., 1990.)

fully answered. In fact, recall and precision can be placed among the many factors that may be associated with ability to complete the task successfully.

The first study by this group using the task-oriented approach compared Boolean versus natural language searching in the textbook *Scientific American Medicine* (Hersh et al., 1994). Thirteen medical students were asked to answer 10 short-answer questions and rate their confidence in their answers. The students were then randomized to one or the other interface and asked to search on the five questions for which they had rated confidence the lowest. The study showed that both groups had low correct rates before searching (average 1.7 correct out of 10) but were mostly able to answer the questions with searching (average 4.0 out of 5). There was no difference in ability to answer questions with one interface or the other. Most answers were found on the first search to the textbook. For the questions that were incorrectly answered, the document with the correct answer was actually retrieved by the user two-thirds of the time and viewed more than half the time.

Another study compared Boolean and natural language searching of MEDLINE with two commercial products, CD Plus (now Ovid) and KF (Hersh et al., 1996). These systems represented the ends of the spectrum in terms of using Boolean searching on human-indexed thesaurus terms (Ovid) versus natural language searching on words in the title, abstract, and indexing terms (KF). Sixteen medical students were recruited and randomized to one of the two systems and given three yes/no clinical questions to answer. The students were able to use each system successfully, answering 37.5 percent correctly before searching and 85.4 percent correctly after searching. There were no significant differences between the systems in time taken, relevant articles retrieved, or user satisfaction. This study demonstrated that both types of systems can be used equally well with minimal training.

The most comprehensive study looked at MEDLINE searching by medical and nurse practitioner (NP) students to answer clinical questions. A total of 66 medical and NP students searched five questions each (Hersh et al., 2002). This study used a multiple-choice format for answering questions that also included a judgment about the evidence for the answer. Subjects were asked to choose from one of three answers:

- Yes, with adequate evidence.
- Insufficient evidence to answer question.
- No, with adequate evidence.

Both groups achieved a presearching correctness on questions about equal to chance (32.3 percent for medical students and 31.7 percent for NP students). However, medical students improved their correctness with searching (to 51.6 percent), whereas NP students hardly did at all (to 34.7 percent).

This study also attempted to measure what factors might influence searching. A multitude of factors, such as age, gender, computer experience, and time taken to search, were not associated with successful answering of questions. Successful answering was, however, associated with answering the question correctly before searching, spatial visualization ability (measured by a validated instrument), searching experience, and EBM question type (prognosis questions easiest, harm questions most difficult). An analysis of recall and precision for each question searched demonstrated a complete lack of association with ability to answer these questions.

19.3.4   Research Directions

A great deal of research is looking at new approaches to IR, a detailed discussion of which is beyond the scope of this chapter. The NLM sponsors biomedical IR research both internally and externally. Its biggest internal project is the **Indexing Initiative**, which is investigating new approaches to automated and semiautomated indexing, mostly based on tools using the UMLS and natural language processing tools (Aronson et al., 2000).

Other approaches to research have focused on improving aspects of automated indexing and retrieval. A number of these have been found to improve retrieval performance in the TREC environment, including:

- Improved approaches to *term weighting*, such as *Okapi* (Robertson and Walker, 1994), *pivoted normalization* (Singhal et al., 1996), and *language modeling* (Ponte and Croft, 1998).
- *Passage retrieval*, where documents are given more weight in the ranking process based on local concentrations of query terms within them (Callan, 1994).
- *Query expansion*, where new terms from highly ranking documents are added to the query in an automated fashion (Srinivasan, 1996; Xu and Croft, 1996).

Additional work has focused on improving the user interface for the retrieval process by organizing the output better. An example of this is Dynacat, a system for consumers that uses UMLS knowledge and MeSH terms to organize search results (Pratt et al., 1999). The goal is to present search results with documents clustered into topical groups, such as the treatments for a disease or the tests used to diagnose it. Another approach is to make the search system vocabulary more understandable in context. The Cat-a-Cone system provides a means to explore term hierarchies by using *cone trees*, which rotate the primary term of interest to the center of the screen and show conelike expansion of other hierarchically related terms nearby (Hearst and Karadi, 1997).

19.4   Digital Libraries

Discussion of IR "systems" thus far has focused on the provision of retrieval mechanisms to access online content. Even with the expansive coverage of some IR systems, such as Web search engines, they are often part of a larger collection of services or activities. An alternative perspective, especially when communities and/or proprietary collections are involved, is the **digital library**. Digital libraries share many characteristics with "brick and mortar" libraries, but also take on some additional challenges. Borgman (1999) notes that libraries of both types elicit different definitions of what they actually are, with researchers tending to view libraries as content collected for specific communities and practitioners alternatively viewing them as institutions or services.

As evidence that digital libraries are a topic of public concern, the **U.S. President's Information Technology Committee (PITAC)** published three reports in 2001, one of which covered the topics of digital libraries (Anonymous, 2001a). The other two focused on the use of information technology to enhance health care (Anonymous, 2001e) and education (Anonymous, 2001f). The digital libraries report stated that the full potential of digital libraries has not been realized, noting that the underlying technologies (particularly the Internet) were developed with federal leadership, that archives face both technical and operational challenges, and that the issue of intellectual property cannot be ignored. The report recommended that support for research be expanded, large-scale testbeds be developed, all federal material be put online, and the government lead efforts to develop digital rights policies.

19.4.1   Functions and Definitions of Libraries

The central function of libraries is to maintain collections of published literature. They may also store nonpublished literature in *archives*, such as letters, notes, and other documents. The general focus on published literature has implications. One of these is that, for the most part, quality control can be taken for granted. At least until the recent past, most published literature came from commercial publishers and specialty societies that had processes such as peer review, which, although imperfect, allowed the library to devote minimal resources to assessing their quality. While libraries can still cede the judgment of quality to these information providers in the Internet era, they cannot ignore the myriad of information published only on the Internet, for which the quality cannot be presumed.

The paper-based nature of traditional libraries carries other implications. For example, items are produced in multiple copies. This frees the individual library from excessive worry that an item cannot be replaced. In addition, items are fairly static, simplifying their cataloging. With digital libraries, these implications are challenged. There is a great deal of concern about archiving of content and managing its change when fewer "copies" of it exist on the file servers of publishers and other organizations. A related problem for digital libraries is that they do not own the "artifact" of the paper journal, book, or other item. This is exacerbated by the fact that when a subscription to an electronic journal is terminated, access to the entire journal is lost; that is, the subscriber does not retain accumulated back issues, as is taken for granted with paper journals.

19.4.2   Access

Probably every Web user is familiar with clicking on a Web link and receiving the error message: *HTTP 404 -File not found*. Digital libraries and commercial publishing ventures need mechanisms to ensure that documents have persistent identifiers so that when the document itself physically moves, it is still obtainable. The original architecture for the Web envisioned by the Internet Engineering Task Force was to have every **uniform resource locator (URL)**, the address entered into a Web browser or used in a Web hyperlink, linked to a **uniform resource name (URN)** that would be persistent (Sollins and Masinter, 1994). The combination of a URN and a URL, a **uniform resource identifier (URI)**, would provide persistent access to digital objects. The resource for resolving URNs and URIs was never implemented on a large scale.

One approach that has begun to see widespread adoption by publishers, especially scientific journal publishers, is the **digital object identifier** (**DOI**, www.doi.org) (Paskin, 1999). The DOI has recently been given the status of a standard by the NISO with the designation Z39.84. The DOI itself is relatively simple, consisting of a prefix that is assigned by the IDF to the publishing entity and a suffix that is assigned and maintained by the entity. For example, the DOI for articles from the *Journal of the American Medical Informatics Association* have the prefix *10.1197* and the suffix *jamia.M####*, where #### is a number assigned by the journal editors. Likewise, all publications in the Digital Library of the Association for Computing Machinery (www.acm.org/dl) have the prefix *10.1145* and a unique identifier for the suffix (e.g., *345508.345539* for the paper Hersh et al., 2000). Publishers are encouraged to facilitate resolution by encoding the DOI into their URLs in a standard way, e.g., http://doi.acm.org/10.1145/345508.345539.

19.4.3   Interoperability

As noted throughout this chapter, metadata is a key component for accessing content in IR systems. It takes on an additional value in the digital library, where there is desire to allow access to diverse but not necessarily exhaustive resources. One key concern of digital libraries is **interoperability** (Besser, 2002). That is, how can resources with heterogeneous metadata be accessed? Arms et al. (2002) note that three levels of agreement must be achieved:

1. Technical agreements over formats, protocols, and security procedures.
2. Content agreement over the data and the semantic interpretation of its metadata.
3. Organizational agreements over ground rules for access, preservation, payment, authentication, and so forth.

One approach to interoperability gaining favor is the **Open Archives Initiative** (**OAI**, www.openarchive.org) (Lagoze and VandeSompel, 2001). This project had its origins in the E-Prints initiative, which aimed to provide persistent access to electronic archives of scientific publications (VandeSompel and Lagoze, 1999). While the OAI effort is rooted in access to scholarly communications, its methods are applicable to a much broader range of content. Its fundamental activity is to promote the "exposure" of archives' metadata such that digital library systems can learn what content is available and how it can be obtained. Each record in the OAI system has an XML-encoded record. The **OAI Protocol for Metadata Harvesting** (**PMH**) then allows selective harvesting of the metadata by systems. Such harvesting can be date-based, such as items added or changed after a certain date, or set-based, such as those belonging to a certain topic, journal, or institution.

19.4.4   Intellectual Property

As with other digital library–related concerns, **intellectual property** issues have already been described at various places in this book (see Chapter 11). Intellectual property is difficult to protect in the digital environment because although the cost of production is not insubstantial, the cost of replication is near nothing. Furthermore, in circumstances such as academic publishing, the desire for protection is situational. For example, individual researchers may want the widest dissemination of their research papers, but each one may want to protect revenues realized from synthesis works or educational products that are developed. The global reach of the Internet has required that intellectual property issues be considered on a global scale. The **World Intellectual Property Organization (WIPO**, www.wipo.org) is an agency of the United Nations attempting to develop worldwide policies, although understandably, there is considerable diversity about what such policies should be.

19.4.5 Preservation

There are a number of issues related to the preservation of digital library materials. Lesk (1997) has compared the longevity of digital materials. He has noted that the longevity for magnetic materials is the least, with the expected lifetime of magnetic tape being 5 to 10 years. Optical storage has somewhat better longevity, with an expected lifetime of 30 to 100 years depending on the specific type. Ironically, paper has a life expectancy well beyond all these digital media. Rothenberg (1999) has referred to the *Rosetta Stone*, which provided help in interpreting ancient Egyptian hieroglyphics and has survived over 20 centuries. He goes on to reemphasize Lesk's description of the reduced lifetime of digital media in comparison with traditional media, and to note another problem familiar to most long-time users of computers, namely, data can become obsolete not only owing to the medium, but also as a result of data format. Both authors note that storage devices as well as computer applications, such as word processors, have seen their formats change significantly over the last couple of decades.

One initiative aiming to preserve content is the **Lots of Copies Keep Stuff Safe (LOCKSS)** project (Reich and Rosenthal, 2001). As the name implies, numerous digital copies of important documents can be maintained. But the project further concerns itself with the ability to detect and repair damaged copies as well as to prevent subversion of the data. This is done via **hashing** schemes that assess the integrity of the data in the multiples caches of content and "fix" altered copies.

Of course, some content such as that on the Web is highly dynamic and undergoes constant change. Kahle (1997) has estimated that the lifetime of an average Web page is 44 days. Koehler has found that the "half-life" of the survival of Web pages may actually be a little longer, at roughly 2 years. He has noted that content pages are more likely to change than navigational pages in the .com top-level domain, whereas the opposite is true in the .edu top-level domain. This likely indicates that commercial pages change because products and information about them come and go whereas persistence is more likely to be desired for pages posted on academic sites. These observations have led Kahle to undertake a project to archive the Internet (www.archive.org) on a periodic basis. A popular feature of this Web site is the Internet Wayback Machine, which allows entry of a URL and its display at different points in time.

Nonetheless, there is an imperative to preserve documents of many types, whatever their medium (Tibbo, 2001). For society in general, there is certainly impetus to preserve historical documents in an unaltered form. And in all of science, certainly health and medicine, there is a need to preserve the archive of scientific discoveries, particularly those presenting original experiments and their data. McCray and Gallagher (2001) have written an overview that describes the various principles of digital library development, with an emphasis on persistent and accessible content. As noted in Chapter 2, a number of initiatives have been undertaken to insure preservation of scientific information. These include the **National Digital Information Infrastructure Preservation Program (NDIIPP)** of the U.S. Library of Congress (Friedlander, 2002) and the **Digital Preservation Coalition** in the United Kingdom (Beagrie, 2002).

19.5   Future Directions for IR Systems and Digital Libraries

There is no doubt that considerable progress has been made in IR and digital libraries. Seeking online information is now done routinely not only by clinicians and researchers, but also by patients and consumers. There are still considerable challenges to make this activity more fruitful to users. They include:

- How do we lower the effort it takes for clinicians to get to the information they need rapidly in the busy clinical setting?
- How can researchers extract new knowledge from the vast quantity that is available to them?
- How can consumers and patients find high-quality information that is appropriate to their understanding of health and disease?
- Can the value added by the publishing process be protected and remunerated while making information more available?
- How can the indexing process become more accurate and efficient?
- Can retrieval interfaces be made simpler without giving up flexibility and power?
- Can we develop standards for digital libraries that will facilitate interoperability but maintain ease of use, protection of intellectual property, and long-term preservation of the archive of science?

Suggested Readings

Baeza-Yates R., Ribeiro-Neto B. (Eds.) (1999). *Modern Information Retrieval*. New York: McGraw-Hill.
A book surveying most of the automated approaches to information retrieval.

Detmer W.M., Shortliffe E.H. (1997). Using the Internet to improve knowledge diffusion in medicine, *Communications of the ACM*, 40:101–108.
An early paper describing the use of the Internet for accessing aggregated resources from "legacy" databases to innovative hypertext collections.

Frakes W.B., Baeza-Yates R. (1992). *Information Retrieval: Data Structures & Algorithms*, Englewood Cliffs, NJ: Prentice-Hall.
A textbook on implementation of information retrieval systems. Covers all of the major data structures and algorithms, including inverted files, ranking algorithms, stop word lists, and stemming. There are plentiful examples of code in the C programming language.

Hersh W.R. (2003). *Information Retrieval, a Health and Biomedical Perspective* (2nd ed.). New York: Springer-Verlag.
A textbook on information retrieval systems in the health and biomedical domain that covers state-of-the-art as well as research systems.

Humphreys B., Lindberg D., et al. (1998). The Unified Medical Language System: An informatics research collaboration. *Journal of the American Medical Informatics Association*, 5:1–11.
A paper describing the motivation and implementation of the National Library of Medicine's Unified Medical Language System.

Miles W.D. (1982). *A History of the National Library of Medicine*, Bethesda, MD: U.S. Department of Health & Human Services.
A comprehensive history of the National Library of Medicine and its forerunners, covering the story of Dr. John Shaw Billings and his founding of *Index Medicus* to the modern implementation of MEDLINE.

Sackett D.L., Richardson W.S., Rosenberg W., Haynes R.B. (2000). *Evidence-Based Medicine: How to Practice and Teach EBM* (2nd ed.). New York: Churchill Livingstone.
An overview of the techniques for practice of evidence-based medicine.

Salton, G. (1991). Developments in automatic text retrieval. *Science*, 253: 974–980.
The most recent succinct exposition of word statistical retrieval systems from the person who originated the approach.

Questions for Discussion

1. With the advent of full-text searching, should the National Library of Medicine abandon human indexing of citations in MEDLINE? Why or why not?
2. Explain why you think PMC is or is not a good idea.
3. How would you aggregate the clinical evidence-based resources described in the chapter into the best digital library for clinicians?
4. Devise a curriculum for teaching clinicians and patients the most important points about searching for health-related information.
5. Find a consumer-oriented Web page and determine the quality of the information on it.
6. What are the limitations of recall and precision as evaluation measures and what alternatives would improve upon them?
7. Select a concept that appears in two or more clinical terminologies and demonstrate how it would be combined into a record in the UMLS Metathesaurus.
8. Describe how you might devise a system that achieves a happy medium between of intellectual property and barrier-free access to the archive of science.

20
Clinical Decision-Support Systems

MARK A. MUSEN, YUVAL SHAHAR, AND EDWARD H. SHORTLIFFE

After reading this chapter, you should know the answers to these questions:

- What are three requirements for an excellent decision-making system?
- What are three decision-support roles for computers in clinical medicine?
- How has the use of computers for clinical decision support evolved since the1960s?
- What is a knowledge-based system?
- What influences account for the gradual improvement in professional attitudes toward use of computers for clinical decision support?
- What are the five dimensions that characterize clinical decision-support tools?
- What are clinical-practice guidelines, and what are the challenges in providing guideline-based decision support?
- What are the principal scientific challenges in building useful and acceptable clinical decision-support tools?
- What legal and regulatory barriers could affect distribution of clinical decision-support technologies?

20.1   The Nature of Clinical Decision-Making

If you ask people what the phrase "computers in medicine" means, they often describe a computer program that helps physicians to make diagnoses. Although computers play numerous important clinical roles, from the earliest days of computing people have recognized that computers might support health-care workrs by helping these people to sift through the vast collection of possible diseases and symptoms. This idea has been echoed in futuristic works of science fiction. In *Star Trek*, for example, medical workers routinely point devices at injured crew members to determine instantly what is the problem and how serious is the damage. The prevalence of such expectations, coupled with a general societal concern about the influence of computers on interpersonal relationships and on job security, has naturally raised questions among health workers. Just what can computers do today to support clinical decision-making? How soon will diagnostic tools be generally available? How good will they be? What will their effects be on the practice of medicine, on medical education, and on relationships among colleagues or between physicians and patients?

We can view the contents of this entire book as addressing clinical data and decision-making. In Chapter 2, we discussed the central role of accurate, complete, and relevant data in supporting the decisions that confront clinicians and other healthcare workers. In

Chapter 3, we described the nature of good decisions and the need for clinicians to understand the proper use of information if they are to be effective and efficient decision-makers. In Chapter 4 we introduced the cognitive issues that underly clinical decision making and that influence the design of systems for decision support. Subsequent chapters have mentioned many real or potential uses of computers to assist with such decision-making. Medical practice *is* medical decision-making, so most applications of computers in health care are intended to have a direct or tangential effect on the quality of healthcare decisions. In this chapter, we bring together these themes by concentrating on systems that have been developed specifically to assist health workers in making decisions.

20.1.1   Types of Decisions

By now, you are familiar with the range of clinical decisions. The classic problem of **diagnosis** (analyzing available data to determine the pathophysiologic explanation for a patient's symptoms) is only one of these. Equally challenging, as emphasized in Chapters 3 and 4, is the **diagnostic process**—deciding which questions to ask, tests to order, or procedures to perform and determining the value of the results relative to associated risks or financial costs. Thus, diagnosis involves not only deciding what is true about a patient but also what data are needed to determine what is true. Even when the diagnosis is known, there often are challenging **management** decisions that test the physician's knowledge and experience: Should I treat the patient or allow the process to resolve on its own? If treatment is indicated, what should it be? How should I use the patient's response to therapy to guide me in determining whether an alternate approach should be tried or, in some cases, to question whether my initial diagnosis was incorrect after all?

Biomedicine is also replete with decision tasks that do not involve specific patients or their diseases. Consider, for example, the biomedical scientist who is using laboratory data to help with the design of her next experiment or the hospital administrator who uses management data to guide decisions about resource allocation in his hospital. Although we focus on systems to assist with clinical decisions in this chapter, we emphasize that the concepts discussed generalize to many other problem areas as well. In Chapter 23, for example, we examine the need for formal decision techniques and tools in creating health policies. The requirements for excellent decision-making fall into three principal categories: (1) accurate data, (2) pertinent knowledge, and (3) appropriate problem-solving skills.

The data about a case must be adequate for making an informed decision, but they must not be excessive. Indeed, a major challenge occurs when decision-makers are bombarded with so much information that they cannot process and synthesize the information intelligently and rapidly (see, for example, Chapter 17). Thus, it is important to know when additional data will confuse rather than clarify and when it is imperative to use tools (computational or otherwise) that permit data to be summarized for easier cognitive management (see Chapter 4). The operating room and intensive-care units are classic settings for this problem; patients are monitored extensively, numerous data are collected, and decisions often have to be made on an emergent basis. Equally important is the quality of the available data. In Chapter 2, we discussed imprecision in terminology, illegibility and inaccessibility of records, and other opportunities for misinterpretation of data. Similarly, measurement instruments or recorded data may simply be erroneous; use of faulty data can have serious adverse effects on patient-care decisions. Thus, clinical data often need to be validated. Even good data are useless if we do not have the basic knowledge necessary to apply them properly. Decision-makers must have broad knowledge of medicine, in-depth familiarity with their area of expertise, and access to information resources that provide pertinent additional information. Their knowledge must be accurate, with areas of controversy well understood and questions of personal choice well distinguished from topics where a dogmatic approach is appropriate. Their knowledge must also be current; in the rapidly changing world of medicine, facts decay just as certainly as dead tissue does.

Good data and an extensive factual knowledge base still do not guarantee a good decision; good problem-solving skills are equally important. Decision-makers must know how to set appropriate goals for a task, how to reason about each goal, and how to make explicit the trade-offs between costs and benefits of diagnostic procedures or therapeutic maneuvers. The skilled clinician draws extensively on personal experience, and new physicians soon realize that good clinical judgment is based as much on an ability to reason effectively and appropriately about what to do as it is on formal knowledge of the field or access to high-quality patient data. Thus, clinicians must develop a strategic approach to test selection and interpretation, understand ideas of sensitivity and specificity, and be able to assess the urgency of a situation. Awareness of biases (see Chapter 3) and of the ways that they can creep into problem-solving also are crucial. This brief review of issues central to clinical decision-making serves as a fitting introduction to the topic of computer-assisted decision-making: Precisely the same topics are pertinent when we develop a computational tool for clinical problem-solving. The programs must have access to good data, they must have extensive background knowledge encoded for the clinical domain in question, and they must embody an intelligent approach to problem-solving that is sensitive to requirements for proper analysis, appropriate cost–benefit trade-offs, and efficiency.

20.1.2   The Role of Computers in Decision Support

A **clinical decision-support system** is any computer program designed to help healthcare professionals to make clinical decisions. In a sense, any computer system that deals with clinical data or knowledge is intended to provide decision support. It is accordingly useful to consider three types of decision-support functions, ranging from generalized to patient specific.

Tools for Information Management

Health-care information systems (Chapter 13) and information-retrieval systems (Chapter 19) are tools that manage information. Specialized knowledge-management workstations are under development in research settings; these workstations provide sophisticated environments for storing and retrieving clinical knowledge, browsing through that knowledge much as we might page through a textbook, and augmenting it with personal notes and information that we may need later for clinical problem-solving. Information-management tools provide the data and knowledge needed by the clinician, but they generally do not help her to apply that information to a particular decision task. Interpretation is left to the clinician, as is the decision about what information is needed to resolve the clinical problem.

Tools for Focusing Attention

Clinical-laboratory systems that flag abnormal values or that provide lists of possible explanations for those abnormalities and pharmacy systems that alert providers to possible drug interactions (Evans et al., 1986; Tatro et al., 1975) are tools that focus the user's attention. Such programs are designed to remind the user of diagnoses or problems that might otherwise have been overlooked. Typically, they use simple logics, displaying fixed lists or paragraphs as a standard response to a definite or potential abnormality.

Tools for Providing Patient-Specific Recommendations

Such programs provide custom-tailored assessments or advice based on sets of patient-specific data. They may follow simple logics (such as algorithms), may be based on decision theory and cost–benefit analysis, or may use numerical approaches only as an adjunct to symbolic problem solving. Some diagnostic assistants (such as DXplain [Barnett et al., 1987] or QMR [Miller et al., 1986]) suggest differential diagnoses or indicate additional information that would help to narrow the range of etiologic possibilities. Other systems (such as the original Internist-1 program [Miller et al., 1982], from which QMR was derived) suggest a single best explanation for a patient's symptomatology. Other systems interpret and summarize the patient's record over time in a manner sensitive to the clinical context (Shahar & Musen, 1996). Still other systems provide therapy advice rather than diagnostic assistance (Musen et al., 1996).

The boundaries among these three categories are not crisp, but the distinctions are useful in defining the range of capabilities that computers can provide to assist clinicians with making decisions. Systems of the first two types are discussed elsewhere in this book. For example, Chapters 12 through 18 describe systems that contain and manipulate patient data that are of importance in reaching good clinical decisions. Chapters 19 and 21 discuss methods for accessing information, knowledge, and the accumulated experience of other professionals. In this chapter, we focus on the third category: patient-specific systems.

20.2   Historical Perspective

Since the earliest days of computers, health professionals have anticipated the time when machines would assist them in the diagnostic process. The first articles dealing with this possibility appeared in the late 1950s (Ledley & Lusted, 1959), and experimental prototypes appeared within a few years (Warner et al., 1964). Many problems prevented the widespread introduction of such systems, however, ranging from the limitations of the scientific underpinnings to the logistical difficulties that developers encountered when encouraging clinicians to use and accept systems that were not well integrated into the practitioners' usual workflow.

Three advisory systems from the 1970s provide a useful overview of the origin of work on clinical decision-support systems: deDombal's system for diagnosis of abdominal pain (de Dombal et al., 1972), Shortliffe's MYCIN system for selection of antibiotic therapy (Shortliffe, 1976), and the HELP system for delivery of inpatient medical alerts (Kuperman et al., 1991; Warner, 1979).

20.2.1   Leeds Abdominal Pain System

Starting in the late 1960s, F. T. deDombal and his associates at the University of Leeds studied the diagnostic process and developed computer-based decision aids using Bayesian probability theory (see Chapter 3). Using surgical or pathologic diagnoses as the gold standard, they emphasized the importance of deriving the conditional probabilities used in Bayesian reasoning from high-quality data that they gathered by collecting information on thousands of patients (Adams et al., 1986). Their system, the Leeds abdominal pain system, used sensitivity, specificity, and disease-prevalence data for various signs, symptoms, and test results to calculate, using Bayes' theorem, the probability of seven possible explanations for acute abdominal pain (appendicitis, diverticulitis, perforated ulcer, cholecystitis, small-bowel obstruction, pancreatitis, and nonspecific abdominal pain). To keep the Bayesian computations manageable, the program made the assumptions of (1) conditional independence of the findings for the various diagnoses and (2) mutual exclusivity of the seven diagnoses (see Chapter 3).

In one system evaluation (de Dombal et al., 1972), physicians filled out data sheets summarizing clinical and laboratory findings for 304 patients who came to the emergency room with abdominal pain of sudden onset. The data from these sheets became the attributes that were analyzed using Bayes' rule. Thus, the Bayesian formulation assumed that each patient had one of the seven conditions and selected the most likely one on the basis of the recorded observations. Had the program been used directly by emergency-room physicians, results could have been available, on average, within 5 minutes after the data form was completed. During the study, however, the cases were run in batch mode; the computer-generated diagnoses were saved for later comparison to (1) the diagnoses reached by the attending clinicians and (2) the ultimate diagnosis verified during surgery or through appropriate tests.

In contrast to the clinicians' diagnoses, which were correct in only 65 to 80 percent of the 304 cases (with accuracy depending on the individual clinician's training and experience), the program's diagnoses were correct in 91.8 percent of cases. Furthermore, in six of the seven disease categories, the computer was more likely to assign the patients to the correct disease category than was the senior clinician in charge of the case. Of particular interest was the program's accuracy regarding appendicitis—a diagnosis that is often made incorrectly (or, less often, is missed or at least delayed). In no cases of appendicitis did the computer fail to make the correct diagnosis, and in only six cases were patients with nonspecific abdominal pain incorrectly classified as having appendicitis. Based on the actual clinical decisions, however, more than 20 patients with nonspecific abdominal pain underwent unnecessary surgery for an incorrect diagnosis of appendicitis, and six patients who did have appendicitis were observed for more than 8 hours before they were finally taken to the operating room.

With the introduction of personal computers, deDombal's system began to achieve widespread use—from emergency departments in other countries to the British submarine fleet. Surprisingly, the system has never obtained the same degree of diagnostic accuracy in other settings that it did in Leeds—even when adjustments were made for differences in prior probabilities of disease. There are several reasons possible for this discrepancy. The most likely explanation is that there may be considerable variation in the way that clinicians interpret the data that must be entered into the computer. For example, physicians with different training or from different cultures may not agree on the criteria for identification of certain patient findings on physical examination, such as "rebound tenderness." Another possible explanation is that there are different probabilistic relationships between findings and diagnoses in different patient populations.

20.2.2 MYCIN

A different approach to computer-assisted decision support was embodied in the **MYCIN** program, a consultation system that de-emphasized diagnosis to concentrate on appropriate management of patients who have infections (Shortliffe, 1976). MYCIN's developers believed that straightforward algorithms or statistical approaches were inadequate for this clinical problem in which the nature of expertise was poorly understood and even the experts often disagreed about how best to manage specific patients, especially before definitive culture results became available. As a result, the researchers were drawn to the field of **artificial intelligence** (AI), a subfield of computer science that has focused on manipulation of abstract symbols rather than on numerical calculations.

Knowledge of infectious diseases in MYCIN was represented as production rules, each containing a "packet" of knowledge derived from discussions with collaborating experts (Figure 20.1). A **production rule** is simply a conditional statement that relates observations to associated inferences that can be drawn. MYCIN's power was derived from such rules in a variety of ways:

- The MYCIN program determined which rules to use and how to chain them together to make decisions about a specific case.
- The rules often formed a coherent explanation of MYCIN's reasoning—those that applied to the current decision were displayed in response to users' questions (Figure 20.2). Although rules were stored in a machine-readable format, English translations could be displayed.
- By removing, altering, or adding rules, system developers could modify the program's knowledge structures rapidly, without explicitly reprogramming or restructuring other parts of the knowledge base. (Making such changes, however, could lead to unintended side effects.)

Rule507

IF:	1)	The infection that requires therapy is meningitis,
	2)	Organisms were not seen on the stain of the culture,
	3)	The type of infection is bacterial,
	4)	The patient does not have a head injury defect, and
	5)	The age of the patient is between 15 years and 55 years
THEN:		The organisms that might be causing the infection are diplococcus-pneumoniae and neisseria-meningitidis

---

Figure 20.1. A typical rule from the MYCIN system. Rules are conditional statements that indicate what conclusions can be reached or actions taken if a specified set of conditions is found to be true. In this rule, MYCIN is able to conclude probable bacterial causes of infection if the five conditions in the premise are all found to be true for a specific patient. Not shown are the measures of uncertainty that are also associated with inference in the MYCIN system.

In this series, how many of the cutures were positive of the e.coli   *(typical system prompt)*
(ORGANISM-1)?

** WHY   *(request from user to determine motivation for question)*

[i.e. WHY is it important to determine the number of cultures which were   *(system's rephrasing of the WHY*
positive for the organism?]   *question, and answer)*

[1.0] This will help to determine whether there is significant disease
associated with this occurrence of the organism.
    It has already been established that
        [1.1] the culture was taken from a sterile source
        [1.2] the number of cultures in the series is greater than 2
    Therefore, if
        [1.3] the number of cultures which were positive for ORGANISM-1
            is greater than 2
    Then there is suggestive evidence (.5) that there is significant disease
            associated with this occurrence of the e.coli (ORGANISM-1).
        [RULE049]
    ** WHY   *(repeated WHY to determine relevance of previous explanation)*

[i.e. WHY is it important to determine if there is significant disease
associated with this occurrence of the organism?]

[2.0] This will help to determine a diagnosis for which the infection should
be treated.
    It has already been established that
        [2.1] the infection is not one of: primary bacteremia, meningitis
        [2.2] for some current culture of the patient it is true that the site
            of the culture is blood
    Therefore, if
        [2.3] there is significant disease associated with this occurrence of
            the organism
    Then
        It is definite (1.0) that the diagnosis for which the infection should
        be treated is secondary-bacterimia
        [RULE103]

Figure 20.2. Two examples of MYCIN's explanation capabilities. User input is shown in boldface capital letters and follows the double asterisks. The system expands each ["WHY"] question (enclosed in square brackets) to ensure that the user is aware of its interpretation of the query.

The developers evaluated MYCIN's performance on therapy selection for patients with blood-borne bacterial infections (Yu 1979b), and for those with meningitis (Yu et al., 1979a]. In the latter study, MYCIN gave advice that compared favorably with that offered by experts in infectious diseases. MYCIN, however, is best viewed as an early exploration of methods for capturing and applying ill-structured expert knowledge to solve important medical problems. Although the program was never used clinically, it paved the way for a great deal of research and development in the 1980s. In fact, the development of knowledge-based systems, and the commercialization of the rule-based approach in a variety of nonmedical fields during the early 1980s, evolved from MYCIN and from related systems developed during the 1970s (Hayes-Roth et al., 1983).

20.2.3   HELP

In the earlier discussion of computer-based patient record systems (Chapter 12), we referred to the HELP system, an integrated hospital information system developed at LDS Hospital in Salt Lake City. HELP has the ability to generate alerts when abnormalities in the patient record are noted, and its impact on the development of the field has been immense, with applications and methodologies that span nearly the full range of activities in biomedical informatics (Kuperman et al., 1991).

HELP adds to a conventional medical-record system a monitoring program and a mechanism for storing decision logic in "HELP sectors" or logic modules. Thus, patient data are available to users who wish to request specific information, and the usual reports and schedules are automatically printed or otherwise communicated by the system. In addition, there is a mechanism for *event-driven* generation of specialized warnings, alerts, and reports. HELP's developers originally created a specialized language named PAL for writing medical knowledge in HELP sectors. Beginning in the 1990s, workers at LDS Hospital, Columbia Presbyterian Medical Center, and elsewhere created and adopted a standard formalism for encoding decision rules known as the **Arden syntax**—a programming language that provides a canonical means for writing rules that relate specific patient situations to appropriate actions for practitioners to follow (Hripcsak et al., 1994). The Arden syntax incorporates many of the features of PAL, as well as those of other frameworks for writing clinical decision rules that other research groups developed during the 1970s and 1980s. In the Arden syntax, each decision rule, or **HELP sector**, is called a **medical logic module** (MLM). Figure 20.3 shows one such MLM and its representation in the Arden syntax.

Whenever new data about a patient become available, regardless of the source, the HELP system checks to see whether the data match the criteria for invoking an MLM. If they do, the system evaluates the MLM to see whether that MLM is relevant for the specific patient. The logic in these MLMs has been developed by clinical experts working with medical information scientists. The output generated by successful MLMs includes, for example, alerts regarding untoward drug actions, interpretations of laboratory tests, or calculations of the likelihood of diseases. This output result is communicated to the appropriate people through the hospital information system's workstations or on written reports, depending on the urgency of the output message and the location and functions of the person for whom the report is intended.

```
penicillin_order :=

    event {medication_order

                where class = penicillin};

/* find allergies */

penicillin_allergy :=

    read last {allergy

            where agent_class = penicillin};

;;

evoke: penicillin_order ;;

logic:

If exist (penicillin_allergy) then conclude true;

endif;

;;

action:

write

"Caution, the patient has the following allergy to penicillin documented:"

|| penicillin_allergy ;;
```

Figure 20.3. This medical logic module (MLM), written in the Arden syntax, prints a warning for healthcare workers whenever a patient who reportedly is allergic to penicillin receives a prescription for a drug in the penicillin class. The **evoke** slot defines a situation that causes the rule to be triggered; the **logic** slot encodes the decision logic of the rule; the **action** slot defines the procedure to follow if the logic slot reaches a positive conclusion.

From the 1970s to the beginning of the current decade, HELP served as a superb example of how the integration of decision support with other system functions can heighten a program's acceptance and encourage its use. Several studies (e.g., Evans et al., 1986) demonstrated the beneficial effect of HELP's decision logic on clinical measurements at LDS Hospital. Alerts and warnings were produced through the normal collection of patient data; transcription of data for reuse in secondary settings were avoided through the full integration of the computing environment. As discussed in Chapter 13, hospital systems have evolved toward more distributed architectures, with desktop or handheld computers serving as workstations and data being shared over local-area networks, sometimes with wireless connectivity. This large project at LDS Hospital has served as an important model of how decision support through integrated data monitoring can bypass many of the traditional barriers to the use of computers for clinical decision support. Ideas from HELP are being incorporated into decision-support components from several commercial vendors of clinical information systems and EHRs.

20.2.4   Lessons from Early Decision-Support Systems

The Leeds abdominal pain system was an important exemplar of the clinical value of Bayesian diagnostic systems. Subsequent Bayesian systems, such as the **Pathfinder** system for diagnosis of lymph-node pathology (Heckerman et al., 1989), built solidly on the foundation laid by deDombal and his co-workers. Similarly, rule-based approaches to clinical decision-making, as pioneered in systems such as MYCIN and HELP, have led to more recent frameworks for representing medical knowledge, such as the Arden syntax. The early decision-support systems demonstrated the feasibility of encoding medical knowledge so that it could be processed by computers. They also have helped researchers in biomedical informatics to clarify both the strengths and limitations of alternative knowledge-representation approaches.

Although the HELP system was a notable exception, most early decision-support tools were rarely used by health personnel and were viewed with skepticism. The subsequent evolution in attitudes has been due in large part to four influences: (1) the emergence of personal workstations, the World Wide Web, and easy-to-use interfaces; (2) the increasing recognition on the part of technology developers that computer systems must meld transparently with the work practices of groups that are asked to adopt new technologies; (3) the growing distress among health professionals and managed-care organizations regarding the amount of information that practitioners need to practice medicine well and to avoid errors; and (4) the increasing fiscal pressure to practice cost-effective, evidence-based medicine, which leads practitioners to consider carefully the clinical utility and reliability of tests, procedures, and therapies—especially when the latter are expensive or risky.

Gradual changes in attitudes and increasing acceptance of the ideas of computer-based decision tools for healthcare professionals are of course not in themselves adequate to ensure developmental progress and the adoption of new information-management facilities. Current enthusiasm will sour rapidly if the products of research are not responsive to real-world needs and are not sensitive to the logistical requirements of the practice settings in which clinicians work.

20.3   A Structure for Characterizing Clinical Decision-Support Systems

If we are to assess adequately any new clinical decision-support tool or to understand the range of issues that can affect the chances for successful implementation, we must have an organizing framework for considering such programs. One approach is to characterize decision-support systems along five dimensions: (1) the system's intended function, (2) the mode by which advice is offered, (3) the consultation style, (4) the underlying decision-making process, and (5) the factors related to human–computer interaction. As this spectrum of considerations suggests, excellent decision-making capabilities alone do not guarantee system utility or acceptance.

20.3.1   System Function

Decision-support programs generally fall into two categories: those that assist health-care workers with determining *what is true* about a patient (usually what the correct diagnosis is—as in the Leeds abdominal-pain system) and those that assist with decisions about *what to do* for the patient (usually what test to order, whether to treat, or what therapy plan to institute—as in MYCIN). Many systems assist clinicians with both activities (e.g., diagnostic programs often help physicians to decide what additional information would be most useful in narrowing the differential diagnosis for a given case), but the distinction is important because advice about what to do for a patient cannot be formulated without balancing the costs and benefits of action. Determination of what is true about a patient, based on a fixed set of data that are already available, can theoretically be made without consideration of cost and risk. Thus, a "pure" diagnostic program leaves to the user the task of deciding what data to gather or requires a fixed set of data for all patients. As all practitioners know, however, it is unrealistic to view making a diagnosis as separable from the process of choosing from the available options for data collection and therapy. Moreover, many physicians believe that the majority of questions about which they seek consultation deal with what they should *do* rather than with what is true about a patient given a fixed data set.

20.3.2   The Mode for Giving Advice

Like the abdominal pain program and MYCIN, most decision-support programs have assumed a passive role in giving advice to clinicians (Reggia & Turhim, 1985). Under this model, the practitioner must recognize when advice would be useful and then must make an explicit effort to access the computer program; the decision-support system waits for the user to come to it. The clinician then describes a case by entering data and requests a diagnostic or therapeutic assessment.

There are also technologies, such as the HELP system, that play a more active role, providing decision support as a byproduct of monitoring or of data-management activities; such systems do not wait for physicians or other health workers specifically to ask for assistance. A great appeal of such systems is their ability to give assistance to health-care workers without requiring laborious data entry by the clinicians themselves. Such capabilities are possible only because the system's decision logic is integrated with a comprehensive database of patient information that is already being gathered from diverse sources within the healthcare enterprise. Because practitioners generally do not request assistance from such systems, but instead receive it whenever monitored patient data warrant it, one challenge is to avoid generating excessive numbers of warnings for minor problems already likely to be understood. Otherwise, such "false-positive" advisory reports can generate antagonistic responses from users and can blunt the usefulness of those warnings that have greater clinical significance.

20.3.3 Style of Communication

Decision-support systems have tended to operate under one of two styles of interaction: the *consulting model* or the *critiquing model*. In the **consulting model**, the program serves as an advisor, accepting patient-specific data, possibly asking questions, and generating advice for the user about diagnosis or management. For example, MYCIN was an early example of a program that adopted the consulting approach. In the **critiquing model**, on the other hand, the clinician has a preconceived idea of what is happening with a patient or what management plan would be appropriate. The computer then acts as a sounding board for the user's own ideas, expressing agreement or suggesting reasoned alternatives. A pioneering example of a critiquing system was **ATTENDING**, a standalone program that critiqued a patient-specific plan for anesthetic selection, induction, and administration after that plan had been proposed by the anesthesiologist who would be managing the case (Miller, 1986). Such critiquing systems meet many physicians' desires to formulate plans on their own but to have those plans double-checked occasionally before acting on them. In the critiquing style, the program focuses more directly on the plan in which the physician is interested.

The critiquing model also can be applied in an active monitoring setting. For example, the HELP system monitored physicians' drug-therapy decisions and suggested alternate approaches that might be preferable (Evans et al., 1986). Similarly, the HyperCritic system (van der Lei & Musen, 1991) offered suggestions regarding how primary-care physicians might improve their management of patients with hypertension by performing a behind-the-scenes analysis of the patients' computer-based record at the time of each clinic visit.

20.3.4 Underlying Decision-Making Process

A wide variety of techniques has been used in the design and implementation of decision-support systems. The simplest logics have involved problem-specific flowcharts designed by clinicians and then encoded for use by a computer. Although such algorithms have been useful for triage purposes and as a didactic technique used in journals and books where an overview for a problem's management has been appropriate, they have been largely rejected by physicians as too simplistic for routine use (Grimm et al., 1975). In addition, the advantage of their implementation on computers has not been clear; the use of simple printed copies of the algorithms generally has proved adequate (Komaroff et al., 1974). A noteworthy exception is a large computer program first described in the early 1970s at the Beth Israel Hospital in Boston (Bleich, 1972); it used a detailed algorithmic logic to provide advice regarding the diagnosis and management of acid–base and electrolyte disorders. Although additional techniques—such as mathematical modeling, pattern recognition, and statistical analysis of large databases—have been used in experimental decision-support systems (Shortliffe et al., 1979), the predominant methods have been drawn from Bayesian modeling, decision analysis, artificial neural networks, and AI.

Because computers were traditionally viewed as numerical calculating machines, people had recognized by the 1960s that they could be used to compute the pertinent probabilities based on observations of patient-specific parameters (as long as each had a known statistical relationship to the possible disease etiologies). Large numbers of **Bayesian diagnosis programs** have been developed in the intervening years, many of which have been shown to be accurate in selecting among competing explanations of a patient's disease state (Heckerman & Nathwani, 1992). As we mentioned earlier, among the largest experiments have been those of deDombal and associates (1972) in England, who adopted a simple Bayesian model that assumed that there are no conditional dependencies among findings (e.g., the fallacioius assumption that the presence of a finding such as *fever* never affects the likelihood of the presence of a finding such as *chills*). More recent work on the use of **belief networks** for automated decision-making has demonstrated that it is practical to develop more expressive Bayesian systems in which conditional dependencies can be modeled explicitly rather than ignored. (Belief networks are described in Chapter 3.)

Because making most decisions in medicine requires weighing the costs and benefits of actions that could be taken in diagnosing or managing a patient's illness, researchers also have developed tools that draw on the methods of decision analysis (Sox et al., 1988; Weinstein & Fineberg, 1980). **Decision analysis** adds to Bayesian reasoning the idea of explicit *decisions* and of **utilities** associated with the various outcomes that could occur in response to those decisions (see Chapter 3). One class of programs is designed for use by the analysts themselves; such programs assume a detailed knowledge of decision analysis and would be of little use to the average clinician (Pauker & Kassirer, 1981). A second class of programs uses decision-analysis concepts within systems designed to advise physicians who are not trained in these techniques. In such programs, the underlying decision models generally have been prespecified—either as decision trees that enumerate all possible decisions and all possible ramifications of those decisions or as belief networks in which explicit decision and utility nodes are added, called **influence diagrams**.

There has been considerable interest in the use of artificial neural networks as the basis for automated medical diagnosis. **Artificial neural networks** (ANNs) are computer programs that perform classification, taking as input a set of findings that describe a given case and generating as output a set of numbers, where each output corresponds to the likelihood of a particular classification that could explain the findings. The program performs this function by propagating carefully calculated **weights** through a network of several layers of nodes. The structure of the network is uniform for any class of decision problem; the weights associated with each of the nodes, however, are tuned so that the network tends to generate the correct classification for any set of inputs. The values for the weights are determined in incremental fashion when a network is trained on a large collection of previously classified examples during a period of **supervised learning**. Like statistical pattern-recognition methods, artificial neural networks translate a set of findings into a set of weighted classifications consistent with those findings. Unfortunately, there is no way that an observer can directly understand why an artificial neural network might reach a particular conclusion. Artificial neural networks may have significant advantages, however, when the correct diagnosis may depend on interactions among the findings that are difficult to predict.

Since the early 1970s, a growing body of researchers have been applying AI techniques to the development of diagnostic and therapy-management systems (Clancey, 1984; Miller, 1988; Szolovits, 1982). We have already discussed the MYCIN system, an important early example of work in this area. Artificial intelligence traditionally has been closely tied to psychology and to the modeling of logical processes by computer (see Chapter 4). Psychological studies of how medical experts perform problem-solving (Elstein et al., 1978; Kupiers & Kassirer, 1984) therefore have been influential in much research in medical AI. Of particular pertinence to the development of decision-support systems is the subfield of AI research that is concerned with knowledge-based systems. A **knowledge-based system** is a program that symbolically encodes concepts derived from experts in a field—in a **knowledge base**—and that uses that knowledge base to provide the kind of problem analysis and advice that the expert might provide.

Clinical decision-making often requires reasoning under uncertainty. Knowledge-based systems in medicine have consequently incorporated either Bayesian or ad hoc schemes for dealing with partial evidence and with uncertainty regarding the effects of proposed interventions. What is most characteristic of a knowledge-based system, however, is that the knowledge base encodes a non-numeric, **qualitative model** of how inferences are related to reach abstract conclusions about a case (e.g., the diseases that a patient might have, the therapy that should be administered, the laboratory tests that should be ordered) (Clancey, 1989). Thus, instead of modeling the relationships among patient findings and possible diagnoses purely in terms of statistical associations or mathematical equations, knowledge-based systems might represent those relationships in terms of qualitative, symbolic structures. Production rules such as those in MYCIN (see Fig. 20.1) often have been used to build knowledge-based systems, as have many other approaches (David et al., 1993). The knowledge in a knowledge-based system may include probabilistic relations, such as between symptoms and underlying diseases. Typically, such relations are augmented by qualitative relations, such as causality and temporal relations.

20.3.5   Human–Computer Interaction

There is perhaps no omission that, historically, accounts more fully for the impracticality of many clinical decision tools than the failure of developers to deal adequately with the logistical, mechanical, and psychological aspects of system use (see also Chapter 4). Often, system builders have concentrated primarily on creating computer programs that can reach good decisions. Yet researchers have shown repeatedly that an ability to make correct diagnoses, or to suggest therapy similar to that recommended by human consultants, is only one part of the formula for system success. Fortunately, there is increasing recognition that decision-support systems should, at the very least, present interfaces to their users that are uncluttered and intuitive, where users can predict in advance the consequences of their actions (and undo those actions, if necessary). At best, the decision-support element should be embedded within some larger computer system that is already part of the users' professional routine—thus making decision support a byproduct of the practitioners' ordinary work practices.

Many potential users of clinical decision-support tools have found their early enthusiasm dampened by programs that are cumbersome to access, slow to perform, and difficult to learn to use. Systems can fail, for example, if they require that a practitioner interrupt the normal pattern of patient care to move to a separate workstation or to follow complex, time-consuming startup procedures. Lengthy interactions, or ones that fail to convey the logic of what is happening on the screen, also discourage use of the program. Health professionals are likely to be particularly frustrated if the decision tool requires the manual reentry of information available on other computers. Solutions to such problems require sensitivity during the design process and, frequently, resolution of inadequacies at the institutional level. For example, linking computers to one another so that they can share data requires implementation of an overall networking and data-sharing strategy for the hospital or clinic. The advent of wireless networks that allow users to roam about a hospital or clinic, writing directly onto a computer tablet with a pen-based interface, offers solutions for both clinical computing in general and for access to decision-support systems in particular. Similarly, novel human–computer interfaces based on speech, gestures, and virtual reality offer new dimensions to the ways in which healthcare workers can interact with decision-support systems (see Chapter 24).

20.4   Construction of Decision-Support Tools

Despite significant research progress since the idea of computer-based medical decision-support systems first emerged, several barriers continue to impede the effective implementation of such tools in clinical settings. As we implied earlier, these obstacles include unresolved questions of both science and logistics.

20.4.1   Acquisition and Validation of Patient Data

As emphasized in Chapter 2, few problems are more challenging than the development of effective techniques for capturing patient data accurately, completely, and efficiently. You have read in this book about a wide variety of techniques for data entry, ranging from keyboard entry, to speech input, to methods that separate the clinician from the computer (such as scannable forms, real-time data monitoring, and intermediaries who transcribe written or dictated data for use by computers). All these methods have limitations, and healthcare workers frequently state that their use of computers will be limited unless they are freed of the task of data entry and can concentrate instead on data review and information retrieval (Shortliffe, 1989). Even if computers could accept unrestricted speech input, there would be serious challenges associated with properly structuring and encoding what was said. Otherwise, spoken input becomes a large free-text database that defies semantic interpretation. Many workers believe that some combination of speech and graphics, coupled with integrated data-management environments that will prevent the need for redundant entry of the same information into multiple computer systems within a hospital or clinic, are the key advances that will attract busy clinicians and other health workers to use computer-based tools.

The problems of data acquisition go beyond entry of the data themselves, however. A primary obstacle is that we lack standardized ways of expressing most clinical situations in a form that computers can interpret. There are several controlled medical terminologies that healthcare workers use to specify precise diagnostic evaluations (e.g., the International Classification of Diseases and SNOMED-CT), clinical procedures (e.g., Current Procedural Terminology), and so on (see Chapter 7). Still, there is no controlled terminology that captures the nuances of a patient's history of present illness or findings on physical examination. There is no coding system that can reflect all the details of physicians' or nurses' progress notes. Given that much of the information in the medical record that we would like to use to drive decision support is not available in a structured, machine-understandable form, there are clear limitations on the data that can be used to assist clinician decision-making. Nevertheless, even when computer-based patient records store substantial information only as free-text entries, those data that are available in coded form (typically, diagnosis codes and prescription data) can be used to significant advantage (van der Lei et al., 1991). Finally, even full electronic medical records may not include all of the relevant patient-specific data (e.g., professional and marital problems) and thus should be viewed realistically as an incomplete source of information.

20.4.2   Modeling of Medical Knowledge

People who have attempted to acquire the knowledge for a medical decision-support system by reading a textbook or several journal articles and by trying to encode the implied knowledge in some program can attest to the complexity of translating from the usual text approach for communicating knowledge to a structure appropriate for the logical application of that knowledge by a computer. The problem is not unlike that of identifying what you as a reader need to do to interpret, internalize, and apply properly the wealth of information in a book such as this. Creation of a computer-based decision-support system thus requires substantial **modeling** activity: deciding what clinical distinctions and patient data are relevant, identifying the concepts and relationships among concepts that bear on the decision-making task, and ascertaining a problem-solving strategy that can use the relevant clinical knowledge to reach appropriate conclusions.

You cannot glean any of this information simply by reading a textbook; clinical experts themselves may not be able to verbalize the knowledge needed to solve even routine cases (Johnson, 1983). Consequently, construction of any decision-support system—regardless of the underlying decision-making methodology—entails development of a model of both the required problem-solving behavior and the clinical knowledge that will inform that problem-solving. Considerable work in biomedical informatics currently concentrates on the design of frameworks that allow system builders to model the knowledge that ultimately will be captured within decision-support tools. Abstract modeling methodologies such as Common KADS (Schreiber et al., 2000) have been widely adopted by commercial developers of decision-support systems, particularly in Europe. Development of computer-based tools that can assist in the modeling of clinical knowledge remains an active area of investigation (Eriksson et al., 1995; Musen et al., 1995; van Heijst et al., 1995).

20.4.3   Elicitation of Medical Knowledge

Researchers are devising methods that will facilitate the development and maintenance of medical knowledge bases (Musen, 1993). The rapid evolution of medical knowledge makes knowledge-base maintenance a particularly important problem. Investigators have developed a variety of computer programs that acquire the knowledge base for a decision-support program by interacting directly with the expert, the goal being to avoid the need for a computer programmer to serve as intermediary (Eriksson & Musen, 1993; Lanzola et al., 1995; Musen et al., 1987). In all these approaches, analysts must first work with clinical experts to model the relevant application area.

For example, early researchers used a special-purpose tool known as **OPAL** (Musen et al., 1987) (Fig. 20.4) to enter and maintain the knowledge base of the cancer-chemotherapy advisor **ONCOCIN** (Shortliffe, 1986); the developers of OPAL built into the tool a comprehensive model of cancer-chemotherapy administration, allowing OPAL to transform the process of knowledge elicitation for ONCOCIN into a matter of filling in the blanks of structured forms and of drawing flowchart diagrams on the computer screen. When creating domain-specific knowledge-elicitation tools such as OPAL, developers create their model of the intended application area for the target decision-support system and then either program that model by hand into the tool (as they did in the case of building the original OPAL program) or enter the model into a **meta-tool** (Eriksson & Musen, 1993), which then generates automatically a special-

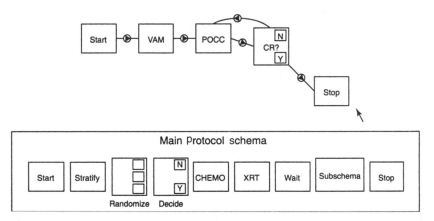

Figure 20.4. A clinical researcher can use OPAL to describe the overall schema of an ONCOCIN cancer-treatment plan using the graphical environment shown here. She creates the individual boxes by making selections from the palette of choices at the bottom of the screen and then positions and joins them as desired. The model of cancer chemotherapy built into OPAL determines that possible selections include chemotherapy (CHEMO in the diagram), X-ray therapy (XRT), as well as the idea of randomization and stratification of patients enrolled in clinical trials. The figure shows a relatively simple protocol in which patients are treated with a three-drug chemotherapy called VAM, followed by a four-drug chemotherapy called POCC, until there is complete response (CR).

purpose knowledge-elicitation tool based on that model. **Protégé** (see Section 20.5.2) is a meta-tool that many developers have used to create automatically domain-specific knowledge-elicitation tools like OPAL by taking as input analysts' models of the relevant application areas (Musen, 1998; Musen et al., 1995).

20.4.4   *Representation of and Reasoning About Medical Knowledge*

Among the ongoing research challenges is the need to refine the computational techniques for encoding the wide range of knowledge used in problem-solving by medical experts. Although well-established techniques such as the use of *frames* or *rules* exist for storing factual or inferential knowledge, several complex challenges remain. For example, physicians use mental models of the three-dimensional relationships among body parts and organs when they are interpreting data or planning therapy. Representing such anatomical knowledge and performing spatial reasoning by computer have proved to be particularly challenging. Similarly, human beings have a remarkable ability to interpret changes in data over time, assessing temporal trends and developing models of disease progression or the response of disease to past therapies. Researchers continue to develop computer-based methods for modeling such tasks.

Another kind of expertise, often poorly recognized but clearly important to optimal knowledge management by computer-based tools, is the human skill inherent in knowing how to use what is known. In medicine, we often call this skill "good clinical judgment," and we properly distinguish it from the memorization of factual knowledge or data from the literature. It is similarly clear that simply giving computers lots of factual knowledge will not make them skilled in a field unless they also are expert in the proper application of that knowledge. It is in this area particularly that improved understanding of the psychology of human problem-solving is helping researchers to develop decision-support tools that more closely simulate the process by which expert clinicians move from observations to diagnoses or management plans (see Chapter 4).

20.4.5   *Validation of System Performance*

Many observers are horrified when they imagine what they might have to do to validate and maintain the currency of large clinical knowledge bases. After all, medical knowledge is advancing at a rapid pace, and an advisory system that uses yesterday's knowledge may fail to provide the best advice available for a patient's problem. Although researchers with limited goals have been willing to take on responsibility for short-term knowledge-base maintenance in support of their scholarly activities, it is likely that professional organizations or other national bodies will in time need to assume responsibility for the currency and integrity of large clinical knowledge bases.

When a knowledge base is well validated, developers still face challenges in determining how best to evaluate the performance of the decision-support tools that use the knowledge. When a gold standard of performance exists, formal studies can compare the program's advice with that accepted standard of "correctness." This technique is especially pertinent for diagnostic tools, where biopsy, surgery, or autopsy data can be used as an appropriate gold standard. In the case of therapy-advice systems, however, the gold standard is more difficult to define. Even experts may disagree about the proper way to treat a specific patient, and there can seldom be a realistic controlled trial that attempts to show which approach is right in any absolute sense. For this reason, workers have experimented with techniques that compare the recommendations of a therapy-management program with those of experts (see Chapter 11). With proper controls, such studies can be useful, although they have shown that even experts in a field generally do not receive perfect marks when assessed by their peers. The problem of evaluation remains a ripe area for further research (Friedman & Wyatt, 1997a).

20.4.6   Integration of Decision-Support Tools

As we have emphasized, the successful introduction of decision-support tools is likely to be tied to these tools' effective integration with routine clinical tasks. We need more innovative research on how best to tie knowledge-based computer tools to programs designed to store, manipulate, and retrieve patient-specific information. We explained how the HELP system included decision-support functions that are triggered to generate warnings or reports whenever an internally specified set of conditions holds for a given patient (Section 20.2.3). As hospitals and clinics increasingly use multiple small machines optimized for different tasks, however, the challenges of integration are inherently tied to issues of networking and systems interfaces. It is in the electronic linking of multiple machines with overlapping functions and data needs that the potential of distributed but integrated patient data processing will be realized.

20.5   Illustrative Examples of Clinical Decision-Support Systems

To illustrate the state of the art and the ways in which new technologies have affected the evolution of decision-support tools, we shall discuss selected features of several well-known decision-support systems in two major areas: diagnosis and patient management. Quick Medical Reference (like its predecessor, Internist-1) supports diagnostic problem solving in general internal medicine, while DXplain is a continuously evolving Web-based diagnostic system. The EON system is a representative example for one of the recent guideline-based decision-support systems, which provide therapeutic recommendations for treatment in accordance with predefined protocols. The systems discussed here in some detail demonstrate widely differing architectures. Quick Medical Reference is used primarily as a standalone system, DXplain is a self-containted system, but currently accessed mostly over the World Wide Web, and EON comprises a set of software components that are designed to be integrated within larger clinical information systems.

20.5.1   Diagnosis: The Internist-1/QMR Project and the DXplain System

We will demonstrate the task of supporting clinical diagnosis using two well known but very different systems: Internist-1, which evolved into the QMR system, and the DXplain system, which is an important Web-based resource.

20.5.1.1   The Internist-1/QMR project

Internist-1 was a large diagnostic program that was developed at the University of Pittsburgh School of Medicine in the 1970s (Miller et al., 1982; Pople, 1982). The Internist-1 program subsequently grew into a decision-support system known as **Quick Medical Reference** (QMR). QMR was marketed commercially for several years, and was used by a large community of practitioners and students. Although currently the system is not actively supported, it has been highly influential and the subject of considerable study by the medical-informatics community.

The goal of the original Internist-1 project was to model diagnosis in general internal medicine. Internist-1 contained knowledge of almost 600 diseases and of nearly 4,500 interrelated *findings*, or *disease manifestations* (signs, symptoms, and other patient characteristics). On average, each disease was associated with between 75 and 100 findings. The task of diagnosis would be straightforward if each disease were associated with a unique set of findings. Most findings, however, such as fever, are associated with multiple disease processes, often with varying levels of likelihood for each disease. Clinicians have long recognized that it is not feasible to perform simple pattern matching to make difficult diagnoses. On the other hand, it is impractical to estimate conditional probabilities (such as those used by the Leeds abdominal pain system) for all the diseases and findings in Internist-1's knowledge base—particularly because many of the 600 disease syndromes are rare and thus are not well described in the clinical literature. For these reasons, the developers of Internist-1 chose to create an ad hoc scoring scheme to encode the relationships between specific findings and diseases.

To construct the Internist-1 knowledge base, the senior physician on the project (a superb senior clinician who had over 50 years of practice experience), other physicians, and medical students worked together, considering each of the encoded diseases. Through careful literature review and case discussions, they determined the list of pertinent findings associated with each disease. For each of these findings, they assigned a **frequency weight** (FW) and an **evoking strength** (ES), two numbers that reflect the strength of the relationship between the disease and the finding (Figure 20.5). The FW is a number between 1 and 5, where 1 means that the finding is seldom seen in the disease and 5 means it is essentially always seen (Table 20.1). The ES reflects the likelihood that a patient with the finding has the disease in question and that the disease is the cause of the finding (Table 20.2). An ES of 0 means that the disease would never be considered as a diagnosis on the basis of this finding alone, whereas an ES of 5 means that the finding is **pathognomonic** for the disease (i.e., all patients with the finding have the disease).

In addition, each finding in the knowledge base is associated with a third number, an **import number** that has a value between 1 and 5 (Table 20.3). The import number

Disease profile for

ECHINOCOCCAL CYST<S> OF LIVER

ES	FW	
1	2	CHEST PERCUSSION DIAPHRAGM ELEVATED UNILATERAL
1	2	COUGH
1	1	FECES LIGHT COLORED
0	2	FEVER
1	3	HEPATOMEGALY PRESENT
1	2	JAUNDICE
1	2	LIVER CONTAINING LARGE PALPABLE MASS<ES>
1	1	LIVER CONTAINING LARGE PALPABLE MASS<ES> FLUCTUANT
1	1	LIVER DISTORTED OR ASYMMETRICAL
1	1	LIVER ENLARGED MASSIVE
1	2	LIVER ENLARGED MODERATE
1	2	LIVER ENLARGED SLIGHT
1	2	LIVER TENDER ON PALPATION
1	1	PRESSURE ARTERIAL DIASTOLIC LESS THAN 60
1	1	PRESSURE ARTERIAL DIASTOLIC LESS THAN 90
1	1	RHONCHI DIFFUSE

Figure 20.5. A sample disease profile from Internist-1. The numbers beside the findings represent the evoking strength ([ES] ranging from 0 [nonspecific] to 5 [pathognomonic]) and the frequency weight ([FW] ranging from 1 [rare] to 5 [always seen]). Only an excerpt from the disease profile for echinococcal cysts is shown here.

Table 20.1. Interpretation of frequency weights.

Frequency weight	Interpretation
1	Listed manifestation occurs rarely in the disease
2	Listed manifestation occurs in a substantial minority of cases of the disease
3	Listed manifestation occurs in roughly one-half of the cases
4	Listed manifestation occurs in the substantial majority of cases
5	Listed manifestation occurs in essentially all cases—that is, it is a prerequisite for the diagnosis

Source: Miller, R.A., Pople, H.E., Myers, J.D. Internist-1: an experimental computer-based diagnostic consultant for general internal medicine. New England Journal of Medicine, 307:468.

Table 20.2. Interpretation of evoking strengths.

Evoking strength	Interpretation
0	Nonspecific—manifestation occurs too commonly to be used to construct a differential diagnosis
1	Diagnosis is a rare or unusual cause of listed manifestation
2	Diagnosis causes a substantial minority of instances of listed manifestation
3	Diagnosis is the most common, but not the overwhelming, cause of listed manifestation
4	Diagnosis is the overwhelming cause of listed manifestation
5	Listed manifestation is pathognomonic for the diagnosis

Source: Miller, R.A., Pople, H.E., Myers, J.D. Internist-1: an experimental computer-based diagnostic consultant for general internal medicine. New England Journal of Medicine, 307:468.

Table 20.3. Interpretation of import values.

Import	Interpretation
1	Manifestation is usually unimportant, occurs commonly in normal persons, and is easily disregarded
2	Manifestation may be of importance but can often be ignored; context is important
3	Manifestation is of moderate importance but may be an unreliable indicator of any specific disease
4	Manifestation is of high importance and can only rarely be disregarded (as, for example, a false-positive result)
5	Manifestation absolutely must be explained by one of the final diagnoses

Source: Miller, R.A., Pople, H.E., Myers, J.D. Internist-1: an experimental computer-based diagnostic consultant for general internal medicine. New England Journal of Medicine, 307:468.

captures the idea that some abnormalities have serious implications and must be explained, whereas others may be safely ignored. Internist-1 uses the import number to handle red herrings (minor problems that are not explained by the current disease process). This familiar clinical-diagnosis problem is not handled well by formal statistical approaches.

Based on these simple measurements, Internist-1 used a scoring scheme that is similar to the hypothetico-deductive approach described in Chapter 2. The physician-user would enter an initial set of findings, and then the program would determine an initial differential diagnosis. Based on the current set of hypotheses, the program would select appropriate questions to ask, choosing from several strategies, depending on how many diseases are under consideration and how closely matched they are to the available patient data. The program considered the cost and risks of tests, as well as the benefits, and asked for simple historical and physical-examination data before recommending laboratory tests or invasive diagnostic procedures. An important feature, not previously implemented in diagnostic programs, was Internist-1's ability to set aside some of the findings not well explained by the current differential diagnosis and to return to them later after making an initial diagnosis. Thus, Internist-1 could diagnose multiple coexistent diseases and did not make the assumptions of mutual exclusivity and completeness that have characterized most Bayesian diagnostic programs.

Using these simple knowledge structures and weighting schemes, Internist-1 demonstrated impressive diagnostic performance. In one study, the developers tested the program on 19 difficult diagnostic cases taken from a major clinical journal (Miller et al., 1982). The 19 patients had a total of 43 diagnoses, of which Internist-1 correctly identified 25. By comparison, the physicians who had cared for the patients in a major teaching hospital made 28 correct diagnoses, and the expert discussants who presented the cases before a large audience before the publication of each case in the journal correctly identified 35 diagnoses. Although Internist-1 missed several of the difficult cases (as did the physicians and discussants), the test patients had problems that were drawn broadly from across all problems in general internal medicine—no other diagnostic program would have been able to deal effectively with more than a small subset of these cases.

Internist-1 was created to run on only large, mainframe computers and therefore was not suited for widespread use by practitioners. In the 1980s, the program was adapted to run on personal computers as QMR (Quick Medical Reference) (Miller et al., 1986). Unlike Internist-1, which was developed to provide only patient-specific diagnostic advice, QMR can serve health professionals in three modes. In its basic mode, QMR is an expert consultation system that provides advice much as Internist-1 did (using essentially the same knowledge base and scoring scheme). Quick Medical Reference can also be used as an **electronic textbook**, listing the patient characteristics reported to occur in a given disease or, conversely, reporting which of its 600 diseases can be associated with a given characteristic. Third, as a **medical spreadsheet**, it can combine a few characteristics or diseases and determine the implications. For example, the user can specify two apparently unrelated medical problems and obtain suggestions about how coexisting diseases could, under the right circumstances, give rise to both problems (Figure 20.6).

The developers of QMR have argued that the system's use as an electronic reference is far more important than its use as a consultation program to help a clinician to clinch a particularly difficult diagnosis (Miller & Masarie, 1990). In fact, in the version of QMR that was available commercially, many of the consultation features of Internist-1 were removed. For example, the QMR product did not ask questions directly of the user in order to pursue a diagnosis and did not attempt to evaluate whether more than one disease might be present at a given time.

20.5.1.2   The DXplain System

DXplain [Barnett et al., 1987; Barnett et al., 1998] is a decision support system developed at the Laboratory of Computer Science at the Massachusetts General Hospital. It was initially described by its developers as a "poor man's Internist-1." Despite this portrayal, the program's capabilities are quite sophisticated. Given a set of clinical findings (signs, symptoms, laboratory data), DXplain produces a ranked list of diagnoses that might explain (or be associated with) the clinical manifestations. DXplain provides justification for why each of these diseases might be considered, suggests what further clinical information would be useful to collect for each disease, and lists what clinical manifestations, if any, would be unusual or atypical for each of the specific diseases. DXplain does not offer definitive medical consultation and, like QMR, is not intended to be used as a substitute for a human clinician. Figure 20.7 demonstrates a part of a typical DXplain session.

DXplain takes advantage of a large data base of the crude probabilities of over 4500 clinical manifestations associated with over 2000 different diseases—a knowledge base considerably larger than that of QMR. The system adopts a modified form of Bayesian reasoning to perform diagnosis using an algorithm that has not been well desribed in the literature. The DXplain system has been implemented both as a stand-alone version and as a server that is accessible over the Internet. The knowledge base and the user interface are continually being improved and adapted as a result of comments from users. DXplain is in use at a number of hospitals and medical schools, mostly for educational purposes, but also for clinical consultation. It is clearly the most extensively used patient-specific decision-support tool available today.

DXplain has the characteristics of both an electronic medical textbook and a medical reference system. In the role of a medical textbook, DXplain can provide

Pulmonary Disease and DIARRHEA Chronic

Pairs of diseases consistent with Entered Finding and Topic

Atelectasis
caused-by Carcinoid Syndrome Secondary to Bronchial Neoplasm

Eosinophilic Pneumonia Acute <LOEFFLER>
caused-by Hookworm Disease

Pulmonary Legionellosis
predisposed-to-by Immune Deficiency Syndrome Acquired <AIDS>

Pleural Effusion Exudative
caused-by Pancreatic Pseudocyst

Pneumoccoccal Pneumonia
predisposed-to-by Immune Deficiency Syndrome Acquired <AIDS>

Pulmonary Hypertension Secondary
caused-by Progressive Systemic Sclerosis
or co-occurring-with Schistosomiasis Chronic Hepatic

Pulmonary Infarction
predisposed-to-by Carcinoma of Body or Tail of Pancreas
or predisposed-to-by Carcinoma of Head of Pancreas
or caused-by Hepatic Vein Obstruction

Pulmonary Lymphoma
coinciding-with Lymphoma of Colon
or coinciding-with Small Intestinal Lymphoma

Figure 20.6. A sample associations list from QMR, a system that permits the physician to request exploratory searches of the knowledge base for associations that might be clinically relevant. For example, as shown here, the physician has asked for pulmonary diseases that may also be associated with chronic diarrhea. The resulting lists, which QMR generates dynamically, can be useful memory joggers for physicians who might otherwise overlook the suggested relationships.

comprehensive descriptions of the more than 2000 diseases in its knowledge base, emphasizing the signs and symptoms that occur in each disease, the etiology, the pathology, and the prognosis. DXplain also provides up to 10 recent bibliographic references that have been selected as being appropriate for each specific disease. In addition, DXplain can provide a list of diseases that should be considered for any one of over

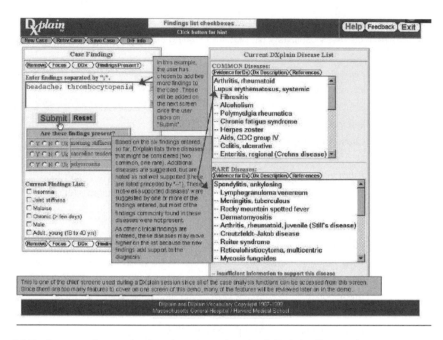

Figure 20.7. A screen from a session demonstrating the DXplain diagnostic system to new users. The user had entered six findings, assisted by a standard medical vocabulary that verifies the free-text strings entered. DXplain then presents a list of the most likely common diseases and the most likely rare diseases fitting these findings. Note that DXplain also points out several pertinent findings that might or might not be present, which would further refine the diagnostic list.

5000 different clinical manifestations (signs, symptoms, and laboraory examinations) known to the system.

20.5.2   Patient Management: Guideline-Based Architectures and The EON System

Clinical practice guidelines are a powerful method for standardization and uniform improvement of the quality of medical care. According to the Institute of Medicine's definition, clinical guidelines are "systematically developed statements to assist practitioner and patient decisions about appropriate health care for specific clinical circumstances" [Field and Lohr., 1992]. Clinical guidelines typically represent a medical expert consensus regarding the screening, diagnosis, or management, over either limited or extended periods of time, of patients who have a particular clinical problem, need, or condition (e.g., *fever of unknown origin*, therapy of *insulin-dependent diabetes*). Clinical guidelines are particularly useful for management of patients over extended periods, as in the management of chronic diseases. The application of clinical guidelines by care providers typically involves collecting and interpreting considerable amounts of data over time, applying standard therapeutic or diagnostic plans in an episodic fashion, and revising those plans when necessary. Thus, reasoning about time-oriented data and actions is essential for guideline-based care.

20.5.2.1   Guideline-Based Patient-Management Systems

It is now agreed that conforming to appropriate clinical practice guidelines is the best way to improve the quality of health care [Grimshaw and Russel, 1993], while reducing the escalating costs of medical care. Clinical guidelines are most useful at the point of care (typically, when the care provider has access to the patient's record), such as at the time of order entry by the care provider. In such a context, even simple reminders and alerts have powerful effects, especially in outpatient contexts. Indeed, investigators have demonstrated significant enhancement of adherance to preventive-care guidelines, such as those for the administration of pneumococcal and influenza vaccinations, by integrating several simple alerts within a hospital's order-entry system [Dexter et al., 2001].

Most clinical guidelines are text-based and not readily accessible to the healthcare workers who most need them. Even when guidelines exist in electronic format, and even when that format is available online, healthcare workers rarely have the time and means to decide which of multiple guidelines best pertains to their patients, and, if so, exactly what does applying that guideline to the particular patient entail. To support the needs of health-care providers as well as administrators, and to ensure continuous quality of care, more sophisticated information processing tools are needed. Due to limitations of current technologies, analyzing unstructured text-based guidelines is not feasible (see Chapter 8). Thus, there is an urgent need to facilitate guideline dissemination and application using machine-readable representations and automated computational methods.

There are several tasks associated with the guideline-based care that would benefit from automation. These tasks include specification (authoring) and maintenance of clinical guidelines, retrieval of guidelines appropriate to each patient, runtime application of guidelines, and retrospective assessment of the quality of the application of the guidelines. Supporting guideline-based care implies creation of a *dialog* between a care provider and an automated support system, each of which has its relative strengths. For example, physicians have better access to certain types of patient-specific clinical information (such as that patient's mental state and likelihood of compliance with therapy) and to general medical and commonsense knowledge. Automated systems have faster and more accurate access to detailed guideline specifications and can detect more easily prespecified complex temporal patterns in the patient's data. Thus, there is great synergy when human beings and machines work cooperatively on the problem of guideline-based care.

Developers often encode the knowledge needed to provide simple decision support for patient management, such as for raising context-sensitive alerts and reminders, as **situation–action rules**. An example is the rule in Figure 20.3, which is expressed in the Arden Syntax [Hripcsak et al., 1994] (Section 2.3), the earliest standard for representation and sharing of medical knowledge. A **rule interpreter** processes such rules—scanning the patient database for situations that trigger relevant rules, evaluating whether the condition part of the rule holds, and, if it does, taking whatever action the rule might specify. Although such rule-based approaches for representing knowledge have been used successfully since the time of MYCIN, development and maintenance of large rule bases can be difficult. Interactions among rules may have unanticipated side effects, leading to unexpected system behaviors when rules are added to or deleted from a previously debugged knowledge base (Bachant & McDermott, 1984; Clancey, 1984; Heckerman & Horvitz, 1986). In general, rule-based approaches to the representation of clinical guidelines, such as the Arden Syntax, do not include an intuitive representation of the guideline's clinical logic, have no semantics for the different types of clinical knowledge represented, and lack the ability to represent and reuse guidelines and guideline components. Such formalisms do not allow for inherent, intended, ambiguities in the therapy algorithm (such as when considerations exist for and against different therapy options, which need to be evaluated by the attending physician, or when the patient's preferences need to be explicitly considered). Most important, approaches such as Arden Syntax do not support the application of guidelines over extended periods of time, as is necessary for the support of the care of patients with chronic disase. Nevertheless, rules are an excellent option when simple, one-time reminders and alerts need to be written and used, without the heavier machinery of more complex guideline representations, and in that sense they complement more expressive guideline-representation formats [Peleg et al., 2001a].

When building comprehensive decision-support systems for clinical practice guidelines, it is often most helpful to view the guidelines as reusable **skeletal plans** [Friedland and Iwasaki, 1985], namely a set of plans at varying levels of abstraction and detail, that, when applied to a particular patient, need to be refined by a care provider over significant time periods, while often leaving considerable room for flexibility in the achievement of particular goals. Another view is that clinical guidelines are a set of *constraints* regarding the *process* of applying the guideline (i.e., care-provider actions) and its desired *outcomes* (i.e., patient health states), constraints that can be viewed as the *intentions* of the guideline authors regarding how care should be administerd and what outcomes from therapy are desirable [Shahar et al., 1998]. These constraints are often *temporal*, or at least have a significant temporal dimension, especially in the case of those clinical practice guidelines that concern the care of patients with chronic problems, or that specify actions to be applied over a significant period.

Numerous workers in biomedical informatics have developed several architectures for the automated application of clinical practice guidelines. Each of these systems assumes an explicit model for representing guideline knowledge. These models are similar, but make different subtle distinctions about guidelines and clinical care. It is impossible to enumerate all of the models that have been suggested, as the automation of guideline-based care remains an area of intensive investigation in biomedical informatics. Some of the best known formalisms include the ProForma language, developed by at the Advanced Computation Laboratory (ACL) of Cancer Research UK [Fox et al., 1998; Fox and Das, 2000]; the GuideLine Interchange Format (GLIF), created as part of collaboration among Columbia, Harvard, and Stanford Universities [Ohno-Machado et al., 1998; Peleg et al., 2000, 2001; Boxwala et al., 2004]; the Asbru guideline language [Miksch et al., 1997], whose focus is on highly expressive time-oriented actions, developed as part of the Asgaard project [Shahar et al., 1998]; the GUIDE model, [Quaglini et al., 2001], which is part of a more general framework, Careflow, developed at the

University of Pavia, Italy, for modeling and applying clinical guidelines in the broad context of general medical care; and the PRODIGY guideline model [Johnson et al., 2000], developed at the University of Newcastle upon Tyne in Britain. Like several of the frameworks mentioned here, the PRODIGY project uses the Protégé suite of tools to acquire and represent a set of clinical guidelines (Musen, 1998; Musen et al., 1995). Peleg and colleagues [2003] provide an excellent review of these alternative guideline-representation approaches.

20.5.2.2   A Guideline-Based Patient-Management Architecture: The EON system

Many of the current approaches for representing the knowledge of clinical-practice guidelines in computer systems build on ideas first explored in a decision-support system known as EON, which has been under development at Stanford University for nearly two decades. EON is a second-generation knowledge-based system (David et al., 1993) that aids practitioners in the care of patients who are being treated in accordance with **protocols** and clinical-practice guidelines (Musen, 1998; Musen et al., 1996). Unlike systems such as MYCIN or QMR, EON cannot be run by itself. Instead, EON constitutes a set of software components that must be embedded within some clinical information systems that healthcare workers use to enter and browse patient-related data. Figure 20.8 shows the major components of EON, which are the following:

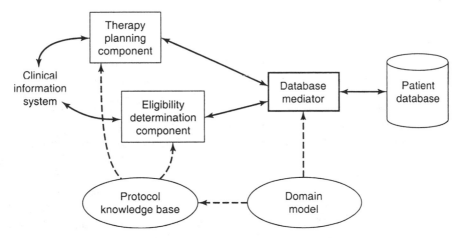

Figure 20.8. The EON architecture. EON consists of a number of problem-solving components (e.g., programs that plan protocol-based therapy and that determine whether a patient potentially is eligible for protocols) that share a common knowledge base of protocol descriptions. The protocol domain model, created with the Proégé system, defines the format of the protocol knowledge base. The same model also defines the schema for the database mediator, a system that channels the flow of patient data between the problem-solving components and an archival relational database. The entire architecture is embedded within a clinical information system.

- **Problem solvers** each address specific tasks (Eriksson et al., 1995), such as (1) determining the treatment that should be given at a particular time if a patient is to receive therapy in accordance with a predefined clinical protocol and (2) determining, for a given patient, whether there are any protocols for which the patient might be eligible.
- Knowledge bases encode descriptions of clinical protocols in a way that all the problem solvers in EON can examine a shared, coherent representation of protocol knowledge, thus using the protocol knowledge bases to solve their particular task. The EON therapy-planning component accesses the protocol knowledge base to identify what are the potential clinical interventions that might be administered to a given patient and what knowledge is needed to determine precisely what treatment is appropriate; the EON **eligibility-determination** component consults the same knowledge base to identify the factors that establish when a given protocol is appropriate and then accesses patient data to see whether the protocol might be a good match.
- A **database mediator** serves as a conduit between all the problem solvers in EON and the database that stores all the patient data (Nguyen et al., 1997). The mediator insulates all the EON problem solvers from many of the logistical problems of querying patient data and making sense out of various time-dependent relationships among the data (e.g., querying the data for the existence of certain trends or patterns). The mediator includes within it a problem solver that addresses the specific task of abstraction of time-oriented patient data into higher-level concepts, the **RÉSUMÉ** system (Shahar & Musen, 1996). Thus, queries such as "Did the patient have more than 2 weeks of bone-marrow toxicity grade II (in a specific context)" can be answered by the mediator directly. The method underlying the RÉSUMÉ solver is the knowledge-based **temporal-abstraction** method (Shahar, 1997).

The components in EON are designed such that they can be mixed and matched to create different decision-support functionalities. For example, EON's therapy-planning component (Tu et al., 1995) and eligibility-determination component (Tu et al., 1993), plus knowledge bases for protocol-based care of AIDS and HIV-related diseases, formed the decision-support elements of a system known as THERAPY-HELPER (or T-HELPER for short) (Musen et al., 1992). T-HELPER contained an electronic patient record with which practitioners could enter patient information at the time of each visit to an outpatient clinic specializing in the care of people with AIDS. T-HELPER would then invoke the EON components to generate specific recommendations regarding patient therapy. If the patient was not currently enrolled in applicable protocols, the T-HELPER system would indicate those protocols for which the patient potentially was eligible. For those protocols in which the patient was already enrolled, the system would indicate what therapy should be administered, given the protocol requirements, the patient's current stage of therapy, and the patient's clinical situation.

In other experiments, the same therapy-planning component and eligibility-determination component were used in conjunction with a knowledge base of breast-cancer protocols (Musen et al., 1996). The EON architecture made it possible to simply "plug in" these previously developed modules and to use them in conjunction with the new breast-cancer knowledge bases. Again, the EON components did not run as a standalone system but were embedded within a computer-based patient-record system that could invoke the EON decision-support components when appropriate.

The EON architecture has been deployed successfully to bring guideline-based decision support to several Veterans Affairs medical centers in the United States. The EON **middleware** forms the basis of the **ATHENA** system for management of hypertension in accordance with national guidelines [Goldstein et al. 2000, 2002]. The ATHENA user interface is integrated with that of **VISTA**, the Veterans Affairs clinical information system, to provide an intuitive overview of the clinical data relevant to treatment of high blood pressure (Figure 20.9). The interface also displays specific suggstions to physicians regarding clinical interventions that they might make to ensure that care is consistent with the hyperternsion guidelines stored in the program's knowledge base. The ATHENA knowledge base stores guideline eligibility criteria, **risk stratification**, blood pressure targets, relevant comorbid diseases, guideline-recommended drugs, and criteria for treatment selection and modification.

The modularity of the EON architecture makes it relatively straightforward to add new problem-solving components in addition to new knowledge bases. For example, developers might design a new problem solver that analyzed the electronic patient record retrospectively to determine whether past treatment was consistent with protocol guidelines. The new module would then be driven by the same shared knowledge bases used by the other components in EON.

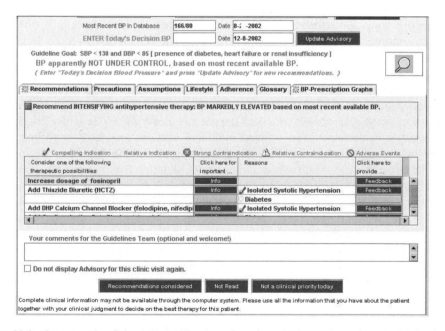

Figure 20.9. An example of the ATHENA system interface. ATHENA provides decision-support for the management of hypertension using the EON architecture. In the screen capture, the provider has entered the patient's most recent blood pressure, and is offered advice based on a relevant clinical-practice guideline. (*Source:* M. K. Goldstein.)

Although it may be easy to apply the EON components to new kinds of protocol knowledge bases, creating such knowledge bases in the first place can be a complex task. Fortunately, knowledge-acquisition for the EON system is greatly facilitated by the previously mentioned knowledge-base-development environment known as Protégé (Musen, 1998; Musen et al., 1995). Protégé provides a set of tools and a principled methodology for building knowledge-based systems, of which EON is only one example. Use of Protégé begins when developers create an abstract model of the application area for which knowledge-based systems are to be built. As shown in Figure 20.8, there is a common model for all the clinical-protocol knowledge bases processed by EON (Tu & Musen, 1996). This protocol model, or **ontology**, specifies the concepts necessary to define clinical protocols in a given domain of medicine. For example, construction of the ATHENA system required creation of a model that defined the concepts common among guidelines for hypertension (drug therapy, laboratory tests, and so on); analogously, construction of the decision-support system for breast-cancer protocols required creation of a somewhat similar model that defined the concepts common among protocols for breast cancer (including concepts such as surgery, radiotherapy, and so on). The terms and relationships of such models when entered into Protégé do more than define the concepts that form the structure of clinical protocols in machine-understandable form: The models serve as the starting point for generation of special-purpose computer-based tools that assist developers in the construction and maintenance of detailed protocol knowledge bases (Musen, 1998; Tu et al., 1995).

In the Protégé approach, developers first create a general model of the concepts and relationships that characterize a particular application area. For example, the model shown in Figure 20.10 represents a small subset of the concepts needed to define clinical protocols. A module in the Protégé system takes as input such a model and generates as output a custom-tailored tool based on that model that developers can use to enter detailed knowledge bases (Eriksson et al., 1994). Protégé thus processes the model for clinical protocols (see Figure 20.10) to construct a tool that knowledge-base authors can use for entry and review of specific protocol descriptions (Figure. 20.11). This tool—because it reflects the predefined model of clinical protocols—can be used by medical experts themselves. Because the tool is produced directly from the protocol model, developers can update and enhance the model and then generate a new knowledge-acquisition tool that reflects the corresponding changes. At the same time, developers can modify their abstract protocol models to reflect modalities of clinical care in new areas of medicine and then generate knowledge-acquisition tools that healthcare workers can use to enter new protocol specifications for these new clinical disciplines.

The EON approach demonstrates several dimensions of modern clinical decision-support systems. EON shows how decision-support systems can be embedded within larger clinical information systems. The architecture also exemplifies the use of emerging standards for network-based communication among software modules—a trend in **software engineering** that will become increasingly important in the years ahead (see Chapter 4). The coupling between the EON decision-support architecture and the Protégé knowledge-acquisition framework exemplifies the use of special-purpose tools for entering and maintaining protocol knowledge bases. As work in the development of clinical decision-support systems evolves, there will be expanding expectations that

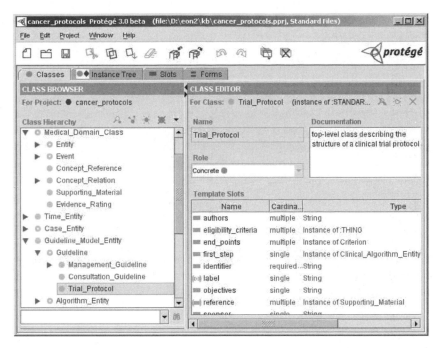

Figure 20.10. A small portion of a generic model of clinical guidelines entered into the PROTÉGÉ system. The hierarchy of entries on the left includes concepts that constitute a starter kit that may be used as building blocks to construct guideline descriptions. The panel on the right shows the attributes of whatever concept is highlighted on the left. Here, dose-information and toxicity list, for example, are attributes of the concept Drug-administration. The domain model entered into Protégé reflects concepts common to all guidelines, but does not include specifications for any guidelines in particular. The complete domain model is used to generate automatically a graphical knowledge-acquisition tool, such as the one shown in Figure 20.9.

decision-makers themselves be able to review and modify the electronic knowledge bases that codify an institution's decision-making policies. As demonstrated by EON, that kind of direct involvement of clinical personnel in knowledge-base management will require increasing use of systems such as Protégé, which can simplify the creation and modification of the necessary knowledge-editing tools.

20.6   Decision Support in the Decade to Come

After more than four decades of research on medical decision-support systems, investigators have learned a great deal about the difficulties inherent in the task and about the complex barriers to successful implementation of programs. In the 1970s and 1980s, researchers made major progress in tackling the scientific questions of computer-based decision support. Technological advances in knowledge representation, knowledge

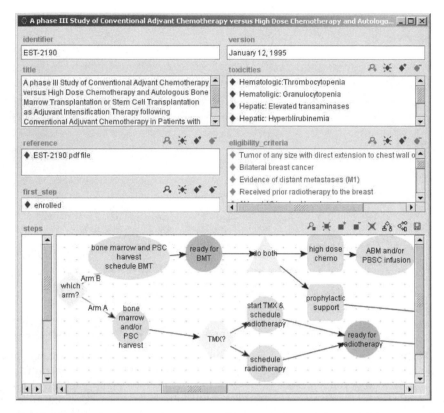

Figure 20.11. A screen from a Protégé-generated knowledge-acquisition tool for entry of breast cancer protocols. This tool is generated automatically from a domain model, part of which appears in Figure 20.8. The protocol depicted specifies the knowledge required to carry out a clinical trial that compares the effects of conventional adjuvant chemotherapy with those of high-dose chemotherapy followed by bone-marrow transplantation.

acquisition, and automated reasoning led to significant new insights related to the modeling, encoding, and dissemination of human expertise in a machine-processable form. Although early workers in biomedical informatics frequently raised concerns that clinicians might always be reluctant to interact with computer-based decision-support systems, the landscape changed radically at the end of the last century.

The advent of managed health care in the United States and growing concerns about the cost and quality of patient care globally have altered the practice of medicine in profound ways (see Chapter 23). Clinical practice guidelines based on empirical medical evidence are now ubiquitous. Practitioners often are highly motivated to follow such guidelines: Not only do physicians inherently want to offer their patients the best care possible based on available evidence in the literature, but often physicians' remuneration and even their medical malpractice premiums depend on their ability to follow predefined guidelines. In an era when there is increasing emphasis on continuous quality improvement via instruments such as clinical practice guidelines, decision-support systems such as those based on the EON architecture are assuming a central role in communicating guideline-based advice to all healthcare workers.

As healthcare organizations were undergoing radical change in the 1990s, computing technology was making an equally radical advance. The advent of the World Wide Web popularized computers in new ways. The World Wide Web demystified computers for many new users while providing connections among distributed processors that had not been imagined just a few year earlier. The Web provided a basis for inexpensive "**thin clients**" that could use a common browser to access a diverse collection of information resources in a uniform manner. Suddenly, it was almost trivial to bring a rich collection of programs directly to the point of care, greatly simplifying access to a variety of information sources and decision-support systems.

The educational potential of decision-support systems has long been recognized (Association of American Medical Colleges, 1986). New pressures to learn best practices coupled with the ubiquity of information technology, however, have greatly encouraged the use of computer-based decision aids in health-professional schools around the world. For the next generation of health-care workers, the use of information technology in most aspects of patient care probably will be taken for granted— much as it is in *Star Trek*.

20.6.1   *Legal and Regulatory Questions*

It may already have occurred to you that there are legal implications inherent in the development and use of such innovations. As mentioned in Chapter 10, formal legal precedents for dealing with clinical decision-support systems are lacking at present. Several observers have noted that a pivotal concern is whether the courts will view the systems under negligence law or product liability law (Miller et al., 1985). Under **negligence law** (which governs medical malpractice), a product or activity must meet reasonable expectations for safety. The principle of **strict liability**, on the other hand, states that a product must not be harmful. Because it is unrealistic to require that decision-support programs make correct assessments under all circumstances—we do not apply such standards to physicians themselves—the determination of which legal principle to apply will have important implications for the dissemination and acceptance of such tools. A related question is the potential liability borne by physicians who could have accessed such a program, and who chose not to do so, and who made an incorrect decision when the system would have suggested the correct one. As with other medical technologies, precedents suggest that physicians will be liable in such circumstances if the use of consultant programs has become the *standard of care* in the community (see Chapter 10). Several guidelines have been suggested for assigning legal liability to builders of knowledge-based medical decision-support systems or to the physicians using them [Allaërt & Dusserne, 1992].

Questions have also arisen regarding the validation of decision-support tools before their release (see Chapter 11). The evaluation of complex decision-support tools is challenging; it is difficult to determine acceptable levels of performance when there may be disagreement even among experts with similar training and experience. There is often no such thing as *the* correct answer to a clinical question. Moreover, component-based architectures such as EON may comprise multiple (potentially fallible) problem-solvers, each of which addresses different clinical problems and which shares a common (potentially fallible) set of knowledge bases. The objective then becomes to isolate the cause of possible errors and to make appropriate modifications to the system overall. Evaluations of medical decision-support tools have suggested a variety of methods for assessing the adequacy of clinical knowledge bases and problem-solving components before such software is introduced for routine use (Friedman & Wyatt, 1997a).

What then should be the role of government in prerelease regulation of medical software? Current policy of the Food and Drug Administration (FDA) in the United States indicates that such tools will not be subject to federal regulation if a trained practitioner is assessing the program's advice and making the final determination of care (Young, 1987). This policy is subject to ongoing reevaluation, however (see Chapter 10). Programs that make decisions directly controlling the patient's treatment (e.g., closed-loop systems that administer insulin or that adjust intravenous infusion rates or respirator settings; see Chapter 17) are viewed as medical devices subject to FDA regulation.

Additional problems arise when considering suggestions to enable access to electronic patient records through the World Wide Web, such as privacy and security. Ease of access versus data security will always constitute a trade-off in clinical information systems.

20.6.2   *Future Directions for Clinical Decision-Support Systems*

Trends for decision-support research and development in the decades ahead are becoming evident. As already mentioned, the World Wide Web will continue to expand the influence of computers in all aspects of society, and the Internet and numerous intranets will link information technologies throughout large healthcare organizations and communities of patients. The Internet will bring decision-support systems designed for patient use directly into those patients' homes and will provide more effective communication among all participants in the healthcare system (see Chapter 14). We already see many communities of patients with illnesses such as coronary-artery disease, AIDS, and breast cancer turning to the Internet to seek out the latest available information and to converse electronically both with healthcare personnel and with other patients.

Research laboratories will continue to explore how new Internet-based media can assist in clinical decision-making and how cyberspace affects both patient and provider information access and use. For example, it is unknown whether many of the information resources available on-line lead to more informed decision-making on the part of patients or whether these resources cause increased confusion and potential patient anxiety about the complexity of clinical problems.

The emerging ubiquity of the Internet in modern culture will affect the underlying technology with which decision-support systems are developed. Many research laboratories already are studying ways in which decision-support software can be assembled from previously created, tested, and debugged components—much like the software components in the EON system. In the future, repositories of such components will be stored in libraries accessible over the Internet. Such libraries will contain, for example, reusable problem-solving modules for tasks such as diagnosis and planning that developers will apply to the construction of new decision aids. Internet-based libraries will contain standard, controlled terminologies, as well as knowledge bases of commonly needed concepts (e.g., anatomical relationships, temporal properties of clinical data, and frequently prescribed medications and their indications and side effects). Construction of clinical decision aids will involve searching the Internet-based libraries for appropriate reusable components and configuring those components into useful problem-solvers. There will be a need for a new kind of information-retrieval technology—one that can help system builders to locate and configure appropriate decision-support software components from the diverse component libraries that research laboratories, healthcare organizations, and a new industry of component vendors will make available.

Considerations of whether specific components happen to use pattern-recognition methods, Bayesian reasoning, or AI techniques will become less important, as researchers create new approaches for combining different reasoning methods to meet the specific requirements of increasingly complex decision-making tasks. Thus, by mixing and matching components, developers will be able to use Bayesian reasoners for performing probabilistic classification, AI techniques for tasks such as planning or constraint satisfaction, and mathematical models for solving problems that can be best understood in terms of systems of equations. There will be enhanced emphasis on modeling the overall task that a decision-support system performs (e.g., tasks such as therapy planning, differential diagnosis, and simulation of surgical interventions). These task models will then inform the selection of appropriate problem-solving components from various libraries.

Concomitantly, heightened understanding of organizational behavior and of clinical workflow will stimulate a new generation of clinical information systems that will integrate smoothly into the practices of healthcare workers of all kinds. Most important, these new information systems will become the vehicles for delivery of decision-support technology in the decade ahead. The very concept of a *decision-support system* itself will fade away, as intelligent assistants that can enhance the judgment of healthcare workers blend into the infrastructure of healthcare delivery. Automated decision support will take place with every practitioner's routine access to clinical data in a manner that is unobtrusive, transparent, and tailored to the specific patient situation.

20.6.3   *Conclusions*

The future of clinical decision-support systems inherently depends on progress in developing useful computer programs and in reducing logistical barriers to implementation. Although ubiquitous computer-based decision aids that routinely assist physicians in most aspects of clinical practice are currently the stuff of science fiction, progress has been real and the potential remains inspiring. Early predictions about the effects such innovations will have on medical education and practice have not yet come to pass (Schwartz, 1970), but growing successes support an optimistic view of what technology will eventually do to assist practitioners with processing of complex data and knowledge. The research challenges have been identified much more clearly, and the implications for health-science education are much better understood. The basic computer literacy of health professional students can be generally assumed, but health-science educators now must teach the conceptual foundations of biomedical informatics if their graduates are to be prepared for the technologically sophisticated world that lies ahead.

Equally important, we have learned much about what is not likely to happen. The more investigators understand the complex and changing nature of medical knowledge, the clearer it becomes that trained practitioners will always be required as elements in a cooperative relationship between physician and computer-based decision tool. There is no evidence that machine capabilities will ever equal the human mind's ability to deal with unexpected situations, to integrate visual and auditory data that reveal subtleties of a patient's problem, or to deal with social and ethical issues that are often key determinants of proper medical decisions. Considerations such as these will always be important to the humane practice of medicine, and practitioners will always have access to information that is meaningless to the machine. Such observations argue cogently for the discretion of healthcare workers in the proper use of decision-support tools.

Suggested Readings

Berg M. (1997). Rationalizing Medical Work: Decision Support Techniques and Medical Practices. Cambridge, MA: MIT Press.
This book, written by a physician who also is a sociologist, examines the difficulty of incorporating decision-support systems into clinical workflow from an organizational perspective. The book analyzes the failures of early automated decision aids and suggests new principles for decision-system design and integration.

Garg, A.X., Adhikari, N.K.J., McDonald, H., Rosas-Arellano, M.P., Devereaux, P.J., Beyene, J., Sam, J., and Haynes, R.B. (2005). Effects of computerized clinical decision support systems in practitioner performance and patient outcomes: A systematic review. *Journal of the American Medical Association*, 293:1223–1238.
The authors provide a comprehensive review of 100 controlled trials of clinical decision-support sytems. Their analysis shows significant affects on the behavior of health-care workers in a majority (64%) of the studies. Demonstration of effects of decision-support systems on patient outcomes is more problematic, however.

Ledley R., Lusted, L. (1959). Reasoning foundations of medical diagnosis. Science, 130:9–21.
This classic article provided the first influential description of how computers might be used to assist with the diagnostic process. The flurry of activity applying Bayesian methods to computer-assisted diagnosis during the 1960s was largely inspired by this provocative article.

Musen, M.A. (2000). Scalable software architectures for decision support. *Methods of Information in Medicine*, 38:229–238.
This paper provides an overview of reusable of ontologies and problem-solving methods as components of current-generation decision support systems.

Schwartz W. (1970). Medicine and the computer: the promise and problems of change. New England Journal of Medicine, 283(23):1257–1264.

A senior clinician from Boston wrote this frequently cited article, which assessed the growing role of computers in health care. Thirty years later, many of the developments anticipated by Schwartz had come to pass, although the rate of change was slower than he predicted.

Staab, S. and Studer, R. eds. (2004). *Hanbook on Ontologies*, Berlin: Springer-Verlag.
This volume provides a collection of papers that describe current work on ontologies for decision support, information management, and Semantic Web applications.

Questions for Discussion

1. Researchers in medical AI have argued that there is a need for more expert knowledge in medical decision-support systems, but developers of Bayesian systems have argued that expert estimates of likelihoods are inherently flawed and that advice programs must be based on solid data. How do you account for the apparent difference between these views? Which view is valid? Explain your answer.

2. Explain the meaning of Internist-1/QMR's frequency weights and evoking strengths. What does it mean for a finding to have a frequency weight of 4 and an evoking strength of 2? How do these parameters relate to the concepts of sensitivity, specificity, and predictive value that were introduced in Chapters 2 and 3?

3. Let us consider how deDombal and other developers of Bayesian systems have used patient-care experience to guide the collection of statistics that they need. For example, consider the database in the following table, which shows the relationship between two findings (f_1 and f_2) and a disease (D) for 10 patients.

Patient	f_1	f_2	D	,D
1	0	1	0	1
2	0	1	1	0
3	0	1	0	1
4	1	1	1	0
5	1	1	1	0
6	1	1	0	1
7	1	0	1	0
8	1	1	1	0
9	1	0	0	1
10	1	1	1	0

In the table, ,D signifies the absence of disease D. A 0 indicates the absence of a finding or disease, and a 1 indicates the presence of a finding or disease. For example, based on the above database, the probability of finding f1 in this population is 7/10570 percent.

Refer back to Chapters 2 and 3 as necessary in answering the following questions:

a. What are the sensitivity and specificity of each of f1 and f2 for the disease D? What is the prevalence of D in this 10-person population?

b. Use the database to calculate the following probabilities:

• $p[f_1 u D]$

• $p[f_1 u, D]$

• $p[f_2uD]$
• $p[f_2u,D]$
• $p[D]$
• $p[,D]$

c. Use the database to calculate $p[Duf_1 \text{ and } f_2]$.

d. Use the probabilities determined in b to calculate $p[Duf1 \text{ and } ,f2]$ using a heuristic method that assumes that findings f1 and f2 are conditionally independent given a disease and the absence of a disease. Why is this result different from the one in c? Why has it generally been necessary to make this heuristic approximation in Bayesian programs?

4. In an evaluation study, the decision-support system ONCOCIN provided advice concerning cancer therapy that was approved by experts in only 79 percent of cases (Hickam et al., 1985b). Do you believe that this performance is adequate for a computational tool that is designed to help physicians to make decisions regarding patient care? What safeguards, if any, would you suggest to ensure the proper use of such a system? Would you be willing to visit a particular physician if you knew in advance that she made decisions regarding treatment that were approved by expert colleagues less than 80 percent of the time? If you would not, what level of performance would you consider adequate? Justify your answers.

5. A large international organization once proposed to establish an independent laboratory—much like Underwriters Laboratory in the United States—that would test medical decision-support systems from all vendors and research laboratories, certifying the effectiveness and accuracy of those systems before they might be put into clinical use. What are the possible dimensions along which such a laboratory might evaluate decision-support systems? What kinds of problems might such a laboratory encounter in attempting to institute such a certification process? In the absence of such a credentialling system for decision-support systems, how can health-care workers feel confident in using a clinical decision aid?

21
Computers in Medical Education

Parvati Dev, Edward P. Hoffer, and G. Octo Barnett

After reading this chapter, you should know the answers to these questions:

- What are the advantages of computer-aided instruction over traditional lecture-style instruction in medical education?
- What are the different learning methods that can be implemented in computer-based education?
- How can computer-based simulations supplement students' exposure to clinical practice?
- What are the issues to be considered when developing computer-based educational programs?
- What are the significant barriers to widespread integration of computer-aided instruction into the medical curriculum?

21.1 The Role of Computers in Medical Education

The goals of medical education are to provide students and graduate clinicians specific facts and information, to teach strategies for applying this knowledge appropriately to the situations that arise in medical practice, and to encourage development of skills necessary to acquire new knowledge over a lifetime of practice. Students must learn about physiological processes and must understand the relationships between their observations and these underlying processes. They must learn to perform medical procedures, and they must understand the effects of different interventions on health outcomes. In addition, student must learn "softer" skills and knowledge, such as interpersonal and interviewing skills and the ethics of medical care. Medical school faculty employ a variety of strategies for teaching, ranging from the one-way, lecture-based transmission of information to the interactive, Socratic method of instruction. In general, we can view the teaching process as the presentation of a situation or a body of facts that contains the essential knowledge that students should learn; the explanations of what the important concepts and relationships are, how they can be derived, and why they are important; and the strategy for guiding interaction with a patient.

As has been discussed throughout this book, information technology is an increasingly important tool for accessing and managing medical information—both patient-specific and more general scientific knowledge. Medical educators are aware of the need for all medical students to learn to use information technology effectively. Computers also can play a direct role in the education process; students may interact with educational computer programs to acquire factual information and to learn and practice problem-solving techniques. In addition, practicing physicians may use computers to expand and reinforce their professional skills throughout their careers. The application of computer technology to education is often referred to as **computer-assisted learning, computer-based education (CBE)**, or **computer-aided instruction (CAI)**.

In this chapter, we present basic concepts that people should consider when they plan the use of computers in medical education.[1] We begin by reviewing the historical use of computers in medical education, describing various modes of computer-based teaching, and giving examples of teaching programs for preclinical students, clinical students, medical professionals, and the lay public. We then present questions and discuss methodologies to consider in the design and development of teaching programs. In closing, we describe evaluation studies that investigate how these programs are used, as well as the efficiency of CBE.

21.1.1   *Advantages of Using Computers in Medical Education*

A computer can be used to augment, enhance, or replace traditional teaching strategies to provide new methods of learning. With its vast storage capacity, a computer can be an extension of the student's memory, providing quick access to reference and new content. Multimedia capabilities allow the computer to present rapidly a much larger number of images than can be accessed through a book or an atlas and to supplement the static images with sounds, video clips, and interactive teaching modules. Immersive interfaces, which present three-dimensional worlds and allow touch and force feedback through a joystick or instrumented glove, promise to support the training environment of tomorrow.

A computer, properly used, can approach the Socratic ideal of a teacher sitting at one end of a log and a student at the other. In contrast to traditional fact-based, lecture-oriented, mass broadcasting of information, computers can support personalized one-on-one education, delivering material appropriate for learners' needs and interests. "Any time, any place, any pace" learning becomes practical. In traditional education, the learner goes to the lecture, which is held at a specific time and location. If it is not possible for the learner to attend the lecture, or if the location is difficult or expensive to reach, the potential experience may be lost. Computer-based learning can take place at the time and location best suited to the needs of the learner. It can also be individualized and interactive; the learner is able to proceed at his or her own pace, independent of the larger group. By placing the student in simulated clinical situations, or in a simulated examination, a computer-based teaching program can exercise the student's knowledge and decision-making capabilities in a nonthreatening environment. Finally, well-constructed computer-based learning can be enjoyable and engaging, maintaining the interest of the student.

---

[1]Although the focus of this chapter is medical education, the underlying concepts and issues apply equally to nursing and health sciences education.

21.1.2   A Historical Look at the Use of Computers in Medical Education

Despite the many advantages, computer-assisted learning programs initially experienced slow growth before gaining acceptance. Piemme (1988) traced the early development of computer-assisted learning in medicine and discussed reasons for the slow acceptance of this technology. Today, computer-assisted learning has become widely available in the medical field.

Pioneering research in computer-assisted learning was conducted in the late 1960s at three primary locations in the United States: Ohio State University (OSU), Massachusetts General Hospital (MGH), and the University of Illinois. Earlier attempts to use computers in medical instruction were hindered by the difficulty of developing programs using low-level languages and the inconvenience and expense of running programs on batch-oriented mainframe computers. With the availability of time-sharing computers, these institutions were able to develop interactive programs that were accessible to users from terminals via telephone lines.

CBE research began at OSU in 1967 with the development of Tutorial Evaluation System (TES). TES programs typically posed true–false, multiple-choice, matching, or ranking questions and then immediately evaluated the student's responses. The programs rewarded correct answers with positive feedback. Incorrect answers triggered corrective feedback, and, in some cases, students were given another opportunity to respond to the question. If a student was not doing well, the computer might suggest additional study assignments or direct the student to review related materials.

In 1969, TES was incorporated into the evolving Independent Study Program, an experimental program that covered the entire preclinical curriculum and was designed to teach basic medical science concepts to medical students (Weinberg, 1973). Although the program did not use CBE in a primary instructional role, students in the program relied heavily on a variety of self-study aids and used the computer intensively for self-evaluation. The use of COURSEWRITER III, a high-level authoring language, facilitated rapid development of programs. By the mid-1970s, TES had a library of over 350 interactive hours worth of instructional programs.

Beginning in 1970, Barnett and coworkers at the MGH Laboratory of Computer Science developed CBE programs to simulate clinical encounters (Hoffer and Barnett, 1986). The most common simulations were case management programs that allowed students to formulate hypotheses, to decide which information to collect, to interpret data, and to practice problem-solving skills in diagnosis and therapy planning. By the mid-1970s, MGH had developed more than 30 case management simulations, including programs for evaluation of comatose patients, for workup of patients with abdominal pain, and for evaluation and therapy management in areas such as anemia, bleeding disorders, meningitis, dyspnea, secondary hypertension, thyroid disease, joint pain, and pediatric cough and fever.

The MGH laboratory also developed several programs that used mathematical or qualitative models to simulate underlying physiological processes and thus to simulate changes in patient state over time and in response to students' therapeutic decisions. The first simulation modeled the effects of warfarin (an anticoagulant drug) and its effects on blood clotting. The system challenged the user to maintain a therapeutic degree of anticoagulation by prescribing daily doses of warfarin to a patient who had a series of complications and who was taking medications that interacted with warfarin. Subsequently, researchers developed a more complex simulation model to emulate a diabetic patient's reaction to therapeutic interventions.

About the same time, Harless et al. (1971) at the University of Illinois were developing a system called Computer-Aided Simulation of the Clinical Encounter (CASE), which simulated clinical encounters between physician and patient. The computer assumed the role of a patient; the student, acting in the role of practicing physician, managed the patient's disease from onset of symptoms through final treatment. Initially, the computer presented a brief description of the patient, and then the student interacted with the program using natural-language queries and commands. The program was able to provide logical responses to most student requests. This feature added greatly to the realism of the interaction, and CASE programs were received enthusiastically by students. The TIME system, later developed by Harless et al. (1986) at the National Library of Medicine (NLM), extended CASE's approach to incorporate videodisk technology.

CBE programs proliferated on a variety of hardware, using a babel of languages. A 1974 survey of the status of medical CAI identified 362 programs written in 23 different computer languages, ranging from BASIC, FORTRAN, and MUMPS to COURSEWRITER III and Programmed Logic for Automated Teaching Operations (PLATO) (Brigham and Kamp, 1974). Little sharing of programs among institutions was possible because the task of transferring programs was typically as large as writing the material de novo. Thus, there was little opportunity to share the substantial costs of developing new CAI programs. The lack of portability of systems and the extreme expense of system development and testing served as barriers to the widespread use of CAI.

The establishment of an NLM-sponsored, nationwide network in 1972 was a significant event in the development of CBE in medicine because it allowed users throughout the country to access CBE programs easily and relatively inexpensively. Previously, the programs created at OSU, MGH, and the University of Illinois were available to users in selected regions over voice-grade telephone lines. Poor quality of transmission and high costs, however, combined to limit access to CBE programs by distant users. Acting on the recommendation of a committee of the Association of American Medical Colleges, the NLM's Lister Hill Center for Biomedical Communications funded an experimental CBE network. Beginning in July 1972, the CBE programs developed at the MGH, OSU, and the University of Illinois Medical College were made available from these institutions' host computers over the NLM network. During the first 2 years of operation, 80 institutions used the programs of one of the three hosts. The high demand for network use prompted the NLM to institute an hourly usage charge, but use continued to rise. Having exhausted the funds set aside for this experiment, the NLM discontinued financial support for the network in 1975.

As a testimony to the value placed on the educational network by its users, MGH and OSU continued to operate the network as an entirely user-supported activity. Beginning in 1983, the MGH programs were offered as the continuing medical education (CME) component of the American Medical Association's Medical Information Network (AMA/NET). AMA/NET provided a variety of services to subscribing physicians in addition to the CME programs, including access to information databases, to the clinical and biomedical literature, to the DXplain diagnostic decision-support tool, and to electronic-mail services. By the mid-1980s, approximately 100,000 physicians, medical students, nurses, and other people had used the MGH CBE programs over a network, with about 150,000 total contact hours.

During the early 1970s, medical schools around the country began to conduct research in CBE. One of the most interesting programs was the PLATO system developed at the University of Illinois. PLATO used a unique plasma-display terminal that allowed presentation of text, graphics, and photographs, singly or in combination. An electrically excitable gas was used to brighten individual points on the screen selectively. The system also included TUTOR, an early authoring language, to facilitate program development. By 1981, authors had created 12,000 hours of instruction in 150 subject areas. The programs received heavy use at the University of Illinois; some of them also were used at other institutions that had access to the system. The high cost of PLATO and the need for specialized terminals and other computer hardware, however, limited the widespread dissemination of the system.

Research on medical applications of artificial intelligence (AI) stimulated the development of systems based on models of the clinical reasoning of experts. The explanations generated by computer-based consultation systems (e.g., why a particular diagnosis or course of management is recommended) can be used in computer-assisted learning to guide and evaluate students' performance in running patient simulations. The GUIDON system was one of the most interesting examples of such an intelligent tutoring system. GUIDON used a set of teaching strategy rules, which interacted with an augmented set of diagnostic rules from the MYCIN expert system (see Chapter 20), to teach students about infectious diseases (Clancey, 1986).

Researchers at the University of Wisconsin applied a different approach to the simulation of clinical reasoning. Their system was used to assess the efficiency of a student's workup by estimating the cost of the diagnostic evaluation (Friedman et al., 1978). In one of the few successful field studies that demonstrated the clinical significance of a simulated diagnosis problem, Friedman (1973) found significant levels of agreement between physicians' performance on simulated cases and actual practice patterns.

As we discuss in Section 21.4, the development of personal computers (PCs), authoring systems, and network technology removed many of the barriers to program development and dissemination, and CBE software proliferated. PCs provide an affordable and relatively standard environment for development, and CBE programs are now widely available via Internet, CD-ROM, and other media. Section 21.3 describes just a few of the many CBE applications now available.

21.2   Modes of Computer-Based Learning

To practice medicine effectively, physicians must have rapid access to the contents of a large and complex medical knowledge base, and they must know how to apply these facts and heuristics to form diagnostic hypotheses and to plan and evaluate therapies. Thus, conveying a body of specific medical facts, teaching strategies for applying this information in medical practice situations, and assisting students in developing skills for lifelong learning are among the goals of medical education. Computers can be used for a wide range of learning methods, from drilling students on a fixed curriculum to allowing students to explore a body of material using methods best suited to their own learning styles.

21.2.1   *Drill and Practice*

Drill and practice was the first widespread use of computer-based learning, developed almost as soon as computers became available. Teaching material is presented to the student, and the student is evaluated immediately via multiple-choice questions. The computer grades the selected answers and, based on the accuracy of the response, repeats the teaching material, or allows the student to progress to new material (Figure 21.1).

Although it can be tedious, drill and practice still has a role in teaching factual material. It allows the educational system to manage the wide variation in ability of students to assimilate material and frees up instructors for more one-on-one interaction where that technique is most effective. It also allows the instructor to concentrate on more advanced material while the computer deals with presenting the routine factual infor-

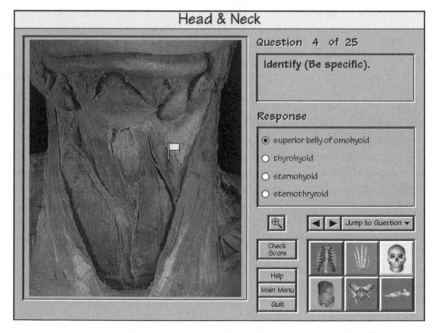

Figure 21.1. Drill and practice. In this image-based quiz, the student is presented with a dissected part and is asked to identify the structure marked with a flag. The question is presented in a multiple-choice format. If he or she wishes, the student can switch to the more difficult option of typing in a textual answer. In typical use, students will use the multiple-choice option while learning the material and the free-text option when evaluating themselves. (*Source*: © 1994, Stanford University, and D. Kim et al. Screen shot from Kim et al., 1995.)

mation. Studies at the elementary school level have found that it is the poorest students who benefit most from computer-based learning, primarily from drill-and-practice work that lets them catch up to their peers (Piemme, 1988).

21.2.2 Didactic: The Lecture

Although much of the focus of computer-based teaching is on the more innovative uses of computers to expand the teaching format, computers can be employed usefully to deliver didactic material, with the advantage of the removal of time and space limitations. A professor can choose to record a lecture and to store, on the computer, the digitized video of the lecture as well as the related slides or other teaching material. This approach has the advantage that relevant background or remedial material can also be made available through links at specific points in the lecture. The disadvantage, of course, is that the professor may not be available to answer questions when the student reviews the lecture (Figure 21.2).

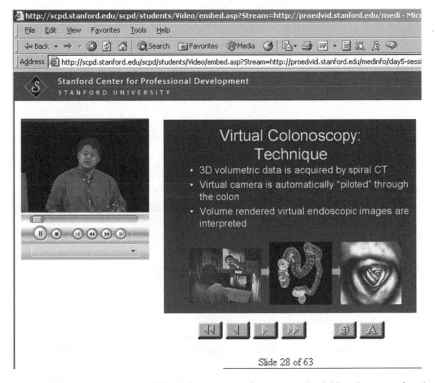

Figure 21.2. Didactic teaching. A digital video lecture is presented within a browser for the Web. The video image in the upper left is augmented with high-resolution images of the lecture slides on the right. Because the whole is presented within a Web browser, additional information, such as links to other Web sites or to study material, could have been added to the Web page. (*Source*: ©2004, Stanford University. Screen shot of a digital video lecture.)

Another use of this method could be the immediate availability on the Internet of presentations from national conferences for interested health students and professionals unable to attend the meetings. With media reports of news from medical meetings often reaching patients the next day as newspaper headlines, physicians can now access the details of the reported news on the Web rather than waiting for published reports, which may lag many months behind the presentations.

An excellent example of how computer-based learning can go beyond the traditional lecture is the Howard Hughes Medical Institute Web site on teaching genetics.[2] This multimedia textbook of genetics uses graphics, hot links, and photographs along with text to present a lively and entertaining series of lectures on genetic disease.

21.2.3   Discrimination Learning

Many clinical situations require the practitioner to differentiate between two apparently similar sets of clinical findings, where subtle differences lead to different diagnoses. **Discrimination learning** is the process that teaches the student to differentiate between the different clinical manifestations. A computer program, through a series of examples of increasing complexity, can train the student to detect the subtle differences. An example is a dermatologic lesion that comprises red rash and inflammation. A rash of the same appearance on different parts of the body can imply different diagnoses. The computer program begins with the differences between a few standard presentations of this lesion and, as the student learns to discriminate between these, presents additional types (Sanford et al., 1996).

21.2.4   Exploration Versus Structured Interaction

Teaching programs differ by the degree to which they impose structure on a teaching session. In general, drill-and-practice systems are highly structured. The system's responses to students' choices are specified in advance; students cannot control the course of an interaction directly. In contrast, other programs create an exploratory environment in which students can experiment without guidance or interference. For example, a neuroanatomy teaching program may provide a student with a fixed series of images and lessons on the brainstem, or it may allow a student to select a brain structure of interest, such as a tract, and to follow the structure up and down the brainstem, moving from image to image, observing how the location and size of the structure changes.

Each of these approaches has advantages and disadvantages. Drill-and-practice programs usually teach important facts and concepts but do not allow students to deviate from the prescribed course or to explore areas of special interest. Conversely, programs that provide an exploratory environment and that allow students to choose any actions in any order encourage experimentation and self-discovery. Without structure or guidance, however, students may waste time following unproductive paths and may fail to learn important material, the result being inefficient learning.

---

[2]Howard Hughes Medical Institute Web site on teaching genetics. http: //www.hhmi.org/GeneticTrail/.

21.2.5   *Constrained Versus Unconstrained Response*

The mechanism for communication between a student and a teaching program can take one of several basic forms. At one extreme, a student, working with a simulation of a patient encounter, may select from a constrained list of responses that are valid in the current situation. The use of a predefined set of responses has two disadvantages: It cues the student (suggests ideas that otherwise might not have occurred to him), and it detracts from the realism of the simulation. On the other hand, simulations that provide students with a list of actions that are allowable and reasonable in a particular situation are easier to write, because the authors do not need to anticipate all responses.

At the opposite extreme, students are free to query the program and to specify actions using unconstrained natural language. Computer recognition of such natural language, however, is just beginning to be feasible. An intermediate approach is to provide a single, comprehensive menu of possible actions, thus constraining choices in a program-specific, but not a situation-specific, manner. The use of a list of actions and a constrained vocabulary is less frustrating to those students who may have difficulty formulating valid interactions.

21.2.6   *Construction*

One of the most effective—but extremely difficult to implement on the computer—ways to teach is the **constructive** approach to learning. A relatively simple example is learning anatomy through reconstructing the human body either by putting together the separated body parts or by placing cross sections at the correct location in the body.

21.2.7   *Simulation*

Many advanced teaching programs use **simulations** to engage the learner (Gaba, 2004). Learning takes place most effectively when the learner is engaged and actively involved in decision making. The use of a simulated patient presented by the computer can approximate the real-world experience of patient care and concentrates the learner's attention on the subject being presented.

Simulation programs may be either **static** or **dynamic**. Figure 21.3 illustrates an interaction between a student and a simulated patient. Under the static simulation model, each case presents a patient who has a predefined problem and set of characteristics. At any point in the interaction, the student can interrupt data collection to ask the computer consultant to display the differential diagnosis (given the information that has been collected so far) or to recommend a data collection strategy. The underlying case, however, remains static. Dynamic simulation programs, in contrast, simulate changes in patient state over time and in response to students' therapeutic decisions. Thus, unlike those in static simulations, the clinical manifestations of a dynamic simulation can be programmed to evolve as the student works through them. These programs help students to understand the relationships between actions (or inactions) and patients' clinical outcomes. To simulate a patient's response to intervention, the programs may explicitly model underlying physiological processes and may use mathematical models.

Immersive simulated environments, with a physical simulation of a patient in an authentic environment such as an operating room, have evolved into sophisticated learning environments. The patient is simulated by an artificial manikin with internal mechanisms that produce the effect of a breathing human with a pulse, respiration, and other vital signs. In high-end simulators, the manikin can be given blood transfusions or medication, and its physiology will alter based on these treatments. These human patient simulators are now used around the world both for skills training and for cognitive training such as crisis management or leadership in a team environment. The environment can represent an operating room, a neonatal intensive care unit, a trauma center, or a physician's office. Teams of learners play roles such as surgeon, anesthetist, or nurse, and practice teamwork, crisis management, leadership, and other cognitive exercises. An extension of the physical human patient simulator is the virtual patient in a virtual operating room or emergency room. Learners are also present virtually, logging in from remote sites, to form a team to manage the virtual patient.

Procedure trainers or *part task trainers* have emerged as a new method of teaching, particularly in the teaching of surgical skills. This technology is still under development, and it is extremely demanding of computer and graphic performance. Early examples have focused on endoscopic surgery and laparoscopic surgery in which the surgeon manipulates tools and a camera inserted into the patient through a small incision. In the simulated environment, the surgeon manipulates the same tool controls, but these tools control simulated instruments that act on computer-graphic renderings of the operative field. Feedback systems inside the tools return pressure and other haptic sensations to the surgeon's hands, further increasing the realism of the surgical experience. Simulated environments will become increasingly useful for all levels of surgery, beginning with training in the basic operations of incision and suturing and going all the way to complete surgical operations. Commercial trainers are now available for some basic surgical tasks and for training eye–hand coordination during laparoscopic procedures.

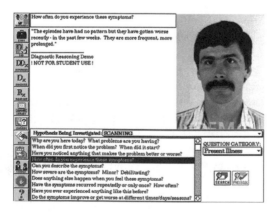

Figure 21.3. A typical interaction screen in a sequential diagnosis problem with a simulated patient. The user interrogates the computer about history, physical findings, and laboratory test results of a simulated patient to reach a diagnosis. (*Source*: © 1993, Diagnostic Reasoning, Illinois. Screen shot from the Diagnostic Reasoning program.)

21.2.8 Feedback and Guidance

Closely related to the structure of an interaction is the degree to which a teaching program provides **feedback** and **guidance** to students. Virtually all systems provide some form of feedback—for example, they may supply short explanations of why answers are correct or incorrect, present summaries of important aspects of cases, or provide references to related materials. Many systems provide an interactive help facility that allows students to ask for hints and advice.

21.2.9 Intelligent Tutoring Systems

More sophisticated systems allow students to take independent action but may intervene if the student strays down an unproductive path or acts in a way that suggests a misconception of fact or inference. Such **mixed-initiative systems** allow students freedom but provide a framework that constrains the interaction and thus helps students to learn more efficiently. Some researchers make a distinction between **coaching** systems and **tutoring** systems. The less proactive coaching systems monitor the session and intervene only when the student requests help or makes serious mistakes. Tutoring systems, on the other hand, guide a session aggressively by asking questions that test a student's understanding of the material and that expose errors and gaps in the student's knowledge. Mixed-initiative systems are difficult to create because they must have models both of the student and of the problem to be solved (Eliot et al., 1996).

21.3 Current Applications

Computer-based learning has been developed for the beginning medical student and the experienced practitioner: for the layperson and the medical expert. In this section, we present examples of actual programs that are being used to support medical education for each of these categories of learners.

21.3.1 Preclinical Applications

Traditional teaching in the preclinical years has been through lectures to large groups and laboratory exercises. With increasing laboratory costs and increasing amounts of information to be imparted to students, the individual, hands-on component of learning has decreased. Computer-based learning has the promise to return the student to individualized, interactive learning while reducing the need to teach in the lecture setting. Teaching programs have been developed for most subjects and using all styles of pedagogy. We describe here a few interesting programs for preclinical learning.

BrainStorm, developed at Stanford University, is an interactive atlas of neuroanatomy, with images of dissections and cross sections, diagrams, and extensive supporting text (Hsu, 1996). The unit of knowledge is a brain structure, such as nucleus, tract, vessel, or subsystem. Each unit has references to three modes of information presentation—image, diagram, and text—each of which contains representations of many structures, the result being a richly connected network of information. When compared with hyperlinks on Web pages, which may lead the student astray from the original learning goal, a named link, such as a cross-reference to an image, contains information that helps the student to decide whether to follow that link and to retrieve the expected information. Multiple-choice quizzes on every image provide thousands of questions for self-evaluation. Animated simulations teach the basics of skills such as performing an examination for a cranial-nerve lesion.

The Digital Anatomist, at the University of Washington, Seattle, uses three-dimensional models of brain and anatomic structures to teach about anatomic structure and localization. A unique aspect of this program is its accessibility over the Internet. Using a client program, the student requests new views of the models. Rotations of the model are performed on the powerful server at the university, and the resulting images are sent to the student for viewing on the client program (Rosse et al., 1998).

The Visible Human male and female are an extraordinary resource available through the NLM.[3] Thousands of cross sections represent the entire bodies of two humans. These data have been licensed freely by numerous sites that then use these images for teaching, for annotation of anatomic structures, for reconstruction of three-dimensional anatomy, for research on image processing and object segmentation, and for research on the development of large image databases.

Developed by researchers at the Harvard Medical School, HeartLab is a simulation program designed to teach medical students to interpret the results of auscultation of (listening to) the heart, a skill that requires regular practice on a variety of patient cases (Bergeron and Greenes, 1989). Physicians can diagnose many cardiac disorders by listening to the sounds made by the movement of the heart valves and the movement of blood in the heart chambers and vessels. HeartLab provides an interactive environment for listening to heart sounds as an alternative to the common practice of listening to audiotapes. A student wearing headphones can compare and contrast similar-sounding abnormalities and can hear the changes in sounds brought on by changes in patient position (sitting versus lying down) and by physician maneuvers (such as changing the location of the stethoscope).

21.3.2   Clinical Teaching Applications

For many years, teaching hospitals usually had numerous patients with diagnostic problems such as unexplained weight loss or fever of unknown origin. This environment allowed for thoughtful "visit rounds," at which the attending could tutor the students and house staff, who could then go to the library to research the subject. A patient might have been in the hospital for weeks, as testing was being pursued and the illness evolved. In the modern era of Medicare's system of lump-sum payment for diagnosis-related groups (DRGs) and of managed care, such a system appears as distant as professors in morning coats. The typical patient in today's teaching hospital is very sick, usually elderly, and commonly acutely ill. The emphasis is on short stays, with diagnos-

---

[3]The Visible Human project: http: // www.nlm.nih.gov/research/ visible/visible_human.html.

tic problems handled on an outpatient basis and diseases evolving at home or in chronic care facilities. Thus, the medical student is faced with few "diagnostic problems" and has little opportunity to see the evolution of a patient's illness over time.

One response of medical educators has been to try to move teaching to the outpatient setting; another has been to use computer-modeled patients. Simulated patients allow rare diseases to be presented and allow the learner to follow the course of an illness over any appropriate time period. Faculty can decide what clinical material must be seen and can use the computer to ensure that this core curriculum is achieved. Moreover, with the use of an indestructible patient, the learner can take full responsibility for decision making, without concern over harming an actual patient by making mistakes. Finally, cases developed at one institution can be shared easily with other organizations. Case libraries are available on the Internet; examples include the AAMC Virtual Patients database[4] and geriatric cases from the University of Florida.[5]

Clinical reasoning tools—such as DXplain, Iliad, and Quick Medical Reference (QMR)—are discussed in Chapter 20. Although not typically thought of as educational in the traditional sense, such diagnostic support systems can provide the ideal educational experience of giving aid to a physician or student when he or she is involved with a real case and thus is most receptive to learning. Literature searching (Chapter 19) confers the same advantages.

The National Board of Medical Examiners (NBME) has had a long-standing interest in using computer-based case simulations for their examinations. These simulations include cost as well as time considerations. The NBME has begun to use these cases in their computer-based examination of medical students.

21.3.3   Continuing Medical Education

Medical education does not stop after the completion of medical school and formal residency training. The science of medicine advances at such a rapid rate that much of what is taught becomes outmoded, and it has become obligatory for physicians to be lifelong learners both for their own satisfaction and, increasingly, as a formal government requirement to maintain licensure.

Although the physician practicing at a major medical center usually has no problem obtaining the required hours of accredited CME, physicians who practice in rural areas or other more isolated locations may face considerable obstacles. Physician CME has become a large industry and is widely available, but often the course fees are high, and attendance also incurs the direct costs of lodging and transportation and the indirect costs of time lost from practice. The cost of CBE is often much lower.

With increasing specialization and subspecialization has come an added difficulty. Traditional lecture-based CME must aim at a broad audience. Therefore, many listeners know as much or more about the topic than the speaker; many others find the material too difficult or of little relevance. A pure subspecialist—even one at a major medical center—may find the majority of CME offerings irrelevant to his or her practice. The

---

[4]AAMC website for Virtual Patients database: http://www.aamc.org/meded/mededportal/vp/
[5]University of Florida Web site on clinical teaching cases: http: //medinfo.ufl.edu/cme/geri/.

ideal form of CME for many physicians would be a preceptorship with a mentor in the same discipline, but the costs of providing such an experience on a wide scale would be prohibitive. With the increasing amount of computer-based material available, including self-assessment examinations from specialty societies, specialists can select topics that are of interest to them. Well-known examples are the Medical Knowledge Self-Assessment Program (MKSAP) from the American College of Physicians, now in its 13th edition, which is available in print and on CD-ROM, and the American College of Cardiology's Self-Assessment Program (ACCSAP), now in its 5th edition, and available in print, on CD-ROM, and online.

Both literature searching (Chapter 19) and use of diagnostic support systems (Chapter 20) are an important part of a physician's continuing education. These aids to the diagnosis and management of complex patient problems reach the physicians when they are most receptive to learning new material. Clinicians must rely on and maintain a very large inventory of rapidly accessible information kept in long-term memory and less accessible resources kept on a bookshelf. To be effective, education need not be formally labeled as such. Often the best education for the practicing clinician occurs in the context of caring for a particular patient. When the "teachable moment" arrives, the education message may be delivered by a colleague or by a consultant, or it may be in the form of a chunk of knowledge delivered by an intelligent computer system. One of the more promising research activities involves the development of a just-in-time (Chueh and Barnett, 1997) approach to delivering knowledge-rich and problem-focused information during the course of routine clinical care.

21.3.4   Consumer Health Education

Today's patients have become health care consumers; they often bring to the health care provider a mass of health-related information (and misinformation) gathered from the media. Medical topics are widely discussed in general interest magazines, in newspapers, on television, and over the Internet. Patients may use the Internet to join disease- or symptom-focused chat groups or to search for information about their own conditions. At the same time that patients have become more sophisticated in their requests for information, practitioners have become increasingly pressed for time under the demands of managed care. Shorter visits allow less time to educate patients. Computers can be used to print information about medications, illnesses, and symptoms so that patients leave the office with a personalized handout that they can read at home. Personal risk profiling can be performed with widely available software, often free from pharmaceutical firms. This type of software clearly illustrates for the patient how such factors as lack of exercise, smoking, or untreated hypertension or hyperlipidemia can reduce life expectation and how changing them can prolong it.

A torrent of consumer-oriented health sites have flowed onto the Web. As we discussed in Chapter 15, one problem that complicates the use of any information site on the Internet is lack of control. Consumers are not readily able to distinguish factual information from hype and snake oil. An important role for the health care provider today is to suggest high-quality Web sites that can be trusted to provide valid information. Many such sites are available from the various branches of the National Institutes of Health (NIH) and from medical professional organizations. The American Medical Association maintains a Web site[6] that includes validated information about such topics as migraine, asthma, human immunodeficiency virus (HIV), and acquired immune deficiency syndrome (AIDS), depression, high blood pressure, and breast cancer. The National Institute of Diabetes and Digestive and Kidney Diseases of the NIH has extensive consumer-oriented material[7] that can be directly accessed by patients. Alternatively, physicians can use the site to print material for distribution to their patients. Most national disease-oriented organizations such as the American Heart Association and the American Diabetes Association now maintain Web sites that can be recommended with confidence. These sites provide additional links to numerous Web sites that have been evaluated for and found to meet a minimum level of quality. A good source of qualified material in a wide variety of topics is available for consumers in NLM's Medline Plus.

21.3.5   *Distance Learning*

The Internet, and in particular the Web, has radically changed the way that we access information. It is now possible to earn university degrees from home at every level from bachelor's to doctorate. Physician CME credit is increasingly available in the same way, in many instances free with pharmaceutical company sponsorship or at modest cost.

A widely used example is Medscape.[8] Their Web site (http: //www.medscape.com/cme-centerdirectory/default) offers hundreds of hours of AMA Category I CME for physicians at no cost. The user must register and endure pharmaceutical advertisements, but has no out-of-pocket costs. Medscape offers detailed reports of papers presented at many major medical meetings, appearing online within hours or days of the presentation.

Numerous Internet sites offer a teaching experience along with CME credit. Helix,[9] sponsored by GlaxoWellcome but without obvious commercial bias, offers articles on nutrition, exercise, and fitness, each of which provides 1 or 1.5 hours of credit after the student completes a test. Grand Rounds on Frontiers in Biomedicine from the George Washington University School of Medicine is also available, in either text or video format. The Marshall University School of Medicine offers the Interactive Patient,[10] a simulated case with which a physician can earn 1 hour of CME credit for a fee of $15. A good source of pointers to online medical education is maintained at the Online Continuing Medical Education site.[11] This site provides a listing of Web educational resources organized by speciality or by topic, with almost 300 sites included.

---

[6]American Medical Association Web site: http:// www.ama-assn.org/.
[7]National Institute of Diabetes and Digestive and Kidney Diseases Web site: http: //www.niddk.nih.gov/.
[8]Medscape Web site: http: //www.medscape.com/ .
[9]GlaxoWellcome's Helix Web site: http: // www.helix.com/.
[10]Marshall University School of Medicine's "Interactive Patient" Web site: http: //medicus.marshall.edu/.
[11]Online Continuing Medical Education Web site: http: //www.cmelist.com/list.htm

Many medical journals, such as the *New England Journal of Medicine* and the *Cleveland Clinic Journal of Medicine* offer online CME tests, with certificates printed immediately after the test is completed.

As we begin a new century, the Internet shows great promise for supporting distance education, but it still has many problems. The challenges facing a physician or a health care provider who is seeking education via the Internet are similar to those of any other user. Technical problems still abound, and the regular user of the Internet is subject to being disconnected in mid-use for no apparent reason. Those people who most need distance learning, such as rural practitioners, are least likely to have high-speed connections, and so are faced with very slow downloading of programs that make extensive use of graphics. In addition to technical problems, the anarchic nature of the Internet means that the environment still dictates caveat emptor. There is no way of telling in advance whether a listed CME program is of high quality, although restricting use to sites that offer AMA Category 1 credit provides some assurance of worthwhile content. Students must also be prepared to find that sites listed in reference guides no longer exist or have changed from the description in the reference guide.

21.4   Design, Development, and Technology

Creation of computer-based learning material requires a systematic process of design and implementation, using technologies appropriate to learning goals. We present some of the issues that arise in this process.

21.4.1   Design of Computer-Based Learning Applications

In the past, each university or group developed its own approach to the design and implementation of its learning software. Developers at each site climbed a learning curve as they determined appropriate designs for pedagogy on the computer and the associated structuring of information. Although no broadly accepted method of design yet exists, a four-level approach to program design appears to be emerging independently at many sites. The four levels are structured content; query, retrieval, and indexing; authoring and presentation; and analysis and reasoning.

Structured Content

Early authoring tools, such as HyperCard and ToolBook, as well as tools for Hypertext Markup Language (HTML) contributed to a development approach in which the learning content, both text and media, was embedded inside the program, along with the code that presented the content and allowed navigation through the program. This intuitive approach to development had the beneficial result that engaging courseware was developed by numerous content experts who did not need to know complex programming languages. On the negative side, the content was difficult to maintain, expand, or modify because the content and its presentation were intermingled throughout the program. Understanding the functionality of a segment of code was also complicated because its operation might depend on many other segments scattered throughout the program. It is therefore desirable that content be maintained separate from the code for its presentation and navigation. Once content is externalized, it is necessary that the content be formatted in a predictable structure such that it can be read and correctly linked by a computer program.

Structured content is different from narrative text. A paragraph of text in a clinical report is narrative text. When the paragraph is broken into subsections, each subsection representing a coherent concept, with the name of the concept used as a tag or keyword to label that subsection, the paragraph has been converted to structured text. A database record, with fields, is a structured item. We can perform computations on a structured item other than simply displaying it. For example, a database can be searched for all occurrences of a specific type of content within a specified field. Another approach to structured content is seen in Extensible Markup Language (XML), a subset of Standardized General Markup Language (SGML) constituting a particular text markup language for interchange of structured data.

Structured content requires more than structuring for layout. It adds labels or tags for semantic structuring (Figure 21.4). The Digital Library Project (Fox and Marchionini, 1998) has developed sample document models and semantic tags for numerous domains, such as environmental engineering and computer science technical reports. Tags that indicate the title of an article, its author, and its date of publication are examples of semantic tags. In clinical material, tags can be developed at many different levels of specificity. A single tag may be used to indicate an entire section on physical examination of the patient. Alternatively, a tag could be used for each step of the examination. Careful design of semantic tags may allow content created for one learning purpose to be reused in other programs.

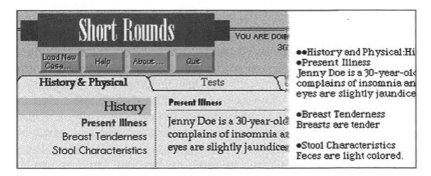

Figure 21.4. Comparison of the final presentation of some clinical content (on the left) with the structured text (on the right) that generated the final view. Simple markup tags (• and ••) are used to indicate header elements and individual feature or findings elements. The program that creates the presentation detects these markup tags and positions the corresponding content appropriately on the page or screen. (*Source*: © 1998, Stanford University. A composite screen shot of the Short Rounds program and of the text file used in the program.)

Query, Retrieval, and Indexing

The second level of design of teaching programs is providing the ability for users to index into and retrieve desired content. Query and retrieval capabilities are rarely used in teaching programs, but indexing is often available. This difference is significant. An index is developed by the author either manually or automatically and is stored along with the program. The student can access only the terms and links made available by the author. Segments of the content that are not indexed cannot be accessed by the student through the index.

In **query and retrieval**, the terms are selected by the student. They can be matched against a predetermined index or, preferably, against a thesaurus that searches for synonyms, more global concepts, and more specific concepts. The system searches the content using the student's terms and any other terms selected through the thesaurus. The entire searchable content can be accessed through this method. Queries that were not conceived of by the program's author, such as one involving an unexpected combination of terms, can be executed by the student.

In unstructured content, searches are executed on the full text. If the content is structured, searches can be applied specifically to certain categories of information. This technique has the potential to increase the specificity of the search because the content is searched in the context (category) specified by the student.

Authoring and Presentation

The third level of teaching program design is programming for author support and for presentation. The ability of subject matter experts to develop courseware within a reasonable time frame depends on the availability of good authoring systems. The ability of the student to understand the program and to make good use of its content depends on the presentation of the content.

An **authoring system** allows the expert to focus on the content of the teaching program and to be unconcerned with the details of writing a computer program. Early teaching programs, using multimedia and hyperlinks, had their content and code intermixed. The content author was also the person programming the navigation and presentation of the content. He or she had to do both even if the programming was at a high level, such as creating flow diagrams for content navigation. An authoring system is based on the recognition that a content domain has a predictable structure—then the author is provided with a template that represents this structure. Content is entered into the template through familiar operations such as typing or importing a digital image. In microbiology, for example, a category of microbes is *bacteria*. For almost every type of bacteria, the following categories are required: description, pathogenesis, laboratory tests, clinical syndromes caused, and other bacteria that can also cause these syndromes. Similarly, every description of a patient's case includes categories such as history, physical examination, tests and procedures, diagnosis, and treatment. A template based on domain structure not only provides a framework for authoring, but also allows multiple authors to create content in parallel, greatly speeding the authoring process.

The *presentation* includes the graphic design of the screen, the location and appearance of the content, the selection of the content to be presented, and the navigation to other content. Although there are numerous resources for guidance in graphic design and content presentation, little is known about how presentation affects the process of learning or the use of the content. Studying the use of the richly linked program for neuroanatomy, BrainStorm, described in Section 21.3.1, Hsu (1996) observed that students who were reviewing the subject made extensive use of annotated cross-section images and the related quizzes. On the other hand, students who were engaged in primary learning made significant use of the many textual resources in the program. The presentation was the same in both cases, but the users' objectives differed, leading to different uses of the program. A further question that has not been studied is whether manipulation of the presentation could have altered the usage. For example, if the program had detected significant study of brainstem nuclei and had prompted the student about the availability of diagrams that had not been examined, would a large number of students have chosen to examine these diagrams?

Teaching content available on the Web is characterized by a large number of links, many leading to material that is distracting for the serious learner. The value of these links lies in making available a large range of content. The student is often, however, unable to judge the quality and value of the content reachable by these links. Navigation support information that indicates the nature of the linked content could increase greatly the value of each such link.

Content-driven automated presentation systems are based on the use of structured content. The selection of content, the layout of the presentation, and the availability of linked information all can be driven by structured content. Figure 21.4 shows the contents of a text file containing structured content and the resulting multimedia presentation. On the one hand, the display program reads and parses the structured content, determining the text and links that will be displayed and the layout that will accommodate the necessary content. On the other hand, because the display is created anew each time, the author has the flexibility to use any terms desired to represent the findings to be displayed. For example, the author may choose to add a finding under the label "Diet," remove the "Stool Characteristics" finding, and change the name of a finding from "Present Illness" to "Chief Complaint." The presentation program will read this file of structured content and will delete the button "Stool Characteristics," add a button for "Diet," and change the name of the "Present Illness" button. The appropriate text will get linked to the new Diet button.

Analysis and Reasoning

The fourth level of design, analysis, and reasoning is frequently not included in a teaching program. A program with built-in automated assessment of students would have analysis capability. A program that observed the student's use of it and identified relevant missed material would be reasoning about the student's possible needs. Intelligent tutoring systems, discussed in Section 21.2.9, have this capability.

21.4.2   Application Development

The process for development of computer-based teaching material is similar to the process for almost any other software project (see Chapter 6). The process begins with identification of a need and a definition of what that need is. This step is followed by a system design and prototyping stage, accompanied by a formative evaluation process. Once the design of the software has been clarified, the software is implemented in the programming language of choice, and the teaching content is entered. The software is then integrated into the teaching process and is evaluated in use. Throughout, the design is guided by available standards for software design as well as for design of content structure.

Definition of the Need

Because the development process for teaching programs is labor-intensive and time-consuming, appropriate planning is essential. Defining the need for computer-based teaching in the curriculum is the first step. Are there difficult concepts that could be explained well through an interactive animated presentation? Is there a need for an image collection that exceeds that which is presented in the context of the lecture? Does the laboratory need support in the form of a guided tour through a library of digitized cross-section images? Could a quantitative concept be explained clearly through a simulation of the physiological or biochemical process, with the student being able to vary the important parameters? Is there a need for a chat group or a newsgroup to supplement the lectures or discussion sections? Would a central repository for course handouts reduce the load on departmental staff?

Assessment of the Resources

The availability and commitment of a content and teaching expert is an obvious necessity. The rich multimedia nature of most computer-based teaching programs implies that graphic, video, and audio media resources must be acquired or be available. Slides or video that are used in the classroom are supplemented by comments from the lecturer, which compensate for their deficiencies. These materials must stand on their own in a software program. Therefore, acquiring media of sufficient quality and comprehensiveness, along with the necessary release of rights, is an important next step in development. Supporting staff for the development process and the necessary funds are additional resources that must be considered.

Prototyping and Formative Evaluation

Significant scholarly work is needed in **prototyping** and **evaluation**, because so little is known about how technology can support medical teaching. Anecdotal results suggest that market research focus groups and small discussion groups with a facilitator can lead to significantly useful design changes in the early stages of development. Participatory development can clarify the focus of the project and modify it so as to make the tool more useful to students (Dev et al., 1998).

Formative evaluation (see Chapter 11) is conducted during the evolution of a project, sometimes at many stages: as the idea is being developed, after the first storyboards are prepared (storyboards are sketches of typical screens, with the interactive behavior indicated), during examination of comparable software, and as segments of the software are developed. During formative evaluation, developers must be prepared to make major changes in direction if such changes will increase the value of the project while retaining the overall goal and keeping the budget within the available resources.

Production

Prototyping determines the form of the teaching program, its goals, the levels of media inclusion and interactivity, the nature of the feedback, and other design parameters. **Production** is the process of executing this design for the entire range of content determined earlier. The requirements during production differ from those of prototyping. Adequate funding and staffing resources must be available at all times. Media must be acquired and processed to the specified standard, and content must be written. Because simultaneous authoring may be needed for different segments and multiple authors may need to review the same section, a method of content collection and version control must be set up. Regular integration of the content into the overall program is required so that any problems of scaling or compatibility will be determined early. Production should be embarked on only if it is very clear that the project is needed and that the resources for completion will be available.

Integration in the Curriculum

An important aspect of courseware development that is often overlooked is the integration of computer-based materials with the curriculum. Currently, most computer-based materials are treated as supplementary material; they are placed in libraries and are used by students or physicians on these users' own initiative. This use is valid, and the programs serve as valuable resources for the students who use them; however, an educator can use such materials more effectively by integrating them into the standard curriculum. For example, programs might be assigned as laboratory exercises or used as the basis of a class discussion.

One of the barriers to integration is the initial high cost of acquiring sufficient computing resources. The cost of the computer equipment has fallen drastically in recent years; even so, the cost of purchasing and supporting enough computers for a whole school to use would be a major item in the curriculum budget of a school. This consideration will become less important as more students purchase their own computers. A second, and important, barrier is the reluctance of faculty to modify their teaching to include references to computer-based material or to operate these programs in the context of their teaching. One of the most effective uses of these programs has been as a lead-in to a small group discussion, such as the presentation of a clinical case on the computer, with students choosing the questions to ask the computer.

Maintenance and Upgrades

Changes in content and changes in the computer operating system or hardware, as well as the discovery of problems with the program, necessitate regular maintenance and upgrades. At the same time, good design requires that any major change in teaching method should trigger iteration through the entire design cycle.

Standards

Maintaining a balance between evolution and standards is difficult but necessary. It is particularly difficult because the publicly acknowledged standards themselves change so rapidly. The standards that apply to teaching programs have to do with the **metadata**: the information that describes the content and thus adds structure to the content. The IMS Learning Resources Meta-data Specification[12] and the Sharable Content Object Reference Model (SCORM)[13] are metadata specifications that have gained widespread acceptance in the learning technology community.

An important value of standardization for sharing among groups is that content created by one group of developers or authors is available for use by another group of authors. Another result of standardization is that presentation and authoring programs can be developed in parallel with content creation. Furthermore, if the standard is upgraded, or if new features are added, programs can be created to convert automatically all material from the old standard to the new.

21.4.3   Technology Considerations

Technology considerations determine the cost and availability of the final teaching product. For example, a program can be delivered on a Web client, or the software designer can choose between developing for the Windows or the Macintosh operating system. True platform independence is a myth, but it is possible to restrict development to a subset of features such that the teaching program has a high probability of running on most computers. The choice of operating over the Internet versus processing on a local machine is a decision that is dependent on the source of the learning content and the performance requirements of the program. Teaching programs that draw on content at many locations on the Internet—such as image collections, digital video, and text reference material—will be restricted by the constraints of a Web client, including a restricted number of display and interaction features. On the other hand, Internet access is more desirable if the program accesses rapidly changing content or bibliographic sources such as Medline.

A need for high performance, or for very large volumes of content, will restrict usage to a local machine. In some cases, such as the use of three-dimensional models in the Virtual Reality Modeling Language (VRML), the model is obtained from a site on the Internet but is then manipulated and displayed locally. The availability of high-capacity storage devices, such as digital video disk (DVD), makes it possible to distribute large quantities of material, with the Internet used for updates, extension of content, and links to additional content.

---

[12]http://www.imsglobal.org/metadata.
[13]http://www.adlnet.org

21.5   Evaluation

Evaluation of a new teaching or training method can measure numerous attributes of success: four levels of evaluation are commonly accepted. The first is the reaction of the student population to the new teaching method and how well the method is assimilated into the existing process of teaching. These measure the *acceptability* of the method. The second level of evaluation is the *usability* of the teaching program. The third level of evaluation measures whether the new teaching method actually had any impact on what the students learned. Here *knowledge acquisition* is measured. The fourth level measures whether the new method results in *behavioral change* because, in the final analysis, content and procedures learned by students should affect how they practice medicine.

21.5.1   Reaction and Assimilation

Many evaluation studies focus on the acceptability of a teaching program to teachers and students. This information is collected through questionnaires, subjective reports, and measurement of actual usage. Without this baseline information, interpretation of more sophisticated analysis may be difficult. These measures do not, however, inform the developer about the effectiveness of a teaching program.

21.5.2   Usability and Cognitive Evaluation

If we wish to measure whether the student understands the operation and capabilities of the program, numerous methods are available. Two complementary methods are the use of the videotaped encounter with the program and the use of the automatically generated log of the student's interaction with the program.

The videotape encounter typically records the actions and words of the student as well as the events on the screen, often presented for analysis in a picture-in-picture format. The video transcript is then segmented into individual events or items. Subsequently, these items are categorized in terms of their cognitive aspects, such as "searching for button" or "selects link to additional information." The researchers use the resultant list of cognitive transactions to identify major categories of usage, sources of success and frustration, and typical information-seeking patterns.

A computer-generated log file can be created if the teaching program is instrumented to record the student's interaction with the program. It may be desirable to be able to select which types of interactions will be recorded. In an analysis of BrainStorm usage (Hsu, 1996), the granularity of recorded information ranged from detecting transfers between pages of information to detecting the selection of every click on a highly detailed annotated image. A computer-generated log file of student interactions can be processed automatically to detect frequency and patterns of usage. Figure 21.5 shows the pattern of transitions between four different types of information in BrainStorm. The students clearly preferred to study the cross-sectional images over all other types of information. A drawback of the automated log is the lack of any information about the student's motives for the interactions. Researchers can gather such information by interrupting

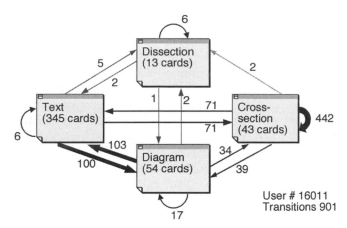

Figure 21.5. Transition graph showing how one student moved between different types of information in the neuroanatomy program BrainStorm. Of the 900 transitions, almost one-half were from one cross-sectional image to another. Even though there were a large number (345) of text screens, with many available hyperlinks between the screens, there was little movement from one text screen to another. Analyses such as these clarify usage and suggest program design strategies. (*Source*: © 1996, Hsu. Adapted from Hsu, 1996.)

selected interactions and requesting the student to type in a comment, but this method is intrusive and breaks the process of information acquisition.

21.5.3   *Knowledge Acquisition*

Evaluation of knowledge acquisition includes the question that is asked most often of developers: Is this computer program more effective than traditional methods of teaching the same material? This question has proved difficult to answer because of the many changes introduced when computer-based teaching is used. One of the most important confounding factors is the renewed attention that the professor pays to preparing teaching material because the course is to be taught in a new format. Perhaps the most interesting evaluation questions are: In what ways is computer-based learning *different from* traditional methods of learning? Can computers enable learning in ways never before possible? Going further, can computers perform evaluations of knowledge acquisition that would be impossible using traditional written or oral examination techniques?

An example of computer-based evaluation is the evaluation of nonverbal knowledge of spatial location in anatomy (Friedman et al., 1993). The rationale was that the better a person knows anatomy, the more accurately he or she will recognize and localize an image of a cross section of the human body. The authors developed a computer game in which the examinee was given an outline of a cross section, with no internal structures displayed, and was asked to position it on a drawing of the human body. The examinee could request additional clues, the clues being pictures of organs in the cross section. After each clue, the examinee was asked to make an attempt to position the slice in the body. Requesting too many clues resulted in a penalty that reduced the maximum possible score. The final score was based on the accuracy of the placement and the number of clues requested. The test differentiated between first-year medical students, fourth-year medical students, and anatomy faculty in their mastery of anatomic knowledge.

21.5.4   Problem Solving and Behavioral Change

The ultimate goal of medical knowledge acquisition is to improve a student's ability to solve problems through application of that knowledge. In some cases, particularly in skill acquisition, such as insertion of an intravenous line, or in interpersonal interaction, such as history taking, the measure is not problem-solving ability but rather behavioral change.

21.6   Conclusion

CBE systems have the potential to help students to master subject matter and to develop problem-solving skills. Properly integrated into the medical school curriculum and into the information systems that serve health care institutions and the greater medical community, computer-based teaching can become part of a comprehensive system for life-long education. The challenge to researchers in computer-based teaching is to develop this potential. The barriers to success are both technical and practical. To overcome them, we require both dedication of support and resources within institutions and a commitment to cooperation among institutions.

Suggested Readings

Chueh H.C., Barnett G.O. (1997). "Just in time" clinical information. *Academic Medicine*, 72(6):512–517.

Gaba D.M. (1997). Simulators in anesthesiology. *Advances in Anesthesia*, 14:55–94.
This article, by the pioneer in human patient simulators, presents many of the uses of this simulation technology.

Kirkpatrick D.L. (1994). *Evaluating Training Programs*. San Francisco: Berrett-Koehler.
This book presents a multilevel system for evaluating training programs.

Lyon H.C., Healy J.C., Bell J.R., O'Donnell J.F., Shultz E.K., Moore-West M., Wigton R.S., Hirai F., Beck J.R. (1992). PlanAlyzer, an interactive computer-assisted program to teach clinical problem solving in diagnosing anemia and coronary artery disease. *Academic Medicine*, 67(12):821–828.
The authors describe their clinical teaching program and present a thoughtful evaluation of its efficacy in learning.

Pugh C.M., Youngblood P. (2002). Development and validation of assessment measures for a newly developed physical examination simulator. *Journal of the American Medical Informatics Association*, 9:448–460.
The authors present a controlled randomized study of the efficacy of a new simulator.

Rosse C., Mejino J.L., Modayur B.R., Jakobovits R., Hinshaw K.P., Brinkley J.F. (1998). Motivation and organizational principles for anatomical knowledge representation: The digital

anatomist symbolic knowledge base. *Journal of the American Medical Informatics Association*, 5(1):17–40.
Rosse's group has developed one of the more comprehensive representations of a domain, in their case, anatomy. Such domain knowledge representation will be necessary for the next generation of educational software systems.

Vosniadou S., DeCorte E., Glaser R., Mandl H. (1996). *International Perspectives on the Design of Technology-Supported Learning Environments*. Mahwah, NJ: Lawrence Erlbaum.
This is a collection of research articles presenting many different aspects of development and assessment in technology-supported learning environments.

Westwood J.D., Hoffman H.M., Stredney D., Weghorst S.J. (1998). *Medicine Meets Virtual Reality*. Amsterdam: IOS Press.
This volume is one in a series of conference proceedings on the emerging area of virtual environments in training and education.

Questions for Discussion

1. What are two advantages and two limitations of including visual material in the following teaching programs:
   a. A simulated case of a patient who is admitted to the emergency unit with a gunshot wound
   b. A lecture-style program on the anatomy of the pelvis
   c. A reference resource on bacteria and fungi
2. You have decided to write a computer-based simulation to teach students about the management of chest pain.
   a. Discuss the relative advantages and disadvantages of the following styles of presentation: (1) a sequence of multiple-choice questions, (2) a simulation in which the patient's condition changes over time and in response to therapy, and (3) a program that allows the student to enter free-text requests for information and that provides responses.
   b. Discuss at least four problems that you would expect to arise during the process of developing and testing the program.
   c. For each approach, discuss how you might develop a model that you could use to evaluate the student's performance in clinical problem solving.
3. Examine two clinical simulation programs. How do they differ in their presentation of history taking or physical examination of the patient?
4. Select a topic in physiology with which you are familiar, such as arterial blood–gas exchange or filtration in the kidney, and construct a representation of the domain in terms of the concepts and subconcepts that should be taught for that topic. Using this representation, design a teaching program using one of the following methods: (1) a didactic approach, (2) a simulation approach, or (3) an exploration approach.
5. Describe at least three challenges you can foresee in dissemination of computer-based medical education programs from one institution to another.
6. Discuss the relative merits and problems of placing the computer in control of the teaching environment, with the student essentially responding to computer inquiries, versus having the student in control, with a much larger range of alternative courses of action.

22
Bioinformatics

Russ B. Altman and Sean D. Mooney

After reading this chapter, you should know the answers to these questions:

- Why is sequence, structure, and biological pathway information relevant to medicine?
- Where on the Internet should you look for a DNA sequence, a protein sequence, or a protein structure?
- What are two problems encountered in analyzing biological sequence, structure, and function?
- How has the age of genomics changed the landscape of bioinformatics?
- What two changes should we anticipate in the medical record as a result of these new information sources?
- What are two computational challenges in bioinformatics for the future?

22.1 The Problem of Handling Biological Information

Bioinformatics is the study of how information is represented and analyzed in biological systems, starting at the molecular level. Whereas clinical informatics deals with the management of information related to the delivery of health care, bioinformatics focuses on the management of information related to the underlying basic biological sciences. As such, the two disciplines are closely related—more so than generally appreciated (see Chapter 1). Bioinformatics and clinical informatics share a concentration on systems that are inherently uncertain, difficult to measure, and the result of complicated interactions among multiple complex components. Both deal with living systems that generally lack straight edges and right angles. Although **reductionist approaches** to studying these systems can provide valuable lessons, it is often necessary to analyze them using **integrative models** that are not based solely on first principles. Nonetheless, the two disciplines approach the patient from opposite directions. Whereas applications within clinical informatics usually are concerned with the social systems of medicine, the cognitive processes of medicine, and the technologies required to understand human physiology, bioinformatics is concerned with understanding how basic biological systems conspire to create molecules, organelles, living cells, organs, and entire organisms. Remarkably, however, the two disciplines share significant methodological elements, so an understanding of the issues in bioinformatics can be valuable for the student of clinical informatics.

The discipline of bioinformatics is currently in a period of rapid growth, because the needs for information storage, retrieval, and analysis in biology—particularly in molecular biology and **genomics**—have increased dramatically in the past decade. History has shown that scientific developments within the basic sciences tend to lag about a decade before their influence on clinical medicine is fully appreciated. The types of information being gathered by biologists today will drastically alter the types of information and technologies available to the health care workers of tomorrow.

22.1.1 Many Sources of Biological Data

There are three sources of information that are revolutionizing our understanding of human biology and that are creating significant challenges for computational processing. The most dominant new type of information is the **sequence information** produced by the **Human Genome Project**, an international undertaking intended to determine the complete sequence of human DNA as it is encoded in each of the 23 chromosomes.[1] The first draft of the sequence was published in 2001 (Lander et al., 2001) and a final version was announced in 2003 coincident with the 50th anniversary of the solving of the Watson and Crick structure of the DNA double helix.[2] Now efforts are under way to finish the sequence and to determine the variations that occur between the genomes of different individuals.[3] Essentially, the entire set of events from conception through embryonic development, childhood, adulthood, and aging are encoded by the DNA blueprints within most human cells. Given a complete knowledge of these DNA sequences, we are in a position to understand these processes at a fundamental level and to consider the possible use of DNA sequences for diagnosing and treating disease.

While we are studying the human genome, a second set of concurrent projects is studying the genomes of numerous other biological organisms, including important experimental animal systems (such as mouse, rat, and yeast) as well as important human pathogens (such as *Mycobacterium tuberculosis* or *Haemophilus influenzae*). Many of these genomes have recently been completely determined by sequencing experiments. These allow two important types of analysis: the analysis of mechanisms of pathogenicity and the analysis of animal models for human disease. In both cases, the functions encoded by genomes can be studied, classified, and categorized, allowing us to decipher how genomes affect human health and disease.

These ambitious scientific projects not only are proceeding at a furious pace, but also are accompanied in many cases by a new approach to biology, which produces a third new source of biomedical information: **proteomics**. In addition to small, relatively focused experimental studies aimed at particular molecules thought to be important for disease, large-scale experimental methodologies are used to collect data on thousands or millions of molecules simultaneously. Scientists apply these methodologies longitudinally over time and across a wide variety of organisms or (within an organism) organs to watch the evolution of various physiological phenomena. New technologies give us the abilities to follow the production and degradation of molecules on **DNA arrays**[4]

---

[1]http://www.genome.gov/page.cfm?pageID=10001694.

[2]http://www.genome.gov/10005139.

[3]http://www.genome.gov/page.cfm?pageID=10001688.

[4]These are small glass plates onto which specific DNA fragments can be affixed and then used to detect other DNA fragments present in a cell extract.

(Lashkari et al., 1997), to study the expression of large numbers of proteins with one another (Bai and Elledge, 1997), and to create multiple variations on a genetic theme to explore the implications of various mutations on biological function (Spee et al., 1993). All these technologies, along with the genome-sequencing projects, are conspiring to produce a volume of biological information that at once contains secrets to age-old questions about health and disease and threatens to overwhelm our current capabilities of data analysis. Thus, bioinformatics is becoming critical for medicine in the twenty-first century.

22.1.2 Implications for Clinical Informatics

The effects of this new biological information on clinical medicine and clinical informatics are difficult to predict precisely. It is already clear, however, that some major changes to medicine will have to be accommodated.

1. *Sequence information in the medical record.* With the first set of human genomes now available, it will soon become cost-effective to consider sequencing or genotyping at least sections of many other genomes. The sequence of a gene involved in disease may provide the critical information that we need to select appropriate treatments. For example, the set of genes that produces essential hypertension may be understood at a level sufficient to allow us to target antihypertensive medications based on the precise configuration of these genes. It is possible that clinical trials may use information about genetic sequence to define precisely the population of patients who would benefit from a new therapeutic agent. Finally, clinicians may learn the sequences of infectious agents (such as of the *Escherichia coli* strain that causes recurrent urinary tract infections) and store them in a patient's record to record the precise pathogenicity and drug susceptibility observed during an episode of illness. In any case, it is likely that genetic information will need to be included in the medical record and will introduce special problems. Raw sequence information, whether from the patient or the pathogen, is meaningless without context and thus is not well suited to a printed medical record. Like images, it can come in high information density and must be presented to the clinician in novel ways. As there are for laboratory tests, there may be a set of nondisease (or normal) values to use as comparisons, and there may be difficulties in interpreting abnormal values. Fortunately, most of the human genome is shared and identical among individuals; less than 1 percent of the genome seems to be unique to individuals. Nonetheless, the effects of sequence information on clinical databases will be significant.

2. *New diagnostic and prognostic information sources.* One of the main contributions of the genome-sequencing projects (and of the associated biological innovations) is that we are likely to have unprecedented access to new diagnostic and prognostic tools. **Single nucleotide polymorphisms (SNPs)** and other genetic markers are used to identify how a patient's genome differs from the draft genome. Diagnostically, the genetic markers from a patient with an autoimmune disease, or of an infectious pathogen within a patient, will be highly specific and sensitive indicators of the subtype of disease and of that subtype's probable responsiveness to different therapeutic agents. For

example, the severe acute respiratory syndrome (SARS) virus was determined to be a corona virus using a gene expression array containing the genetic information from several common pathogenic viruses.[5] In general, diagnostic tools based on the gene sequences within a patient are likely to increase greatly the number and variety of tests available to the physician. Physicians will not be able to manage these tests without significant computational assistance. Moreover, genetic information will be available to provide more accurate prognostic information to patients. What is the standard course for this disease? How does it respond to these medications? Over time, we will be able to answer these questions with increasing precision, and will develop computational systems to manage this information.

Several **genotype**-based databases have been developed to identify markers that are associated with specific **phenotypes** and identify how genotype affects a patient's response to therapeutics. The *Human Gene Mutations Database* (HGMD) annotates mutations with disease phenotype.[6] This resource has become invaluable for genetic counselors, basic researchers, and clinicians. Additionally, the *Pharmacogenomics Knowledge Base* (PharmGKB) collects genetic information that is known to affect a patient's response to a drug.[7] As these data sets, and others like them, continue to improve, the first clinical benefits from the genome projects will be realized.

3. *Ethical considerations*. One of the critical questions facing the genome-sequencing projects is "Can genetic information be misused?" The answer is certainly yes. With knowledge of a complete genome for an individual, it may be possible in the future to predict the types of disease for which that individual is at risk years before the disease actually develops. If this information fell into the hands of unscrupulous employers or insurance companies, the individual might be denied employment or coverage due to the likelihood of future disease, however distant. There is even debate about whether such information should be released to a patient even if it could be kept confidential. Should a patient be informed that he or she is likely to get a disease for which there is no treatment? This is a matter of intense debate, and such questions have significant implications for what information is collected and for how and to whom that information is disclosed (Durfy, 1993; see Chapter 10).

22.2   The Rise of Bioinformatics

A brief review of the biological basis of medicine will bring into focus the magnitude of the revolution in molecular biology and the tasks that are created for the discipline of bioinformatics. The genetic material that we inherit from our parents, that we use for the structures and processes of life, and that we pass to our children is contained in a sequence of chemicals known as **deoxyribonucleic acid (DNA)**.[8] The total collec-

---

[5]http://www.cdc.gov/ncidod/sars/.

[6]http://archive.uwcm.ac.uk/uwcm/mg/hgmd0.html.

[7]http://pharmgkb.org.

[8]If you are not familiar with the basic terminology of molecular biology and genetics, reference to an introductory textbook in the area would be helpful before you read the rest of this chapter.

tion of DNA for a single person or organism is referred to as the **genome**. DNA is a long polymer chemical made of four basic subunits. The sequence in which these subunits occur in the polymer distinguishes one DNA molecule from another, and the sequence of DNA subunits in turn directs a cell's production of proteins and all other basic cellular processes. **Genes** are discreet units encoded in DNA and they are transcribed into **ribonucleic acid (RNA)**, which has a composition very similar to DNA. Genes are transcribed into *messenger RNA* (mRNA) and a majority of mRNA sequences are translated by ribosomes into protein. Not all RNAs are messengers for the translation of proteins. *Ribosomal RNA*, for example, is used in the construction of the ribosome, the huge molecular engine that translates mRNA sequences into protein sequences.

Understanding the basic building blocks of life requires understanding the function of genomic sequences, genes, and proteins. When are genes turned on? Once genes are transcribed and translated into proteins, into what cellular compartment are the proteins directed? How do the proteins function once there? Equally important, how are the proteins turned off? Experimentation and bioinformatics have divided the research into several areas, and the largest are: (1) genome and protein sequence analysis, (2) macromolecular structure–function analysis, (3) gene expression analysis, and (4) proteomics.

22.2.1   Roots of Modern Bioinformatics

Practitioners of bioinformatics have come from many backgrounds, including medicine, molecular biology, chemistry, physics, mathematics, engineering, and computer science. It is difficult to define precisely the ways in which this discipline emerged. There are, however, two main developments that have created opportunities for the use of information technologies in biology. The first is the progress in our understanding of how biological molecules are constructed and how they perform their functions. This dates back as far as the 1930s with the invention of **electrophoresis**, and then in the 1950s with the elucidation of the structure of DNA and the subsequent sequence of discoveries in the relationships among DNA, RNA, and protein structure. The second development has been the parallel increase in the availability of computing power. Starting with mainframe computer applications in the 1950s and moving to modern workstations, there have been hosts of biological problems addressed with computational methods.

22.2.2   The Genomics Explosion

The Human Genome Project was completed and a nearly finished sequence was published in 2003.[9] The benefit of the human genome sequence to medicine is both in the short and in the long term. The short-term benefits lie principally in diagnosis: The availability of sequences of normal and variant human genes will allow for the rapid identification of these genes in any patient (e.g., Babior and Matzner, 1997). The

---

[9]http://www.genome.gov/10005139.

long-term benefits will include a greater understanding of the proteins produced from the genome: how the proteins interact with drugs; how they malfunction in disease states; and how they participate in the control of development, aging, and responses to disease.

The effects of genomics on biology and medicine cannot be understated. We now have the ability to measure the activity and function of genes within living cells. Genomics data and experiments have changed the way biologists think about questions fundamental to life. Where in the past, reductionist experiments probed the detailed workings of specific genes, we can now assemble those data together to build an accurate understanding of how cells work. This has led to a change in thinking about the role of computers in biology. Before, they were optional tools that could help provide insight to experienced and dedicated enthusiasts. Today, they are required by most investigators, and experimental approaches rely on them as critical elements.

22.3   Biology Is Now Data-Driven

Twenty years ago, the use of computers was proving to be useful to the laboratory researcher. Today, computers are an essential component of modern research. This is because advances in research methods such as **microarray chips**, drug screening robots, **X-ray crystallography**, **nuclear magnetic resonance spectroscopy**, and DNA sequencing experiments have resulted in massive amounts of data. These data need to be properly stored, analyzed, and disseminated.

The volume of data being produced by genomics projects is staggering. There are now more than 22.3 million sequences in GenBank comprising more than 29 billion digits.[10] But these data do not stop with sequence data: PubMed contains over 15 million literature citations, the PDB contains three-dimensional structural data for over 40,000 protein sequences, and the Stanford Microarray Database (SMD) contains over 37,000 experiments (851 million data points). These data are of incredible importance to biology, and in the following sections we introduce and summarize the importance of sequences, structures, gene expression experiments, systems biology, and their computational components to medicine.

22.3.1   *Sequences in Biology*

Sequence information (including DNA sequences, RNA sequences, and protein sequences) is critical in biology: DNA, RNA, and protein can be represented as a set of sequences of basic building blocks (bases for DNA and RNA, amino acids for proteins). Computer systems within bioinformatics thus must be able to handle biological sequence information effectively and efficiently.

One major difficulty within bioinformatics is that standard database models, such as relational database systems, are not well suited to sequence information. The basic problem is that sequences are important both as a set of elements grouped together and

---

[10]http://www.ncbi.nlm.nih.gov/Genbank/GenbankOverview.html.

treated in a uniform manner and as individual elements, with their relative locations and functions. Any given position in a sequence can be important because of its own identity, because it is part of a larger subsequence, or perhaps because it is part of a large set of overlapping subsequences, all of which have different significance. It is necessary to support queries such as, "What sequence motifs are present in this sequence?" It is often difficult to represent these multiple, nested relationships within standard relational database schema. In addition, the neighbors of a sequence element are also critical, and it is important to be able to perform queries such as, "What sequence elements are seen 20 elements to the left of this element?" For these reasons, researchers in bioinformatics are developing **object-oriented databases** (see Chapter 6) in which a sequence can be queried in different ways, depending on the needs of the user (Altman, 2003).

22.3.2 *Structures in Biology*

The sequence information mentioned in Section 22.3.1 is rapidly becoming inexpensive to obtain and easy to store. On the other hand, the **three-dimensional structure information** about the proteins that are produced from the DNA sequences is much more difficult and expensive to obtain, and presents a separate set of analysis challenges. Currently, only about 30,000 three-dimensional structures of biological macromolecules are known.[11] These models are incredibly valuable resources, however, because an understanding of structure often yields detailed insights about biological function. As an example, the structure of the ribosome has been determined for several species and contains more atoms than any other to date. This structure, because of its size, took two decades to solve, and presents a formidable challenge for functional annotation (Cech, 2000). Yet, the functional information for a single structure is vastly outsized by the potential for comparative genomics analysis between the structures from several organisms and from varied forms of the functional complex, since the ribosome is ubiquitously required for all forms of life. Thus a wealth of information comes from relatively few structures. To address the problem of limited structure information, the publicly funded structural genomics initiative aims to identify all of the common structural scaffolds found in nature and grow the number of known structures considerably. In the end, it is the physical forces between molecules that determine what happens within a cell; thus the more complete the picture, the better the functional understanding. In particular, understanding the physical properties of therapeutic agents is the key to understanding how agents interact with their targets within the cell (or within an invading organism). These are the key questions for structural biology within bioinformatics:

1. How can we analyze the structures of molecules to learn their associated function? Approaches range from detailed molecular simulations (Levitt, 1983) to statistical analyses of the structural features that may be important for function (Wei and Altman, 1998).

---

[11]For more information see http://www.rcsb.org/pdb/.

2. How can we extend the limited structural data by using information in the sequence databases about closely related proteins from different organisms (or within the same organism, but performing a slightly different function)? There are significant unanswered questions about how to extract maximal value from a relatively small set of examples.

3. How should structures be grouped for the purposes of classification? The choices range from purely functional criteria ("these proteins all digest proteins") to purely structural criteria ("these proteins all have a toroidal shape"), with mixed criteria in between. One interesting resource available today is the **Structural Classification of Proteins** (SCOP),[12] which classifies proteins based on shape and function.

22.3.3   *Expression Data in Biology*

The development of DNA microarrays has led to a wealth of data and unprecedented insight into the fundamental biological machine. The premise is relatively simple; up to 40,000 gene sequences derived from genomic data are fixed onto a glass slide or filter. An experiment is performed where two groups of cells are grown in different conditions, one group is a control group and the other is the experimental group. The control group is grown normally, while the experimental group is grown under experimental conditions. For example, a researcher may be trying to understand how a cell compensates for a lack of sugar. The experimental cells will be grown with limited amounts of sugar. As the sugar depletes, some of the cells are removed at specific intervals of time. When the cells are removed, all of the mRNA from the cells is separated and converted back to DNA, using special enzymes. This leaves a pool of DNA molecules that are only from the genes that were turned on (expressed) in that group of cells. Using a chemical reaction, the experimental DNA sample is attached to a red fluorescent molecule and the control group is attached to a green fluorescent molecule. These two samples are mixed and then washed over the glass slide. The two samples contain only genes that were turned on in the cells, and they are labeled either red or green depending on whether they came from the experimental group or the control group. The labeled DNA in the pool sticks or hybridizes to the same gene on the glass slide. This leaves the glass slide with up to 40,000 spots and genes that were turned on in the cells are now bound with a label to the appropriate spot on the slide. Using a scanning confocal microscope and a laser to fluoresce the linkers, the amount of red and green fluorescence in each spot can be measured. The ratio of red to green determines whether that gene is being turned off (downregulated) in the experimental group or whether the gene is being turned on (upregulated). The experiment has now measured the activity of genes in an entire cell due to some experimental change. Figure 22.1 illustrates a typical gene expression experiment from SMD.[13]

Computers are critical for analyzing these data, because it is impossible for a researcher to comprehend the significance of those red and green spots. Currently scientists are using gene expression experiments to study how cells from different organ-

---

[12]See http://scop.mrc-lmb.cam.ac.uk/scop/.
[13]http://genome-www5.stanford.edu/MicroArray/SMD/.

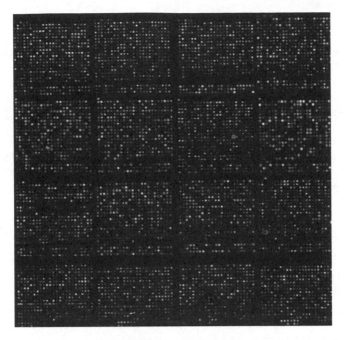

Figure 22.1. Measuring global levels of gene expression. Genomics has created a new need for bioinformatics tools. In this experiment (from the Stanford Microarray Database), stress-induced changes in the gene expression pattern for bakers yeast (*S. cerevisae*) are shown.

isms compensate for environmental changes, how pathogens fight antibiotics, and how cells grow uncontrollably (as is found in cancer). A new challenge for biological computing is to develop methods to analyze these data, tools to store these data, and computer systems to collect the data automatically.

22.3.4   Systems Biology

With the completion of the human genome and the abundance of sequence, structural, and gene expression data, a new field of systems biology that tries to understand how proteins and genes interact at a cellular level is emerging. The basic algorithms for analyzing sequence and structure are now leading to opportunities for more integrated analysis of the pathways in which these molecules participate and ways in which molecules can be manipulated for the purpose of combating disease. A detailed understanding of the role of a particular molecule in the cell requires knowledge of the context—of the other molecules with which it interacts—and of the sequence of chemical transformations that take place in the cell. Thus, major research areas in bioinformatics are elucidating the key pathways by which chemicals are transformed, defining the molecules that catalyze these transformations, identifying the input compounds and the output compounds, and linking these pathways into networks that we can then represent computationally and analyze to understand the significance of a particular molecule. The Alliance for Cell Signaling is generating large amounts of data related to how signal molecules interact and affect the concentration of small molecules within the cell.

22.4   Key Bioinformatics Algorithms

There are a number of common computations that are performed in many contexts within bioinformatics. In general, these computations can be classified as sequence alignment, structure alignment, pattern analysis of sequence/structure, gene expression analysis, and pattern analysis of biochemical function.

22.4.1   Early Work in Sequence and Structure Analysis

As it became clear that the information from DNA and protein sequences would be voluminous and difficult to analyze manually, algorithms began to appear for automating the analysis of sequence information. The first requirement was to have a reliable way to align sequences so that their detailed similarities and distances could be examined directly. Needleman and Wunsch (1970) published an elegant method for using **dynamic programming** techniques to align sequences in time related to the cube of the number of elements in the sequences. Smith and Waterman (1981) published refinements of these algorithms that allowed for searching both the best global alignment of two sequences (aligning all the elements of the two sequences) and the best local alignment (searching for areas in which there are segments of high similarity surrounded by regions of low similarity). A key input for these algorithms is a matrix that encodes the similarity or substitutability of sequence elements: When there is an inexact match between two elements in an alignment of sequences, it specifies how much "partial credit" we should give the overall alignment based on the similarity of the elements, even though they may not be identical. Looking at a set of evolutionarily related proteins, Dayhoff et al. (1974) published one of the first matrices derived from a detailed analysis of which amino acids (elements) tend to substitute for others.

Within structural biology, the vast computational requirements of the experimental methods (such as X-ray crystallography and nuclear magnetic resonance) for determining the structure of biological molecules drove the development of powerful structural analysis tools. In addition to software for analyzing experimental data, graphical display algorithms allowed biologists to visualize these molecules in great detail and facilitated the manual analysis of structural principles (Langridge, 1974; Richardson, 1981). At the same time, methods were developed for simulating the forces within these molecules as they rotate and vibrate (Gibson and Scheraga, 1967; Karplus and Weaver, 1976; Levitt, 1983).

The most important development to support the emergence of bioinformatics, however, has been the creation of databases with biological information. In the 1970s, structural biologists, using the techniques of X-ray crystallography, set up the Protein Data Bank (PDB) of the Cartesian coordinates of the structures that they elucidated (as well as associated experimental details) and made PDB publicly available. The first release, in 1977, contained 77 structures. The growth of the database is chronicled on the Web:[14] the PDB now has over 30,000 detailed atomic structures and is the primary source of information about the relationship between protein sequence and protein structure. Similarly, as the ability to obtain the sequence of DNA molecules became widespread, the need for a database of these sequences arose. In the mid-1980s, the GENBANK database was formed as a repository of sequence information. Starting with 606 sequences and 680,000 bases in 1982, the GENBANK has grown by much more than 2 million sequences and 100 billion bases. The GENBANK database of DNA sequence information supports the experimental reconstruction of genomes and acts as a focal point for experimental groups.[15] Numerous other databases store the sequences of protein molecules[16] and information about human genetic diseases.[17]

Included among the databases that have accelerated the development of bioinformatics is the Medline[18] database of the biomedical literature and its paper-based companion *Index Medicus* (see Chapter 19). Including articles as far back as 1953 and brought online free on the Web in 1997, Medline provides the glue that relates many high-level biomedical concepts to the low-level molecule, disease, and experimental methods. In fact, this "glue" role was the basis for creating the Entrez and PubMed systems for integrating access to literature references and the associated databases.

22.4.2   *Sequence Alignment and Genome Analysis*

Perhaps the most basic activity in computational biology is comparing two biological sequences to determine (1) whether they are similar and (2) how to align them. The problem of alignment is not trivial but is based on a simple idea. Sequences that perform a similar function should, in general, be descendants of a common ancestral sequence, with mutations over time. These mutations can be replacements of one amino acid with another, deletions of amino acids, or insertions of amino acids. The goal of **sequence alignment** is to align two sequences so that the evolutionary relationship between the sequences becomes clear. If two sequences are descended from the same ancestor and have not mutated too much, then it is often possible to find corresponding locations in each sequence that play the same role in the evolved proteins. The problem of solving correct biological alignments is difficult because it requires knowledge about the evolution of the molecules that we typically do not have. There are now, however, well-established algorithms for finding the mathematically optimal alignment of two sequences. These algorithms require the two sequences and a scoring system based on (1) *exact matches* between amino acids that have not mutated in the two sequences and can be aligned perfectly; (2) *partial matches* between amino acids that have mutated in ways that have preserved their overall biophysical properties; and (3) *gaps in the alignment* signifying places where one sequence or the other has undergone a deletion or

---

[14]See http://www.rcsb.org/pdb/holdings.html.

[15]http://gdbwww.gdb.org/.

[16]The Protein Identification Resource: http://pir.georgetown.edu; Swiss-Prot at http://www.expasy.ch/sprot/.

[17]Online Mendelian Inheritance in Man: http://www3.ncbi.nlm.nih.gov/omim/.

[18]See http://www.ncbi.nlm.nih.gov/PubMed/.

insertion of amino acids. The algorithms for determining optimal sequence alignments are based on a technique in computer science known as **dynamic programming** and are at the heart of many computational biology applications (Gusfield, 1997). Figure 22.2 shows an example of a Smith-Waterman matrix.

Unfortunately, the dynamic programming algorithms are computationally expensive to apply, so a number of faster, more heuristic methods have been developed. The most popular algorithm is the **Basic Local Alignment Search Tool (BLAST)** (Altschul et al., 1990). BLAST is based on the observations that sections of proteins are often conserved without gaps (so the gaps can be ignored—a critical simplification for speed) and that there are statistical analyses of the occurrence of small subsequences within larger sequences that can be used to prune the search for matching sequences in a large database. Another tool that has found wide use in mining genome sequences is BLAT (Kent, 2003). BLAT is often used to search long genomic sequences with significant performance increases over BLAST. It achieves its 50-fold increase in speed over other tools by storing and indexing long sequences as nonoverlapping k-mers, allowing efficient storage, searching, and alignment on modest hardware.

22.4.3   *Prediction of Structure and Function from Sequence*

One of the primary challenges in bioinformatics is taking a newly determined DNA sequence (as well as its translation into a protein sequence) and predicting the structure of the associated molecules, as well as their function. Both problems are difficult, being fraught with all the dangers associated with making predictions without hard experimental data. Nonetheless, the available sequence data are starting to be sufficient to allow good predictions in a few cases. For example, there is a Web site devoted to the assessment of biological macromolecular structure prediction methods.[19] Recent results suggest that when two protein molecules have a high degree (more than 40 percent) of sequence similarity and one of the structures is known, a reliable model of the other can be built by analogy. In the case that sequence similarity is less than 25 percent, however, performance of these methods is much less reliable.

When scientists investigate biological structure, they commonly perform a task analogous to sequence alignment, called **structural alignment**. Given two sets of three-dimensional coordinates for a set of atoms, what is the best way to superimpose them so that the similarities and differences between the two structures are clear? Such computations are useful for determining whether two structures share a common ancestry and for understanding how the structures' functions have subsequently been refined during evolution. There are numerous published algorithms for finding good structural alignments. We can apply these algorithms in an automated fashion whenever a new structure is determined, thereby classifying the new structure into one of the protein families (such as those that SCOP maintains).

One of these algorithms is MinRMS (Jewett et al., 2003).[20] MinRMS works by finding the minimal root-mean-squared-distance (RMSD) alignments of two protein

---

[19]http://predictioncenter.org/.
[20]http://www.cgl.ucsf.edu/Research/minrms/.

a) Pairwise alignment between human chymotrypsin and human trypsin.

```
CTRB_HUMAN    MAFLWLLSCWALLGTTFGCGVPAIHPVLSGLSRIVNGEDAVPGSWPWQVSLQDKTGFHFC
TRY1_HUMAN    MNPLLILTFVA----------AALAAPFDDDDKIVGGYNCEENSVPYQVSLN--SGYHFC

CTRB_HUMAN    GGSLISEDWVVTAAHCGVRTSDVVVAGEFDQGSDEENIQVLKIAKVFKNPKFSILTVNND
TRY1_HUMAN    GGSLINEQWVVSAGHC-YKSRIQVRLGEHNIEVLEGNEQFINAAKIIRHPQYDRKTLNND

CTRB_HUMAN    ITLLKLATPARFSQTVSAVCLPSADDDFPAGTLCATTGWGKTKYNANKTPDKLQQAALPL
TRY1_HUMAN    IMLIKLSSRAVINARVSTISLPTAPP--ATGTKCLISGWGNTASSGADYPDELQCLDAPV

CTRB_HUMAN    LSNAECKKSWGRRITDVMICAG--ASGVSSCMGDSGGPLVCQKDGAWTLVGIVSWGSDTC
TRY1_HUMAN    LSQAKCEASYPGKITSNMFCVGFLEGGKDSCQGDSGGPVVCNG----QLQGVVSWGDGCA

CTRB_HUMAN    STSSPGVYARVTKLIPWVQKILAAN-
TRY1_HUMAN    QKNKPGVYTKVYNYVKWIKNTIAANS
```

b) Smith Waterman matrix illustrating the aligned region in A, using the BLOSUM62 mutation matrix (Henikoff and Henikoff, 1994).

	G	F	L	E	G	G	K	D	S	C	Q	G	D	S	G	G	P	V	V	C	N	G	Q	L	Q
G	6	-3	-4	-2	6	6	-2	-1	0	-3	-2	6	-1	0	6	6	-2	-3	-3	-3	0	6	-2	-4	-2
A	0	-2	-1	-1	0	0	-1	-2	1	0	-1	0	-2	1	0	0	-1	0	0	0	-2	0	-1	-1	-1
S	0	-2	-2	0	0	0	0	0	4	-1	0	0	0	4	0	0	-1	-2	-2	-1	1	0	0	-2	0
G	6	-3	-4	-2	6	6	-2	-1	0	-3	-2	6	-1	0	6	6	-2	-3	-3	-3	0	6	-2	-4	-2
V	-3	-1	1	-2	-3	-3	-2	-3	-2	-1	-2	-3	-3	-2	-3	-3	-2	4	4	-1	-3	-3	-2	1	-2
S	0	-2	-2	0	0	0	0	0	4	-1	0	0	0	4	0	0	-1	-2	-2	-1	1	0	0	-2	0
S	0	-2	-2	0	0	0	0	0	4	-1	0	0	0	4	0	0	-1	-2	-2	-1	1	0	0	-2	0
C	-3	-2	-1	-4	-3	-3	-3	-3	-1	9	-3	-3	-3	-1	-3	-3	-3	-1	-1	9	-3	-3	-3	-1	-3
M	-3	0	2	-2	-3	-3	-1	-3	-1	-1	0	-3	-3	-1	-3	-3	-2	1	1	-1	-2	-3	0	2	0
G	6	-3	-4	-2	6	6	-2	-1	0	-3	-2	6	-1	0	6	6	-2	-3	-3	-3	0	6	-2	-4	-2
D	-1	-3	-4	2	-1	-1	-1	6	0	-3	0	-1	6	0	-1	-1	-1	-3	-3	-3	1	-1	0	-4	0
S	0	-2	-2	0	0	0	0	0	4	-1	0	0	0	4	0	0	-1	-2	-2	-1	1	0	0	-2	0
G	6	-3	-4	-2	6	6	-2	-1	0	-3	-2	6	-1	0	6	6	-2	-3	-3	-3	0	6	-2	-4	-2
G	6	-3	-4	-2	6	6	-2	-1	0	-3	-2	6	-1	0	6	6	-2	-3	-3	-3	0	6	-2	-4	-2
P	-2	-4	-3	-1	-2	-2	-1	-1	-1	-3	-1	-2	-1	-1	-2	-2	7	-2	-2	-3	-2	-2	-1	-3	-1
L	-4	0	4	-3	-4	-4	-2	-4	-2	-1	-2	-4	-4	-2	-4	-4	-3	1	1	-1	-3	-4	-2	4	-2
V	-3	-1	1	-2	-3	-3	-2	-3	-2	-1	-2	-3	-3	-2	-3	-3	-2	4	4	-1	-3	-3	-2	1	-2
C	-3	-2	-1	-4	-3	-3	-3	-3	-1	9	-3	-3	-3	-1	-3	-3	-3	-1	-1	9	-3	-3	-3	-1	-3
Q	-2	-3	-2	2	-2	-2	1	0	0	-3	5	-2	0	0	-2	-2	-1	-2	-2	-3	0	-2	5	-2	5
K	-2	-3	-2	1	-2	-2	5	-1	0	-3	1	-2	-1	0	-2	-2	-1	-2	-2	-3	0	-2	1	-2	1
D	-1	-3	-4	2	-1	-1	-1	6	0	-3	0	-1	6	0	-1	-1	-1	-3	-3	-3	1	-1	0	-4	0
G	6	-3	-4	-2	6	6	-2	-1	0	-3	-2	6	-1	0	6	6	-2	-3	-3	-3	0	6	-2	-4	-2
A	0	-2	-1	-1	0	0	-1	-2	1	0	-1	0	-2	1	0	0	-1	0	0	0	-2	0	-1	-1	-1
W	-2	1	-2	-3	-2	-2	-3	-4	-3	-2	-2	-2	-4	-3	-2	-2	-4	-3	-3	-2	-4	-2	-2	-2	-2
T	-2	-2	-1	-1	-2	-2	-1	-1	1	-1	-1	-2	-1	1	-2	-2	-1	0	0	-1	0	-2	-1	-1	-1
L	-4	0	4	-3	-4	-4	-2	-4	-2	-1	-2	-4	-4	-2	-4	-4	-3	1	1	-1	-3	-4	-2	4	-2
V	-3	-1	1	-2	-3	-3	-2	-3	-2	-1	-2	-3	-3	-2	-3	-3	-2	4	4	-1	-3	-3	-2	1	-2

Figure 22.2. Example of sequence alignment using the Smith Waterman algorithm.

structures as a function of matching residue pairs. MinRMS generates a family of alignments, each with different number of residue position matches. This is useful for identifying local regions of similarity in a protein with multiple domains. MinRMS solves two problems. First, it determines which structural *superpositions*, or alignment, to evaluate. Then, given this superposition, it determines which residues should be considered "aligned" or matched. Computationally, this is a very difficult problem. MinRMS reduces the search space by limiting superpositions to be the best superposition between four atoms. It then exhaustively determines all potential four-atom-matched superpositions and evaluates the alignment. Given this superposition, the number of aligned residues is determined, as any two residues with C-alpha carbons (the central atom in all amino acids) less than a certain threshold apart. The minimum average RMSD for all matched atoms is the overall score for the alignment. In Figure 22.3, an example of such a comparison is shown.

A related problem is that of using the structure of a large biomolecule and the structure of a small organic molecule (such as a drug or cofactor) to try to predict the ways in which the molecules will interact. An understanding of the structural interaction between a drug and its target molecule often provides critical insight into the drug's mechanism of action. The most reliable way to assess this interaction is to use experimental methods to solve the structure of a drug–target complex. Once again, these experimental approaches are expensive, so computational methods play an important role. Typically, we can assess the physical and chemical features of the drug molecule and can use them to find complementary regions of the target. For example, a highly electronegative drug molecule will be most likely to bind in a pocket of the target that has electropositive features.

Prediction of function often relies on use of sequential or structural similarity metrics and subsequent assignment of function based on similarities to molecules of known

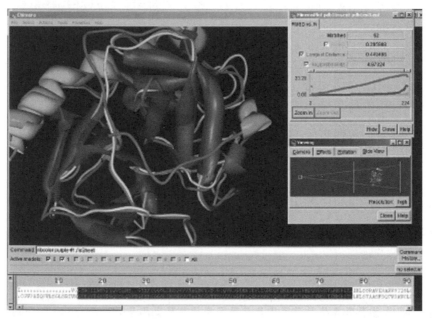

Figure 22.3. Example of structural comparison. Comparison of the chymotrypsin and trypsin protein structures using Chimera and MinRMS (http://www.cgl.ucsf.edu/chimera).

function. These methods can guess at general function for roughly 60 to 80 percent of all genes, but leave considerable uncertainty about the precise functional details even for those genes for which there are predictions, and have little to say about the remaining genes.

22.4.4   Clustering of Gene Expression Data

Analysis of gene expression data often begins by clustering the expression data. A typical experiment is represented as a large table, where the rows are the genes on each chip and the columns represent the different experiments, whether they be time points or different experimental conditions. Within each cell is the red to green ratio of that gene's experimental results. Each row is then a vector of values that represent the results of the experiment with respect to a specific gene. Clustering can then be performed to determine which genes are being expressed similarly. Genes that are associated with similar expression profiles are often functionally associated. For example, when a cell is subjected to starvation (fasting), ribosomal genes are often downregulated in anticipation of lower protein production by the cell. It has similarly been shown that genes associated with neoplastic progression could be identified relatively easily with this method, making gene expression experiments a powerful assay in cancer research (see Guo, 2003, for review). In order to cluster expression data, a distance metric must be determined to compare a gene's profile with another gene's profile. If the vector data are a list of values, Euclidian distance or correlation distances can be used. If the data are more complicated, more sophisticated distance metrics may be employed. Clustering methods fall into two categories: supervised and unsupervised. Supervised learning methods require some preconceived knowledge of the data at hand. Usually, the method begins by selecting profiles that represent the different groups of data, and then the clustering method associates each of the genes with the representative profile to which they are most similar. Unsupervised methods are more commonly applied because these methods require no knowledge of the data, and can be performed automatically.

Two such unsupervised learning methods are the hierarchical and K-means clustering methods. Hierarchical methods build a dendrogram, or a tree, of the genes based on their expression profiles. These methods are agglomerative and work by iteratively joining close neighbors into a cluster. The first step often involves connecting the closest profiles, building an average profile of the joined profiles, and repeating until the entire tree is built. K-means clustering builds k clusters or groups automatically. The algorithm begins by picking k representative profiles randomly. Then each gene is associated with the representative to which it is closest, as defined by the distance metric being employed. Then the *center of mass* of each cluster is determined using all of the member gene's profiles. Depending on the implementation, either the center of mass or the nearest member to it becomes the new representative for that cluster. The algorithm then iterates until the new center of mass and the previous center of mass are within some threshold. The result is k groups of genes that are regulated similarly. One drawback of K-means is that one must chose the value for k. If k is too large, logical "true" clusters may be split into pieces and if k is too small, there will be clusters that are merged. One way to determine whether the chosen k is correct is to estimate the average distance from any member profile to the center of mass. By varying k, it is best to choose the lowest k where this average is minimized for each cluster. Another drawback of K-means is that different initial conditions can give different results, therefore it is often prudent to test the robustness of the results by running multiple runs with different starting configurations (Figure 22.4).

The future clinical usefulness of these algorithms cannot be understated. In 2002, van't Veer et al. (2002) found that a gene expression profile could predict the clinical outcome of breast cancer. The global analysis of gene expression showed that some can-

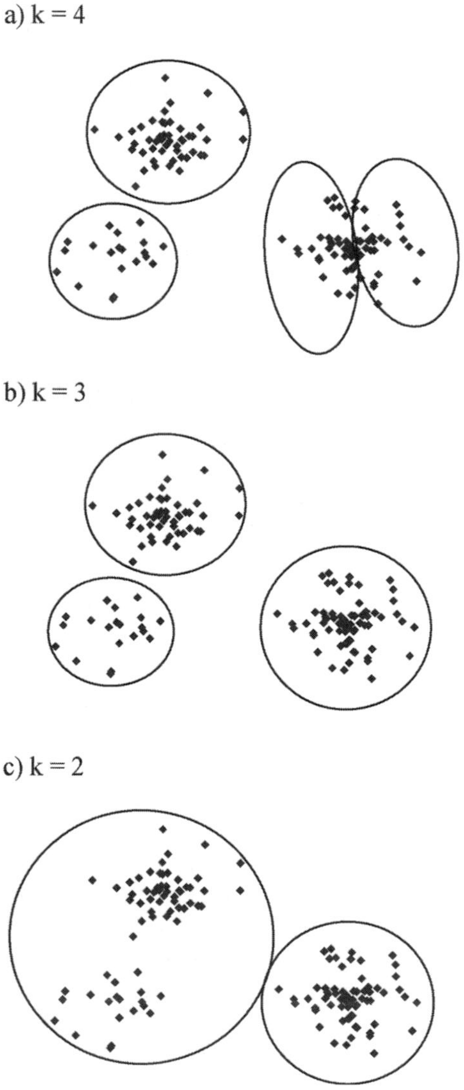

a) k = 4

Figure 22.4. K-means clustering example with varying k. In this case, $k = 3$ is the most reasonable.

b) k = 3

c) k = 2

cers were associated with different prognosis, not detectable using traditional means. Another exciting advancement in this field is the potential use of microarray expression data to profile the molecular effects of known and potential therapeutic agents. This molecular understanding of a disease and its treatment will soon help clinicians make more informed and accurate treatment choices.

22.5   Current Application Successes from Bioinformatics

Biologists have embraced the Web in a remarkable way and have made Internet access to data a normal and expected mode for doing business. Hundreds of databases curated by individual biologists create a valuable resource for the developers of computational methods who can use these data to test and refine their analysis algorithms. With standard Internet search engines, most biological databases can be found and accessed within moments. The large number of databases has led to the development of meta-databases that combine information from individual databases to shield the user from the complex array that exists. There are various approaches to this task.

The *Entrez* system from the National Center for Biological Information (NCBI) gives integrated access to the biomedical literature, protein, and nucleic acid sequences, macromolecular and small molecular structures, and genome project links (including both the Human Genome Project and sequencing projects that are attempting to determine the genome sequences for organisms that are either human pathogens or important experimental model organisms) in a manner that takes advantages of either explicit or computed links between these data resources.[21] The *Sequence Retrieval System* (SRS) from the European Molecular Biology Laboratory allows queries from one database to another to be linked and sequenced, thus allowing relatively complicated queries to be evaluated.[22] Newer technologies are being developed that will allow multiple heterogeneous databases to be accessed by search engines that can combine information automatically, thereby processing even more intricate queries requiring knowledge from numerous data sources.

22.5.1   Sequence and Genome Databases

The main types of sequence information that must be stored are DNA and protein. One of the largest **DNA sequence databases** is *GENBANK*, which is managed by NCBI.[23] GENBANK is growing rapidly as genome-sequencing projects feed their data (often in an automated procedure) directly into the database. Figure 22.5 shows the logarithmic growth of data in GENBANK since 1982. Entrez Gene curates some of the many genes within GENBANK and presents the data in a way that is easy for the researcher to use (Figure 22.6).

---

[21]See http://www3.ncbi.nlm.nih.gov/Entrez/.

[22]See http://www.lionbioscience.com/solutions/products/srs/.

[23]http://www.ncbi.nlm.nih.gov/.

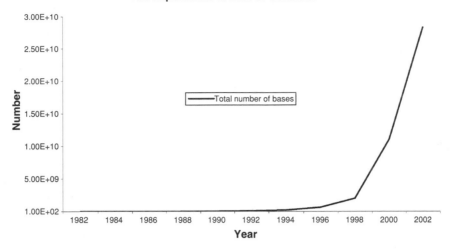

Figure 22.5. The exponential growth of GENBANK. This plot shows that since 1982 the number of bases in GENBANK has grown by five full orders of magnitude and continues to grow by a factor of 10 every 4 years.

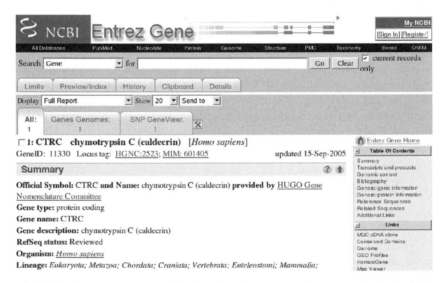

Figure 22.6. The Entrez Gene entry for the digestive enzyme chymotrypsin. Basic information about the original report is provided, as well as some annotations of the key regions in the sequence and the complete sequence of DNA bases (a, g, t, and c) is provided as a link. (Courtesy of NCBI)

In addition to GENBANK, there are numerous special-purpose DNA databases for which the curators have taken special care to clean, validate, and annotate the data. The work required of such curators indicates the degree to which raw sequence data must be interpreted cautiously. GENBANK can be searched efficiently with a number of algorithms and is usually the first stop for a scientist with a new sequence who wonders "Has a sequence like this ever been observed before? If one has, what is known about it?" There are increasing numbers of stories about scientists using GENBANK to discover unanticipated relationships between DNA sequences, allowing their research programs to leap ahead while taking advantage of information collected on similar sequences.

A database that has become very useful recently is the University of California Santa Cruz genome assembly browser[24] (Figure 22.7). This data set allows users to search for specific sequences in the UCSC version of the human genome. Powered by the similarity search tool BLAT, users can quickly find annotations on the human genome that contain their sequence of interest. These annotations include known variations (mutations and SNPs), genes, comparative maps with other organisms, and many other important data.

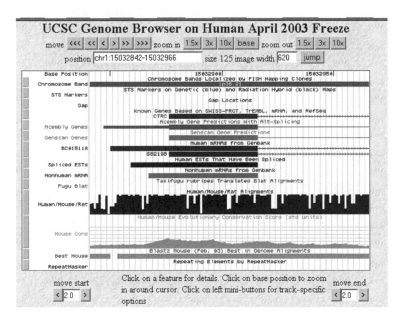

Figure 22.7. Screen from the UC Santa Cruz genome browser showing chymotrypsin. The rows in the browser show annotations on the gene sequence. The browser window here shows a small segment of human chromosome 15, as if the sequence of a, g, c and t are represented from left to right (5 to 3). The annotations include gene predictions and annotations as well as an alignment of the similarity of this region of the genome when compared with the mouse genome.

---

[24]http://genome.ucsc.edu/.

22.5.2   Structure Databases

Although sequence information is obtained relatively easily, structural information remains expensive on a per-entry basis. The experimental protocols used to determine precise molecular structural coordinates are expensive in time, materials, and human power. Therefore, we have only a small number of structures for all the molecules characterized in the sequence databases. The two main sources of structural information are the Cambridge Structural Database[25] for small molecules (usually less than 100 atoms) and the PDB[26] for macromolecules (see Section 22.3.2), including proteins and nucleic acids, and combinations of these macromolecules with small molecules (such as drugs, cofactors, and vitamins). The PDB has approximately 20,000 high-resolution structures, but this number is misleading because many of them are small variants on the same structural architecture (Figure 22.8). If an algorithm is applied to the database to filter out redundant structures, less than 2,000 structures remain.

There are approximately 100,000 proteins in humans; therefore many structures remain unsolved (e.g., Burley and Bonanno, 2002; Gerstein et al., 2003). In the PDB,

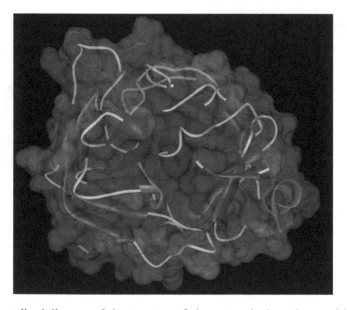

Figure 22.8. A stylized diagram of the structure of chymotrypsin, here shown with two identical subunits interacting. The red portion of the protein backbone shows α-helical regions, while the blue portion shows β-strands, and the white denotes connecting coils, while the molecular surface is overlaid in gray. The detailed rendering of all the atoms in chymotrypsin would make this view difficult to visualize because of the complexity of the spatial relationships between thousands of atoms.

---

[25]http://www.ccdc.cam.ac.uk/.
[26]http://www.rcsb.org/.

each structure is reported with its biological source, reference information, manual annotations of interesting features, and the Cartesian coordinates of each atom within the molecule. Given knowledge of the three-dimensional structure of molecules, the function sometimes becomes clear. For example, the ways in which the medication methotrexate interacts with its biological target have been studied in detail for two decades. Methotrexate is used to treat cancer and rheumatologic diseases, and it is an inhibitor of the protein dihydrofolate reductase, an important molecule for cellular reproduction. The three-dimensional structure of dihydrofolate reductase has been known for many years and has thus allowed detailed studies of the ways in which small molecules, such as methotrexate, interact at an atomic level. As the PDB increases in size, it becomes important to have organizing principles for thinking about biological structure. SCOP[27] provides a classification based on the overall structural features of proteins. It is a useful method for accessing the entries of the PDB.

22.5.3   Analysis of Biological Pathways and Understanding of Disease Processes

The *ECOCYC* project is an example of a computational resource that has comprehensive information about biochemical pathways.[28] ECOCYC is a knowledge base of the metabolic capabilities of *E. coli*; it has a representation of all the enzymes in the *E. coli* genome and of the compounds on which they work. It also links these enzymes to their position on the genome to provide a useful interface into this information. The network of pathways within ECOCYC provides an excellent substrate on which useful applications can be built. For example, they could provide: (1) the ability to guess the function of a new protein by assessing its similarity to *E. coli* genes with a similar sequence, (2) the ability to ask what the effect on an organism would be if a critical component of a pathway were removed (would other pathways be used to create the desired function, or would the organism lose a vital function and die?), and (3) the ability to provide a rich user interface to the literature on *E. coli* metabolism. Similarly, the Kyoto Encyclopedia of Genes and Genomes (KEGG) provides pathway datacets for organism genomes.[29]

22.5.4   Postgenomic Databases

A **postgenomic database** bridges the gap between molecular biological databases with those of clinical importance. One excellent example of a postgenomic database is the *Online Mendelian Inheritance in Man* (OMIM) database,[30] which is a compilation of known human genes and genetic diseases, along with manual annotations describing the state of our understanding of individual genetic disorders. Each entry contains links to special-purpose databases and thus provides links between clinical syndromes and basic molecular mechanisms (Figure 22.9).

---

[27]See http://scop.mrc-lmb.cam.ac.uk/scop/.
[28]http://www.ecocyc.org/.
[29]http://www.genome.ad.jp/kegg/.
[30]http://www3.ncbi.nlm.nih.gov/omim/.

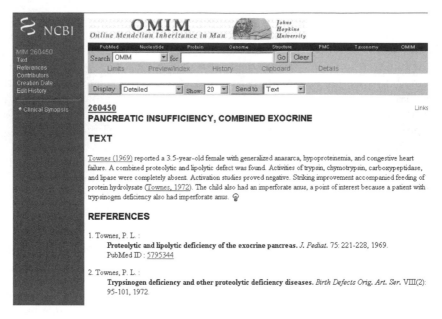

Figure 22.9. Screen from the Online Mendelian Inheritance in Man (OMIM) database showing an entry for pancreatic insufficiency, an autosomal recessive disease in which chymotrypsin (LocusLink entry shown in Figure 22.2) is totally absent (as are some other key digestive enzymes). (Courtesy of NCBI)

The SMD is another example of a postgenomic database that has proven extremely useful, but has also addressed some formidable challenges. As discussed previously in several sections, expression data are often represented as vectors of data values. In addition to the ratio values, the SMD stores images of individual chips, complete with annotated gene spots (see Figure 22.1). Further, the SMD must store experimental conditions, the type and protocol of the experiment, and other data associated with the experiment. Arbitrary analysis can be performed on different experiments stored in this unique resource.

A critical technical challenge within bioinformatics is the interconnection of databases. As biological databases have proliferated, researchers have been increasingly interested in linking them to support more complicated requests for information. Some of these links are natural because of the close connection of DNA sequence to protein structure (a straightforward translation). Other links are much more difficult because the semantics of the data items within the databases are fuzzy or because good methods for linking certain types of data simply do not exist. For example, in an ideal world, a protein sequence would be linked to a database containing information about that sequence's function. Unfortunately, although there are databases about protein function, it is not always easy to assign a function to a protein based on sequence information alone, and so the databases are limited by gaps in our understanding of biology. Some excellent recent work in the integration of diverse biological databases has been done in connection with the NCBI Entrez/PubMed systems,[31] the SRS resource,[32] DiscoveryLink,[33] and the Biokleisli project.[34]

22.6   Future Challenges as Bioinformatics and Clinical Informatics Converge

The human genome sequencing projects will be complete within a decade, and if the only *raison d'etre* for bioinformatics is to support these projects, then the discipline is not well founded. If, on the other hand, we can identify a set of challenges for the next generations of investigators, then we can more comfortably claim disciplinary status for the field. Fortunately, there is a series of challenges for which the completion of the first human genome sequence is only the beginning.

22.6.1   Completion of Multiple Human Genome Sequences

With the first human genome in hand, the possibilities for studying the role of genetics in human disease multiply. A new challenge immediately emerges, however: collecting individual sequence data from patients who have disease. Researchers estimate that more than 99 percent of the DNA sequences within humans are identical, but the remaining sequences are different and account for our variability in susceptibility to and development of disease states. It is not unreasonable to expect that for particular disease syndromes, the detailed genetic information for individual patients will provide valuable information that will allow us to tailor treatment protocols and perhaps let us make more accurate prognoses. There are significant problems associated with obtaining, organizing, analyzing, and using this information.

22.6.2   Linkage of Molecular Information with Symptoms, Signs, and Patients

There is currently a gap in our understanding of disease processes. Although we have a good understanding of the principles by which small groups of molecules interact, we are not able to fully explain how thousands of molecules interact within a cell to create both normal and abnormal physiological states. As the databases continue to accumulate information ranging from patient-specific data to fundamental genetic information, a major challenge is creating the conceptual links between these databases to create an audit trail from molecular-level information to macroscopic phenomena, as manifested in disease. The availability of these links will facilitate the identification of important targets for future research and will provide a scaffold for biomedical knowledge, ensuring that important literature is not lost within the increasing volume of published data.

---

[31]http://www.ncbi.nlm.nih.gov/PubMed/.

[32]http://srs.embl-heidelberg.de:8000/.

[33]http://www.research.ibm.com/journal/sj/402/haas.html.

[34]http://www.geneticxchange.com/.

22.6.3   Computational Representations of the Biomedical Literature

An important opportunity within bioinformatics is the linkage of biological experimental data with the published papers that report them. Electronic publication of the biological literature provides exciting opportunities for making data easily available to scientists. Already, certain types of simple data that are produced in large volumes are expected to be included in manuscripts submitted for publication, including new sequences that are required to be deposited in GENBANK and new structure coordinates that are deposited in the PDB. However, there are many other experimental data sources that are currently difficult to provide in a standardized way, because the data either are more intricate than those stored in GENBANK or PDB or are not produced in a volume sufficient to fill a database devoted entirely to the relevant area. Knowledge base technology can be used, however, to represent multiple types of highly interrelated data.

Knowledge bases can be defined in many ways (see Chapter 20); for our purposes, we can think of them as databases in which (1) the ratio of the number of tables to the number of entries per table is high compared with usual databases, (2) the individual entries (or records) have unique names, and (3) the values of many fields for one record in the database are the names of other records, thus creating a highly interlinked network of concepts. The structure of knowledge bases often leads to unique strategies for storage and retrieval of their content. To build a knowledge base for storing information from biological experiments, there are some requirements. First, the set of experiments to be modeled must be defined. Second, the key attributes of each experiment that should be recorded in the knowledge base must be specified. Third, the set of legal values for each attribute must be specified, usually by creating a controlled terminology for basic data or by specifying the types of knowledge-based entries that can serve as values within the knowledge base.

The development of such schemes necessitates the creation of terminology standards, just as in clinical informatics. The RiboWeb project is undertaking this task in the domain of RNA biology (Chen et al., 1997). RiboWeb is a collaborative tool for ribosomal modeling that has at its center a knowledge base of the ribosomal structural literature. RiboWeb links standard bibliographic references to knowledge-based entries that summarize the key experimental findings reported in each paper. For each type of experiment that can be performed, the key attributes must be specified. Thus, for example, a *cross-linking experiment* is one in which a small molecule with two highly reactive chemical groups is added to an ensemble of other molecules. The reactive groups attach themselves to two vulnerable parts of the ensemble. Because the molecule is small, the two vulnerable areas cannot be any further from each other than the maximum stretched-out length of the small molecule. Thus, an analysis of the resulting reaction gives information that one part of the ensemble is "close" to another part. This experiment can be summarized formally with a few features—for example, target of experiment, cross-linked parts, and cross-linking agent.

The task of creating connections between published literature and basic data is a difficult one because of the need to create formal structures and then to create the necessary content for each published article. The most likely scenario is that biologists will write and submit their papers along with the entries that they propose to add to the knowledge base. Thus, the knowledge base will become an ever-growing communal store of scientific knowledge. Reviewers of the work will examine the knowledge-based elements, perhaps will run a set of automated consistency checks, and will allow the knowledge base to be modified if they deem the paper to be of sufficient scientific merit. RiboWeb in prototype form can be accessed on the Web.[35]

22.6.4   A Complete Computational Model of Physiology

One of the most exciting goals for computational biology and bioinformatics is the creation of a unified computational model of physiology. Imagine a computer program that provides a comprehensive simulation of a human body. The simulation would be a complex mathematical model in which all the molecular details of each organ system would be represented in sufficient detail to allow complex "what if?" questions to be asked. For example, a new therapeutic agent could be introduced into the system, and its effects on each of the organ subsystems and on their cellular apparatus could be assessed. The side-effect profile, possible toxicities, and perhaps even the efficacy of the agent could be assessed computationally before trials are begun on laboratory animals or human subjects. The model could be linked to visualizations to allow the teaching of medicine at all grade levels to benefit from our detailed understanding of physiological processes—visualizations would be both anatomic (where things are) and functional (what things do). Finally, the model would provide an interface to human genetic and biological knowledge. What more natural user interface could there be for exploring physiology, anatomy, genetics, and biochemistry than the universally recognizable structure of a human that could be browsed at both macroscopic and microscopic levels of detail? As components of interest were found, they could be selected, and the available literature could be made available to the user.

The complete computational model of a human is not close to completion. First, all the participants in the system (the molecules and the ways in which they associate to form higher-level aggregates) must be identified. Second, the quantitative equations and symbolic relationships that summarize how the systems interact have not been elucidated fully. Third, the computational representations and computer power to run such a simulation are not in place. Researchers are, however, working in each of these areas. The genome projects will soon define all the molecules that constitute each organism. Research in simulation and the new experimental technologies being developed will give us an understanding of how these molecules associate and perform their functions. Finally, research in both clinical informatics and bioinformatics will provide the computational infrastructure required to deliver such technologies.

22.7   Conclusion

Bioinformatics is closely allied to clinical informatics. It differs in its emphasis on a reductionist view of biological systems, starting with sequence information and moving

---

[35]http://smi-web.stanford.edu/projects/helix/riboweb.html.

to structural and functional information. The emergence of the genome sequencing projects and the new technologies for measuring metabolic processes within cells is beginning to allow bioinformaticians to construct a more synthetic view of biological processes, which will complement the whole-organism, top-down approach of clinical informatics. More importantly, there are technologies that can be shared between bioinformatics and clinical informatics because they both focus on representing, storing, and analyzing biological data. These technologies include the creation and management of standard terminologies and data representations, the integration of heterogeneous databases, the organization and searching of the biomedical literature, the use of machine learning techniques to extract new knowledge, the simulation of biological processes, and the creation of knowledge-based systems to support advanced practitioners in the two fields.

Suggested Readings

Altman R.B., Dunker A.K., Hunter L., Klein T.E. (2003). *Pacific Symposium on Biocomputing '03*. Singapore: World Scientific Publishing.
The proceedings of one of the principal meetings in bioinformatics, this is an excellent source for up-to-date research reports. Other important meetings include those sponsored by the International Society for Computational Biology (ISCB, http://www.iscb.org/), Intelligent Systems for Molecular Biology (ISMB, http://iscb.org/conferences.shtml.35), and the RECOMB meetings on computational biology (http://www.ctw-congress.de/recomb/). ISMB and PSB have their proceedings indexed in Medline.

Baldi P., Brunak S. (1998). *Bioinformatics: The Machine Learning Approach*. Cambridge, MA: MIT Press.
This introduction to the field of bioinformatics focuses on the use of statistical and artificial intelligence techniques in machine learning.

Baldi P., Hatfield, G.W. (2002). *DNA Microarrays and Gene Expression*. Cambridge: Cambridge University Press.
Introduces the different microarray technologies and how they are analyzed.

Bishop M., Rawlings C. (Eds.) (1997). *DNA and Protein Sequence Analysis—A Practical Approach*. New York: IRL Press at Oxford University Press.
This book provides an introduction to sequence analysis for the interested biologist with limited computing experience.

Durbin R., Eddy R., Krogh A., Mitchison G. (1998). *Biological Sequence Analysis: Probabilistic Models of Proteins and Nucleic Acids*. Cambridge: Cambridge University Press.
This edited volume provides an excellent introduction to the use of probabilistic representations of sequences for the purposes of alignment, multiple alignment, and analysis.

Gribskov M., Devereux J. (1991). *Sequence Analysis Primer*. New York: Stockton Press.
This primer provides a good introduction to the basic algorithms used in sequence analysis, including dynamic programming for sequence alignment.

Gusfield D. (1997). *Algorithms on Strings, Trees and Sequences: Computer Science and Computational Biology*. Cambridge: Cambridge University Press.

Gusfield's text provides an excellent introduction to the algorithmics of sequence and string analysis, with special attention paid to biological sequence analysis problems.

Hunter L. (1993). *Artificial Intelligence and Molecular Biology*. Menlo Park, CA: AAAI Press/MIT Press.
This volume shows a variety of ways in which artificial intelligence techniques have been used to solve problems in biology.

Malcolm S., Goodship, J. (Eds.) (2001) *Genotype to Phenotype* (2nd ed.). Oxford: BIOS Scientific Publishers.
This volume illustrates the different efforts to understand how diseases are linked to genes

Salzberg S., Searls D., Kasif S. (Eds.) (1998). *Computational Methods in Molecular Biology*. New York: Elsevier Science.
This volume offers a useful collection of recent work in bioinformatics.

Setubal J., Medianis J. (1997). *Introduction to Computational Molecular Biology*. Boston: PWS Publishing.
Another introduction to bioinformatics, this text was written for computer scientists.

Stryer L. (1995). *Biochemistry*. New York: W.H. Freeman.
The textbook by Stryer is well written, and is illustrated and updated on a regular basis. It provides an excellent introduction to basic molecular biology and biochemistry.

Questions for Discussion

1. In what ways will bioinformatics and medical informatics interact in the future? Will the research agendas of the two fields merge, or will they always remain separable?
2. Will the introduction of DNA and protein sequence information change the way that medical records are managed in the future? Which types of systems will be most affected (laboratory, radiology, admission and discharge, financial, order entry)?
3. It has been postulated that clinical informatics and bioinformatics are working on the same problems, but in some areas one field has made more progress than the other. Identify three common themes. Describe how the issues are approached by each sub-discipline.
4. Why should an awareness of bioinformatics be expected of clinical informatics professionals? Should a chapter on bioinformatics appear in a clinical informatics textbook? Explain your answers.
5. One major problem with introducing computers into clinical medicine is the extreme time and resource pressure placed on physicians and other health care workers. Will the same problems arise in basic biomedical research?
6. Why have biologists and bioinformaticians embraced the Web as a vehicle for disseminating data so quickly, whereas clinicians and clinical informaticians have been more hesitant to put their primary data online?

Unit III
Biomedical Informatics in the Years Ahead

23
Health Care Financing and Information Technology: A Historical Perspective

Sara J. Singer, Alain C. Enthoven, and Alan M. Garber

After reading this chapter, you should know the answers to these questions:

- How did health care insurance contribute to rapid growth in health care spending during the 1970s through the 1980s? What helped to stem the growth of health care spending in the mid-1990s? What new and old causes contributed to accelerated growth again in the late 1990s and early 2000s?
- How has health care financing influenced the development of health care information technology?
- What are health maintenance organizations (HMOs), prepaid group practices, preferred-provider organizations (PPOs), point-of-service (POS) plans, and high deductible plans? How do these groups provide incentives to reduce health care costs?
- How have employers and managed care organizations acted to improve health care quality and to reduce health care spending?
- How have changes in fiscal designs and incentives affected the development and adoption of health care information technology?
- How can health care information systems help health care institutions to respond to the changing financial environment?

23.1 Introduction

Why is a chapter on health care financing and delivery included in a book about computer applications in medicine? In much the same way that financing is an important factor in determining the organization of health care delivery in general, financing may be the single most important driver of developments in the field of health care information.

Fiscal issues have become increasingly important to the study of medical informatics, with growing pressures on hospitals and other health care providers to deliver care more efficiently, to generate and use information more effectively, and to deal optimally with a complex array of reimbursement schemes. Information technology has become an essential part of these functions, and new approaches to collecting and using data and to providing information will have a profound effect on the ability of the health care community to respond to this increasingly challenging financial environment.

In this chapter, we provide an overview of the U.S. health care economy and describe how health care institutions are reimbursed for the services that they provide. We describe how the public and private health care financing and delivery systems have evolved from an era of open-ended spending through a series of attempted public and private reforms in the decades of the 1980s, 1990s, and 2000s to its current financing and organizational forms. The remainder of the chapter explores the relationships among health care finance, health care delivery, and health care information technology. We address the implications of changes in health care financing on health care information technology and how these changes have affected both its introduction and its use. We also examine the implications of new information technology for health care delivery, management, and administrative functions and conclude by acknowledging the challenges health care organizations face in implementing and capturing value from technological innovation.

23.2   The Era of Open-Ended Spending

The period from 1960 to 1980 can be characterized as the era of open-ended financing in health care. During those two decades, national health care spending increased from about $27 billion to nearly $250 billion (Table 23.1), from about 5 percent of the gross domestic product (GDP) to nearly 9 percent (Table 23.1). Public-sector spending on health care increased from $6.6 billion to nearly $105 billion. Aggregate private health care insurance premiums increased from $1.2 billion to $12.1 billion. In this section, we consider the ways in which patients managed to pay for their care as costs soared dramatically during the 20-year period.

Table 23.1. National health expenditures (NHE) by year.[a]

Spending category	1960	1970	1980	1990	1993	1999	2000	2001
In billions National health expenditures	26.9	73.1	245.8	696.0	888.1	1219.7	1310.0	1424.5
Public	6.6	27.6	104.8	282.5	390.4	550.0	591.3	646.7
Private	20.2	45.4	140.9	413.5	497.7	669.7	718.7	777.9
Cost of private health insurance	1.2	2.8	12.1	40.0	53.3	73.2	80.7	89.7
As a percentage of the gross domestic product (GDP)								
NHE as percent of GDP	5.1	7.0	8.8	12.0	13.4	13.2	13.3	14.1
Average annual percent change in NHE	—	10.5	12.9	11.0	8.5	5.4	7.4	8.7
GDP	$527	$1,040	$2,796	$5,803	$6,642	$9,274	$9,825	$10,082
Average annual percent change in GDP	—	7.0	10.4	7.6	4.6	5.7	5.9	3.6

[a]Table 23.1 tracks the dramatic growth of NHE and its relationship to the growth in GDP.
(*Source*: HCFA Office of the Actuary: National Health Statistics. Levit K. [2001]. Trends in U.S. Health Spending, 2001, Health Affairs, January/February 2003.)

23.2.1   Private (Employer-Paid) Health Care Insurance

Although the antecedents to modern health insurance began in the nineteenth century, and several formative decisions were made in the 1930s, health insurance in the United States did not become a large-scale enterprise until World War II. About 12 million people had insurance for health care expenses in 1940; nearly 77 million had insurance by 1950 (Figure 23.1) (Health Insurance Association of America, 1991, 2002). Most were insured through their employers. Several trends encouraged this development. Collective bargaining was an important factor, as union leaders considered employer-paid health insurance to be an attractive bargaining prize. Employers of nonunionized personnel also generally were willing to provide insurance because they wished to avoid grievances that would encourage unionization. Perhaps the most influential factor was that employer-paid health insurance was excluded from the taxable incomes of employees; thus, health insurance was a form of tax-free compensation. Health insurance as a fringe benefit continued to grow rapidly in the 1950s. In 1959, legislation was enacted to cover all federal employees. By 1960, about 123 million people were covered, at least for hospital expenses.

During this period, health insurance generally was of two types. Commercial insurance companies offered **indemnity insurance**, modeled on casualty insurance. The typical form was payment of a specified amount for a hospital day or for each of a list of surgical procedures. Commercial insurance companies had no contractual link to providers. Their role was to indemnify patients for medical expenses as part of a package that included group life and disability insurance. As time went by, coverage became more comprehensive. Frequently, it was backed up by **major medical insurance** that paid 80 percent of all the patient's outlays after the patient had paid a specified amount or **deductible**.

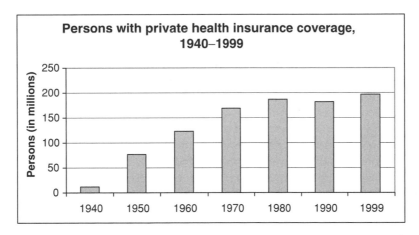

Figure 23.1. Persons with private health insurance coverage. Health insurance, through a variety of favorable incentives, became widespread after World War II. (*Source*: Health Insurance Association of America.)

The other type of health insurance was called **service benefit**, offered by Blue Cross and Blue Shield. Blue Cross plans were independent local nonprofit insurance companies sponsored by hospital associations. Blue Shield plans were sponsored by medical societies. These organizations were created to ensure that the providers would be paid in the manner most acceptable to those providers—that is, they could choose to be paid through cost reimbursement or through payment of billed charges to hospitals and fee-for-service (FFS) payment to physicians. Most hospitals and physicians participated in Blue Cross and Blue Shield (the "Blues"). In the former case, participation usually meant that hospitals would give Blue Cross a discount from the fees charged for patients who were insured by other carriers. In the latter case, it usually meant physicians would agree to accept Blue Shield fees as payment in full.

These insurance systems shared certain features. First, they reimbursed physicians for services based on **usual, customary, and reasonable fees**. They paid hospitals on the basis of billed charges or of retrospective cost reimbursement. Thus, they assigned providers no responsibility for the total cost of care. They did not create incentives to analyze or control costs. On the contrary, they paid providers more for doing more whether or not more is necessary or beneficial to the patient. If outlays exceeded premium revenues, future premiums were raised to make up the difference. Second, these insurance systems were based on the principle that at all times the patient must have free choice of provider. It was even against the law for the insurer to influence the patient's choice of provider. In such an arrangement, the insurer has no bargaining power with providers and thus no way to control prices or costs. Third, these financing systems generally covered entire employee groups. They were not conceived as competitors in situations in which individual employees would have a choice among health care–financing plans.

During the era of open-ended spending, the number of persons covered and the scope of private health insurance coverage increased markedly. The number of people with private insurance protection increased from 123 million in 1960 to 187 million by 1980 (Health Insurance Association of America, 1991) (Figure 23.1). This increase was encouraged by federal and state tax laws. The inflation that started in the late 1960s and intensified in the 1970s pushed people into higher and higher income-tax brackets. As this shift occurred, it became increasingly advantageous for employers and employees to agree that an employer would pay for comprehensive health insurance with before-tax dollars rather than paying the same amount in cash to employees and letting them pay for the insurance with net after tax dollars.

By 1980, the average taxpayer was in about the 40 percent marginal tax bracket, counting both income and payroll taxes, i.e., of the final dollar earned by an average taxpayer, about 40 percent went to federal and state income and payroll taxes. In 1981, this tax subsidy for health insurance (in which employers used nontaxed dollars to purchase insurance for employees) cost the federal government about $20 billion in foregone tax revenues (Figure 23.2) (Ginsburg, 1982). The same subsidy continues today and was calculated to reduce federal income and payroll tax revenues by $120 billion in 2001 (Congressional Budget Office, Budget Options, February 2001).

In the 1970s, high interest rates made it more advantageous for large employers to self-insure. Instead of paying a premium to an insurance company that would keep the money for perhaps 3 or 4 months before paying the bills, a growing number of large

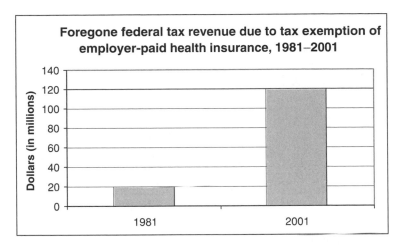

Figure 23.2. Foregone federal tax revenue. By allowing employers to purchase tax-free health insurance, the government foregoes billions of dollars in tax revenues. (*Source*: Ginsburg P. [1982]. Containing Medical Care Costs Through Market Forces, and Congressional Budget Office [2001] Budget Options.)

employers decided to pay their employees' medical bills directly, to hire insurance companies to perform claims processing or **administrative services only (ASO)**, and perhaps to buy insurance for only truly catastrophic cases. Under the Employee Retirement Income Security Act (ERISA) of 1974, these **self-insured plans** were also exempted from state regulation of insurance, which could be cumbersome and expensive. In effect, being self-insured means the employer takes on the health insurance function and risk directly. Although most practical for large employers, the availability of reinsurance or **stop-loss coverage**, which shifts the risk of a catastrophic case to an insurance company, has made it possible for small employers to self-insure as well. In 2002, about 66 percent of all employees, including 62 percent of employees in firms with between 200 and 999 workers and 12 percent of employees in firms with 3 to 199 workers, were covered by self-insured conventional indemnity plans (Kaiser Family Foundation 2002) (Figure 23.3).

The most important exception to the private-sector FFS system of health care finance was **prepaid group practice**, in which members paid an annual fee set in advance and received comprehensive health care during the year. In 1960, membership in prepaid group practice plans was small (about 1 million nationwide). The plans' importance lay in the concepts on which they were based. Kaiser Permanente, the largest and most successful of these organizations, adopted the following principles (Somers, 1971):

- Multispecialty group practice.
- Integrated inpatient and outpatient facilities.
- Direct prepayment to the medical care organization.
- Reversal of economics: providers are better off if the patients remain well or have their medical problems solved promptly.

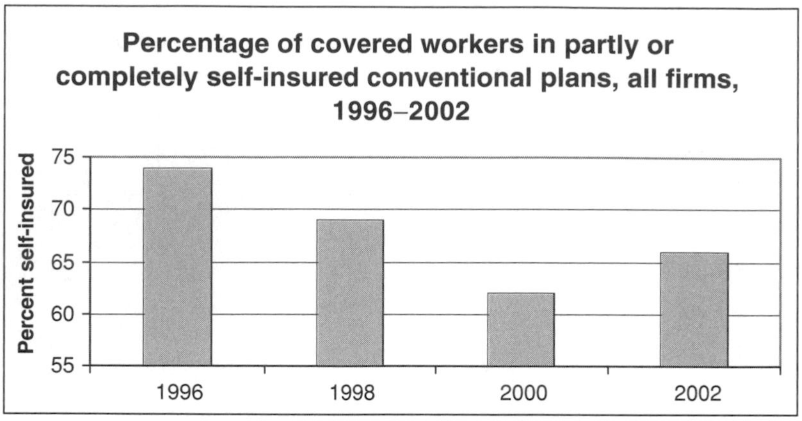

Percentage of covered workers in partly or completely self-insured conventional plans, all firms, 1996–2002

Figure 23.3. Percentage of covered workers in partly or completely self-insured conventional plans in 1996–2002. To realize the benefits from interest accrued on insurance premiums rather than handing it over to insurance companies and to avoid state regulation, many employers choose to self-insure. (*Source*: The Kaiser Family Foundation and Health Research and Educational Trust [2002]. Employer Health Benefits.)

- Voluntary enrollment: every enrollee should have a choice among competing alternatives.
- Physician responsibility for quality and cost of care.

The principle of voluntary enrollment was the beginning of the competition among health care financing and delivery plans that became widespread by the mid-1980s. Direct prepayment could reflect the overall efficiency of the provider organization, as well as the health risks and problems present in the enrolled population. Direct prepayment implies a reversal of the economic incentives in the FFS system, such that doctors prosper by keeping patients healthy and by diagnosing and solving their patients' medical problems promptly and effectively. Tertiary care (e.g., open heart surgery and organ transplants, which are usually done in regional referral centers), seen as a major profit center in the traditional system, became a cost center. Under the traditional paradigm, filled beds were an indicator of success; under the new paradigm, it was better to minimize hospital utilization. In theory, direct prepayment holds providers accountable for costs and for the costs of poor quality. If a procedure is done poorly and leads to complications and the need for more treatment, providers, rather than insurers or patients, pay the extra costs.

23.2.2 *Public-Sector Insurance*

In 1965, Congress enacted the Medicare and Medicaid programs in Titles XVIII and XIX of the Social Security Act. **Medicare** is the federal program of hospital and medical insurance for Social Security retirees. In 1972, legislation added coverage for the long-term disabled and for patients suffering from chronic renal failure. By 1980, Medicare covered 25.5 million aged and 3 million disabled persons (Figure 23.4).

Medicare was based on the same principle of payment as the Blue Cross and Blue Shield plans: reimbursement of reasonable cost to hospitals and fees to physicians. Patients were given unlimited free choice of provider, so a Medicare beneficiary received no financial advantage from going to a less costly hospital. The Medicare law did provide for certain deductibles and coinsurance to be paid by the patient who was receiving services. For example, under the Medicare system as of 2003, the hospitalized patient was charged a deductible that approximates 1 day's cost at the average hospital's per diem rate. After an annual deductible, Medicare paid 80 percent of the doctor's usual and customary fee; the patient is responsible for the rest. The coinsurance was the remaining 20 percent that the Medicare beneficiary was responsible for paying. However, any cost consciousness that cost sharing might encourage was attenuated, because almost 90 percent of Medicare beneficiaries have some form of supplemental insurance that offsets or removes the cost sensitivity intended by the cost-sharing features of Medicare. Of those with supplemental coverage, 72 percent have employer-sponsored or individually purchased private supplemental insurance that helps to pay the coinsurance and deductibles. Another 27 percent have private or Medicare health maintenance organization (HMO) coverage, which generally provides comprehensive benefits and low out-of-pocket costs. Finally, 9 percent of beneficiaries with supplemental insurance are considered to fall below the federally defined poverty level and thus are jointly covered by Medicaid, which has no coinsurance, and deductibles (Medicare Current Beneficiary Survey, 1999). **Medicaid** is a program of federal grants to help states pay for the medical care of welfare recipients and of other people who resemble welfare recipients (people in welfare categories, above the welfare income line). Only about one-half of the population below the poverty line is covered by Medicaid. For example, care for medically indigent adults has

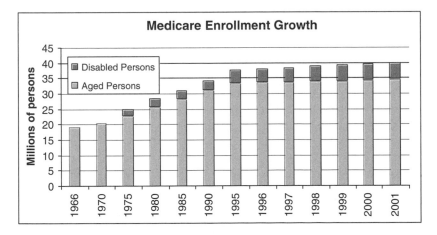

Figure 23.4. Growth of Medicare enrollment. With the enactment of the Medicare program, elderly Americans were ensured access to health care. (*Source*: Centers for Medicare and Medicaid Services, "Medicare Enrollment; National Trends 1966-2003" available at http://www.cms.hhs.gov/statistics/enrollment/natltrends/default.asp, accessed September 15, 2005.)

remained the responsibility of local—usually county—governments. Under Medicaid, the federal government sets elaborate standards that a state program must meet to be eligible for federal subsidies. The federal government pays a share of the cost (minimum 50 percent; average 57 percent as of 2001), depending on the state's per capita income. Like Medicare, Medicaid was based on the principles of FFS, cost reimbursement, and free choice of provider. Many physicians, however, choose not to participate in Medicaid because reimbursement is low.

In an effort to slow the growth of federal and state health care outlays for Medicare and Medicaid, the federal government imposed numerous regulatory restraints during the 1970s, with little success. Examples include institution of reimbursement limits on daily routine hospital care, creation of local nonprofit physicians' organizations called Professional Standards Review Organizations (PSROs) to review use of Medicare and Medicaid services and to deny payment for unnecessary services, and tying of the growth in reimbursable physician fees to an index of wages. These restraints were ineffective; Medicare and Medicaid outlays grew by about 17 percent per year through the 1970s.

23.3   Cost Growth and Strategies for Reform in the 1980s and 1990s

The cost-increasing incentives in the FFS model, fueled by information and medical technology, continued to increase the costs of health care in the 1980s at rates faster than inflation. National health expenditures increased as a percentage of GDP from nearly 9 to 12 percent, from nearly $250 billion in 1980 to nearly $700 billion in 1990—an average annual increase of 11 percent (see Table 23.1). Private-sector spending on health care increased from about $141 billion to $413.5 billion, and public-sector spending increased from nearly $105 billion to $282.5 billion. From 1980 to 1990, Medicare outlays grew from $37.4 billion to $110.2 billion, or 11.4 percent per year (Table 23.2).

Table 23.2. Medicare and Medicaid expenditures aggregate (in billions) by year.[a]

Spending category	1960[b]	1970[c]	1980	1990	1993	1999	2000	2001
Medicare	NA	7.7	37.4	110.2	148.3	213.6	224.4	241.9
Average annual percent change in Medicare	NA	NA	17.1	11.4	10.4	6.3	5.1	7.8
Medicaid[d]	NA	5.2	26.0	73.6	121.6	186.0	202.4	224.2
Average annual percent change in Medicaid	NA	NA	17.5	11.0	18.2	7.3	8.8	10.8
Average annual percent change in GDP	NA	7.0	10.4	7.6	4.6	5.7	5.9	3.6

[a]Medicare and Medicaid expenditures have grown faster than the gross domestic product (GDP) in every year except 2000.
[b]NA=not applicable; Medicare and Medicaid became effective in July 1966.
[c]Average annual growth, 1960–1970.
[d]Includes SCHIP (Title XXI).
(*Source*: HCFA Office of the Actuary: National Health Statistics Group. Levit, K. (2003). Trends in U.S. Health Spending, 2001, Health Affairs, January/February 2003.

Medicaid outlays grew from $26 billion to $73.6 billion, or 11 percent per year between 1980 and 1990. By comparison, the GDP grew about 7.6 percent per year between 1980 and 1990.

Despite the similarities in the problems they faced, the public and private sectors responded differently. Legislators attempted to control spending in the Medicare and Medicaid programs by making changes to the existing programs but leaving their FFS incentives intact, whereas private-sector purchasers more willingly embraced the logic of the incentives inherent in the prepaid group practice model.

23.3.1 Public-Sector Reform

Fiscal pressure in the early 1980s led to legislative activity designed to change the government's commitment from open-ended, cost-unconscious retrospective payment to alternatives that placed providers at greater financial risk for the costs of care. The most significant changes were the adoption of prospective payment and, for the Medicaid program in particular, limited choice of provider. These efforts, however, were not generally successful.

The Omnibus Budget Reconciliation Act of 1981 (OBRA, 1981) included many changes in Medicare and Medicaid. Two changes in Medicaid were particularly significant. First, federal matching payments to each state were reduced. States could avoid part of these reductions if they took certain actions to control costs. Second, Congress granted states more discretion in changing the features of their Medicaid programs to control costs. In particular, the law provided that the Secretary of Health and Human Services (HHS) could waive the provision for freedom of choice of provider in Medicaid law and could thus allow states to engage in selective provider contracting. This flexibility led certain states, such as California, to enact legislation to require their Medicaid programs to contract selectively on the basis of price and to seek competitive bids from hospitals.

The Tax Equity and Fiscal Responsibility Act (TEFRA) of 1982 put two new constraints on the all-inclusive cost per case for Medicare. First, it placed a limit on total inpatient operating costs, applied on a cost-per-case basis, adjusted for each hospital's severity of case mix. Second, it placed a new limit on each hospital's rate of increase in cost per case, based on an index of the wages and prices that hospitals pay. The same law provided that Medicare could contract with HMOs or with other "competitive medical plans" to care for Medicare beneficiaries. Medicare paid these plans on the basis of a fixed prospective per capita payment equal to 95 percent of the adjusted average per capita cost to Medicare of similar patients who remained with FFS providers.

In the Social Security Amendments of 1983, Congress enacted the **prospective payment system (PPS)** for Medicare inpatient cases. Under PPS, Medicare pays hospitals a uniform national fixed payment per case based on about 468 **diagnosis-related groups (DRGs)**, adjusted for area hospital wage levels. The DRG classification system was derived empirically; diagnoses were assigned to a group based on major diagnostic category, secondary diagnosis, surgical procedure, age, and types of services required. The DRG classification system was intended to produce homogeneous groups from the point of view of resource use. Within each DRG, the average length of stay was expected to be similar. The PPS created hospital responsibility for effectively integrating the pieces of the inpatient care process and powerful incentives to reduce the cost of inpatient cases. The PPS thus successfully slowed the growth of cost of inpatient services, but its introduction was followed by a rapid acceleration in the growth of outpatient services and, later on, home health agency services.

In the Omnibus Budget Reconciliation Act of 1989 (OBRA, 1989), Congress embarked on the **Resource-Based Relative Value Scale** (RBRVS) and **Volume Performance Standard** (VPS) systems for paying for Medicare physicians' services. RBRVS was intended to correct the large inequities and perverse incentives in Medicare's "customary, prevailing, and reasonable" (CPR) payment system. Medicare's CPR payment system reimbursed practitioners generously for doing procedures but poorly for providing cognitive services such as history taking and advice giving. RBRVS was intended to produce relative prices for physicians' services that approximated what would exist in an effective market system—that is, prices proportional to marginal costs. The intention of RBRVS was to diminish the incentives that providers had to perform expensive procedures. VPS was intended to control volume but may have instead motivated an increase in physician services as doctors sought to protect their real incomes in the face of controlled prices and a surplus of doctors.

The legislative changes in the 1980s did little to stem growth in the overall costs of Medicare and Medicaid. From 1990 to 1993, Medicare expenditures continued to grow at 10.4 percent—almost the same rate as the previous decade—to $148.3 billion. Medicaid outlays increased faster than they had in the 1980s, by 18.2 percent between1990 and 1993, to $121.6 billion by 1993. In contrast, the GDP slowed during this period, growing by only 4.6 percent per year (see Table 23.2).

23.3.2   Private-Sector Reform

Pressure for changes in the private sector intensified as costs increased. Rather than trying to improve on the inherently flawed incentives intrinsic in the existing FFS model, the private sector turned to managed care for cost relief.

Managed care was intended to be a complex bundle of innovative solutions to the problems of the traditional FFS system. There was great variation among individual managed care organizations in the extent to and success with which principles were applied in practice, and ultimately most managed care organizations, with the notable exception of Kaiser Permanente, abandoned many of these strategies in the face of pressure from consumers and physicians. The essential principles of managed care were as follows.

- *Selective provider contracting.* Insurers selected providers for quality and economy. Quality was important because people demanded high quality of care; employers cared about the health and satisfaction of their employees (if they did not, their trade unions were likely to care); because insurers cared about their reputations; and because mistakes cost money. Historically, quality and economy have often gone hand in hand. That is, many efforts to improve quality and to reduce rework and mistakes resulted in lower costs. Providers were also chosen for their willingness to cooperate with the managed care organization's quality and utilization management programs and reporting requirements.

- *Utilization management.* This principle varied from the crude to the sophisticated. For example, some managed care organizations retained actuarial consulting firms to develop guidelines for how long various types of patients should be hospitalized, and these guidelines were translated into limits on what the insurance would pay. Many employed **primary care gatekeepers**—primary care physicians who controlled referrals to specialists. Many managed care organizations dealing with doctors from the FFS sector who were thought to be overutilizers required prior authorization before a patient with a nonemergent problem could be hospitalized. An insurance contract might have included, for example, a $200 deductible for hospitalizations, waived if the patient obtained authorization. Some managed care organizations employed concurrent review, whereby utilization management professionals checked regularly on the hospital inpatient's condition and planned prompt discharges.

  The more advanced form of utilization management was based on the recognition that medical uncertainty is often great and practice variations are wide. Teams of physicians studied particular medical conditions, reviewed the medical literature, analyzed and studied their own data, and developed recommended practice guidelines based on professional consensus within the team. Typically, the guidelines reflected the least costly way of achieving the best obtainable outcomes.

- *Negotiated payment.* The basic idea of negotiated payment was to trade higher patient volume for lower prices. Compared with the usual and customary fees in the FFS system, managed care organizations typically obtained discounts in the range of 20 to 40 percent. These negotiated payments often included some bundling of services—for example, all-inclusive payments per inpatient day (for different types of patient) or per inpatient hospital case.

- *Quality management.* For example, a managed care organization might have surveyed patients about their satisfaction and rewarded with bonuses those providers who scored well. Providers who scored poorly might not have been offered a renewal of their contracts. Sophisticated organizations attempted to measure outcomes of care, or performance of processes of care, and reported these measurements to consumers and purchasers.

In some communities, prepaid group practices, such as Kaiser Permanente, were successful and growing during this period. The term **health maintenance organization (HMO)** was coined in 1970 by Paul Ellwood to describe prepaid group practices, which were the earliest form of managed care (Ellwood et al., 1971).

In general, an HMO is a health insurance carrier that covers a comprehensive list of health care services: physician, hospital, laboratory, diagnostic imaging, and usually prescription drugs. The coverage provides for nominal copayments at the point-of-service (POS) (e.g., $10 per doctor office visit), but there is no deductible and in general, no limit on the amount that the HMO will pay. Copayments are not supposed to be so large as to constitute a barrier to care.

HMOs contract with employers and individual subscribers on the basis of per capita prepayment. In this contract, the HMO bears the full risk for the cost of medical care. The amount and type of risk sharing that the HMO then arranges with providers varies widely, but usually the HMO shares some risk, explicitly or implicitly. An explicit risk-sharing arrangement might be a contract with a medical group to provide all necessary professional services for a fixed per capita payment. An implicit risk-sharing arrangement might pay individual doctors on a discounted FFS basis, but the HMO would then keep track of the per patient costs of each doctor, adjusted for age, gender, and possibly diagnosis; doctors whose costs consistently exceed norms might receive extra counseling on practice patterns or might not have their contracts renewed (Table 23.3).

Originally, HMOs were of several types. **Group-model HMOs** were based on contracts between physicians organized in a medical group and the HMO. The medical group accepted risks of costs of care and usually rewarded the partners if the group was successful in managing costs. **Staff-model HMOs**, in contrast, retained doctors on staff and paid them as salaried employees. Although the two are usually considered to be substantially similar organizational forms, there is an important difference. The doctors in group-model HMOs were more likely to see themselves as part owners of the enterprise and to feel more responsible for its success. Both types attempted to organize comprehensive care systems. Their doctors cared exclusively for patients enrolled in their affiliated health insurance plan. They generally cared for patients in HMO-owned or HMO-leased facilities.

Doctors in FFS solo practice, feeling competitive pressure from prepaid group practices, formed **individual practice associations (IPAs)**, also known as **network-model HMOs**, through which they could offer patients the financial equivalent of the prepaid group practices. Independent medical group practices and individual doctors generally contracted with several insurance carrier IPA HMOs to see the patients enrolled with those carriers while also continuing to see patients enrolled in traditional insurance, Medicare, Medicaid, other, or no coverage. The doctors continued to practice in their own offices. The medical groups were paid on a per capita basis for professional services under contracts that included incentives for efficient hospital use. A typical contract might have provided a fixed-dollar monthly amount per enrolled person for professional services plus a risk-sharing arrangement for hospital costs. Individual doctors were paid negotiated FFSs, with incentives for economical behavior, and were usually monitored for the economy of their practice patterns. A typical contract might have paid primary care doctors 80 percent of their fees soon after delivery of services, with the other 20 percent withheld to be sure that there was enough money in the pool. At the end of the year, the doctors were paid in proportion to their billings if there was money left over. In addition, the pool of primary care doctors may have shared in the savings from efficient specialist referrals and hospital use.

Table 23.3. Comparisons between fee-for-service and managed care.[a]

Fee-for-service	Managed care
Providers are paid a fee for each service provided	Providers are paid a fixed payment per member per month
Potential incentive for unnecessary services	Potential incentive for underprovision of services
Patients see any provider	Patients see selected providers
Little or no quality or utilization management	Features quality and utilization management

[a]Managed care constitutes a reversal of the economic incentives in fee-for-service insurance.

In response to the early development and acceptance of HMOs, in 1973 Congress passed the HMO Act. The HMO Act (1) defined HMOs as being of either the group practice or the individual practice variety; (2) provided grants and loans to help start nonprofit HMOs; and (3) required that all employers of 25 or more employees, subject to the Fair Labor Standards Act, who were offering traditional insurance, also offer to their employees the choice of one group-practice and one individual-practice HMO as alternatives to traditional health insurance if such HMOs served the areas where their employees lived and asked to be offered; and (4) overruled state laws that inhibited HMO growth.

The HMO Act had an important effect in opening up the market to competition. These provisions also helped to expand access to HMOs and thus the number of HMOs. By 1978, there were 7.3 million members in 195 operating HMOs. At that time, the HMO industry was made up almost entirely of local nonprofit HMOs and of Kaiser Permanente, which was then a large national organization serving 3.5 million enrollees in six states—a multistate or national HMO. By 1996, 623 mostly for-profit HMO firms served 60.6 million enrollees (Table 23.4). Between 1978 and 1996, HMO annual enrollment growth exceeded 12.5 percent.

Some employers wanted to be able to offer employees health insurance based on selective provider contracting—that is, insurance that resembled the traditional model except that employees would be offered preferential terms of coverage if they used contracting providers. Then, employers and insurers would be able to negotiate prices and utilization controls with providers. Until 1982, however, in compliance with the principle of free choice of independently practicing providers, this kind of insurance was illegal under the insurance codes in most states. In 1982, a major legislative battle erupted in California. Employers, insurers, and labor unions teamed up to defeat the California Medical Association and to secure the enactment of new legislation permitting insurers to contract selectively and to pass on the savings to the insured. Most other states followed. Thus, the states authorized **preferred-provider insurance (PPI)**, another form of managed care.

PPI represented less change from the traditional FFS model than did HMOs. Some people used the term **preferred-provider organization (PPO)** to parallel the better-established term "HMO." These entities were not, however, medical care organizations; they were insurance companies that contracted with large numbers of providers that were not otherwise related to one another (Boland, 1985). The typical preferred-provider insurer

Table 23.4. Health maintenance organization (HMO) growth by year.[a]

	1978	1985	1996	1999	2001
HMOs	195	485	623	617	533
Members (millions)	7.3	21.0	60.6	80.0	78.1
Members by model type (millions)					
Staff	—	3.0	0.7	0.4	0.2
Individual practice association (IPA)	0.6	6.4	26.5	32.4	32.3
Network	—	5.0	3.6	6.9	7.8
Group	6.7	6.6	8.7	7.5	7.1
Mixed	—	—	20.9	32.7	30.1

[a]Both the number of and enrollment in HMOs grew rapidly since 1978, but started to decline in the late 1990s. (*Source*: InterStudy Publications.)

contracted with a large number of doctors, hospitals, laboratories, home health agencies, and so on. It created incentives for insured patients to choose contracting providers. For example, the insurance contract might have paid in full the negotiated fee for the services of contracting providers but paid only 80 percent of what it would have paid contracting providers for the services of noncontracting providers, with the patient liable to pay the rest. The insurer negotiated discounted fees, and the provider agreed to accept those fees as payment in full from contracting patients; that is, providers agreed to no balance billing. Finally, the insurer adopted utilization management tools, such as prior authorization for hospital admissions, length-of-stay guidelines, and review of provider credentials.

Some preferred-provider insurers covered comprehensive health care services. Others specialized, carving out a subset of comprehensive services, such as mental health, pharmacy, cardiology, or radiology. They served as subcontractors to insurers that covered comprehensive services. They could offer greater detailed knowledge of their particular specialty. They might also have contracted with several insurers that covered comprehensive care and subcontracted the components.

HMO providers differed from contracting PPI providers in that the former bore the financial risk associated with members' use of services, whereas the latter did not. The HMO agreed to provide all necessary services for a comprehensive per capita payment set in advance, independent of the number of services actually used. Contracting PPI providers did not suffer financially if the use of services increased, and they were not directly rewarded for reducing the use of services or for treating patients in less costly ways (Table 23.5).

Table 23.5. Characteristics of managed care organizations.[a]

Plan characteristic	Health maintenance organization (HMO)	Preferred-provider organization (PPO)	Point-of-service (POS) plan	High deductible plan
Financing Arrangement	Insures via prepayment for comprehensive health services	Arranges discounted fee-for-service rates with contracted providers	Adds PPO option to HMO plan	• Requires a high deductible • Offers a health spending account to pay deductible and cost sharing • Functions like a PPO above the deductible
Provider Access	Choice of provider limited to those within HMO	Offers incentives for enrollees to use contracted providers	Allows for free choice of provider with financial incentive to use HMO providers	
Risk Bearing	Providers bear risk for the cost of care	Providers do not bear risks for the cost of care		

[a]Different organizational forms present trade-offs between cost and access.

In the 1980s, PPI was introduced at a rapid rate, and participation in PPI grew continuously through the 1990s. By 1998, 98 million people were enrolled in PPOs (Aventis Pharmaceuticals, 2000).

In the long run, PPI are expected to be less effective at reducing costs than HMOs because the providers retained FFS incentives and were not financially constrained by a per capita budget. The PPI format did not reward providers for keeping patients out of the hospital, and keeping them out may be the single most important source of cost savings in health care. PPI did not organize the health care system for efficiency; it merely tried to shop for the lowest price in an inefficient system.

PPI was initially viewed as an important part of the transition from the traditional unmanaged FFS system to HMOs that use per capita prepayment. A group of doctors may have begun with a discounted FFS contract, acquired experience on which they could base a per capita payment, and then eventually converted to per capita prepayment.

For consumers, managed care, especially HMOs, required a change in patterns of access to doctors, from complete free choice to choice limited to the managed care plan's contracting providers. People who were accustomed to the traditional system often did not understand this change and the reasons for it. In addition, when they were seriously ill, some patients wanted to be able to go to a famous regional or national referral center and to take their insurance with them. In the mid-1980s, HMOs introduced the **point-of-service (POS)** plan to address this concern.

A POS HMO functioned as an HMO for those who wished to stay with the medical group that they chose within their HMO but added a PPI plan that the member could access by paying a deductible (typically, the first several hundred dollars of expense) and a fraction of each medical bill, and also a traditional insurance plan with an even stronger financial disincentive. This plan gave the covered person the full range of choice of provider but offered more favorable financial terms for sticking to the HMO primary physician network. Most people in these arrangements stayed with their primary care group for more than 90 percent of the services that they used. POS options were popular when introduced. It appeared that people simply wanted the comfort of knowing they had the option to choose. In March 1987, 11 HMOs reported POS enrollment of nearly 400,000. By July 1995, 318 HMOs served over 5 million enrollees in POS plans (American Association of Health Plans, 1995).

Some HMOs worked to improve customer service. For example, they tried to offer convenient access to **advice nurses** who could help patients to make good decisions about the care they sought. Some HMOs developed call centers to shorten telephone waiting time and to expedite appointments. Their standard of access to doctors was same-day appointments (with a doctor, if not with your own doctor) for people who thought they needed immediate care. Some HMOs designed open-access insurance plans that allowed members to see a doctor of any specialty within an HMO network without a referral. Innovations in information systems that allowed plans to keep the primary care physicians informed of interactions throughout the delivery system made feasible such open-access plans. As was the experience with POS plans, there seemed to be less-than-expected use of the open-access option among customers.

23.4   The Era of Managed Care: Adoption, Backlash, and Beyond

Employers responded to rapidly increasing health care costs and the threat of increased government regulation to control health care spending in the mid-1990s by turning to managed care, which promised to be a lower cost alternative (Table 23.6). Managed care plans, competing for customers, responded by lowering their prices and increasing their utilization and care management. During the 1990s, national health expenditures increased from nearly $700 in 1990 to more than $1.3 trillion in 2000, from 12 to 13.3 percent of the GDP (Table 23.1). The increase in overall private national health expenditures between 1990 and 2000 was greatly reduced compared with that in the previous decade. Private expenditures grew from $413.5 billion in 1990 to $718.7 billion in 2000—an annual average growth rate of 5.6 percent, just slightly faster than the GDP. Between 1993 and 1999, private health expenditures declined slightly as a percentage of the GDP from 7.5% in 1993 to 7.2% in 1999. Public-sector expenditures grew from $282.5 billion to $591.3 billion between 1990 and 2000. Medicare outlays grew from $110.2 billion to $224.4 billion, and Medicaid outlays grew from $73.6 billion to $202.4 billion, growth rates of 7.4 and 10.6 percent per year, respectively (Levit et al., 2003) (Table 23.2).

23.4.1   Medicare and Medicaid

The component of the health care system most resistant to change has been the Medicare program. Medicare built in virtually no quality management or improvement and required little accountability on the part of doctors, hospitals, or other providers. Although Medicare's risk basis contracting program has made HMO alternatives available to some beneficiaries, the government's reimbursement policy of 95 percent of the average adjusted per capita fee-for-service costs (AAPCCs) deprives the government of potential savings. If an HMO can provide Medicare's standard benefit package at lower cost than 95 percent of the AAPCC, the HMO must provide more benefits rather than offering a lower price. In addition, if the HMO enrolls a healthier-than-average population, government payments may greatly exceed 95 percent of the expenditures that the HMO enrollees would have generated if they had chosen the FFS option. If Medicare's reimbursement increases do not keep pace with medical inflation, as in the late 1990s, the government's policy drives plans to withdraw, depriving consumers of the choice to pay the extra cost if they believe a plan is worth the additional expense. As of 1998, 5.8 million, or 17 percent of, Medicare beneficiaries were enrolled in managed care plans compared with 64 percent of the total U.S. population (Figure 23.5). The pace of Medicare

Table 23.6. Comparison of fee-for-service and HMO insurance.[a]

Fee-for-service insurers	Health maintenance organizations
Traditionally not cost accountable	Theoretically accountable for cost and quality
Providers are paid more for their services	Fixed reimbursement regardless of service quantity

[a]HMOs attempted to create accountability for cost and quality by decoupling the financing from the quantity of services provided.

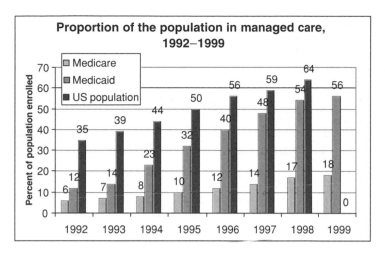

Figure 23.5. Proportion of the population in managed care. Enrollment in managed care plans has grown sharply for Medicaid recipients, but slowly for the Medicare population. (*Source*: Health Care Financing Review [1996–2001]. Medicare and Medicaid Statistical Supplements. InterStudy Publications [1996–2001], and Aventis Pharmaceuticals, Managed Care Digest Series Publications [1995–2000].)

managed care enrollment accelerated between 1995 and 1999 before declining again through 2001 (Levit, 2001; Cawley et al., 2002).

In contrast to Medicare, Medicaid has seen a rapid expansion of managed care, particularly in the form of risk-based programs. In 2001, Medicaid managed care enrollment was 20.7 million, up 28 percent per year from 3.7 million in 1992 (Health Care Financing Review, 2001). As of 2002, only three states—Alaska, Mississippi, and Wyoming—had no Medicaid managed care.

In 1997, Congress enacted the State Children's Health Insurance Program, or S-CHIP, through the Balanced Budget Act to provide funds to states to initiate and expand child health assistance to uninsured, low-income children. State approaches to S-CHIP implementation vary. Some states expanded eligibility to children through Medicaid programs, other states established separate child health programs, and some states did both. Initial approaches to payment and delivery included FFS, managed care, primary care case management, and mixed systems. Forty-three states had a managed care delivery system, though managed care was dominant in 20, and the sole system in 8 states (Thompson, 2002). Enrollment of children in S-CHIP doubled from approximately 1 million in 1998 to 2 million in 1999 and reached 5.3 million in 2002.

By 1996, there was a consensus that the Medicare program was in dire need of reform. The trustees of the program predicted the impending expiration of the Medicare Trust Funds (Medicare Board of Trustees Reports, 1996). Federal outlays for Medicare were expected almost to double as a percentage of the nation's GDP, to 4.2 percent by 2010 (the year 78 million baby boomers start to become eligible for Medicare benefits), up from 2.3 percent in 1995 (Federal Hospital Insurance Trust Fund, 1996; Congressional Budget Office, 1996). Medicare would thus become the federal government's single largest expense.

By 2015, the elderly population will have increased to 43.7 million. By 2030 there will be just over two workers to support the costs of each beneficiary; in 1997, there were four. The proportion of elderly in the population is expected to be 20 percent—more than twice the proportion when the program was initiated (U.S. Bureau of the Census) (Figure 23.6).

In response to these grave predictions, Congress enacted major reforms to the Medicare program through the Balanced Budget Act of 1997 and the Medicare Prescription Drug Improvement and Modernization Act of 2003. The Balanced Budget Act introduced many provider and private health plan payment changes and established the Medicare+Choice program, which expanded private plan options to Medicare beneficiaries. Although this legislation should have encouraged beneficiaries' transition to managed care, it was not expected to solve the long-run problems of the program. In addition, when government payment rate increases did not keep pace with medical inflation, many managed care plans withdrew from or limited their participation in Medicare. Managed care plan departures resulted in a 10% drop in Medicare managed care enrollment in 2001 (Levit, Jan/Feb 2003). The Medicare Modernization Act added a drug benefit to fee for service Medicare, revised and expanded the managed care program now called Medicare Advantage, and created demonstration projects in chronic care, disease management and pay for performance to reward health plans that meet performance standard (http://www.cms.hhs.gov/medicarereform). These reforms, whose goals and features are diverse, in some cases promote value, but in their totality do not represent a systematic strategy to promote value-based purchasing in medicare.

23.4.2 Managed Competition and Purchaser Initiatives

Employer interventions to reduce costs in a cost-unconscious environment dominated by forms of FFS insurance included requiring employees to pay a share of the cost for

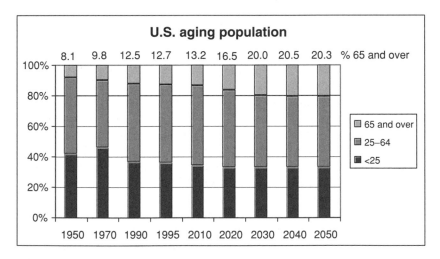

Figure 23.6. U.S. aging population. As the baby-boom generation approaches retirement age, problems with Medicare will grow dramatically. (*Source*: U.S. Bureau of Census, International Data Base http://www.census.gov/cgi-bin/ipc/idbsprd (last accessed July 17, 2003) for historical data and National Population Projections Summary Files: http://www.census.gov/population/www/* projections/natsum-T3.html (last accessed July 16, 2003) for projections.)

health insurance, consolidating the number of plans an employer offered so as to consolidate purchasing clout, and using self-insurance to eliminate administrative costs and to maximize the time value of money. Although these interventions may have reduced employer health care costs in the short term, they had no effect on health delivery and therefore could not reduce health care costs in the long run.

Dissatisfaction with these methods led many employers to embrace managed care. Initial efforts were only modestly effective at reducing costs, because most employers were unwilling or unable to make their employees responsible for premium price differences. Managed care organizations that competed with FFS plans recognized that they could attract customers by offering better service or benefits rather than by charging lower prices. Thus costs declined only modestly.

In contrast, some employers chose to hold health plans accountable for both the cost and the quality of the care delivered, thus intervening in ways that could affect care delivery and long-term costs if enough employers adopted these practices. **Managed competition** (Enthoven, 1993) is a strategy used to varying degrees by some purchasers of health care services intended (1) to create health services delivery organizations capable of acquiring appropriate health care resources, obtaining value for money, deploying the resources to care for an enrolled population, designing and executing care processes that produce good outcomes and value for money, and measuring and monitoring performance (outcomes, satisfaction, and cost) and continuously improving it (i.e., managing care); (2) to create a framework of incentives for such organizations to improve quality and reduce cost; and (3) to use market forces to transform the health care delivery system from its former fragmented, nonaccountable mode to efficient integrated comprehensive care organizations constantly striving to improve. In brief, managed competition refers to the rules of the game within which managed care organizations play (Table 23.7).

To manage competition, a "sponsor," either an employer or a group of employers, continuously structures and adjusts the market to overcome attempts by health plans to avoid price competition. The sponsor offers its members a choice of standardized health care coverage options and provides them with information and incentives to choose a health plan that provides them the greatest value for money. The sponsor selects the managed care organizations or insurance carriers that compete; sets equitable rules for pricing and enrollment within which all health plans must compete and monitors compliance; organizes a coordinated annual open enrollment during which members have an opportunity to consider alternative health plans; and provides comparative information about health plan prices, performance, quality, and service.

Table 23.7. Principles of managed competition.

Sponsor establishes equitable rules within which multiple plans compete and administers an open enrollment process
Individual is responsible for premium difference among competing plans
Standardizes coverage contracts between sponsored groups
Provides for individual choice of plan rather than group choice
Information on quality, plans, and providers is accessible and understandable
Risk selection is managed by providing a single point of entry and standard coverage contracts, and by risk-adjusting premiums

Under managed competition, sponsors also require members to pay the full premium differences if they choose a plan whose premium is higher than the low-priced plan. This gives members an incentive to seek value for money and, more importantly, gives plans an incentive to offer the greatest value. In practice, few sponsors employ the principles of managed competition. Of employees offered a choice of carriers in 1997, about one-quarter received a fixed-dollar contribution from the employer, and only about 6 percent of the insured workforce had a cost-conscious choice of carriers. Even among Fortune 500 companies, fewer than 10 percent of employers offered such a cost-conscious choice (Enthoven, 2003). A complicating factor in creating subscriber premium responsibility is the fact that employer-based health insurance contributions are still tax-free without limit to the employee. The effect is that, at the margin, choices of more costly health plans are subsidized by the government. This could be corrected by a limit on the tax-free amount, set at the premium of the low-priced plan.

The sponsor should also design solutions to offset the profitability of "risk selection" to ensure that health care organizations focus on giving better care at lower cost rather than selecting only healthy enrollees.

Managed competition was introduced most extensively in California, mainly led by a few large employers and **purchasing coalitions**—groups of employers that together structured their health care benefits program and negotiated with health plans. Most employers, even in California, have not applied all or even most of the principles outlined here. Examples of each component of the strategy, however, do exist. The Pacific Business Group on Health, a private large-employer purchasing coalition, negotiates health plan premiums on behalf of member employers and requires participating health plans to meet performance standards on quality of care, customer service, and data provision. The HMOs each put a total of 2 percent of premiums at risk for all performance standards, weighted according to each health plan's relative weaknesses. Pacific Health Advantage, formerly the Health Insurance Plan of California, a small-employer purchasing coalition, adjusts payments to health plans based on average risk profiles of enrollees, using diagnostic information to ensure that health plans that attract higher risk populations will be compensated for their additional costs. Several large employers are also now employing mechanisms that adjust for health status as well as demographic differences among the populations enrolled in the health plans serving their employees.

The California Public Employees Retirement System provides comparative price and quality information to state and other California agency employees. It has also done special analyses of the people who had been hospitalized or were frequent users of care to see if they were as satisfied as the healthy customers. Some California universities require their employees who choose a more expensive plan to pay the full premium difference. All these sponsors offer a choice of health plans and provide an annual open enrollment during which members choose plans. In response to these employer initiatives, competition among managed care plans became active in California, and health care costs decreased. In inflation-adjusted terms, the 1997 premiums for competitive HMOs were about 13 percent below their 1992 levels. These efforts, however, did not stave off premium increases for long.

Employers in other states also took an active role. Some formed coalitions to bargain collectively for health insurance premiums. Others supported the National Committee for Quality Assurance, and other organizations that measure the outcomes of care provided by health plans to provide information about quality. Increasing numbers of employers offered their employees a choice of health plans, and, although most do not require their employees to pay the full difference in price, many make their employees aware of price differences and require them to pay a portion of the difference. As a result, in the mid-1990s, national average HMO premium growth flattened. According to one survey, HMO average premiums fell by 0.2 percent between 1995 and 1996, down consistently from a 12.1 percent increase between 1990 and 1991 (Kaiser Family Foundation, 1999). Managed competition, however, was never implemented on a scale sufficient to reform health care delivery, and premiums began increasing again.

23.4.3   Managed Care and Provider Opportunities

Important gains in quality and economy of health care delivery could have been realized, given enough pressure from greater competition. At least seven forms of integration could be achieved through contractual relationship or ownership (Table 23.8). Selected managed care organizations attempted to integrate in some of these ways in the mid-1990s. However, most of these efforts were not sustained for a variety of reasons described below. Thus, these opportunities to integrate largely persist.

The first integration is between financial responsibility and delivery of care. It occurs with per capita prepayment by the purchaser to the chosen medical care organization. HMOs translated the broad incentive of **capitated** payment into payment to doctors in a great variety of ways. Some paid salaries. Others paid salaries with bonuses for productivity, patient satisfaction, and overall economic success. Others paid various forms of FFS with management controls. Some HMOs empirically tuned their methods, trying to discover what worked in their marketplaces. Some IPAs tried to select doctors and drive hard bargains with them as well as with the insurers with which they contracted. The best IPAs evaluated their primary care providers continuously and paid them in a manner that provided appropriate financial incentives. Good performers won cash bonuses; IPAs tried to drop poor performers from their programs. Some IPAs contracted with selected specialists on a discounted FFS basis and gave the primary care doctors as a group a financial incentive to control specialist referrals. More recently, HMOs participated in pay-for-performance initiatives, which reward physician groups that meet specified performance standards.

Table 23.8. Seven integrations of managed care.[a]

Financing and delivery: responsibility for costs of health care delivery
Providers and populations: population-based medicine
Full spectrum of health care services: care provided in least costly appropriate setting
Doctors and other health care professionals: right numbers and types
Doctors and hospitals: vertical integration
Hospitals: horizontal integration
Information: information management

[a]Greater integration can lead to better quality and lower costs.

Embedded in these reimbursement schemes were often incentives to improve quality. They motivated providers to "do it right the first time" because mistakes cost money. Patients with unsolved or poorly managed problems continued to impose costs on the health care system. Per capita prepayment facilitated the alignment of incentives of doctors with the interests of patients in high-quality economical care. It paid for and rewarded cost-effective preventive services, such as more outreach of prenatal care to reduce the costs of neonatology, or more effective management of chronic diseases to minimize acute episodes. It provided a framework for cost–benefit analysis, which helped to determine the most effective place to spend limited resources. It also rewarded cost-reducing innovation, such as the many incremental changes that reduced the length of hospital stays for total hip replacement operations from an average of 17 days in 1983 to 8 days in 1993, with several facilities achieving 3- or 4-day average stays (Keston and Enthoven, 1996).

The second integration is between providers and populations. This integration facilitated and encouraged population-based medicine that added an epidemiological perspective to encounter-based medicine. Providers looked behind the encounters with patients to the underlying causes of the patients' complaints to see whether there were effective methods of prevention. One of the enduring legends of Kaiser Permanente is that the founding doctor, Sidney Garfield, who was treating construction site workers with nail-puncture wounds in their feet, went to the site with a hammer and pounded down the offending nails. Some HMOs gave children bicycle helmets and videotapes explaining why the helmets should always be used. Thus, HMOs could allocate resources to maximize the wellness of their enrolled populations through preventive and patient education services. Also, the defined population base enabled HMOs to match the numbers and types of doctors in their groups, and also other resources, to the needs of the enrolled population.

The third integration is the full spectrum of health care services: inpatient, outpatient, doctor offices, home nursing, and so on, as well as drugs and other services. HMOs put resources into improved preventive services and outpatient care and were compensated by reduced inpatient cost. They sought to deliver care in the least costly appropriate setting. They were motivated to organize seamless comprehensive care so that patients were not left to their own devices when they left the hospital. In the best-managed HMOs, committees of doctors and pharmacists chose drug regimens to produce the best outcomes and to minimize total costs of care rather than merely minimizing the cost of drugs.

The fourth integration is among doctors and other health professionals. The goal was the right numbers and types of professionals, the right specialty mix to ensure that patients had good access and to ensure that the specialists were proficient in caring for their patients. It included rational referral patterns and efficient specialist–generalist division of labor. For example, specialists might have served as consultants to generalists who delivered the care. It included efficient use of paramedicals, such as nurse practitioners and social workers, who might have worked in teams with primary care physicians.

The fifth integration is between doctors and hospitals: giving doctors a serious interest in reducing hospital costs. Aligning doctors' and hospitals' interests is difficult because most doctors are not employed by the hospitals in which they see patients. In a well-integrated system, doctors developed practice patterns that facilitated efficient hospital operations. They worked with hospitals to reduce unnecessary record keeping, they supported "value for money" investment decisions.

The sixth integration is horizontal integration among hospitals. Groups of hospitals in a region combined to share administrative support functions, including management personnel, and tended to consolidate volume-sensitive clinical services, such as open-heart surgery and neonatology and laboratories.

The seventh integration is information. We describe this integration and its benefits in the remainder of this chapter. We argue that information, both clinical and financial, and its management are fundamental to successful integration of the delivery system.

In the mid-1990s, employers struggled with health care costs and believed that managed care organizations had the potential to offer increased value. As a result, managed care penetrated the markets of many states. By 1996, health plan enrollments in the private sector included 31 percent in HMOs and another 14 percent in POS plans (Kaiser Family Foundation, 2002) (Table 23.9). With the growth of managed care organizations, traditional, unmanaged FFS disappeared almost entirely in many areas. Even FFS insurers began managing their plans to avail themselves of the same purchasing preferences for buying large quantities and other economies of scale. By 2002, health plan enrollments in the private sector included only 5 percent in conventional FFS plans (Table 23.9) (Kaiser Family Foundation, 2002).

23.4.4   The Managed Care Backlash and Its Aftermath

Employers were only temporarily successful in their efforts to use managed care to control costs. Many managed care organizations moderated premium growth by squeezing provider payments and shortening hospital stays, not by fundamentally reforming health care organization and delivery. Consumers resented attempts to limit their care, and doctors and hospitals resisted attempts to limit their use of resources. Consumers became wary of providers who had real or imaginary financial incentives to limit service delivery. As patients, they began to demand greater responsibility for decisions about their care. The managed care backlash was accompanied by an intense onslaught from lawyers, politicians, consumers, and doctors. As a result, efforts to manage care were cut back or abandoned. The breakdown of managed care, in combination with other factors such as

Table 23.9. Health plan enrollments by year (in percent).[a]

Health plan type	1988[b]	1993	1996	1998	2000	2002
Health maintenance organization (HMO)	16	21	31	27	29	26
Preferred-provider organization (PPO)	11	26	28	35	41	52
Point-of-service (POS)	NA	7	14	24	22	18
Conventional with precertification	73	46	27	14	8	5

[a]Enrollments in conventional fee-for-service plans decreased and in managed care plans increased in the 1990s and early 2000s.
[b]NA=not applicable.
(*Source*: The Kaiser Family Foundation and Health Research and Education Trust, Employer Health Benefits [2002].)

the diffusion of expensive new technologies, caused health care inflation to resume and annual premium increases to take off. Average health insurance premiums increased 8.3 percent in 2000, 11.0 percent in 2001, and 12.7 percent in 2002 (Kaiser Family Foundation and Health Research and Eductional Trust, 2002). Premium increases are expected to continue.

Two forms of HMO became distinguished during the mid-1990s. The first is "delivery system HMOs," which provide health insurance for populations and deliver services through their own dedicated medical groups that are primarily paid on a capitated basis. These differ from "carrier HMOs," which are insurance companies that offer a comprehensive benefit package, characteristic of HMOs, but deliver the services by contracting with independent doctors or medical groups whose main mode of payment remains FFS. Physicians contracting with carrier HMOs typically contract with many organizations, so many of their patients are insured by traditional plans with FFS reimbursement. Efforts by carrier HMOs to integrate failed, and introduction of rules and requirements, such as drug formularies and care guidelines, were lost among the competing policies issued by other carrier HMOs to the same providers. Physicians typically had little involvement in the design and development of these policies, limiting their effectiveness in controlling cost and raising quality of care. The comprehensive benefits offered by carrier HMOs, however, removed the financial restraint on consumers' demands. By continuing to pay FFS, they perpetuated rewards for doctors to do more. When the carriers alone tried to restrain costs, against the desires of doctors and patients, they lost, if not immediately in practice, then through the court of public opinion and ultimately often through courts of law. Further, providers in many areas formed large groups to enhance their bargaining power and successfully negotiated large payment increases from carrier HMOs.

As a result, the promise of the seven integrations remains largely unrealized. The U.S. health care system remains oriented toward treatment of acute episodes rather than toward chronic disease management, despite the fact that some 60 to 75 percent of health expenditures are associated with people with chronic conditions (Hoffman et al., 1996). In the long run, chronic disease management could reduce complications, improve quality of life, and increase life expectancy at relatively low cost (Diabetes Control and Complications Trial Research Group, 1996). There remain wide variations in medical practice, which suggests much overuse and underuse. There is also evidence that care not only is variable but is often not compliant with guidelines (Wennberg and Cooper, 1999; McGlynn et al., 2003). Underuse can add to costs in the long run. Finally, costly problems of poor quality are rampant in our health care system, and there is a chasm between what our quality is and what it could reasonably be expected to be (Kohn et al., 1999; Institute of Medicine, 2001; Leape, 2005).

Employers retreated away from HMOs to less managed forms of health insurance. Enrollment in HMOs declined from a high of 31 percent in 1996 to 26 percent by 2002. POS enrollment also declined from 24 percent in 1998 to 18 percent in 2002. In contrast, PPI continued to experience gains in enrollment, reaching 52 percent of employees in 2002 (Table 23.9). Employers had no strategy to deal with the explosion in expenditures. Many, especially small employers, simply stopped offering health insurance to workers, sixty percent of U.S. employers offered health insurance in 2005, compared to 69% in 2000. (Kaiser Family Foundation and HRET 2005) Others sought to reduce premiums, by reducing benefits and increasing cost sharing by employees. While increased cost sharing reduces utilization, particularly among poor people, excluding benefits and services is difficult, and significant premium savings cannot be achieved through minor increases in copayment and deductibles (Newhouse, 1993). Higher premiums have also encouraged some employers to turn to new PPI entrants offering high deductibles and medical spending accounts, and promising to empower and make consumers cost-conscious shoppers. **High deductible plans** combine a catastrophic insurance component with medical savings accounts and other features, designed to simultaneously make enrollees sensitive to costs while giving them the resources to pay for care when they need it. These high deductible or consumer-driven models are unlikely to stem health care inflation because health expenses are concentrated among high-cost patients whose personal expenses exceed deductibles. In 1998, 22 percent of the U.S. population with employment-based insurance who spent $2,000 or more on health care accounted for 77 percent of employee-based insurance spending (Fronstin, 2002). For many people a high deductible provides little or no incentive to be cost-conscious consumers of medical care because a high-cost episode or a chronic illness will quickly absorb their deductible.

Large employers that continue to offer a choice of plans, comparative information, risk-adjusted contributions, and some incentive for selecting a plan that offers a high value are a minority. Collective action among purchasers through organizations such as the Leapfrog Group and the National Committee for Quality Assurance and initiatives including pay for performance supported by a series of Institute of Medicine reports documenting the quality chasm in the U.S. health care system and providing a prescription for reform have tried to create a more central role for value-based purchasing. Innovations in information technologies could facilitate value-based purchasing. For example, a stronger and more organized evidence base could facilitate the adoption of best practices, as well as the development of valid and reliable quality measures for priority conditions that could be used for both internal quality improvement and external accountability (IOM, 2001). However, without financial and organizational incentives better aligned toward this goal, its achievement will be difficult.

23.5 Relationships Among Health Care Financing, Health Care Delivery, and Health Care Technology

Health care financing, health care delivery, and health care technology are directly linked. The way in which health care professionals and health care organizations are paid creates incentives that have consequences both in the way they act and in the information that they seek.

23.5.1 Technology During the Era of Open-Ended Spending

The open-ended, third-party reimbursement that was widespread in both the public and the private sectors from the 1960s through the 1980s resulted, as we have said, in payments to doctors and hospitals for each service rendered. Logically, this system created an incentive for doctors and hospitals to maximize their incomes by performing—or at least billing for—as many services as possible, especially highly paid services. As a result of this incentive, health care providers purchased computer applications for tracking and maximizing charges and for billing payers. Hospital financial systems that could do so thrived.

FFS reimbursement also gave hospitals an incentive to attract as many physicians as possible to use their facilities. More physicians admitted more patients. Each day that a hospital bed was filled, it generated additional income for the hospital. Thus, hospitals invested money and effort in pursuit of physicians who would keep their beds filled. More highly specialized physicians were more highly prized, because hospital charges for the admissions that their services required were higher. Hospitals often enticed specialists to use their facilities by acquiring high-technology equipment.

With the emphasis on reimbursement and high technology, administrative systems received limited attention and financial resources. Unlike most industries, which spend significant proportions of their budgets on quality control and administration, medical care viewed administration as wasteful. Selling, general, and administrative expenses in other industries range up to 44 percent of total expenditures (CFO, 1996). To this day, those who accuse HMOs of having high administrative costs fail to acknowledge the legitimate need for "administrative" expenditure on quality improvement and on cost and utilization management (Woolhandler and Himmelstein, 1997).

Some people view the health care information technology of this era as unsophisticated. By the 1980s, however, information technology, in general, had become much more sophisticated. Computer systems in the banking industry, for example, reported trades of shares of public companies on a stock exchange almost immediately all around the world and allowed bankers to track the performance of multiple stocks over time at a glance. By the mid-1980s, at least one, and often many, computer terminals sat atop the desks of most investment bankers.

Certain health care information technology was also extremely advanced. Medical devices and equipment used some of the most advanced technology in existence. Computer systems designed to track charges were extremely sophisticated. These technologies were perceived at the time as offering the greatest financial returns, so money and resources flowed in their direction. As the financial incentives in the health care system changed, these technologies became less central. Similarly, technologies that enabled health care organizations to respond to today's incentives were unnecessary in an era of open-ended spending and thus were underfunded or not developed at all.

As interest shifted toward cost management, information systems that tracked charges became less useful because the relationship between charges and costs is inexact at best (Table 23.10). An emphasis on charges was acceptable in the 1980s when cost reduction was not an issue. Charge-based systems were also less useful when government and employer demands focused on quality because charge-based systems

Table 23.10. Fee-for-service and managed care systems generate different information needs.

Fee-for-service	Managed care
Bill charges for services without awareness of costs	Need to understand and be accountable for the costs of delivering services
Charge-based information systems	Cost- and encounter-based information systems

did not track information about provider performance. Patient outcomes were limited to crude measures, such as in-hospital mortality. Hospital computer systems could not assist in answering questions like whether a particular course of treatment improved a patient's functioning or whether a particular physician had greater success performing a procedure than one of his or her colleagues. Physicians staunchly refused to allow disclosure of physician-specific information and fought proposals that would do so (Millenson, 1997). Even hospital-level information was difficult to obtain (Singer, 1991).

23.5.2 New Incentives and Requirements Created by Managed Care, Value-Based Purchasing, and Responsible and Empowered Consumers

With a shift from loosely organized care toward managed care, value-based purchasing, and responsible and empowered consumers, the health care financing and delivery system faces a new set of incentives. These new incentives create a need for new types of technology and performance. The strength of these incentives has varied through the 1990s and into the 2000s.

The most important incentives created by these transitions fall into four broad categories: (1) incentives for purchasers and consumers to seek value and information, (2) incentives for health plans and providers to improve quality and to reduce costs, (3) potential incentives for providers to underserve patients, and (4) an incentive for health plans to attract the healthiest possible populations. The first two incentives are desirable and require information to implement; the second two conflict with social goals and require information to counteract.

Incentives for Purchasers and Consumers to Seek Value and Information

A variety of incentives have caused consumers to seek information more actively. Increasingly, individuals contribute directly to health insurance premiums and bear more of the costs of care out-of-pocket when they are insured. Many have also lost trust in the physician–patient relationship and seek independent information about their medical condition. Individuals with a choice of health plans need information with which to compare plans. Individuals responsible for cost sharing and those taking a more active role in their health and medical treatment also seek comparative price, volume, and quality information about doctors and hospitals. Large employers, seeking to reduce their own health care costs, also have an incentive to provide comparative information for their employees.

Information currently available includes measures of satisfaction of members enrolled in health plans; measures of access to providers, whether for scheduled appointments, on the telephone, or on an unscheduled basis; measures of quality as perceived by patients; and measures of compliance with guidelines for preventive services, such as providing immunizations for children or mammograms for women. Risk-adjusted, condition-specific, and population-based measures of outcomes are more desirable, yet more difficult to obtain. Although strong purchasers may demand this information, most providers have not yet been able to put in place systems that can track outcomes (other than death) of the care that they provide or the health of the population that they serve.

Patients can get a variety of information over the Internet about their health plan's reimbursement rules, etc. about participating providers, and about general self-help and health maintenance activities. However, detailed information about provider quality is not generally available, and consumers often find it hard to identify trustworthy sources of information about specific conditions. Therefore, to date the Internet has only partially met their information needs.

Incentives for Health Plans and Providers to Improve Quality and Reduce Costs

In response to demands for better quality and value from purchasers and the public, health plans and providers need the ability to measure cost and quality. These incentives make it necessary to collect information that was not required in the past.

First, information is required for process improvement. For example, measuring variation and improvement in processes, outcomes, and costs among physicians and their practices would enable these physicians to compare themselves with their colleagues, to seek help from colleagues who have better results in certain areas, and to improve their practice patterns. In addition, the measurement of inputs and outputs would allow health care managers to track and improve productivity. Availability of this type of information would open up new areas for improved care management processes, such as closer monitoring of patients who have chronic conditions and case management of patients who have catastrophic illnesses.

Second, to improve continuity of care, it is no longer adequate to track patients within a single hospital stay; providers need to track patients in different care settings across the health system. If a patient visits a primary care physician in a clinic, has a series of outpatient visits, and is then admitted to the hospital for a procedure weeks later, information about that patient—including results of previous laboratory tests, prescription drugs, and so on—should be available to ensure continuity of care.

Third, to improve the health of the population they serve, health plans need information about enrollees even before those people receive medical care. This information is important not only to make health plan comparisons but also to identify enrollees at high risk of illness and disease. Quality would be enhanced and costs reduced if problems could be identified early or avoided completely because preventive measures are taken. Thus, health plans should want to have good information on the presence of chronic conditions even before patients present with complaints.

Fourth, information is required to enable the assessment of new technologies. Before the introduction of new technologies, payers should consider both the costs and the benefits. This process requires detailed information on operating costs and productivity in practice. Technologies that are not cost-effective or that do not provide benefit relative to technology that is already available should not be introduced.

Fifth, health care managers should conduct make-versus-buy analyses to evaluate, for example, whether they can obtain a test at less cost by contracting with an outside laboratory rather than by purchasing the testing equipment and running the tests themselves. Information about the costs associated with providing services, equipment, and facilities in-house is vital for negotiating appropriate contracts with external vendors. Again, detailed information on operating costs would be needed.

Finally, health plans and providers should evaluate both physicians and health care facilities to determine where consolidation is appropriate. For example, the American College of Cardiology recommends that teams of physicians at any particular health care facility perform a minimum of 200 to 300 open-heart surgeries per year (California Office of Statewide Health Planning and Development, 1992). At a lower quantity, surgeons may not be proficient, and the facility is more likely to provide low-quality care. Thus, hospitals performing open-heart surgeries should track the number and outcomes of their procedures and should seek ways to concentrate such procedures at high-volume, high-quality centers.

Potential Incentive for Providers to Underserve Patients

Per capita prepayment is a double-edged sword. It gives providers an incentive to hold down costs. Ideally, providers would respond to this incentive by finding ways to become more productive, to keep people healthy, to avoid mistakes, and so on. Because capitation places providers at financial risk for services that enrollees consume, however, capitated providers may also have an incentive to underserve. Patients who need the most care are most vulnerable to underprovision of care not only because plans or providers may save money by holding back services but also because plans benefit if such patients "vote with their feet" by leaving for another health plan. This is a widespread and important fear among consumers.

In response to this fear, health plans and providers experimented with a variety of financial incentives designed to control costs while preserving quality. For example, to mitigate the intensity of the incentive to underserve, some plans based capitation payments on populations of patients rather than on individual patients. They also spread capitation across groups of providers so they would share the risk of a few expensive cases. They created tiered coverage categories to encourage enrollees to use low cost and high quality hospitals, provider networks, and drugs. In addition, plans used combinations of per capita prepayment with bonuses for high-quality care to prevent abuses.

Many provider organizations found it difficult to manage these population risks and, as they gained market power, many providers rejected global capitation, which provided perperson prepayment for all services, including prescription drugs. While some large provider organizations continue to accept capitation for outpatient services, many have returned to other forms of payment, including FFS and payments per day or per episode of care.

Capitation and related forms of payment created a host of information technology needs, including the need to track blatant abuses (a possible role for government), the need to monitor provider use patterns and outcomes, and also the need to provide access to information relevant to consumers, such as treatment options and provider characteristics. Technologies such as video and CD-ROM could be used to describe the costs and benefits of particular procedures to consumers to aid in their decisions.

Incentive for Health Plans to Attract the Healthiest Populations Possible

Health insurers have an incentive to attract to their plans those individuals and families who are likely to use the least medical care. One of the easiest ways to minimize health plan costs is to enroll a healthier population that has less total need for medical services. Plans that fail at this strategy may end up with the sickest or highest risk population. In this situation, even the most efficient plan may not be able to survive. Competition exacerbates this problem.

Assuming quality is constant, it would be best if the most efficient health plans were also the most successful. This outcome requires that health plans with a sicker and higher risk population than average be compensated for the additional expected cost of care. This requires a reliable risk adjustment mechanism; several have been developed and some of them have been applied in practice. The successful implementation of a risk adjustment mechanism requires substantial diagnostic and demographic information and coordination of information, which in turn requires large databases, analytical capability, and the ability to combine information from multiple technology platforms. The best-performing risk adjustment models are notable for their comprehensive data requirements; they use both inpatient and outpatient data and repeated observations on the same individual over time.

23.5.3   *Implications of Developing Information Technology for Health Care Financing and Delivery*

Just as the needs of the health care financing and delivery system direct development of new health care information technologies, the maturation of information technologies enables significant improvements in health care financing and delivery. In this section, we describe a few of the most important advances in information technology and discuss the progress that they will permit.

Cost-Accounting Systems

Based on cost-accounting applications in other industries, health care cost-accounting systems, adapted from cost-accounting applications in other industries, have been adopted widely. In health care, accounting for costs is extremely complicated because there are so many costs in even the simplest hospital stay and so many ways to account for them. In addition, health care organizations have not traditionally accounted for costs and so lack a time-tested, broadly accepted basis for defining costs. Difficulties in defining costs may be compounded by the large fixed costs of hospitals, which use expensive capital heavily, and the presence of joint production. Some resources are used for multiple activities, so allocation of their costs to any single activity is difficult and often arbitrary. Without a defined cost for items, even the most sophisticated cost-accounting systems cannot provide satisfactory answers to the most basic questions. For a typical hospital, the process of defining costs accurately may take years.

Cost-accounting systems enable the measurement of costs—the first step toward being able to manage costs. They enable the assessment of technologies on the basis of costs relative to benefits, so decisions can be made about which technologies are cost-effective and which should be used sparingly or not at all. Cost-accounting systems enable organizations to profile and compare the utilization patterns of physicians, clinics, and hospitals on the basis of which they can target practice improvements, select a network, and determine bonuses. They empower organizations with information on the basis of which to negotiate contracts that cover at least variable costs. They enable organizations to determine that the costs of providing a service are higher than those of contracting it out. The better the ability to measure costs, the greater the capacity of the health care organization to survive in a competitive managed care environment. Cost-accounting systems, still new to many organizations, are an essential and important tool.

Internet or Intranet

The advent of the information superhighway expanded the possibilities for information and communication in the health care industry, as it did in other industries (National Research Council, 2000). The Internet, and its proprietary counterpart—intranets—enable new forms of interaction that promise to have a profound effect on health care delivery and administration. About half of the adult U.S. population used the Internet as of 2001, and about 40 percent of Internet users (20 percent of the entire adult population in the United States) used the Internet for health care purposes (Baker et al., 2003). The Internet provides an open, widely accepted standard for transferring information. In general, health care information technologies, not unlike information technologies in other sectors, have used proprietary technology, much of which has been unable to communicate with other technologies. The result is great difficulty in sharing information across organizations—a function that is vitally important in health care as patients move among organizations. In contrast, health care information technologies based on the Internet standard can more easily communicate with one another.

Health care is a global concern; health care delivery is a local business. The Internet has real limitations: there are concerns about inaccurate information, and potential difficulties with the confidentiality of personal information. Nevertheless, the Internet promises to offer a means to disseminate information about health and health care, enhance communication, and facilitate a wide range of interactions between patients and the health care delivery system. These kinds of changes could produce important improvements in health care and, ultimately, the health of the population. The Internet gives health care organizations the potential to communicate at low cost, because the Internet infrastructure is already built and is publicly available. Physicians and health care organizations can communicate with other physicians in different settings; they can also communicate with patients where the patients live and work. This ability enhances home health care, HMO–patient communication, physician–patient communication, and internal communications within increasingly large and decentralized health care organizations (see Chapter 13). Additional Internet applications currently in use to some extent include consumer and clinician access to the medical literature, creation of communities of patients and clinicians with shared interests, consumer access to information on health plans, participating providers, eligibility for procedures, and covered drugs in a formulary, and videoconferencing among public health officials during an emergency (IOM, 2001). In addition, telemedicine (see Chapter 24) has become much more practical with Internet technologies.

Comprehensive Longitudinal Clinical Databases

Theoretically, patient medical records include detailed information about every interaction an individual has with the health care delivery system. In practice, paper-based information is difficult to retrieve, and too often it is lost. Over time, and for individuals with complex problems, medical records can become thick documents of loose notes from multiple sources, test results, and images (see Chapter 2). For decades, most of the reports included in medical records were handwritten. Subsequently, many organizations added transcription departments or relied on outsourced services to type medical records.

Paper-based medical records do not support continuity of care across physicians and across health care institutions. Health care organizations do not share medical records. Thus, an individual may have multiple, but incomplete, medical records in different doctors' offices, clinics, and hospitals, representing different portions of the patient's medical history. Even if medical records are shared in a multispecialty-group practice setting, paper records may be missing when they are needed. Finding relevant information in even the best-organized medical records is a difficult and time-consuming task. Using medical record information for learning about patterns of care across multiple patients can be a Herculean task.

Comprehensive, longitudinal, clinical databases—in effect, a paperless, complete medical record—have been viewed by many people as the holy grail in health care information technology (see Chapters 1 and 12). Integrated delivery of care requires comprehensive longitudinal records for each patient so that each provider who contacts patients as well as the patients themselves can have a complete picture of the patients' medical history, access that helps to avoid duplicate tests and unfavorable drug interactions. In addition, the information can serve as a basis for research on the relationships among diagnoses, treatments, and outcomes. Comprehensive patient records would also enable outcomes measurement, technology assessment, physician profiling, measurement of practice variation, identification of best practices, continuous quality improvement, utilization management, continuity of care, measurement of compliance with guidelines, and risk adjustment.

Projects to develop comprehensive, computer-based medical records were common in the 1980s; they still persist. (Refer to Chapter 12 for a detailed discussion of computer-based patient records.) They raised concern among consumer advocates about the confidentiality of information, prompting adoption and implementation of comprehensive privacy legislation through the Health Insurance Portability and Accountability Act in 1996. Privacy concerns created yet another opportunity for health care information technology development: systems to address data security concerns (see Chapters 5 and 10).

Longitudinal databases are also being used to achieve slightly less ambitious aims. Some information technology companies focus on tracking courses of treatment for particular conditions or in single settings, such as hospitals. Clinical information systems focus on six major functions: computerized physician order entry and alerts, clinical documentation, decision support, results reporting, messaging, and data analysis. Automated drug order-entry systems, when used in hospitals, eliminate handwriting errors and call attention to potentially harmful drug interactions. These have the potential to reduce serious medication errors in hospitals by 50 percent (Leapfrog Group). Clinical documentation systems facilitate comprehensive and consistent physician notetaking with common orders, forms, and structured templates, which may be electronically searched. Decision-support systems can alert physicians to potential errors and facilitate adherence to evidence-based practices. Results reporting systems make laboratory and imaging findings available to clinicians by linking them to orders and providing alerts when results, particularly abnormal results, become available. Electronic messaging within a clinical information system not only facilitates communication between patients, physicians, and care teams, but also self-documents contacts, which become part of the patient record. Finally, by linking clinical records to a central data repository, clinical information systems provide opportunities far beyond those presented by paper records for data analysis and information about the relative efficacy and efficiency of all approaches to care. These technologies represent a great improvement in health care management and information and offer the potential to make care more affordable, higher quality, and more satisfying for patients.

In addition, better analytic methods have rendered information based on readily available hospital inpatient administrative data more useful. For example, the Agency for Healthcare Research and Quality's quality and safety indicators enable hospitals to flag potential opportunities for prevention and improvement. (http://www.quality indicators.ahrq.gov/).

There are a variety of reasons why hospitals and physicians have been slow to adopt electronic medical records, although some form of this technology has been available for years (Bates, 2003). Key reasons for not adopting include:

1. Providers do not want to get locked in to proprietary systems; the vendors may not survive so that the large investment becomes a waste after a period of years. This problem would be mitigated by widespread adoption of standards (see below) or the emergence of one or more credible vendors whose longevity is not in doubt. There are large vendors now but some providers are still skeptical.
2. Data exchange is not yet standardized; many providers are waiting for imminent standardization, including agreement on Extensible Markup Language (XML) standards and medical terminology (see Chapter 7). Integration of systems thus remains extremely complex and costly.
3. Data entry in these systems is often costly. Current user interfaces may be slow and cumbersome, so they fail to save providers' time.
4. Total costs of maintaining the systems may still be high. Although the cost of hardware, quality-adjusted, has plummeted, the maintenance costs are another matter.
5. The hospital/physician may feel that they bear all the costs but do not capture all the benefits from use of the technology, i.e., incentives are misaligned.
6. Providers often cite limitations in the features offered in these systems. Everyone expects features to improve in the future, so they may rationally choose to wait longer to invest.

Increasing numbers of organizations are adopting electronic medical records despite these impediments, and adoption will likely increase as barriers are addressed.

Information exchange across health care settings is more difficult. The likely evolution of a comprehensive computer-based medical record will include several phases: The first phase will be the capability to exchange electronically enrollment and eligibility information through the development of universal identifiers for enrollees and providers. The second phase will be the capability to exchange pharmacy, laboratory, and encounter records through standardization and expanded coding. This intermediate stage will represent a tremendous step forward, facilitating quality improvement and performance measurement. The third phase of evolution will be the comprehensive computer-based medical record systems originally envisioned.

23.5.4   The Challenge of Implementation

The era of open-ended spending left many health care organizations with a legacy of substantial but antiquated infrastructure. Data management systems are also typically plagued by incomplete data and a lack of quality control. Both the management systems and the information technologies associated with FFS reimbursement were ingrained through years of development and use. In general, technology that predates the 1990s was proprietary to particular institutions and therefore incompatible with technology in other institutions. This situation makes difficult not only the transfer of information across institutions but also the modernization of existing technology. The transition to new integrated systems and new technologies therefore is extremely challenging and costly. Converting or replacing existing systems requires substantial investment (see Chapter 13). Health care organizations, which face ongoing cost pressures, require champions to demonstrate a business case for information technology. Active purchaser demand, through organizations such as the Leapfrog Group, the National Committee for Quality Assurance, and pay for performance initiatives.

Health care institutions today must constantly balance the trade-off between the cost of upgrading information capabilities and collecting and disseminating information and the value that the additional information can provide. While organizations continue to debate the size and timing of information technology investments, changing circumstances including movement toward standardization, the influx of trainees and young physicians who demand technological capabilities for their clinical care, pressure from purchasers, and patient expectations, are adding to the pressure to adopt these capabilities. Evolution of these systems will support future quality and patient safety improvement, performance measurement, improved efficiency, and restoration of consumer confidence.

Suggested Readings

Ellwood P.M. (1988). Shattuck lecture—Outcomes management: A technology of patient experience. *New England Journal of Medicine*, 318(23):1549–1556.
The author describes the destabilizing and democratizing effects in terms of choices and decisions of HMOs on patients, payers, and health care organizations. He coins the term "health maintenance organization" and makes the case for outcomes measurement.

Enthoven A.C. (1993). The history and principles of managed competition. *Health Affairs*, 12(Suppl):24–48.

The author articulates the principles of managed competition, a plan for comprehensive health reform that combines microeconomics with careful observation and analysis of what works. Managed competition relies on a sponsor to structure and adjust the market for competing health plans, to establish equitable rules, to create price-elastic demand, and to avoid uncompensated risk selection.

Fuchs V.R. (1983). *Who Shall Live?* (2nd ed.). New York: Basic Books.
The author presents an excellent introduction to the structure of the health care delivery system. The roles of the main players and the relationship between medical care and health are discussed.

Fuchs V.R. (1993). *The Future of Health Policy*. Cambridge, MA: Harvard University Press.
The author provides the reader with the necessary concepts, facts, and analyses to clarify complicated issues of health policy. The book addresses cost containment, managed competition, technology assessment, poverty and health, children's health, and national health insurance.

Institute of Medicine Committee on Quality of Health Care in America (2001). *Crossing the Quality Chasm: A New Health System for the 21st Century*. Washington, D.C.: National Academy Press.
Available online at http://www.nap.edu/openbook/0309072808/html.
This book responds to evidence of quality problems in America's health care system by providing a strategy to achieve substantial improvement in the quality of health care over the next decade.

Weller C.D. (1984). "Free choice" as a restraint of trade in American health care delivery and insurance. *Iowa Law Review*, 69(5):1351–1378, 1382–1392.
This article explains in simple yet powerful terms many of the issues raised by the fundamental restructuring of the health care industry from the era of open spending to the era of accountability by providing a historical account of the transition from "guild free choice," which prevented doctors from organizing into groups and offering discounts, to "market free choice," which permits competition.

Questions for Discussion

1. Define the following terms, each of which is relevant to current health care financing:
   a. Usual, customary, and reasonable fees
   b. Health maintenance organization
   c. Diagnosis-related group
   d. Preferred-provider insurance
2. Compare HMOs, PPOs, POS plans, and high deductible plans. What are the strengths and potential limitations of each with respect to cost and quality of care?
3. How will the differences in incentives for providers under each of the following payment systems affect providers' assessments of new medical technologies, such as patient-monitoring systems?
   a. An HMO
   b. An individual physician participating in a PPO arrangement
   c. A hospital with a large number of patients treated under Medicare's prospective payment system
   d. A standard fee-for-service arrangement
4. Compare information system needs in a hospital that treats mostly private-pay patients with those in one that accepts capitated payments.

5. You are the new administrator of the Center for Medicare and Medicaid Services, the agency responsible for Medicare and for the federal component of Medicaid. You are about to authorize a new program for health care financing for the elderly. The program offers elderly beneficiaries a choice of all health plans on the market.
   a. With what information do you think it is important to provide beneficiaries so that they can choose among plans?
   b. What data would you want to collect to evaluate the performance of plans?
   c. What mechanisms would you implement to collect these data?
6. Describe at least three ways in which health care organizations can use the Internet to improve patient care.

24
The Future of Computer Applications in Biomedicine

Lawrence M. Fagan and Edward H. Shortliffe

After reading this chapter, you should know the answers to these questions:

- What are possible future directions for biomedical informatics?
- What are the forces that are driving these changes?

In this book, we have summarized the current state of biomedical informatics in a variety of application areas and have reflected on the development of the field during the past 50 years. To provide a background for our discussions, we opened the book with a glimpse into the future—a vision of medical practice when individual physicians routinely and conveniently use computers and electronic health records to help with information management, communication, and clinical decision making. In this chapter, we again look forward, this time concentrating on likely trends in biomedical applications of computers, on current avenues of research, and on the issues that will determine along which paths biomedical informatics will develop.

24.1 Progress in Biomedical Computing

We begin by looking back at the changes in biomedical computing since the first edition of this book was published in 1990. Then we look ahead to the not-too-distant future—presenting a few scenarios that we can extrapolate from the current trends in the field. These scenarios provide perspective on the ways that computers may pervade clinical practice and the biological science laboratory. A key aspect of the clinical scenarios is the extent to which, unlike most specialized medical paraphernalia of today, medical computing applications are integrated into routine medical practice rather than used on an occasional basis. In much the same way, computers are becoming a crucial part of the analysis of data in the research laboratory, especially in the areas of genomics and proteomics, where the amount of incoming data is very large (see Chapter 22). The realization of a highly integrated environment depends on the solution of technological challenges, such as integrating information from multiple data sources and making the integrated information accessible to professionals when, where, and in the form that it is needed. Integration of medical and biological information also encompasses social issues, such as defining the appropriate role of computers in the workplace, resolving questions of legal liability and ethics related to biomedical computing, and assessing the effects of computer-based technology on health care costs. The chance that our hypothetical scenarios will become reality thus depends on the resolution of a number of technological and social issues that will be debated during the coming years.

24.1.1 Looking Back to 1990

In the first edition of our book, the closing chapter included two future scenarios of medical care and discussed emerging topics such as the Unified Medical Language System (UMLS), integrated academic information management systems (IAIMS), and the medical information bus (MIB). Today the UMLS is employed in information retrieval systems as a tool for converting textual medical information into standardized terms taken from coding schemes and terminologies such as MeSH, SNOMED, and ICD and to help translate from one vocabulary to another (McCray and Miller, 1998). IAIMS sites are now scattered around the country with many different models being implemented. The MIB has been approved as the IEEE 1073 family of standards for medical device interconnection (Stead, 1997b) and has been incorporated into multiple instruments at the bedside (see Chapter 17).

The scenarios we discussed in the first edition included computer-based support during both cardiac bypass surgery and long-term care of a patient with a chronic disease. Although the information-support capabilities have changed considerably in the decade since the first version of this chapter was written, it is possible that the practice of medicine has changed just as much. For example, less invasive alternatives to open-chest bypass surgery have become more common. Stricter criteria for admission to the hospital and shorter lengths of stay once hospitalized mean that sicker patients are routinely cared for in outpatient settings. In such situations, the need for computer-based tracking of a patient's medical status is increased. This need has led to experiments such as the use of wireless pen-based computers by home health care nurses for logging patient conditions and Internet-based disease management interactions between clinicians and patients in their homes. Major attention to data protection and patient data confidentiality has significantly altered the technological solutions to such data management and access tasks (see Chapter 10).

Significant advances have been made in raw computing power (e.g., hardware and software for the manipulation of three-dimensional images); interconnectivity (e.g., high-speed network backbones and wireless connections to palm-sized handheld computing devices); the ability to store very large amounts of data (e.g., the terabyte data storage device shown in Figure 24.1); and the development of infrastructure—particularly in the area of communication standards (e.g., health level 7 (HL7) and object broker architectures). On the other hand, the anticipated level of seamless integration between applications, highly interconnected medical databases with embedded decision-support tools, and ubiquitous computing support have remained elusive but are an increasing focus of policy as well as technical emphasis.

24.1.2 Looking to the Future

During testimony before the U.S. House of Representatives Committee on Science in 1997 concerning the future role of the Internet, one of the authors (EHS) laid out a set

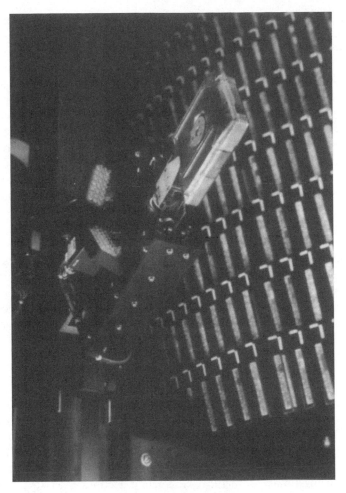

Figure 24.1. Multi-terabyte mass storage in a tape robot facility. (*Source*: Reprinted by permission from StorageTek, Louisville, CO. 1998.)

of long-term goals for medical informatics. Like the scenarios we depicted nearly a decade ago, these goals depend on the occurrence of both technical and social changes for their fulfillment. If the assumptions identified in Section 24.1.3 prove valid, medical practice in the future will incorporate aspects of the following scenarios:

- *Low-cost, high-quality telemedicine*: The telemedicine experiments of the mid-1990s were dependent on specialized equipment and expensive special-use communications lines. This has evolved such that the Internet is a common vehicle for linking medical experts with other clinicians and patients at a distance (National Research Council, 2000; Shortliffe, 2000). In the future, the Internet will be able to support clear video images routinely, with high-fidelity audio links to support listening to the heart and lungs, and common computing platforms at both ends of the links to make telemedicine a cost-effective form of medical practice. Patients will avoid unnecessary travel from rural settings to major medical centers, primary care clinicians will have expert consultation delivered to them in their offices in a highly personalized fashion, and patients will accomplish in single office visits what now often requires multiple visits and major inconvenience. There is reason to believe that such applications will become commonplace soon, with several successful demonstration projects under way to demonstrate cost-effectiveness and a positive benefit for patients (see Chapter 14).

- *Remote consultation*: Quick and easy electronic access between clinical providers to discuss patient cases will improve access to expert patient care and enhance patient satisfaction. For example, an attending physician, residents, and medical students in a community clinic who treat a patient with an unusual skin lesion will obtain immediate teleconsultation with a dermatologist at a regional medical center. The remote medical team will learn from the dermatologist, the expert will receive clear, diagnostic-quality images of the lesion, and the patient will promptly receive a specialist's assessment. All too often today, patients, when referred to major centers, experience significant delays or fail to keep their appointments due to travel problems. Instead of sending patients to the experts, we will improve their care by using the Internet to bring the experts to them. Current demonstration projects in a handful of locations have shown the feasibility of such remote access to expertise; it remains to make the applications commonplace, well integrated with routine care, and generally accepted as reimbursable clinical activities.

- *Integrated health records*: We envision the day when citizens no longer will have multiple records of their health care encounters scattered throughout the offices of numerous physicians and the medical record rooms of multiple hospitals. Instead, their records will be linked electronically over the Internet so that each person has a single "virtual health record"—the distributed, but unified, summary of all the health care they have received in their lives. Furthermore, this record will be secure, treated with respect and confidentiality, and released to providers only with the patient's permission or during times of medical emergency according to strictly defined and enforced criteria (National Research Council, 1997). Important steps have been taken recently to make this scenario more likely to happen. The development of a National Health Information Infrastructure and adoption of nomenclature standards such as SNOMED-CT, and privacy rules such as Health Insurance Portability and Accountability Act (HIPAA) are contributing toward this goal. In 2004, President Bush announced a federal goal to implement ubiquitous electronic health records for all citizens within a decade. In addition, the U.S. armed services are actively pursing electronic dog-tags that will contain abstracts of the electronic medical record of each participant in the military.

- *Computer-based learning*: Soon, medical students on their orthopedics rotation, preparing to observe their first arthroscopic knee surgery, will be able to go the school's electronic learning center and use the Internet to access and manipulate a three-dimensional "virtual reality" model of the knee on a computer at the National Institutes of Health. They will use new immersive technologies to "enter" the model knee, to look from side to side to view and learn the anatomic structures and their spatial relationships, and to manipulate the model with a simulated arthroscope, thus getting a surgeon's-eye view of the procedure before experiencing the real thing. Using the experimental Next-Generation Internet, remote access to medical dissections is becoming available in a limited way. In the near future, many hard-to-learn procedures, such as female pelvic examination, will be routinely taught to medical students on a computer simulation/mannikin with immediate feedback rather than with patients or living models.

- *Patient and provider education*: Health science schools are starting to provide distance-learning experiences via the Internet for postgraduate education, refresher courses, and home study by health science students. Eventually, clinicians will be able to prescribe specially selected video educational programs for patients that will be delivered to home television sets by a direct Internet connection. Our hospitals and clinics will use video servers over the Internet not only to deliver such materials to patients but also to provide continuing medical and nursing education to their staffs. Providers are beginning to make patient-oriented versions of the electronic medical records available online along with relevant online information tailored to the patient's problems (Cimino et al., 2002).

- *Disease management*: High-speed Internet access via Digital Subscriber Line (DSL), cable, or satellite is now being offered to most families in the United States and more than 50 million households now have broadband connectivity. Soon, clinicians will move beyond the simple use of telephones for managing patient problems at a distance to using their visual senses as well via two-way video links. The infirm will receive "home visits" via video links, thus avoiding unnecessary office or emergency room visits, and care managers will have important new tools for monitoring patients that emphasize prevention rather than crisis management. Early experiments show remarkable enthusiasm by patients when familiar physicians and nurses provide such videoconferencing interactions in the home (see Chapter 14).

Over these last 5 years since these goals were elucidated, we have made significant progress toward meeting these long-term objectives for computer-assisted learning, provider and patient communication, and medical care utilizing high-speed networks and fast, commodity computers. Similar changes have been taking place in the collection, interpretation, and dissemination of biological information. For example with the advent of very fast, multiprocessor supercomputers, researchers can begin to model biological processes such as the folding of a protein or the binding of a drug to a receptor site. Some of this modeling work can be done using the high-speed Internet and distant computers, such as the biologically focused supercomputers in San Diego, California, and Pittsburgh, Pennsylvania. One scientist working in this area has suggested some of the major challenges and opportunities facing the field of computational biology:[1]

- *A computational model of physiology*: Can we create a simulation of the human body and estimate of the effects of medications on the diseased and nondiseased portions

---

[1]R.B. Altman in a presentation entitled "Final thoughts: Further opportunities in bioinfomatics and computational biology", presented at a conference on Bioinformatics Methods and Techniques, Stanford, CA. June 23–25, 2003.

of the body with sufficient fidelity to avoid most animal and early human testing of drugs? Having this simulation model would bring a tremendous benefit by reducing the number of years of testing that occurs for most drugs. However, the complexity of the task is daunting. Much of the pathophysiology needed to build this model is unknown, and even the parts that are known would create such a complex set of relationships that the computers models may be intractable given near-term computational capabilities. Furthermore, the genetic variation between individuals that is being studied in pharmacogenetics experiments greatly increases the complexity of the modeling process.

- *Design of new compounds for medical and industrial use*: Can we design a protein or nucleic acid to have a specified function? The determination that a particular drug can be used to treat a medical condition has traditionally been done by testing a large collection of substances in the laboratory to see if any show in vitro activity. This step is then followed by extensive animal testing. Now that we have a better understanding of protein structure, and a clearer model of how to modify the disease process, can the drug creation process be switched to build biological custom materials to reverse or deter a pathological process?

- *Engineering new biological pathways*: Can we devise methods for designing and implementing new metabolic capabilities for treating disease? The biological metabolic pathways of various species are being mapped out quite rapidly. It is interesting to observe the variation from species to species in pathways that perform similar metabolic functions for the animals. This suggests the possibility of building new metabolic pathways in areas such as inborn metabolic diseases. Some diseases, such as sickle cell anemia, have a single flaw that must be overcome. In other genetic diseases multiple elements of the pathways may be missing, and there will be a need to construct an alternative pathway that takes into account the particular manifestations of the disease.

- *Data mining for new knowledge*: Can we ask computer programs to examine data (in the context of our models) and create new knowledge? As we create large databases of measurements taken during clinical care, the question arises about finding new patterns in those data. Exactly what effects does a drug have on various laboratory tests and measurements? If we have enough data collected across different patients but in similar situations, will we have enough statistical power to recognize unknown relationships? A large number of statistical approaches are being employed to perform a structured analysis of large data sets to learn new relationships.

These biological challenges are still likely to be unanswered as we approach the 10th edition of this textbook. Because they require the development of considerable biological knowledge, computational techniques, and new methodologies for analysis, they likely represent distant goals of biomedical computation.

24.1.3   *Assumptions Underlying the Scenarios*

To help you to evaluate these scenarios of the future, we must make explicit the assumptions on which these speculations are based. In particular, we assume that health care workers and life scientists will work increasingly with computers in their daily lives and that improvements in computer technology will continue, independent of technological advances in biomedical science. Furthermore, we assume that concerns about health care cost containment and the threat of malpractice litigation will continue to be unresolved issues for the near term.

The technological development of medical computing depends in large part on advances in general computing capabilities. Except in the area of medical imaging, little computer technology is first developed for medical applications and then applied to the rest of industry. This is especially true now that a few general-purpose microprocessors and operating systems have become standard for all personal computers. Specialized computer chips will continue to be created for computationally intensive medical applications, such as signal processing. In these image-processing applications, rotation, filtering, enhancement, and reconstruction algorithms must handle more data than can be processed with the standard microprocessors; thus, a market exists for specialized machines.

It is difficult to predict whether the development of new general-purpose computer products will continue to follow an evolutionary trend or will undergo a *paradigm shift*—defined by Kuhn in his book on the nature of scientific discovery as a complete change in perspective, such as occurred with the revelation that the Earth is not flat (Kuhn, 1962). Computer processing has gone through some major shifts in direction over the last 40 years: from single-user batch processing, to timesharing on a central resource, and then back to single-user processing, this time on local machines with access to specialized machines through a network. As more and more people try to access key Internet sites, we have moved back to a version of the timesharing model of 30 years ago.

The human–machine interaction style has changed dramatically, with graphical interfaces for novices almost completely replacing command-line interfaces. Pen, speech, and three-dimensional interfaces have been built but have not been widely deployed, except in the case of pen-based datebook applications and spoken systems for very defined tasks such as airline reservations or banking. For example, Figure 24.2 shows one approach for using three-dimensional representations for literature retrieval. This application built at the Palo Alto Research Center (PARC) uses the three-dimensional spatial information to show complex trees in much greater detail than in most two-dimensional layouts. There also has been a significant change from electrical to optical methods of network transmission (fiberoptic cables) as well as a steady progression from analog to digital recording of information, best illustrated by the switch from film to digital images in radiology, the widespread introduction of high-speed fiber networks, and the development of satellite communication networks. For the purposes of this chapter, we shall assume the continued progression of current trends rather than a significant paradigm shift. An unanticipated discovery that is just around the corner could, of course, quickly invalidate the assumptions.

Another subtle, but pervasive, assumption underlies this book, much of which is written by researchers in biomedical informatics. We tend to believe that more technology, thoughtfully introduced, is usually better and that computers can enhance almost any aspect of clinical practice and biomedical research—especially information access, the

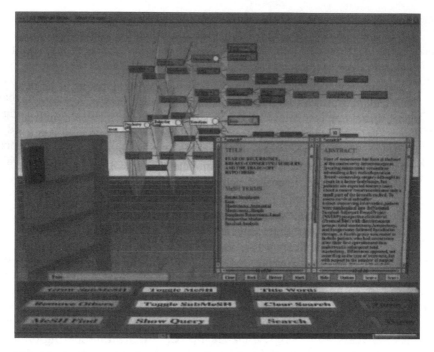

Figure 24.2. Three-dimensional representation of the MeSH tree using the Information Visualizer Toolkit created at Xerox PARC. A portion of a citation about breast cancer is shown in the foreground. (*Source*: Reprinted from Hearst/Karadi, SIGIR'97, courtesy of ACM.)

diagnostic and therapeutic components of the decision-making process, and the analysis of huge amounts of biological data. For example, paper documents are still the mainstay of medical records in many medical settings. Still, we strive to eliminate the paper-based components and assume that a well-designed interface (e.g., one that allows handwritten or continuous-speech input) applied to a sufficiently fast computer can significantly improve the overall process of recording and retrieving clinical data. Although this assumption has yet to be formally verified, there is a groundswell of development and investment activity based on successful experiments that encourage the belief that electronic records will positively transform the way in which we provide patient care and monitor health.

People frequently criticize medical professionals for being technocrats—for encouraging an increase in mechanization and electronic gadgetry that tends to alienate both workers and patients. Such increases fuel the concern that modern medicine is becoming increasingly impersonal and sterile. How do we meld the automated environments proposed in this chapter's introductory scenarios with our wistful memories of kindly family doctors making house calls and attending their patients' weddings, christenings, bar mitzvahs, and the like? The reality, of course, is that the trend away from such traditional images predated the introduction of computers in medicine and has resulted more from modern pressures on health care financing and the need for subspecialization to deal with an increasingly complex subject area. The role for computers and other information technologies results as much from these pressures as it does from a blind faith that all technology is good, useful, and worth the associated costs. Many argue, in fact, that the prudent use of computing technology will introduce the kinds of efficiencies needed if clinicians are to return to an era in which more relaxed time spent with patients is feasible.

Once medical computing applications have been shown to be effective, the technologies will need to be evaluated carefully and consistently before their routine adoption. We need to know that the benefits exceed the costs, both financial and sociological. The debate about where and how computers should be used is even more complex in developing countries, where advanced technology might partially compensate for shortages in medical expertise but where scarce health care resources might be more effectively employed to provide sanitation, antibiotics, and basic medical supplies. Nonetheless, the scenarios above were painted with the assumptions that there will be an increased application of computers in all aspects of medicine and that the key difference between the future and today will be that computers will become ubiquitous and that they will have a high degree of interconnection and an increased ability to interoperate.

24.2   Integration of Computer-Based Technologies

Most of the individual capabilities described in the preceding scenarios exist today in prototype form. What does not exist is an environment that brings together a large variety of computer-based support tools. The removal of barriers to integration requires both technological advances, such as the development of standards for data sharing and communication (see Chapter 7), and a better understanding of sociological issues, such as when computer use may be inappropriate or how the need for coordinated planning can overcome logistical barriers to connecting heterogeneous resources in a seamless fashion.

We can begin to assess the degree of connectivity in a medical center by asking simple questions. Can the laboratory computer communicate results to the computer that provides decision support, without a person having to reenter the data? Do the programs that provide decision support use the same terms to describe symptoms as do those that professionals use to perform electronic searches of citation databases? Do physicians and other health personnel use computers to get information without thinking about the fact that they are using a computer system, just as they pick up a medical chart and use it without first thinking about the format of the paper documents?

Computer systems must be integrated into the medical setting in three ways. First, applications must fit the existing information flow in the settings where they are to be used. If the machine sits in a corner of the clinic, out of the normal traffic flow, and if there is another way to accomplish the specific task, then the computer system is likely to be ignored. Likewise, programs that arbitrarily constrain physicians to unnatural procedures for entering and accessing information are less likely to be used. User interfaces should be flexible and intuitive; just as the fields of a paper medical form can be completed in an arbitrary order, data-entry programs should allow users to enter information in any order.

Surgeons attempting so-called telepresence surgery over the Internet, bringing special-ized expertise to an operating room possibly hundreds of miles away, will be unable to assist in the procedure if the movements they make with hand devices at one end are not instantly reflected in what they see happening with the actual instruments at the other end of the link. How do we ensure interoperability across the many networks that now span our coun-try (National Research Council, 2000)? Can we guarantee adequate response time for the telesurgery application not only on the major backbone networks but also on the last seg-ments of wire, cable, or wireless network that come into offices and other remote settings?

Second, computer systems should provide common access to all computer-based resources, so a user cannot tell where one program ends and another starts. In this book, we have described such diverse applications as computed tomographic scanning and bibliographic searching. Many of these systems have been developed independ-ently, and most are completely incompatible. In the future, the radiologists' picture archiving and communications system (PACS) workstation (see Chapter 18) should deliver more than just images—for example, a radiologist may wish also to search eas-ily for references on unusual presentations of a specific disease process and to include these references in a paper being composed with a text editor. Ideally, users should not have to switch between computers, to stop one program and to start another, or even to use different sets of commands to obtain all the information they need. That the desired information resources may exist on multiple machines in different parts of the medical center or the country should be invisible to the user.

Third, the user interface must be both consistent across applications and easy to use, which may require multiple interface modalities, such as pointing, flexible spoken natural-language interfaces, and text input. Both at the user interface and internally, programs should use a common terminology to refer to frequently used concepts, such as a diagnosis, a symptom, or a laboratory test value.

We are seeing increasing amounts of medical information packed into smaller, more powerful computers, such as hand-sized personal digital assistants (PDAs). The config-uration of computers is starting to change. Figure 24.3 shows a computer system that is worn attached to the body. Using spoken input or a keypad mounted on the arm along with a heads-up display, the computer is inherently as mobile as the person using the system. Although this device may seem far in the future for medical care, a less sophis-ticated version of this equipment is used everyday in the rental car business to check-in returning cars and print receipts. Although the rental car business is far more structured than medical practice, the example shows that this type of technological change can be successfully integrated into the workplace.

Figure 24.4 is a fanciful figure from Wired Magazine that hints at the future effects of nanotechnology. Technology is not quite at the Fantastic Voyage level where miniature robots flow through the body repairing problems, but the field of microelectromechan-ical systems (MEMS) has created methods to build very small sensors and miniature mechanical devices. In the figure, the illustrator imagines miniature devices being used as an intervention to remove "smart dust" household sensors that might have been acci-dentally inhaled. Certainly, the ability to build sensors and treatment devices at such a small scale will influence future medical care, especially in the management of chronic diseases such as diabetes.

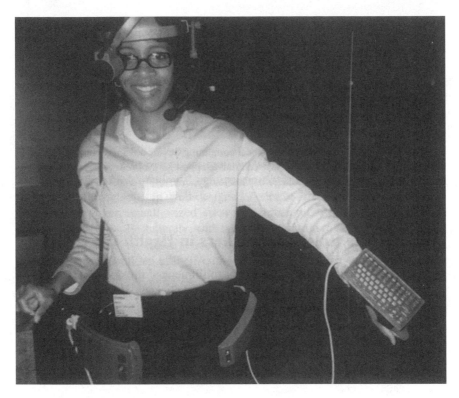

Figure 24.3. A wearable computer, including monacle display, voice input, belt-mounted central processing unit, and hand-mounted keypad. (*Source*: Photograph by Lawrence M. Fagan. Xybernaut, Mobile Assistant, and MA IV are registered trademarks of Xybernaut Corporation.)

24.3   Future Role of Computers in Health Care and Biomedicine

As we discussed in the previous section, fulfillment of the opening scenarios in this chapter will require significant technological changes. Equally important are the organizational and attitudinal changes that will be necessary to implement the new technologies as they emerge. Health professionals, health institutions, medical system developers, and society as a whole must carefully consider the appropriate role of computers in medicine and assess the potential benefits of computers in terms of improved access to information, enhanced communication, increased efficiency of health care delivery, and higher quality of medical care.

Although the potential benefits of using computers are many, there are also potential costs, only some of which are monetary. For example, computer-based medical record systems will never exactly replicate the flexibility of current paper-based systems. This flexibility includes the ability to create progress notes about patients, using any words in any order and in any format, with or without diagrams, to record the information.

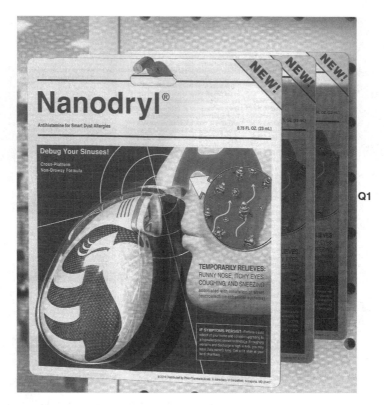

Figure 24.4. Amusing illustration of miniature robotic devices used as a treatment of accidental inhalation of "smart dust" robotic sensors. (*Source*: Illustration by Chuck Henderson. *Reprinted by permission from Wired Magazine. This illustration appeared in the April, 2004 issue.*)

Computer-based systems limit flexibility in return for increased legibility and access to the information and for the ability to use the information for other purposes, such as clinical research studies that use multiple patient databases. We see the same pattern in the use of automated bank-teller machines. There are only a few ways to complete a cash withdrawal transaction through a sequence of button pushes, but there are a large number of ways in which we can make this request of a human teller. Automated tellers are available at 3:00 A.M. in the morning, however; human tellers are not.

The idea that computer approaches would require the additional structuring of medical records was perceived by Lawrence Weed more than 30 years ago (Weed, 1969). Weed noted that, for medical records to be useful, they had to be indexed such that important information could be extracted. In particular, he proposed that the medical record be organized according to the patient's current problems—the problem-oriented medical record (POMR). Variations of the POMR have become a standard feature of medical record keeping, regardless of whether computers are used. In the problem-oriented medical information system (PROMIS), a computer-based implementation of the POMR, such rigid and time-consuming indexing of patient problems was required that clinicians ultimately proved reluctant to use the system. Standardization provides benefits but exacts costs in terms of decreased flexibility; it makes information more accessible but restricts freedom to pursue alternate means to accomplish the same result. It is unlikely that new computer innovations will ever eliminate this trade-off.

Similarly, the use of computers requires trade-offs with respect to confidentiality of medical information. Legitimate users can more conveniently access computer-based records in well-designed systems. Without sufficient security and policy measures, however, unauthorized users may threaten the confidentiality and integrity of databases. Fortunately, with adequate attention to security issues, modern methods backed by effective security policies can ensure that patient data are kept with greater confidentiality in computer systems than they are in the paper charts of hospital wards. The growing volume of clinical data stored electronically, widespread remote access capabilities, and the trend toward secondary and tertiary uses of clinical information result in the need for ongoing attention to concerns of security and confidentiality (see Chapter 10).

Earlier fears that computers could replace physicians have not been borne out, and computers are likely to remain decision-support tools rather than substitute decision makers (Shortliffe, 1989). It is more likely that computers will be used increasingly to monitor the quality of health care delivered and to help evaluate physician performance. Greater automation will therefore change the nature of medical practice in nontrivial ways. The challenge for system developers and users will be to identify the solution that provides the optimal balance between flexibility and standardization.

Computers in the future are likely to have even a greater influence on the practice of biology in the research laboratory. Exponential increases in the availability of experimental data necessitate computational support. Examples include cross-species investigation of DNA sequences, analysis of microarray data, and simulation of cellular function. Just as clinicians need to adjust their practice to accommodate computational support, biologists need to provide a computational infrastructure for the collection, analysis, and dissemination of laboratory data. An exceptional illustration of the power of computers is in the field of pharmacogenetics, where clinical and biological data are combined to determine individual responses to drug therapy. This requires the development of terminologies to support these disparate data sources, a complex database schema to store the information, and intelligent searching function to highlight the key relationships. It is likely that these types of biological and clinical applications will be a focus of research and development in the coming decades.

24.4 Forces Affecting the Future of Medical Computing

In this book, we have identified several important factors that affect the current and future role of computers in medicine. These factors include advances in biotechnology and computer hardware and software, changes in the background of health professionals, changes in the medicolegal climate, and changing strategies for health care reimbursement. The relative strengths of these forces will determine how likely it is that the scenarios we proposed will take place and how quickly we can expect such changes to occur.

24.4.1   Changes in Computers and Biomedical Technology

Modern computers are smaller, less expensive, and more powerful than were their predecessors. Although microchip designers are approaching the physical limits on how close together electronic elements can be placed, these trends will continue. By the time a new microprocessor chip or memory chip is adapted for use in new computer systems, manufacturers are creating samples of the next generation of chips. The most important ramification of current trends in microcomputer technology is that it is now possible to include a microprocessor and memory in most pieces of medical equipment.

The ability to connect multiple devices over high-speed networks has enabled a dramatic change in the way medical computer systems are designed. It is now practical to develop systems in which multiple data storage devices are accessed by complex computers that sort and abstract the numerous patient data that are generated. This design contrasts with the traditional approach in which health professionals would need to gather information from many different devices or locations in the medical center to obtain a complete picture of a patient's status. Relatively low-cost computer workstations or network-based terminals now allow information to be manipulated at each patient's bedside, as well as at other work areas in medical centers and ambulatory clinics.

High-speed networks and private intranets allow physicians in private offices to connect to computers in the hospitals where they admit patients or to repositories of data from multiple care settings and systems.

We have much more data to transmit over the network, such as those from digitized radiology images, online reports, and computer-based charting of the patient's condition. In the future, even faster networks and larger storage devices will be necessary to manage the overwhelming volume of data that will be created by all-digital clinical data systems.

24.4.2   Changes in the Background of Health Professionals and Biologists

Computers will continue to be made faster and less expensive and will have more features; however, sufficient computing power now exists for most applications. Thus, the limitations on the pervasiveness of computers in medicine do not hinge as crucially on the development of new hardware as they did in the past. The availability of relatively inexpensive and powerful computers is changing health care workers' familiarity with machines by exposing these people to computers in all aspects of their daily lives. This increased familiarity in turn increases acceptance of computers in the workplace, another crucial determinant of how computers will fare in the next 15 years.

Since the early 1970s, people have increasingly interacted with computers in their daily lives to perform financial transactions, to make travel arrangements, and even to purchase groceries. In many situations, people do not use the computer themselves but rather talk to an intermediary, such as an airline reservation agent or bank clerk. Large computer systems are so deeply integrated into many business practices that it is not uncommon to hear, "I can't help you—the computer is down." This switch to computer-based record keeping for most financial transactions is so pervasive that you would be surprised and concerned if you were to receive a monthly bank statement that was written out in longhand. Within the last 10 years, many mediated computer-based transactions have been replaced by direct contact between a consumer and a computer system. We can withdraw cash from automated bank tellers, request a trip routing from a computer at the rental car stand, or obtain an account balance by a touch-tone telephone. As described in almost every chapter in this book, the acceptance of the Internet model of interaction is cutting out intermediary steps and allowing users to access large online databases directly from home or work.

Young health care workers today have been exposed to computers throughout their education. Many college courses assign projects that must be carried out using the computer. It is difficult to determine how the current hodgepodge of computers in the medical setting will bias these users. It may be that, when the integrated system becomes available, health care professionals will not use the system fully because of previous negative experiences in less sophisticated environments. On the other hand, familiarity with computers and with their operation may prepare users to accept well-designed, easy-to-use systems.

24.4.3   Legal Considerations

The number of malpractice lawsuits and the sizes of the settlements have increased in recent years. Today, the specter of potential legal action hangs over every medical interaction. Computers can either exacerbate or alleviate this situation. The computer-based diagnostic system may provide a reminder of a rare but life-threatening disease that might have been overlooked in the differential diagnosis. On the other hand, decision-support systems might generate warnings that, if ignored by health care workers, could be used as evidence against those workers in a court action (see Chapter 10).

During the last few years, there has been a national-level focus on the cause of medical errors during the diagnostic and treatment process. The Institute of Medicine (IOM) has performed several key studies in this area (Kohn, 1999; Committee on Quality of Health Care in America, 2001; Aspden, 2003). These studies showed a series of issues with the medical process that can lead to medical errors. One of the results of these studies has been new requirements to track errors and near misses. The second IOM report suggested that the number of errors would be reduced by the widespread introduction of information technology. The 2003 IOM report laid out possible data standards that would help to increase patient safety. In 2004, the government increased its efforts to promote a National Health Information Infrastructure that will provide mechanisms to interlink medical records at diverse institutions, and thus decrease the possibilities of errors or repeated tests because of increased access to clinical information.

24.4.4   Health Care Financing

Some people assume that the continuing evolution of computer hardware and software is the most important force influencing the development of medical computing. Social issues such as health care financing and the legal aspects of medicine, however, probably outweigh the technological factors. Perhaps the strongest force at work today is the pressure to control health care costs. Health care financing influences all choices regarding the acquisition and maintenance of high-technology equipment and information systems.

Current schemes for health care financing have been designed to slow the rate of growth of health care costs. These policies translate into pressure to reduce costs in every aspect of medical diagnosis and treatment, such as to substitute ambulatory care for hospitalizations, to shorten hospital stays, to select less expensive surgical procedures, and to order fewer laboratory tests. As incentives for making optimal decisions in these areas increase, there is a greater need for computers that can collect, store, interpret, and present data during the decision-making process.

Order-entry systems routinely screen test orders against criteria for test ordering and question or cancel tests that do not meet the criteria. A more sophisticated clinical decision-support system might serve as an adjunct to an order management system, assessing which tests are most appropriate to order for specific patients who require expensive workups (e.g., custom-tailored evaluation of thyroid function). Such a system might also evaluate drug orders and suggest less expensive substitutes that are equally effective while checking for drug–drug interactions, and so on.

It is now common that computers are used by health plans to enforce a particular style of care through concurrent or post hoc review of the medical decision-making process, including decisions about length of stay and tests performed. Thus, one force promoting the use of computers by clinicians is the knowledge that computers are often used by insurers to review these clinicians' decisions after the fact. The clinicians may prefer to know what the computer system will advise beforehand so that they can be prepared to justify intentional deviations from the norm. Increasingly, health care administrators and medical practice directors are requiring use of clinical systems by clinicians to understand and manage clinical interventions and outcomes in response to decreasing reimbursement for services and managed care contracting arrangements.

In the United States, an entire new and thriving industry has evolved in response to efforts to manage health care costs more effectively: **pharmacy benefits managers (PBMs)**. Highly dependent on computer technology to manage their business functions, the PBMs manage the prescription benefits for insured individuals, working with retail pharmacies but also providing mail-order options and encouraging appropriate conversion to generic equivalents that can greatly reduce the cost of care for insurers (and for the employers who are the PBM's clients). Note that the PBMs, like managed care organizations, must distinguish between their customers (generally employers) and their members (employees and their families who receive their medical insurance through the employee's work). PBMs are only one example of new industries that have evolved in part because of the unusual nature of health care financing in the United States when compared with other parts of the world (see Chapter 23).

Although the use of computer technology can help health professionals to cope with the growing complexity of medical practice, it also contributes to the increasing cost of health care. Studies are beginning to show the benefits of outpatient computerized patient order entry (Johnston, 2003). Some computers are so embedded in the clinical environment, especially in complex environments such as operating rooms or intensive care units, that it is hard to show a decrease in patient morbidity or mortality due to the computers alone. Large numbers of devices are already being used in these settings, and patients are often treated for multiple concurrent problems. Even if patient-monitoring equipment could help health care workers to recognize potentially dangerous situations earlier than they otherwise would, showing that the computer system affected the outcome would be difficult. At the other extreme are devices that can be shown to make a difference, but whose cost is very high, such as computed tomography and magnetic resonance imaging systems. Because they replace invasive techniques (which have a significant potential for causing harm) or provide information that is available from no other source, there has been little debate about the utility of these new modalities. Instead, the high cost of this equipment has focused attention on how best to distribute these new resources. Demonstrating the return on investment in computer technology is a major challenge to widespread implementation of health care computer systems in light of their often staggering capital cost and the expense of staff resources required to support the many clinical users and to implement, integrate, manage, and maintain increasingly complex distributed systems and networks. No matter how computer systems are used in the future, we will need to evaluate the influence of the computer application on health care financing and to assess the new technology in light of alternative uses of resources.

24.5   Looking Back: What Have We Learned?

An introductory book can only scratch the surface of a field as varied and complex as biomedical informatics. In each chapter, we have examined technical questions about how a system works (or ought to work); we must also view each area in light of the health care trends and the social and fiscal issues that shape the ways in which clinical care is delivered now and in the future. In this chapter, we have emphasized the rich social and technological context in which biomedical informatics moves ahead both as a scientific discipline and as a set of methodologies, devices, and complex systems that serve health care workers and, through them, their patients. One of the most important changes is the increase in the use of computers to help with the analysis of biological data. As more clinically important genetic data come online, new application areas such as pharmacogenetics are influencing clinical care. This type of new application that spans clinical and biological data is clearly the start of a new trend in informatics. Glimpses of the future can be at once both exciting and frightening—exciting when we see how emerging technologies can address the frequently cited problems that confound current health care practices but frightening when we realize that methodologies must be applied wisely and with sensitivity if patients are to receive the humane and cost-sensitive health care that they have every right to expect. The question is not whether computer technologies will play a pervasive role in the health care environment of the future, but how we can ensure that future systems are designed and implemented effectively to optimize technology's role as a stimulus and support for the health care system and for individual practitioners. The outcomes of the process will depend as much on health care planners, practitioners, and policymakers as they will on the efforts of system developers and biomedical informatics professionals. It is to all such individuals that this book has been dedicated.

Suggested Readings

Altman R.B. (2001). Challenges for intelligent systems in biology. *IEEE Intelligent Systems*, 16(2): 2001, 14–18.
In this summary article, R.B. Altman lays out some major future challenges for biocomputation.

http: //www.citl.org/research/ ACPOE_Executive_Preview.pdf (Web site accessed July 9, 2004).
This Web site provides an executive summary of the cost/ benefits of Ambulatory Computerized Provider Order Entry. See Johnston (2003) for the full report.

Committee on Quality of Health Care in America, Institute of Medicine, *Crossing the Quality Chasm: A New Health System for the 21st Century*. Washington, D.C.: National Academies Press.
This report discussed structural changes to the practice of medicine to address some of the issues discussed in the IOM report, To Err is Human.

Stead W.W., et al. (Eds.) (1998). Focus on an agenda for biomedical informatics. *Journal of the American Medical Informatics Association*, 5(5):395–420. Special Issue.
The 1998 Scientific Symposium of the American College of Medical Informatics (ACMI) was devoted to developing visions for the future of health care and biomedicine and a strategic agenda for health and biomedical informatics in support of those visions. The first five articles contained in this special issue illustrate these findings and continue to be timely.

Questions for Discussion

1. Select an area of biomedicine with which you are familiar. Based on what you have learned in this book, propose a scenario for that area that takes place 20 years in the future. Be sure to think about how issues of system integration, networking, and changes in workflow will affect the evolution of computers in the setting you describe.
2. Imagine that you are a patient visiting a health care facility at which the physicians have made a major commitment to computer-based tools. How would you react to the following situations?
   a. Before you are ushered into the examining room, the nurse takes your blood pressure and pulse in a work area and then enters the information into a computer terminal located in the nursing station adjacent to the waiting room.
   b. While the physician interviews you, he or she occasionally types information into a computer workstation that is facing the physician; you cannot see the screen.
   c. While the physician interviews you, he or she occasionally uses a mouse-pointing device to enter information into a computer workstation located such that, when facing the physician, you cannot see the screen.
   d. While the physician interviews you, he or she occasionally uses a mouse-pointing device to enter information into a computer workstation that you both can see. While doing so, the physician explains the data being reviewed and entered.
   e. While the physician interviews you, he or she enters information into a clipboard-sized computer terminal that responds to finger touch and requires no keyboard typing.

f. While the physician interviews you, he or she occasionally stops to dictate a phrase. A speech-understanding interface processes what is being said and stores the infor   mation in a medical record system.

g. There is no computer in the examining room, but you notice that between visits, the physician uses a workstation in the office to review and enter patient data.

Now imagine that you are the physician in each situation. How would you react in each case? What do your answers to these questions tell you about the potential effect of computers on patient–physician rapport? What insight have you gained regarding how interactive technologies could affect the patient–physician encounter? Did you have different reactions to scenarios c and d? Do you believe that most people would respond to these two situations as you did?

3. You are the medical director of a 30-physician multispecialty group practice. The practice is physician-owned and managed and maintains a tight affiliation with a nearby academic medical center. You are considering implementing an ambulatory medical record system to support your practice operations. Discuss at least eight significant challenges you will face, considering technology, user, legal, and financial factors. How will you address each issue?

4. Defend or refute the following proposition: "Knowledge-based clinical systems will be widely used and generally accepted by clinician users within the next 5 years."

5. You are asked to design a pharmacogenetic system that can help to understand which patients will respond to particular medicines. You need to design a database of studies that relate descriptions of the medical conditions, medications, and genetic sequences. Which terminologies would you choose for each of these data types? What are some key elements that would need to be included in the database schemas? What problems do you anticipate having in the design of the data structures for this task?

Bibliography

3M Health Information Systems (updated annually). *AP-DRGs: All Patient Diagnosis Related Groups.* Wallingford, CT: 3M Health Care.

A. Foster Higgins & Co. Inc. (1997). *Foster Higgins National Survey of Employer-sponsored Health Plans.*

Abbey, L.M., Zimmerman, J. (eds.) (1991). *Dental Informatics, Integrating Technology into the Dental Environment.* New York: Springer-Verlag.

Abromowitz, K. (1996). *HMO's: Cycle Bottoming; Secular Opportunity Undiminished.*: Berstein Research.

Ackerman, M.J. (1991). The Visible Human Project. *Journal of Biocommunication,* 18(2):14.

ADAM (1995). *ADAM Software* [CD-ROM]: ADAM Scholar Series.

Adams, I.D., Chan, M., Clifford, P.C., Cooke, W.M., Dallos, V., de Dombal, F.T., Edwards, M.H., Hancock, D.M., Hewett, D.J., McIntyre, N. (1986). Computer aided diagnosis of acute abdominal pain: A multicenter study. *British Medical Journal,* 293(6550):800–804.

Adderley, D., Hyde, C., Mauseth, P. (1997). The computer age impacts nurses. *Computers in Nursing,* 15(1):43–46.

Adhikari, N., Lapinsky, S.E. (2003). Medical Informatics in the intensive care unit: Overview of technology assessment. *J Crit Care* 18(1):41–47

Afrin, J. N. & Critchfield, A. B. (1997). Low-cost telepsychiatry for the deaf in South Carolina. *Proceeding of the AMIA Fall Symposium, p.* 901.

Agrawal, M., Harwood, D., Duraiswami, R., Davis, L. S., & Luther, P. W. (2000). Three-dimensional ultrastructure from transmission electron micropscope tilt series, *Proceedings, Second Indian Conference on Vision, Graphics and Image Processing.* Bangalore, India.

Ahrens, E. T., Laidlaw, D. H., Readhead, C., Brosnan, C. F., & Fraser, S. E. (1998). MR microscopy of transgenic mice that spontaneously acquire experimental allergic encephalomyelitis. *Magnetic Resonance in Medicine,* 40(1):119–132.

Aine, C.J. (1995). A conceptual overview and critique of functional neuroimaging techniques in humans: I. MRI/fMRI and PET. *Critical Reviews in Neurobiology* 9(2-3):229–309.

Akin, O. (1982). *The Psychology of Architecture Design.* London: Pion.

Allaërt F.A., Dusserne L. (1992). Decision support systems and medical liability. *Proceedings of the 16th Annual Symposium on Computer Applications in Medical Care,* Baltimore, MD., pp. 750–753.

Allard, F., & Starkes, J. L. (1991). Motor-skill experts in sports, dance, and other domains. In K.A. Ericsson & J. Smith (eds.), *Toward a General Theory of Expertise: Prospects and Limits.* New York: Cambridge University Press, pp. 126–152.

Allen, J. (1995). *Natural Language Understanding* (2nd Edition). Redwood City, CA: Benjamin Cummings.

Alpert, S.A. (1998). Health care information: access, confidentiality, and good practice. In Goodman K.W. (ed.), *Ethics, Computing, and Medicine: Informatics and the Transformation of Health Care.* Cambridge: Cambridge University Press, pp.75–101.

Altman, R.B. (1997). Informatics in the care of patients: Ten notable challenges. *Western Journal of Medicine* 166(6):118–122.

Altman, RB. (2003). Complexities of managing biomedical information. *OMICS* 7(1):127–9.

Altman, R.B., Dunker, A.K., Hunter, L., Klein T.E. (eds.) (1998). *Pacific Symposium on Biocomputing '98.* Singapore: World Scientific Publishing.

Altman, R.B., Dunker, A.K., Hunter, L., Klein, T.E. (2003). *Pacific Symposium on Biocomputing '03.* Singapore: World Scientific Publishing.

Altschul, S.F., Gish, W., Mille,r W., Myers, E.W., Lipman, D.J. (1990). Basic local alignment search tool. *Journal of Molecular Biology* 215(3):403–410.

American Association of Health Plans (1995). AAHP HMO and PPO Trends Report. *AMCRA Census Database and AAHP Sample Survey of HMOs and PPOs.*

American College of Pathologists (1982). *SNOMED.* Skokie, IL: College of American Pathology.

American Medical Association (updated annually). *Current Procedural Terminology.* Chicago, IL: The American Medical Association.

American Nurses Association (1995). *Scope of practice for nursing informatics.* Washington, DC: American Nurses Publishing.

American Nurses Association (1997). *NIDSEC standards and scoring guidelines.* Washington, DC: American Nurses Publishing.

American Psychiatric Association Committee on Nomenclature and Statistics (1987). *Diagnostic and Statistical Manual of Mental Disorders.* (Rev. 3rd ed.). Washington, D.C.: The American Psychiatric Association.

American Psychiatric Association Committee on Nomenclature and Statistics (1994). *Diagnostic and Statistical Manual of Mental Disorders.* (4th ed.). Washington, D.C.: The American Psychiatric Association.

American Society for Testing and Materials (1999). *Standard Guide for Properties of a Universal Healthcare Identifier (UHID).* (E1714-95.) West Conshohocken, PA: American Society for Testing and Materials.

Amir, M., Shabot, M.M., Karlan, B.Y. (1997). Surgical intensive care unit care after ovarian cancer surgery: An analysis of indications. *American Journal of Obstetrics and Gynecology,* 176(6):1389–93.

Anderson, J.G., Aydin, C.E. (1994). Overview: Theoretical perspectives and methodologies for the evaluation of health care information systems. In Anderson J.G., Aydin C.E., Jay S.J. (eds.), *Evaluating Health Care Information Systems: Methods and Applications.* Thousand Oaks, CA: Sage.

Anderson, J.G., Aydin, C.E. (1998). Evaluating medical information systems: social contexts and ethical challenges. In Goodman K.W. (ed.), *Ethics, Computing, and Medicine: Informatics and the Transformation of Health Care.* (, pp.57–74) Cambridge: Cambridge University Press.

Anderson, J.G., Aydin, C.E., Jay, S.J. (eds.) (1994). *Evaluating Health Care Information Systems: Methods and Applications.* Thousand Oaks, CA: Sage Publications.

Anderson, J.G., Aydin, C.E., Jay, S.J. (eds.) (1995). *Computers in health care: research and evaluation.* Newbury Park, CA: Sage Publications.

Anderson, J.G., Jay, S.J. (eds.) (1987). *Use and Impact of Computers in Clinical Medicine.* New York: Springer-Verlag.

Anderson, J.R. (1983). *The Architecture of Cognition.* Mahwah, N.J.: L. Erlbaum Associates.

Anderson, J.R. (1985). *Cognitive Psychology and its Implications.* New York: W.H. Freeman.

Anderson, J., Rainey, M., et al. (2003). The impact of CyberHealthcare on the physician-patient relationship. *Journal of Medical Systems,* 27: 67–84.

Anderson, R. E. (1998). Imagery and spatial representation. In W. Bechtel & G. Graham (eds.), *A Companion to Cognitive Science*. Malden, MA: Blackwell Publishers.

Anonymous (1879). Practice by Telephone. *Lancet* 2, 819.

Anonymous (1993a). *Draft Application Protocol for Electronic Exchange in Health Care Environments*. (Vol. Version 2.2, HL7).

Anonymous (1993b). *Standard for Health Care Data Interchange – Information Model Methods*. Draft P1157.1, IEEE.

Anonymous (1994). *NCPDP Data Dictionary*. June 1, 1994.

Anonymous (1999). *Dublin Core Metadata Element Set*, Version 1.1: Reference Description. Dublin Core Metadata Initiative. (Accessed 2005 at: http://www.dublincore.org/documents/dces/)

Anonymous (2000a). *Cataloging Practices*. National Library of Medicine. (Accessed 2005 at: http://www.nlm.nih.gov/mesh/catpractices2004.html)

Anonymous (2000b). *Features of the MeSH Vocabulary*. National Library of Medicine. (Accessed 2005 at: http://www.nlm.nih.gov/mesh/intro_features2005.html)

Anonymous (2000c). *Organization of National Library of Medicine Bibliographic Databases*. National Library of Medicine. (Accessed 2005 at: http://www.nlm.nih.gov/pubs/techbull/mj00/mj00_buckets.html)

Anonymous (2001a). *Digital Libraries: Universal Access to Human Knowledge*. President's Information Technology Advisory Committee. (Accessed 2005 at: http://www.nitrd.gov/pubs/pitac/pitac-dl-9feb01.pdf)

Anonymous (2001b). *The Dublin Core Metadata Element Set*. Dublin Core Metadata Initiative. (Accessed 2005 at: http://www.niso.org/standards/resources/Z39-85.pdf)

Anonymous (2001c). The future of the electronic scientific literature. *Nature*, 413:1–3.

Anonymous (2001d). *PubMed Help*. National Library of Medicine. (Accessed 2005 at: http://www.ncbi.nlm.nih.gov/entrez/query/static/help/pmhelp.html)

Anonymous (2001e). *Transforming Health Care Through Information Technology*. President's Information Technology Advisory Committee. (Accessed 2005 at: http://www.nitrd.gov/pubs/pitac/pitac-hc-9feb01.pdf)

Anonymous (2001f). *Using Information Technology to Transform the Way We Learn*. President's Information Technology Advisory Committee. (Accessed 2005 at: http://www.nitrd.gov/pubs/pitac/pitac-tl-9feb01.pdf)

Arenson, R.L. (1984). Automation of the radiology management function. *Radiology*, 153:65–68.

Arenson, R.L., Gitlin, J.N., London, J.W. (1982). The formation of a radiology computer consortium. *Proceedings of the 7th Conference on Computer Applications in Radiology*, Boston, MA, 153–164, April.

Arenson, R.L., Seshadri, S., Kundel, H.L., DeSimone, D., Van der Voorde, F., Gefter, W.B., Epstein, D.M., Miller, W.T., Aronchick, J.M., Simson, M.B. (1988). Clinical evaluation of a medical image management system for chest images. *American Journal of Roentgenology*, 150(1):55–59.

Arms, W., Hillmann, D., et al. (2002). A spectrum of interoperability: the site for science prototype for the NSDL. *D-Lib Magazine*, 8. (Accessed 2005 at: http://www.dlib.org/dlib/january02/arms/0Aarms.html)

Aronow, D.B., Cooley, J.R., Soderland, S. (1995). Automated identification of episodes of asthma exacerbation for quality measurement in a computer-based medical record. *Proc Annu Symp Comput Appl Med Care*, pp.309–313.

Aronow, D.B., Soderland, S., Ponte, J.M., Feng, F., Croft, W.B., Lehnert, W.G. (1995). Automated classification of encounter notes in a computer based medical record. *Proceedings of Medinfo 1995*, Pt 1:8–12.

Aronow, D.B., Feng, F., Croft, W.B. (1999). Ad hoc classification of radiology reports. *Journal of the American Medical Informatics Association*, 6(5):343–411.

Aronson, A.R. (2001). Effective mapping of biomedical text to the UMLS metathesaurus: the MetaMap program. *Proceedings of the AMIA Annual Symposium*: Hanley & Belfus, pp. 17–21.

Aronson, A., Bodenreider, O., et al. (2000). The NLM indexing initiative. *Proceedings of the AMIA Annual Symposium*, Los Angeles, CA. Hanley & Belfus, pp. 17–21.

Arroll, B., Pandit, S., et al. (2002). Use of information sources among New Zealand family physicians with high access to computers. *Journal of Family Practice*, 51:8.

Ascioli, G. A. (1999). Progress and perspectives in computational neuroanatomy. *Anatomical Record (New Anat.)*, 257(6),195–207.

Ash, J. (1997). Organizational factors that influence information technology diffusion in academic health centers. *Journal of the American Medical Informatics Association*, 4(2):102–111.

Ash, J. S., Gorman, P. N., Lavelle, M., Payne, T. H., Massaro, T. A., Frantz, G. L., Lyman JA. (2003). A cross-site qualitative study of physician order entry. *Journal of the American Medical Informatics Association*, 10(2),188–200.

Ashburner, J., & Friston, K. J. (1997). Multimodal image coregistration and partitioning - a unified framework. *Neuroimage*, 6(3),209–217.

Aspden, P., Corrigan, J.M., Wolcott, J., Erickson, S.M. (editors) and the Committee on Data Standards for Patient Safety (2004). *Patient Safety: Achieving a New Standard for Care*, National Academies Press (Issued November 20, 2003).

Association of American Medical Colleges (1986). *Medical Education in the Information Age, Proceedings of the Symposium on Medical Informatics*. Washington D.C.: Association of American Medical Colleges.

ASTM (1989). *Standard Guide for Nosologic Standards and Guides for Construction of New Biomedical Nomenclature*. (Standard E1284-89.) Philadephia: ASTM.

ASTM (1994). *A Standard Specification for Representing Clinical Laboratory Test and Analyte Names*. (Standard E3113.2 (Draft).) Philadelphia: ASTM.

Atkinson W, Orenstein W, Krugman S (1992). The resurgence of measles in the United States, 1989-90. *Annual Rev Med* 43:451– 463.

Atkinson, R., & Shiffrin, R. (1968). Human memory: A proposed system and its control processes. In *Spence, K.W and Spence, J.T., The Psychology of Learning and Motivation: II.*

Axford, R., Carter, B. (1996). Impact of clinical information systems on nursing practice: Nurses' perspectives. *Computers in Nursing*, 14(3):156–163.

Ayers, S. (1983). NIH consensus conference. Critical care medicine. *Journal of the American Medical Association*, 250(6):798–804.

Babior, B.M., Matzner, Y. (1997). The familial Mediterranean fever gene—cloned at last. *New England Journal of Medicine*, 337(21):1548–1549.

Bachant, J., McDermott, J. (1984). R1 revisited: Four years in the trenches. *AI Magazine*, 5:3.

Bachrach, C., Charen, T. (1978). Selection of MEDLINE contents, the development of its thesaurus, and the indexing process. *Medical Informatics*, 3(3):237–254.

Bader, S. (1993). Recognition of computer-based materials in the promotion guidelines of U.S. medical schools. *Academic Medicine*, 68:S16–S17.

Baeza-Yates, R. and Ribeiro-Neto, B., eds. (1999). *Modern Information Retrieval*. New York: McGraw-Hill.

Bahls, C., Weitzman, J., et al. (2003). Biology's models. *The Scientist*, 17: 5.

Bai, C., Elledge, S.J. (1997). Gene identification using the yeast two-hybrid system. *Methods of Enzymology*, 283:141–56.

Baker, E.L., Friede, A., Moulton, A.D., Ross, D.A. (1995). CDC's information network for public health officials (INPHO): A framework for integrated public health information and practice. *Journal of Public Health Management and Practice*, 1:43– 47.

Baker, L., Wagner, T., et al. (2003). Use of the Internet and e-mail for health care information: Results from a national survey. *Journal of the American Medical Association*, 289:2400–2406.

Bakken, S., Cimino, J. J., Haskell, R., Kukafka, R., Matsumoto, C., Chan, G. K., Huff, S. MK.(2000) Evaluation of the clinical LOINC (Logical Observation Identifiers, Names, and Codes) semantic structure as a terminology model for standardized assessment measures. *Journal of the American Medical Informatics Association,* 7(6):529–538.

Bakken, S., Curran, C., Delaleu-McIntosh, J., Desjardins, K., Hyun, S., Jenkins, M., John, R., Ramirez, A-M., Tamayo, R. (2003). Informatics for evidence-based nurse practitioner practice at the Columbia University School of Nursing. *Proceedings of NI 2003.* Rio de Janeiro, Brazil.

Balas, E.A., Austin, S.M., Mitchell, J.A., Ewigman, B.G., Bopp, K.D., Brown, G.D. (1996). The clinical value of computerized information services: A review of 98 randomized clinical trials. *Archives of Family Medicine,* 5(5):271–278.

Balas, E.A. and Boren, S.A. (2000). Managing clinical knowledge for health care improvement. *IMIA Yearbook of Medical Informatics* (R. Haux and A.T. McCray, eds), pp.65–70, Stuttgart, Germany: Schattauer Publishing Company.

Baldi, P., Brunak, S. (1998). *Bioinformatics: The Machine Learning Approach.* Cambridge, MA: MIT Press.

Baldi, P, Hatfield, G.W. (2002) *DNA Microarrays and Gene Expression.* Cambridge University Press.

Ball, M. (ed.) (1995). *Introduction to Nursing Informatics.* New York: Springer.

Bansler, J.P., Bødker, K. (1993). A reappraisal of structured analysis: Design in an organizational context. *Proceedings of the ACM Transactions on Information Systems,* 11:165–193.

Barfield, W., Furness, T. (eds.) (1995). *Virtual Environments and Advanced Interface Design.* New York: Oxford University Press.

Barnett, G.O. (1976). *Computer-Stored Ambulatory Record (COSTAR).* (DHEW (HRA) 76-3145.): Department of Health, Education, and Welfare.

Barnett, G.O. (1984). The application of computer-based medical-record systems in ambulatory practice. *New England Journal of Medicine,* 310(25):1643–1650.

Barnett, G.O., Cimino, J.J., Hupp, J.A., Hoffer, E.P. (1987). DXplain: An evolving diagnostic decision-support system. *Journal of the American Medical Association,* 258(1):67–74.

Barrows Jr., R.C., Clayton, P.D. (1996). Privacy, confidentiality, and electronic medical records. *Journal of the American Medical Informatics Association,* 3(2):139–148.

Barnett, GO, Famiglietti, KT, Kim, RJ, Hoffer, EP, Feldman, MJ. (1998). DXplain on the Internet. *Proceedings of the AMIA Annual Fall Symposium,* pp. 607–611.

Bashshur, R.L., Mandil, S.H., Shannon, G.W. (eds). Telemedicine/telehealth: An international perspective. (2002) *Telemedicine Journal and e-Health.* 8(1):95–107.

Bashshur, R., Sanders, J., & Shannon, G. (1997). *Telemedicine: Theory and Practice* Charles C. Thomas, Springfield,IL.

Bass, D.M., McClendon, M.J., Brennan, P.F., McCarthy, C. (1998). The buffering effect of a computer support network on caregiver strain. *Journal of Aging and Health,* 10(1):20–43.

Bass, D.M., McClendon, M.J., Brennan, P.F., McCarthy, C. (1998) The buffering effect of a computer support network on caregiver strain. *Journal of Aging & Health.* 10(1):20–43.

Bates, D.W. (2000). Using information technology in hospitals to reduce rates of medication errors in hospitals. *BMJ* 320:788–91.

Bates, D.W., Ebell, M., Gotlieb, E., Zapp, J., Mullins, H.C., (2003). A proposal for electronic medical records in U.S. primary care. *J Am Med Inform Assoc.* 10(1):1–10.

Bates, D.W., Evans, R.S., Murff, H., Stetson, P.D., Pizziferri, L., Hripcsak, G.(2003). Detecting adverse events using information technology. *J Am Med Inform Assoc;* 10(2):115–128.

Bates, D.W., Gawande, A.A. (2003). Patient safety: improving safety with information technology. *The New England Journal of Medicine,* 348(25):2526–34.

Bates, D.W., Leape, L.L., Cullen, D.J., et al (1998). Effect of computerized physician order entry and a team intervention on prevention of serious medication errors. *Journal of the American Medical Association* 280(15):1311–1316.

Bates, D.W., Spell, N., Cullen, D.J., Burdick, E., Laird, N., Petersen, L.A., Small, S.D., Sweitzer, B.J., Leape, L.L. (1997). The costs of adverse drug events in hospitalized patients. *Journal of the American Medical Association*, 277(4):307–311.

Baud, R., Lovis, C., Rassinoux, A.M., Michel, P.A., Scherrer, J.R. Automatic extraction of linguistic knowledge from an international classification (1998). *Medinfo 1998* Pt 1:581–5.

Bauman, R.A., Arenson, R.L., Barnett, G.O. (1975a). Computer-based master folder tracking and automated file room operations. *Proceedings of the 4th Conference on Computer Applications in Radiology*, Las Vegas, NV, 469– 480.

Bauman, R.A., Arenson, R.L., Barnett, G.O. (1975b). Fully automated scheduling of radiology appointments. *Proceedings of the 4th Conference on Computer Applications in Radiology*, Las Vegas, NV, 461– 46.

Bauman, R.A., Gell, G., Dwyer, 3rd S.J. (1996). Large picture archiving and communication systems of the world-Part 2. *Journal of Digital Imaging*, 9(4):172–177.

Bauman, R.A., Pendergrass, H.P., Greenes, R.A. (1972). Further development of an on-line computer system for radiology reporting. *Proceedings of the Conference on Computer Applications in Radiology*, 409– 422.

Baxevanis, A. (2003). The Molecular Biology Database Collection: 2003 update. *Nucleic Acids Research*, 31: 1–12.

Beagrie, N. (2002). An update on the Digital Preservation Coalition. *D-Lib Magazine*, 8. (Accessed 2005 at: http://www.dlib.org/dlib/april02/beagrie/04beagrie.html)

Bechtel, W., Abrahamsen, A., & Graham, G. (1998). Part I: The life of cognitive science. In W. Bechtel, G. Graham & D.A. Balota (eds.), *A Companion to Cognitive Science* (Blackwell Companions to Philosophy , Vol. 13, pp. 2–104). Malden, MA: Blackwell.

Bechtel, W., Graham, G., & Balota, D. A. (1998). *A Companion to Cognitive Science*. Malden, Mass.: Blackwell.

Beck, J.R., Pauker, S.G. (1983). The Markov process in medical prognosis. *Medical Decision Making*, 3(4):419–58.

Beckett, D., Miller, E., et al. (2000). Using Dublin Core in XML. *Dublin Core Metadata Initiative*. (Accessed 2005 at: http://dublincore.org/documents/dcmes-xml/)

Bell, D.S., Greenes, R.A. (1994). Evaluation of UltraSTAR: Performance of a collaborative structured data entry system. *Proceedings of the 18th Annual Symposium on Computer Applications in Medical Care*, Washington, D.C., pp. 216–221.

Benko, L.B. (2003). Back to the drawing board; Cedars-Sinai's physician order-entry system suspended. *Modern Healthcare*, 12.

Benson, D.A., Karsch-Mizrachi, I, Lipman, DJ, Ostell, J, Wheeler, DL. GenBank. *Nucleic Acids Res.* 2003;31(1):23–7.

Bentt, L.R., Santora, T.A., Leyerle, B.J., LoBue, M., Shabot, M.M. (1990). Accuracy and utility of pulse oximetry in a surgical ICU. *Current Surgery*, 47(4):267–268.

Berenson, R. (1984). *Health Technology Case Study 28: Intensive Care Units (ICUs)-Clinical Outcomes, Costs and Decisionmaking*. Washington, DC: Office of Technology Assessment.

Berg, M. (1997). *Rationalizing Medical Work: Decision Support Techniques and Medical Practices*. Cambridge, MA: MIT Press.

Berg, M. (1999). Patient care information systems and health care work: a sociotechnical approach. *International Journal of Medical Informatics*, 55(2),87–101.

Bergeron, B.P., Greenes, R.A. (1989). Clinical skill-building simulations in cardiology: HeartLab and EKGLab. *Computer Methods and Programs in Biomedicine*, 30(2-3):111–126.

Berland, G., Elliott, M., et al. (2001). Health information on the Internet: Accessibility, quality, and readability in English and Spanish. *Journal of the American Medical Association*, 285:2612–2621.

Berman, J.J., Edgerton, M.E., Friedman, B.A. (2003). The tissue microarray data exchange specification: A community-based, open source tool for sharing tissue microarray data. *BMC Med Inform Decis Mak*. 3(1):5.

Berners-Lee, T., Cailliau, R., Luotonen, A., Nielsen, H., Secret, A. (1994). The World-Wide-Web. *Communications of the Association for Computing Machinery*, 37:76–82.

Bero, L., Rennie, D. (1996). The Cochrane Collaboration: Preparing, maintaining, and disseminating systematic reviews of the effects of health care. *Journal of the American Medical Association*, 274:1935–1938.

Besser, H. (2002). The next stage: Moving from isolated digital collections to interoperable digital libraries. *First Monday*, 7: 6. (Available 2005 at: http://www.firstmonday.dk/issues/issue7_6/besser/)

Bickel, R.G. (1979). The TRIMIS concept. *Proceedings of the 3rd Annual Symposium for Computer Applications in Medical Care*, Washington, DC, pp. 839–842.

Bidgood, W.D. Jr.(1998). Clinical importance of the DICOM structured reporting standard. *Int J Card Imaging*. 14(5):307–15.

Bidgood, W.D., Horii, S.C., Prior, F.W., Van Syckle, D.E. (1997). Understanding and using DICOM, the data interchange standard for biomedical imaging. *Journal of the American Medical Informatics Association*, 4(3):199–212.

Biondich, P.G., Anand, V., Downs, S.M., McDonald, C.J. (2003). *Proceedings AMIA Annu Symp*, pp. 86–90.

Bishop, M., Rawlings, C. (eds.) (1997). *DNA and Protein Sequence Analysis—A Practical Approach*: IRL Press at Oxford University Press.

Blaine, G.J., Hill, R.L., Cox, J.R. (1983). PACS workbench at Mallinckrodt Institute of Radiology (MIR). *Proceedings of the SPIE (Society of Photo-optical Instrumentation Engineers)*, Kansas City, MO, 418 (PACSII):80–86.

Blake, J.A., Richardson, J.E., Bult, C.J., Kadin, J.A., Eppig, J.T., and the members of the Mouse Genome Database Group (2003). MGD: The Mouse Genome Database. *Nucleic Acids Res*, 31:193–195.

Bleich, H. (1972). Computer-based consultation: Electrolyte and acid-base disorders. *American Journal of Medicine*, 53:285–291.

Bleich, H.L., Beckley, R.F., Horowitz, G.L., Jackson, J.D., Moody, E.S., Franklin, C., Goodman, S.R., McKay, M.W., Pope, R.A., Walden, T., Bloom, S.A., Slack, W.V. (1985). Clinical computing in a teaching hospital. *New England Journal of Medicine*, 312(12):756–764.

Bleich, H.L., Safra,n C., Slack, W.V. (1989). Departmental and laboratory computing in two hospitals. *MD Computing*, 6(3):149–155.

Bliss-Holtz, J. (1995). Computerized support for case management: ISAACC. *Computers in Nursing*, 13(6):289–294.

Blois, M.S. (1984). *Information and Medicine: The Nature of Medical Descriptions*. Berkeley: University of California Press.

Bloom, F.E., & Young, W.G. (1993). *Brain Browser* (Scripps, Trans.). New York: Academic Press.

Blum, B. (1992). *Software Engineering, A Holistic Approach*: Oxford University Press.

Blum, B.I. (1986a). *Clinical Information Systems*. New York: Springer-Verlag.

Blum, B.I. (1986b). Clinical Information Systems: A review. *Western Journal of Medicine*, 145(6):791–797.

Boeckmann B., Bairoch A., Apweiler R., Blatter M.-C., Estreicher A., Gasteiger E., Martin M.J., Michoud K., O'Donovan C., Phan I., Pilbout S., Schneider M. (2003). The SWISS-PROT protein knowledgebase and its supplement TrEMBL in 2003. *Nucleic Acids Res* 31:365–370.

Boehm, B. (1999): Managing software productivity and reuse; *IEEE Computer*, 31(9):111–113.

Boehm, B., Egyed, A., Kwan, J., Port, D., Shah, A., Madachy, R. (1998). Using the Win Win Spiral Model: A Case Study. *IEEE Computer*, 31(7):33– 44.

Boland, P. (1985). *The New Healthcare Market: A Guide to PPOs for Purchasers, Payers and Providers*. Homewood, Illinois: Dow Jones Irwin.

Bone, R.C. (1995). Standards of evidence for the safety and effectiveness of critical care monitoring devices and related interventions. *Critical Care in Medicine*, 23(10):1756–1763.

Booch, G. (1994). *Object-Oriented Design with Applications*. (2nd ed.): Benjamin-Cummins.

Bookstein, F.L. (1989). Principal warps: thin-plate splines and the decomposition of deformations. *IEEE Transactions on Pattern Analysis and Machine Intelligence*, 11(6):567–585.

Bookstein, F.L. (1997). Biometrics and brain maps: The promise of the morphometric synthesis. In: Koslow SH, Huerta MF, editors. *Neuroinformatics: An Overview of the Human Brain Project*. pp. 203–254. Mahwah, New Jersey: Lawrence Erlbaum Associates.

Bookstein, F.L., Green, W.D.K. (2001). *The Edgewarp 3D Browser*. Accessed 2005 from http://vhp.med.umich.edu/edgewarpss.html.

Bopp, K. (2000). Information services that make patients co-producers of quality health care. *Studies in Health Technology and Informatics*, 76:93–106.

Borgman, C. (1999). What are digital libraries? Competing visions. *Information Processing and Management*, 35:227–244.

Bowden, D.M., Martin, R.F. (1995). Neuronames brain hierarchy. *Neuroimage*, 2:63–83.

Bowie, J., Barnett G.O. (1976). MUMPS: An economical and efficient time-sharing system for information management. *Comput Programs Biomed* 6:11–22.

Bowker, G. C., Star, S. L. (1999). *Sorting Things Out: Classification and its Consequences*. Cambridge, Mass.: MIT Press.

Boxwala, A.A., Peleg, M., Tu, S, Ogunyemi, O., Zeng, Q.T., Wang, D., Patel, V.L., Greenes, R., and Shortliffe, E.H. (2004). GLIF3: A representation format for sharable computer-interpretable clinical practice guidelines. *Journal of Biomedical Informatics,* 37(3):147–161.

Boyd, S. and Herkovic, A. (1999). *Crisis in Scholarly Publishing: Executive Summary*. Stanford Academic Council Committee on Libraries. (Accessed 2005 at: http://www.stanford.edu/~boyd/schol_pub_crisis.html)

Boynton, J., Glanville, J., et al. (1998). Identifying systematic reviews in MEDLINE: developing an objective approach to search strategy design. *Journal of Information Science*, 24:137–157.

Bradshaw, K.E., Gardner, R.M., Clemmer, T.P., Orme, J.F., Thomas, F., West, B.J. (1984). Physician decision-making: Evaluation of data used in a computerized ICU. *International Journal of Clinical Monitoring and Computing*, 1(2):81–91.

Bradshaw, K.E., Sittig, D.F., Gardner, R.M., Pryor, T.A., Budd, M. (1988). Improving efficiency and quality in a computerized ICU. *Proceedings of the 12th Annual Symposium on Computer Applications in Medical Care*, Washington, D.C., 763–767.

Brahams, D., Wyatt, J.C. (1989). Decision aids and the law. *Lancet*, 2(8663):632–634.

Brailer, D.J. (2002). Personal Communication.

Brain Innovation, B.V. (2001). *Brain Voyager*. Accessed 2005 at http://www.BrainVoyager.de/

Brannigan V.M. (1991). Software quality regulation under the safe medical devices act of 1990: Hospitals are now the canaries in the software mine. *Proceedings of the 15th Annual Symposium on Computer Applications in Medical Care*, Washington, DC, 238–242.

Bransford, J.D.E., Brown, A.L.E., & Cocking, R.R.E. (1999). *How People Learn: Brain, Mind, Experience, and School*. Washington, DC: National Academies Press.

Brazma, A, Hingamp, P, Quackenbush, J, et. al. (2001). Minimum information about a microarray experiment (MIAME): Toward standards for microarray data. *Nat Genet*. 29(4):365–71.

Brennan, P.F. (1996). The future of clinical communication in an electronic environment. *Holistic Nursing Practice*, 11(1):97–104.

Brennan, P.F. (1998). Computer network home care demonstration: A randomized trial in persons living with AIDS. *Computers in Biology and Medicine,* 28(5):489–508.

Brennan, P.F., Moore, S.M., Bjornsdottir, G., Jones, J., Visovsky, C., Rogers, M. (2001). HeartCare: an Internet-based information and support system for patient home recovery after coronary artery bypass graft (CABG) surgery. *Journal of Advanced Nursing.* 35(5):699–708.

Brennan, P.F., Moore, S.M., Smyth, K.A. (1995). The effects of a special computer network on caregivers of persons with Alzheimer's Disease. *Nursing Research,* 44(3):166–172.

Brennan, P.F., Ripich, S. (1994). Use of a home care computer network by persons with AIDS. *International Journal of Technology Assessment in Health Care,* 10(2):258–272.

Brennan, P., Strombom, I. (1998). Improving health care by understanding patient preferences: The role of computer technology. *Journal of the American Medical Informatics Association,* 5:257–262.

Brenner, S. McKinin, E. (1989). CINAHL and MEDLINE: a comparison of indexing practices. *Bulletin of the Medical Library Association,* 77:366–371.

Brin, S., Page, L. (1998). The anatomy of a large-scale hypertextual Web search engine. *Computer Networks,* 30:107–117.

Brigham, C.R., Kamp, M. (1974). The current status of computer-assisted instruction in the health sciences. *Journal of Medical Education,* 49(3):278–279.

Brimm, J. (1987). Computers in critical care. *Critical Care Nursing Quarterly,* 9(4):53.

Brin, S. and Page, L. (1998). The anatomy of a large-scale hypertextual Web search engine. *Computer Networks,* 30:107–117.

Brinkley, J. F. (1985). Knowledge-driven ultrasonic three-dimensional organ modelling. *PAMI,* 7(4):431–441.

Brinkley, J.F. (1991). Structural informatics and its applications in medicine and biology. *Academic Medicine,* 66:589–591.

Brinkley, J. F. (1992). Hierarchical geometric constraint networks as a representation for spatial structural knowledge (UW, Trans.), *Proceedings of the 16th Annual Symposium on Computer Applications in Medical Care,* pp. 140–144.

Brinkley, J. F. (1993a). A flexible, generic model for anatomic shape: Application to interactive two-dimensional medical image segmentation and matching. *Computers and Biomedical Research, 26,* 121–142.

Brinkley, J.F. (1993b). The potential for three-dimensional ultrasound. In Chervenak F.A., Isaacson G.C., Campbell S. (eds.), *Ultrasound in Obstetrics and Gynecology.* Boston: Little, Brown and Company.

Brinkley, J. F., Bradley, S. W., Sundsten, J. W., & Rosse, C. (1997). The Digital Anatomist information system and its use in the generation and delivery of Web-based anatomy atlases. *Computers and Biomedical Research,* 30:472–503.

Brinkley, J.F., Moritz, W.E., Baker, D.W. (1978). Ultrasonic three-dimensional imaging and volume from a series of arbitrary sector scans. *Ultrasound in Medicine and Biology,* 4:317–327.

Brinkley, J.F., Myers, L.M., Prothero, J.S., Heil, G.H., Tsuruda, J.S., Maravilla, K.R., Ojemann, G.A., Rosse, C. (1997). A structural information framework for brain mapping. In Koslow S.H., Huerta M.F. (eds.), *Neuroinformatics: An Overview of the Human Brain Project,* pp.309–334. Mahwah, NJ: Lawrence Erlbaum.

Brinkley, J.F., Rosse, C. (1997). The Digital Anatomist distributed framework and its applications to knowledge based medical imaging. *Journal of the American Medical Informatics Association,* 4(3):165–183.

Brinkley, J. F., Rosse, C. (2002). Imaging and the Human Brain Project: a review. *Methods of Information in Medicine,* 41:245–260.

Brinkley, J. F., Wong, B. A., Hinshaw, K. P., & Rosse, C. (1999). Design of an anatomy information system. *Computer Graphics and Applications,* 19(3):38–48.

Brody, B.A. (1989). The ethics of using ICU scoring systems in individual patient management. *Problems in Critical Care*, 3:662–670.

Brown, C.L., Howarth, S.P. (2004). The power of picture archiving and communication systems: Strategic hospital considerations. *J Health Inf Manag*. 18(4):19–26.

Brown, SH, Lincoln, MJ, Groen, PJ, Kolodner, RM. (2003). VistA–U.S. Department of Veterans Affairs national-scale HIS. *Int J Med Inf*. 69(2-3):135–56.

Bruer, J. T. (1993). *Schools for Thought: A Science of Learning in the Classroom*. Cambridge, MA: MIT Press.

Bryant, G.D., Norman, G.R. (1980). Expressions of probability: Words and numbers. *The New England Journal of Medicine*, 302:411.

Buchman, T.G. (1995). Computers in the intensive care unit: Promises yet to be fulfilled. *Journal of Intensive Care Medicine*, 10:234–240.

Bulecheck, G.M., McCloskey, J.C., Donahue, W.J. (1995). Nursing Interventions Classification (NIC): A language to describe nursing treatments, *Nursing Data Systems: The Emerging Framework,* pp.115-131. Washington, D.C.: American Nurses Publishing.

Burley, S.K., Bonanno, J.B. (2002). Structuring the universe of proteins. *Annual Review of Genomics and Human Genetics*. 3:243–62.

Byrne, MD. (2003). Cognitive architecture. In J. Jacko & A. Sears (Eds), *Human-Computer Interaction Handbook* (pp. 97–117). Mahwah, N.J.: Lawrence Erlbaum Associates.

California Managed Health Care Improvement Task Force (1998). Public perceptions and experiences with managed care, *Improving Managed Health Care in California*. (Vol. 2:13– 42 & Vol. 3:207–212), Sacramento, CA.

California Office of Statewide Health Planning and Development (1992). *Volume of Coronary Artery Bypass Grafts for 1989–1992 from the Patient Discharge Data Set*.

Callan, J. (1994). Passage level evidence in document retrieval. *Proceedings of the 17th Annual International ACM SIGIR Conference on Research and Development in Information Retrieval*, Dublin, Ireland: Springer-Verlag, pp. 302–310.

Campbell, J.R., Carpenter, P., Sneiderman, C., Cohn, S., Chute, C.G., Warren, J. (1997). Phase II evaluation of clinical coding schemes: Completeness, taxonomy, mapping, definitions, and clarity. CPRI Work Group on Codes and Structures. *Journal of the American Medical Informatics Association*, 4(3):238–251.

Campbell, K.E., Tuttle, M.S., Spackman, K.A. (1998). A "lexically-suggested logical closure" metric for medical terminology maturity. *Proceedings of the 1998 AMIA Annual Fall Symposium*, Orlando, FL, pp. 785–789.

Capin, T.K., Noser, H., Thalmann, D., Pandzic, I.S., Thalmann, N.M. (1997). Virtual human representation and communication in VLNet. *IEEE Computer Graphics and Applications*, 17(2):42–53.

Card, S. K., Mackinlay, J. D., Shneiderman, B. (1999). *Readings in Information Visualization: Using Vision to Think*. San Francisco, Calif.: Morgan Kaufmann Publishers.

Card, S. K., Moran, T. P., & Newell, A. (1983). *The Psychology of Human-Computer Interaction*. Hillsdale, N.J.: L. Erlbaum Associates.

Carroll, J. M. (1997). Human-computer interaction: Psychology as a science of design. *Annual Review of Psychology,* 48(1):61–83.

Carroll, J. M. (ed.) (2002). *Human-Computer Interaction in the New Millenium*. New York: Addison-Wesley.

Carroll, J. M. (2003). *HCI Models, Theories, and Frameworks: Toward a Multidisciplinary Science*. San Francisco, Calif.: Morgan Kaufmann.

Caruso, D. (2000). Digital Commerce; If the AOL-Time Warner deal is about proprietary content, where does that leave a noncommercial directory it will own? *New York Times*. January 17, 2000.

Caviness, V. S., Meyer, J., Makris, N., & Kennedy, D. N. (1996). MRI-based topographic parcellation of human neocortex: an anatomically specified method with estimate of reliability. *Journal of Cognitive Neuroscience,* 8(6):566–587.

Cawley, J., Chernew, M., McLaughlin, C. (2002). CMS payments necessary to support HMO participation in Medicare Managed Care. In Alan M. Garber, ed., *Frontiers in Health Policy Research,* Volume 5, pp1–25. Cambridge, MA: MIT Press,.

Cech, TR. (2000) Structural Biology. The ribosome is a ribozyme. *Science* 289(5481):878–879.

Centers for Disease Control and Prevention (1997). *Community Immunization Registries Manual.* (Accessed 2005 at: http://www.cdc.gov/nip/registry/cir-manual.htm)

Centers for Disease Control and Prevention (2002). Immunization Registry Progress —United States, 2002. *Morbidity and Mortality Weekly Report.* August 30, 2002 / 51(34):760–762.

Centers for Disease Control and Prevention (2003). *Public Health Information Network Conference.*

Centers for Medicare & Medicaid Services (1999). *Medicare Current Beneficiary Survey.*

CFO (1996). The Third Annual Survey: Holding the Line on SG&A. *CFO,* December 1996:28–36.

Chalmers, I., Altman D. (eds.) (1995). *Systematic Reviews.* London: BMJ Publishing Group.

Chandler, P., & Sweller, J. (1991). Cognitive load theory and the format of instruction. *Cognition and Instruction,* 8(4):293–332.

Chandra, M., Wagner, W.H., Shabot, M.M. (1995). ICU care after infrainguinal arterial surgery: A critical analysis of outcomes. *The American Surgeon,* 61(10):904–907.

Channin, D.S. (2002). Integrating the healthcare enterprise: a primer. Part 6: the fellowship of IHE. *Radiographics,* 22(6):1555–60.

Chapman, K.A., Moulton, A.D. (1995). The Georgia Information Network for Public Health Officials: A demonstration of the CDC INPHO concept. *Journal of Public Health Management & Practice,* 1(2):39–43.

Charen, T. (1976). *MEDLARS Indexing Manual, Part I: Bibliographic Principles and Descriptive Indexing.* Springfield, VA: National Technical Information Service.

Charen, T. (1983). *MEDLARS Indexing Manual, Part II.* Springfield, VA: National Technical Information Service.

Charniak, E. (1993). Statistical Language Learning. Cambridge: MIT Press.

Chase, W. G., Simon, H. A. (1973). Perception in chess. *Cognitive Psychology,* 4(1):55–81.

Chen, R., Felciano, R., Altman, R.B. (1997). RIBOWEB: Linking structural computations to a knowledge base of published experimental data. *Intelligent Systems for Molecular Biology,* 5:84–87.

Cheung, N.T., Fung, K.W., Wong, K.C., Cheung, A., Cheung, J., Ho, W., Cheung, C., Shung, E., Fung, V., Fung, H. (2001). Medical informatics – the state of the art in the Hospital Authority. *Int J Med Inf.* 62:113–119.

Chi, M.T.H., Feltovich, P.J., Glaser, R. (1981). Categorization and representation of physics problems by experts and novices. *Cognitive Science,* 5:121–152.

Chi, M.T.H., Glaser, R. (1981). Categorization and representation of physics problems by experts and novices. *Cognitive Science,* 5:121–152.

Chi, M.T.H., Glaser, R., Farr, M.J. (1988). *The Nature of Expertise.* Hillsdale, N.J.: L. Erlbaum Associates.

Chin, T (2003). February 17, 2003. *American Medical News.*

Chinchor, N.A. (1998). Overview of MUC-7/MET-2. Proceedings of the 7th Message Understanding Conference, April 1998.

Choi, H.S., Haynor, D.R., & Kim, Y. (1991). Partial volume tissue classification of multichannel magnetic resonance images -a mixel model. *IEEE Trans. Med. Imaging,* 10(3):395–407.

Christensen, L., Haug, P., Fiszman, P. (2002). MPLUS: A probabilistic medical language understanding system. *Natural Language Processing in the Biomedical Domain.* Association for Computational Linguistics.

Christensen, G.E., Miller, M.I., Vannier, M.W. (1996). Individualizing neuroanatomical atlases using a massively parallel computer. *IEEE Computer*, 29(1):32–38.

Christensen, G. E., Rabbitt, R. D., & Miller, M. I. (1996). Deformable templates using large deformation kinematics. *IEEE Trans. Image Processing*, 5(10):1435–1447.

Chu, S., Cesnik, B. (2000). A three-tier clinical information systems design model. *Int J Med Inform*. 57(2-3):91–107.

Chuang, J.H., Friedman, C., Hripcsak, G. (2002). A comparison of the Charlson comorbidities derived from medical language processing and administrative data. *Proc AMIA Fall Symp*, pp. 160–164.

Chueh, H.C., Barnett, G.O. (1997) "Just In Time" Clinical Information. *Academic Medicine*, 72(6):512–517

Chute, C.G. (2000). Clinical classification and terminology: Some history and current observations. *J Am Med Inform Assoc*. 7(3):298–303.

Chute, C.G., Cohn, S.P., Campbell, K.E., Oliver, D.E., Campbell, J.R. (1996). The content coverage of clinical classifications. *Journal of the American Medical Informatics Association*, 3:224–233.

Cimino, J. (1996). Linking patient information systems to bibliographic resources. *Methods of Information in Medicine*, 35:122–126.

Cimino, J.J. (1998). Desiderata for controlled medical vocabularies in the twenty-first century. *Methods Inf Med*. 37(4-5):394–403.

Cimino, J.J., Elhanan, G., Zeng, Q. (1997). Supporting infobuttons with terminological knowledge. *Proc AMIA Annual Fall Symp*, pp. 528–532.

Cimino, J.J., Huang, X., Patel, V., Sengupta, S., Kushniruk, A. (1998). PatCIS: Support for informed patient decision-making. *Proceeding of the AMIA Fall Symposium*, p. 47.

Cimino, J.J., Johnson, S.B., Aguirre, A., Roderer, N., Clayton, P.D. (1992). The MEDLINE button. *Proceedings of the 16th Annual Symposium on Computer Applications in Medical Care*, Baltimore, MD, pp. 81–85.

Cimino, J.J., Li, J.,Bakken, S., Patel, V (2002). Theoretical, empirical, and practical approaches to resolving the unmet information needs of clinical information systems users. *Proceedings of the AMIA Symposium*, pp.170– 4.

Cimino, J.J., Li, J., Mendonca, E.A., Sengupta, S., Patel, V.L., Kushniruk, A.W. (2000). An evaluation of patient access to their electronic medical records via the World Wide Web. *Proc AMIA Fall Symp*, pp. 151–155.

Cimino, J.J., Li, J., Graham, M., Currie, L.M., Allen, M., Bakken, S., Patel, V.L., (2003). Use of online resources while using a clinical information system. *Proceedings AMIA Annu Sym* pp. 175–179.

Cimino, J.J., Patel, V.L., Kushniruk, A.W. (2002). The patient clinical information system (PatCIS): Technical solutions for and experience with giving patients access to their electronic medical records. *Int J Med Inf*. 18;68(1-3):113–27.

Clancey, W.J. (1984). The epistemology of a rule-based expert system: A framework for explanation. *Artificial Intelligence*, 20:215–251.

Clancey, W. J. (1986). From GUIDON to NEOMYCIN and HERACLES in twenty short lessons: ORN final report 1979-1985. *AI Magazine*, 7(3):40–60.

Clancey W.J. (1989). Viewing knowledge bases as qualitative models. *IEEE Expert*, 4(2):9–23.

Clancey, W.J., Shortliffe, E.H. (1984). *Readings in Medical Artificial Intelligence: The First Decade*. Reading, Mass: Addison-Wesley.

Clark, J., Lang, N.M. (1992). Nursing's next advance: An international classification for nursing practice. *International Nursing Review*, 39(4):109–112.

Clarysse, P., Friboulet, D., Magnin, I.E. (1997). Tracking geometrical descriptors on 3-D deformable surfaces: application to the left-ventricular surface of the heart. *IEEE Transactions on Medical Imaging*, 16(4):392– 404.

Classen, D.C., Pestotnik, S.L., Evans, R.S., Lloyd, J.F., Burke, J.P. (1997). Adverse drug events in hospitalized patients. Excess length of stay, extra costs, and attributable mortality. *Journal of the American Medical Association*, 277(4):301–306.

Clemmer, T.P., Spuhler, V.J., Oniki, T.A., Horn, S.D. (1999) Results of a collaborative quality improvement program on outcomes and costs in a tertiary critical care unit. *Crit Care Med*, 27(9):1768–1774.

Coenen, A., McNeil, B., Bakken, S., Bickford, C., Warren, J.J. and the American Nurses Association Committee on Nursing Practice Information Infrastructure (2001). Toward comparable nursing data: American Nurses Association criteria for data sets, classification systems, and nomenclatures. *Comput Nurs,* 19(6):240–6.

Cohen, J.D. (2001). *FisWidgets*. University of Pittsburgh. (Accessed 2005 at: http://neurocog. lrdc.pitt.edu/fiswidgets/)

Cohen, P.R. (1995). *Empirical Methods for Artificial Intelligence*. Cambridge, MA: MIT Press.

Cole, M., Engestroem, Y. (1997). A cultural-historical approach to distributed cognition. In G. Salomon (ed.), *Distributed Cognitions: Psychological and Educational Considerations (Learning in Doing: Social, Cognitive, and Computational Perspectives)*, pp. 1– 46. Cambridge University Press.

Cole, W.G., Stewart, J.G. (1994). Human performance evaluation of a metaphor graphic display for respiratory data. *Methods of Information in Medicine,* 33:390–396.

College of American Pathologists (1971). *Systematized Nomenclature of Pathology*. Chicago: The College of American Pathologists.

Collen, M.F. (1983). The functions of an HIS: An overview. *Proceedings of MEDINFO 83*, Amsterdam: North Holland, pp. 61–64.

Collen, M.F. (1995). *A History of Medical Informatics in the United States: 1950 to 1990*. Bethesda, MD: American Medical Informatics Association, Hartman Publishing.

Coletti, M., Bleich, H. (2001). Medical subject headings used to search the biomedical literature. *Journal of the American Medical Informatics Association*, 8:317–323.

Collins, D.L., Holmes, D J., Peters, T.M., & Evans, A.C. (1995). Automatic 3-D model-based neuroanatomical segmentation. *Hum Brain Mapp,* 3:190–208.

Collins, D.L., Neelin, P., Peters, T.M., Evans, A.C. (1994). Automatic 3-D intersubject registration of MR volumetric data in standardized Talairach space. *Journal of Computer Assisted Tomography*, 18(2):192–205.

Commission on Professional and Hospital Activities (1978). *International Classification of Diseases, Ninth Revision, with Clinical Modifications (ICD-9-CM)*. Ann Arbor: American Hospital Association.

Committee on Quality of Health Care in America, Institute of Medicine (2001). *Crossing the Quality Chasm: A New Health System for the 21st Century*, Washington, DC: National Academies Press.

Committee on Ways and Means (1997). *Medicare and Health Care Chartbook*. U.S. House of Representatives.

Congressional Budget Office (1996). *Reducing the Deficit: Spending and Revenue Options*. Washington, D.C.: U.S. Government Printing Office.

Congressional Budget Office, *Budget Options*, February 2001.

Conley, D.M., Sundsten, J.W., Ratiu, P., Rauschning, W., Rosse, C. (1995). The Digital Anatomist series: 3-D, segmented, dynamic atlases of body regions. *Proceedings of the 19th Symposium on Computer Applications in Medical Care*, New Orleans, p. 1016.

Connolly, D. (ed.) (1997). *XML: Principles, Tools, and Techniques*. Cambridge, MA: O'Reilly & Associates.

Cooke, J.T., Barie, P.S. (1998). Information management and decision support systems in the intensive care unit. *Surgical Technology International*, VI.

Corina, D.P., Poliakov, A.V., Steury, K., Martin, R.F., Brinkley, J.F., Mulligan, K.A., Ojemann, G.A. (2000). Correspondences between language cortex identified by cortical stimulation mapping and fMRI. *Neuroimage (Human Brain Mapping Annual Meeting, June 12-16)*, 11(5), S295.

Côté, R.A., Robboy, S. (1980). Progress in medical information management: Systematized nomenclature of medicine (SNOMED). *Journal of the American Medical Association*, 243:756.

Côté, R.A., Rothwell, D.J. (1993). *The Systematised Nomenclature of Human and Veterinary Medicine*. Northfield, IL: College of American Pathologists.

Côté, R.A., Rothwell, D.J., Palotay, J.L., Beckett, R.S., Brochu, L. (eds.) (1993). *The Systematized Nomenclature of Medicine: SNOMED International*. Northfield, IL: College of American Pathologists.

Council, N.R. (1997). *Assessment of Performance Measures for Public Health, Substance Abuse, and Mental Health*. Washington, DC: National Academy Press.

Covell, D.G., Uman, G.C., Manning, P.R. (1985). Information needs in office practice: are they being met? *Annals of Internal Medicine*, 103(4):596–599.

Covitz, P.A., Hartel, F., Schaefer, C., De Coronado, S., Fragoso, G., Sahni, H., Gustafson, S., Buetow, K.H. (2003). caCORE: A common infrastructure for cancer informatics. *Bioinformatics*. 19(18):2404–12.

Cox Jr., J. (1972). Digital analysis of the electroencephalogram, the blood pressure wave, and the electrocardiogram. *Proceedings of the IEEE*, 60:1137.

Cox, R.W. (1996). AFNI: Software for analysis and visualization of functional magnetic resonance neuroimages. *Computers and Biomedical Research, 29*, 162–173.

CPR Systems Evaluation Work Group (1994). *Draft CPR Project Evaluation Criteria.*: (Available from the Computer-based Patient Record Institute, 919 N. Michigan Ave., Chicago, IL 60611).

Crocco, A., Villasis-Keever, M., et al. (2002). Analysis of cases of harm associated with use of health information on the internet. *Journal of the American Medical Association*, 287:2869–2871.

Crowley, R.S., Naus, G.J., Stewart, J., Friedman, C. P. (2003). Development of visual diagnostic expertise in pathology – an information-processing study. *Journal of the American Medical Informatics Association,* 10(1):39–51.

Cunneen, S.A., Shabot, M.M., Wagner, W.H. (1998). Outcomes from abdominal aortic aneurysm resection: Does SICU length of stay make a difference? *American Surgeon*, 64(2):196–199.

Curran, W.J., Stearns, B., Kaplan, H. (1969). Privacy, confidentiality, and other legal considerations in the establishment of a centralized health-data system. *New England Journal of Medicine*, 281(5):241–248.

Cushing, H. (1903). On routine determination of arterial tension in operating room and clinic. *Boston Medical Surgical Journal*, 148:250.

Dacey, D. (1999). Primate retina: cell types, circuits and color opponency. *Prog Retin Eye Res,* 18(6):737–763.

Dager, S.R., Steen, R.G. (1992). Applications of magnetic resonance spectroscopy to the investigation of neuropsychiatric disorders. *Neuropsychopharmacology*, 6(4):249–266.

Dale, A.M., Fischl, B., Sereno, M.I. (1999). Cortical surface-based analysis. I. Segmentation and surface reconstruction. *Neuroimage, 9*(2):179–194.

Dalto, J.D., Johnson, K.V., Gardner, R.M., Spuhler, V.J., Egbert, L. (1997). Medical Information Bus usage for automated IV pump data acquisition: evaluation of usage patterns. *International Journal of Clinical Monitoring and Computing*, 14(3):151–154.

Dansky, K.H., Palmer, L., Shea, D., & Bowles, K.H. (2001). Cost analysis of telehomecare. *Telemed J E Health,* 7(3):225–232.

Darmoni, S., Leroy, J., et al. (2000). CISMeF: a structured health resource guide. *Methods of Information in Medicine*, 9:30–35.

Davatzikos, C. (1997). Spatial transformation and registration of brain images using elastically deformable models. *Computer Vision and Image Understanding,* 66(2):207–222.

Davatzikos, C., Bryan, R.N. (1996). Using a deformable surface model to obtain a shape representation of the cortex. *IEEE Trans. Medical Imaging,* 15(6):785–795.

David, J.M., Krivine, J.P., Simmons, R. (eds.) (1993). *Second Generation Expert Systems.* Berlin: Springer-Verlag.

Davis, R., Buchanan, B.G., Shortliffe, E.H. (1977). Production rules as a representation for a knowledge-based consultation program. *Artificial Intelligence,* 8:15–45.

Davis, W.S. (1994). *Business Systems Design and Analysis.* Belmont, CA: Wadsworth Publishing.

Day, H. (1963). An intensive coronary care area. *Diseases of the Chest,* 44:423.

Dayhoff, M.O. (1974). Computer analysis of protein sequences. *Federal Proceedings,* 33(12):2314–2316.

Dayhoff, M.O., Barker ,W.C., McLaughlin, P.J. (1974). Inferences from protein and nucleic acid sequences: Early molecular evolution, divergence of kingdoms and rates of change. *Origins of Life,* 5(3):311–330.

DeBakcy, M. (1991). The National Library of Medicine: Evolution of a premier information center. *Journal of the American Medical Association,* 266:1252–1258.

de Bliek, R., Friedman, C.P., Blaschke, T.F., France, C.L., Speedie, S.M. (1988). Practitioner preferences and receptivity for patient-specific advice from a therapeutic monitoring system. *Proceedings of the 12th Annual Symposium on Computer Applications in Medical Care,* Washington, DC, pp. 225–228.

de Dombal, F.T. (1987). Ethical considerations concerning computers in medicine in the 1980s. *Journal of Medical Ethics,* 13(4):179–84.

de Dombal, F.T., Leaper, D.J., Staniland, J.R., McCann, A.P., Horrocks, J.C. (1972). Computer-aided diagnosis of acute abdominal pain. *British Medical Journal,* 1:376–380.

Dean, A.G., Dean, J.A., Burton, A.H., Dicker, R.C. (1991). EpiInfo: a general purpose microcomputer program for public health information systems. *American Journal of Preventitive Medicine,* 7(3):178–182.

Degoulet, P., Phister, B., Fieschi, M. (1997). *Introduction to Clinical Informatics.* New York: Springer-Verlag.

deGroot, A.D. (1965). *Thought and Choice in Chess.* The Hague: Mouton.

Deibel, S.R., Greenes, R.A. (1995). An infrastructure for the development of health care information systems from distributed components. *Journal of the American Society for Information Science,* 26:765–771.

Deibel, S.R., Greenes, R.A. (1996). Radiology systems architectures. In Greenes, R.A. & Bauman, R.A. (eds.) Imaging and information management: computer systems for a changing health care environment. *The Radiology Clinics of North America,* 34(3):681–696.

Department of Health and Human Services (1994). Essential Public Health Functions. *Public Health in America.* (Accessed 2005 at: http://www.health.gov/phfunctions/public.htm)

Department of Health and Human Services (2000). Immunization and Infectious Diseases. *Healthly People 2010 – Conference Edition,* Objective 14-26: Immunization Registries. (Accessed 2005 at: http://www.cdc.gov/nip/registry/hp2010.htm)

Department of Health and Human Services (2003). *Building the National Health Information Infrastructure.* (Accessed 2005 at: http://aspe.hhs.gov/sp/nhii/)

DeQuardo, J.R., Keshavan, M.S., Bookstein, F.L., Bagwell, W.W., Green, W.D.K., Sweeney, J.A., Haas, G.L., Tandon, R., Schooler, N.R., Pettegrew, J.W. (1999). Landmark-based morphometric analysis of first-episode schizophrenia. *Biological Psychiatry,* 45(10):1321–1328.

Detmer,, W.M., Barnett, G.O., Hersh, W.R. (1997). MedWeaver: integrating decision support, literature searching, and Web exploration using the UMLS Metathesaurus. *Proceedings of the 1997 AMIA Annual Fall Symposium,* Nashville, TN, pp. 490–494.

Detmer, W.M., Friedman, C.P. (1994). Academic physicians' assessment of the effects of computers on health care. *Proceedings of the 18th Annual Symposium on Computer Applications in Medical Care*, Washington, D.C., pp. 558–562.

Detmer, W.M., Shortliffe, E.H. (1995). A model of clinical query management that supports integration of biomedical information over the World Wide Web. *Proceedings of the 19th Annual Symposium on Computer Applications in Medical Care*, New Orleans, LA, pp. 898–902.

Detmer, W.M., Shortliffe, E.H. (1997). Using the Internet to improve knowledge diffusion in medicine. *Communications of the ACM*, 40:101–108.

Dev, P., Pichumani, R., Walker, D., Heinrichs, W.L., Karadi, C., Lorie, W. (1998). Formative design of a virtual learning environment, *Medicine Meets Virtual Reality*, p. 6. Amsterdam: IOS Press.

Dexter, P.R., Perkins, S., Overhage, J.M., Maharry, K., Kohler, R.B., McDonald, C.J.(2001). A computerized reminder system to increase the use of preventive care for hospitalized patients. *N Engl J Med*, 345(13): 965–970.

Dhenain, M., Ruffins, S.W., Jacobs, R.E. (2001). Three-dimensional digital mouse atlas using high-resolution MRI. *Dev. Biol.,* 232(2):458– 470.

Diabetes Control and Complications Trial Research Group (1996). Lifetime benefits and costs of intensive therapy as practiced in the diabetes control and complications trial. *JAMA*, 276(17):1409–15.

Dick, R., Steen, E. (eds.) (1991 (Revised 1997)). *The Computer-Based Patient Record: An Essential Technology for Health Care*. Washington, D.C.: Institute of Medicine, National Academy Press.

Dohi, T., Kikinis, R. (Eds.) (2002). *Proceedings of Medical Image Computing and Computer-Assisted Intervention - MICCAI 2002*, 5th International Conference, Tokyo, Japan, September 25-28, Parts I and II.

Dolin, R., Alschuler, L., et al. (2001). The HL7 Clinical Document Architecture. *Journal of the American Medical Informatics Association*, 8:552–569.

Donabedian, A. (1996). Evaluating the quality of medical care. *Millbank Memorial Quarterly*, 44:166–206.

Doolan, D.F., Bates, D.W., James, B.C. (2003). The use of computers for clinical care: A case series of advanced U.S. sites. *Journal of the American Medical Informatics Association*, 10(1), 94 –107.

Dowell, R.D., Jokerst, R.M., Day, A., Eddy, S.R., Stein, L. (2001). The distributed annotation system. *BMC Bioinformatics.* 2(1):7.

D'Orsi, C.J., Kopans, D.B. (1997). Mammography interpretation: the BI-RADS method. *American Family Physician*, 55(5):1548–1550.

Downs, S.M., Carroll, A.E., Anand, V., Biondich, P.G. (2005). Human and system errors: Using adaptive turnaround documents to capture data in a busy practice. *Proceedings AMIA Annu Symp*. pp. 211–215.

Drazen, E., Metzger, J. (1999). *Strategies for Integrated Health Care: Emerging Practices in Information Management and Cross-Continuum Care*. San Francisco: Jossey-Bass Publishers.

Dhenain, M., Ruffins, S.W., Jacobs, R.E. (2001). Three-dimensional digital mouse atlas using high-resolution MRI. *Dev. Biol.,* 232(2), 458– 470.

Drury, H.A., Van Essen, D.C. (1997). Analysis of functional specialization in human cerebral cortex using the visible man surface based atlas. *Hum Brain Mapp,* 5:233–237.

Duda, R.O., Shortliffe, E.H. (1983). Expert systems research. *Science*, 220(4594):261–268.

Duncan, R.G., Saperia, D., Dulbandzhyan, R., Shabot, M.M., Polaschek, J.X., Jones, D.T. (2001). Integrated web-based viewing and secure remote access to a clinical data repository and diverse clinical systems. *Proc AMIA Fall Symp*, pp. 149–53.

Durbin, R.., Eddy, R., Krogh, A., Mitchison, G. (1998). *Biological Sequence Analysis: Probabilistic Models of Proteins and Nucleic Acids.* Cambridge, UK: Cambridge University Press.

Durfy, S.J. (1993). Ethics and the Human Genome Project. *Archives of Pathology and Laboratory Medicine*, 117(5):466– 469.

Dwyer, S.J. (1996). Imaging system architectures for picture archiving and communication systems. In Greenes, R.A. & Bauman, R.A. (eds.) Imaging and information management: computer systems for a changing health care environment. *The Radiology Clinics of North America*, 34(3):495–503.

East, T.D., Bohm, S.H., Wallace, C.J., Clemmer, T.P., Weaver, L.K., Orme Jr., J.F., Morris, A.H. (1992). A successful computerized protocol for clinical management of pressure control inverse ration ventilation. *Chest*, 101(3):697–710.

Eddy, D.M. (1992). *A Manual for Assessing Health Practices and Designing Practice Policies: The Explicit Approach.* Philadelphia: American College of Physicians.

Editorial (1997). Electronic threats to medical privacy. *The New York Times*: March 11, 1997, A14.

Egan, D., Remde, J., Gomez, L., Landauer, T., Eberhardt, J., Lochbaum, C. (1989). Formative design-evaluation of Superbook. *ACM Transactions on Information Systems*, 7:30–57.

Eisner, E.W. (1991). *The Enlightened Eye: Qualitative Inquiry and the Enhancement of Educational Practice.* New York: McMillan Publishing Co.

Eliot, C.R., Williams, K.A., Woolf, B.P. (1996). An intelligent learning enviornment for advanced cardiac life support. *Proceedings of the AMIA Annual Fall Symposium*, Washington, DC, pp. 7–11.

Elkin, P L., Sorensen, B., De Palo, D., Poland, G., Bailey, K.R., Wood, D.L., et al. (2002). Optimization of a research Web environment for academic internal medicine faculty. *J Am Med Inform Assoc,* 9(5):472– 478.

Ellwood Jr., P.M., Anderson, N.N., Billings, J.E., Carlson, R.J., Hoagberg, E.J., McClure, W. (1971). Health maintenance strategy. *Medical Care*, 9(3):291–298.

Ellwood, P.M. (1988). Shattuck lecture—Outcomes management: A technology of patient experience. *New England Journal of Medicine*, 318(23):1549–1556.

Elstein A.S., Shulman L.S., Sprafka S.A. (1978). *Medical Problem Solving: An Analysis of Clinical Reasoning.* Cambridge, MA: Harvard University Press.

Elting, L., Martin, C., Cantor, S.B., & Rubenstein, E.B. (1999). Influence of data display on physician investigators' decisions to stop trials: Prospective trial with repeated measures. *British Medical Journal,* 317:1527–1531.

Ely, J., Osheroff, J., et al. (1999). Analysis of questions asked by family doctors regarding patient care. *British Medical Journal*, 319:358–361.

Ely, J., Osheroff, J., et al. (2002). Obstacles to answering doctors' questions about patient care with evidence: Qualitative study. *British Medical Journal*, 324:710–713.

Employee Benefit Research Institute (EBRI) (1995). *Sources of Health Insurance and Characteristics of the Uninsured: Analysis of the March 1994 Current Population Survey.*

Employer Health Benefits (2002). *Annual Survey*, Menlo Park, CA and Chicago, IL: Henry J. Kaiser Family Foundation and Health Research and Educational Trust.

Enthoven, A.C. (1993). The history and priciples of managed competition. *Health Affairs*, 12(Supplement):24– 48.

Enthoven, A.C. (1997). Market based reform of US health care financing and delivery: Managed care and managed competition. *Innovations in Health Care Financing: Proceedings of a World Bank Conference*, March 10–11, pp. 195–214, .

Enthoven, A.C. (2003). Employment-based health insurance is failing: Now what? *Health Affairs*, W3:237-249, 28 May.

Enthoven A.C., Singer S.J. (1997). *Reforming medicare before it's too late.* (Research Paper Series, No. 1411): Stanford University Graduate School of Business.

Ericsson, K.A (ed.) (1996). *The Road to Excellence: The Acquisition of Expert Performance in the Arts and Sciences, Sports and Games.* Hillsdale, NJ: Lawrence Erlbaum Publishers.

Ericsson, K. A., Simon, H. A. (1993). *Protocol Analysis: Verbal Reports as Data* (Revised ed.). Cambridge, Mass: MIT Press.

Ericsson, K. A., Smith, J. (1991). *Toward a General Theory of Expertise: Prospects and Limits.* New York: Cambridge University Press.

Eriksson, H., Musen, M.A. (1993). Metatools for knowledge acquisition. *IEEE Software*, 10(3):23–29.

Eriksson H., Puerta A.R., Musen M.A. (1994). Generation of knowledge-acquisition tools from domain ontologies. *International Journal of Human-Computer Studies*, 41:425– 453.

Eriksson, H., Shahar, Y., Tu, S.W., Puerta, A.R., Musen, M.A. (1995). Task modeling with reusable problem-solving methods. *Artificial Intelligence*, 79(2):293–326.

Estes, W.K. (1975). *Handbook of Learning and Cognitive Processes.* Hillsdale, N.J.: L. Erlbaum Associates.

EUCLIDES Foundation International (1994). *EUCLIDES Coding System Version 4.0*: The EUCLIDES Foundation.

Evans, D.A., Cimino, J.J., Hersh, W., Huff, S.M., Bell D.S. (1994). Toward a medical-concept representation language. The Canon Group. *J Am Med Inform Assoc.* 1(3):207–217.

Evans, A.C., Collins, D.L., Neelin, P., MacDonald, D., Kamber, M., Marrett, T.S. (1994). Three-dimensional correlative imaging: applications in human brain mapping. In R.W. Thatcher, M. Hallett, T. Zeffiro, E.R. John, M. Heurta (eds.), *Functional Neuroimaging: Technical Foundations*, pp. 145-162. San Diego: Academic Press.

Evans, D.A., Gadd, C.S. (1989). Managing coherence and context in medical problem-solving discourse. In D. A. Evans & V. L. Patel (eds.), *Cognitive Science in Medicine:* pp. 211–255. Cambridge, Mass: MIT Press.

Evans, D., Patel, V. (eds.) (1989). *Cognitive Science in Medicine: Biomedical Modeling.* Cambridge, Mass: MIT Press.

Evans, R.S., Larson, R.A., Burke, J.P., Gardner, R.M., Meier, F.A., Jacobson, J.A., Conti, M.T., Jacobson, J.T., Hulse, R.K. (1986). Computer surveillance of hospital-acquired infections and antibiotic use. *Journal of the American Medical Association*, 256(8):1007–1011.

Evans, R.S., Pestotnik, S.L., Classen, D.C., Burke, J.P. (1999). Evaluation of a computer-assisted antibiotic-dose monitor. *Ann Pharmacother.* 33(10):1026–1031.

Evans, R.S., Pestotnik, S.L., Classen, D.C., Clemmer, T.P., Weaver, L.K., Orme Jr., J.F., Lloyd, J.F., Burke, J.P. (1998). A computer-assisted management program for antibiotics and other antiinfective agents. *New England Journal of Medicine*, 338(4):232–238.

Eysenbach, G., Diepgen, T. (1998). Towards quality management of medical information on the internet: evaluation, labelling, and filtering of information. *British Medical Journal*, 317: 1496–1502.

Eysenbach, G,. Powell, J., Kuss, O., Su, E.R.(2002) Empirical studies assessing the quality of health information for consumers on the world wide web: A systematic review. *JAMA*, 287(20):2691–700.

Eysenbach, G., Su, E., et al. (1999). Shopping around the internet today and tomorrow: Towards the millennium of cybermedicine. *British Medical Journal*, 319:1294–1298.

Fafchamps, D., Young, C.Y., Tang, P.C. (1991). Modelling work practices: Input to the design of a physician's workstation. *Proceedings of the 15th Annual Symposium on Computer Applications in Medical Care*, Washington, D.C., pp. 788–792.

Federative Committee on Anatomical Terminology (1998). *Terminologia Anatomica.* Stuttgart: Thieme.

Feinstein, A.R. (1995). Meta-analysis: Statistical alchemy for the 21st century. *Journal of Clinical Epidemiology*, 48(1):71–79.

Feltovich, P.J., Ford, K.M., Hoffman, R.R. (eds.) (1997). *Expertise in Context.* Cambridge, Mass.: MIT Press.

Feltovich, P.J., Johnson, P.E., Moller, J H., Swanson, D.B. (1984). LCS: The role and development of medical knowledge in diagnostic expertise. In W.J. Clancey & E.H. Shortliffe (eds.),

Readings in Medical Artificial Intelligence: The First Decade, pp. 275–319. Reading, Mass: Addison-Wesley.

Ferguson, T. (2002). From patients to end users: quality of online patient networks needs more attention than quality of online health information. *British Medical Journal*, 324:555–556.

Fiala, J.C., Harris, K.M. (2001). Extending unbiased stereology of brain ultrastructure to three-dimensional volumes. *J Am Med Ass,* 8(1),1–16.

Field M.J. (ed.) (1996). *Telemedicine: A Guide to Assessing Telecommunications in Health Care.* Washington, D.C.: National Academy Press.

Field, M.J., Lohr K.N. (1992). *Clinical Practice Guidelines: Directions for a New Program.* Washington, DC: National Academies Press.

Fielding, N.G., Lee R.M. (1991). *Using Computers in Qualitative Research.* Newbury Park, CA: Sage Publications.

Finkel, A. (ed.) (1977). *CPT4: Physician's Current Procedural Terminology* (4th ed.). Chicago: American Medical Association.

Fischl, B., Sereno, M.I., Dale, A.M. (1999). Cortical surface-based analysis. II: Inflation, flattening, and a surface-based coordinate system. *Neuroimage,* 9(2),195–207.

Flexner, A. (1910). *Medical Education in the United States and Canada: A Report to the Carnegie Foundation for the Advancement of Teaching.* Boston, MA: Merrymount Press.

Flickner, M., Sawhney, H., Niblack, W., Ashley, J., Huang, Q., Dom, B., Gorkani, M., Hafner, J., Lee, D., Petkovic, D., Steele, D., Yanker, P. (1995). Query by image and video content: The QBIC system. *IEEE Computer*, 28(9):23–32.

The FlyBase Consortium (2003). The FlyBase database of the Drosophila genome projects and community literature. *Nucleic Acids Research;*31:172–175.

FMRIDB Image Analysis Group (2001). *FSL -The FMRIB Software Libarary*. (Accessed 2005 at: http://www.fmrib.ox.ac.uk/fsl/index.html)

Foley, J.D. (2001). *Computer Graphics: Principles and Practice.* Reading, Mass.: Addison-Wesley.

Foley, DD., Van Dam, A., Feiner, S.K., Hughes, J.F. (1990). *Computer Graphics: Principles and Practice.* Reading, MA: Addison-Wesley.

Force, U.S.P.S.T. (1996). *Guide to Clinical Preventive Services.* (2nd. ed.). Baltimore: Williams & Williams.

Forrey, A.W., McDonald, C.J., DeMoor, G., Huff, S.M., Leavelle, D., Leland, D., Fiers, T., Charles, L., Griffin, B., Stalling, F., Tullis, A., Hutchins, K., Baenziger, J. (1996). Logical observation identifier names and codes (LOINC) database: A public use set of codes and names for electronic reporting of clinical laboratory test results. *Clinical Chemistry*, 42(1):81–90.

Forsythe, D.E. (1992). Using ethnography to build a working system: Rethinking basic design assumptions. *Proceedings of the 16th Annual Symposium on Computer Applications in Medical Care,* Baltimore, MD, pp. 505–509.

Forsythe, D.E., Buchanan, B.G. (1992). Broadening our approach to evaluating medical information systems. *Proceedings of the 16th Annual Symposium on Computer Applications in Medical Care,* Baltimore, MD, pp. 8–12.

Fougerousse, F., Bullen, P., Herasse, M., Lindsay, S., Richard, I., Wilson, D., Suel, L., Durand, M., Robson, S., Abitbol, M., Beckmann, J. S., & Strachan, T. (2000). Human-mouse differences in the embryonic expression of developmental control genes and disease genes. *Human Molecular Genetics,* 9(2),165–173.

Fox, C. (1992). Lexical analysis and stop lists. In Frakes, W. and Baeza-Yates, R., eds. *Information Retrieval: Data Structures and Algorithms*, pp. 102-130. Englewood Cliffs, NJ: Prentice-Hall.

Fox, E.A., Marchionini, G. (1998). Toward a worldwide digital library. *Communications of the ACM*, 41(4):29–98.

Fox, J., Das, S. (2000). *Safe and Sound: Artificial Intelligence in Hazardous Applications.* Cambridge, MA: AAAI and MIT Press.

Fox, J., Johns, N., Rahmanzadeh, A. (1998). Disseminating medical knowledge: The PROforma approach. *Artificial Intelligence in Medicine*, 14:157–181.

Fox, M. (2001). Seal of approval issued to 13 health web sites. *Reuters*. (Accessed 2005 at: http://www.cancerpage.com/news/article.asp?id=3743)

Fox, P.T. (ed.) (2001). *Human Brain Mapping.* New York: John Wiley & Sons.

Frackowiak, R.S.J., Friston, K.J., Frith, C.D., Dolan, R.J., Mazziotta, J.C. (eds.) (1997). *Human Brain Function.* New York: Academic Press.

Frakes, W. (1992). Stemming algorithms. In Frankes, W. and Baeza-Yates, R., eds. *Information Retrieval: Data Structures and Algorithms*, pp.131-160. Englewood Cliffs, NJ. Prentice-Hall.

Frakes, W.B., Baeza-Yates, R. (1992). *Information Retrieval: Data Structures and Algorithms.* Englewood Cliffs, NJ: Prentice-Hall.

Frank, S.J. (1988). What AI practitioners should know about the law. *AI Magazine*, Part One, 9:63–75 & Part Two, 9109–114.

Franklin, K.B.J., Paxinos, G. (1997). *The Mouse Brain in Stereotactic Coordinates.* San Diego: Academic Press.

Frederiksen, C.H. (1975). Representing logical and semantic structure of knowledge acquired from discourse. *Cognitive Psychology,* 7(3):371– 458.

Freiman, J.A., Chalmers, T.C., Smith, H., Kuebler, R.R. (1978). The importance of beta, the Type II error and sample size in the design and interpretation of the randomized controlled trial. *New England Journal of Medicine*, 299:690–694.

Friede, A., Freedman, M.A., Paul, J.E., Rizzo, N.P., Pawate, V.I., Turczyn, K.M. (1994). DATA2000: A computer system to link HP2000 objectives, data sources, and contacts. *American Journal of Preventive Medicine*, 10:230–234.

Friede A., McDonald M.C., Blum H. (1995). Public health informatics: How information-age technology can strengthen public health. *Annual Review Public Health*, 16:239–252.

Friede, A., O'Carroll, P.W. (1996). CDC and ATSDR Electronic Information Resources for Health Officers. *Journal of Public Health Practice Management*, 2:10–24

Friede, A, O'Carroll, PW (1998). Public health informatics. In Last JM (ed.), *Last Public Health and Preventive Medicine, 14th Edition.* Norwalk, CT: Appleton & Lange, pp. 59-65.

Friede, A., O'Carroll, P.W., Thralls, R.B., Reid, J.A. (1996). CDC WONDER on the Web. *Proceedings of the AMIA Annual Fall Symposium*, Washington, DC, pp. 408– 412.

Friede, A., Rosen, D.H., Reid, J.A. (1994). CDC WONDER: Cooperative processing for public health informatics. *Journal of the American Medical Informatics Association*, 1(4):303–312.

Friedlander, A. (2002). The National Digital Information Infrastructure Preservation Program: Expectations, realities, choices, and progress to date. *D-Lib Magazine*, 8. (Accessed 2005 at: http://www.dlib.org/dlib/april02/friedlander/04friedlander.html)

Friedman, B., Dieterle, M. (1987). The impact of the installation of a local area network on physicians and the laboratory information system in a large teaching hospital. *Proceedings of the 11th Annual Symposium on Computer Applications in Medical Care*, Washington, D.C., pp. 783–788.

Friedman, C. (ed.) (2002). Special Issue: Biomedical Sublanguage. *J Biomed Inf.*:35(4).

Friedman, C., Alderson, P.O., Austin, J., Cimino, J.J., Johnson, S.B. (1994). A general natural language text processor for clinical radiology. *JAMIA,* 1(2):161–174.

Friedman, C.P., Dev, P., Dafoe, B., Murphy, G., Felciano, R. (1993). Initial validation of a test of spatial knowledge in anatomy. *Proceedings of the 17th Annual Symposium of Computer Applications in Medical Care*, Washington, DC, pp. 791–795.

Friedman, C., Hripcsak, G. (1997). Evaluating natural language processors in the clinical domain. In Chute CG, editor, *Proceedings of the Conference on Natural Language and Medical Concept Representation* (IMIA WG6) Jacksonville, Fl, pp. 41–52.

Friedman, C., Hripcsak, G., Johnson, S.B., Cimino, J.J., Clayton, P.D.(1990). A generalized relational schema for an integrated clinical patient database. *Proceedings of the 14th Annual Sympoisum on computer Applications in Medical Care*. CA: IEEE Computer Soc. Press, pp. 335–339.

Friedman, C., Huff, S.M., Hersh, W.R., Pattison-Gordon, E., Cimino, J.J..(1995). The Canon group's effort: working toward a merged model. *JAMIA* ; 2(1):4 –18.

Friedman, C., Kra, P., Krauthammer, M., Yu, H., Rzhetsky, A.(2001). GENIES: A naturallangauge processing system for the extraction of molecular pathways from journal articles. *Bioinformatics* :suppl:S74–82.

Friedman, C., Shagina, L., Lussier, Y., Hripcsak, G. (2004). Automated encoding of clinical documents based on natural language processing. *J Am Med Inform Assoc*. 11(5):392–402.

Friedman C.P. (1995). Where's the science in medical informatics? *Journal of the American Medical Informatics Association*, 2(1):65–67.

Friedman, C.P., Abbas, U.L. (2003). Is medical informatics a mature science? A review of measurement practice in outcome studies of clinical systems. *Intl J Med Inf*. 69, 261–272.

Friedman, C.P., Wyatt, J.C. (1997a). *Evaluation Methods in Medical Informatics*. New York: Springer-Verlag.

Friedman, C.P., Wyatt, J.C. (1997b). Studying clinical information systems. In Friedman C.P., & Wyatt, J.C., (ed.), *Evaluation Methods in Medical Informatics*, pp.41–64 New York: Springer-Verlag.

Friedland, P., Iwasaki, Y. (1985). The concept and implementation of skeletal plans, *Journal of Automated Reasoning*, 1(2),161–208.

Friedman, R.B. (1973). A computer program for simulating the patient-physician encounter. *Journal of Medical Education*, 48(1):92–97.

Friedman, R.B., Gustafson, D.H. (1977). Computers in clinical medicine: A critical review. *Computers and Biomedical Research*, 10(3):199–204.

Friedman, R.B., Korst, D.R., Schultz, J.V., Beatty, E., Entine, S. (1978). Experience with the simulated patient-physician encounter. *Journal of Medical Education*, 53(10):825–830.

Fries, J.F. (1974). Alternatives in medical record formats. *Medical Care*, 12(10):871–881.

Frisse, M.E., Braude, R.M., Florance, V., Fuller, S. (1995). Informatics and medical libraries: changing needs and changing roles. *Academic Medicine*, 70(1):30–35.

Friston, K.J., Holmes, A.P., Worsley, K.J., Poline, J.P., Frith, C.D., Frackowiak, R.S.J. (1995). Statstical parametric maps in functional imaging: a general linear approach. *Hum Brain Mapp*, 2,189–210.

Fronstin, P. (2002). Can `Consumerism' Slow the Rate of Health Benefit Cost Increases?" Issue Brief no. 247, Washington: Employee Benefit Research Institute, July.

Fuchs, V.R. (1983). *Who Shall Live?* New York: Basic Books.

Fuchs, V.R. (1993). *The Future of Health Policy*. Cambridge, MA: Harvard University Press.

Fuchs, V.R., Garber A.M. (1990). The new technology assessment. *New England Journal of Medicine*, 323(20):673–677.

Fuller, S. (1997). Regional health information systems: Applying the IAIMS model. *Journal of the American Medical Informatics Association*, 4(2):S47–S51.

Funk, M.E., Reid, C.A., McGoogan, L.S. (1983). Indexing consistency in MEDLINE. *Bulletin of the Medical Library Association*, 71(2):176–183.

Gaasterland, T., Karp, P., Karplus, K., Ouzounis, C., Sander C., Valencia, A. (eds.) (1997). *Proceedings of the Fifth International Conference on Intelligent Systems for Molecular Biology*. Menlo Park, CA: AAAI Press.

Gabrieli, E.R. (1989). A new electronic medical nomenclature. *Journal of Medical Systems*, 13(6):355–373.

Gaba, D.M. (2004). The future vision of simulation in health care. *Qual Saf Health Care*, 13 Suppl 1:i2–i10.

Garber, A.M., Owens, D.K. (1994). Paying for evaluative research. In Gelijns A.C., Dawkins H.V. (eds.), *Medical Innovations at the Crossroads, Volume IV: Adopting New Medical Technology*, pp.172–192. Washington, D.C.: National Academy Press.

Garcia-Molina, H., Ullman, J.D., Widom, J.D. (2002). *Database Systems: The Complete Book*, New York: Prentice-Hall.

Gardner, H. (1985). *The Mind's New Science: A History of the Cognitive Revolution*. New York: Basic Books.

Gardner, R.M. (1989). *Personal Communication.* : LDS Hospital, Salt Lake City, UT.

Gardner, R.M. (1997). Fidelity of recording: Improving the signal-to-noise ratio. In Tobin M.J. (ed.), *Principals and Practice of Intensive Care Monitoring*, pp.123–132. New York: McGraw-Hill.

Gardner, R.M., Hawley, W.H., East, T.D., Oniki, T.A., Young, H.F. (1992). Real time data acquisition: Recommendations for the medical information bus (MIB). *International Journal of Clinical Monitoring and Computing*, 8(4):251–258.

Gardner, R.M., Lundsgaarde, H.P. (1994). Evaluation of user acceptance of a clinical expert system. *Journal of the American Medical Informatics Association*, 1(6):428– 438.

Gardner, R.M., Monis, S., Oehler, P. (1986). Monitoring direct blood pressure: Algorithm enhancements. *IEEE Computers in Cardiology*, 13:607.

Gardner, R.M., Shabot, M.M. (2001). Patient-monitoring systems. In E. H. Shortliffe & L. E. Perreault (eds.), *Medical Informatics* (2nd ed), pp. 443– 485. New York: Springer Verlag.

Gardner, R.M., Sittig, D.F., Clemmer, T.P. (1995). Computers in the intensive are unit: A match meant to be! In Shoemaker W.C. (ed.), *Textbook of Critical Care.* (3rd ed.), pp.1757–1770. Philadelphia, PA: W.B. Saunders.

Garg, A.X., Adhikari, N.K.J., McDonald, H., Rosas-Arellano M.P., Devereaux, P.J., Beyene, J., Sam, J., Haynes, R.B. (2005). Effects of computerized clinical decision support systems on practitioner performance and patient outcomes: A systematic review. *JAMA* 293(10):1223–1238.

Garibaldi, R.A. (1998). Editorial: Computers and the quality of care: A clinician's perspective. *New England Journal of Medicine*, 338(4):259–260.

Gazmararian, J., Baker, D., et al. (1999). Health literacy among Medicare enrollees in a managed care organization. *Journal of the American Medical Association*, 281:545–551.

Gee, J.C., Reivich, M., Bajcsy, R. (1993). Elastically deforming 3D atlas to match anatomical brain images. *J. Computer Assisted Tomography*, 17(2), 225–236.

Geissbuhler, A., Miller R.A. (1996). A new approach to the implementation of direct careprovider order entry. *Proceedings of the AMIA Annual Fall Symposium*, pp. 689–693.

Geissbuhler, A.J., Miller, R.A. (1997). Desiderata for product labeling of medical expert systems. *International Journal of Medical Informatics*, 47(3):153–163.

Gelfand, M. (1995). Prediction of function in DNA sequence analysis. *Journal of Computational Biology*, 2(1):87–115.

The Gene Ontology Consortium (2003). Gene Ontology: tool for the unification of biology. *Nature Genet,* 25: 25–29.

George, J.S., Aine, C.J., Mosher, J.C., Schmidt, D.M., Ranken, D.M., Schlitz, H.A., Wood, C.C., Lewine, J.D., Sanders, J.A., Belliveau, J.W. (1995). Mapping function in human brain with magnetoencephalography, anatomical magnetic resonance imaging, and functional magnetic resonance imaging. *Journal of Clinical Neurophysiology*, 12(5):406– 431.

Gerstein, M., Edwards, A., Arrowsmith, C.H., Montelione, G.T. (2003). Structural genomics: Current progress. *Science*. 298(5595):948–950.

Gibson, K., Scheraga, H. (1967). Minimization of polypeptide energy. I. Preliminary structures of bovine pancreatic ribonuclease S-peptide. *Proceedings of the National Academy of Sciences*, 58(2):420– 427.

Giger M., MacMahon H. (1996). Image processing and computer-aided diagnosis. In Greenes, R.A. & Bauman, R.A. (eds.) Imaging and information management: computer systems for a changing health care environment. *The Radiology Clinics of North America*, 34(3):565–596.

Gillan, D.J., Schvaneveldt, R.W. (1999). Applying cognitive psychology: Bridging the gulf between basic research and cognitive artifacts. In F. T. Durso, R.S. Nickerson (eds.), *Handbook of Applied Cognition*, pp. 3–31. New York: Wiley.

Gilman, AG., Simon, MI., Bourne, HR., Harris, BA., Long, R., Ross, EM., Stull, JT., Taussig, R., Bourne, HR., Arkin, AP., Cobb, MH., Cyster, JG., Devreotes, PN., Ferrell, JE., Fruman, D., Gold, M., Weiss, A., Stull, JT., Berridge, MJ., Cantley, LC., Catterall, WA., Coughlin, SR., Olson, EN., Smith, TF., Brugge, JS., Botstein, D., Dixon, JE., Hunter, T., Lefkowitz, RJ., Pawson, AJ., Sternberg, PW., Varmus, H., Subramaniam, S., Sinkovits, RS., Li, J., Mock, D., Ning, Y., Saunders, B., Sternweis, PC., Hilgemann, D., Scheuermann, RH., DeCamp, D., Hsueh, R., Lin, KM., Ni, Y., Seaman, WE., Simpson, PC., O'Connell, TD., Roach, T., Simon, MI., Choi, S., Eversole-Cire, P., Fraser, I., Mumby, MC., Zhao, Y., Brekken, D., Shu, H., Meyer, T., Chandy, G., Heo, WD., Liou, J., O'Rourke, N., Verghese, M., Mumby, SM., Han, H., Brown, HA., Forrester, JS., Ivanova, P., Milne, SB., Casey, PJ., Harden, TK., Arkin, AP., Doyle, J., Gray, ML., Meyer, T., Michnick, S., Schmidt, MA., Toner, M., Tsien, RY., Natarajan, M., Ranganathan, R., Sambrano, GR. (2003). Overview of the Alliance for Cellular Signaling. *Nature*. 420(6916):703–6.

Ginsburg, P. (1982). *Containing Medical Care Costs Through Market Forces*. Washington, D.C.: Congressional Budget Office.

Ginzton, L.E., Laks, M.M. (1984). Computer aided ECG interpretation. *M.D. Computing*, 1(3):36– 44.

Giuse, D.A., Mickish, A. Increasing the availability of the computerized patient record. *Proc AMIA Annu Fall Symp.* 1996, pp. 633–7.

Glowniak, J.W., Bushway, M.K. (1994). Computer networks as a medical resource: Accessing and using the Internet. *Journal of the American Medical Association*, 271(24):1934–1940.

Gold, M.R., Siege,l J.E., Russell, L.B., Weinstein, M.C. (eds.) (1996). *Cost Effectiveness in Health and Medicine*. New York: Oxford University Press.

Goldberg, M.A. (1996). Teleradiology and telemedicine. In Greenes, R.A. & Bauman, R.A. (eds.) Imaging and information management: computer systems for a changing health care environment. *The Radiology Clinics of North America*, 34(3):647–665.

Goldstein, B., McNames, J., McDonald, B.A., et al. (2003). Physiological data acquisition system and database for the study of disease dynamics in the intensive care unit. *Crit Car Med*, 31(2):433–441

Goldstein, M.K., Hoffman, B.B., Coleman, R.W., Musen, M.A., Tu, S.W., Advani, A., Shankar, R.D., O'Connor, M. (2000). Implementing clinical practice guidelines while taking account of evidence: ATHENA, an easily modifiable decision-support system for management of hypertension in primary care. *Proceedings of the Annual AMIA Fall Symposium*, pp. 300-304, Hanley & Belfus, Philadelphia.

Goldstein, M.K., Hoffman, B.B., Coleman, R.W., Musen, M.A., Tu, S.W., Shankar, R.D., O'Connor, M., Martins, S., Advani, A., Musen, M.A. (2002). Patient safety in guideline-based decision support for hypertension management: ATHENA DSS. *Journal of the American Medical Informatics Association* 9(6 Suppl): S11–16.

Gonzales, R., Bartlett, J., et al. (2001). Principles of appropriate antibiotic use for treatment of acute respiratory infections in adults: background, specific aims, and methods. *Annals of Internal Medicine*, 134:479– 486.

Goodman, K.W. (1996). Ethics, genomics and information retrieval. *Computers in Biology and Medicine*, 26(3):223–229.

Goodman, K.W. (ed.) (1998a). *Ethics, Computing, and Medicine: Informatics and the Transformation of Health Care*. Cambridge and New York: Cambridge University Press.

Goodman, K.W. (1998b). Bioethics and health informatics: An introduction. In Goodman K.W. (ed.), *Ethics, Computing, and Medicine: Informatics and the Transformation of Health Care*, pp.1-31. Cambridge and New York: Cambridge University Press.

Goodman, K.W. (1998c). Outcomes, futility, and health policy research. In Goodman K.W. (ed.), *Ethics, Computing, and Medicine: Informatics and the Transformation of Health Care*, pp. 116-138. Cambridge: Cambridge University Press.

Goodwin, J.O., Edwards, B.S. (1975). Developing a computer program to assist the nursing process: Phase I-From systems analysis to an expandable program. *Nursing Research*, 24(4):299–305.

Gordon, M. (1982). Historical perspective: The National Conference Group for Classification of Nursing Diagnoses. *Proceedings of the Classification of Nursing Diagnoses: Proceedings of the Third and Fourth National Conferences*.

Gorman, P.N. (1995). Information needs of physicians. *Journal of the American Society for Information Science*, 46:729–736.

Gorman, P.N., Ash, J., Wykoff, L. (1994). Can primary care physicians' questions be answered using the medical literature? *Bulletin of the Medical Library Association*, 82(2):140–146.

Gorman, P.N., Helfand, M. (1995). Information seeking in primary care: how physicians choose which clinical question to pursue and which to leave unanswered. *Medical Decision Making*, 15(2):113–119.

Gould, M.K., Kushner, W.G., Rydzak, C.E., Maclean, C.C., Demas, A.N., Shigemitsu, H., Chan, J.K., Owens, D.K. (2003). Test performance of positron emission tomography and computed tomography for mediastinal staging in patients with non-small cell lung cancer: A meta analysis. *Annals of Internal Medicine* 139:879–892.

Graves, J.R., Corcoran, S. (1989). The study of nursing informatics. *Image: Journal of Nursing Scholarship*, 21:227–231.

Gray, J.E., Safran, C., Davis, R.B., Pompilio-Weitzner, G., Stewart, J.E., Zaccagnini, L., Pursley, D. (2000). Baby CareLink: using the internet and telemedicine to improve care for high-risk infants. *Pedriatrics* 106,1318–1324.

Greenes, R.A. (1982). OBUS: A microcomputer system for measurement, calculation, reporting, and retrieval of obstetrical ultrasound examinations. *Radiology*, 144:879–883.

Greenes, R.A. (1989). The radiologist as clinical activist: A time to focus outward. *Proceedings of the First International Conference on Image Management and Communication in Patient Care: Implementation and Impact (IMAC 89)*, Washington, D.C., pp. 136–140.

Greenes, R.A., Barnett, G.O., Klein, S.W., Robbins, A., Prior, R.E. (1970). Recording, retrieval, and review of medical data by physician-computer interaction. *New England Journal of Medicine*, 282(6):307–315.

Greenes, R.A., Bauman, R.A., Robboy, S.J., Wieder, J.F., Mercier, B.A., Altshuler, B.S. (1978). Immediate pathologic confirmation of radiologic interpretation by computer feedback. *Radiology*, 127(2):381–383.

Greenes, R.A., Bauman, R.A. (1996). Imaging and information management: Computer systems for a changing health care environment. *The Radiology Clinics of North America*, 34(3):463–697.

Greenes, R.A., Brinkley, J.F. (2001). Radiology Systems. In E.H. Shortliffe & L.E. Perreault (eds.), *Medical Informatics* (2nd ed.), pp. 485-538. New York: Springer Verlag.

Greenes, R.A., Deibel, S.R. (1996). Constructing workstation applications: Component integration strategies for a changing health-care system. In Van Bemmel J.H., McCray A.T. (eds.), *IMIA Yearbook of Medical Informatics '96*, pp.76-86. Rotterdam, The Netherlands: IMIA.

Greenes, R.A., Shortliffe, E.H. (1990). Medical informatics: An emerging academic discipline and institutional priority. *Journal of the American Medical Association*, 263(8):1114–1120.

Greenlick, M.R. (1992). Educating physicians for population-based clinical practice. *Journal of the American Medical Association*, 267(12):1645–1648.

Greeno, J.G., Simon, H.A. (1988). Problem solving and reasoning. In R.C. Atkinson & R.J. Herrnstein (eds.), *Stevens' Handbook of Experimental Psychology* (2nd ed., Vol. 1: Perception and Motivation), pp. 589–672. Oxford, England: John Wiley & Sons.

Gribskov, M., Devereux, J. (1991). *Sequence Analysis Primer*. New York: Stockton Press.

Griffith, H.M., Robinson, K.R. (1992). Survey of the degree to which critical care nurses are performing current procedural terminology-coded services. *American Journal of Critical Care*, 1(2):91–98.

Grigsby, J., Sanders, J.H. (1998). Telemedicine: Where it is and where it's going. *Annals of Internal Medicine*, 129(2):123–127.

Grimm, R.H., Shimoni, K., Harlan, W.R., Estes, E.H.J. (1975). Evaluation of patient-care protocol use by various providers. *New England Journal of Medicine*, 282(10):507–511.

Grimshaw, J.M. Russel, I.T. (1993). Effect of clinical guidelines on medical practice: A systematic review of rigorous evaluations. *Lancet*, 342:1317–1322.

Grishman,R., Kittredge R.(eds.) (1986), *Analyzing Language in Restricted Domains: Sublanguage Description and Processing*. Hillsdale, New Jersey: Erlbaum Associates.

Grobe, S.J. (1996). The nursing intervention lexicon and taxonomy: Implications for representing nursing care data in automated records. *Holistic Nursing Practice*, 11(1):48–63.

Gross, M.S., Lohman, P. (1997). The technology and tactics of physician integration. *Journal of the Healthcare Information and Management Systems Society*, 11(2):23–41.

Grosz, B, Joshi, A, Weinstein, S. (1995). Centering: A framework for modeling the local coherence of discourse. *Computational Linguistics*; 2(21):203–225.

Guo, Q.M.. (2003). DNA microarray and cancer. *Current Opinion in Oncology*. 15(1):36–43.

Gupta, L., Ward, J.E., Hayward, R.S. (1997). Clinical practice guidelines in general practice: A national survey of recall, attitudes and impact. *Med J Aust* 166(2):69–72.

Gusfield, D. (1997). *Algorithms on Strings, Trees, and Sequences: Computer Science and Computational Biology*. Cambridge, England: Cambridge University Press.

Gustafson, D.H., Hawkins, R.P., Boberg, E.W., McTavish, F., Owens, B., Wise, M., Berhe, H., Pingree, S. (2002). CHESS: 10 years of research and development in consumer health informatics for broad populations, including the underserved. *International Journal of Medical Informatics*. 65(3):169–77.

Gustafson, D.H., Taylor, J.O., Thompson, S., Chesney, P. (1993). Assessing the needs of breast cancer patients and their families. *Quality Management in Health Care*, 2(1):6–17.

Guyatt, G. Rennie, D. et al. (2001). *Users' Guide to the Medical Literature: Essentials of Evidence-Based Clinical Practice*. Chicago. American Medical Association.

Hagen, P.T., Turner, D., Daniels, L., Joyce, D. (1998). Very large-scale distributed scanning solution for automated entry of patient information. *TEPR Proceedings (Toward an Electronic Patient Record)*, One:228–32.

Hahn, U.; Romacker, M.; Schulz, S. (1999) Discourse structures in medical reports – watch out! The generation of referentially coherent and valid text knowledge bases in the medSynDiKATe system.: *International Journal of Medical Informatics*, 53(1):1–28.

Halamka, J.D., Safran, C. (1998). CareWeb: A web-based medical record for an integrated healthcare delivery system. *Proceedings of Medinfo 1998*; pt 1:36–39.

Hamilton, D., Macdonald, B., King, C., Jenkins, D., Parlett, M. (eds.) (1977). *Beyond the Numbers Game*. Berkeley, CA: McCutchan Publishers.

Hammond, W.E., Stead, W.W., Straube, M.J., Jelovsek, F.R. (1980). Functional characteristics of a computerized medical record. *Methods of Information in Medicine*, 19(3):157–162.

Hanlon, W.B., Fene, E.F., Davi, S.D., Downs, J.W. (1996). Project BRAHMS: PACS implementation at Brigham and Women's Hospital. *Proceedings of the SICAR96*, Denver, CO, pp. 489–490.

Hansen, L.K., Nielsen, F.A., Toft, P., Liptrot, M.G., Goutte, C., Strother, S.C., Lange, N., Gade, A., Rottenberg, D.A., & Paulson, O.B. (1999). Lyngby-modeler's Matlab toolbox for spatio-temporal analysis of functional neuroimages. *Neuroimage,* 9(6), S241.

Haralick, R.M. (1988). *Mathematical Morphology*: Seattle: University of Washington.

Haralick, R.M., Shapiro, L.G. (1992). *Computer and Robot Vision.* Reading, MA: Addison-Wesley.

Hardiker, N.R., Hoy, D., Casey, A. Standards for nursing terminology. *Journal of the American Medical Informatics Association,* 7:6,523–528.

Harless, W.G., Drennon, G.G., Marxer, J.J., Root, J.A., Miller, G.E. (1971). CASE: A computer-aided simulation of the clinical encounter. *Journal of Medical Education,* 46(5):443–448.

Harless, W.G., Zier, M.A., Duncan, R.C. (1986). Interactive videodisc case studies for medical education. *Proceedings of the 10th Annual Symposium on Computer Applications in Medical Care,* Washington, DC, pp. 183–187.

Harnad, S. (1998). On-line journals and financial firewalls. *Nature,* 395:127–128.

Harris, J.R., Caldwell, B., Cahill, C. (1998). Measuring the public's health in an era of accounta-bility: Lessons from HEDIS (Health Plan Employer Data and Information Set). *American Journal of Preventive Medicine,* 14(3 suppl):9–13.

Harris, MA, Clark, J, Ireland, A, et al. for the Gene Ontology Consortium (2004). The Gene Ontology (GO) database and informatics resource. *Nucleic Acids Res.* 32(Database issue):D258-6.

Harris, Z. (1991), *A Theory of Language and Information: A Mathematical Approach,* Oxford University Press, New York.

Harris, Z, Gottfried, M, Ryckmann, T, Mattick, Jr P, Daladier, A, Harris, TN, Harris, S. (1989). *The Form of Information in Science: Analysis of an Immunology Sublanguage.* Boston, MA: Reidel Dordrecht Studies in the Philosophy of Science.

Harter, S. (1992). Psychological relevance and information science. *Journal of the American Society for Information Science,* 43: 602–615.

Hayes-Roth, F., Waterman, D., Lenat, D. (eds.) (1983). *Building Expert Systems.* Reading, MA: Addison-Wesley.

Haynes, R. (2001). Of studies, syntheses, synopses, and systems: The "4S" evolution of services for finding current best evidence. *ACP Journal Club,* 134:A11–A13.

Haynes, R., Devereaux, P., et al. (2002). Clinical expertise in the era of evidence-based medicine and patient choice. *ACP Journal Club,* 136:A11.

Haynes, R., McKibbon, K., et al. (1985). Computer searching of the medical literature: An eval-uation of MEDLINE searching systems. *Annals of Internal Medicine,* 103:812–816.

Haynes, R.B., McKibbon, K.A., Walker, C.J., Ryan, N., Fitzgerald, D., Ramsden, M.F. (1990). Online access to MEDLINE in clinical settings. *Annals of Internal Medicine,* 112(1):78–84.

Haynes, R., Walker, C., et al. (1994). Performance of 27 MEDLINE systems tested by searches with clinical questions. *Journal of the American Medical Informatics Association,* 1:285–295.

Haynes, R.B., Wilczynski, N., McKibbon, K.A., Walker, C.J., Sinclair, J.C. (1994). Developing optimal search strategies for detecting clinically sound studies in MEDLINE. *Journal of the American Medical Informatics Association,* 1(6):447–458.

Health Care Financial Management Association (1992). *Implementation Manual for the 835 Health Care Claim Payment/Advice*: The Health Care Financial Management Association.

Health Care Financial Management Association (1993). *Implementation Manual for the 834 Benefit Enrollment and Maintenance.* : The Health Care Financial Management Association.

Health Care Financing Administration (1980). *The International Classification of Diseases 9th Revision, Clinical Modification, ICD-9-CM.* (PHS 80-1260.) Washington, D.C.: U.S. Department of Health and Human Services.

Health Care Financing Review (1996). *Medicare and Medicaid Statistical Supplement.* Baltimore: U.S. Department of Health and Human Services.

Health Devices (anon) (2003). Next-generation pulse oximetry. *Health Devices*, 32(2):49–103

Health Insurance Association of America (HIAA) (1983). *Source Book of Health Insurance Data 1982–1983*. Washington, D.C.: HIAA.

Health Level 7 (2003). *Arden Syntax*. (Accessed 2005 at: http://www.hl7.org/Special/committees/Arden/arden.htm)

Health Level Seven (HL7) (2004). *Technical Committees and Special Interest Groups*. http://www.hl7.org.

Hearst, M., Karadi, C. (1997). Cat-a-Cone: An interactive interface for specifying searches and viewing retrieval results using a large category hierarchy. *Proceedings of the 20th Annual International ACM SIGIR Conference on Research and Development in Information Retrieval*, Philadelphia, PA. ACM Press, pp. 246–255.

Heath, C., Luff, P. (2000). *Technology in Action*. New York: Cambridge University Press.

Heathfield, H.A., Wyatt, J.C. (1993). Philosophies for the design and development of clinical decision-support systems. *Methods of Information in Medicine*, 32(1):1–8.

Heathfield H.A., Wyatt J.C. (1995). The road to professionalism in medical informatics: A proposal for debate. *Methods of Information in Medicine*, 34(5):426–433.

Heckerman, D., Horvitz, E. (1986). The myth of modularity in rule-based systems for reasoning with uncertainty. In Lemmer J., Kanal L. (eds.), *Uncertainty in Artificial Intelligence 2*. Amersterdam, Netherlands: North Holland.

Heckerman, D., Horvitz, E., Nathwani, B. (1989). Update on the Pathfinder project. *Proceedings of the Thirteenth Annual Symposium on Computer Applications in Medical Care*, Washington, DC, pp. 203–207.

Heckerman D., Nathwani B. (1992). An evaluation of the diagnostic accuracy of Pathfinder. *Computers and Biomedical Research*, 25:56–74.

Heiss, W.D., Phelps, M.E. (eds.) (1983). *Positron Emission Tomography of the Brain*. Berlin; New York: Springer-Verlag.

Helfand, M., & Redfern, C. (1998). Screening for thyroid disease. *Annals of Internal Medicine, 129*(2):144–158.

Hellmich, M., Abrams, K.R., Sutton, A.J. (1999). Bayesian approaches to meta-analysis of ROC curves. *Medical Decision Making* 19:252–264.

Henchley, A. (2003). *Understanding Version 3: A Primer on the HL7 Version 3 Communication Standard*. Munich, Germany: Alexander Moench Publishing Co.

Henderson, M. (2003). *HL7 Messaging*. Silver Spring, Maryland OTech Inc.

Henderson, S. Crapo, R.O., Wallace, C.J., East, T.D., Morris, A.H., Gardner, R.M. (1991). Performance of computerized protocols for the management of arterial oxygenation in an intensive care unit. *International Journal of Clinical Monitoring and Computing*, 8(4):271–280.

Henikoff, S, Henikoff, JG. (1992). *Amino acid substitution matrices from protein blocks*. Proceedings of the National Academy of the Sciences. 89(22):10915–9.

Henley, R.R., Wiederhold, G. (1975). *An Analysis of Automated Ambulatory Medical Record Systems*. (AAMRS Study Group, Technical Report 13(1).): Laboratory of Medical Information Science, University of California, San Francisco.

Hennessy, J.L., Patterson, D.A. (1994). *Computer Architecture, A Quantitative Approach*. (2nd ed.). San Francisco: Morgan Kaufmann.

Henry (Bakken), S.B., Holzemer, W.L., Randell, C., Hsieh, S.F., Miller, T.J. (1997). Comparison of nursing interventions classification and current procedural terminology codes for categorizing nursing activities. *Image: Journal of Nursing Scholarship*, 29(2):133–138.

Henry (Bakken), S.B., Holzemer, W.L., Reilly, C.A., Campbell, K.E. (1994). Terms used by nurses to describe patient problems: Can SNOMED III represent nursing concepts in the patient record? *Journal of the American Medical Informatics Association*, 1(1):61–74.

Henry (Bakken), S.B., Holzemer, W.L., Tallberg, M., Grobe, S. (1995). Informatics: infrastructure for quality assessment and improvement in nursing. *Proceedings of the 5th International Nursing Informatics Symposium (NI94) Post-Conference*, Austin, TX.

Henry (Bakken), S.B., Mead, C.N. (1997). Nursing classification systems: Necessary but not sufficient for representing "what nurses do" for inclusion in computer-based patient record systems. *Journal of the American Medical Informatics Association*, 4(3):222–232.

Hersh, W.R. (1991). Evaluation of Meta-1 for a concept-based approach to the automated indexing and retrieval of bibliographic and full-text databases. *Medical Decision Making*, 11 (4 Suppl):S120–S124.

Hersh, W.R. (1994). Relevance and retrieval evaluation: perspectives from medicine. *Journal of the American Society for Information Science*, 45:201–206.

Hersh, W.R. (1996). *Information Retrieval: A Health Care Perspecive*. New York: Springer-Verlag.

Hersh, W.R. (1999). "A world of knowledge at your fingertips": The promise, reality, and future directions of on-line information retrieval. *Academic Medicine*, 74:240–243.

Hersh, W.R. (2001). Interactivity at the Text Retrieval Conference (TREC). *Information Processing and Management*, 37: 365–366.

Hersh, W.R. (2003). *Information Retrieval, A Health and Biomedical Perspective (Second Edition)*, New York: Springer-Verlag.

Hersh, W.R., Brown, K.E., Donohoe, L.C., Campbell, E.M., Horacek, A.E. (1996). CliniWeb: managing clinical information on the World Wide Web. *Journal of the American Medical Informatics Association*, 3:273–280.

Hersh, W.R., Crabtree, M., et al. (2002). Factors associated with success for searching MEDLINE and applying evidence to answer clinical questions. *Journal of the American Medical Informatics Association*, 9:283–293.

Hersh, W.R., Elliot, D., et al. (1994). Towards new measures of information retrieval evaluation. *Proceedings of the 18th Annual Symposium on Computer Applications in Medical Care*, Washington, DC. Hanley & Belfus, pp. 895–899.

Hersh, W.R., Elliot, D.L., Hickam, D.H., Wolf, S.L., Molnar, A., Leichtenstein, C. (1995). Towards new measures of information retrieval evaluation. *Proceedings of the 18th Annual International ACMSIGIR Conference on Research and Development in Information Retrieval*, Seattle, WA, .

Hersh, W.R., Hickam, D. (1994). Use of a multi-application computer workstation in a clinical setting. *Bulletin of the Medical Library Association*, 82(4):382–389.

Hersh, W.R., Hickam, D. (1998). How well do physicians use electronic information retrieval systems? A framework for investigation and review of the literature. *Journal of the American Medical Association*, 280: 1347–1352.

Hersh, W.R., Pentecost, J., Hickam, D. (1996). A task-oriented approach to information retrieval evaluation. *Journal of the American Society for Information Science*, 47:50–56.

Hersh, W.R. and Rindfleisch, T.C. (2000). Electronic publishing of scholarly communication in the biomedical sciences. *Journal of the American Medical Informatics Association*, 7:324 –325.

Hersh, W.R., Turpin, A., et al. (2000). Do batch and user evaluations give the same results? *Proceedings of the 23rd Annual International ACM SIGIR Conference on Research and Development in Information Retrieval*, Athens, Greece. ACM Press, pp. 17–24.

Hickam, D.H., Shortliffe, E.H., Bischoff, M.B., Scott, A.C., Jacobs, C.D. (1985). The treatment advice of a computer-based cancer chemotherapy protocol advisor. *Annals of Internal Medicine*, 103(6 Pt 1):928–936.

Hickam, D.H., Sox, H.C., Sox, C.H. (1985). Systematic bias in recording the history in patients with chest pain. *Journal of Chronic Diseases*, 38:91.

Hilgard, E.R., Bower, G.H. (1975). *Theories of Learning* (4th ed.). Englewood Cliffs, N.J.: Prentice-Hall.

Hillestad, R., Bigelow, J., Bower, A., Girosi, F., Meili, R., Scoville, R., Taylor, R. (2005). Can electronic medical record systems transform health care? Potential health benefits, savings, and costs. *Health Affairs* 24:1103–1117.

Hillman, B.J. (2002). Current clinical trials of the American College of Radiology Imaging Network. *Radiology* 224(3):636–637.

Hinshaw, K.P., Brinkley, J.F. (1997). Using 3-D shape models to guide segmentation of MR brain images. *Proceedings of the 1997 AMIA Annual Fall Symposium*, Nashville, TN, pp. 469–478.

Hinshaw, K.P., Poliakov, A.V., Martin, R.F., Moore, E.B., Shapiro, L.G., & Brinkley, J.F. (2002). Shape-based cortical surface segmentation for visualization brain mapping. *Neuroimage*, 16(2), 295–316.

Hobbs, J.R., Appelt, D.E., Bear, J., Israel, D., Kameyama, M., Stickel, M. et al. (1996). FASTUS: A cascaded finite-state transducer for extracting information from natural-language text. In *Finite State Devices for Natural Language Processing*, Cambridge, MA: MIT Press.

Hodge, M.H. (1990). History of the TDS medical information system. In B.I. Blum & K. Duncan (ed.), *A History of Medical Informatics*, pp.328–344. New York: ACM Press.

Hoey, J. (1998). When the physician is the vector. *CMAJ* 159(1):45–46.

Hoffer, E.P., Barnett, G.O. (1986). Computer-aided instruction in medicine: 16 years of MGH experience. In Salamon R., B. Blum, & M. Jorgensen, (ed.), *MEDINFO 86*. Amsterdam: Elsevier North-Holland.

Hoffman, C., Rice, D., Sung, H.Y. (1996). Persons with chronic conditions: Their prevalence and costs, *JAMA*, 276,1473–1479.

Hoffman, R.R. (ed.) (1992). *The Psychology of Expertise: Cognitive Research and Empirical AI*. Hilldale, NJ: Lawrence Erlbaum Associates, Publishers.

Hoffman, R.R., Schadbolt, N.R., Burton, A.M., Klein, G. (1995). Eliciting knowledge from experts: A methodological analysis. *Organizational Behavior & Human Decision Processes*, 62(2),129–158.

Hohne, K., Bomans, M., Pommert, A., Riemer, M., Schiers, C., Tiede, U., & Wiebecke, G. (1990). 3-D visualization of tomographic volume data using the generalized voxel model. *The Visual Computer*, 6(1), 28–36.

Hohne, K.H., Bomans, M., Riemer, M., Schubert, R., Tiede, U., Lierse, W. (1992). A volume-based anatomical atlas. *IEEE Computer Graphics and Applications*, 72–78.

Hohne, K.H., Pflesser, B., Riemer, M., Schiemann, T., Schubert, R., Tiede, U. (1995). A new representation of knowledge concerning human anatomy and function. *Nature Medicine*, 1(6):506–510.

Honeyman-Buck, J. (2003). PACS adoption. *Semin Roentgenol.* 38(3):256–269.

Hopf, HW. (2003). Molecular diagnostics of injury and repair responses in critical illness: What is the future of "monitoring" in the intensive care unit? *Crit Care Med*; 31(8)[Suppl.]:S518–523

Horii, S.C. (1996). Image acquisition: Sites, technologies and approaches. In Greenes, R.A. & Bauman, R.A. (eds.) Imaging and information management: computer systems for a changing health care environment. *The Radiology Clinics of North America*, 34(3):469–494.

Horne, P, Saarlas, K, Hinman, A (2000). Costs of immunization registries. Experience from the All Kids Count II Projects. *Am J Prev Med*, 18:262–267.

Horsky, J., Kaufman, D.R., Oppenheim, M.I., Patel, V.L. (2003). A framework for analyzing the cognitive complexity of computer-assisted clinical ordering. *Journal of Biomedical Informatics*, 36(1-2),4–22.

Horsky, J., Kaufman, D.R., Patel, V.L. (2003). The cognitive complexity of a provider order entry interface *Proceedings of the AMIA Annual Fall Symposium*, Washington, DC, pp. 294–298.

House, E.R. (1980). *Evaluating with Validity*. Beverly Hills, CA: Sage Publications.

Hoy, J.D., Hyslop, A.Q. (1995). Care planning as a strategy to manage variation in practice: From care planning to integrated person-based record. *Journal of the American Medical Informatics Association*, 2(4):260–266.

Hripcsak, G., Austin, J.H., Alderson, P.O., Friedman, C. (2002). Use of natural language processing to translate clinical information from a database of 889,921 chest radiographic reports. *Radiology*, 224(1):157–163.

Hripcsak, G., Cimino, J.J., Sengupta, S. (1999). WebCIS: Large scale deployment of a Web-based clinical information system. *Proceedings of the Annual AMIA Symposium*, pp. 804–808.

Hripcsak, G., Ludemann, P., Pryor, T.A., Wigertz, O.B., Clayton, P.D. (1994). Rationale for the Arden syntax. *Computers and Biomedical Research*, 27:291–324.

Hripcsak, G, Wilcox, A. (2002). Reference standards, judges, and comparison subjects: roles for experts in evaluating system performance. *J Am Med Inform Assoc*; 9(1):1–15.

Hsu, H.L. (1996). *Interactivity of Human-Computer Interaction and Personal Characteristics in a Hypermedia Learning Environment.* Unpublished doctoral dissertation, Stanford University.

Huang, H.K. (2003). Enterprise PACS and image distribution. *Comput Med Imaging Graph,* 27 (2-3):241–53

Hucka, M., Finney, A., Sauro, H.M., et al. (2003). The systems biology markup language (SBML): A medium for representation and exchange of biochemical network models. *Bioinformatics*, 19(4):524–31.

Hudson, L. (1985). Monitoring of critically ill patients. Conference summary. *Respiratory Care*, 30:628.

Huff, S.M, Rocha, R.A., McDonald, C.J., DeMoor, G.J., Fiers, T., Bidgood, W.D. Jr., Forrey, A.W., Francis, W.G., Tracy, W.R., Leavelle, D., Stalling, F., Griffin, B., Maloney, P., Leland, D., Charles, L., Hutchins, K., Baenziger, J. (1998). Development of the Logical Observation Identifier Names and Codes (LOINC) vocabulary. *J Am Med Inform Assoc* 5(3):276–292.

Human Brain Project. (2003). *Home page.* (Accessed 2005 at: http://www.nimh.nih.gov/neuroinformatics/index.cfm)

Humphreys, B.L. (2000). Electronic health record meets digital library: A new environment for achieving an old goal. *Journal of the American Medical Informatics Association,* 7: 444–452.

Humphreys, B.L. (ed.) (1990). *UMLS Knowledge Sources – First Experimental Edition Documentation.* Bethesda, MD: National Library of Medicine.

Humphreys, B.L., Lindberg, D.A. (1993). The UMLS project: making the conceptual connection between users and the information they need. *Bulletin of the Medical Library Association*, 81(2):170–177.

Humphreys, BL, Lindberg, DA, Schoolman, HM, Barnett, GO (1998). The Unified Medical Language System: An informatics research collaboration. *J Am Med Inform Assoc.* 5(1):1–11.

Hunt, L.T., Dayhoff, M.O. (1974). Table of abnormal human globins. *Annual of the New York Academy of Science*, 241:722–735.

Hunt, D.L., Haynes, R.B., Hanna, S.E., Smith, K. (1998). Effects of computer-based clinical decision support systems on physician performance and patient outcomes: A systematic review. *JAMA*; 280:1339–1346.

Hunter, L. (1993). *Artificial Intelligence and Molecular Biology.* Menlo Park: AAAI Press/MIT Press.

Hurdal, M.K., Stephenson, K., Bowers, P., Sumners, D.W., Rottenberg, D.A. (2000). Coordinate systems for conformal cerebellar flat maps. *Neuroimage,* 11(5), S467.

Hussein, R., Engelmann, U., Schroeter, A., Meinzer, H.P. (2004). DICOM structured reporting: Part 2. Problems and challenges in implementation for PACS workstations. *Radiographics*, 24(3):897–909.

Hutchins, E. (1995). *Cognition in the Wild.* Cambridge, Mass: MIT Press.

IAIMS (1996). *Proceedings of the 1996 IAIMS Symposium.* Nashville, TN: Vanderbilt University.

International Anatomical Nomenclature Committee. (1989). *Nomina Anatomica* (6th ed.). Edinburgh: Churchill Livingstone.

Institute of Medicine (1985). *Assessing Medical Technologies.* Washington, D.C.: National Academy Press.

Institute of Medicine (1988). *The Future of Public Health*. Washington, DC: National Academy Press.

Institute of Medicine (1991). *The Computer-Based Patient Record: An Essential Technology for Patient Care*. Washington, DC: National Academy Press.

Institute of Medicine (1996). *Healthy Communities: New Partnerships for the Future of Public Health*. Washington, DC: National Academy Press.

Institute of Medicine (1997**a**). *Improving Health in the Community: A Role for Performance Monitoring*. Washington, DC: National Academy Press.

Institute of Medicine (1997**b**). *Managing Managed Care: Qualtiy Improvement in Behavioral Health*. Washington, DC: National Academy Press.

Institute of Medicine (1997**c**). *The Computer-Based Patient Record: An Essential Technology for Health Care*. (2nd ed.). Washington, D.C.: National Academy Press.

Institute of Medicine (2000a). *To Err Is Human: Building a Safer Health Care System*. Washington, DC: National Academy Press.

Institute of Medicine (2000b). *Calling the Shots — Immunization Finance Policies and Practices*. Washington, DC: National Academy Press.

Institute of Medicine (2001) *Crossing the Quality Chasm: A New Health System for the Twenty-First Century*, Washington: National Academies Press.

Institute of Medicine (2002). *Priority Areas for National Action: Transforming Health Care Quality*. Washington DC: National Academies Press.

Institute of Medicine (2003). *Patient Safety: Achieving a New Standard for Care*. Washington, DC: National Academies Press.

International Standards Organization (1987). *Information processing systems-Concepts and terminology for the conceptual schema and the information base*. (ISO TR 9007:1987.): International Standards Organization.

International Standards Organization. (2003). *Integration of a Reference Terminology Model for Nursing* (ISO 18104:2003). International Standards Organization.

Interstudy (1995). *The Interstudy Competitive Edge, Part II: Industry Report*. Excelsior, Minn.

Issel-Tarver, L., Christie, K.R., Dolinski, K., Andrada, R., Balakrishnan, R., Ball, C.A., Binkley, G., Dong, S., Dwight, S.S., Fisk, D.G., Harris, M., Schroeder, M., Sethuraman, A., Tse, K., Weng, S., Botstein, D., Cherry, J.M. (2001). Saccharomyces genome database. *Methods Enzymol*; 350:329–46.

Ivers, M.T., Timson, G.F. (1985). The applicability of the VA integrated clinical CORE information system to the needs of other health care providers. *MUG Quarterly*, 14:19–21.

Jacky, J. (1989). Programmed for disaster. *The Sciences*, 29(5):22–27.

Jadad, A. (1999). Promoting partnerships: Challenges for the Internet age. *British Medical Journal*, 319:761–764.

Jain, R. (1991). *The Art of Computer Systems Performance Analysis: Techniques for Experimental Design, Measurement, Simulation, and Modeling*. New York: John Wiley & Sons, Inc.

Jakobovits, R.M., Modayur, B., Brinkley, J.F. (1996). A Web-based manager for brain mapping data. *Proceedings of the 1996 AMIA Annual Fall Symposium*, Washington, DC, pp. 309–313.

Jakobovits, R.M., Brinkley, J.F., Rosse, C., Weinberger, E.(2001). Enabling clinicians, researchers, and educators to build custom web-based biomedical information systems. *Proc AMIA Annual Fall Symposium*; pp. 279–283.

Jakobovits, R.M., Rosse, C., Brinkley, J.F.(2002). An open source toolkit for building biomedical web applications. *J Am Med Info. Ass.*;9(6):557–590.

Jewett, A.I., Huang, C.C., Ferrin, T.E. (2003). MINRMS: An efficient algorithm for determining protein structure similarity using root-mean-squared-distance. *Bioinformatics*. 19(5):625–34.

John, B.E. (2003). Information processing and skilled behavior. In J. M. Carroll (ed.), *HCI Models, Theories and Frameworks: Toward a Multidisciplinary Science*. San Francisco, CA: Morgan Kaufmann.

Johnson, K.A., Becker, J.A. (2001). *The Whole Brain Atlas*. Harvard University. (Accessed 2005 at: http://www.med.harvard.edu/AANLIB/home.html)

Johnson, P. (1983). What kind of expert should a system be? *Journal of Medicine and Philosophy*, 8:77–97.

Johnson, P.D., Tu, S.W., Booth, N., Sugden, B., Purves, I.N. (2000). Using scenarios in chronic disease management guidelines for primary care. *Proceedings of the AMIA Annual Symposium,* Los Angeles, CA, Hanley & Belfus, Philadelphia.

Johnson, S.B. (2000). Natural language processing in biomedicine. In: Bronzino JD. *The Handbook of Biomedical Engineering*. Boca Raton, FL: CRC Press, pp. 188–196.

Johnson, S.B., Friedman, C., Cimino, J.J., Clark, T., Hripcsak, G., Clayton, P.D. (1991). Conceptual data model for a central patient database. *Proceedings of the Fifteenth Symposium on Computer Applications in Medical Care*. Washington, D.C., pp. 381–385.

Johnston, D., Pan, E., Walker, J., Bates, D.W., Middleton, B. (2003). *The Value of Computerized Provider Order Entry in Ambulatory Settings*. Boston: Center for Information Technology Leadership, Partners HealthCare.

Johnston, M.C., Langton, K.B., Haynes, R.B., Mathieu, A. (1994). Effects of computer-based clinical decision support systems on clinician performance and patient outcome. A critical appraisal of research. *Annals of Internal Medicine*, 120(2):135–142.

Jolesz, F.A. (1997). 1996 RSNA Eugene P. Pendergrass New Horizons Lecture. Image-guided procedures and the operating room of the future. *Radiology*, 204(3):601–612.

Jollis, J.G., Ancukiewicz, M., DeLong, E.R., Pryor, D.B., Muhlbaier, L.H., Mark, D.B. (1993). Discordance of databases designed for claims payment versus clinical information systems. Implications for outcomes research. *Annals of Internal Medicine*, 119(8):844–850.

Jurafsky, D, Martin, JH. (2000a). *Speech and Language Processing: An Introduction to Natural Language Processing, Computational Linguistics and Speech Recognition*. New York: Prentice Hall.

Jydstrup R.A., Gross M.J. (1966). Cost of information handling in hospitals. *Health Services Research*, 1(3):235–271.

Kahle, B. (1997). Preserving the Internet. *Scientific American*, 276(3):82–83.

Kahn, M.G. (1994). Clinical databases and critical care research. *Critical Care Clinics*, 10(1):37–51.

Kaiser Family Foundation and Health Research and Educational Trust (2005). *Employer Health Benefits 2005 Annual Survey*. Menlo Park, CA.

Kalet, I.J., Austin-Seymour, M.M. (1997). The use of medical images in planning and delivery of radiation therapy. *Journal of the American Medical Informatics Association*, 4(5):327–339.

Kalinski, T., Hofmann, H., Franke, D.S., Roessner, A. (2002). Digital imaging and electronic patient records in pathology using an integrated department information system with PACS. *Pathol Res Pract*, 198(10):679–84.

Kane, B. Sands, D.Z. (1998). Guidelines for the clinical use of electronic mail with patients. *J Am Med Inform Assoc* 5,104–111.

Kaplan, B. (1997). Addressing organizational issues into the evaluation of medical systems. *Journal of the American Medical Informatics Association*, 4(2):94–101.

Kaplan, B., Duchon, D. (1988). Combining qualitative and quantitative methods in information systems research: A case study. *MIS Quarterly*, 4:571–586.

Karat, C.M. (1994). A business case approach to usability cost justification. In R. G. Bias & D.J. Mayhew (eds.), *Cost Justifying Usability*, pp. 45-70. New York: Academic Press.

Karplus, M., Weaver, D.L. (1976). Protein-folding dynamics. *Nature*, 260(5550):404–406.

Kass, B. (2001). Reducing and preventing adverse drug events to decrease hospital costs. *Research in Action, Issue 1*. AHRQ Publication Number 01-0020. (Accessed 2005 at: http://www.ahrq.gov/qual/aderia/aderia.htm)

Kass, M., Witkin, A., Terzopoulos, D. (1987). Snakes: Active contour models. *International Journal of Computer Vision*, 1(4):321–331.

Kassirer, J.P., Gorry, G.A. (1978). Clinical problem solving: A behavioral analysis. *Annals of Internal Medicine*, 89(2):245–255.

Kastor, J.A.. (2001). *Mergers of Teaching Hospitals in Boston, New York, and Northern California*. Ann Arbor: University of Michigan Press.

Kaufmann, A, Meltzer, M, Schmid, G. (1997). The economic impact of a bioterrorist attack: Are prevention and post-attack intervention programs justifiable? *Emerg Infect Dis* 3(2):83–94.

Kaufman, D.R., Patel, V.L., Hilliman, C., Morin, P.C., Pevzner,J., Weinstock,R., et al. (2003). Usability in the real world: Assessing medical information technologies in the patient's home. *Journal of Biomedical Informatics.* 36(1-2), 45–60.

Kaufman, D.R., Patel, V.L., Magder, S. (1996). The explanatory role of spontaneously generated analogies in reasoning about physiological concepts. *International Journal of Science Education,* 18(3),369–386.

Kaushal, R., Shojania, K.G., Bates, D.W. (2003). Effects of computerized physician order entry and clinical decision support systems on medication safety: A systematic review. *Archives of Internal Medicine*, 163(12):1409–16.

Keen, P.G.W. (1981). Information systems and organizational change. *Communications of the ACM*, 24:24.

Kennedy, D. (2001). *Internet Brain Segmentation Repository*. Massachusetts General Hospital. (Accessed 2005 at: http://neuro-www.mgh.harvard.edu/cma/ibsr)

Kennelly, R.J., Gardner, R.M. (1997). Perspectives on development of IEEE 1073: The Medical Information Bus (MIB) standard. *International Journal of Clinical Monitoring and Computing*, 14(3):143–149.

Kenny, N.P. (1997). Does good science make good medicine? Incorporating evidence into practice is complicated by the fact that clinical practice is as much art as science. *CMAJ* 157(1):33–36.

Kent, W.J. (2003). BLAT – the BLAST-like alignment tool. *Genome Research.* 12(4):656–64.

Keston, V., Enthoven, A.C. (1996). Total hip replacement: A history of innovations to improve quality while reducing costs. *Stanford University Working Paper Number 1411*: October 29, 1996.

Kevles, B. (1997). *Naked to the Bone: Medical Imaging in the Twentieth Century*. New Brunswick, NJ: Rutgers University Press.

Khorasani, R., Hanlon, W.B., Fener, E.F., Lester, J.M., Dreyer, K., Seltzer, S.E., Holman, B.L. (1997). Exploiting the Internet and the world wide web for rapid and inexpensive distribution of digital images and radiology reports. Unpublished technical report, Brigham and Women's Hospital..

Khorasani, R., Lester, J.M., Davis, S.D., Hanlon, W.B., Fener, E.F., Seltzer, S.E., Adams, D.F., Holman, B.L. (1998). Web-based digital radiology teaching file: Facilitating case input at time of interpretation. *AJR American Journal of Roentgenology*, 170(5):1165–1167.

Kikinis, R., Shenton, M.E., Iosifescu, D.V., McCarley, R.W., Saiviroonporn, P., Hokama, H.H., Robatino, A., Metcalf, D., Wible, C.G., Portas, C.M., Donnino, R., Jolesz, F. (1996). A digital brain atlas for surgical planning, model-driven segmentation, and teaching. *IEEE Trans. Visualization and Computer Graphics,* 2(3), 232–241.

Kim, D., Constantinou, P.S., Glasgow, E. (1995). *Clinical Anatomy: Interactive Lab Practical.* St. Louis: Mosby-Year Book. CD-ROM., .

Kimborg, D.Y., Aguirre, G.K. (2002). *A Flexible Architecture for Neuroimaging Data Analysis and Presentation.* (Accessed 2005 at: http://www.nimh.nih.gov/neuroinformatics/kimberg.cfm)

King, W., Proffitt, J., Morrison, L., Piper, J., Lane, D., Seelig, S. (2000). The role of fluorescence in situ hybridization technologies in molecular diagnostics and disease management. *Mol Diagn,* 5(4),309–319.

Kingsland, L.C., Harbourt, A.M., Syed, E.J., Schuyler, P.L. (1993). Coach: Applying UMLS knowledge sources in an expert searcher environment. *Bulletin of the Medical Library Association*, 81(2):178–183.

Kintsch, W. (1988). The role of knowledge in discourse comprehension: A construction-integration model. *Psychological Review,* 95(2), 163–182.

Kirby, M., Miller, N. (1986). MEDLINE searching on Colleague: Reasons for failure or success of untrained users. *Medical Reference Services Quarterly*, 5:17–34.

Kirkpatrick, D.L. (1994). *Evaluating Training Programs.* San Francisco, CA: Berrett-Koehler Publishers.

Kittredge, R. J. Lehrberger (eds.) (1982). *Sublanguage: Studies of Language in Restricted Semantic Domains*, New York: De Gruyter.

Kjems, U., Strother, S.C., Anderson, J.R., Law, I., Hansen, L.K. (1999). Enhancing the multivariate signal of ^{15}O water PET studies with a new nonlinear neuroanatomical registration algorithm. *IEEE Trans. Med. Imaging,* 18, 301–319.

Kleinmuntz, B. (1968). *Formal Representation of Human Judgement.* New York: Wiley.

Kleinmuntz, D.N., Schkade, D.A. (1993). Information displays in decision making. *Psychological Science,* 4, 221–227.

Knaus, W.A., Draper, E.A., Wagner, D.P., Zimmerman, J.E. (1986). An evaluation of outcome from intensive care in major medical centers. *Annals of Internal Medicine*, 104(3):410–418.

Knaus, W.A., Wagner, D.P., Lynn, J. (1991). Short-term mortality predictions for critically ill hospitalized adults: Science and ethics. *Science*, 254(5030):389–394.

Knight, E., Glynn, R., et al. (2000). Failure of evidence-based medicine in the treatment of hypertension in older patients. *Journal of General Internal Medicine*, 15:702–709.

Koedinger, K.R., Anderson, J.R. (1992). Abstract planning and perceptual chunks. *Cognitive Science,* 14(4), 511–550.

Kohn, L.T., Corrigan, J.M., Donaldson,M.S. (eds) (1999). *To Err is Human: Building A Safer Health System*, Washhington, DC: National Academy Press.

Kolodner, R.M., Douglas, J.V. (eds) (1997). *Computerizing Large Integrated Health Networks: The VA Success.* New York: Springer.

Komaroff, A. (1979). The variability and inaccuracy of medical data. *Proceedings of the IEEE*, 67:1196.

Komaroff, A., Black, W., Flatley, M. (1974). Protocols for physician assistants: Management of diabetes and hypertension. *New England Journal of Medicine*, 290:370–312.

Koo, D, O'Carroll, PW, LaVenture, M (2001). Public health 101 for informaticians. *Journal of the American Medical Informatics Association* 8(6):585–97.

Kosara, R., Miksch, S. (2002). Visualization methods for data analysis and planning in medical applications. *Int J Med Inf,* 68(1-3),141–153.

Koski, E.M., Makivirta, A., Sukuvaara, T., Kari, A. (1995). Clinicians' opinions on alarm limits and urgency of therapeutic responses. *Int J Clin Monit Comput* 12(2):85–88

Koslow, S.H., Huerta, M.F. (1997). *Neuroinformatics: An Overview of the Human Brain Project.* Mahwah, NJ: Lawrence Erlbaum.

KPMG Peat Marwick (1996). Health Benefits in 1996. *KPMG Survey of Employer Sponsored Health Benefits.*

Kuhn, I.M., Wiederhold, G., Rodnick, J.E., Ramsey-Klee, D.M., Benett, S., Beck, D.D. (1984). Automated ambulatory medical record systems in the U.S. In B. Blum (ed.), *Information Systems for Patient Care*, pp.199-217. New York: Springer-Verlag.

Kuhn, T. (1962). *The Structure of Scientific Revolutions.* Chicago: University of Chicago Press.

Kulikowski, C.A. (1997). Medical imaging informatics: Challenges of definition and integration. *Journal of the American Medical Informatics Association*, 4(3):252–253.

Kulikowski, C.A., Jaffe, C.C. (1997). Focus on Imaging Informatics. *Journal of the American Medical Informatics Association*, 4(3).

Kuperman, G., Gardner, R., Pryor, T.A. (1991). *HELP: A Dynamic Hospital Information System.* New York: Springer-Verlag.

Kuperman, G.J., Gibson, R.F. (2003). Computer physician order entry: benefits, costs, issues. *Ann Intern Med.* 139(1):31–39.

Kupiers, B., Kassirer, J. (1984). Causal reasoning in medicine: Analysis of a protocol. *Cognitive Science*, 8:363–385.

Kurtzke, J.F. (1979). ICD-9: A regression. *American Journal of Epidemiology*, 108(4):383–393.

Kushniruk, A.W., Kaufman, D.R., Patel, V.L., Levesque, Y., Lottin, P. (1996). Assessment of a computerized patient record system: A cognitive approach to evaluating medical technology. *MD Computing, 13*(5), 406– 415.

Lagoze, C., VandeSompel, H. (2001). The Open Archives Initiative: Building a low-barrier interoperability framework. *Proceedings of the First ACM/IEEE-CS Joint Conference on Digital Libraries*, Roanoke, VA.: ACM Press. 54–62.

Lancaster, J.L., Woldorff, M.G., Parsons, L.M., Liotti, M., Freitas, C.S., Rainey, L., Kochunov, P.V., Nickerson, D., Mikiten, S.A., Fox, P.T. (2000). Automated Talairach atlas labels for functional brain mapping. *Hum Brain Mapp, 10*(3), 120–131.

Lander, E.S., Linton, L.M., Birren, B., and colleagues (2001). Initial sequencing and analysis of the human genome. *Nature*. 409(6822):860–921.

Lange, L.L. (1996). Representation of everyday clinical nursing language in UMLS and SNOMED. *Proceedings of the 1996 AMIA Annual Fall Symposium*, Washington, D.C., pp. 140–144.

Langridge, R. (1974). Interactive three-dimensional computer graphics in molecular biology. *Federal Proceedings*, 33(12):2332–2335.

Lanzola, G., Quaglini, S., Stefanelli, M. (1995). Knowledge-acquisition tools for medical knowledge-based systems. *Methods of Information in Medicine*, 34(1-2):25–39.

Larkin, J.H., McDermott, J., Simon, D.P., Simon, H.A. (1980). Expert and novice performance in solving physics problems. *Science, 208*,1335–1342.

Larkin, J.H., Simon, H.A. (1987). Why a diagram is (sometimes) worth ten thousand words. *Cognitive Science*, 11(1), 65–99.

Lashkari, D.A., DeRisi, J.L., McCusker, J.H., Namath, A.F., Gentile, C., Hwang, S.Y., Brown, P.O., Davis, R.W. (1997). Ycast microarrays for genome wide parallel genetic and gene expression analysis. *Proc Natl Acad Sci.* 94(24):13057–1362.

Lassila, O., Hendler, J., et al. (2001). The Semantic Web. *Scientific American, 284*(5):34 – 43.

Lawrence, S. (2001). Online or invisible? *Nature*, 411: 521.

Lawrence, S., Giles, C., et al. (1999). Digital libraries and autonomous citation indexing. *IEEE Computer*, 32: 67–71.

Leape, L.L. & Berwick, D.M. (2005). Five years after "To Err is Human": What have we learned? *JAMA* 239(19):2384–2390.

Leatherman, S., Berwick, D., Iles, D., Lewin, L.S., Davidoff, F., Nolan, T., Bisognano, N. (2003). The business case for quality: Case studies and an analysis. *Health Affairs*, 22(2):17–30.

Le Bihan, D., Mangin, J.F., Poupon, C., Clark, C.A., Pappata, S., Molko, N., Chabriat, H. (2001). Diffusion tensor imaging: concepts and applications. *J. Magnetic Resonance Imaging*, 13(4),534 –546.

Lederberg, J. (1978). Digital communications and the conduct of science: The new literacy. *Proceedings of the IEEE*, 66(11):1314–1319.

Ledley, R., Lusted L. (1959). Reasoning foundations of medical diagnosis. *Science*, 130:9–21.

Lee, C.C., Jack, C.R.J., Riederer, S.J. (1996). Use of functional magnetic resonance imaging. *Neurosurgery Clinics of North America*, 7(4):665–683.

Lee, D.H. (2003). Magnetic resonance angiography. *Adv Neurol,* 92:43–52.

Leeming, B.W.A., Simon, M. (1982). CLIP: A 1982 update. *Proceedings of the 7th Conference on Computer Applications in Radiology,* Boston, MA, pp. 273–289.

Lehr, J.L., Lodwick, G.S., Nicholson, B.F., Birznieks, F.B. (1973). Experience with MARS (Missouri Automated Radiology System). *Radiology,* 106(2):289-294.

Leiner, F., Haux, R. (1996). Systematic planning of clinical documentation. *Methods of Information in Medicine,* 35:25–34.

Leitch, D. (1989). Who should have their cholesterol measured? What experts in the UK suggest. *British Medical Journal,* 298:1615–1616.

Lenert ,L.A., Michelson, D., Flowers, C., Bergen, M.R. (1995). IMPACT: An object-oriented graphical environment for construction of multimedia patient interviewing software. *Proceedings of the Annual Symposium of Computer Applications in Medical Care,* Washington, DC, pp. 319–323.

Lenhart, A., Horrigan, J., et al. (2003). *The Ever-Shifting Internet Population: A New Look at Internet Access and the Digital Divide.* Pew Internet & American Life Project. (Accessed 2005 at: http://www.pewinternet.org/reports/toc.asp?Report=88)

Lesgold, A., Rubinson, H., Feltovich, P., Glaser, R., Klopfer, D., Wang, Y. (1988). Expertise in a complex skill: Diagnosing x-ray pictures. In M. T. H. Chi & R. Glaser (eds.), *The Nature of Expertise,* pp. 311-342. Hillsdale, NJ: Lawrence Erlbaum Associates.

Lesgold, A.M. (1984). Acquiring expertise. In J. R. Anderson & S. M. Kosslyn (eds.), *Tutorials in Learning and Memory: Essays in Honor of Gordon Bowe, pp.* 31-60. San Francisco, CA: W.H. Freeman.

Lesk, M. (1997). *Practical Digital Libraries: Books, Bytes, & Bucks.* San Francisco. Morgan Kaufmann.

Levit, KR. et al. (2003). Trends in U.S. health care spending, *Health Affairs,* 22(1): 154 –64.

Levit, K.R., Lazenby, H.C., Braden, B.R., Cowan, C.A., McDonnell, P.A., Sivarajan, L., Stiller, J.M., Won, D.K., Donham, C.S., Long, A.M., Stewart, M.W. (1996). Data view: National health expenditures, 1995. *Health Care Financing Review,* 18:175–214.

Levitt, M. (1983). Molecular dynamics of native protein. I. Computer simulation of trajectories. *Journal of Molecular Biology,* 168(3):595–617.

Leymann, F., Roller, D. (2000). *Production Workflow: Concepts and Techniques;* New York: Prentice-Hall.

Liberman, L., Menell, J.H. (2002). Breast imaging reporting and data system (BI-RADS). *Radiol Clin North Am.* 40(3):409–430.

Libicki, M.C. (1995). *Information Technology Standards: Quest for the Common Byte:* Digital Press.

Lichtenbelt, B., Crane, R., Naqvi, S. (1998). *Introduction to Volume Rendering.* Upper Saddle River, N.J.: Prentice Hall.

Lin, L., Isla, R., Doniz, K., Harkness, H., Vicente, K.J., Doyle, D. J. (1998). Applying human factors to the design of medical equipment: Patient-controlled analgesia. *Journal of Clinical Monitoring & Computing,* 14(4),253–263.

Lin, L., Vicente, K.J., Doyle, D.J. (2001). Patient safety, potential adverse drug events, and medical device design: a human factors engineering approach. *Journal of Biomedical Informatics.,* 34(4),274 –284.

Lincoln, Y.S., Guba, E.G. (1985). *Naturalistic Inquiry.* Beverly Hills, CA: Sage Publications.

Lindberg, D.A.B. (1965). Operation of a hospital computer system. *Journal of the American Veterinary Medical Association,* 147(12):1541–1544.

Lindberg, D.A.B., Humphreys, B.L., McCray, A.T. (1993). The Unified Medical Language System. *Methods of Information in Medicine,* 32(4):281–291.

Lipton, E, Johnson, K (2001): The Anthrax Trail; Tracking Bioterror's Tangled Course. *New York Times,* Section A, p. 1, 12/26/2001.

Lorensen, W.E., Cline, H.E. (1987). Marching cubes: A high resolution 3-D surface construction algorithm. *ACM Computer Graphics,* 21(4):163–169.

Lorenzi, N.M., Riley, R.T., Blyth, A.J., Southon, G., Dixon, B.J. (1997). Antecedents of the people and organizational aspects of medical informatics. *Journal of the American Medical Informatics Association,* 4(2):79–93.

Lou, S.L., Huang, H.K., Arenson, R.L. (1996). Workstation design: Image manipulation, image set handling, and display issues. In Greenes, R.A. & Bauman, R.A. (eds.) Imaging and information management: computer systems for a changing health care environment. *The Radiology Clinics of North America,* 34(3):525–544.

Lowe, H.J., Barnett, G.O. (1994). Understanding and using the medical subject headings (MeSH) vocabulary to perform literature searches. *Journal of the American Medical Association,* 271(14):1103–1108.

Lusignan, S.D., Stephens, P.N., Adal, N., Majeed, A. (2002) Does feedback improve the quality of computerized medical records in primary care. *Journal of American Medical Informatics Association,* 9,395– 401.

Lussier, Y, Shagina, L, Friedman, C. (2001). Automating SNOMED coding using medical language understanding: A feasibility study. *Proceedings of the AMIA Annual Symposium,* pp. 418– 422. Phila: Hanley&Belfus.

Lyon Jr., H.C., Healy, J.C., Bell, J.R., O'Donnell, J.F., Shultz, E.K., Moore-West, M., Wigton, R.S., Hirai, F., Beck, J.R. (1992). PlanAlyzer: An interactive computer-assisted program to teach clinical problem solving in diagnosing anemia and coronary artery disease. *Academic Medicine,* 67(12):821–828.

Maas, M.L., Johnson, M., Moorhead, S. (1996). Classifying nursing-sensitive patient outcomes. *Image: Journal of Nursing Scholarship,* 28(4):295–301.

Macklin, R. (1992). Privacy and control of genetic information. In Annas G.J., Elias S. (eds.), *Gene Mapping: Using Law and Ethics as Guides.* New York: Oxford University Press.

Mahon, BE, Rosenman, MB, Kleiman, MB. (2001). Maternal and infant use of erythromycin and other macrolide antibiotics as risk factors for infantile hypertrophic pyloric stenosis. *J Pediat,* 139(3):380–384.

Major, K., Shabot, M.M., Cunneen, S. (2002). Wireless clinical alerts and patient outcomes in the surgical intensive care unit. *Am Surg.* 68(12):1057–60.

Malcolm, S., Goodship, J. (eds.) (2001). *Genotype to Phenotype* (2nd Edition). BIOS Scientific Publishers Ltd.

Malet, G., Munoz, F., et al. (1999). A model for enhancing Internet medical document retrieval with "medical core metadata". *Journal of the American Medical Informatics Association,* 6:183–208.

Maloney Jr., J. (1968). The trouble with patient monitoring. *Annals of Surgery,* 168(4):605–619.

Managed Care Trends Digest (2000). Managed Care Digest Series 2000,. Parsippany, NJ: Aventis Pharmaceuticals, Inc.

Manning, C.D., Schütze, H. (1999). *Foundations of Statistical Natural Language Processing.* Cambridge: MIT Press.

Mant, J., Hicks, N. (1995). Detecting differences in quality of care: The sensitivity of measures of process and outcome in treating acute myocardial infarction. *British Medical Journal,* 311(7008):793–796.

Margulies, S.I., Wheeler, P.S. (1972). Development of an automated reporting system. *Proceedings of the Conference on Computer Applications in Radiology,* Columbia, MO, pp. 423– 440.

Maroto, M., Reshef, R., Munsterberg, A.E., Koester, S., Goulding, M., Lassar, A.B. (1997). Ectopic Pax-3 activates MyoD and Myf-5 expression in embryonic mesoderm and neural tissue. *Cell,* 89:139– 48.

Marrone, T.J., Briggs, J.M., McCammon, J.A. (1997). Structure-based drug design: Computational advances. *Annual Review of Pharmacology and Toxicology,* 37:71–90.

Marshall, E. (1996). Hot property: biologists who compute [news]. *Science*, 272(5269):1730–1732.

Marti,n K.S., Scheet, N.J. (1992). *The Omaha System: Applications for Community Health Nursing*. Philadelphia: WB Saunders.

Martin, K.S., Scheet, N.J. (eds.) (1995). *The Omaha System: Nursing diagnoses, Interventions, and Client Outcomes*. Washington, D.C.: American Nurses Publishing.

Martin, R.F., Bowden, D.M. (2001). *Primate Brain Maps: Structure of the Macaque Brain*. New York: Elsevier Science.

Martin, R.F., Mejino, J.L.V., Bowden, D.M., Brinkley, J.F., Rosse, C. (2001). Foundational model of neuroanatomy: Implications for the Human Brain Project, *Proc AMIA Annu Fall Symp*, pp. 438– 442. Washington, DC.

Martin, R.F., Poliakov, A.V., Mulligan, K.A., Corina, D.P., Ojemann, G.A., Brinkley, J.F. (2000). Multi-patient mapping of language sites on 3-D brain models. *Neuroimage* (Human Brain Mapping Annual Meeting, June 12–16), 11(5),S534.

Massoud, T.F., Gambhir, S.S. (2003). Molecular imaging in living subjects: seeing fundamental biological processes in a new light. *Genes and Development,* 17,545–580.

Masys, D.R. (1992). An evaluation of the source selection elements of the prototype UMLS information sources map. *Proceedings of the 16th Annual Symposium on Computer Applications in Medical Care*, Baltimore, MD, pp. 295–298.

Masys, D.R. (2001). Knowledge Management: Keeping Up with the Growing Knowledge. *Speech given at the IOM Annual Meeting 2001*. (Accessed 2005 at: http://www.iom.edu/subpage. asp?id=7774

Mayes, R.T., Draper, S.W., McGregor, A.M., Oatley, K. (1988). Information flow in a user interface: The effect of experience of and context on the recall of MacWrite screens. In D. M. Jones & R. Winder (eds.), *People and Computers IV*, pp. 257–289. Cambridge, England: Cambridge University Press.

Mazziotta, J., Toga, A., Evans, A., Fox, P., et al. (2001). A four-dimensional probabilistic atlas of the human brain. *J Am Med Inform Ass,* 8(5), 401– 430.

McAlister, F.A., Laupacis, A., Teo, K.K., Hamilton, P.G., Montague, T.J. (1997). A survey of clinician attitudes and management practices in hypertension. *J Hum Hypertens,* 11(7), 413–419.

McAlister, F.A., Teo, K.K., Lewanczuk, R.Z., Wells, G., Montague, T.J. (1997). Contemporary practice patterns on the management of newly diagnosed hypertension. *Canadian Medical Association Journal,* 157(1), 23–30.

McCloskey, J.C., Bulecheck, G.M. (1996). *Nursing Interventions Classification*. (2nd ed.). St. Louis: C.V. Mosby.

McCormick, K.A., Lang, N., Zielstorff, R., Milholland, D.K., Saba, V., Jacox, A. (1994). Toward standard classification schemes for nursing language: Recommendations of the American Nurses Association Steering Committee on Databases to Support Clinical Nursing Practice. *Journal of the American Medical Informatics Association*, 1(6):421– 427.

McCray, A., Gallagher, M. (2001). Principles for digital library development. *Communications of the ACM*, 44:49–54.

McCray, A.T., Miller, R.A. (1998). Focus on the Unified Medical Language System. *Journal of the American Medical Informatics Association*, 5(1):1–138.

McDaniel, A.M. (1997). Developing and testing a prototype patient care database. *Computers in Nursing*, 15(3):129–136.

McDonald, C.J. (1973). Computer applications to ambulatory care, *Proceedings of the IEEE Conference on Systems, Man, and Cybernetics*. Boston, MA.

McDonald, C.J. (1976). Protocol-based computer reminders, the quality of care and the non-perfectibility of man. *New England Journal of Medicine*, 295(24):1351–1355.

McDonald, C.J. (1984). The search for national standards for medical data exchange. *MD Computing*, 1(1):3–4.

McDonald, C.J. (ed.) (1987). *Tutorials (M.D. Computing: Benchmark Papers)*. New York: Springer-Verlag.

McDonald, C.J. (1988). Computer-stored medical record systems. *M.D. Computing*, 5(5):1–62.

McDonald, C.J. (1997). The barriers to electronic medical record systems and how to overcome them. *Journal of the American Medical Informatics Association*, 4(3):213–221.

McDonald, C.J., Bhargava, B., Jeris, D.W. (1975). A clinical information system (CIS) for ambulatory care. *Proc AFIPS Natl Comput Conf*, Anaheim, California.

McDonald, C.J., Dexter, P., Schadow, G., Chueh, H.G., Abernathy, G., Hook, J., Blevins, L., Overhage, J.M., Berman, J.J. (2005). SPIN Query tools for de-identified research on a humongous database. *Proceedings AMIA Annu Symp*, pp. 515–519.

McDonald, C.J., Huff, S.M., Suico, J.G., Hill, G., Leavelle, D., Aller, R., Forrey, A., Mercer, K., DeMoor, G., Hook, J., Williams, W., Case, J., Maloney, P. (2003). LOINC, a universal standard for identifying laboratory observations: A 5-year update. *Clinical Chemistry*, 49(4):624–633.

McDonald, C.J., Hui, S.L., Smith, D.M., Tierney, W.M., Cohen, S.J., Weinberger, M., McCabe, G.P. (1984). Reminders to physicians from an introspective computer medical record. A two year randomized trial. *Annals of Internal Medicine*, 100(1):130–138.

McDonald, C.J., Overhage, J.M., Dexter, P., Takesue, B.Y., Dwyer, D.M. (1997). A framework for capturing clinical data sets from computerized sources. *Annals of Internal Medicine*, 127(8):675–682.

McDonald, C.J., Overhage, J.M., Tierney, W.M., et al. (1999). The Regenstrief Medical Record System: A quarter century experience. *Int J Med Inf.* 54(3):225–53.

McDonald, C.J., Overhage, J.M., Barnes, M., Schadow, G., Blevins, L., Dexter, P.R., Mamlin, B, and the INPC management committee (2005). The Indiana network for patient care: A working local health information infrastructure. *Helth Aff* (Millwood). 24(5):1214–1220.

McDonald, C.J., Tierney, W.M. (1986a). Research uses of computer-stored practice records in general medicine. *Journal of General Internal Medicine*, 1(4 supplement):S19–S24.

McDonald, C.J., Tierney, W.M. (1986b). The medical gopher: A microcomputer system to help find, organize and decide about patient data. *The Western Journal of Medicine*, 145(6):823–829.

McDonald, C.J., Tierney, W.M., Overhage, J.M., Martin, D.K., Wilson, G.A. (1992). The Regenstrief Medical Record System: 20 years of experience in hospitals, clinics, and neighborhood health centers. *MD Computing*, 9(4):206–217.

McDonald, C.J., Schadow, G., Barnes, M., Dexter, P., Overhage, J.M., Mamlin, B., McCoy, J.M. (2003). Open Source software in medical informatics: Why, how and what. *Int J Med Inform*, 69:175–184.

McDonald, C.J., Wiederhold, G., Simborg, D., Hammond, W.E., Jelovsek, F., Schneider, K. (1984). A discussion of the draft proposal for data exchange standards for clinical laboratory results. *Proceedings of the 8th Annual Symposium on Computer Applications in Medical Care*, pp. 406–413.

MacDonald, D. (1993). *Register*: McConnel Brain Imaging Center, Montreal Neurological Institute.

MacDonald, D., Kabani, N., Avis, D., Evans, A. C. (2000). Automated 3-D extraction of inner and outer surfaces of cerebral cortex from MRI. *Neuroimage, 12*(3),340–356.

McFarland, G.K., McFarlane, E.A. (1993). *Nursing Diangosis & Intervention: Planning for Patient Care*. (2nd ed.). St. Louis: Mosby.

McGlynn, E.A., Asch, S.M., Adams, J.. et al (2003): The quality of health care delivered to adults in the United States. *NEJM* 348:2635–2645.

McGrath, J.C., Wagner, W.H., Shabot, M.M. (1996). When is ICU care warranted after carotid endarterectomy? *The American Surgeon*, 62(10):811–814.

McIntosh, N. (2002). Intensive care monitoring: Past, present, future. *Clin Med*, 2(4):349–355

McKibbon, K., Haynes, R., et al. (1990). How good are clinical MEDLINE searches? A comparative study of clinical end-user and librarian searches. *Computers and Biomedical Research*, 23(6):583–593.

McKinin, E.J., Sievert, M.E., Johnson, E.D., Mitchell, J.A. (1991). The Medline/full-text research project. *Journal of the American Society for Information Science*, 42:297–307.

McKnight, L, Wilcox, AB, Hripcsak, G. (2002). The effect of sample size and disease prevalence on supervised machine learning of narrative data. *Proceedings of the AMIA Annual Symp*, pp. 519–522.

McLaughlin, P.J., Dayhoff, M.D. (1970). Eukaryotes versus prokaryotes: An estimate of evolutionary distance. *Science*, 168(938):1469–1471.

McNeer, J.F., Wallace, A.G., Wagner, G.S., Starmer, C.F., Rosati, R.A. (1975). The course of acute myocardial infarction: Feasibility of early discharge of the uncomplicated patient. *Circulation*, 51:410–413.

McPhee, S.J., Bird, J.A., Fordham, D., Rodnick, J.E., Osborn, E.H. (1991). Promoting cancer prevention activities by primary care physicians: results of a randomized, controlled trial. *Journal of the American Medical Association*, 266(4):538–544.

Medicare Board of Trustees (1996). *1996 Annual Report of the Board of Trustees of the Federal Hospital Insurance Trust Fund and of the Federal Supplementary Medical Insurance Trust Fund*. Washington, DC.

Meek, J. (2001). Science world in revolt at power of the journal owners. The Guardian.

Mehta, T.S., Raza, S., Baum, J.K. (2000). Use of Doppler ultrasound in the evaluation of breast carcinoma. *Semin Ultrasound CT MR*, 21(4),297–307.

Meigs, J., Barry, M., Oesterling, J., Jacobsen, S. (1996). Interpreting results of prostate-specific antigen testing for early detection of prostate cancer. *Journal of General Internal Medicine*, 11(9):505–512.

Mejino, J.L.V., Noy, N.F., Musen, M.A., Brinkley, J.F., Rosse, C. (2001). Representation of structural relationships in the foundational model of anatomy, *Proceedings of the AMIA Fall Symposium*, p. 973. Washington, DC.

Melton III, L.J. (1996). History of the Rochester Epidemiology Project. *Mayo Clin Proc*; 71: 266–274.

Michaelis, J., Wellek, S., Willems, J.L. (1990). Reference standards for software evaluation. *Methods of Information in Medicine*, 29(4):289–297.

Michel, A., Zorb, L., Dudeck, J. (1996). Designing a low-cost bedside workstation for intensive care units. *Proceedings of the AMIA Annual Fall Symposium*, Washington, DC, pp. 777–781.

Miettinen, O.S. (1998). Evidence in medicine: Invited commentary. *CMAJ* 158(2):215–221.

Miksch, S., Shahar, Y., Johnson, P. (1997). Asbru: A task-specific, intention-based, and time-oriented language for representing skeletal plans. *Proceedings of the Seventh Workshop on Knowledge Engineering Methods and Languages* (KEML-97) (Milton Keynes, UK).

Miles, W.D (1982). *A History of the National Library of Medicine: The Nation's Treasury of Medical Knowledge*. Bethesda, MD: U.S. Department of Health and Human Services.

Millenson, M. (1997) *Demanding Medical Evidence: Doctors and Accountability in the Information Age*, Chicago: University of Chicago Press.

Miller, E. (1998). An introduction to the Resource Description Framework. *D-Lib Magazine*.

Miller, G.A., Galanter, E., Pribram, K.H. (1986). *Plans and the Structure of Behavior*. New York: Adams-Bannister-Cox.

Miller, N., Lacroix, E., et al. (2000). MEDLINEplus: Building and maintaining the National Library of Medicine's consumer health Web service. *Bulletin of the Medical Library Association*, 88:11–17.

Miller, P.L. (1986). *Expert Critiquing Systems: Practice-Based Medical Consultation by Computer*. New York: Springer-Verlag.

Miller, P.L. (1988). *Selected Topics in Medical Artificial Intelligence.* New York: Springer-Verlag.

Miller, P.L., Frawley SJ, Sayward FG (2001). Exploring the utility of demographic data and vaccination history data in the deduplication of immunization registry patient records. *J Biomed Inform,* 34(1):37–50.

Miller, R.A., Masarie, F. (1990). The demise of the Greek oracle model for medical diagnosis systems. *Methods of Information in Medicine,* 29:1–2.

Miller, R.A., Pople Jr., H., Meyers, J. (1982). INTERNIST-1: An experimental computer-based diagnostic consultant for general internal medicine. *New England Journal of Medicine,* 307:468–476.

Miller, R., Schaffner, K., Meisel, A. (1985). Ethical and legal issues related to the use of computer programs in clinical medicine. *Annals of Internal Medicine,* 102(4):529–537.

Miller, R.A. (1989). Legal issues related to medical decision support systems. *International Journal of Clinical Monitoring and Computing,* 6:75–80.

Miller, R.A. (1990). Why the standard view is standard: people, not machines, understand patients' problems. *Journal of Medicine and Philosophy,* 15(6):581–591.

Miller, R.A., Gardner, R.M. (1997a). Summary recommendations for responsible monitoring and regulation of clinical software systems. *Annals of Internal Medicine,* 127(9):842–845.

Miller, R.A., Gardner, R.M. (1997b). Recommendations for responsible monitoring and regulation of clinical software systems. *Journal of the American Medical Informatics Association,* 4(6):442–457.

Miller, R.A., Gieszczykiewicz F.M., Vries J.K., Cooper G.F. (1992). CHARTLINE: Providing bibliographic references relevant to patient charts using the UMLS Metathesaurus knowledge sources. *Proceedings of the 16th Annual Symposium on Computer Applications in Medical Care,* Baltimore, MD, pp. 86–90.

Miller, R.A., Goodman, K.W. (1998). Ethical challenges in the use of decision-support software in clinical practice. In Goodman K.W. (ed.), *Ethics, Computing, and Medicine: Informatics and the Transformation of Health Care.* Cambridge: Cambridge University Press.

Miller, R.A., McNeil, M.A., Challinor, S.M., Masarie Jr., F.E., Myers, J.D. (1986). The INTERNIST-1/Quick Medical Reference project: Status report. *Western Journal of Medicine,* 145(6):816–822.

Modayur, B., Portero, J., Ojemann, G., Maravilla, K., Brinkley, J. (1997). Visualization-based mapping of language function in the brain. *Neuroimage,* 6(4):245–258.

Mohr, D.N., Offord, K.P., Owen, R.A., Melton, L.J. (1986). Asymptomatic microhematuria and urologic disease. A population-based study. *Journal of the American Medical Association,* 256(2):224–229.

Morris, AH. (2003). Treatment algorithms and protocolized care. *Curr Opin Crit Care* 9:236–240

Morris, A.H. (2001). Rational use of computerized protocols in the intensive care unit. *Crit Care,* 5(5):249–254

Mortensen, R.A., Nielsen, G.H. (1996). *International Classification of Nursing Practice (Version 0.2).* Geneva, Switzerland: International Council of Nursing.

Moses, L.E., Littenberg, B., Shapiro, D. (1993). Combining independent studies of a diagnostic test into a summary ROC curve: Data-analytic approaches and some additional considerations. *Statistics in Medicine,* 12(4):1293–1316.

Muller, H., Michoux, N., Bandon, D., Geissbuhler, A. (2004). A review of content-based image retrieval systems in medical applications: Clinical benefits and future directions. *Int J Med Inform.* 73(1):1–23.

Mulrow, C.D. (1987). The medical review article: State of the science. *Annals of Internal Medicine,* 106:485–488.

Mulrow, C., Cook, D., et al. (1997). Systematic reviews: Critical links in the great chain of evidence. *Annals of Internal Medicine,* 126: 389–391.

Munnecke, T., Kuhn, I. (1989). Large-scale portability of hospital information system software within the Veterans Administration. In H. Orthner and B. Blum (ed.), *Implementing Health Care Information Systems.* New York: Springer-Verlag.

Murphy, P. (1994). Reading ability of parents compared with reading level of pediatric patient education materials. *Pediatrics,* 93: 460–468.

Musen M.A. (1993). An overview of knowledge acquisition. In David J.M., Krivine J.P., Simmons R. (eds.), *Second Generation Expert Systems,* pp.415-438. Berlin: Springer-Verlag.

Musen, M.A. (1997). Modeling for decision support. In van Bemmel, J., Musen, M. (eds.), *Handbook of Medical Informatics,* pp.431–448. Heidelberg: Springer-Verlag.

Musen, M.A.. (1998). Domain ontologies in software engineering: Use of PROTÉGÉ with the EON architecture. *Methods of Information in Medicine,* 37(4-5):540–550.

Musen, M.A., Carlson, R.W., Fagan, L.M., Deresinski S.C. (1992). T-HELPER: Automated support for community-based clinical research. *Proceedings of the 16th Annual Symposium on Computer Applications in Medical Care,* Baltimore, MD, pp. 719–723.

Musen, M.A., Fagan, L.M., Combs, D.M., Shortliffe, E.H. (1987). Use of a domain model to drive an interactive knowledge-editing tool. *International Journal of Man-Machine Studies,* 26(1):105–121.

Musen, M.A., Gennari, J.H., Eriksson, H., Tu, S.W., Puerta, A.R. (1995). PROTÉGÉ-II: Computer support for development of intelligent systems from libraries of components. *Proceedings of the MEDINFO 1995,* Vancouver, British Columbia, pp. 766–770.

Musen, M.A., Tu, S.W., Das, A.K., Shahar, Y. (1996). EON: A component-based approach to automation of protocol-directed therapy. *Journal of the American Medical Informatics Association,* 3(6):367–388.

Mutalik, P.G., Deshpande, A., Nadkarni, P.M. (2001). Use of general-purpose negation detection to augment concept indexing of medical documents: A quantitative study using the UMLS. *J Am Med Inform Assoc*; 8(6):598–609.

Mynatt, B., Leventhal, L., et al. (1992). Hypertext or book: Which is better for answering questions? *Proceedings of Computer-Human Interface 92,* pp.19–25.

Nadkarni, P, Chen, R, Brandt, C. (2001). UMLS concept indexing for production databases: A feasibility study. *J Am Med Inform Assoc*; 8(1):80–91.

Napoli, M., Nanni, M., Cimarra, S., Crisafulli, L., Campioni, P., Marano, P. (2003). Picture archiving and communication in radiology. *Rays,* 28(1):73–81.

National Committee for Quality Assurance (1997). *HEDIS 3.0.* Washington, DC: National Committee for Quality Assurance.

National Committee on Vital and Health Statistics (2000). NCVHS Report to the Secretary on Uniform Standards for Patient Medical Record Information. *NCVHS Reports and Recommendations.* (Accessed 2005 at: http://www.ncvhs.hhs.gov/hipaa000706.pdf)

National Committee on Vital and Health Statistics (2001). Information for Health: A Strategy for Building the National Health Information Infrastructure. *NCVHS Reports and Recommendations.* (Accessed 2005 at: http://www.ncvhs.hhs.gov/nhiilayo.pdf)

National Council for Prescription Drug Programs (1994). *Data Dictionary.*

National Equipment Manufacturers Association (NEMA) (2004). *DICOM 3.0 Specification.* http://www.nema.org/prod/med/dicom.cfm.

National League for Nursing (1987). *Guidelines for Basic Computer Education in Nursing.* New York: National League for Nursing.

National Library of Medicine. (1999, updated annually). *Medical Subject Headings -Annotated Alphabetic List.* Bethesda, MD: U.S. Department of Health and Human Services, Public Health Service.

National Priority Expert Panel on Nursing Informatics (1993). *Nursing Informatics: Enhancing Patient Care.* Bethesda, MD: U.S. Department of Health and Human Services, U.S. Public Health Service, National Institutes of Health.

National Research Council (1997). *For the Record: Protecting Electronic Health Information.* Washington, D.C.: National Academy Press.

National Research Council (2001). *Networking Health: Prescriptions for the Internet.* Washington, DC: National Academy Press.

National Vaccine Advisory Committee (1999). *Development of Community- and State-Based Immunization Registries.* (Accessed 2005 at: http://www.cdc.gov/nip/registry/nvac.htm)

Nease Jr, R.F., Kneeland, T., O'Connor, G.T., Sumner, W., Lumpkins, C., Shaw, L., Pryor, D., Sox, H.C. (1995). Variation in patient utilities for the outcomes of the management of chronic stable angina. Implications for clinical practice guidelines. *Journal of the American Medical Association,* 273(15):1185–1190.

Ncase Jr, R.F., Owens, D.K. (1994). A method for estimating the cost-effectiveness of incorporating patient preferences into practice guidelines. *Medical Decision Making,* 14(4):382-92.

Nease Jr., R.F., Owens, D.K. (1997). Use of influence diagrams to structure medical decisions. *Medical Decision Making,* 17(13):263–275.

Nease Jr., R. F., Tsai, R., Hynes, L.H., Littenberg, B. (1996). Automated utility assessment of global health. *Quality of Life Research,* 5(1):175–182.

Needleman, S.B., Wunsch, C.D. (1970). A general method applicable to the search for similarities in the amino acid sequence of two proteins. *Journal of Molecular Biology,* 48(3):443–453.

Neisser, U. (1967). *Cognitive Psychology.* New York,: Appleton-Century-Crofts.

Nelson, S.J., Brown, S.H., Erlbaum, M.S., Olson, N., Powell, T., Carlsen, B., Carter, J., Tuttle, M.S., Hole, W.T.(2002) A semantic normal form for clinical drugs in the UMLS: Early experience with the VANDF. *Proceedings of the AMIA Fall Symposium;* pp 557–561.

Newell, A. (1990). *Unified Theories of Cognition.* Cambridge, Mass.: Harvard University Press.

Newell, A., Simon, H.A. (1972). *Human Problem Solving.* Englewood Cliffs, N.J.: Prentice-Hall.

Newhouse, J. (1993) *Free for All? Lessons from the Rand Health Insurance Experiment,* Cambridge, MA: Harvard University Press.

New York Academy of Medicine (1961). *Standard Nomenclature of Diseases and Operations.* (5th ed.). New York: McGraw-Hill.

Nguyen, J.H., Shahar, Y., Tu, S.W., Das, A.K., Musen, M.A. (1997). A temporal database mediator for protocol-based decision support. *Proceedings of the AMIA Annual Fall Symposium,* Nashville, TN, pp. 298–302.

NHS Centre for Coding and Classification (1994a). *Read Codes, Version 3.* (April ed.). London: NHS Management Executive, Department of Health.

NHS Centre for Coding and Classification (1994b). *Read Codes and the Terms Projects: A Brief Guide.* (April ed.). Leicestershire, Great Britain: NHS Management Executive, Department of Health.

Nielsen, G.H., Mortensen, R.A. (1996). The architecture for an International Classification of Nursing Practice (ICNP). *International Nursing Review,* 43(6):175–182.

Nielsen, J. (1993). *Usability Engineering.* Boston: Academic Press.

Nielsen, J. (1994). Heuristic evaluation. In J. Nielsen & R. L. Mack (eds.), *Usability Inspection Methods,* pp. 25-62. New York: Wiley & Sons, Inc.

Norman, D.A. (1986). Cognitive engineering. In D. A. Norman & S. W. Draper (eds.), *User Centered System Design: New Perspectives on Human-Computer Interaction,* pp. 31–61. Hillsdale, NJ: Lawrence Erlbaum Associates.

Norman, D.A. (1988). *The Psychology of Everyday Things.* New York: Basic Books.

Norman, D.A. (1993). *Things That Make Us Smart: Defending Human Attributes in the Age of the Machine*. Reading, Mass.: Addison-Wesley Pub. Co.

Norman, F. (1996). Organizing medical networked information: OMNI. *Medical Informatics*, 23: 43–51.

O'Carroll, P.W., Friede, A., Noji, E.K., Lillebridge, S.R., Fries, D.J., Atchison, C.G. (1995). The rapid implementation of a statewide emergency health information system during the 1993 Iowa flood. *American Journal of Public Health*, 85(4):564–567.

O'Carroll, P.W., Yasnoff, W.A., Ward, M.E., Ripp, L.H., Martin, E.L. (eds.) (2003). *Public Health Informatics and Information Systems*. New York: Springer-Verlag.

O'Connell, E.M., Teich, J.M., Pedraza, L.A., Thomas, D. (1996). A comprehensive inpatient discharge system. *Proceedings of the AMIA Annual Fall Symposium*, Washington, D.C., pp. 699-703.

O'Donnell-Maloney, M.J., Little, D.P. (1996). Microfabrication and array technologies for DNA sequencing and diagnostics. *Genetic Analysis*, 13(6):151–157.

Office of Technology Assessment (OTA) (1980). *The Implications of Cost-Effectiveness Analysis of Medical Technology*. Washington D.C.: Congress of the United States, U.S. Government Printing Office.

Ohno-Machado, L., Gennari, J.H., Murphy, S.N., et al. (1998). The guideline interchange format: A model for representing guidelines. *Journal of the American Medical Informatics Association*, 5:357–72.

Ohta, T., Tateisi, Y., Mima, H,., Tsujii, J. (2002). GENIA Corpus: An annotated research abstract corpus in molecular biology domain. *Proceedings of the Human Language Technology Conference (HLT 2002)*, pp. 73–77.

Ojemann, G., Ojemann, J., Lettich, E., Berger, M. (1989). Cortical language localization in left, dominant hemisphere: an electrical stimulation mapping investigation in 117 patients. *J. Neurosurgery*, 71, 316–326.

Oldendorf, W.H., Oldendorf Jr., W.H. (1991). *MRI Primer*. New York: Raven Press.

Oniki, T.A., Clemmer, T.P., Pryor, T.A. (2003). The effect of computer-generated reminders on charting deficiencies in the ICU. *Journal of the American Medical Informatics Association*, 10:177–187

Ono, M.S., Kubik, S., Abernathy, C.D. (1990). *Atlas of the Cerebral Sulci*. New York: Thieme Medical Publishers.

Organization for Human Brain Mapping. (2001). *Proceedings of the Annual Conference on Human Brain Mapping*. Brighton, United Kingdom.

Orthner, H.F., Blum, B.I. (eds.) (1989). *Implementing Health Care Information Systems*. New York: Springer-Verlag.

Osheroff, J. (ed.) (1995). *Computers in Clinical Practice. Managing Patients, Information, and Communication*. Philadelphia, PA: American College of Physicians.

O'Sullivan, J., Franco, C., Fuchs, B., Lyke, B., Price, R., Swendiman, K. (1997). *Medicare Provisions in the Balanced Budget Act of 1997*. Congressional Research Service Report for Congress BBA 97, P.L. 105–33.

Overhage, J.M. (ed.) (1998). *Proceedings of the Fourth Annual Nicholas E. Davies CPR Recognition Symposium*. Schaumburg, IL: Computer-based Patient Record Institute.

Overhage, J.M. (2002). Personal Communication.

Overhage, J.M., Dexter, P.R., Perkins, S.M., Cordell, W.H., McGoff, J., McGrath, R., McDonald, C.J. (2002). A randomized, controlled trial of clinical information shared from another institution. *Ann Emerg Med*; 39(1):14–23.

Overhage, J.M., Suico, J., McDonald, C.J. (2001). Electronic laboratory reporting: barriers, solutions and findings. *J Public Health Manag Prac*; 7(6):60–6.

Owens, D., Harris, R., Scott, P., Nease Jr., R.F. (1995). Screening surgeons for HIV infection: A cost-effectiveness analysis. *Annals of Internal Medicine*, 122(9):641–652.

Owens, D.K. (1998a). Patient preferences and the development of practice guidelines. *Spine*, 23(9):1073–1079.

Owens D.K. (1998b). Interpretation of cost-effectiveness analyses. *Journal of General Internal Medicine*, 13(10):716–717.

Owens, D.K., Holodniy, M., Garber, A.M., Scott, J., Sonnad, S., Moses, L., Kinosian, B., Schwartz, J.S. (1996). The polymerase chain reaction for the diagnosis of HIV infection in adults: A meta-analysis with recommendations for clinical practice and study design. *Annals of Internal Medicine*, 124(9):803–15.

Owens, D.K., Holodniy, M., McDonald, T.W., Scott, J., Sonnad, S. (1996). A meta-analytic evaluation of the polymerase chain reaction (PCR) for diagnosis of human immunodeficiency virus (HIV) infection in infants. *Journal of the American Medical Association*, 275(17):1342–1348.

Owens, D.K., Nease Jr., R.F. (1993). Development of outcome-based practice guidelines: A method for structuring problems and synthesizing evidence. *Joint Commission Journal on Quality Improvement*, 19(7):248–263.

Owens, D.K., Nease Jr., R.F. (1997). A normative analytic framework for development of practice guidelines for specific clinical populations. *Medical Decision Making*, 17(4):409–426.

Owens, D.K., Sanders, G.D., Harris, R.A., McDonald, K.M., Heidenreich, P.A., Dembitzer, A.D., Hlatky, M.A. (1997). Cost-effectiveness of implantable cardioverter defibrillators relative to amiodarone for prevention of sudden cardiac death. *Annals of Internal Medicine*, 126(1):1–12.

Owens, D.K., Shachter, R.D., Nease Jr., R.F. (1997). Representation and analysis of medical decision problems with influence diagrams. *Medical Decision Making*, 17(3):241–262.

Ozbolt, J.F., Schultz II, S., Swain, M.A., Abraham, I.I. (1985). A proposed expert system for nursing practice: A springboard to nursing science. *Journal of Medical Systems*, 9(1–2):57–68.

Ozbolt, J.G. (1996). From minimum data to maximum impact: Using clinical data to strengthen patient care. *Advanced Practice Nursing Quarterly*, 1(4):62–69.

Ozbolt, J.G., Fruchnicht, J.N., Hayden, J.R. (1994). Toward data standards for clinical nursing information. *Journal of the American Medical Informatics Association*, 1(2):175–185.

Ozbolt, J.G., Russo, M., Stultz, M.P. (1995). Validity and reliability of standard terms and codes for patient care data. *Proceedings of the 19th Symposium on Computer Applications in Medical Care*, New Orleans, pp. 37–41.

Ozbolt, J. (2000). Terminology standards for nursing: Collaboration at the Summit. *Journal of the American Medical Informatics Association, 7:6*, 517–522.

Ozbolt, J. (2003). Reference terminology for therapeutic goals: A new approach. *Proceedings of the AMIA Fall Symposium*, pp. 504–08.

Ozbolt, J., Brennan G., Hatcher I. (2001). PathworX: An informatics tool for quality improvement. *Proceedings of the AMIA Fall Symposium*, pp 518–22.

Ozdas, A., Speroff, T., Waitman, L.R., Ozbolt, J., Butler, J., Miller, R.A. (2006). Integrating "best of care" protocols into clinicians' workflow via care provider order entry: Impact of quality of care indicators for acute myocardial infarction. *J Amer Med Informatics Assoc*, 13(2) [in press].

Pabst, M.K., Scherubel, J.C., Minnick, A.F. (1996). The impact of computerized documentation on nurses' use of time. *Computers in Nursing*, 14(1):25–30.

Paddock, S.W. (1994). To boldly glow: Applications of laser scanning confocal microscopy in developmental biology. *Bioessays*, 16(5):357–365.

Palda, V.A., Detsky, A.S. (1997). Perioperative assessment and management of risk from coronary artery disease. *Annals of Internal Medicine*, 127(4):313–328.

Palmer, S. (1978). Fundamental aspects of cognitive representation. In E. Rosh & B. B. Lloyd (eds.), *Cognition and Categorization*. Hillsdale, NJ: Lawrence Erlbaum Associates.

Paskin, N. (1999). DOI: Current status and outlook. *D-Lib Magazine*, 5. (Accessed 2005 at: http://www.dlib.org/dlib/may99/05paskin.html)

Patel, V.L. (1998). Individual to collaborative cognition: A paradigm shift? *Artif Intell Med*, 12(2), 93–96.

Patel, V.L., Allen, V.G., Arocha, J.F., Shortliffe, E.H. (1998). Representing clinical guidelines in GLIF: Individual and collaborative expertise. *Journal of the American Medical Informatics Association*, 5(5),467– 483.

Patel, V.L., Arocha, J.F. (1995). Cognitive models of clinical reasoning and conceptual representation. *Methods of Information in Medicine.*, 34(1–2),47–56.

Patel, V.L., Arocha, J.F., Diermeier, M., How, J., Mottur-Pilson, C. (2001). Cognitive psychological studies of representation and use of clinical practice guidelines. *International Journal of Medical Informatics*, 63(3), 147–167.

Patel, V.L., Arocha, J.F., Diermeier, M., Greenes, R.A., Shortliffe, E.H. (2001). Methods of cognitive analysis to support the design and evaluation of biomedical systems: The case of clinical practice guidelines. *Journal of Biomedical Informatics*, 34(1):52–66.

Patel, V.L., Arocha, J.F., Kaufman, D.R. (1994). Diagnostic reasoning and medical expertise. In D. L. Medin (ed.), *The Psychology of Learning and Motivation: Advances in Research and Theory* (Vol. 31), pp. 187–252. San Diego, CA: Academic Press, Inc.

Patel, V.L., Arocha, J.F., Kaufman, D.R. (2001). A primer on aspects of cognition for medical informatics. *Journal of the American Medical Informatics Association*, 8(4),324–343.

Patel, V.L., Branch, T, Arocha, J.F. (2002). Errors in interpreting quantities as procedures: The case of pharmaceutical labels. *International Journal of Medical Informatics*, 65(3),193–211.

Patel, V.L. Frederiksen, C.H. (1984). Cognitive processes in comprehension and knowledge acquisition by medical students and physicians. In H.G. Schmidt and M.C. de Volder (eds.), *Tutorials in Problem-Based Learning*, pp. 143–157. Assen, Holland: van Gorcum.

Patel, V.L., Groen, G.J. (1986). Knowledge-based solution strategies in medical reasoning. *Cognitive Science*, 10:91–116.

Patel, V.L., Groen, G.J. (1991). The general and specific nature of medical expertise: A critical look. In K. A. Ericsson & J. Smith (eds.), *Toward a General Theory of Expertise: Prospects and Limits*, pp. 93–125. New York, NY: Cambridge University Press.

Patel, V.L., Groen, G.J., Arocha, J.F. (1990). Medical expertise as a function of task difficulty. *Memory & Cognition*, 18(4), 394 – 406.

Patel, V.L., Groen, G.J., Frederiksen, C.H. (1986). Differences between students and physicians in memory for clinical cases. *Medical Education*, 20,3–9.

Patel, V.L., Kaufman, D. R. (1998). Medical informatics and the science of cognition. *JAMIA*, 5(6),493–502.

Patel, V.L., Kaufman, D.R., Arocha, J.F. (2000). Conceptual change in the biomedical and health sciences domain. In R. Glaser (ed.), *Advances in Instructional Psychology: Educational Design and Cognitive Science* (5th ed., Vol. 5), pp. 329–392. Mahwah, NJ: Lawrence Erlbaum Associates.

Patel, V.L., Kaufman, D.R., Arocha, J.F. (2002). Emerging paradigms of cognition in medical decision-making. *Journal of Biomedical Informatics*, 35,52–75.

Patel, V.L., Kaufman, D.R., Magder, S.A. (1996). The acquisition of medical expertise in complex dynamic environments. In K.A. Ericsson (ed.), *The Road to Excellence: The Acquisition of Expert Performance in the Arts and Sciences, Sports, and Games*, pp. 127–165. Hillsdale, NJ: Lawrence Erlbaum Associates, Inc.

Patel, V.L., Kushniruk, A.W., Yang, S., Yale, J.F. (2000). Impact of a computer-based patient record system on data collection, knowledge organization, and reasoning. *Journal of the American Medical Informatics Association.* 7(6), 569–585.

Patel, V.L., Ramoni, M.F. (1997). Cognitive models of directional inference in expert medical reasoning. In Feltovich, P.J., Ford, K.M., Hoffman, R.R. (eds.). *Expertise in Context*, pp. 67–99. Cambridge, MA: The MIT Press.

Patten, S.F., Lee, J.S., Nelson, A.C. (1996). NeoPath, Inc. NeoPath AutoPap 300 Automatic Pap Screener System. *Acta Cytologica*, 40(1):45–52.

Pauker, S.G., Gorry, G.A., Kassirer, J.P., Schwartz, W.B. (1976). Towards the simulation of clinical cognition. Taking a present illness by computer. *American Journal of Medicine*, 60(7):981–996.

Pauker, S.G., Kassirer, J.P. (1980). The threshold approach to clinical decision making. *New England Journal of Medicine*, 302(20):1109–1117.

Pauker, S.G., Kassirer, J.P. (1981). Clinical decision analysis by computer. *Archives of Internal Medicine*, 141(13):1831–1837.

Biondich, P.G., Anand, V., Downs, S.M., McDonald, C.J. (2003). Using adaptive turnaround documents to electronically acquire structured data in vlinical dettings. Proceedings of the AMIA Annual Symposium, pp. 86–90.

Paxinos, G., Watson, C. (1986). *The Rat Brain in Stereotaxic Coordinates*. San Diego: Academic Press.

Payne, S.H. (2003). User's mental models: The very idea. In J. M. Carroll (ed.), *HCI Models, Theories and Frameworks*, pp. 135–156. San Francisco, CA: Morgan Kauffman Publishers.

Peabody, G. (1922). The physician and the laboratory. *Boston Medical Surgery Journal*, 187:324.

Peleg, M., Boxwala, A., Bernstam, E., Tu, S.W., Greenes, R.A., Shortliffe, E.H. (2001). Sharable representation of clinical guidelines in GLIF: Relationship to the Arden syntax. *Journal of Biomedical Informatics,* 34:170–181.

Peleg, M, Boxwala, A.A., Omolola, O., Zeng, Q., Tu, S.W, Lacson, R., Bernstam, E., Ash, N., Mork, P., Ohno-Machado, L., Shortliffe, E.H., Greenes, R.A. (2000). GLIF3: The evolution of a guideline representation format. *Proceedings of the AMIA Annual Symposium*, pp. 645–649. Philadelphia: Hanley & Belfus.

Peleg, M, Boxwala, A.A., Tu, S., Zeng, Q., Ogunyemi, O, Wang, D, Patel, VL, Greenes, RA, Shortliffe, EH (2004). The InterMed approach to sharable computer-interpretable guidelines: A review. *Journal of the American Medical Informatics Association*, 11:1–10.

Perkins, D.N., Schwartz, S., Simmons, R. (1990). A view from programming. In M. Smith (ed.), *Toward a Unified Theory of Problem Solving: Views from Content Domains*. Hillsdale, NJ: Lawrence Erlbaum Associates.

Perkins, G., Renken, C., Martone, M.E., Young, S.J., Ellisman, M., Frey, T. (1997). Electron tomography of neuronal mitochondria: Three-dimensional structure and organization of cristae and menbrane contacts. *J. Structural Biology,* 119(3),260–272.

Peleg, M, Tu, S, Bury, J, Ciccarese, P., Fox, J., Greenes, R.A., Hall, R., Johnson, P.D., Jones, N., Kumar, A., Miksch, S., Quaglini, S., Seyfang,A., Shortliffe, E.H., Stefanelli, M. (2003). Comparing computer-interpretable guideline models: A case-study approach. *J Am Med Inform Asso,* 10(1):52–68

Perreault, L.E., Metzger, J.B. (1999). A pragmatic framework for understanding clinical decision support. *Healthcare Information Management,* 13(2);5–21.

Perry, M. (2003). Distributed cognition. In J. M. Carroll (ed.), *HCI Models, Theories, and Frameworks : Toward a Multidisciplinary Science*. San Francisco, Calif.: Morgan Kaufmann.

Peterson, W., Birdsall, T. (1953). *The Theory of Signal Detectability.* (Technical Report No. 13.): Electronic Defense Group, University of Michigan, Ann Arbor.

Piemme, T.E. (1988). Computer-assisted learning and evaluation in medicine. *Journal of the American Medical Association*, 260(3):367–372.

Pigoski, T.M. (1997): *Practical Software Maintenance: Best Practices for Managing Your Software Investment*, IEEE Computer Society Press.

Pinciroli, F. (1995). Virtual Reality for Medicine. *Computers in Biology and Medicine*, 25(2):81–83.

Polson, P.G., Lewis, C.H., Rieman, J., Wharton, C. (1992). Cognitive walkthroughs: A method for theory-based evaluation of user interfaces. *International Journal of Man-Machine Studies*, 36(5),741–773.

Ponte, J., Croft, W. (1998). A language modeling approach to information retrieval. *Proceedings of the 21st Annual International ACM SIGIR Conference on Research and Development in Information Retrieval*, Melbourne, Australia. ACM Press, pp. 275–281.

Poon, E.G., Kuperman, G.J., Fiskio, J., Bates, D.W. (2002). Real-time notification of laboratory data requested by users through alphanumeric pagers. *JAMIA*; 9(3):217–222.

Pople, H. (1982). Heuristic methods for imposing structure on ill-structured problems: The structuring of medical diagnosis. In Szolovits P. (ed.), *Artificial Intelligence in Medicine*. Boulder, CO: Westview Press.

Potchen, E. J. (2000). Prospects for progress in diagnostic imaging. *J. Internal Medicine*, 247(4), 411–424.

Pouratian, N., Sheth, S.A., Martin, N.A., Toga, A.W. (2003). Shedding light on brain mapping: Advances in human optical imaging. *Trends in Neurosciences*, 26(5):277–282.

Pratt, W., Hearst, M., et al. (1999). A knowledge-based approach to organizing retrieved documents. *Proceedings of the 16th National Conference on Artificial Intelligence*, pp 80–85. Orlando, FL.: AAAI.

President's Information Technology Advisory Committee (2001). *Transforming Health Care Through Information Technology*. (*President's Information Technology Advisory Committee: Panel on Transforming Health Care*).. (Accessed 2005 at: http://www.itrd.gov/pubs/pitac/pitac-hc-9feb01.pdf)

Prothero, J.S., Prothero, J.W. (1982). Three-dimensional reconstruction from serial sections: I. A portable microcomputer-based software package in Fortran. *Computers and Biomedical Research*, 15:598–604.

Prothero, J.S., Prothero, J.W. (1986). Three-dimensional reconstruction from serial sections IV. The reassembly problem. *Computers and Biomedical Research*, 19(4):361–373.

Pruitt, K.D., Maglott, D.R.. (2001). RefSeq and LocusLink: NCBI gene-centered resources. *Nucleic Acids Res*;29(1):137–140.

Pryor, T.A. (1988). The HELP medical record system. *MD Computing*, 5(5):22–33.

Pryor, T.A., Gardner, R.M., Clayton, P.D., Warner, H.R. (1983). The HELP system. *Journal of Medical Informatics* 7(2):87–102.

Public Health Service (1991). *Healthy People 2000: National Health Promotion and Disease Prevention Objectives: Full Report, with Commentary*. (DHHS publication no. (PHS)91–50212.): Washington, DC: U.S. Department of Health and Human Services, Public Health Service.

Pyper, C., Amery, J., Watson, M., Crook, C., Thomas, B. (2002). Patients' access to their online electronic health records. *J Telemed Telecare*. 8(Suppl 2):103–5.

Quaglini, S., Stefaneli, M., Lanzola, G., Caporusso, V., Panzarasa, S. (2001). Flexible guideline-based patient careflow systems. *Artificial Intelligence in Medicine* 22:65–80

Quarterman, J.S. (1990). *The Matrix: Computer Networks and Conferencing Systems Worldwide*: Digital Press.

Raiffa, H. (1970). *Decision Analysis: Introductory Lectures on Choices Under Uncertainty*. Reading, MA: Addison-Wesley.

Ransohoff, D.F., Feinstein, A.R. (1978). Problems of spectrum and bias in evaluating the efficacy of diagnostic tests. *New England Journal of Medicine*, 299(17):926–930.

Read, J.D. (1990). Computerizing medical language. In DeGlanville H., Roberts J. (eds.), *Current Perspectives in Health Computing HC90. British Journal of Health Care Computing*, pp.203–208.

Read, J.D., Benson, T.J. (1986). Comprehensive coding. *British Journal of Health Care Computing*, pp.:22–25.

Rector, A.L., Glowinski, A.J., Nowlan, W.A., Rossi-Mori, A. (1995). Medical-concept models and medical records: an approach based on GALEN and PEN & PAD. *Journal of the American Medical Informatics Association*, 2(1):19–35.

Rector, A.L., Nowlan, W.A., Glowinski, A. (1993). Goals for concept representation in the GALEN project. *Proceedings of the 17th Annual Symposium on Computer Applications in Medical Car, pp.* 414 – 418. New York: McGraw Hill.

Redman, P., Kelly, J., et al. (1997). Common ground: The HealthWeb project as a model for Internet collaboration. *Bulletin of the Medical Library Association*, 85: 325–330.

Reddy, M.C., Pratt, W., Dourish, P., Shabot, M. (2002). Asking questions: Information needs in a surgical intensive care unit. *Proc AMIA Symp.* pp. 647–651.

Reggia, J., Turhim, S. (eds.) (1985). *Computer-Assisted Medical Decision Making.* New York: Springer-Verlag.

Reich, V., Rosenthal, D. (2001). LOCKSS: A permanent Web publishing and access system. *D-Lib Magazine*, 7. (Accessed 2005 at: http://www.dlib.org/dlib/june01/reich/06reich.html)

Reiser, S. (1991). The clinical record in medicine. Part 1: Learning from cases. *Annals of Internal Medicine*, 114(10):902–907.

Reiser, S.J., Anbar, M. (eds.) (1984). *The Machine at the Bedside: Strategies for Using Technology in Patient Care.* Cambridge, MA: Cambridge University Press.

Richardson, J.S. (1981). The anatomy and taxonomy of protein structure. *Advances in Protein Chemistry*, 34:167–339.

Rimoldi, H.J.A. (1961). The test of diagnostic skills. *Journal of Medical Education,* 36:73–79.

Ringold, D.J.,et al., (2000). ASHP national survey of pharmacy practice in acute care settings: Dispensing and administration – 1999," *Am J Health Syst Pharm*, 57(19):1759–75.

Ritchie, C.J., Edwards, W.S., Cyr, D.R., Kim, Y. (1996). Three-dimensional ultrasonic angiography using power-mode Doppler. *Ultrasound in Medicine and Biology*, 22(3):277–286.

Robb, R.A. (2000). *Biomedical Imaging, Visualization, and Analysis.* New York: Wiley-Liss.

Robbins, A.H., Vincent, M.E., Shaffer, K., Maietta, R., Srinivasan, M.K. (1988). Radiology reports: Assessment of a 5,000-word speech recognizer. *Radiology*, 167(3):853–855.

Robertson, S., Walker, S. (1994). Some simple effective approximations to the 2-Poisson model for probabilistic weighted retrieval. *Proceedings of the 17th Annual International ACM SIGIR Conference on Research and Development in Information Retrieval*, pp. 232–241. Dublin, Ireland. Springer-Verlag.

Roethligsburger, F.J., Dickson, W.J. (1939). *Management and the Worker.* Cambridge, MA: Harvard University Press.

Rogers, W.A. (ed.). (2002). *Human Factors Interventions for the Health Care of Older Adults.* Mahwah, NJ: Lawrence Erlbaum Associates.

Rogers, Y. (2004). New theoretical approaches for HCI. *Annual Review of Information Science and Technology,* 38:87–143.

Rose, M.T. (1989). *The Open Book: A Practical Perspective on OSI.* New Jersey: Prentice Hall.

Rosen, G. (1993). *History of Public Health.* Baltimore, MD: Johns Hopkins University Press.

Rosen, G.D., Williams, A.G., Capra, J.A., Connolly, M.T., Cruz, B., Lu, L., Airey, D.C., Kulkarni, K., Williams, R.W. (2000). The Mouse Brain Library @ www.mbl.org, *Int. Mouse Genome Conference,* 14:166.

Ross, B., Bluml, S. (2001). Magnetic resonance spectroscopy of the human brain. *Anatomical Record (New Anat.),* 265(2),54–84.

Rosse, C. (2000). Terminologia Anatomica: Considered from the perspective of next-generation knowledge sources. *Clinical Anatomy*, 14:120–133.

Rosse, C., Mejino, J.L.V. (2003). A reference ontology for bioinformatics: The Foundational Model of Anatomy. *Journal of Bioinformatics*, 36(6),478–500.

Rosse, C., Mejino, J.L., Jakobovits, R.M., Modayur, B.R., Brinkley, J.F. (1997). Motivation and organizational principles for anatomical knowledge representation: The digital anatomist symbolic knowledge base. *Journal of the American Medical Informatics Association*, 5(1):17–40.

Rosse, C., Shapiro, L.G., Brinkley, J.F. (1998). The Digital Anatomist foundational model: principles for defining and structuring its concept domain, *Proceedings of the AMIA Fall Symposium*, pp. 820–824. Orlando, Florida.

Rossi, P.H., Freeman, H.E. (1989). *Evaluation: A Systematic Approach*. (4th ed.). Newbury Park, CA: Sage Publications.

Roth, E.M., Patterson, E.S., Mumaw, R.J. (2002). Cognitive engineering: Issues in user-centered system design. In J. J. Marciniak (ed.), *Encyclopedia of Software Engineering*, 2nd edition, pp. 163–179. New York: John Wiley & Sons.

Rothenberg, J. (1999). *Ensuring the Longevity of Digital Information*. RAND Corporation. (Accessed 2005 at: http://www.clir.org/pubs/archives/ensuring.pdf)

Rothschild, M.A., Wett, H.A., Fisher, P.R., Weltin, G.G., Miller, P.L. (1990). Exploring subjective vs. objective issues in the validation of computer-based critiquing advice. *Computer Methods and Programs in Biomedicine*, 31(1):11–18.

Rothwell, D.G., Côté, R.A., Cordeau, J.P., Boisvert, M.A. (1993). Developing a standard data structure for medical language: The SNOMED proposal. *Proceedings of the 17th Annual Symposium for Computer Applications in Medical Care*, Washington, DC, pp. 695–699.

Rothwell, D.J., Côté, R.A. (1996). Managing information with SNOMED: Understanding the model. *Proceedings of the AMIA Annual Fall Symposium*, Washington, DC, pp. 80–83.

Rotman, B.L., Sullivan, A.N., McDonald, T.W., Brown, B.W., DeSmedt, P., Goodnature, D., Higgins, M.C., Suermondt, H.J., Young, C., Owens, D.K. (1996). A randomized controlled trial of a computer-based physician workstation in an outpatient setting: Implementation barriers to outcome evaluation. *Journal of the American Medical Association*, 3(5):340–348.

Rowen, L., Mahairas, G., Hood, I. (1997). Sequencing the human genome. *Science*, 278(5338):605–607.

Rubin, RD (2003). The community health information movement: Where it's been, where it's going. In O'Carroll, P.W., Yasnoff, W.A., Ward, M.E., Ripp, L.H., Martin, E.L. (eds.), *Public Health Informatics and Information Systems*. New York: Springer-Verlag, p. 605.

Ruland, C.M. (2002). Handheld technology to improve patient care. *Journal of the American Medical Informatics Association*, 9:192–200.

Saba, V.K. (1992). The classification of home health care nursing: Diagnoses and interventions. *Caring Magazine*, 11(3):50–56.

Saba, V.K. (1994). *Home Health Care Classification of Nursing Diagnoses and Interventions*. Washington, DC: Georgetown University.

Saba, V.K. (1995). Home Health Care Classifications (HHCCs): Nursing diagnoses and nursing interventions, In *Nursing Data Systems: The Emerging Framework*, pp.61–103. Washington, D.C.: American Nurses Publishing.

Saba, V.K., McCormick, K. (1996). *Essentials of Computers for Nurses*. New York: McGraw-Hill.

Sackett, D.L., Richardson, W.S., Rosenberg, W.M., Haynes, R.B. (eds.) (1997). *Evidence-Based Medicine: How to Practice and Teach EBM*. New York: Churchill Livingstone.

Sackett, D.L., Richardson, W.S., Rosenberg, W., Haynes, R.B.(2000) *Evidence-Based Medicine: How to Practice and Teach EBM (Second Edition)*, New York: Churchhill Livingstone..

Safran, C, Using routinely collected data for clinical research. *Stat Med*; 10:559–564.

Safran, C., Porter, D., Lightfoot, J., Rury, C.D., Underhill, L.H., Bleich, H.L., Slack, W.V. (1989). ClinQuery: A system for online searching of data in a teaching hospital. *Annals of Internal Medicine*, 111(9):751–6.

Safran, C., Rind, D.M., Davis, R.B., Ives, D., Sands, D.Z., Currier, J., Slack, W.V., Makadon, H.J., Cotton, D.J. (1995). Guidelines for management of HIV infection with computer-based patient's record. *Lancet*, 346(8971):341–346.

Safran, C., Rury, C., Rind, D.M., Taylor, W.C. (1991). A computer-based outpatient medical record for a teaching hospital. *MD Computing*, 8(5):291–299.

Safran, C., Slack, W.V., Bleich, H.L. (1989). Role of computing in patient care in two hospitals. *MD Computing*, 6(3):141–148.

Sager, N, Friedman, C, Lyman, MS. (1987). *Medical Language Processing: Computer Management of Narrative Data*. New York: Addison-Wesley.

Sailors, R.M., East, T.D. (1997). Role of computers in monitoring. In Tobin M.J. (ed.), *Principals and Practice of Intensive Care Monitoring*, pp.1329–1354. New York: McGraw-Hill.

Salomon, G., Perkins, D.N., Globerson, T. (1991). Partners in cognition: Extending human intelligence with intelligent technologies. *Educational Researcher*, 20(3):2–9.

Salpeter, S.R., Sanders, G.D., Salpeter, E.E., Owens, D.K. (1997). Monitored isoniazid prophylaxis for low-risk tuberculin reactors older than 35 years of age: A risk-benefit and cost-effectiveness analysis. *Annals of Internal Medicine*, 127(12):1051–1061.

Salton, G. (1983). *Introduction to Modern Information Retrieval*. New York: McGraw-Hill.

Salton, G. (1991). Developments in automatic text retrieval. *Science*, 253:974 –980.

Salton, G., Buckley, C. (1990). Improving retrieval performance by relevance feedback. *Journal of the American Society for Information Science*, 41:288–97.

Salton, G., Fox, E., et al. (1983). Extended Boolean information retrieval. *Communications of the ACM*, 26:1022–1036.

Salton, G., Lesk, M. (1965). The SMART automatic document retrieval system: An illustration. *Communications of the ACM*, 8: 391–398.

Salzberg, S., Searls, D., Kasif, S. (eds.) (1998). *Computational Methods in Molecular Biology*. New York: Elsevier Science.

Sanders, G.D., Hagerty, C.G., Sonnenberg, F.A., Hlatky, M.A., Owens, D.K. (1999). Distributed dynamic decision support using a web-based interface for prevention of sudden cardiac death. *Medical Decision Making*, 19(2):157–66.

Sanders, D.L., Miller, R.A. (2001). The effects on clinician ordering patterns of a computerized decision support system for neuroradiology imaging studies. *Proceedings of the AMIA Annual Fall Symposium*, pp. 583–587.

Sandor, S., Leahy, R. (1997). Surface-based labeling of cortical anatomy using a deformable atlas. *IEEE Trans. Med. Imaging*, 16(1), 41–54.

Sanford, M.K., Hazelwood, S.E., Bridges, A.J., Cutts 3rd, J.H., Mitchell, J.A., Reid, J.C., Sharp, G. (1996). Effectiveness of computer-assisted interactive videodisc instruction in teaching rheumatology to physical and occupational therapy students. *Journal of Allied Health*, 25(2):141–148.

Saracevic, T. (1991). Individual differences in organizing, searching, and retrieving information. *Proceedings of the 54th Annual Meeting of the American Society for Information Science*, Washington, D.C.

Sarkar, I.N. Starren, J. (2002). Desiderata for personal electronic communications in clinical systems. *J Am Med Inform Assoc* 9:209–216.

Sartorius, N. (1976). I. Methodologic problems of common terminology, measurement, and classification. II. Modifications and new approaches to taxonomy in long-term care: Advantages and limitations of the ICD. *Medical Care*, 14(4 Suppl):109–15.

Scaife, M., Rogers, Y. (1996). External cognition: How do graphical representations work? *International Journal of Human-Computer Studies*, 45(2),185–213.

Schaltenbrand, G., Warren, W. (1977). *Atlas for Stereotaxy of the Human Brain*. Stuttgart: Thieme.

Scherrer, J.R., Baud, R.H., Hochstrasser, D., Ratib, O. (1990). DIOGENE: An integrated hospital information system in Geneva. *MD Computing*, 7(2):81–89.

Scherrer, J.R., Lovis, C., Borst, F. (1995). DIOGENE 2: A distributed hospital information system with an emphasis on its medical information content. In J.H. van Bemmel and A.T. McCray (ed.), *Yearbook of Medical Informatics*, pp.86–97. Stuttgart: Schattauer.

Schmidt, H.G., Boshuizen, H.P. (1993). On the origin of intermediate effects in clinical case recall. *Memory & Cognition*, 21(3):338–351.

Schneiderman, B. (1992). *Designing the User Interface: Strategies for Effective Human-Computer Interaction*. Don Mills, ON: Addison-Wesley Publishing Company.

Schreiber, A.T., Akkermans, J., Anjewierden, A., De Hoog, R., Shadbolt, N., Van De Velde, W., Wielinga, B. (2000). *Knowledge Engineering and Management: The Common KADS Methodology*. Cambridge, MA: The MIT Press.

Schreiber, G., Wielinga, B., Breuker, J. (eds.) (1993). *KADS: A Principled Approach to Knowledge-Based System Development*. London: Academic Press.

Schulz, K.F., Chalmers, I., Hayes, R.J., Altman, D.G. (1995). Empirical evidence of bias:. Dimensions of methodological quality associated with estimates of treatment effects in controlled trials. *Journal of the American Medical Association*, 273(5):408–412.

Schulze-Kremer, S. (1994). *Advances in Molecular Bioinformatics*. Washington, D.C.: IOS Press.

Schultz, E.B., Price, C., Brown, P.J.B. (1997). Symbolic anatomic knowledge representation in the Read Codes Version 3: Structure and application. *J. Am. Med. Inform. Assoc.*, 4:38–48.

Schwartz, R.J., Weiss, K.M., Buchanan, A.V. (1985). Error control in medical data. *MD Computing*, 2(2):19–25.

Schwartz, W.B. (1970). Medicine and the computer: The promise and problems of change. *New England Journal of Medicine*, 283(23):1257–1264.

Science (1997). Special issue on bioinformatics. *Science*, 278(Oct. 24):541–768.

Scriven, M. (1973). Goal free evaluation. In House E.R. (ed.), *School Evaluation*. Berkeley, CA: McCutchan Publishers.

Seiver, A. (2000). Critical care computing: Past, present, future. *Crit Care Clin,* 17(4):601–621.

Selden, C., Humphreys, B.L., Friede, A., Geisslerova, Z. (1996). *Public Health Informatics, January 1980 through December 1995: 471 Selected Citations*. Bethesda, MD: National Institutes of Health, National Library of Medicine, pp. 1–21.

Senior Medical Review (1987). Urinary tract infection. *Senior Medical Review*.

Sensor Systems Inc. (2001). *MedEx*. (Accessed 2005 at: http://medx.sensor.com/products/medx/index.html)

Setubal, J., Medianis, J. (1997). *Introduction to Computational Molecular Biology*. Boston: PWS Publishing Company.

Severinghaus, J.W., Astrup, P.B. (1986). History of blood gas analysis IV. Oximetry. *Journal of Clinical Monitoring*, 2(4):270–288.

Sewell, W., Teitelbaum, S. (1986). Observations of end-user online searching behavior over eleven years. *Journal of the American Society for Information Science*, 37(4):234–245.

Shabot, M.M. (1982). Documented bedside computation of cardiorespiratory variables with an inexpensive programmable calculator. In DeAngelis J. (ed.), *Debates and Controversies in the Management of High Risk Patients*, pp.153–163. San Diego, CA: Beach International.

Shabot, M.M. (1989). Standardized acquisition of bedside data: The IEEE P1073 medical information bus. *International Journal of Clinical Monitoring and Computing*, 6(4):197–204.

Shabot, M.M. (1995). Computers in the intensive care unit: Was Pogo correct? *Journal of Intensive Care Medicine*, 10:211–212.

Shabot, M.M. (1997a). Automated clinical pathways for surgical services. *Surgical Services Management*, June:19–23.

Shabot, M.M. (1997b). The HP CareVue clinical information system. *International Journal of Clinical Monitoring and Computing*, 14(3):177–184.

Shabot, M.M., Gardner, R.M. (eds.) (1994). *Decision Support Systems in Critical Care*. Boston: Springer-Verlag.

Shabot, M.M., Leyerle, B.J., LoBue, M. (1987). Automatic extraction of intensity-intervention scores from a computerized surgical intensive care unit flowsheet. *American Journal of Surgery*, 154(1):72–78.

Shabot, M.M., LoBoe, M. (1995). Real-time wireless decision support alerts on a palmtop PDA. *Proceedings of the 19th Annual Symposium on Computer Applications in Medical Care*, New Orleans, LA, pp. 174 –177.

Shabot, M.M., Shoemaker, W.C., State, D. (1977). Rapid bedside computation of cardiorespiratory variables with a programmable calculator. *Critical Care Medicine*, 5(2):105–111.

Shabot, MM. (2003). Closing address: Breaking free of the past: Innovation and technology in patient care. *Nurs Outlook*, 51(3):S37–38

Shahar, Y. (1997). A framework for knowledge-based temporal abstractions. *Artificial Intelligence*, 90:79–133.

Shahar, Y., Miksch, S., Johnson, P.D. (1988). The Asgaard Project: A task-specific framework for the application and critiquing of time-oriented clinical guidelines. *Artificial Intelligence in Medicine*, 14:29–51.

Shahar, Y., Musen, M.A. (1996). Knowledge-based temporal abstractions in clinical domains. *Artificial Intelligence in Medicine*, 8(3):267–298.

Shan, M.C., Davis, J.W. (1996). Business process flow management and its application in the telecommunications management network. *HP-Journal*, October 1996.

Shapiro, L.G., Stockman, G.C. (2001). *Computer Vision*. Upper Saddle River, N.J.: Prentice Hall.

Shaughnessy, A., Slawson, D., et al. (1994). Becoming an information master: A guidebook to the medical information jungle. *Journal of Family Practice*, 39: 489–499.

Shea, S., DuMouchel, W., Bahamonde, L. (1996). A meta-analysis of 16 randomized controlled trials to evaluate computer-based clinical reminder systems for preventive care in the ambulatory setting. *Journal of the American Medical Informatics Association*, 3(6):399– 409.

Shea, S., Starren, J., Weinstock, R.S., Knudson, P.E., Teresi, J., Holmes, D., et al. (2002). Columbia University's Informatics for Diabetes Education and Telemedicine (IDEATel) project: Rationale and design. *J Am Med Inform Assoc*, 9(1),49–62.

Sheppard, L.C., Kouchoukos, N.T., Kurtts, M.A., Kirklin, J.W. (1968). Automated treatment of critically ill patients following operation. *Annals of Surgery*, 168(4):596–604.

Shlaer, S., Mellor, S.J. (1992). *Object Life Cycles, Modeling the World in States*: New York: Prentice-Hall.

Shortell, S.M., Gillies, R.R., Anderson, D.A. (2000). *Remaking Health Care In America: The Evolution of Organized Delivery Systems* (2nd ed.). San Francisco. Jossey-Bass Publishers.

Shortliffe, E.H. (1976). *Computer-Based Medical Consultations: MYCIN*. New York: Elsevier/North Holland.

Shortliffe, E.H. (1984). Coming to terms with the computer. In Reiser S., Anbar M. (eds.), *The Machine at the Bedside: Strategies for Using Technology in Patient Care*, pp.235–239. Cambridge, MA: Cambridge University Press.

Shortliffe, E.H. (1986). Medical expert systems: Knowledge tools for physicians. *The Western Journal of Medicine*, 145:830–839.

Shortliffe, E.H. (1989). Testing reality: The introduction of decision-support technologies for physicians. *Methods of Information in Medicine*, 28:1–5.

Shortliffe, E.H. (1993). Doctors, patients, and computers: Will information technology dehumanize healthcare delivery? *Proceedings of the American Philosophical Society*, 137(3):390–398.

Shortliffe, E.H. (1994). Dehumanization of patient care: Are computers the problem or the solution. *Journal of the American Medical Informatics Association*, 1(1):76–78.

Shortliffe, E.H. (1995a). Medical informatics meets medical education. *Journal of the American Medical Association*, 273(13):1061–1065.

Shortliffe, E.H. (1995b). Medical informatics training at Stanford University School of Medicine. In van Bemmel J.H., McCray A.T. (eds.), *IMIA Yearbook of Medical Informatics.* (Vol. 1995), pp.105–110. Stuttgart, Germany: Schattauer Publishing Company.

Shortliffe, E.H. (1998a). Health care and the Next Generation Internet (editorial). *Annals of Internal Medicine*, 129(2):138–140.

Shortliffe, E.H. (1998b). The Next Generation Internet and health care: A civics lesson for the informatics community. *Proceedings of the AMIA Annual Fall Symposium*, Orlando, FL, pp. 8–14.

Shortliffe, E.H. (1998c). The evolution of health-care records in the era of the Internet, *Proceedings of Medinfo 98*. Seoul, Korea: Amsterdam: IOS Press.

Shortliffe, E.H. (2000). Networking health: Learning from others, taking the lead. *Health Affairs* 19(6):9–22.

Shortliffe, E.H., Blois, M.S. (2000). The Computer meets medicine and biology: Emergence of a discipline. In E. H. Shortliffe & L. E. Perreault (eds.), *Medical Informatics: Computer Applications in Health Care and Biomedicine* (2nd ed.), pp. 3–40. New York: Springer Verlag.

Shortliffe, E.H., Buchanan, B.G., Feigenbaum, E. (1979). Knowledge engineering for medical decision making; A review of computer-based clinical decision aids. *Proceedings of the IEEE*, 67:1207–1224.

Shortliffe, E.H., Johnson, S.B. (2002). Medical informatics training and research at Columbia University. In *IMIA Yearbook of Medical Informatics* (R. Haux and A.T. McCray, eds), pp 173–180. Stuttgart, Germany: Schattauer Publishing Company.

Shortliffe, E.H., Sondik, E. (2004). The informatics infrastructure: Anticipating its role in cancer surveillance. *Proceedings of the C-Change Summit on Cancer Surveillance and Information: The Next Decade*, Phoenix, Arizona.

Shubin, H., Weil, M.H. (1966). Efficient monitoring with a digital computer of cardiovascular function in seriously ill patients. *Annals of Internal Medicine*, 65(3):453–460.

Siegel, E., Cummings, M., Woodsmall, R. (1990). Bibliographic Retrieval Systems. In E. Shortliffe & L. Perreault (ed.), *Medical Informatics: Computer Applications in Health Care* (1st ed), pp.434–465. Reading, MA: Addison-Wesley.

Siegel, E.L., Protopapas, Z., Reiner, B.I., Pomerantz, S.M. (1997). Patterns of utilization of computer workstations in a filmless environment and implications for current and future picture archiving and communication systems. *Journal of Digital Imaging*, 10(3 Suppl 1):41–43.

Silberg, W.M., Lundberg, G.D., Musacchio, R.A. (1997). Assessing, controlling, and assuring the quality of medical information on the Internet: Caveat lector et viewor — let the reader and viewer beware. *Journal of the American Medical Association*, 277(15):1244–1245.

Simborg, D.W. (1984). Networking and medical information systems. *Journal of Medical Systems*, 8(1–2):43–47.

Simborg, D.W., Chadwick, M., Whiting-O'Keefe, Q.E., Tolchin, S.G., Kahn, S.A., Bergan, E.S. (1983). Local area networks and the hospital. *Computers and Biomedical Research*, 16(3):247–259.

Simmons, D.A. (1980). *A Classification Scheme for Client Problems in Community Health Nursing: Nurse Planning Information Series.* (Volume 14, Pub No.[HRP] 501501). Springfield, VA: National Technical Information Service.

Simon, D.P., Simon, H. A. (1978). Individual differences in solving physics problems. In R. Siegler (ed.), *Children's Thinking: What Develops?* Hillsdale, NJ: Lawrence Erlbaum Associates, Publishers.

Singer, S.J. (1991). Problems in gaining access to hospital information. *Health Affairs*, 10(2):148–151.

Singer, S.J., Hunt, K., Gabel, J., Liston, D., Enthoven, A.C. (1997). New research shows how to save money on employee health benefits. *Managing Employee Health Benefits*, 5(4):1–9.

Singhal, A., Buckley, C., et al. (1996). Pivoted document length normalization. *Proceedings of the 19th Annual International ACM SIGIR Conference on Research and Development in Information Retrieval*, Zurich, Switzerland. ACM Press, pp. 21–29.

Sinha, U., Bui, A., Taira, R., Dionisio, J., Morioka, C., Johnson, D., Kangarloo, H. (2002). A review of medical imaging informatics. *Ann N Y Acad Sci,* 980:168–97

Sittig, D. (1987). Computerized management of patient care in a complex, controlled clinical trial in the intensive care unit. *Proceedings of the 11th Annual Symposium on Computer Applications in Medical Care*, Washington, D.C., pp. 225–232.

Slack, W.V., Bleich, H.L. (1999). The CCC system in two teaching hospitals: A progress report. *Int J Med Inf,* 54(3):183–96.

Sloboda, J. (1991). Musical expertise. In K. A. Ericsson & J. Smith (eds.), *Toward a General Theory of Expertise: Prospects and Limits*, pp. 153–171. New York: Cambridge University Press.

Smith, D. (1994). *Biocomputing: Informatics and Genome Projects*. New York: Academic Press.

Smith, L. (1985). Medicine as an art. In Wyngaarden J., Smith L. (eds.), *Cecil Textbook of Medicine*. Philadelphia: W. B. Saunders.

Smith, L.D. (1986). *Behaviorism and Logical Positivism : A Reassessment of the Alliance*. Stanford, Calif.: Stanford University Press.

Smith, R. (1992). Using a mock trial to make a difficult clinical decision. *British Medical Journal*, 305(6864):1284–1287.

Smith, T., Waterman, M. (1981). Identification of common molecular subsequences. *Journal of Molecular Biology*, 147(1):195–197.

Snow, V., Lascher, S., & Mottur-Pilson, C. (2000). Pharmacologic treatment of acute major depression and dysthymia. *Annals of Internal Medicine, 132*(9):738–742.

Sollins, K. and Masinter, L. (1994). *Functional Requirements for Uniform Resource Names*. Internet Engineering Task Force. (Accessed 2005 at: http://www.w3.org/Addressing/rfc1737.txt)

Somers, A.R. (1971). *The Kaiser Permanente Medical Care Program*, New York: Commonwealth Fund.

Sonnenberg, F.A., Beck, J.R. (1993). Markov models in medical decision making: A practical guide. *Medical Decision Making*, 13(4):322–338.

Soto, G.E., Young, S.J., Martone, M.E., Deerinck, T.J., Lamont, S.L., Carragher, B.O., Hamma, K., Ellisman, M.H. (1994). Serial section electron tomography: A method for three-dimensional reconstruction of large structures. *Neuroimage*, 1:230–243.

Southon, F.C., Sauer, C., Dampney, C.N. (1997). Information technology in complex health services: Organizational impediments to successful technology transfer and diffusion. *Journal of the American Medical Informatics Association*, 4(2):112–124.

Sowa, J.F. (1983). *Conceptual Structures: Information Processes in Mind and Machine*. Reading, MA: Addison-Wesley.

Sowa, J.F. (2000). *Knowledge Representation: Logical, Philosophical, and Computational Foundations*. Pacific Grove: Brooks/Cole.

Sox, H.C. (1986). Probability theory in the use of diagnostic tests. An introduction to critical study of the literature. *Annals of Internal Medicine*, 104(1):60–66.

Sox, H.C. (1987). Probability theory in the use of diagnostic tests: Application to critical study of the literature. In Sox H.C. (ed.), *Common Diagnostic Tests: Use and Interpretation*, pp.1–17. Philadelphia: American College of Physicians.

Sox, H.C., Blatt, M.A., Higgins, M.C., Marton, K.I. (1988). *Medical Decision Making*. Boston, MA: Butterworth Publisher.

Spackman, K.A. (2000) SNOMED RT and SNOMEDCT. Promise of an international clinical terminology. *MD Comput*, 17(6):29.

Spackman, K.A., Campbell, K.E., Cote, R.A. (1997). SNOMED RT: A reference terminology for health care. *Proc AMIA Annu Fall Symp*, pp. 640–644. Philadelphia:Hanley and Belfus.

Spee, J.H., de Vos, W.M., Kuipers, O.P. (1993). Efficient random mutagenesis method with adjustable mutation frequency by use of PCR and dITP. *Nucleic Acids Research*, 21(3):777–778.

Spellman, P.T., Miller, M., Stewart, J., et al. (2002). Design and implementation of microarray gene expression markup language (MAGE-ML). *Genome Biol*, 23;3(9):RESEARCH0046. Epub 2002 Aug 23.

Spitzer, V., Ackerman, M., et al. (1996). The visible human male: A technical report. *Journal of the American Medical Informatics Association*, 3: 118–130.

Spitzer, V.M., Whitlock, D.G. (1998). The Visible Human Dataset: The anatomical platform for human simulation. *Anat Rec,* 253(2),49–57.

Srinivasan, P. (1996). Query expansion and MEDLINE. *Information Processing and Management*, 32: 431– 444.

Stallings, W. (1987a). *The Open Systems Interconnection (OSI) Model and OSI-Related Standards*. (Vol. 1). New York: Macmillian.

Stallings, W. (1987b). *Handbook of Computer-Communications Standards*. New York: Macmillan Publishing Company.

Stallings, W. (1997). *Data and Computer Communications*. New Jersey: Prentice Hall.

Starr P. (1982). *The Social Transformation of American Medicine*. New York: Basic Books.

Starr, P. (1983). *Social Transformation of American Medicine.* Basic Books.

Starren, J., Hripcsak, G., Sengupta, S., Abbruscato, C.R., Knudson, P., Weinstock, R.S., Shea, S. (2002). Columbia University's Informatics for Diabetes Education and Telemedicine (IDEATel) project: Technical implementation. *J Am Med Inform Assoc,* 9, 25–36.

Starren J., Johnson, S.B. (2000). An object-oriented taxonomy of medical data presentations. *J American Medical Informatics Association*; 7(1):1–20.

Stavri, P. (2001). Personal health information seeking: a qualitative review. *Proceedings of Medinfo 2001*. London, England. IOS Press, pp. 1484–1488.

Stead, W.W. (1997a). Building infrastructure for integrated health systems: Proceedings of the 1996 IAIMS Symposium. *Journal of the American Medical Informatics Association*, 4(2 Suppl):S1–76.

Stead, W.W. (1997b). The evolution of the IAIMS: Lessons for the next decade. *Journal of the American Medical Informatics Association*, 4(2 Suppl):S4–9.

Stead, W.W., Borden, R., Bourne, J., Giuse, D., Giuse, N., Harris, T.R., Miller, R.A., Olsen, A.J. (1996). The Vanderbilt University fast track to IAIMS: Transition from planning to implementation. *Journal of the American Medical Informatics Association*, 3(5):308–317.

Stead, W.W., Hammond, W.E. (1988). Computer-based medical records: The centerpiece of TMR. *MD Computing*, 5(5):48–62.

Steedman, D. (1990). *Abstract Syntax Notation One: The Tutorial and Reference*. Great Britain: Technology Appraisals Ltd.

Steen, E.B. (ed.) (1996). *Proceedings of the Second Annual Nicholas E. Davies CPR Recognition Symposium*. Schaumburg, IL: Computer-Based Patient Record Institute.

Sternberg, R.J., Horvarth, J.A. (1999). *Tacit Knowledge in Professional Practice. Researcher and Practitioner Perspectives*. Mahwah, NJ: Lawrence Erlbaum Associates.

Stensaas, S.S., Millhouse, O.E. (2001). *Atlases of the Brain*. University of Utah. (Accessed 2005 at: http://medstat.med.utah.edu/kw/brain_atlas/)

Stewart, B.K., Lange,r S.G., Hoath, J.I., Tarczy-Hornuch, P. (1997). DICOM image integration into a Web-browsable electronic medical record, *RSNA 1997 Scientific Program Supplement to Radiology.*, p.205.

Stringer, W.A. (1997). MRA image production and display. *Clinical Neuroscience*, 4(3):110–116.

Strong, D.M., Lee, Y.W., Wang, R.T. (1997). 10 potholes in the road to information quality. *IEEE Computer*, 31:38– 46.

Stryer, L. (1995). *Biochemistry*. New York: WH Freeman.

Subramaniam, B., Hennessey, J.G., Rubin, M.A., Beach, L.S., Reiss, A.L. (1997). Software and methods for quantitative imaging in neuroscience: The Kennedy Krieger Institute Human Brain Project. In S. H. Koslow & M. F. Huerta (eds.), *Neuroinformatics: An Overview of the Human Brain Project*, pp. 335–360. Mahwah, New Jersey: Lawrence Erlbaum.

Suchman, L. (1987). *Plans and Situated Actions: The Problem of Human/Machine Communication*. Cambridge: Cambridge University Press.

Sumner, W., Nease Jr., R.F., Littenberg, B. (1991). U-titer: A utility assessment tool. *Proceedings of the 15th Annual Symposium on Computer Applications in Medical Care*, Washington, DC, pp. 701–5.

Sundheim, B. (1991). *Proceedings of the Third Message Understanding Conference (MUC-3)*. San Mateo, CA: Morgan Kaufmann.

Sundheim, B. (1992). *Proceedings of the Fourth Message Understanding Conference (MUC-4)*. San Mateo, CA: Morgan Kaufmann.

Sundheim, B. (1994). *Proceedings of the Fifth Message Understanding Conference (MUC-5)*. San Mateo, CA.: Morgan Kaufmann.

Sundheim, B. (1996). *Proceedings of the Sixth Message Understanding Conference (MUC-6)*. San Mateo, CA.: Morgan Kaufmann.

Sundsten, J.W., Conley, D.M., Ratiu, P., Mulligan, K.A., Rosse, C. (2000). *Digital Anatomist web-based interactive atlases*. (Accessed 2005 at: http://www9.biostr.washington.edu/da.html)

Sussman, S.Y. (2001). *Handbook of Program Development for Health Behavior Research & Practice*. Thousand Oaks, Calif.: Sage.

Swanson, D. (1988). Historical note: Information retrieval and the future of an illusion. *Journal of the American Society for Information Science*, 39: 92–98.

Swanson, L.W. (1992). *Brain Maps: Structure of the Rat Brain*. Amsterdam; New York: Elsevier.

Swanson, L.W. (1999). *Brain Maps: Structure of the Rat Brain* (2nd ed.). Amsterdam; New York: Elsevier Science.

Sweeney, L. (1996). Replacing personally-indentifying information in medical records: The SCRUB system. *Proceedings of the AMIA Annual Fall Symposium*, Washington, DC, pp. 333–337.

Swets, J.A. (1973). The relative operating characteristic in psychology. *Science*, 182:990.

Szolovits, P. (ed.) (1982). *Artificial Intelligence in Medicine*. Boulder, CO: Westview Press.

Szolovits, P., Pauker, S.G. (1979). Computers and clinical decision making: Whether, how much, and for whom? *Proceedings of the IEEE*, 67:1224–1226.

Tagare, H.D., Jaffe, C.C., Duncan, J. (1997). Medical image databases: A content-based retrieval approach. *Journal of the American Medical Informatics Association*, 4(3):184–198.

Tagare, H.D., Vos, F.M., Jaffe, C.C., Duncan, J.S. (1995). Arrangement: a spatial relation between parts for evaluating similarity of tomographic section. *IEEE Transactions on Pattern Analysis and Machine Intelligence*, 17(9):880–893.

Talairach, J., Tournoux, P. (1988). *Co-Planar Stereotaxic Atlas of the Human Brain*. New York: Thieme Medical Publishers.

Tanenbaum, A.S. (1987). *Computer Networks*. (2nd ed.). Englewood Cliffs, NJ: Prentice Hall.

Tanenbaum, A.S. (1996). *Computer Networks*. (3rd ed.). Englewood Cliffs, NJ: Prentice-Hall.

Tang, PC. (2003). *Key Capabilities of an Electronic Health Record System* (Letter Report). Committee on Data Standards for Patient Safety. Board on Health Care Services, Institute of Medicine.

Tang, P.C., Annevelink, J., Suermondt, H.J., Young, C.Y. (1994). Semantic integration in a physician's workstation. *International Journal of Bio-Medical Computing*, 35(1):47–60.

Tang, P.C., Fafchamps, D., Shortliffe, E.H. (1994). Traditional medical records as a source of clinical data in the outpatient setting. *Proceedings of the 18th Annual Symposium on Computer Applications in Medical Care*, Washington, DC, pp. 575–579.

Tang, P.C., Marquardt, W.C., Boggs, B., et al. (1999). NetReach: Building a clinical infrastructure for the enterprise. In Overhage JM (ed.) *Fourth Annual Proceedings of the Davies CPR Recognition Symposium*, pp. 25–68. Chicago: McGraw-Hill.

Tang, P.C., McDonald, C J. (2001). Computer-Based Patient-Record Systems. In E.H. Shortliffe & L.E. Perreault (eds.), *Medical Informatics* (2nd ed)., pp. 327–358. New York: Springer Verlag.

Tang, P., Newcomb, C., et al. (1997). Meeting the information needs of patients: Results from a patient focus group. *Proceedings of the 1997 AMIA Annual Fall Symposium*, Nashville, TN. Hanley & Belfus, pp. 672–676.

Tang, P.C., Patel, V.L. (1993). Major issues in user interface design for health professional workstations: Summary and recommendations. *International Journal of Bio-Medical Computing*, 34(104):139–148.

Tarczy-Hornuch, P., Kwan-Gett, T.S., Fouche, L., Hoath, J., Fuller, S., Ibrahim, K.N., Ketchell, D.S., LoGerfo, J.P., Goldberg, H. (1997). Meeting clinician information needs by integrating access to the medical record and knowledge sources via the Web. *Proceedings of the 1997 AMIA Annual Fall Symposium*, Nashville, TN, pp. 809–813.

Tatro, D., Briggs, R., Chavez-Pardo, R., Hannigan, J., Moore, T., Cohen, S. (1975). Online drug interaction surveillance. *American Journal of Hospital Pharmacy*, 32:417.

Taylor, H., Leitman, R. (2001). *The Increasing Impact of eHealth on Physician Behavior.* Harris Interactive. (Accessed 2005 at: http://www.harrisinteractive.com/news/newsletters/healthnews/HI_HealthCareNews2001Vol1_iss31.pdf)

Teach, R.L., Shortliffe, E.H. (1981). An analysis of physician attitudes regarding computer-based clinical consultation systems. *Computers and Biomedical Research*, 14(6):542–558.

Teich, J.M. (ed.) (1997). *Proceedings of the Third Annual Nicholas E. Davies CPR Recognition Symposium.* Schaumburg, IL: Computer-based Patient Record Institute.

Teich, J.M., Glaser, J.P., Beckley, R.F. (1996). Toward cost-effective, quality care: the Brigham Integrated Computing System. In E.B. Steen (ed.), *Proceedings of the Second Annual Nicholas E. Davies CPR Recognition Symposium.* (Vol. 2), pp.3–34. Schaumburg, IL: Computer-Based Patient Record Institute.

Teich, JM, Glaser, JP, Beckley, RF, et al. (1999). The Brigham integrated computing system (BICS): Advanced clinical systems in an academic hospital environment. *Int J Med Inf,* 54(3):197–208.

Teich, J.M., Kuperman, G.J., Bates, D.W. (1997). Clinical decision support: Making the transition from the hospital to the community network. *Healthcare Information Management*, 11(4):27–37.

Teich, J.M., Merchia, P.R., Schmiz, J.L., Kuperman, G.J., Spurr, C.D., Bates, D.W. (2000). Effects of computerized physician order entry on prescribing practices. *Arch Intern Med*, 160(18):2741–2747.

Telecommunication N. (1992). *NCPDP Telecommunication Standard Format.* (Version 3.2).

Templeton, A.W., Dwyer, S.J., Johnson, J.A., Anderson, W.H., Hensley, K.S., Rosenthal, S.J., Lee, K.R., Preston, D.F., Batnitzky, S., Price, H.I. (1984). An on-line digital image management system. *Radiology*, 152(2):321–325.

Terry, K. (2002). Beam it up, Doctor: Inexpensive wireless networking technology, now available on PDAs and tablet computers, can connect you with clinical and scheduling data throughout your office. *Med Econ.* 79(13):34–6.

Thompson, P., Toga, A.W. (1996). A surface-based technique for warping three-dimensional images of the brain. *IEEE Transactions on Medical Imaging*, 15(4):402–417.

Thompson, P.M., Mega, M.S., Toga, A.W. (2001). Disease-specific brain atlases. In J.C. Mazziotta & A. W. Toga (eds.), *Brain Mapping III: The Disorders*. New York: Academic Press.

Thompson, P.M., Toga, A.W. (1997). Detection, visualization and animation of abnormal anatomic structure with a deformable probalistic brain atlas based on random vector field transformations. *Med Image Anal,* 1, 271–294.

Thompson, Tommy G. (2002). *The State Children's Health Insurance Program: A Summary Evaluation of States' Early Experience with SCHIP.* Washington, DC: Dept of Health and Human Services.

Tibbo, H. (2001). Archival perspectives on the emerging digital library. *Communications of the ACM,* 44(5): 69–70.

Tierney, W.M., McDonald, C.J. (1991). Practice databases and their uses in clinical research. *Stat Med,* 10(4):541–57.

Tierney, W.M., Miller, M.E., Overhage, J.M., McDonald, C.J. (1993). Physician inpatient order writing on microcomputer workstations: Effects on resource utilization. *Journal of the American Medical Association,* 269(3):379–383.

Todd, W., Harris, R.L., Schwarz, E., Bradnam, K., Lawson, D., Chen, W., Blasier, D., Kenny, E., Cunningham, F., Kishore, R., Chan, J., Muller, H.M., Petcherski, A., Thorisson, G., Day, A., Bieri, T., Rogers, A., Chen, C.K., Spieth, J., Sternberg, P., Durbin, R., Stein, L.D. (2003). WormBase: A cross-species database for comparative genomics. *Nucleic Acids Research;* 31:133–137.

Toga, A.W. (2001a). *Brain Atlases.* (Accessed 2005 at: http://www.loni.ucla.edu/Atlases/)

Toga, A.W. (2001b). *UCLA Laboratory for Neuro Imaging (LONI).* (Accessed 2005 at: http://www.loni.ucla.edu/)

Toga, A.W., Ambach, K.L., Schluender, S. (1994). High-resolution anatomy from in situ human brain. *Neuroimage,* 1(4), 334–344.

Toga, A.W., Frackowiak, R.S.J., Mazziotta, J.C. (eds.). (2001). *Neuroimage: A Journal of Brain Function.* New York: Academic Press.

Toga, A.W., Santori, E.M., Hazani, R., Ambach, K. (1995). A 3-D digital map of rat brain. *Brain Research Bulletin,* 38(1), 77–85.

Toga, A.W., Thompson, P.W. (2001). Maps of the brain. *Anatomical Record (New Anat.),* 265, 37–53.

Tolbert, S., Pertuz, A. (1977). Study shows how computerization affects nursing activities in ICU. *Hospitals,* 51(17):79.

Torrance, G.W., Feeny, D. (1989). Utilities and quality-adjusted life years. *International Journal of Technology Assessment in Health Care,* 5(4):559–75.

Tsien, C.L., Fackler, J.C. (1997). Poor prognosis for existing monitors in the intensive care unit. *Critical Care Medicine,* 25(4):614–619.

Tsui, F.C., Espino, J.U., Dato, V.M., Gesteland, P.H., Hutman, J., Wagner, M.M. (2003). Technical Description of RODS: A Real-time Public Health Surveillance System. *J Am Med Inform Assoc,* 10(5):399–408.

Tu, S., Musen, M.A. (1996). The EON model of intervention protocols and guidelines. *Proceedings of the AMIA Annual Fall Symposium,* Washington, DC, pp. 587–591.

Tu, S.W., Ericsson, H., Gennari, J.H., Shahar, Y., Musen, M.A. (1995). Ontology-based configuration of problem-solving methods and generation of knowledge-acquisition tools: Application of PROTÉGÉ-II to protocol-based decision support. *Artificial Intelligence in Medicine,* 7(3):257–289.

Tu, S.W., Kemper, C.A., Lane, N.M., Carlson, R.W., Musen, M.A. (1993). A methodology for determining patients' eligibility for clinical trials. *Methods of Information in Medicine,* 32(4):317–325.

Tunis, S.R., Hayward, R.S., Wilson, M.C., Rubin, H.R., Bass, E.B., Johnston,M., et al. (1994). Internists' attitudes about clinical practice guidelines. *Ann Intern Med,* 120(11), 956–963.

Turing, A.M. (1950). Computing machinery and intelligence. *Mind,* 59:433–460.

Tversky, A., Kahneman, D. (1974). Judgment under uncertainty: Heuristics and biases. *Science*, 185:1124–1131.

Tysyer, D.A. (1997). Copyright law: databases. *Bitlaw*, (Accessed 2005 at: http://www.bitlaw.com/copyright/database.html)

Ullman, J.D., Widom, J. (1997). *A First Course in Database Systems*. New Jersey: Prentice Hall.

U.S. Bureau of the Census (continuously updated), Population Estimates and Population Projections, *www.census.gov.*

United States General Accounting Office (1993). *Automated Medical Records: Leadership Needed to Expedite Standards Development: Report to the Chairman/Committee on Governmental Affairs*. Washington, D.C.: U.S. Senate, USGAO/IMTEC-93-17.

van der Lei, J., Musen, M.A. (1991). A model for critiquing based on automated medical records. *Computers and Biomedical Research*, 24(4):344–378.

van der Lei, J., Musen, M.A., van der Does, E., Man in 't Veld, A.J., van Bemmel, J.H. (1991). Comparison of computer-aided and human review of general practitioners' management of hypertension. *Lancet*, 338(8781):1504–1508.

van Heijst, G., Falasconi, S., Abu-Hanna, A., Schreiber, G., Stefanelli, M. (1995). A case study in ontology library construction. *Artificial Intelligence in Medicine*, 7(3):227–255.

vanBemmel, J.H., Musen, M.A. (1997). *Handbook of Medical Informatics*. Heidelberg/New York: Bohn Stafleu Van Loghum, Houten, and Springer-Verlag.

van Dijk, T.A., & Kintsch, W. (1983). *Strategies of Discourse Comprehension*. New York: Academic.

Van Essen, D.C. (2002). Windows on the brain. The emerging role of atlases and databases in neuroscience. *Curr. Op. Neurobiol.*, 12:574–579.

Van Essen, D.C., Drury, H.A. (1997). Structural and functional analysis of human cerebral cortex using a surface-basec atlas. *J. Neuroscience*, 17(18):7079–7102.

Van Essen, D.C., Drury, H.A., Dickson, J., Harwell, J., Hanlon, D., Anderson, C.H. (2001). An integrated software suite for surface-based analysis of cerebral cortex. *J Am Med Ass*, 8(5):443–459.

Van Essen, D.C., Drury, H.A., Joshi, S., Miller, M.I. (1998). Functional and structural mapping of human cerebral cortex: solutions are in the surfaces. *Proc. National Academy of Sciences*, 95:788–795.

VandeSompel, H., Lagoze, C. (1999). The Santa Fe Convention of the Open Archives Initiative. *D-Lib Magazine*, 5. (Accessed 2005 at: http://www.dlib.org/dlib/february00/vandesompel-oai/02vandesompel-oai.html)

Vannier, M.W., Marsh, J.W. (1996). Three-dimensional imaging, surgical planning, and image-guided therapy. In Greenes, R.A. and Bauman, R.A. (eds.) Imaging and information management: computer systems for a changing health care environment. *The Radiology Clinics of North America*, 34(3):545–563.

Van Noorden, S. (2002). Advances in immunocytochemistry. *Folia Histochem Cytobiol*, 40(2): 121–124.

vanRijsbergen, C. (1979). *Information Retrieval*. London. Butterworth.

van 't Veer, L.J., Dai, H., van de Vijver, M.J., et al. (2002). *Gene expression profiling predicts clinical outcome of breast cancer. Nature*. 415(6871):484–485.

Varmus, H. (1999). *PubMed Central: A Proposal for Electronic Publication in the Biomedical Sciences*. National Institutes of Health. (Accessed 2005 at: http://www.nih.gov/welcome/director/ebiomed/ebi.htm)

Varon, J., Marik, P.E. (2002). Clinical information systems and the electronic medical record in the intensive care unit. *Curr Opin Crit Care*, 8(6):614–624

Vetterli, M., Kovarevic, J. (1995). *Wavelets and Subband Coding*. Englewood Cliffs, NJ: Prentice Hall.

Vicente, K.J. (1999). *Cognitive Work Analysis: Toward Safe, Productive & Healthy Computer-Based Work*. Mahwah, N.J.: Lawrence Erlbaum Associates.

Vogel, L.H. (2003). Finding value from information technology investments: Exploring the elusive ROI in healthcare. *Journal for Health Information Management*, 17(4):20–28.

Voorhees, E. (1998). Variations in relevance judgments and the measurement of retrieval effectiveness. *Proceedings of the 21st Annual International ACM SIGIR Conference on Research and Development in Information Retrieval,* Melbourne, Australia, pp.315–323. ACM Press.

Voorhees, E., Harman, D. (2000). Overview of the Sixth Text REtrieval Conference (TREC). *Information Processing and Management*, 36: 3–36.

Voorhees, E., Harman, D. (2001). Overview of TREC 2001. *Proceedings of the Text Retrieval Conference 2001*, Gaithersburg, MD, pp. 1–15.

Vosniadou, S. (1996). *International Perspectives on the Design of Technology-Supported Learning Environments.*: Mahwah, NJ: Lawrence Erlbaum Associates.

Wachter, S.B., Agutter, J., Syroid, N., Drews, F., Weinger, M.B., Westenskow, D. (2003). The employment of an iterative design process to develop a pulmonary graphical display. *J Am Med Inform Assoc,* 10(4):363–372.

Wagner, M.M., Dato, V., Dowling, J.N., Allswede, M. (2003). Representative threats for research in public health surveillance. *J Biomed Informatics*, 36(3):177–88.

Wake, M.M., Murphy, M., Affara, F.A., Lang, N.M., Clark, J., Mortensen, R. (1993). Toward an international classification for nursing practice: A literature review and survey. *International Nursing Review*, 40(3):77–80.

Walker, J., Pan, E., Johnston, D., Adler-Milstein, J., Bates, D.W., Middleton, B. (2004). *The Value of Healthcare Information Exchange and Interoperability*. Boston, MA: Centre for Information Technology Leadership.

Wang, A.Y., Sable, J.H., Spackman, K.A. (2002). The SNOMED clinical terms development process: Refinement and analysis of content. *Proceedings of the AMIA Annual Symp*, pp. 845–9.

Ware, C. (2003). Design as applied perception. In J. M. Carroll (ed.), *HCI Models, Theories and Frameworks*, pp. 11–26. San Francisco, CA: Morgan Kaufmann.

Warner, H.R. (1979). *Computer-Assisted Medical Decision-Making*. New York: Academic Press.

Warner, H.R., Gardner, R.M., Toronto, A.F. (1968). Computer-based monitoring of cardiovascular function in postoperative patients. *Circulation*, 37(4 Suppl):II68–II74.

Warner, H.R., Toronto, A.F., Veasy, L. (1964). Experience with Bayes' theorem for computer diagnosis of congenital heart disease. *Annals of the New York Academy of Science*, 115:2–16.

Warren, J.J., Hoskins, L.M. (1995). NANDA's nursing diagnosis taxonomy: A nursing database, In *Nursing Data Systems: The Emerging Framework*, pp.49–59 Washington, D.C.: American Nurses Publishing.

Watson, J., Crick, F. (1953). A structure for deoxyribose nucleic acid, *Nature*, 171:737.

Watson, R.J. (1977). A large-scale professionally oriented medical information system: Five years later. *Journal of Medical Systems*, 1:3–16.

Wang, A.Y., Sable, J.H., Spackman, K.A. (2002). The SNOMED clinical terms development process: Refinement and analysis of content. *Proc AMIA Annual Symposium*, pp. 845–849.

Webster, J.G. (ed.) (1988). *Encyclopedia of Medical Devices and Instrumentation*, New York: Wiley.

Weed, L.L. (1969). *Medical Records, Medical Education and Patient Care: The Problem-Oriented Record as a Basic Tool*. Chicago, IL: Year Book Medical Publishers.

Weed, L.L. (1975). Problem-Oriented Medical Information System (PROMIS) Laboratory. In G.A. Giebin & L.L. Hurst (ed.), *Computer Projects in Health Care*. Ann Arbor, MI: Health Administration Press.

Wei, L., Altman, R.B. (1998). Recognizing protein binding sites using statistical descriptions of their 3D environments. *Proceedings of the Pacific Symposium on Biocomputing '98*, Singapore, pp. 497–508.

Weibel, S. (1996). The Dublin Core: A simple content description model for electronic resources. *ASIS Bulletin*, 24(1): 9–11.

Weibel, W.R. (1979). *Stereological Methods*. New York: Academic Press.

Weil, T.P. (2001) *Health Networks: Can They Be the Solution?*, Ann Arbor, Michigan, University of Michigan Press.

Weinberg, A.D. (1973). CAI at the Ohio State University College of Medicine. *Computers in Biology and Medicine*, 3(3):299–305.

Weiner, J., Parente, S., et al. (1995). Variation in office-based quality: A claims-based profile of care provided to Medicare patients with diabetes. *Journal of the American Medical Association*, 273:1503–1508.

Weinfurt, P.T. (1990). Electrocardiographic monitoring: An overview. *Journal of Clinical Monitoring*, 6(2):132–138.

Weinger, M.B., Slagle, J. (2001). Human factors research in anesthesia patient safety. *Proc AMIA Annual Fall Symp*, pp. 756–760.

Weinstein, M.C., Fineberg, H. (1980). *Clinical Decision Analysis*. Philadelphia: W. B. Saunders.

Weissleder, R., Mahmood, U. (2001). Molecular imaging. *Radiology, 219*,316–333.

Wellcome Department of Cognitive Neurology. (2001). *Statistical Parametric Mapping*. (Accessed 2005 at: http://www.fil.ion.ucl.ac.uk/spm/)

Weller, C.D. (1984). "Free Choice" as a restraint of trade in American health care delivery and insurance. *Iowa Law Review*, 69(5):1351–1378 and 1382–1392.

Wennberg, J. (1998). *The Dartmouth Altas of Health Care in the United States*. Dartmouth Medical School: American Hospital Publishing Inc.

Wennberg, J.E, Cooper, M.M. (eds) (1999). *The Quality of Medical Care in the United States: A Report on the Medicare Program*, Chicago: American Hospital Association.

Wennberg, J., Gittelsohn, A. (1973). Small area variations in health care delivery. *Science*, 182(117):1102–1108.

Werley, H.H., Lang, N.M. (eds.) (1988). *Identification of the Nursing Minimum Data Set*. New York: Springer.

Westwood, J.D., Hoffman, H.M., Stredney, D., Weghorst, S.J. (1998). *Medicine Meets Virtual Reality*. Amsterdam: IOS Press.

White, B.Y., Frederiksen, J.R. (1990). Causal model progressions as a foundation for intelligent learning environments. In W. J. Clancey & E. Soloway (eds.), *Artificial Intelligence and Learning Environments* (Special issues of *Artificial Intelligence*), pp. 99–157.

White House (1997). Remarks by President Clinton in Announcement on Immunization-Child Care.

Whitely, W.P., Rennie, D., Hafner, A.W. (1994). The scientific community's response to evidence of fraudulent publication: The Robert Slutsky case. *Journal of the American Medical Association*, 272(2):170–173.

Whiting-O'Keefe, Q.E., Simborg, D.W., Epstein, W.V. (1980). A controlled experiment to evaluate the use of a time-oriented summary medical record. *Medical Care*, 18(8):842–852.

Whiting-O'Keefe, Q.E., Simborg, D.W., Epstein, W.V., Warger, A. (1985). A computerized summary medical record system can provide more information than the standard medical record. *Journal of the American Medical Association*, 254(9):1185–1192.

Widman, L.E., Tong, D.A. (1997). Requests for medical advice from patients and families to health care providers who publish on the World Wide Web. *Archives of Internal Medicine*, 15(2):209–212.

Wiederhold, G. (1981). *Databases for Health Care*. New York: Springer-Verlag.

Wiederhold, G., Bilello, M., Sarathy, V., Qian, X. (1996). A security mediator for health care information. *Proceedings of the AMIA Annual Fall Symposium*, Washington, DC, pp. 120–124.

Wiederhold, G., Clayton, P.D. (1985). Processing biological data in real time. *M.D. Computing*, 2(6):16–25.

Wilcox, A, Hripcsak, G.(1999) Classification algorithms applied to narrative reports. *Proc AMIA Annual Symposium*, pp. 455–59.

Wildemuth, B., deBliek, R., et al. (1995). Medical students' personal knowledge, searching proficiency, and database use in problem solving. *Journal of the American Society for Information Science*, 46:590–607.

Williams, D., Counselman, F., et al. (1996). Emergency department discharge instructions and patient literacy: a problem of disparity. *American Journal of Emergency Medicine*, 14:19–22.

Williams, R.M., Baker, L.M., Marshall, J.G. (1992). *Information Searching*. Thorofare, NJ: Slack.

Wilson, M.C., Hayward, R.S., Tunis, S.R., Bass, E.B., Guyatt, G. (1995). User's guides to the medical Literature. VIII.: How to use clinical practice guidelines. *JAMA* 274(20):1630–1632.

Wilson, T. (1990). *Confocal Microscopy*. San Diego: Academic Press Ltd.

Wilson, A.L., Hill, J.J., Wilson, R.G., Nipper, K., Kwon, I.W. (1997). Computerized medication administration records decrease medication occurrences. *Pharm Pract Manag Q,* 17(1):17–29.

Winograd, T., Flores, F. (1987). *Understanding Computers and Cognition: A New Foundation for Design*. Reading, MA: Addison-Wesley.

Winston, P.H., Narasimhan, S. (1996). *On to Java*. Reading, MA: Addison Wesley.

Wittenber, J., Shabot, M.M. (1990). Progress report: The medical device data language for the IEEE 1073 medical information bus. *International Journal of Clinical Monitoring and Computing*, 7(2):91–98.

Wong, B.A., Rosse, C., & Brinkley, J.F. (1999). Semi-automatic scene generation using the Digital Anatomist Foundational Model (UW, Trans.). *Proceedings of the AMIA Annual Symposium*, pp. 637–641. Washington, D.C.

Wong, S.T., Tjandra, D., Wang, H., Shen, W. (2003). Workflow-enabled distributed component-based information architecture for digital medical imaging enterprises. *IEEE Trans Inf Technol Biomed.* 7(3):171–183.

Wood, E.H. (1994). MEDLINE: The options for health professionals. *Journal of the American Medical Informatics Association*, 1(5):372–380.

Woods, R.P., Cherry, S.R., Mazziotta, J.C. (1992). Rapid automated algorithm for aligning and reslicing PET images. *J. Comp. Assisted Tomogr.,* 16:620–633.

Woods, R.P., Mazziotta, J.C., Cherry, S.R. (1993). MRI-PET registration with automated algorithm. *J. Comp. Assisted Tomogr.,* 17:536–546.

Woods, J.W. (ed.) (1991). *Subband Image Coding*. Boston, MA: Kluwer Academic Computer Publishers.

Woolhandler, S., Himmelstein D.U. (1997). Costs of care and administration at for-profit and other hospitals in the United States. *New England Journal of Medicine*, 336(11):769–774.

World Health Organization (1977). *Ninth Edition. International Classification of Diseases Index. Manual for the International Statistical Classification of Diseases*. Geneva: The World Health Organization.

World Health Organization (1992). *International Classification of Diseases Index. Tenth Revision. Volume 1: Tabular List*. Geneva: The World Health Organization.

Wright, P.C., Fields, R.E., Harrison, M.D. (2000). Analyzing human-computer interaction as distributed cognition: The resources model. *Human-Computer Interaction,* 15(1),1–41.

Wyatt, J.C. (1989). Lessons learned from the field trial of ACORN, an expert system to advise on chest pain. *Proceedings of Medinfo 1989*, Singapore, pp. 111–115.

Wyatt, J.C. (1991a). *A Method for Developing Medical Decision-Aids Applied to ACORN, a Chest Pain Advisor.* Unpublished DM thesis, Oxford University.

Wyatt, J.C. (1991b). Use and sources of medical knowledge. *Lancet,* 338(8779):1368–1373.

Wyatt, J.C., Altman, D.G. (1995). Prognostic models: clinically useful, or quickly forgotten? *British Medical Journal,* 311:1539–1541.

Wyatt, J.C., Spiegelhalter, D. (1990). Evaluating medical expert systems: What to test and how? *Medical Informatics,* 15(3):205–217.

Wyatt, J, Wyatt, S. (2003). When and how to evaluate health information systems? *Int J Med Inf,* 69: 251–9.

Xu, J., Croft, W. (1996). Query expansion using local and global document analysis. *Proceedings of the 19th Annual International ACM SIGIR Conference on Research and Development in Information Retrieval,* Zurich, Switzerland. ACM Press, pp. 4–11.

Yamazaki, S, Satomura, Y. (2000). Standard method for describing an electronic patient record template: Application of XML to share domain knowledge. *Methods Inf Med,* 39(1):50–5.

Yasnoff, W.A. (2003). Case study: An immunization data collection system for private providers. In O'Carroll, P.W., Yasnoff, W.A., Ward, M.E., Ripp, L.H., Martin, E.L. (eds.): *Public Health Informatics and Information Systems.* New York: Springer-Verlag, pp. 691–709.

Yasnoff, W.A., Miller, P.L. (2003). Decision support and expert systems in public health. In O'Carroll, P.W., Yasnoff, W.A., Ward, M.E., Ripp, L.H., Martin, E.L. (eds.): *Public Health Informatics and Information Systems.* New York: Springer-Verlag, pp.494–512.

Yasnoff, W.A., Humphreys, B.L., Overhage, J.M., Detmer, D.E., Brennan, P.F., Morris, R.W., Middleton, B., Bates, D.W., Fanning, J.P. (2004). A consensus action agenda for achieving the national health information infrastructure. *J Am Med Informatics Assoc* 11(4):332–338.

Yasnoff, W.A., O'Carroll, P.W., Koo, D., Linkins, R.W., Kilbourne, E.M. (2000). Public Health Informatics: Improving and transforming public health in the information age. *Journal of Public Health Management & Practice,* 6(6):67–75.

Young, D.W. (1980). An aid to reducing unnecessary investigations. *British Medical Journal,* 281(6225):1610–1611.

Young, F. (1987). Validation of medical software: Present policy of the Food and Drug Administration. *Annals of Internal Medicine,* 106:628.

Young, W.H., Gardner, R.M., East, T.D., Turne,r K. (1997). Computerized ventilator charting: Artifact rejection and data reduction. *International Journal of Clinical Monitoring and Computing,* 14(3):165–176.

Youngner, S.J. (1988). Who defines futility? *Journal of the American Medical Association,* 260(14):2094 –2095.

Yu, V.L., Buchanan, B.G., Shortliffe, E.H., Wraith, S.M., Davis, R., Scott, A.C., Cohen, S.N. (1979). Evaluating the performance of a computer-based consultant. *Computer Programs in Biomedicine,* 9(1):95–102.

Yu ,V.L., Fagan, L.M., Wraith, S.M., Clancey, W.J., Scott, A.C., Hannigan, J., Blum, R.L., Buchanan, B.G., Cohen, S.N. (1979). Antimicrobial selection by a computer. A blinded evaluation by infectious disease experts. *Journal of the American Medical Association,* 242(12):1279–1282.

Zachary, W.W., Strong, G.W., Zaklad, A. (1984). Information systems ethnography: Integrating anthropological methods into system design to insure organizational acceptance. In Hendrick, H.W., Brown, O. (eds.), *Human Factors in Organizational Design and Management,* pp.223–227. Amsterdam: North Holland Press.

Zhang, J. (1997a). Distributed representation as a principle for the analysis of cockpit information displays. *International Journal of Aviation Psychology,* 7(2):105–121.

Zhang, J. (1997b). The nature of external representations in problem solving. *Cognitive Science,* 21(2):179–217.

Zhang, J., Johnson, T.R., Patel, V.L., Paige, D.L., Kubose, T. (2003). Using usability heuristics to evaluate patient safety of medical devices. *Journal of Biomedical Informatics*, 36(1–2):23–30.

Zhang, J., Norman, D.A. (1994). Representations in distributed cognitive tasks. *Cognitive Science*, 18:87–122.

Zhang, J., Patel, V.L., Johnson, K.A., Malin, J. (2002). Designing human-centered distributed information systems. *IEEE Intelligent Systems*, 17(5):42–47.

Zhang, J., Patel, V.L., Johnson, T.R. (2002). Medical error: Is the solution medical or cognitive? *Journal of the American Medical Informatics Association*, 9(6 Suppl):75–77.

Zielstorff, R.D., Barnett, G.O., Fitzmaurice, J.B., Estey, G., Hamilton, G., Vickery, A., Welebob, E., Shahzad, C. (1996). A decision support system for prevention and treatment of pressure ulcers based on AHCPR guidelines. *Proceedings of the AMIA Annual Fall Symposium*, Washington, DC, pp. 562–566.

Zielstorff, R.D., Hudgings, C.I., Grobe, S.J. (1993). *Next-Generation Nursing Information Systems: Essential Characteristics for Nursing Practice*. Washington, DC: American Nurses Publishing.

Zijdenbos, A.P., Evans, A.C., Riahi, F., Sled, J., Chui, J., Kollokian, V. (1996). Automatic quantification of multiple sclerosis lesion volume using stereotactic space, *Proc. 4th Int. Conf. on Visualization in Biomedical Computing*, pp. 439–448. Hamburg.

Zuriff, G.E. (1985). *Behaviorism: A Conceptual Reconstruction*. New York: Columbia University Press.

Zweigenbaum, P, Courtois, P. (1998).Acquisition of lexical resources from SNOMED for medical language processing. *Proceedings of Medinfo 1998*; Pt 1:586–90.

Glossary

[Key chapters in which a term is used are indicated in square brackets.]

Abstraction: A level of medical data encoding that entails examining the recorded data and selecting an item from a terminology with which to label the data. [7]

Accountability: Security function that ensures users are responsible for their access to, and use of, information based on a documented need and right to know. [5]

Acquired immunodeficiency syndrome (AIDS):   A disease of the immune system caused by a retrovirus and transmitted chiefly through blood or blood products, characterized by increased susceptibility to opportunistic infections, to certain cancers, and to neurological disorders. [3,15,21]

Active storage: In a hierarchical data storage scheme, the devices used to store data that have long-term validity and that must be accessed rapidly. [5]

Address: In a computer system, a number or symbol that identifies a particular cell of memory. [5]

Administrative services only (ASO):   The practice by employers of paying their employees' medical bills directly (self-insurance), and hiring insurance companies only to process claims. [23]

Admission-discharge-transfer (ADT):   The core component of a hospital information system that maintains and updates the hospital census, including bed assignments of patients. [13]

Advanced Research Projects Agency Network (ARPANET):   A large wide-area network created in the 1960s by the U.S. Department of Defense Advanced Research Projects Agency (DARPA) for the free exchange of information among universities and research organizations; the precursor to today's Internet. [1,5]

Advice nurse: A health professional, typically trained in nursing, who is available by telephone to answer patients' questions and to help them to make appropriate use of health services. [23]

Aggregate content: Information from multiple sources, which can be viewed within an information retrieval system using a single interface. [19]

Alert message: A computer-generated warning that is generated when a record meets pre-specified criteria; e.g., receipt of a new laboratory test result with an abnormal value. [12]

Algorithm: A well-defined procedure or sequence of steps for solving a problem. [1]

Allocation bias: Overestimation of the effects of an intervention caused by systematic assignment of favorable subjects to the study group by investigators. [11]

Alphabetic ranking: A common ranking criterion used by information retrieval systems; for a particular field in the database, results are output based on the order of the field's first word in the alphabet. [19]

Alphanumeric: Descriptor of data that are represented as a string of letters and numeric digits, without spaces or punctuation. [19]

Ambulatory medical record system (AMRS):   A clinical information system designed to support all information requirements of an outpatient clinic, including registration, appointment scheduling, billing, order entry, results reporting, and clinical documentation. [13]

American Standard Code for Information Interchange (ASCII):   A 7-bit code for representing alphanumeric characters and other symbols. [5]

Analog signal: A signal that takes on a continuous range of values. [5]

Analog-to-digital conversion (ADC):   Conversion of sampled values from a continuous-valued signal to a discrete-valued digital representation. [5,17]

Anchoring and adjustment: A heuristic used when estimating probability, in which a person first makes a rough approximation (the anchor) and then adjusts this estimate to account for additional information. [3]

Angiography: A technique used to increase the contrast resolution of X-ray images of the blood vessels by injection of radiopaque contrast material into the vessels. [9,18]

Antibiotic-assistant program: A computer program developed to assist physicians in ordering antibiotics for patients who have, or who are suspected of having, an infection. [17]

Applets: Small computer programs that can be embedded in an HTML document and that will execute on the user's computer when referenced. [5]

Application program: A computer program designed to accomplish a user-level task. [5]

Applications research: Systematic investigation or experimentation with the goal of applying knowledge to achieve practical ends. [1]

Arc (in an influence diagram): A diagrammatic element that appears between two chance nodes and indicates that a probabilistic dependency relationship may exist between them. [3]

Archival storage: In a hierarchical data storage scheme, the devices used to store data for long-term backup, documentary, or legal purposes. [5]

Arden Syntax: A coding scheme or language that provides a canonical means for writing rules (Medical Logic Modules), which relate specific patient situations to appropriate actions for practitioners to follow. The Arden Syntax standard is maintained by HL7. [7,20]

Art criticism approach: An evaluation approach that relies on the review and opinions of an experienced and respected critic to highlight an information resource's strengths and weaknesses. [11]

Artificial intelligence (AI): The branch of computer science concerned with endowing computers with the ability to simulate intelligent human behavior. [1,20,21]

Artificial neural network (ANN): A computer program that performs classification by taking as input a set of findings that describe a given situation, propagating calculated weights through a network of several layers of interconnected nodes, and generating as output a set of numbers, where each output corresponds to the likelihood of a particular classification that could explain the findings. [20]

Assembler: A computer program that translates assembly-language programs into machine-language instructions. [5]

Assembly language: A low-level language for writing computer programs using symbolic names and addresses within the computer's memory. [5]

Assessment bias: Overestimation (or underestimation) of the effects of an intervention caused by systematic favorable (or unfavorable) evaluations of results by the investigators. [11]

Asynchronous transfer mode (ATM): A network protocol designed for sending streams of small, fixed-length cells of information over very high-speed, dedicated connections, often digital optical circuits. [5]

ATTENDING: A standalone decision-support program that critiqued a patient-specific plan for anesthetic selection, induction, and administration after that plan had been proposed by the anesthesiologist who would be managing the case. [20]

Audit trail: A chronological record of all accesses and changes to data records, often used to promote accountability for use of, and access to, medical data. [5]

Augmented reality: A user-interface method in which a computer-generated scene is superimposed on the real world, usually by painting the scene on semi-transparent goggles that track the motion of the head. [21]

Authentication: A process for positive and unique identification of users, implemented to control system access. [5]

Authoring system: In computer-aided instruction, a specialized, high-level language used by educators to create computer-based teaching programs. [21]

Authorization: Within a system, a process for limiting user activities only to actions defined as appropriate based on the user's role. [5]

Automated indexing: The most common method of full-text indexing; words in a document are stripped of common suffixes, entered as items in the index, then assigned weights based on their ability to discriminate among documents (see **vector-space model**). [19]

Availability: In decision making, a heuristic method by which a person estimates the probability of an event based on the ease with which he can recall similar events. [3] In security systems, a function that ensures delivery of accurate and up-to-date information to authorized users when needed. [5]

Averaging out at chance nodes: The process by which each chance node of a decision tree is replaced in the tree by the expected value of the event that it represents. [3]

Backbone links: Sections of high-capacity trunk (backbone) network that interconnect regional and local networks. [5]

Backbone network: A high-speed communication network that carries major traffic between smaller networks. [1]

Background question: A question that asks for general information on a topic (see also **foreground question**). [19]

Back-projection: A method for reconstructing images, in which the measured attenuation along a path is distributed uniformly across all pixels along the path. [9]

Bandwidth: The capacity for information transmission; the number of bits that can be transmitted per unit of time. [1,5]

Baseband transmission: A data transmission technique in which bits are sent without modulation (see modem). [5]

Baseline measurement: An observation collected prior to an intervention and used for comparison with an associated study observation. [11]

Baseline rate, population: The prevalence of the condition under consideration in the population from which the subject was selected; **individual:**   The frequency, rate, or degree of a condition before an intervention or other perturbation. [2]

Basic Linear Alignment and Search Technique (BLAST):   An algorithm for determining optimal genetic sequence alignments based on the observations that sections of proteins are often conserved without gaps and that there are statistical analyses of the occurrence of small subsequences within larger sequences that can be used to prune the search for matching sequences in a large database. [22]

Basic research: Systematic investigation or experimentation with the goal of discovering new knowledge, often by proposing new generalizations from the results of several experiments. [1]

Basic science: The enterprise of performing basic research. [1]

Batch mode: A noninteractive mode of using a computer, in which users submit jobs for processing and receive results on completion (see time-sharing mode). [5]

Baud rate: The rate of information transfer; at lower speeds, baud rate is equal to the number of bits per second being sent. [5]

Bayes' theorem: An algebraic expression often used in clinical diagnosis for calculating posttest probability of a condition (e.g., a disease) if the pretest probability (prevalence) of the condition, as well as the sensitivity and specificity of the test, are known (also called Bayes' rule). Bayes' theorem also has broad applicability in other areas of biomedical informatics where probabilistic inference is pertinent, including the interpretation of data in bioinformatics. [3]

Bayesian diagnosis program: A computer-based system that uses Bayes' theorem to assist a user in developing and refining a differential diagnosis. [20]

Before–after study: An experiment that compares study measurements to the same (baseline) measurements collected prior to introduction of the resource of interest (see historically controlled experiment). [11]

Behaviorism: A social science framework for analyzing and modifying behavior. [4]

Belief network: A diagrammatic representation used to perform probabilistic inference; an influence diagram that has only chance nodes. [3,20]

Bias: A systematic difference in outcome between groups that is caused by a factor other than the intervention under study. [3,11]

Binary: The condition of having only two values or alternatives. [5]

Bibliographic content: In information retrieval, information abstracted from the original source. [19]

Bibliographic database: A collection of citations or pointers to the published literature. [19]

Biocomputation: The field encompassing the modeling and simulation of tissue, cell, and genetic behavior; see **biomedical computing**. [1]

Bioinformatics: The study of how information is represented and transmitted in biological systems, starting at the molecular level. [10,22]

Biomed Central: An independent publishing house specializing in the publication of electronic journals in biomedicine (see www.biomedcentral.com). [19]

Biomedical computing: The use of computers in biology or medicine. [1]

Biomedical engineering: An area of engineering concerned primarily with the research and development of biomedical instrumentation and biomedical devices. [1]

Biomedical informatics: A field of study concerned with the broad range of issues in the management and use of biomedical information, including biomedical computing and the study of the nature of biomedical information itself. Formerly called **medical informatics**, the new name is intended to clarify that the domain encompasses biological and biomolecular informatics as well as clinical, imaging, and public health informatics. [1]

Biomedical Information Science and Technology Initiative (BISTI):   An initiative launched by the NIH in 2000 to make optimal use of computer science, mathematics, and technology to address problems in biology and medicine. It includes a consortium of senior-level representatives from each of the NIH institutes and centers plus representatives of other Federal agencies concerned with biocomputing. (see http://www.bisti.nih.gov). [1]

Biometric identifier: A measurable physical attribute of an organism (usually, a human being) that helps to establish that individual's identity; examples include fingerprints and retinal scans. [6]

Bit map: A digital representation of an image in memory, in which there is a one-to-one correspondence between groups of bits (one or more bytes) and pixels of a displayed image. [9]

Bit rate: The rate of information transfer; a function of the rate at which signals can be transmitted and the efficacy with which digital information is encoded in the signal. [5]

Bit: A digit that can assume the value of either 0 or 1. [5]

Bit-mapped display: A display screen that is divided into a grid of tiny areas (pixels), each associated with a bit that indicates whether the area is on (black) or off (white). [9]

Body (of e-mail):   The portion of a simple electronic mail message that contains the free-text content of the message. [5]

Boolean operators: The mathematical operators AND, OR, and NOT, which are used to combine index terms in information retrieval searching. [19]

Boolean searching: A search method in which search criteria are logically combined using AND, OR, and NOT operators. [19]

Bootstrap: A small set of initial instructions that is stored in read-only memory and executed each time a computer is turned on. Execution of the bootstrap is called *booting* the computer. By analogy, the process of starting larger computer systems. [5]

Bound morpheme: A morpheme that creates a different form of a word but must always occur with another morpheme (e.g., -ed, -s). [8]

Bridge: A device that links or routes signals from one network to another. [5]

Broadband transmission: A data transmission technique in which multiple signals may be transmitted simultaneously, each modulated within an assigned frequency range. [5]

Browser: A user interface to the World Wide Web that allows users to search for and display remote information resources in a suitable format. [6]

Browsing: Scanning a database, a list of files, or the Internet, either for a particular item or for anything that seems to be of interest. [5]

Business services: Remote network services that are designed for controlled or contractual user access (also see **informational services**). [6]

Business logic layer: A conceptual level of system architecture that insulates the applications and processing components from the underlying data and the user interfaces that access the data. [13]

Buttons: Graphic elements within a dialog box or user-selectable areas within an HTML document that, when activated, perform a specified function (such as invoking other HTML documents and services). [5]

Byte: A sequence of 8 bits, often used to store an ASCII character. [5]

Canonical form: A preferred string or name for a term or collection of names; the canonical form may be determined by a set of rules (e.g., "all capital letters with words sorted in alphabetical order") or may be simply chosen arbitrarily. [19]

Capitated system: System of health care reimbursement in which providers are paid a fixed amount per patient to take care of all the health needs of a population of patients. [12,23]

Capitation: In health care financing, the payment of premiums or dues directly to the provider organization in the form of a fixed periodic payment for comprehensive care, set in advance (also called per capita payment). [23]

Case manager: A health professional assigned to monitor and coordinate a patient's care across care providers and health settings throughout an episode of treatment. [16]

Cathode-ray tube (CRT): A data output device that displays information by projecting streams of electrons onto a fluorescent screen to create programmed patterns of light and dark or color. [5,17]

Centering theory: A theory that attempts to explain what entities are indicated by referential expressions (such as pronouns) by noting how the center (focus of attention) of each sentence changes across the text. [8]

Centers for Disease Control (and Prevention) **(CDC):** The U.S. government health agency responsible for monitoring and reporting incidences and trends in infectious disease, bacterial-resistance patterns, and other public health information. [2,15]

Central computer system: A single system that handles all computer applications in an institution using a common set of databases and interfaces. [13]

Central monitor: Computer-based monitoring system with waveform analysis capabilities and high-capacity data storage. [17]

Central processing unit (CPU): The "brain" of the computer. The CPU executes a program stored in main memory by fetching and executing instructions in the program. [5]

Certificate: Coded authorization information that can be verified by a certification authority to grant system access. [5]

Chance node: A symbol that represents a chance event. By convention, a chance node is indicated in a decision tree by a circle. [3]

Charge coupled device (CCD) camera: A device used to convert light directly to digital form without the need for film. [9]

Charges: In a health care institution, the established prices for services; charges often do not reflect the cost of providing the service. [23]

Check tag: In MeSH, terms that represent certain facets of medical studies, such as age, gender, human or nonhuman, and type of grant support; check tags provide additional indexing of bibliographic citations in databases such as Medline. [19]

Checklist effect: The improvement observed in decision making due to more complete and better structured data collection when paper- or computer-based forms are used to collect patient data. [11]

Chronology: The primary ranking criterion in many information retrieval systems, in which the most recent entries are output first. [19]

CINAHL Subject Headings: A set of terms based on MeSH, with additional domain-specific terms added, used for indexing the Cumulative Index to Nursing and Allied Health Literature (CINAHL). [19]

Citation database: A database of citations found in scientific articles, showing the linkages among articles in the scientific literature. [19]

Classification (of features):   In image processing, the categorization of segmented regions of an image based on the values of measured parameters, such as area and intensity. [9]

Client–server: Information processing interaction that distributes application processing between a local computer (the client) and a remote computer resource (the server). [5]

Clinical data repository (CDR):   Clinical database optimized for storage and retrieval for individual patients and used to support patient care and daily operations. [13]

Clinical decision-support system: A computer-based system that assists physicians in making decisions about patient care. [20]

Clinical Document Architecture (CDA):   An HL7 standard for naming and structuring clinical documents, such as reports. [19]

Clinical expert system: A computer program designed to provide decision support for diagnosis or therapy planning at a level of sophistication that an expert physician might provide. [10,20]

Clinical guidelines: Systematically developed statements to assist practitioner and patient decisions about appropriate health care for specific clinical circumstances. [1,20]

Clinical informatics: The application of biomedical informatics methods in the patient care domain; a combination of computer science, information science, and clinical science designed to assist in the management and processing of clinical data, information, and knowledge to support clinical practice. [1,16]

Clinical information system (CIS):   The components of a health care information system designed to support the delivery of patient care, including order communications, results reporting, care planning, and clinical documentation. [13]

Clinical judgment: Decision making by clinicians that incorporates professional experience and social, ethical, psychological, financial, and other factors in addition to the objective medical data. [10]

Clinical modifications: A published set of changes to the International Classification of Diseases (ICD) that provides additional levels of detail necessary for statistical reporting in the United States. [7]

Clinical pathway: Disease-specific plan that identifies clinical goals, interventions, and expected outcomes by time period. [13,16]

Clinical practice guidelines: See **clinical guidelines**. [4,20]

Clinical prediction rule: A rule derived from statistical analysis of clinical observations that is used to assign a patient to a clinical subgroup with a known probability of disease. [3]

Clinical research: The collection and analysis of medical data acquired during patient care, to improve medical science and the knowledge clinicians use in caring for patients. [10]

Clinical subgroup: A subset of a population in which the members have similar characteristics and symptoms, and therefore similar likelihood of disease. [3]

Clinical trials: Experiments in which data from specific patient interactions are pooled and analyzed in order to learn about the safety and efficacy of new treatments or tests and to gain insight into disease processes that are not otherwise well understood. [1]

Clinically relevant population: The population of patients that is seen in actual practice. In the context of estimating the sensitivity and specificity of a diagnostic test, that group of patients in whom the test actually will be used. [3]

Closed-loop control: Regulation of a physiological variable, such as blood pressure, by monitoring the value of the variable and altering therapy without human intervention. [17]

Coaching system: A computer-based education system that monitors the session and intervenes only when the student requests help or makes serious mistakes (see **tutoring system**). [21]

Coaxial cable: A cable typically used in the cable television industry that has a concentric arrangement of conductors and insulators, usually with a solid wire core, an insulator sheath, and an outer web of conductor wires. [18]

COBOL: COmmon Business Oriented Language. A programming language designed for business data processing and the first ANSII standard programming language. [7]

Coded: Form of data that has been standardized and classified for processing by a computer. [12]

Coding scheme: A system for classifying objects and entities (such as diseases, procedures, or symptoms) using a finite set of numeric or alphanumeric identifiers. [2]

Coercion: A function of a computer language that provides for automatic conversion of data types when a mismatch is identified. [5]

Cognitive artifacts: Human-made materials, devices, and systems that extend people's abilities in perceiving objects, encoding and retrieving information from memory, and problem solving. [4]

Cognitive heuristics: Mental processes by which we learn, recall, or process information; rules of thumb. [3]

Cognitive load: An excess of information that competes for limited cognitive resources, creating a burden on working memory. [4]

Cognitive science: Area of research concerned with studying the processes by which people think and behave. [1,4]

Cognitive walkthrough: An analytic method for characterizing the cognitive processes of users performing a task. The method is performed by an analyst or group of analysts "walking through" the sequence of actions necessary to achieve a goal, thereby seeking to identify potential usability problems that may impede the successful completion of a task or introduce complexity in a way that may frustrate users. [4]

Coinsurance: The percentage of charges that is paid by the insuree rather than by the insurance company once the deductible has been satisfied. [23]

Color resolution: A measure of the ability to distinguish among different colors (indicated in a digital image by the number of bits per pixel). Three sets of multiple bits are required to specify the intensity of red, green, and blue components of each pixel color. [5]

Communication (computer):   Data transmission and information exchange between computers using accepted protocols via an exchange medium such as a telephone line or fiberoptic cable. [5]

Community Health Information Network (CHIN):   A computer network developed for exchange of sharable health information among independent participant organizations in a geographic area (or community). [10,15]

Compact disk (CD):   A round, flat piece of material used to encode data through the use of a laser that alters the material's reflectivity. [5]

Compact-disk read-only memory (CD-ROM):   An optical-disk technology for storing and retrieving large numbers of prerecorded data. Data are permanently encoded through the use of a laser that marks the surface of the disk, then can be read an unlimited number of times using a finely focused semiconductor laser that detects reflections from the disk. [5]

Comparison-based approach: Evaluation approach that studies an experimental resource in contrast to a control resource or placebo. [11]

Compiler: A program that translates a program written in a high-level programming language to a machine-language program, which can then be executed. [5]

Comprehensibility and control: Security function that ensures that data owners and data stewards have effective control over information confidentiality and access. [5]

Computability theory: The foundation for assessing the feasibility and cost of computation to provide the complete and correct results to a formally stated problem. Many interesting problems cannot be computed in a finite time and require heuristics. [1]

Computed check: Procedure applied to entered data that verifies values based on calculation of a correct mathematical relationship; for example, white blood cell differential counts (reported as percentages) must sum to 100. [12]

Computed radiography: An imaging technique in which a latent image is recorded on a specially coated cassette that is then scanned by a computer to capture the image in digital form. [9]

Computed tomography (CT):   An imaging modality in which X-rays are projected through the body from multiple angles and the resultant absorption values are analyzed by a computer to produce cross-sectional slices. [5,9,12,18]

Computer architecture: The basic structure of a computer, including memory organization, a scheme for encoding data and instructions, and control mechanisms for performing computing operations. [5]

Computer interpretation: Translation by computer of voice input into appropriate text, codes, or commands. [12]

Computer program: A set of instructions that tells a computer which mathematical and logical operations to perform. [5]

Computer system: An integrated arrangement of computer hardware and software, operated by users to perform prescribed tasks. [6]

Computer-aided instruction (CAI):   The application of computer technology to education (also called **computer-assisted learning** and **computer-based education**). [21]

Computer-assisted learning: See **computer-aided instruction**. [21]

Computer-based education (CBE):   See **computer-aided instruction**. [21]

Computer-based monitoring: Use of computers to acquire, process, and evaluate analog physiological signals captured from patients. [17]

Computer-based patient monitor: A patient monitoring device that supports other data functions, such as database maintenance, report generation, and decision making. [17]

Computer-based patient record (CPR):   See **electronic health record (EHR)**.

Computer-based patient record system: See **electronic health record system.**

Computer-based physician order entry (CPOE):   A clinical information system that allows physicians and other clinicians to record patient-specific orders for communication to other patient care team members and to other information systems (such as test orders to laboratory systems or medication orders to pharmacy systems). Sometimes called **provider order entry** or **practitioner order entry** to emphasize such systems' uses by clinicians other than physicians. [13]

Concept: An abstract idea generalized from specific instances of objects that occur in the world. [19]

Conceptual knowledge: Knowledge about **concepts**. [4]

Concordant (test results):   Test results that reflect the true patient state (true-positive and true-negative results). [3]

Conditional independence: Two events, A and B, are conditionally independent if the occurrence of one does not influence the probability of the occurrence of the other, when both events are conditioned on a third event C. Thus, $p[A \mid B,C] = p[A \mid C]$ and $p[B \mid A,C] = p[B \mid C]$. The conditional probability of two conditionally independent events both occurring is the product of the individual conditional probabilities: $p[A,B \mid C] = p[A \mid C] \times p[B \mid C]$. For example, two tests for a disease are conditionally independent when the probability of the result of the second test does not depend on the result of the first test, given the disease state. For the case in which disease is present, p[second test positive | first test positive and disease present] = p[second test positive | first test negative and disease present] = p[second test positive | disease present]. More succinctly, the tests are conditionally independent if the sensitivity and specificity of one test do not depend on the result of the other test (see **independence**). [3]

Conditional probability: The probability of an event, contingent on the occurrence of another event. [3]

Conditioned event: A chance event, the probability of which is affected by another chance event (the **conditioning event**). [3]

Conditioning event: A chance event that affects the probability of occurrence of another chance event (the **conditioned event**). [3]

Confidentiality: The ability of data owners and data stewards to control access to, or release of, private information. [5,10]

Consensus opinion: With respect to medical care, general agreement regarding proper action. [11]

Consistency check: Procedure applied to entered data that detects errors based on internal inconsistencies; e.g., recognizing a problem with the recording of *cancer of the prostate* as the diagnosis for a female patient. [12]

Constructive (approach to learning):   An approach to teaching in which students learn through reassembly of separated parts;e.g., learning anatomy by putting together body parts or by placing cross sections at the correct location in the body. [21]

Consulting model: A style of interaction in a decision-support system, in which the program serves as an adviser, accepting patient-specific data, asking questions, and generating advice for the user about diagnosis or management. [20]

Consulting system: A computer-based system that develops and suggests problem-specific recommendations based on user input (see **critiquing system**). [20]

Consumer health informatics (CHI):   Applications of medical informatics technologies that focus on patients or healthy individuals as the primary users. [10,14]

Content structuring: The process by which distinct semantic regions of content, such as title, author names, and abstract, are identified. [19]

Content: In information retrieval, media developed to communicate information or knowledge. [19]

Context: The placement of a word in text that helps determine the intended meaning of the word. [19]

Context deficit: A lack of clues in a document that might help a human being or natural language processor infer the intended meaning of words in the document. [19]

Context-free grammar: A mathematical model of a set of strings whose members are defined as capable of being generated from a starting symbol, using rules in which a single symbol is expanded into one or more symbols. [8]

Contingency table: A 2×2 table that shows the relative frequencies of true-positive, true-negative, false-positive, and false-negative results. [3]

Continuity of care: The coordination of care received by a patient over time and across multiple health care providers. [2]

Continuous-speech recognition: Translation by computer of voice input, spoken using a natural vocabulary and cadence, into appropriate text, codes, and commands. [12]

Continuum of care: The full spectrum of health services provided to patients, including health maintenance, primary care, acute care, critical care, rehabilitation, home care, skilled nursing care, and hospice care. [16]

Contract-management system: A computer system used to support managed care contracting by estimating the costs and payments associated with potential contract terms and by comparing actual with expected payments based on contract terms. [13]

Contrast radiography: A technique used to increase the contrast resolution of X-ray images by injection of radiopaque contrast material into a body cavity or blood vessels. [9]

Contrast resolution: A measure of the ability to distinguish among small differences in intensity (indicated in a digital image by the number of bits per pixel). [5,9]

Controlled terminology: A finite, enumerated set of terms intended to convey information unambiguously. [7]

Controls: In an experiment, subjects who are not affected by the intervention of interest. [11]

Convolution: In image processing, a mathematical edge-enhancement technique used to sharpen blurred computed tomographic images. [9]

Copyright law: Protection of written materials and intellectual property from being copied verbatim. [10]

Cost center: An organizational department that does not have revenue associated with the services it provides (e.g., administration, data processing, billing, and house-keeping). [23]

Cost–benefit analysis (CBA):   An analysis of the costs and benefits associated with alternative courses of action that is designed to identify the alternative that yields the maximum net benefit. CBA is generally used when it is possible to assign dollar values to all relevant costs and benefits. [11]

Cost-effectiveness analysis (CEA):   An analysis of alternative courses of action, the objective of which is to identify either the alternative that yields the maximum effectiveness achievable for a given amount of spending, or the alternative that minimizes the cost of achieving a stipulated level of effectiveness. CEA is generally used when it is not possible to measure benefits in dollar units. [11]

Cost-effectiveness threshold: Threshold level in a cost-effectiveness analysis that reflects a decision maker's value judgment regarding a maximum (or minimum) value; e.g., the maximum value of a quality-adjusted life year to be used in an analysis. [11]

Credentialing: Certification of an individual or resource's quality by a recognized body such as a clinical professional association. [14]

Critical care: Monitoring and treatment of patients with unstable physiologic systems, with life-threatening conditions, or at high-risk of developing life-threatening conditions, typically in an intensive care or coronary care unit. [10]

Critiquing model: A style of interaction in a decision-support system, in which the program acts as a sounding board for the user's ideas, expressing agreement or suggesting reasoned alternatives. [20]

Critiquing system: A computer-based system that evaluates and suggests modifications for plans or data analyses already formed by a user (see **consulting system**). [20]

Cross validation: Verification of the accuracy of data by comparison of two sets of data collected by alternate means. [17]

Cryptographic encoding: Scheme for protecting data based on use of keys for encrypting and decrypting information (see secret-key and private-key cryptography). [5]

Cumulative Index to Nursing and Allied Health Literature (CINAHL):   A non-NLM bibliographic database that covers nursing and allied health literature, including physical therapy, occupational therapy, laboratory technology, health education, physician assistants, and medical records. [19]

Cursor: A blinking region of a display monitor, or a symbol such as an arrow, that indicates the currently active position on the screen. [5]

Customary, prevailing, and reasonable: The payment system used by Medicare (prior to implementation of the Resource-Based Relative Value Scale and Volume Performance Standard) that reimbursed practitioners generously for doing procedures and relatively poorly for providing cognitive services such as history taking and advice giving. [23]

Custom-designed system: A computer system designed and developed within an institution to meet the special needs of that institution. [6]

Customer: The user who interacts with the software and hardware of a computer system and uses the results. [6]

Data acquisition: The input of data into a computer system through direct data entry, acquisition from a medical device, or other means. [16]

Data bus: An electronic pathway for transferring data; e.g., between a CPU and memory. [5]

Data capture: The acquisition or recording of information. [12]

Data compression: A mathematical technique for reducing the number of bits needed to store data, with or without loss of information. [18]

Data Encryption Standard (DES):   A widely used method for securing information storage and communications that uses a private (secret) key for encryption and requires the same key for decryption (see also public key cryptography). [5]

Data flow: The input, processing, storage, and output of information in a computer system. [6]

Data flow diagram (DFD):   A graphical representation for the sources, transformation processes, storage, and presentation of data in a computer system. [6]

Data independence: The insulation of applications programs from changes in data storage structures and data access strategies. [5]

Data interchange standards: Adopted formats and protocols for exchange of data between independent computer systems. [7]

Data layer: A conceptual level of system architecture that isolates the data collected and stored in the enterprise from the applications and user interfaces used to access those data. [13]

Data overload: The inability to access or use crucial information due to an overwhelming number of irrelevant data or due to the poor organization of data. [17]

Data processing: The manipulation of data to convert it to some desired result (also called **data transformation**). [16]

Data recording: The documentation of information for archival or future use through mechanisms such as handwritten text, drawings, machine-generated traces, or photographic images. [2]

Data standard: A set of syntactic and semantic rules for defining elements of information to be recorded or exchanged. [7,16]

Data storage: The methods, programs, and structures used to organize data for subsequent use. [16]

Data transcription: The transfer of information from one data-recording system to another. Typically, the entry into a computer by clerical personnel of the handwritten or dictated notes or datasheets created by a health professional. [12]

Data transformation: The manipulation of data to convert it to some desired result (also called **data processing**). [16]

Data warehouse: Database optimized for long-term storage, retrieval, and analysis of records aggregated across patient populations, often serving the longer-term business and clinical analysis needs of an organization. [13]

Database: A collection of stored data—typically organized into fields, records, and files—and an associated description (schema). [2,5]

Database management system (DBMS):   An integrated set of programs that manages access to databases. [5]

Database mediator: A software component that serves as a conduit between one or more other client software components and a database server. The mediator insulates the client components from logistical issues associated with accessing the database server. [20]

Datum: Any single observation of fact. A medical datum generally can be regarded as the value of a specific parameter (e.g., red blood cell count) for a particular object (e.g., a patient) at a given point in time. [2]

Debugger: A system program that provides traces, memory dumps, and other tools to assist programmers in locating and eliminating errors in their programs. [5]

Decision analysis: A methodology for making decisions by identifying alternatives and assessing them with regard to both the likelihood of possible outcomes and the costs and benefits of those outcomes. [20]

Decision node: A symbol that represents a choice among actions. By convention, a decision node is represented in a decision tree by a square. [3]

Decision tree: A diagrammatic representation of the outcomes associated with chance events and voluntary actions. [3]

Decision facilitation approach: A formative evaluation approach designed to resolve issues important to system developers and administrators by asking and answering successive questions during the course of resource development. [11]

Decryption: The process of transforming encrypted information back to its original form; see **encryption**. [1]

Deductible: A set dollar amount of covered charges that must be paid by the insuree before the insurance company begins to reimburse for outlays or to make direct payments to providers of service. [23]

Deformable model: In image processing, a generic shape that is close in shape to a structure of interest, and which can be reshaped (deformed) until it matches the imaged structure. The deformation is controlled by an optimization procedure that minimizes a cost function. [9,18]

Delta check: Procedure applied to entered data that compares the values of new and previous results to detect large and unlikely differences in value; e.g., a recorded weight change of 100 pounds in 2 weeks. [12]

Demonstration study: An experiment designed to draw inferences about performance, perceptions, or effects of an information resource. [11]

Deoxyribonucleic acid (DNA):   The genetic material that is the basis for heredity. DNA is a long polymer chemical made of four basic subunits. The sequence in which these subunits occur in the polymer distinguishes one DNA molecule from another and in turn directs a cell's production of proteins and all other basic cellular processes. [22]

Departmental system: A system that focuses on a specific niche area in the health care setting, such as a laboratory, pharmacy, radiology department, etc. [13]

Dependent variable: In a statistical analysis, the variable that measures experimental outcome. Its value is assumed to be a function of the experimental conditions (**independent variables**). [11]

Derivational morpheme: A morpheme that changes the meaning or part of the speech of a word (e.g., -ful as in painful, converting a noun to an adjective). [8]

Derived parameter: A parameter that is calculated indirectly from multiple parameters that are measured directly. [17]

Descriptive (or **uncontrolled**) **study:** Experiment in which there is no control group for comparison. [11]

Diagnosis: The process of analyzing available data to determine the pathophysiologic explanation for a patient's symptoms. [1,10,20]

Diagnosis-related group (DRG): One of almost 500 categories based on major diagnosis, length of stay, secondary diagnosis, surgical procedure, age, and types of services required. Used to determine the fixed payment per case that Medicare will reimburse hospitals for providing care to elderly patients. [21,23]

Diagnostic process: The activity of deciding which questions to ask, which tests to order, or which procedures to perform, and determining the value of the results relative to associated risks or financial costs. [20]

DICOM (Digital Imaging and Communications in Medicine): A standard developed by the National Equipment Manufacturers Association for the electronic exchange of medical images and the data associated with the image, related to the patient, the study, the series, the image acquisition and presentation method, annotations, and associated reports. This multipart standard has been widely adopted and is one of the most successful examples of the benefits of standardization. [18]

Differential diagnosis: The set of active hypotheses (possible diagnoses) that a physician develops when determining the source of a patient's problem. [2]

Digital acquisition of images: Medical images may be acquired from a number of image generation devices. Digital acquisition refers to the process of obtaining the image data in electronic form, usually in the form of an array of picture elements (pixels) or for three-dimensional images, volume elements (voxels). Digital acquisition may be primary through a variety of digital image capture technologies, or secondary, through scanning of film-based images. [18]

Digital computer: A computer that processes discrete values based on the binary digit or bit. Essentially all modern computers are digital, but **analog computers** also existed in the past. [5]

Digital image: An image that is stored as a grid of numbers, where each picture element (pixel) in the grid represents the intensity, and possibly color, of a small area. [9,18]

Digital Imaging and Communications in Medicine: See **DICOM.**

Digital library: Organized collections of electronic content, intended for specific communities or domains. [19]

Digital object identifier (DOI):   A system for providing unique identifiers for published digital objects, consisting of a prefix that is assigned by the International DOI Foundation to the publishing entity and a suffix that is assigned and maintained by the entity. [19]

Digital Preservation Coalition: An initiative in the United Kingdom directed at insuring the preservation of scientific information. [19]

Digital radiography: The process of producing X-ray images, which are stored in digital form in computer memory, rather than on film. [9]

Digital radiology: The use of digital radiographic methods for medical imaging to support the clinical interpretation of those images. [18]

Digital signal processing (DSP) chip: An integrated circuit designed for high-speed data manipulation and used in audio communications, image manipulation, and other data acquisition and control applications. [5]

Digital signal: A signal that takes on discrete values from a specified range of values. [5]

Digital subscriber line (DSL):   A digital telephone service that allows high-speed network communication using conventional (twisted pair) telephone wiring. [5]

Digital subtraction angiography (DSA):   A radiologic technique for imaging blood vessels in which a digital image acquired before injection of contrast material is subtracted pixel by pixel from an image acquired after injection. The resulting image shows only the differences in the two images, highlighting those areas where the contrast material has accumulated. [9]

Digital versatile disk (DVD):   A plastic-and-metal disk that is used to store data optically, at a very high density; also called a **digital video disk**. [5]

Digital video disk (DVD):   Next generation optical disk storage technology that allows encoding and high-volume storage of video, audio, and computer data on a compact disk. [5,21]

Direct cost: A cost that can be directly assigned to the production of goods or services. For example, direct costs in the laboratory include the cost of the technician's salary, equipment, and supplies. [11]

Direct entry: The entry of data into a computer system by the individual who personally made the observations. [12]

Discounting: Calculation that accounts for time preference by reducing the value of expenditures and payments that accrue in the future relative to those that occur immediately. [11]

Discrimination learning: An approach to teaching in which students are presented with a series of examples of increasing complexity, thereby learning to detect subtle differences. [21]

Display monitor: A device for presenting output to users through use of a screen (see also **cathode-ray tube**). [5]

Display: In information retrieval, the last step of the information retrieval process, in which the final result set is shown to the user. [19]

Distributed cognition: A view of cognition that considers groups, material artifacts, and cultures and that emphasizes the inherently social and collaborative nature of cognition. [4]

Distributed computer system: A collection of independent computers that share data, programs, and other resources. [13]

DNA arrays: Small glass plates onto which specific DNA fragments can be affixed and then used to detect other DNA fragments present in a cell extract. [22]

DNA sequence database: A searchable, stored collection of known DNA sequences (GENBANK is one of the largest). Individual databases may also contain information about the biological source of the sequence, reference information, and annotations regarding the data. [22]

Domain Name System (DNS):   A hierarchical name management system used to translate computer names to Internet protocol (IP) addresses. [5]

Domain: A unique corporate or institutional address that designates one or multiple hosts on the Internet. [1]

Doppler shift: A perceived change in frequency of a signal as the signal source moves toward or away from a signal receiver. [18]

Double-blind: A clinical study methodology in which neither the researchers nor the subjects know to which study group a subject has been assigned. [2]

Drill and practice: An approach to teaching in which students are presented with a small amount of information, and then asked questions about the material, and thus receive immediate feedback to support the learning process. [21]

Dublin Core Metadata Initiative (DCMI):   A standard metadata model for indexing published documents. [19]

DXplain: A diagnostic decision-support system produced by the Massachusetts General Hospital that maintains profiles of findings for over 2000 diseases and generates differential diagnoses when sets of findings are entered. [19,20]

Dynamic (simulation program attribute):   A simulation program that models changes in patient state over time and in response to students' therapeutic decisions. [21]

Dynamic programming: A computationally intensive computer science technique used, for example, to determine optimal sequence alignments in many computational biology applications. [22]

EBM database (evidence-based medicine database):   A highly organized collection of clinical evidence to support medical decisions based on the results of controlled clinical trials. [19]

Edge-detection technique: A method, such as application of an edge-following algorithm, used to identify a region of interest from an overall image by delineating the borders of the region. [9]

Efficacy: The capacity for producing a desired result. [11]

Electrocardiogram (ECG):   The graphic recording of minute differences in electric potential caused by heart action. Also often called **EKG**. [5,7,17]

Electroencephalography (EEG):   A method for measuring the electromagnetic fields generated by the electrical activity of the neurons using scalp sensors, the outputs of which may be processed to localize the source of the electrical activity inside the brain. [9]

Electronic Data Interchange (EDI):   Electronic exchange of standard data transactions, such as claims submission and electronic funds transfer. [7,13]

Electronic health record (EHR):   A repository of electronically maintained information about an individual's lifetime health status and health care, stored such that it can serve the multiple legitimate users of the record. [12]

Electronic health record system: The addition to an electronic health record of information management tools that provide clinical alerts and reminders, linkages with external health knowledge sources, and tools for data analysis. [12]

Electronic textbook: An online reference containing nonpatient-specific information. [20]

Electronic-long, paper-short system (ELPS):   A publication method that provides on the Web site supplemental material that did not appear in the print version of the journal. [19]

Electrophoresis: A method of separating substances based on the rate of movement of each component in a colloidal suspension while under the influence of an electric field, for the purpose of analyzing molecular structure. [22]

EMBASE: A commercial biomedical and pharmacological database from Excerpta Medica that provides information about medical and drug-related subjects. [19]

Emergent: Experimental design whereby the results of earlier stages of investigation are used to identify future issues for evaluation. [11]

Empiricism: The view that experience is the only source of knowledge. [4]

EMTREE: A hierarchically structured, controlled vocabulary used for subject indexing, used to index **EMBASE**. [19]

Encrypted: Data that have been rendered unreadable through the process of **encryption**. [1]

Encryption: The process of transforming information such that its meaning is hidden, with the intent of keeping it secret, such that only those who know how to decrypt it can read it; see **decryption**. [1,5]

Enterprise master patient index (EMPI):   An architectural component that serves as the name authority in a health care information system composed of multiple independent systems; the EMPI provides an index of patient names and identification numbers used by the connected information systems. [13]

Entrez: A search engine from the National Center for Biotechnology Information (NCBI), at the National Library of Medicine; Entrez can be used to search a variety of life sciences databases, including PubMed. [19]

Entry term: A synonym form for a subject heading in the Medical Subject Headings (MeSH) controlled, hierarchical vocabulary. [19]

Epidemiology: The study of the incidence, distribution, and causes of disease in a population. [1,15]

Escrow: Use of a trusted third party to hold cryptographic keys, computer source code, or other valuable information to protect against loss or inappropriate access. [5]

Ethernet: A network standard that uses a bus or star topology and regulates communication traffic using the Carrier Sense Multiple Access with Collision Detection (CSMA/CD) approach. [5]

Ethics: A system of moral principles; the rules of conduct recognized in respect to a particular class of human actions or a particular group or culture. [10]

Ethnography: A branch of anthropology dealing with the scientific description of individual cultures. [11]

Evaluation: Data collection and analysis designed to appraise a situation, answer a question, or judge the success of an intervention. [11,19,21]

Evidence-based guidelines: Consensus approaches for handing recurring health management problems aimed at reducing practice variability and improving health outcomes. Clinical guideline development emphasizes using clear evidence from the existing literature, rather than expert opinion alone, as the basis for the advisory materials. [1]

Evidence-based medicine (EBM):   An approach to medical practice whereby the best possible evidence from the medical literature is incorporated in decision making. Generally such evidence is derived from controlled clinical trials. [10,19]

Evoking strength (ES):   One of two numbers used by the Internist-1 decision-support system to reflect the strength of the relationship between a disease and a finding; the evoking strength is a number between 0 and 5 that reflects the likelihood that a patient with the finding has the disease in question (see **frequency weight**). [20]

Exact-match searching: A search method that looks for a literal match of the search term, allowing precise control over the items retrieved. [19]

Excerpta Medica: A collection of life sciences databases published by Elsevier Science Publishers. [19]

Expected value: The value that is expected on average for a specified chance event or decision. [3]

Expected-value decision making: A method for decision making in which the decision maker selects the option that will produce the best result on average (i.e., the option that has the highest expected value). [3]

Experimental science: Systematic study characterized by posing hypotheses, designing experiments, performing analyses, and interpreting results to validate or disprove hypotheses and to suggest new hypotheses for study. [1]

Expert system: See **knowledge-based system.**

Expert witness: A person, such as a physician, who provides testimony at a legal proceeding in the form of professional opinions. [10]

Explosion: In information retrieval systems, the process in which a general vocabulary term and the more specific terms beneath it in the hierarchy are combined using the OR Boolean operator. [19]

Extended Binary Coded Decimal Interchange Code (EBCDIC):   An 8-bit code for representing alphanumeric characters and other symbols. [7]

Extensible Markup Language (XML):   A subset of the **Standard Generalized Markup Language (SGML)** from the World Wide Web Consortium (W3C), designed especially for Web documents. It allows designers to create their own custom-tailored tags, enabling the definition, transmission, validation, and interpretation of data between applications and between organizations. [19]

External router: A computer that resides on multiple networks and that can forward and translate message packets sent from a local or enterprise network to a regional network beyond the bounds of the organization. [5]

External validity: Characteristic of a well-founded study methodology, such that the study conclusions can be generalized from the specific setting, subjects, and intervention studied to the broader range of settings that other people will encounter. [11]

Factual knowledge: Knowledge of facts without necessarily having any in-depth understanding of their origin or implications. [4]

False-negative rate (FNR):   The probability of a negative result, given that the condition under consideration is true—e.g., the probability of a negative test result in a patient who has the disease under consideration. [3]

False-negative result (FN):   A negative result when the condition under consideration is true—e.g., a negative test result in a patient who has the disease under consideration. [3]

False-positive rate (FPR):   The probability of a positive result, given that the condition under consideration is false—e.g., the probability of a positive test result in a patient who does not have the disease under consideration. [3]

False-positive result (FP):   A positive result when the condition under consideration is false—e.g., a positive test result in a patient who does not have the disease under consideration. [3]

Feature detection: In image processing, determination of parameters, such as volume or length, from segmented regions of an image. In signal processing, identification of specific waveforms or other patterns of interest in a signal. [9,17]

Feature extraction: Computer processing to identify patterns of interest and characteristics within imaged, waveforms, and other signals (see **feature detection**). [17]

Feedback: In a computer-based education program, system-generated responses, such as explanations, summaries, and references, provided to further a student's progress in learning. [21]

Fee-for-service model: Unrestricted system of health care reimbursement in which payers pay providers for those services the provider has deemed necessary. [12]

Fiber-optic cable: A communication medium that uses thin glass fibers to guide light waves to transmit information signals. [5,18]

Field qualification: In information retrieval systems, the designation of which index or field should be searched. [19]

Field: The smallest named unit of data in a database. Fields are grouped together to form records. [5] In the context of an evaluation study, the setting or settings in which the activity under study is carried out. [11]

File server: A computer that is dedicated to storing shared or private data files. [5]

File Transfer Protocol (FTP): The protocol used for copying files to and from remote computer systems on a network using **TCP/IP**. [5]

File: In a database, a collection of similar records. [5]

Filtering algorithm: A defined procedure applied to input data to reduce the effect of noise. [5]

Finite state automaton: See finite state machine. [8]

Finite state machine: A mathematical model of a set of strings whose members are defined by following transitions (characters of a given alphabet) among a finite number of states, until arriving at a designated final state. [8]

Firewall: A security system intended to protect an organization's network against external threats by preventing computers in the organization's network from communicating directly with computers external to the network, and vice versa. [5]

Fixed cost: A cost that does not vary with the volume of production during a given period. Examples are expenses for plant, equipment, and administrative salaries. [23]

Fixed fee: Restricted system of health care reimbursement in which payers pay providers a set amount for health services approved by the payer. [12]

Flash card: A portable electronic storage medium that uses a semiconductor chip with a standard physical interface; a convenient method for moving data between computers. [5]

Floppy disk: An inexpensive magnetic disk that can be removed from the disk-drive unit and thereby used to transfer or archive files. [5]

Flowsheet: A tabular summary of information that is arranged to display the values of variables as they change over time. [12]

Fluoroscopy: An imaging method in which a screen coated with a fluorescent substance is used for viewing objects by means of X-ray or other radiation. [9]

Food and Drug Administration (FDA):   Division of the Department of Health and Human Services that regulates medical devices, as well as food, drugs, and cosmetics. [10,17,20]

Foreground question: Question that asks for general information related to a specific patient (see also **background question**). [19]

Formal systems analysis: A methodology for evaluating requirements and generating specifications for developing computer systems and other information resources. [11]

Formative decision: A decision made as a result of a study undertaken while a resource is being developed and that can affect future development of the resource. [11]

Formative evaluation: An assessment of a system's behavior and capabilities conducted during the development process and used to guide future development of the system. [21]

Fortran (also FORTRAN):   A computer programming language developed in the 1950s and used for scientific and numerical computation. The name stands for Formula Translator/Translation. [5]

Fourier transform: A mathematical method for analyzing complex electrical or sound signals to extract intensities of multiple frequencies over time. [18]

Frame relay: A high-speed network protocol designed for sending digital information over shared wide-area networks using variable length packets of information. [5]

Free morpheme: A morpheme that is a word and that does not contain another morpheme (e.g., arm, pain). [8]

Free text: Unstructured, uncoded representation of information in text format; e.g., sentences describing the results of a patient's physical examination. [12]

Frequency weight (FW):   One of two numbers used by the Internist-1 decision-support system to reflect the strength of the relationship between a disease and a finding; the FW is a number between 1 and 5, where 1 means that the finding is seldom seen in the disease and 5 means it is essentially always seen (see **evoking strength**). [20]

Frequency modulation: A method of encoding information in which changes in input signal amplitude are encoded as frequency changes in a corresponding transmitted signal around the base frequency of a carrier wave. Because the input amplitude is encoded as a frequency shift, the encoded signal is less subject to outside interference, which primarily affects the amplitude of transmitted signals. [5]

Front-end application: In database applications, a front-end application is a program, often with a graphical user interface, that helps a user manipulate information in the database without having to know details of the database design or how to program queries. [5]

Full disclosure: In ECG monitoring, a process whereby all data regarding the full set of leads are stored and available for reconstruction of the complete cardiogram as it would have appeared during a period of abnormal rhythms. [17]

Full-text content: The complete textual information contained in a bibliographic source. [19]

Full-text database: A bibliographic database that contains the entire text of journal articles, books, and other literature, rather than only citations and abstracts. [19]

Functional image: An image, such as a computed tomographic image or a digital subtraction angiogram image, which is computed from derived quantities, rather than being measured directly. [9]

Functional magnetic resonance imaging (fMRI):   A **magnetic resonance imaging** method that reveals changes in blood oxygenation that occur following neural activity. [9]

Functional mapping: An imaging method that relates specific sites on images to particular physiologic functions. [9,18]

Gateway: A computer that resides on multiple networks and that can forward and translate message packets sent between nodes in networks running different protocols. [5]

Gene: A hereditary unit consisting of a sequence of DNA that occupies a specific location on a chromosome and determines a particular characteristic in an organism. [22]

Genetic data: Information regarding a person or organism's genome and heredity. [10]

Genome: The total collection of DNA for a person or other organism. [22]

Genomics: The study of all of the nucleotide sequences, including structural genes, regulatory sequences, and noncoding DNA segments, in the chromosomes of an organism. [22]

Genomics database: An organized collection of information from gene sequencing, protein characterization, and other genomic research. [19]

Genotype: The genetic makeup, as distinguished from the physical appearance, of an organism or a group of organisms. [22]

Gigabits per second (Gbps):   A common unit of measure for data transmission over high-speed networks. [5]

Gigabyte: 2^{30} or 1,073,741,824 bytes. [5]

Global processing: Any image-enhancement technique in which the same computation is applied to every pixel in an image. [9]

Goal-free approach: An evaluation approach in which evaluators are purposely unaware of the intended effects of an information resource and collect evidence to enable identification of all effects, intended or not. [11]

Gold-standard test: The test or procedure whose result is used to determine the true state of the subject—e.g., a pathology test such as a biopsy used to determine a patient's true disease state. [3]

Google: A commercial search engine that provides free searching of documents on the World Wide Web. [19]

Grammar: A mathematical model of a potentially infinite set of strings. [8]

Granularity: The level of detail of a search strategy, ranging from general topics to very specific concepts. [19]

Graphic editor: A program used to create and manipulate drawings or images for storage as computer files. [5]

Graphical user interface (GUI):   A type of environment that represents programs, files, and options by means of icons, menus, and dialog boxes on the screen. [4, 5]

Gray scale: A scheme for representing intensity in a black-and-white image. Multiple bits per pixel are used to represent intermediate levels of gray. [5]

Group-model HMO: A type of HMO that is based on contracts between physicians organized in a medical group and the HMO; the medical group accepts risks of costs of care and usually rewards the partners if the group is successful in managing costs (see **staff-model HMO**). [23]

Guidance: In a computer-based education program, proactive feedback, help facilities, and other tools designed to assist a student in learning the covered material. [21]

Haptic feedback: A user interface feature in which physical sensations are transmitted to the user to provide a tactile sensation as part of a simulated activity. [18]

Hard disk: A magnetic disk used for data storage and typically fixed in the disk-drive unit. [5]

Hardware: The physical equipment of a computer system, including the central processing unit, memory, data storage devices, workstations, terminals, and printers. [5,6]

Hashing: A method of transforming a search key into an address for the purpose of efficiently storing and retrieving items of data. [19]

Hawthorne effect: The tendency for humans to improve their performance if they know it is being studied. [11]

Header (of email):   The portion of a simple electronic mail message that contains information about the date and time of the message, the address of the sender, the addresses of the recipients, the subject, and other optional information. [5]

Health information infrastructure: The set of public and private resources, including networks, databases, and policies, for collecting, storing and transmitting health information. [15]

Health Insurance Portability and Accountability Act (HIPPA):   A law enacted in 1996 to protect health insurance coverage for workers and their families when they change or lose their jobs. An "administrative simplification" provision requires the Department of Health and Human Services to establish national standards for electronic health care transactions and national identifiers for providers, health plans, and employers. It also addresses the security and privacy of health data. [5]

Health Level 7 (HL7):   An ad hoc standards group formed to develop standards for exchange of health care data between independent computer applications; more specifically, the health care data messaging standard developed and adopted by the HL7 standards group. [1,7,12,]

Health on the Net (HON):   A private organization establishing ethical standards for health information published on the World Wide Web. [19]

Health Security Act: The 1994 proposal (by then President Clinton) drafted to overhaul the health care financing and delivery system and to provide universal health insurance coverage for all Americans. [23]

Health care information system (HCIS):   An information system used within a health care organization to facilitate communication, to integrate information, to document health care interventions, to perform record keeping, or otherwise to support the functions of the organization. [13]

Health care organizations (HCO):   Any organization, such as a physician's practice, hospital, or health maintenence organization, that provides care to patients. [13]

Health care team: A coordinated group of health professionals including physicians, nurses, case managers, dieticians, pharmacists, therapists, and other practitioners who collaborate in caring for a patient. [2]

Health maintenance organization (HMO):   A group practice or affiliation of independent practitioners that contracts with patients to provide comprehensive health care for a fixed periodic payment specified in advance. [7,23]

Hearsay evidence: Testimony based on what a witness has heard from another source rather than on direct personal knowledge or experience. [10]

HELP sector: A decision rule encoded in the HELP system, a clinical information system that was developed by researchers at LDS Hospital in Salt Lake City. [20]

Helpers (plug-ins):   Applications that are launched by a Web browser when the browser downloads a file that the browser is not able to process itself. [5]

Heuristic: A mental "trick" or rule of thumb; a cognitive process used in learning or problem solving. [2]

Heuristic evaluation: A usability inspection method, in which the system is evaluated on the basis of a small set of well-tested design principles such as visibility of system status, user control and freedom, consistency and standards, flexibility and efficiency of use. [4]

High-level process: A complex process comprising multiple lower-level processes. [1]

Histogram equalization: An image-enhancement technique that spreads the image's gray levels throughout the visible range to maximize the visibility of those gray levels that are used frequently. [9,18]

Historically controlled experiment: A study that makes and compares the same measurements before and after the introduction of the resource of interest (see **before–after study**). [11]

Hospital information system (HIS):   Computer system designed to support the comprehensive information requirements of hospitals and medical centers, including patient, clinical, ancillary, and financial management. [1,5,6,7,12,13,16,18]

Human–computer interaction (HCI):   Formal methods for addressing the ways in which human beings and computer programs exchange information. [4]

Human Genome Project: An international undertaking, the goal of which is to determine the complete sequence of human deoxyribonucleic acid (DNA), as it is encoded in each of the 23 chromosomes. [22]

Human immunodeficiency virus (HIV):   A retrovirus that invades and inactivates helper T cells of the immune system and is a cause of AIDS and AIDS-related complex. [5,7,15,21]

Hypertext: Text linked together in a nonsequential web of associations. Users can traverse highlighted portions of text to retrieve additional related information. [5,19]

HyperText Markup Language (HTML):   The document specification language used for documents on the World Wide Web. [5,6,19,20,21]

HyperText Transfer Protocol (HTTP):   The client–server protocol used to access information on the World Wide Web. [5,19]

Hypothetico-deductive approach: In clinical medicine, an iterative approach to diagnosis in which physicians perform sequential, staged data collection, data interpretation, and hypothesis generation to determine and refine a differential diagnosis. [2]

ICD-9-CM: see **Ninth International Classification of Diseases–Clinical Modification (ICD-9-CM).** [7]

Icon: In a graphical interface, a pictorial representation of an object or function. [5]

IDF*TF weighting: A simple weighting measure used for document retrieval based on term frequency (TF) and inverse document frequency (IDF); terms that occur often in only a small number of documents are given the highest weighting. [19]

Image database: An organized collection of clinical image files, such as X-rays, photographs, and microscopic images. [19]

Image enhancement: The use of global processing methods to improve the appearance of an image, either for human viewing or for subsequent processing by computer. [9,18]

Image generation: The process of producing images. [9,18]

Image integration: The combination of images with other information needed for interpretation, management, and other tasks. [9]

Image management: The application of methods for storing, transmitting, displaying, retrieving, and organizing images. [9,18]

Image manipulation: The use of pre- and postprocessing methods to enhance, visualize, or analyze images. [9,18]

Image processing: The transformation of one or more input images, either into one or more output images, or into an abstract representation of the contents of the input images. [9,18]

Imaging informatics: A subdiscipline of bioedical informatics concerned with the common issues that arise in all image modalities, relating to the acquisition of images in or conversion to digital form, and the analysis, manipulation, and use of those images once they are in digital form. [1, 9, 18]

Imaging modality: A method for producing images. Examples of medical applications are X-ray imaging, computed tomography, ultrasonography, magnetic resonance imaging, and photography. [9,18]

Immersive simulated environment: A teaching environment in which a student manipulates tools to control simulated instruments, producing visual, pressure, and other feedback to the tool controls and instruments. [21]

Immunization registries: Confidential, population based, computer-based information systems that contain data about children and vaccinations. [15]

Impact printer: Output device that uses typewriter, print chain, or drum technologies to contact a paper, thus producing a character or mark. [5]

Implementation phase: A major step in the system life cycle in which the system is constructed based on its design specifications. [6]

Import number: A number used by the Internist-1 decision-support system; the import number captures the notion that some abnormalities have serious implications and must be explained, whereas others may be safely ignored. [20]

Inaccessibility: Unavailability; a limitation of traditional medical records, which can be used by only one person at a time. [12]

Incremental cost-effectiveness ratio: The difference in the costs between two interventions or options divided by the difference in benefits. [11]

Incrementalist: Person who is able to make changes gradually, by degrees. [11]

Indemnity insurance: A type of insurance modeled on casualty insurance. Typically, an insuree is reimbursed a specified amount for a hospital day, or for each of a list of surgical procedures. [23]

Independence: Two events, A and B, are considered independent if the occurrence of one does not influence the probability of the occurrence of the other. Thus, $p[A \mid B] = p[A]$. The probability of two independent events A and B both occurring is given by the product of the individual probabilities: $p[A, B] = p[A] \times p[B]$. (See **conditional independence**.) [3]

Independent variable: A variable believed to affect the outcome (dependent variable) of an experiment. [11]

Index: In information retrieval, a shorthand guide to the content that allows users to find relevant content quickly. [19,21]

Index attribute: A term that describes some aspect of an index item, such as the document numbers where the item appears or the frequency of the item within a document. [19]

Index item: A unit of information used for matching with a query during searching. [19]

Index Medicus: The printed index used to catalog the medical literature. Journal articles are indexed by author name and subject heading, and then aggregated in bound volumes. The Medline database was originally constructed as an online version of the Index Medicus. [19]

Index test: The diagnostic test whose performance is being measured. [3]

Indexing: In information retrieval, the assignment to each document of specific terms that indicate the subject matter of the document and that are used in searching. [19]

Indexing Initiative: An effort from the National Library of Medicine to investigate methods whereby automated indexing methods can partially or completely substitute for current (manual) indexing practices. [19]

Indirect care: Activities of health professionals that are not directly related to patient care, such as teaching and supervising students, continuing education, and attending staff meetings. [16]

Individual practice association (IPA):   A group of individual physicians that has joined together to contract with one or more insurance carriers to see patients enrolled with those carriers. The physicians continue to practice in their own offices and continue to see patients with other forms of insurance coverage. The group is paid on a per capita basis for services delivered by member physicians under the IPA contracts. Individual physician members agree to fee schedules, management controls, and risk-sharing arrangements (also known as **network-model HMOs**). [23]

Inflectional morpheme: A morpheme that creates a different form of a word without changing the meaning of the word or the part of speech (e.g., -ed, -s, -ing as in activated, activates, activating.) [8]

Influence diagram: A belief network in which explicit decision and utility nodes are also incorporated. [3,20]

InfoMastery: For Information Mastery, a set of methods from evidence-based medicine for determining the value and validity of information. [19]

Information: Organized data or knowledge that provide a basis for decision making. [2]

Information extraction: Methods that process text to capture and organize specific information in the text and also to capture and organize specific relations between the pieces of information. [8]

Information need: In information retrieval, the searchers' expression, in their own language, of the information that they desire. [19]

Information resources: In biomedical informatics, computer systems developed to collect, process, and disseminate health information. [11]

Information retrieval (IR):   Methods that efficiently and effectively search and obtain data, particularly text, from very large collections or databases. It is also the science and practice of identification and efficient use of recorded media. [8,19]

Information retrieval (IR) database: An organized collection of stored bibliographic data, which typically contains both an index and the full original content. [19,8]

Information science: The field of study concerned with issues related to the management of both paper-based and electronically stored information. [1]

Information Sources Map (ISM):   One component of the Unified Medical Language System, the Information Sources Map (ISM) is a database of available databases, indexed by terms in the Metathesaurus. [19]

Information theory: The theory and mathematics underlying the processes of communication. [1]

Informational services: Remote network services that are designed to be broadly accessible (see also **business services**). [6]

Ink-jet printer: Output device that uses a moveable head to spray liquid ink on paper; the head moves back and forth for each line of pixels. [5]

Input: The data that represent state information, to be stored and processed to produce results (output). [6]

Institute of Electrical and Electronics Engineers (IEEE):   An international organization through which many of the world's standards in telecommunications, electronics, electrical applications, and computers have been developed. [7,17]

Institutional review board (IRB):   A committee responsible for reviewing an institution's research projects involving human subjects in order to protect their safety, rights, and welfare. [5,8]

Integrated circuit (IC):   A circuit of transistors, resistors, and capacitors constructed on a single chip and interconnected to perform a specific function. [5]

Integrated delivery network (IDN):   A large conglomerate health care organization developed to provide and manage comprehensive health care services. [10,13,18]

Integrated Services Digital Network (ISDN):   An international communications standard for sending digital information over telephone lines. ISDN supports data transfer rates of 64 Kbps. [5]

Integrative model: Model for understanding a phenomenon that draws from multiple disciplines and is not necessarily based on first principles. [22]

Intellectual property: Software programs, knowledge bases, Internet pages, and other creative assets that require protection against copying and other unauthorized use. [10]

Intensive care unit (ICU):   A hospital unit in which critically ill patients are monitored closely. [1,7,17]

Interdisciplinary care: A patient care approach that recognizes and coordinates the complementary contributions of multiple clinicians, including physicians, nurses, dieticians, pharmacists, physical therapists, etc. [16]

Interface engine: A computer system that translates and formats data for exchange between independent (sending and receiving) computer systems. [12, 13]

Intermittent monitoring: The periodic measurement of a physiological parameter. [17]

Internal validity: Characteristic of a well-founded experiment; the ability to have confidence in an experiment's conclusions due to the quality of its methodology. [11]

Internet: A worldwide collection of gateways and networks that communicate with each other using the TCP/IP protocol, collectively providing a range of services including electronic mail and World Wide Web access. [5]

Internet 2:   The initial project of the University Consortium for Advanced Internet Development (UCAID), Internet 2 is a test bed for high-bandwidth communications to support research and education that builds on existing federally funded or experimental networks. [1]

Internet (or IP) address: A 32-bit number, written as a sequence of four 8-bit numbers, that identifies uniquely a device attached to the Internet. IP addresses are often written as a dotted sequence of numbers: a.b.c.d. Although not assigned geographically, the first number identifies a region, the second a local area, the third a local net, and the fourth a specific computer. [5]

Internet Control Message Protocol (ICMP):   A network-level Internet protocol that provides error correction and other information relevant to processing data packets. [5]

Internet Corporation for Assigned Names and Numbers (ICANN):   The organization responsible for managing Internet domain name and IP address assignments. [5]

Internet Mail Access Protocol (IMAP):   A protocol used by electronic mail programs to access messages stored on a mail server. [5]

Internet Protocol (IP):   The protocol within **TCP/IP** that governs the creation and routing of data packets and their reassembly into data messages. [5]

Internet service provider (ISP):   A commercial communications company that supplies fee-for-service Internet connectivity to individuals and organizations. [5]

Internet standards: The set of conventions and protocols all Internet participants use to enable effective data communications. [5]

Interoperability: The ability for systems to exchange data and operate in a coordinated, seamless manner. [19]

Interpreter: A program that converts each statement in a high-level program to a machine-language representation and then executes the binary instruction(s). [5]

Interventional radiology: The use of needles, catheters, biopsy instruments, or other invasive methodologies with the aim of producing a diagnostic or therapeutic, or possibly palliative, effect. Examples are balloon angioplasty for coronary stenosis and cyst aspiration and drainage. [18]

Intranet: An enterprise-wide network that is managed and controlled by an organization for communication and information access within the organization by authorized users. [1]

Intuitionist-pluralist: A philosophical orientation whereby an observation depends on both the resource under study and the perspective of the observer. [11]

Invasive monitoring technique: A method for measuring a physiological parameter that requires breaking the skin or otherwise entering the body. [17]

Inverse document frequency (IDF):   A measure of how infrequently a term occurs in a document collection. $IDF_i = \log\left(\dfrac{\text{number of documents.}}{\text{number of documents with term i}}\right) + 1$. [19]

Inverted index: In information retrieval, a simple guide to the content that includes items (such as words) and item attributes (such as documents that contain the words). [19]

Ionizing radiation: X-rays and other forms of radiation that penetrate cells, and, when sufficiently intense, inhibit cell division, thereby causing cell death. [9]

IP address: A 32-bit number that uniquely identifies a computer connected to the Internet. [5]

Job: A set of tasks submitted by a user for processing by a computer system. [5]

Joystick: A lever-like device (like the steering stick of an airplane) that a user moves to control the position of a cursor on a screen. [5]

"Just in time" information model: An approach to providing necessary information to a user at the moment it is needed, usually through anticipation of the need. [19]

Kernel: The core of the operating system that resides in memory and runs in the background to supervise and control the execution of all other programs and direct operation of the hardware. [5]

Key field: A field in the record of a file that uniquely identifies the record within the file. [5]

Keyboard: A data input device used to enter alphanumeric characters through typing. [5]

Kilobyte: 2^{10} or 1024 bytes. [5]

Knowledge: Relationships, facts, assumptions, heuristics, and models derived through the formal or informal analysis (or interpretation) of data. [2]

Knowledge base: A collection of stored facts, heuristics, and models that can be used for problem solving. [2,20]

Knowledge-based information: Information that has been derived and organized from observational or experimental research. [19]

Knowledge-based system: A program that symbolically encodes, in a knowledge base, facts, heuristics, and models derived from experts in a field and uses that knowledge to provide problem analysis or advice that the expert might have provided if asked the same question. Also known as *expert system.* [10, 20]

Large-Scale Networking: A federal initiative to coordinate advanced network components, technologies, security, infrastructure, and middleware; grid and collaboration networking tools and services; and engineering, management, and use of large-scale networks for science and engineering research and development. It is the successor to the **Next Generation Internet** program that was active in the 1990s (see http://www.nitrd.gov/subcommittee/lsn.html). [1]

Laser printer: Output device that uses an electromechanically controlled laser beam to generate an image on a xerographic surface, which is then used to produce paper copies. [5]

Latency: The time required for a signal to travel between two points in a network. [1]

Legacy system: A computer system that remains in use and is difficult to phase out after an organization installs new systems. [13]

Legal issues: The aspects of using software applications in clinical practice and in biomedical research that are defined by law, including liability under tort law, legislation governing privacy and confidentiality, and intellectual property issues. [10]

Level: One of a set of discrete values that can be assumed by a categorical variable. [11]

Lexeme: A minimal lexical unit in a language that represents different forms of the same word. [8]

Lexical-statistical retrieval: Retrieval based on a combination of word matching and relevance ranking. [19]

Lexicography: The study of analyzing electronic dictionaries and creating lexical resources. [8]

Light pen: A penlike photosensitive device with which a user can select and enter data by pointing at the screen of a video display terminal. [5]

Light: Electromagnetic radiation that can be detected by the organs of sight. [9]

Likelihood ratio (LR):   A measure of the discriminatory power of a test. The LR is the ratio of the probability of a result when the condition under consideration is true to the probability of a result when the condition under consideration is false (e.g., the probability of a result in a diseased patient to the probability of a result in a nondiseased patient). The LR for a positive test is the ratio of true-positive rate (TPR) to false-positive rate (FPR). [3]

Link-based indexing: An indexing approach that gives relevance weight to web pages based on how often they are cited by other pages. [19]

Liquid crystal display (LCD):   A display technology that uses rod-shaped molecules to bend light and alter contrast and viewing angle to produce images. [5,17]

Listserve: A distribution list for electronic mail messages. [5]

Literature reference database: See **bibliographic database**. [19]

Local-area network (LAN):   A network for data communication that connects multiple nodes, all typically owned by a single institution and located within a small geographic area. [5,18]

Logical link control (LLC): A sublayer of the data link layer of the ISO Open Systems Interconnection model. [7]

Logical positivism: The view that all statements are analytic (true by logical deduction), verifiable by observation, or meaningless. [4]

Logical-positivist: A philosophical orientation that holds factual only that which has verifiable consequences in experience. [11]

Long-term memory: The part of memory that acquires information from short-term memory and retains it for long periods of time. [4]

Lossless compression: A mathematical technique for reducing the number of bits needed to store data while still allowing for the re-creation of the original data. [18]

Lossy compression: A mathematical technique for reducing the number of bits needed to store data but which results in loss of information. [18]

Lots of Copies Keep Stuff Safe (LOCKSS): An initiative that seeks to preserve important documents by making numerous digital copies, combined with the ability to detect and repair damaged copies as well as to prevent subversion of the data. [19]

Low-level process: An elementary process that has its basis in the physical world of chemistry or physics. [1]

Machine code: The set of primitive instructions to a computer represented in binary code (machine language). [5]

Machine language: The set of primitive instructions represented in binary code. [5]

Machine translation: Automatic mapping of text written in one natural language into text of another language. [8]

Macro: In assembly language, a set of instructions, often with parameters that specify arguments or conditions for assembly, that provide a higher level operator for programming above the machine instruction. As with subroutines, macros make programming easier and facilitate reuse of common program segments (like saving a block of registers to the stack). [5]

Magnetic disk: A round, flat plate of material that can accept and store magnetic charge. Data are encoded on magnetic disk as sequences of charges on concentric tracks. [5]

Magnetic resonance imaging (MRI): A modality that produces images by evaluating the differential response of atomic nuclei in the body when the patient is placed in an intense magnetic field and perturbed by an orthogonal radiofrequency pulse. [5,9,18]

Magnetic tape: A long ribbon of material that can accept and store magnetic charge. Data are encoded on magnetic tape as sequences of charges along longitudinal tracks. [5]

Magnetism: The properties of attraction possessed by magnets. Many atomic nuclei within the body act like tiny magnets, a characteristic that is used in the creation of images through methods such as nuclear magnetic resonance spectroscopy. [9]

Magnetoencephalography (MEG):   A method for measuring the electromagnetic fields generated by the electrical activity of the neurons using a large arrays of scalp sensors, the outputs of which are processed in a similar way to CT in order to localize the neuronal activity. [9]

Mailing list: A set of mailing addresses used for bulk distribution of electronic or physical mail. [5]

Mainframe computer: A large, expensive, multiuser computer, typically operated and maintained by professional computing personnel. [5]

Maintenance phase: The final step in the system life cycle during which the system is in routine use and is periodically modified based on changing requirements. [6]

Major medical insurance: Comprehensive insurance for medical expenses. Typically, the insurer pays a certain percentage of covered charges once the insuree has satisfied the deductible. [23]

Malpractice: Class of litigation in health care based on negligence theory; failure of a health professional to render proper services in keeping with the standards of the community. [10]

Managed competition: A strategy used by health services purchasers intended to use market forces to transform the health care delivery system; to create integrated, efficient provider organizations capable of delivering high-value health services and good health outcomes; and to create incentives for continuous quality improvement and cost reduction. [23]

Management: The process of treating a patient (or allowing the condition to resolve on its own) once the medical diagnosis has been determined. [20]

Manual indexing: The process by which human indexers, usually using standardized terminology, assign indexing terms and attributes to documents, often following a specific protocol. [19]

Marginal cost: The increase in total cost associated with the production of one more unit of a good or service. [23]

Marginal cost-effectiveness ratio: The relative value of two interventions, calculated as the difference in the measured costs of the two interventions divided by the difference in the measured benefits of the interventions. [11]

Markov cycle: The period of time specified for a transition probability within a Markov model. [3]

Markov model: A mathematical model of a set of strings in which the probability of a given symbol occurring depends on the identity of the immediately preceding symbol or the two immediately preceding symbols. Processes modeled in this way are often called **Markov processes.** [3,8]

Markup language: A document specification language that identifies and labels the components of the document's contents. [6]

Markup: Labeling of distinct semantic regions of content in a document. [19]

Master patient index (MPI): The module of a health care information system used to identify a patient uniquely within the system. Typically, the MPI stores patient identification information, basic demographic data, and basic encounter-level data such as dates and locations of service. [13]

Matching: The first step of the information retrieval process, in which a query is compared against an index to create a result set. [19]

Mean average precision (MAP): A method for measuring overall retrieval precision in which precision is measured at every point at which a relevant document is obtained, and the MAP measure is found by averaging these points for the whole query. [19]

Measurement study: An experiment that seeks to determine how accurately an attribute of interest can be measured in a population of objects. [11]

Measurement: The process of assigning a value corresponding to presence, absence, or degree of a specific attribute in a specific object. [11]

Measures of concordance: Measures of agreement in test performance: the true-positive and true-negative rates. [3]

Measures of discordance: Measures of disagreement in test performance: the false-positive and false-negative rates. [3]

Medicaid: A program of federal grants to help states pay for the medical care of welfare recipients and of other individuals who fall into special categories of support for their health care needs. [23]

Medical computer science: The subdivision of computer science that applies the methods of computing to medical topics. [1]

Medical computing: The application of methods of computing to medical topics (see **medical computer science**). [1]

Medical datum: Any single observation of medical fact; the value of a specific parameter (e.g., red blood cell count) for a particular object (e.g., a patient) at a given point in time. [2]

Medical informatics: Former name for **biomedical informatics**, now generally viewed as a synonym for **clinical informatics**, although these definitions and conventions are in transition. [1]

Medical information bus (MIB): A data communication system that supports data acquisition from a variety of independent devices. [7,17]

Medical information science: The field of study concerned with issues related to the management and use of biomedical information (see also **biomedical informatics**). [1]

Medical Literature Analysis and Retrieval System (MEDLARS): The initial electronic version of Index Medicus developed by the National Library of Medicine. [19]

Medical logic module (MLM): A single chunk of medical reasoning or decision rule, typically encoded using the **Arden Syntax**. [20]

Medical management: Process employed by a health plan or integrated delivery network to manage patient care proactively and to ensure delivery of (only) appropriate health services. [13]

Medical record: A paper-based or computer-stored document in which are recorded the data gathered during a patient's encounters with the health care system. [12]

Medical spreadsheet: A tool within the Quick Medical Reference decision-support system used to determine how coexisting diseases might give rise to a user-specified combination of diseases or findings. [20]

Medical Subject Headings (MeSH): Some 18,000 terms used to identify the subject content of the biomedical literature. The National Library of Medicine MeSH vocabulary has emerged as the de facto standard for biomedical indexing. [7,19]

Medical technology: Techniques, drugs, equipment, and procedures used by health care professionals in delivering medical care to individuals, and the system within which such care is delivered. [11]

Medical record committee: An institutional panel charged with ensuring appropriate use of medical records within the organization. [10]

Medicare: The federal program of hospital and medical insurance for Social Security retirees, the long-term disabled, and patients suffering from chronic renal failure. [23]

MEDLARS Online (MEDLINE):   The National Library of Medicine's electronic catalog of the biomedical literature, which includes information abstracted from journal articles, including author names, article title, journal source, publication date, abstract, and medical subject headings. [19]

MEDLINEplus: An online resource from the National Library of Medicine that contains health topics, drug information, medical dictionaries, directories, and other resources, organized for use by health care consumers. [19]

MedWeaver: A Web application that was designed to integrate functions from the DXplain decision-support system, the WebMedline literature search system, and the CliniWeb clinical Web search system using the UMLS Metathesaurus for vocabulary translation. [19]

Megabit: One million bits; usually used in reference to transmission speed, as in "megabits per second". [5]

Megabits per second (Mbps):   A common unit of measure for specifying a rate of data transmission. [5]

Megabyte: 2^{20} or 1,048,576 bytes. [5]

Member checking: Step in a subjectivist study during which the investigator shares emerging thoughts and beliefs with the participants themselves in order to validate and reorganize the structure of the study. [11]

Memorandum of understanding: Document that represents the general goals, scope, methods, conditions, and expected outcomes of a research study. [11]

Memory stick: A portable electronic storage medium that uses a semiconductor chip with a standard physical interface; a convenient method for moving data between computers. [5]

Memory: Areas that are used to store programs and data. The computer's working memory comprises read-only memory (ROM) and random-access memory (RAM). [5]

Mental models: A form of mental representation that enables one to understand how something in the world works. One can "run" a mental model to predict future states of a system (e.g., what happens when I click on this link?) or to explain the cause of a change in state of a system (e.g., why did my computer crash?). [4]

Menu: In a user interface, a displayed list of valid commands or options from which a user may choose. [5]

Merck Medicus: An aggregated set of resources, including Harrison's Online, MDConsult, and DXplain. [19]

MeSH: See **Medical Subject Headings.**

MeSH subheading: One of 76 qualifier terms that can be added to an MeSH entry term to specify the meaning further. [19]

Metadata: Literally, data about data, describing the format and meaning of a set of data. [5,19]

Meta-analysis: A summary study that combines quantitatively the estimates from individual studies. [3]

Meta data: In database applications, abstract descriptors of record structures and their interrelationships that facilitate locating records and fields and manipulating their contents. If programs use meta data to access and process database information, they can achieve data independence in that changes to a database structure can be made and reflected in the meta data in such a way that the program continues to operate without reprogramming. [5]

Metacontent: Information that describes the content of an information resource and thus adds structure to the content. [21]

Meta-tool: A computer program used to generate automatically a domain-specific knowledge-elicitation tool based on a model of the intended application area for a decision-support system. [20]

Metathesaurus: One component of the Unified Medical Language System, the Metathesaurus contains linkages between terms in Medical Subject Headings (MeSH) and in dozens of controlled vocabularies. [19]

Microarray chip: A microchip that holds DNA probes that can recognize DNA from samples being tested. [22]

Middleware: Software that resides between, and translates information between, two or more types of software. For example, middleware components may support access, processing, analysis, and composition of lower-level resources available through basic services, such as access to image data or clinical data. [18]

Mixed-initiative system: An educational program in which user and program share control of the interaction. Usually, the program guides the interaction, but the student can assume control and digress when new questions arise during a study session. [21]

Model organism database: Organized reference databases that combine bibliographic databases, full text, and databases of sequences, structure, and function for organisms whose genomic data has been highly characterized, such as the mouse, fruit fly, and Sarcchomyces yeast. [19]

Modeling: Task in the creation of a computer-based decision-support system that entails deciding what distinctions and data are relevant, identifying the concepts and relationships among concepts that bear on the decision-making task, and ascertaining a problem-solving strategy that can use the relevant knowledge to reach appropriate conclusions. [20]

Modem: A device used to modulate and demodulate digital signals for transmission to a remote computer over telephone lines; converts digital data to audible analog signals, and vice versa. [5]

Modular computer system: A system composed of separate units, each of which performs a specific set of functions. [13]

Molecular imaging: A technique for capturing images at the cellular and subcellular level by marking particular chemicals in ways that can be detected with image or radiodetection. [9]

Morpheme: The smallest unit in the grammar of a language that has a meaning or a linguistic function; it can be a root of a word (e.g., -arm), a prefix (e.g., re-), or a suffix (e.g., -it/-is). [8]

Morphology: The study of meaningful units in language and how they combine to form words. [8, 19]

Morphometrics: The quantitative study of growth and development, a research area that depends on the use of imaging methods. [9,18]

Mouse (input device):   A small boxlike device that is moved on a flat surface to position a cursor on the screen of a display monitor. A user can select and mark data for entry by depressing buttons on the mouse. [5]

Multi-axial terminology: A terminology that seperates terms into multiple "axes" (usually, seperate hierarchies) for the purposes of selecting terms from more than one axis to express meaning (see **postcoordination**). [7]

Multidisciplinary care: A system of patient care characterized by the collaboration of health professionals, including physicians, nurses, therapists, technicians, dieticians, pharmacists, and other care providers. [16]

Multimedia content: Information sources that encompass all common computer-based forms of information, including texts, graphics, images, video, and sound. [19]

Multimodality image fusion: Image processing that uses multiple techniques of image manipulation to generate a composite visualization that combines images from more than one source. [9]

Multiprocessing: The use of multiple processors in a single computer system to increase the power of the system (see **parallel processing**). [5]

Multiprogramming: A scheme by which multiple programs simultaneously reside in the main memory of a single central processing unit. [5]

Multipurpose Internet Mail Extensions (MIME):   An extended standard for exchange of electronic mail that allows the direct transmission of video, sound, and binary data files by Internet electronic mail. [5]

Multiuser system: A computer system that shares its resources among multiple simultaneous users. [5]

MUMPS: Massachusetts General Hospital Utility Multi-Programming System; a specialized programming language (the second ANSII standard programming language, after **COBOL**) developed for use in medical applications; also known as **M**. [1]

Mutually exclusive: State in which one, and only one, of the possible conditions is true;e.g., either A or not A is true, and one of the statements is false. When using Bayes' theorem to perform medical diagnosis, we generally assume that diseases are mutually exclusive, meaning that the patient has exactly one of the diseases under consideration and not more. [3]

MYCIN: A computer-assisted decision support system developed in the 1970s that used artificial intelligence techniques (production rules) to recommend appropriate therapy for patients with infections. [20]

Name authority: The component of a health care information system that uniquely identifies a patient within the system. [13]

Name-server: In networked environments such as the Internet, computers that convert a host name into an IP address before the message is placed on the network. [5]

National Digital Information Infrastructure Preservation Program (NDIIPP):   A program of the U.S. Library of Congress intended to help assure preservation of scientific information through a preservation program that will evolve with technical storage modalities. [19]

National Center for Biotechnology Information (NCBI): Established in 1988 as a national resource for molecular biology information, the NCBI is a component of the National Library of Medicine that creates public databases, conducts research in computational biology, develops software tools for analyzing genome data, and disseminates biomedical information. [19]

National Guidelines Clearinghouse: A public resource, coordinated by the Agency for Health Research and Quality, that collects and distributes evidence-based clinical practice guidelines (see www.guideline.gov). [19]

National Health Information Infrastructure (NHII): A comprehensive knowledge-based network of interoperable systems of clinical, public health, and personal health information that is intended to improve decision making by making health information available when and where it is needed. [1]

National Information Standards Organization (NISO): A nonprofit association accredited by the American National Standards Institute (ANSI) that identifies, develops, maintains, and publishes technical standards to manage information (see www.niso.org). [19]

National Institute for Standards and Technology (NIST): A nonregulatory federal agency within the U.S. Commerce Department's Technology Administration; its mission is to develop and promote measurement, standards, and technology to enhance productivity, facilitate trade, and improve the quality of life (see www.nist.gov). [19]

Natural-language query: A question expressed in unconstrained text, from which meaning must somehow be extracted or inferred so that a suitable response can be generated. [19]

Naturalistic: In evaluation studies, an environment that is drawn from the real world and not constrained or externally controlled as a part of the study design. [11]

Negative Dictionary: A list of **stop words** used in information retrieval. [19]

Negative predictive value (PV–): The probability that the condition of interest is absent if the result is negative—e.g., the probability that a specific disease is absent given a negative test result. [3]

Negligence law: Laws, such as those governing medical malpractice, that are based on negligence theory. [20]

Negligence theory: A concept from tort law that states that providers of goods and services are expected to uphold the standards of the community, thereby facing claims of negligence if individuals are harmed by substandard goods or services. [10]

Net present value (NPV):   The difference between the present value of benefits and the present value of costs (see **present value**). [11]

Network access provider: A company that builds and maintains high-speed networks to which customers can connect, generally to access the Internet (see also **Internet service provider**). [5]

Network-based hypermedia: The mechanism by which media of all types (text, graphics, images, audio, and video) are integrated, interlinked, and delivered via networks. [19]

Network-model HMO: A model whereby groups of physicians in private practice band together to offer contracted services, generally simulating a prepaid group practice approach (see also **individual practice associations**). [23]

Network node: One of the interconnected computers or devices linked in a communications network. [5]

Network protocol: The set of rules or conventions that specifies how data are prepared and transmitted over a network and that governs data communication among the nodes of a network. [5]

Network stack: The method within a single machine by which the responsibilities for network communications are divided into different levels, with clear interfaces between the levels, thereby making network software more modular. [5]

Network topology: The configuration of the physical connections among the nodes of a communications network. [5]

Neuroinformatics: An emerging subarea of biomedical informatics in which the discipline's methods are applied to the management of neurological data sets and the modeling of neural structures and function. [9]

Next Generation Internet: A federally funded research program in the late 1990s and early in the current decade that sought to provide technical enhancements to the Internet to support future applications, which currently are infeasible or are incapable of scaling for routine use. [1]

Ninth International Classification of Diseases–Clinical Modification (ICD-9-CM):   A coding system for medical diagnoses, symptoms, and nonspecific complaints. It is frequently used on insurance claim forms to identify the reasons for providing medical services. [7]

Node: In networking topologies, a machine on the network that sits at the intersection of incoming and outgoing communications channels. [5]

Noise: The component of acquired data that is attributable to factors other than the underlying phenomenon being measured (e.g., electromagnetic interference, inaccuracy in sensors, or poor contact between sensor and source). [5]

Nomenclature: A system of terms used in a scientific discipline to denote classifications and relationships among objects and processes. [2,4,7]

Noninvasive monitoring technique: A method for measuring a physiological parameter that does not require breaking the skin or otherwise entering the body. [17]

Nonionizing radiation: Radiation that does not cause damage to cells; e.g., the sound waves used in ultrasonography (see **ionizing radiation**). [9]

Nonquantifiable benefits and costs: In a cost-benefit analysis, those elements that are important to consider but may defy formal numeric measurements. [23]

Notifiable disease: In communicable disease management, a disease that must be reported to a public health agency when a new case occurs. [15]

NP hard: A complexity class of problems, which are intrinsically harder than those that can be solved in polynomial time. When a definitive version of a combinatorial optimization problem is proven to belong to a class of well-known complex problems such as satisfiability, traveling salesman, and bin packing, an optimization version is said to be NP hard. [11]

Nuclear magnetic resonance (NMR) spectroscopy: A spectral technique used in chemistry to characterize chemical compounds by measuring magnetic characteristics of their atomic nuclei. [9]

Nuclear-medicine imaging: A modality for producing images by measuring the radiation emitted by a radioactive isotope that has been attached to a biologically active compound and injected into the body. [9]

Null hypothesis: In evaluation studies, the negatively stated hypothesis that is the subject of study, generally because of a suspicion that the hypothesis is incorrect. [11]

Nursing care plan: A proposed series of nursing interventions based on nursing assessments and nursing diagnoses. It identifies nursing care problems, states specific actions to address the problems, specifies the actions taken, and includes an evaluation of a client's response to care. [16]

Nursing informatics: The application of biomedical informatics methods and techniques to problems derived from the field of nursing. Viewed as a subarea of clinical informatics. [16]

Nursing information system (NIS):   A computer-based information system that supports nurses' professional duties in clinical practice, nursing administration, nursing research, and education. [16]

Nursing intervention: Any of a variety of interactions between nurse and client, including physical care, emotional support, and client education. [16]

Nyquist frequency: The minimum sampling rate necessary to achieve reasonable signal quality. In general, it is twice the frequency of the highest-frequency component of interest in a signal. [5]

Object-oriented database: A database that is structured around individual objects (concepts) that generally include relationships among those objects and, in some cases, executable code that is relevant to the management and or understanding of that object. [22]

Object-oriented programming: An approach to computer programming in which individual concepts are modeled as objects that are acted upon by incoming messages and that act upon other objects by outgoing messages. [6]

Objectives-based approach: An evaluation methodology in which a study seeks to determine whether a resource meets its designers' objectives. [11]

Objectivist: A philosophy of evaluation that suggests that the merit and worth of an information resource—the attributes of most interest in evaluation—can in principle be measured with all observations yielding the same result. [11]

Occam's razor: A philosophical and scientific rule that the simpler explanation is preferred to a more complicated one, all else being equal. [2]

Odds: An expression of the probability of the occurrence of an event relative to the probability that it will not occur. [3]

Odds-likelihood form: See **odds-ratio form**. [3]

Odds-ratio form: An algebraic expression for calculating the posttest odds of a disease, or other condition of interest, if the pretest odds and **likelihood ratio** are known (an alternative formulation of **Bayes' theorem**, also called the **odds-likelihood form**). [3]

Offline device: A device that operates independently of the processor; e.g., a photographic printer with input from storage devices such as flash memory cards or memory sticks. [5]

ONCOCIN: An expert system built in the 1980s to assist physicians with the management of patients enrolled in cancer chemotherapy clinical trials. [20]

Online bibliographic searching: The use of computers to search electronically stored databases of indexed literature references. [19]

Online device: A device that is under the direct control of a computer's processor; e.g., a magnetic-disk drive. [5]

Ontology: A description (like a formal specification of a program) of the concepts and relationships that can exist for an agent or a community of agents. In biomedicine, such ontologies typically specify the meanings and hierarchical relationships among terms and concepts in a domain. [9, 20]

OPAL: A knowledge acquisition program, related to **ONCOCIN**, designed to allow clinicians to specify the logic of cancer clinical trials using visual-programming techniques. [20]

Open Archives Initiative: An effort to provide persistent access to electronic archives of scientific (and other) publications; its fundamental activity is to promote the specification of archives' metadata such that digital library systems can learn what content is available and how it can be obtained. [19]

Open-loop control: A computer system that assists in regulation of a physiological variable, such as blood pressure, by monitoring the value of the variable and reporting measured values or therapy recommendations. Health care personnel retain responsibility for therapeutic interventions (see **closed-loop control**). [17]

Open policy: In standards group, a policy that allows anyone to become involved in discussing and defining the standard. [7]

Open source: An approach to software development in which programmers can read, redistribute, and modify the source code for a piece of software, resulting in community development of a shared product. [12]

Operating system (OS):   A program that allocates computer hardware resources to user programs and that supervises and controls the execution of all other programs. [5]

Opportunity cost: The value of the alternatives foregone that might have been produced with those resources (also called the **economic cost**). [23]

Optical disk: A round, flat plate of plastic or metal that is used to store information. Data are encoded through the use of a laser that marks the surface of the disk. [5]

Order entry: In a hospital or health care information system, online entry of orders for drugs, laboratory tests, and procedures, usually by nurses or physicians. [13]

Order-entry systems: See **computer-based physician order-entry (CPOE) systems.** [1]

Orienting issues: Initial investigations that help to define the issues of interest in a subjectivist study design. [11]

Orienting questions: The aims of a study, defined at the outset and sometimes contractually mandated. [11]

Original content: Online information created and provided by the same organization. [19]

Outcomes: In a study, the events or measurements that reflect the possible influences of the interventions being studied. [11]

Outcomes data: Formal information regarding the results of interventions. [10]

Outcome measure: A parameter for evaluating the success of a system; the parameter reflects the top-level goals of the system. [11]

Outcome variable: See **outcome measure**. [11]

Output: The results produced when a process is applied to input. Some forms of output are hardcopy documents, images displayed on video display terminals, and calculated values of variables. [5,6]

Overhead: See **indirect cost**. [23]

Packet: In networking, a variable-length message containing data plus the network addresses of the sending and receiving nodes, and other control information. [5]

Page: A partitioned component of a computer user's programs and data that can be kept in temporary storage and brought into main memory by the operating system as needed. [5]

PageRank (PR) indexing: In indexing for information retrieval on the Internet, an algorithmic scheme for giving more weight to a Web page when a large number of other pages link to it. [19]

Parallel processing: The use of multiple processing units running in parallel to solve a single problem (see **multiprocessing**). [5]

Parse tree: The representation of structural relationships that results when using a grammar (usually context-free) to analyze a given sentence. [8]

Part of speech tagging: Assignment of syntactic classes to a given sequence of words, e.g., determiner, adjective, noun and verb. [8]

Partial-match searching: An approach to information retrieval that recognizes the inexact nature of both indexing and retrieval, and attempts to return the user content ranked by how close it comes to the user's query. [19]

Patent: A specific legal approach for protecting methods used in implementing or instantiating ideas (see **intellectual property**). [10]

Pathfinder: A computer program that uses Bayesian methods in the diagnosis of lymph node pathology. [20]

Pathognomonic: Distinctively characteristic, and thus, uniquely identifying a condition or object (100 percent specific). [2,20]

Pathways: See **clinical pathways**. [1]

Patient care system: Comprehensive computer systems used by health workers in the management of individual patients, usually in hospital settings. [16]

Patient chart: Another name for the medical record of a patient. [12]

Patient monitor: An instrument that collects and displays physiological data, often for the purpose of watching for, and warning against, life-threatening changes in physiological state. [17]

Patient monitoring: Repeated or continuous measurement of physiological parameters for the purpose of guiding therapeutic management. [17]

Patient record: Another name for the medical record, but one often preferred by those who wish to emphasize that such records often need to contain information about patients that extends beyond the details of their diseases and medical or surgical management. [12]

Patient-specific information: Clinical information about a particular patient (as opposed to general knowledge of a disease, syndrome, relationship, etc.). [19]

Patient-tracking application: A computer system used to monitor and manage the movement of patients through multistep processes, such as in the emergency department or imaging department. [13]

Patient triage: A computer system that helps health professionals to classify new patients and direct them to appropriate health resources. [13]

Pattern check: A method for verifying the accuracy of an identifier by assuring that it follows a predefined pattern (e.g., that a Social Security Number must be of the form xxx-yy-zzzz where x, y, and z are digits). [12]

Pattern recognition: The process of organizing visual, auditory, or other data and identifying meaningful motifs. [17]

Peer review: In scientific publication, the process of requiring that articles be reviewed by other scientists who are peers of the author and that, before acceptance for publication, the author subsequently revise the paper in response to comments and criticisms from such reviewers. [19]

Per capita payment: See **capitation**. [23]

Perimeter definition: Specification of the boundaries of trusted access to an information system, both physically and logically. [5]

Personal computer (PC): A small, relatively inexpensive, single-user computer. [5,21]

Personal digital assistant (PDA): A small, relatively inexpensive, handheld device with electronic schedule and contact list capabilities, possibly with handwriting recognition and other productivity tools. [13]

Phantom: In image processing, an object of known shape, used to calibrate imaging machines. The reconstructed image is compared to the object's known shape. [9]

Pharmacokinetic parameters: The drug-specific and patient-specific parameters that determine the shape of the mathematical models used to forecast drug concentrations as a function of drug regimen. [20]

Pharmacokinetics: The study of the routes and mechanisms of drug disposition over time, from initial introduction into the body, through distribution in body tissues, biotransformation, and ultimate elimination. [1,20]

Pharmacy benefits managers (PBMs): A product of the U.S. health care financing system, PBMs are hired by health plans, insurers, and large employers to fulfill the prescription benefits that are due to their members. A PBM generally negotiates for bulk discounts in purchasing drugs from pharmaceutical companies, and seeks to reduce the total drug cost to the payers, while often providing other services such as mail-order pharmacy deliveries. [24]

Pharmacy information system: A computer-based information system that supports pharmacy personnel. [13]

Phased installation: The incremental introduction of a system into an institution. [6]

Phenotype: The observable physical characteristics of an organism, produced by the interaction of **genotype** with environment. [22]

Physician-hospital organization (PHO): An approach wherein one or a group of hospitals team up with their medical staffs to offer subscribers comprehensive health services for a per capita prepayment. [23]

Picture-archiving and communication system (PACS): An integrated computer system that acquires, stores, retrieves, and displays digital images. [18]

Picture-archiving and communication system (PACS) workbench: A set of tools to study PACS design and to conduct experiments related to image acquisition, transmission, archiving, and viewing. [7,18]

Pixel: One of the small picture elements that makes up a digital image. The number of pixels per square inch determines the spatial resolution. Pixels can be associated with a single bit to indicate black and white or with multiple bits to indicate color or gray scale. [5,9,18]

Placebo effect: In some drug trials, simply giving patients an inactive tablet or other placebo can cause a measurable improvement in some clinical variables because patients feel good about receiving attention and potentially useful medication. This placebo effect may be more powerful than the drug effect itself, and may obscure a complete absence of pharmaceutical benefit. [11]

Plug-ins: Software components that are added to Web browsers or other programs to allow them a special functionality, such as an ability to deal with certain kinds of media (e.g., video or audio). [5]

Point-of-care system: A hospital information system that includes bedside terminals or other devices for capturing and entering data at the location where patients receive care. [13]

Point of service (POS):   A type of health plan introduced by HMOs in the mid-1980s to allow patients, at some expense, to seek care outside of the network that includes their contracted providers. [23]

Pointing device: A manual device, such as a mouse, light pen, or joystick, that can be used to specify an area of interest on a computer screen. [5]

Polysemy: The characteristic of a word having multiple possible meanings. [19]

Population-based atlas: An atlas that encodes the anatomy and variation from a group of individuals constituting some relevant population. Compare with a template atlas that is created from a single individual. [9]

Portable Document Format (PDF):   Invented by Adobe, Inc., PDF is a published specification used for secure, reliable electronic document distribution and exchange. When converted to PDF, a document maintains its original look and integrity. [19]

Positive predictive value (PV+):   The probability that the condition of interest is true if the result is positive—e.g., the probability that a disease is present given a positive test result. [3]

Positron emission tomography (PET):   A tomographic imaging method that measures the uptake of various metabolic products (generally a combination of a positron-emitting tracer with a chemical such as glucose), e.g., by the functioning brain, heart, or lung. [9]

Postcoordination: Coding of data by using multiple terms, as needed, to express meaning that cannot be accurately captured by any single term. [7]

Postgenomic database: A database that combines molecular and genetic information with data of clinical importance or relevance. *Online Mendelian Inheritance in Man* (OMIM) is a frequently cited example of such a database. [22]

Postgenomic era: The coming period in which genomic information will be combined with other types of clinical or patient-specific data to provide new approaches to diagnosis and therapy. [9]

Post Office Protocol (POP):   A protocol used in the delivery of electronic mail services to any of a number of client software packages used to read e-mail from a central server. [5]

Posterior probability: The updated probability that the condition of interest is present after additional information has been acquired. [3]

Post-test probability: The updated probability that the disease or other condition under consideration is present after the test result is known (more generally, the **posterior probability**). [3]

Practice management system (PMS):   A computer information system designed to support all information requirements of a physician office or group practice, including registration, appointment scheduling, billing, and clinical documentation. [13]

Pragmatics: The study of how contextual information affects the interpretation of the underlying meaning of the language. [8]

Precision: The degree of accuracy with which the value of a sampled observation matches the value of the underlying condition, or the exactness with which an operation is performed. In information retrieval, a measure of a system's performance in retrieving relevant information (expressed as the fraction of relevant records among total records retrieved in a search). [5,19]

Precoordination: Expansion of a terminology, as needed, to express meanings with single terms, without needing to resort to the use of multiple terms (see **postcoordination**). [7]

Predicate calculus: The branch of symbolic logic that uses symbols for quantifiers and for arguments and predicates of propositions as well as for unanalyzed propositions and logical connectives. [4]

Predictive model: In evaluation studies, the unusual situation in which investigators have a mechanism to tell them what would have happened to patients if they had not intervened. Such models allow comparisons of what actually happens with what is predicted. [11]

Predictive value: The posttest probability that a condition is present based on the results of a test (see positive predictive value and negative predictive value). [2]

Preferred-provider insurance (PPI):   In managed care, an insurance plan in which companies contract with large numbers of providers that are not otherwise related to one another. [23]

Preferred-provider organization (PPO):   A method of health care financing based on selective contracting in advance for the services of health care providers. A PPO typically is composed of a panel of providers, a negotiated fee schedule that providers agree to accept as payment in full for their services, a mechanism for utilization control, and incentives for consumers to select providers from the panel, usually in the form of reduced coinsurance. [7,23]

Prepaid group practice: An affiliation of health care providers that agrees to provide comprehensive health care to members for a fixed annual fee set in advance. [23]

Present value (PV):   The current value of a payment or stream of payments to be received in the future. The concept of present value generally reflects the fact that $1 received 1 year from now is not worth as much as $1 received today both because of inflation and because that dollar is not available to earn interest over the course of the year. [23]

Presentation: The forms in which information is delivered to the end user after processing. [16]

Presentation layer: In software systems, the components that interact with the user. The term generally connotes an architecture in which the system components are modular and *layered* between the underlying data structures and the uscr interface. [18]

President's Information Technology Advisory Committee (PITAC):   A federal advisory body, comprising individuals from academia and industry in the private sector, which was created under the High Performance Computing and Communications initiative of the 1990s and provides advice to the White House on matters related to information technology, including its role in science and health care. [19]

Pressure transducer: A device that produces electrical signals proportional in magnitude to the level of a pressure reading. [17]

Pretest probability: The probability that the disease or other condition under consideration is present before the test result is known (more generally, the **prior probability**). [3]

Prevalence: The frequency of the condition under consideration in the population. For example, we calculate the prevalence of disease by dividing the number of diseased individuals by the number of individuals in the population. Prevalence is the prior probability of a specific condition (or diagnosis), before any other information is available. [2,3]

Primary care: The level of care normally provided by a personal physician or walk-in clinic. The point of entry to the health care system. [12]

Primary care gatekeepers: In managed care settings, those primary care physicians who provide all initial care and then make determinations about when referral of a patient to a specialist is necessary or appropriate. [23]

Primary knowledge-based information: The original source of knowledge, generally in a peer-reviewed journal article that reports on a research project's results. [19]

Primary literature: Scientific articles that present the initial research results, as opposed to review articles or textbooks that synthesize such studies into general coverage of a topic. [19]

Prior probability: The probability that the condition of interest is present before additional information has been acquired. In a population, the prior probability also is called the **prevalence**. [3]

Privacy: A concept that applies to people, rather than documents, in which there is a presumed right to protect that individual from unauthorized divulging of personal data of any kind. [5,10]

Privacy-Enhanced Mail protocol (PEM): A protocol whereby electronic mail is encrypted to assure that only the sender and intended receiver can read it. [5]

Private branch exchange (PBX): A telephone switching center. PBXs can be extended to provide a local-area network in which digital data are converted to analog signals and are transmitted over an existing telephone system. [5]

Probabilistic context-free grammar: A context-free grammar in which the possible ways to expand a given symbol have varying probabilities rather than equal weight. [8]

Probabilistic relationship: Exists when the occurrence of one chance event affects the probability of the occurrence of another chance event. [3]

Probability: Informally, a means of expressing belief in the likelihood of an event. Probability is more precisely defined mathematically in terms of its essential properties. [3]

Problem-oriented medical record (POMR): A clinical record in which the data collected, the physician's assessment, and the proposed therapeutic plans are grouped by association with the patient's specific medical problems. [12]

Problem solver: A program designed to address a certain class of problems using a defined methodology. [20]

Problem space: The range of possible solutions to a problem. [4]

Procedural knowledge: Knowledge of how to perform a task (as opposed to factual knowledge about the world). [4]

Process measure: A parameter for evaluating the success of a system; the parameter measures a byproduct of the system's function. [11]

Product: An object that goes through the processes of design, manufacture, distribution, and sale. [10]

Production: The process of executing a product's design in an ongoing, maintained manner. [21]

Production rule: A conditional statement that relates premise conditions to associated actions or inferences. [20]

Productivity cost: Costs that accrue because of changes in productivity due to illness or death. [11]

Professional-developed: A reference to educational and other resources created by health professionals and their organizations for direct use by patients. [14]

Professional–patient relationship: Refers to a set of assumptions regarding the primacy of patient well-being rather than other external factors in the determination of actions by health professionals. [10]

Professional-review approach: An approach to evaluation in which panels of experienced peers spend several days in the environment where the resource or activity to be assessed is operational. [11]

Professional Standards Review Organization (PSRO): A physicians' organization created to review use of Medicare and Medicaid services and to deny payment for unnecessary services. [23]

Prognostic scoring system: An approach to prediction of patient outcomes based on formal analysis of current variables, generally through methods that compare the patient in some way with large numbers of similar patients from the past. [10]

Projection: In imaging systems, a measured attenuation or superposition. [9]

Proposition: An expression, generally in language or other symbolic form, that can be believed, doubted, or denied or is either true or false. [4]

Prospective payment: A method of health care reimbursement in which providers receive a set payment specified in advance for providing a global unit of care, such as hospitalization for a specified illness or a hospital day. [23]

Prospective payment system (PPS):   A scheme for health care financing enacted by Congress in 1983, in which hospitals receive from Medicare a fixed payment per hospital admission, adjusted for **diagnosis-related group**. [23]

Prospective study: An experiment in which researchers, before collecting data for analysis, define study questions and hypotheses, the study population, and data to be collected. [2,12]

PROTÉGÉ: A software meta-tool used by developers to create automatically domain-specific knowledge-elicitation tools by taking as input analysts' models of the relevant applications areas. [20]

Protein-sequence database: A database that contains the known sequences of amino acids of proteins. [22]

Proteomics: By analogy with **genomics**, and the study of genes, the study of the structure and function of proteins. [22]

Protocol: A standardized method or approach. [5,20]

Protocol analysis: In cognitive psychology, methods for gathering and interpreting data that are presumed to reveal the mental processes used during problem solving (e.g., analysis of "think-aloud" protocols). [4]

Protocol for Metadata Harvesting (PMH):   A method for harvesting summary information from metadata, which are stored with archival materials (see Open Archive Initiative). [19]

Prototype system: A working model of a planned system that demonstrates essential features of the operation and interface. [6,21]

Provider-profiling system: Computer system used to manage utilization of health resources by tracking and comparing physicians' resource utilization (e.g., cost of drugs prescribed, laboratory tests ordered) compared to severity-adjusted outcomes of the providers' patients. [13]

Proximity searching: A technique used with full-text databases that retrieves documents containing the specified words when they are adjacent in the text, or when they occur within a certain number of words of each other. [19]

PubMed: A software environment for searching the Medline database, developed as part of the suite of search packages, known as **Entrez**, by the NLM's **National Center for Biotechnology Information (NCBI)**. [19]

PubMed Central: An effort by the National Library of Medicine to gather the full text of scientific articles in a freely accessible database, enhancing the value of Medline by providing the full articles in addition to titles, authors, and abstracts. [19]

Public health: The field that deals with monitoring and influencing trends in habits and disease in an effort to protect or enhance the health of the population. [10,15]

Public Health Informatics: An application area of biomedical informatics in which the field's methods and techniques are applied to problems drawn from the domain of public health. [1]

Publication type: One of several classes of articles or books into which a new publication will fall (e.g., review articles, case reports, original research, textbook, etc.). [19]

Public-key cryptography: In data encryption, a method whereby two keys are used, one to encrypt the information and a second to decrypt it. Because two keys are involved, only one needs to be kept secret. [5]

Purchasing coalitions: Groups of employers that together structure their health care benefits program and negotiate with health plans. [23]

QRS wave: In an electrocardiogram (ECG), the portion of the waveform that represents the time it takes for depolarization of the ventricles. [5]

Qualitative arrangement: An approach to image retrieval that looks at the relative relationships of regions in the image, without trying to identify them, and retrieves images that have similar relationships. [18]

Qualitative model: A method for capturing the characteristics of a process or phenomenon in descriptive terms without attempting to define or simulate it quantitatively. [20]

Quality-adjusted life year (QALY):   A measure of the value of a health outcome that reflects both longevity and morbidity; it is the expected length of life in years, adjusted to account for diminished quality of life due to physical or mental disability, pain, and so on. [3]

Quality assurance: A means for monitoring and maintaining the goodness of a service, product, or process. [23]

Quality management: A specific effort to let quality of care be the goal that determines changes in processes, staffing, or investments. [16]

Quantitation: In imaging, global processing and segmentation to characterize meaningful regions of interest. [9]

Quasi-legal approach: An evaluation method that establishes a *mock trial*, or other formal adversarial proceeding, to judge a resource. [11]

Query: In a database system, a request for specific information that is stored in the computer. By extension, updates to the database. [12,19]

Query formulation: The process of stating information needs in terms of queries. Also the process by which information needs are translated into queries suitable for searching. [19]

Query and retrieval: An approach to information retrieval in which the user selects the terms. Terms can be matched against a predetermined index or against a thesaurus that searches for synonyms, more global concepts, and more specific concepts. [21]

Queue: In a computer system, an ordered set of jobs waiting to be executed. [5]

Quick Medical Reference (QMR):   A decision-support system that grew out of the Internist-1 program. QMR has been marketed commercially for use by both students and practitioners. [20,21]

Radioactive isotope: Chemical compounds used in nuclear medicine imaging techniques. Specific compounds are selected because they tend to concentrate in specific types of tissues. [9]

Radiography: The process of making images by projecting X-rays through the patient onto X-ray-sensitive film. [9]

Radiology: The medical field that deals with the definition of health conditions through the use of visual images that reflect information from within the human body. [9,18]

Radiology information system (RIS):   Computer-based information system that supports radiology department operations; includes management of the film library, scheduling of patient examinations, reporting of results, and billing. [7,18]

Random-access memory (RAM):   The portion of a computer's working memory that can be both read and written into. It is used to store the results of intermediate computation, and the programs and data that are currently in use (also called **variable memory** or **core memory**). [5,18]

Randomization: A research technique for assigning subjects to study groups without a specific pattern. Designed to minimize experimental bias. [11]

Randomized clinical trial (RCT):   A prospective experiment in which subjects are randomly assigned to study subgroups to compare the effects of alternate treatments. [2]

Randomly: Without bias. [2]

Range check: Verification that a clinical parameter falls in an expected (normal) range. [12]

Ranking: In information retrieval, the specification of a retrieved item's match to the query, based on some kind of sorting criteria. [19]

Raster-scan display: A pattern of closely spaced rows of dots that forms an image on the cathode-ray tube of a video display monitor. [9]

Readability: In information retrieval, the notion of identifying and displaying an information resource that uses words, concepts, and sentence structures that will be understandable to the typical user of the search tool in question. [19]

Read-only memory (ROM):   The portion of a computer's working memory that can be read, but not written into. [5,17]

Real-time acquisition: The continuous measurement and recording of electronic signals through a direct connection with the signal source. [5]

Recall: In information retrieval, the ability of a system to retrieve relevant information (expressed as the ratio of relevant records retrieved to all relevant records in the database). [19]

Receiver: In data interchange, the program or system that receives a transmitted message. [7]

Receiver operating characteristic (ROC) curve: A curve that depicts the trade-off between the sensitivity and specificity of a test as the criteria for when that test is to be judged abnormal are varied. [3]

Record: In a data file, a group of data fields that collectively represent information about a single entity. [5]

Reductionist approach: An attempt to explain phenomena by reducing them to common, and often simple, first principles. [22]

Region-detection techniques: A technique in which structures are delineated by their composition on the image. [9]

Regional network: A network that provides regional access from local organizations and individuals to the major backbone networks that interconnect regions. [5]

Reference Information Model (RIM):   The data model for HL7 version 3.0. [7]

Referent: A person, object or event referenced by a given linguistic expression, e.g., the pronoun "she" in clinical text typically has the patient as its referent. [8]

Referential expression: A sequence of one or more words that refers to a particular person, object or event, e.g., "she," "Dr. Jones, " or "that procedure". [8]

Referral bias: In evaluation studies, a bias that is introduced when the patients entering a study are in some way atypical of the total population, generally because they have been referred to the study based on criteria that reflect some kind of bias by the referring physicians. [3]

Refinement: In information retrieval, the adjustment of a search query in order to obtain more appropriate information than was initially retrieved. [19]

Region-detection technique: A method, such as application of a connected-components algorithm, used to identify a region of interest from an overall image by grouping together pixels that are both adjacent and have similar intensities. [9]

Regional Health Information Network (RHIN):   A public–private alliance among health care providers, pharmacies, public health departments and payers, designed to share health information among all health participants, thereby improving community health and heath care (see also **CHIN**). [13,15]

Regional Health Information Organization (RHIO):   An organization that works to create a **RHIN**. [15]

Register: In a computer, a group of electronic switches used to store and manipulate numbers or text. [5]

Registration: One of the problems to solve in multimodality image fusion, specifically the alignment of separately acquired image volumes. [9]

Regular expression: A mathematical model of a set of strings, defined using characters of an alphabet and the operators concatenation, union and closure (zero or more occurrences of an expression). [8]

Relative recall: An approach to measuring recall when it is unrealistic to enumerate all the relevant documents in a database. Thus the denominator in the calculation of **recall** is redefined to represent the number of relevant documents identified by multiple searches on the query topic. [19]

Relevance feedback: The process that allows a searcher to obtain more relevant documents by designating retrieved documents as relevant and adding terms from them into a new query. [19]

Relevance ranking: The degree to which the results are relevant to the information need specified in a query. [19]

Reliability: In networking, the ability of a networked resource to be available and to meet expectations for performance, as related to network bandwidth and quality of service. [1]

Reminder systems: A decision-support system that monitors a patient's care over time and uses encoded logic to generate warnings and reminders to clinicians when situations arise that require clinical attention. [20]

Remote access: Access to a system or to information therein, typically by telephone or communications network, by a user who is physically removed from the system. [5]

Remote-presence health care: The use of video teleconferencing, image transmission, and other technologies that allow clinicians to evaluate and treat patients in other than face-to-face situations. [10]

Report generation: A mechanism by which users specify their data requests on the input screen of a program that then produces the actual query, using information stored in a database schema, often at predetermined intervals. [5]

Representation: A level of medical data encoding, the process by which as much detail as possible is coded. [7]

Representativeness: A heuristic by which a person judges the chance that a condition is true based on the degree of similarity between the current situation and the stereotypical situation in which the condition is true. For example, a physician might estimate the probability that a patient has a particular disease based on the degree to which the patient's symptoms matches the classic disease profile. [3]

Requirements analysis: An initial analysis performed to define a problem clearly and to specify the nature of the proposed solution (e.g., the functions of a proposed system). [6]

Research protocol: In clinical research, a prescribed plan for managing subjects that describes what actions to take under specific conditions. [2]

Resource-based relative value scale (RBRVS):   A system authorized by Congress for paying for Medicare physician's services, intended to correct the large inequities and perverse incentives in Medicare's "customary, prevailing, and reasonable" payment system (see also **volume performance standard**). [23]

Resource Description Framework (RDF):   An emerging standard for cataloging metadata about information resources (such as Web pages) using the **Extensible Markup Language (XML)**. [19]

Responsive-illuminative approach: An approach to evaluation that seeks to represent the viewpoints of both users of the resource and the people who are an otherwise significant part of the clinical environment where the resource operates. [11]

Results reporting: In a hospital or health care information system, online access to the results of laboratory tests and other procedures. [13]

Retrieval: A process by which queries are compared against an index to create results for the user who specified the query. [19]

Retrospective chart review: Extraction and analysis of data from medical records to investigate a question that was not a subject of study at the time the data were collected. [2]

Retrospective payment: A method of health care financing in which providers are reimbursed based on charges for the services actually delivered. [23]

Retrospective study: An analysis of pre-existing sets of data to answer experimental questions. [12]

Revenue center: In a health care institution, a department that charges patients directly for the services provided (see also **cost center**). [13]

Review of systems: The component of a typical history and physical examination in which the physician asks general questions about each of the body's major organ systems to discover problems that may not have been suggested by the patient's chief complaint. [2]

Risk attitude: A person's willingness to take risks. [3]

Risk-neutral: Having the characteristic of being indifferent between the expected value of a gamble and the gamble itself. [3]

Role-limited access: The mechanism by which an individual's access to information in a database, such as a medical record, is limited depending upon that user's job characteristics and their need to have access to the information. [5]

Router: In networking, a device that is connected between multiple networks and receives messages from a network and forwards them to another connected network according to their intended destination. [5]

RS-232-C: A commonly used standard for serial data communication that defines the number and type of the wire connections, the voltage, and the characteristics of the signal, and thus allows data communication among electronic devices produced by different manufacturers. [5]

Rule interpreter: The software component of a rule-based system that assesses individual rules and determines their applicability in a specific case or situation. [20]

Sample attrition rate: The proportion of the sample population that drops out before the study is complete. [11]

Sampling rate: The rate at which the continuously varying values of an analog signal are measured and recorded. [5]

Schema: In a database management system, a machine-readable definition of the contents and organization of a database. [5]

Schema (cognitive science):   A mental structure that represents an aspect of the world. Schemas are used to organize categories of knowledge and enable understanding. [4]

Screening: The use of global processing, segmentation, feature detection, and classification to determine whether an image should be flagged for careful review by a human being who is an expert in an image-processing domain. [9]

Script: In software systems, a keystroke-by-keystroke record of the actions performed for later reuse. [5]

Search intermediary: In information retrieval, a specially trained information specialist who interprets users' requests for information, formulates search requests in terms of the commands and vocabulary of the search systems, and carries out the search. [19]

Secondary care: The level of care normally provided by a typical hospital. [13]

Secondary knowledge-based information: Writing that reviews, condenses, and/or synthesizes the primary literature (see **primary knowledge-based information**). [19]

Secret-key cryptography: In data encryption, a method whereby the same key is used to encrypt and to decrypt information. Thus, the key must be kept secret, known to only the sender and intended receiver of information. [5]

Secure Sockets Layer (SSL):   a protocol developed by Netscape for transmitting private documents via the Internet. By convention, URLs that require an SSL connection start with 'https:' instead of 'http:'. [5]

Security: The process of protecting information from destruction or misuse, including both physical and computer-based mechanisms. [5]

Segmentation: In image processing, the extraction of selected regions of interest from an image using automated or manual techniques. [9]

Selection bias: An error in the estimates of disease prevalence and other population parameters that results when the criteria for admission to a study produce systematic differences between the study population and the clinically relevant population. [11]

Selectivity: In data collection and recording, the process that accounts for individual styles, reflecting an ongoing decision-making process, and often reflecting marked distinctions among clinicians. [2]

Self-insured plans: The system whereby (large) employers pay their employees' medical bills directly, hire insurance companies to perform claims processing, and perhaps buy outside insurance for only truly catastrophic cases. [23]

Semantic analysis: The study of how symbols or signs are used to designate the meaning of words and the study of how words combine to form or fail to form meaning. [8]

Semantic grammar: A mathematical model of a set of sentences based on patterns of semantic categories, e.g., patient, doctor, medication, treatment, and diagnosis. [8]

Semantic pattern: The study of the patterns formed by the co-occurrence of individual words in a phrase of the co-occurrence of the associated semantic types of the words. [8]

Semantic relation: A classification of the meaning of a linguistic relationship, e.g., "treated in 1995" signifies time while "treated in ER" signifies location. [8]

Semantics: The meaning of individual words and the meaning of phrases or sentences consisting of combinations of words. [5,8,19,20]

Semantic type: The categorization of words into semantic classes according to meaning. Usually, the classes that are formed are relevant to specific domains. [8]

Semantic Web: A future view that envisions the Internet not only as a source of content but also as a source of intelligently linked, agent-driven, structured collections of machine-readable information. [19]

Semi-structured interview: The process whereby an investigator specifies in advance a set of topics that he would like to address, but is flexible as to the order in which these topics are addressed and is open to discussion of topics not on the prespecified list. [11]

Sender: In data interchange, the program or system that sends a transmitted message. [7]

Sensitivity (of a test):   The probability of a positive result, given that the condition under consideration is present—e.g., the probability of a positive test result in a person who has the disease under consideration (also called the **true-positive rate**). [2,3]

Sensitivity analysis: A technique for testing the robustness of a decision analysis result by repeating the analysis over a range of probability and utility estimates. [3]

Sensitivity calculation: An analysis to determine which parameters, scenarios, and uncertainties affect a decision, and by how much. [3]

Sequence alignment: An arrangement of two or more sequences (usually of DNA or RNA), highlighting their similarity. The sequences are padded with gaps (usually denoted by dashes) so that wherever possible, columns contain identical or similar characters from the sequences involved. [22]

Sequence information: Information from a database that captures the sequence of component elements in a biological structure (e.g., the sequence of amino acids in a protein or of nucleotides in a DNA segment). [22]

Server: A computer that shares its resources with other computers and supports the activities of many users simultaneously within an enterprise. [5]

Service: An intangible activity provided to consumers, generally at a price, by a (presumably) qualified individual or system. [10]

Service benefit: A type of health insurance benefit, created to ensure that the providers are paid in the manner most acceptable to them—i.e., they can choose to be paid through cost reimbursement, or through payment of billed charges to hospitals and fee-for-service payment to physicians. [23]

Service bureau: A data-processing business that produces bills, third-party invoices, and financial reports for medical practices from information recorded on encounter forms. [13]

Set-based searching: Constraining a search to include only documents in a given class or set (e.g., from a given institution or journal). [19]

Shadowgraph: In radiology, a superposition of all the structures traversed by each X-ray beam. Various body tissues differentially absorb the beams, and the X-rays produce shadows on the radiographic film. [9]

Short-run cost: The cost of producing a good or service when the levels of some inputs (e.g., plant and equipment) remain fixed (see **long-run cost**). [23]

Signal artifact: A false feature of the measured signal caused by noise or other interference. [17]

Simple Mail Transport Protocol (SMTP):   The standard protocol used by networked systems, including the Internet, for packaging and distributing email so that it can be processed by a wide variety of software systems. [5]

Simulation: A system that behaves according to a model of a process or another system; for example, simulation of a patient's response to therapeutic interventions allows a student to learn which techniques are effective without risking human life. [21]

Simultaneous access: Access to shared, computer-stored information by multiple concurrent users. [5]

Simultaneous controls: In an evaluation study, subjects who are not subject to the intervention under consideration but who are subject to the other influences of the clinical environment in question. [11]

Single nucleotide polymorphism (SNP):   A DNA sequence variation, occurring when a single nucleotide in the genome is altered. For example, an SNP might change the nucleotide sequence AAGCCTA to AAGCTTA. A variation must occur in at least 1% of the population to be considered an SNP. [22]

Single-user system: Computers designed for use by single individuals, such as personal computers, as opposed to servers or other resources that are designed to be shared by multiple people at the same time. [5]

Site visit: An evaluation method whereby experts visit the site of a study or experiment in order to assess the detailed local components of the study as well as the relevant expertise of the investigators. [11]

Situation-action rules: Rules in software environments that propose a specific action that should be taken when a situation arises (see **production rules**). [20]

Skeletal plans: A general approach to a problem, generally expressed as a set of steps, which can be used as the basis for developing a custom-tailored approach by adjusting one or more steps in the skeletal plan. [20]

Software: Computer programs that direct the **hardware** how to carry out specific automated processes. [5,6]

Software engineering: The discipline concerned with organizing and managing the software development process (the process of creating computer programs and documentation) to facilitate production of high-quality systems in a timely and cost-effective manner. [6]

Software-oversight committees: Groups within organizations that are constituted to oversee computer programs and to assess their safety and efficacy in the local setting. [10]

Spamming: The process of sending unsolicited e-mail to large numbers of unwilling recipients, typically to sell a product or make a political statement. [5]

Spatial resolution: A measure of the ability to distinguish among points that are close to each other (indicated in a digital image by the number of **pixels** per square inch). [5,9]

Specialist Lexicon: one of three UMLS Knowledge Sources, this lexicon is intended to be a general English lexicon that includes many biomedical terms and supports natural-language processing. [19]

Specialized registry: A bibliographic database containing documents that may extend beyond those found in the scientific literature. The **National Guideline Clearinghouse** is one such example. [19]

Specification phase: In system design, the stage during which general system requirements are analyzed and formalized. [6]

Specificity (of a test):   The probability of a negative result, given that the condition under consideration is absent—e.g., the probability of a negative test result in a person who does not have a disease under consideration (also called the **true-negative rate**). [2,3]

Spectrum bias: Systematic error in the estimate of a study parameter that results when the study population includes only selected subgroups of the clinically relevant population—e.g., the systematic error in the estimates of sensitivity and specificity that results when test performance is measured in a study population consisting of only healthy volunteers and patients with advanced disease. [3]

Speech understanding: The field of computer science related to the development of computer programs that appropriately interpret and act upon information that is entered using human speech through a microphone. [5]

Speech recognition: The process of taking as input a spoken utterance (generally entered via a microphone) and translating it into a corresponding text representation in natural language. [5]

Spelling check: The software process whereby a specified selection of text is assessed for accuracy of the spelling of its words. [12]

Spiral model: A software engineering model in which an initial prototype is presented to the customers, who assess it, and expand and modify requirements in an ongoing iterative process. [6]

Spirometry: Evaluation of the air capacity and physiologic function of the lungs. [17]

Staff-model HMOs: A health maintenance organization in which doctors are retained as salaried employees on the organization's staff (see also **group-model HMOs**). [23]

Staged evaluation: Incremental evaluation of a system, in which different criteria for success are applied at successive stages of development. [11]

Standard-gamble: A technique for utility assessment that enables an analyst to determine the utility of an outcome by comparing an individual's preference for a chance event when compared with a situation of certain outcome. [3]

Standard of care: The community-accepted norm for management of a specified clinical problem. [10]

Standardized coding and classification (SCC):   A generic term describing any system that is used to define a standard for data coding. [16]

Standards development organization (SDO):   An organization charged with developing a standard that is accepted by the community of affected individuals. [7]

Static: In patient simulations, a program that presents a predefined case in detail but that does not vary in its response depending on the actions taken by the learner. [21]

Statistical error: In a model relating x to y, the portion of the variance in the dependent variable that cannot be explained by variance in the independent variables. [11]

Statistical life: An anonymous individual, such as a person affected by a policy that saves "one life in a thousand" (see **identified life**). [11]

Statistical package: A collection of programs that implement statistical procedures. Used to analyze data and report results. [11]

Stop-loss coverage: Reinsurance, which shifts the risk of a catastrophic case to an insurance company, thereby making it possible for small employers to self-insure (as large employers do). [23]

Stop-word list: In full-text indexing, a list of words that are low in semantic content (e.g., "the", "a", "an") and are generally not useful as mechanisms for retrieving documents. [19]

Stemmed: The process of converting a word to its root form by removing common suffixes from the end. [19]

Strict product liability: The principle that states that a product must not be harmful. [10,20]

String: A sequence of like items, such as bits, characters, or words. [19]

Structural alignment: In biological sequences, the task of aligning a new structure against a database of known structures, to determine regions of identity or similarity. [22]

Structural informatics: The study of methods for organizing and managing diverse sources of information about the physical organization of the body and other physical structures. [1,9]

Structured data: Data that are organized according to a particular format. [8]

Structured encounter form: A form for collecting and recording specific information during a patient visit. [12]

Structured Query Language (SQL):   A commonly used syntax for retrieving information from relational databases. [5]

Structured content: The organization and labeling of text (or other information) according to subsections that represent coherent concepts. [21]

Structured programming: The composition of computer programs using only sequences of statements and formal constructs for iteration (*do while*) and selection (*if...then...else*); implies modularity, absence of *go to* statements, and the use of stylistic conventions, such as indentation and the use of meaningful variable and subroutine names. [6]

Structured interview: An evaluation method that uses a schedule of questions that are always presented in the same words and in the same order. [11]

Study population: The population of subjects—usually a subset of the clinically relevant population—in whom experimental outcomes (e.g., the performance of a diagnostic test) are measured. [3]

Study protocol: A prescribed plan for managing experimental subjects that describes what actions to take under what conditions. [11]

Subject: An individual about whom data are collected during the conduct of a study. [11]

Subject heading: In information retrieval, the standardized terms used to categorize documents in order to facilitate their retrieval when appropriate. [19]

Subjectivist: A philosophy of evaluation that suggests that what is observed about a resource depends in fundamental ways on the observer. [11]

Subheading: In **MeSH**, qualifiers of subject headings that narrow the focus of a term. [19]

Sublanguage: Language of a specialized domain, such as medicine, biology, or law. [8]

Summary ROC curve: A composite **ROC curve** developed by using estimates from many studies. [3]

Summative decision: A decision made after a resource is installed in its envisioned environment; deals explicitly with how effectively the resource performs in that environment. [11]

Superbill: An itemized bill that summarizes the financial transactions occurring during a patient–physician encounter, including specification of the type of visit and a listing of the procedures performed and drugs administered; also, a checklist form for generating such a bill. [20]

Supervised learning: In automated neural networks, a process by which the values for weights are determined in an incremental fashion as the network is trained on a large collection of previously classified examples. [20]

Surface-based warping: A method for aligning 3-D surface models of anatomical structures extracted from image volumes by establishing a non-linear transformation (warp) that relates the two surface models. (see also **volume-based warping**). [9]

Surface rendering: A visualization technique that provides an alternative to volume rendering. This is the primary technique used in computer graphics, and has been applied widely in the entertainment industry for movies such as *Toy Story*. Surface rendering requires that the surface of interest be segmented from the image volume, after which rendering speeds on standard workstations are much faster than those possible with volume rendering. [9]

Surveillance: In a computer-based medical record system, systematic review of patients' clinical data to detect and flag conditions that merit attention. [12] In public health, the ongoing collection, analysis, interpretation, and dissemination of data on health conditions and threats to health [15]

Switch: In networking, a device that joins multiple computers or LAN segments together. A switch operates at the Data Link Layer and can inspect data packets to forward them only to the intended connected device, thereby conserving network bandwidth. [5]

Symbolic programming language: A programming language in which a programmer defines variables to represent abstract entities and can specify arithmatic, logical, and/or symbolic operations without worrying about the details of how the hardware performs these operations. Symbolic languages may support mathematical operations, text or string processing, database retrievals, logical operations involved in decision processes, and so on. [5]

Syndromic surveillance: An ongoing process for monitoring of clinical data, generally from public health, hospital, or outpatient resources, whereby the goal is early identification of outbreaks, epidemics, new diseases, or, in recent years, bioterrorist events. [10]

Synonymy: Occurs when two words have identical meanings. [19]

Synoptic content: Information in computer systems and databases that is created by extracting important observations and principles from sources of original content, as well as from personal experience. [19]

Syntactic: That which relates to the *structure* of words, phrases, or sentences (as opposed to their meanings). [19]

Syntax: The grammatical structure of language describing the relations among words in a sentence. [5,8]

System: A set of integrated entities that operates as a whole to accomplish a prescribed task. [6]

System integration: The process by which software systems and components are brought together to work as a coherent whole. [6]

System programs: The operating system, compilers, and other software that are included with a computer system and that allow users to operate the hardware. [5]

System review form: A paper form used during a physical examination to record findings related to each of the body's major systems. [2,12]

Systematic Classification of Proteins (SCOP):   A currently available online resource that classifies proteins based on shape and function. [22]

Systematic review: A type of journal article that reviews the literature related to a specific clinical question, analyzing the data in accordance with formal methods to assure that data are suitably compared and pooled. [19]

Systematized Nomenclature Of MEDicine (SNOMED):   The expanded form of the diagnostic coding scheme, formerly known as **SNOP (Systematized Nomenclature of Pathology)**. A multiaxial nomenclature system for the coding of several aspects of a diagnosis or other clinical entity. [2,7]

Systematized Nomenclature Of Pathology (SNOP):   A widely used diagnostic coding scheme, developed by pathologists. A nomenclature system of the College of American Pathologists based on four coding axes: topography, morphology, etiology, and function. A predecessor to SNOMED. [2,7]

Systems aggregation: A situation in which functions from disparate and widely distributed information systems are brought together in one application. [19]

Tactile feedback: In virtual or **telepresence** environments, the process of providing (through technology) a sensation of touching an object that is imaginary or otherwise beyond the user's reach (see also **haptic feedback**). [5]

Task: An activity of study, when computers or people solve problems or work through clinical cases. [11]

Taxonomy: An orderly classification, reflecting natural relationships among objects. [4]

Technical characteristics: The first stage in a technology assessment, in which the formal capabilities of a studied technology are defined and assessed. [11]

Technology assessment: Any process of examining and reporting properties of a medical technology used in health care, such as safety, efficacy, feasibility, and indication for use, cost, and cost-effectiveness, as well as social, economic, and ethical consequences, whether intended or unintended. [11]

Teledermatology: The application of **telemedicine** methods to dermatology, in which an expert dermatologist examines skin lesions on a patient at a distance by the use of photography and networked communication. [18]

Telemedicine: A broad term used to describe the delivery of health care at a distance, increasingly but not exclusively by means of the Internet. [1,10,14]

Telepathology: Use of telecommunication technologies to transmit data and images to and from a remote site for diagnosis, education, and research in pathology. [18]

Telepresence: A technique of telemedicine in which a viewer can be physically removed from an actual medical procedure or surgery, viewing the abnormality through a video monitor that displays the patient or operative field and allows the observer to participate in the procedure. [18]

Teleradiology: The provision of remote interpretations, increasing as a mode of delivery of radiology services. [18]

Telerobotics: A technique of telemedicine in which the manipulation of a biomedical device (e.g., a robot arm, a microscope, or an endoscope) is controlled at a distance by the hand movements of a remote operator. [18]

Template atlas: A (usually 3-D) labeled and segmented anatomical model from a single individual, to which the anatomy of other individuals is registered [9]

Temporal resolution: The time between acquisition of each of a series of images. Limited by the time needed to produce each image. [9,18]

Temporal subtraction: A technique of image enhancement that subtracts a reference image from later images that are registered to the first. A common use of temporal subtraction is **digital-subtraction angiography (DSA)**, in which a background image is subtracted from an image taken following the injection of contrast material. [9]

Term: In information retrieval, a word or phrase that forms part of the basis for a search request. [19]

Term frequency (TF):   In information retrieval, a measurement of how frequently a term occurs in a document. [19]

Term weighting: The assignment of metrics to terms so as to help specify their utility in retrieving documents well matched to a query. [19]

Terminal: A simple device that has no processing capability of its own but allows a user to access a server. [5]

Terminal interface processor (TIP):   A utility communications computer that is used to attach video display terminals and other communications devices to a LAN. [5]

Terminology: A set of terms representing the system of concepts of a particular subject field. [7]

Terminology authority: The component of a health care information system that defines the vocabulary standard and valid terms within the system; the medical entities dictionary. [13]

Terminology services: A set of functions provided by a health care information system and used to link, translate, and cross-reference diverse vocabulary terms for consistent use within the system. [13]

Tertiary care: The level of care normally provided by a specialized medical center. [13]

Test interpretation bias: Systematic error in the estimates of sensitivity and specificity that results when the index and gold standard test are not interpreted independently. [3]

Test referral bias: Systematic error in the estimates of **sensitivity** and **specificity** that results when subjects with a positive index test are more likely to receive the **gold standard test**. [3]

Testing: The process of formally running a newly developed computer system or set of programs to exercise them fully and to determine their reliability, accuracy, and freedom from programming errors. [6]

Text editor: A program used to create files of character strings, such as other computer programs and documents. [5]

Text generation: Methods that create coherent natural-language text from structured data or from textual documents in order to satisfy a communication goal. [8]

Text parsing: Conversion of unstructured text into a structured representation, using a given grammar. [8]

Text REtrieval Conference (TREC): Organized by **NIST**, an annual conference on text retrieval that has provided a test bed for evaluation and a forum for presentation of results (see trec.nist.gov). [19]

Text-scanning devices: A mechanical device that scans a paper document and converts text into computer-interpretable elements. [5]

Text-word searching: In an information retrieval, retrieval of relevant articles based on the words that appear in titles and abstracts, rather than the index terms that have been assigned to each entry. [19]

TF*IDF weighting: A specific approach to term weighting that combines the **inverse document frequency (IDF)** and **term frequency (TF)**. [19]

Thesaurus: A set of subject headings or descriptors, usually with a cross-reference system for use in the organization of a collection of documents for reference and retrieval. [19]

Thin client: A program on a local computer system that mostly provides connectivity to a larger resource over a computer network, thereby providing access to computational power that is not provided by the machine, which is local to the user. [20]

Think-aloud protocols: In cognitive science, the generation of descriptions of what a person is thinking or considering as they solve a problem. [4]

Three-dimensional reconstruction and visualization: The process of producing three-dimensional models from uniform data (typically from slices through a structure) and rendering them for computer visualization and manipulation. [9]

Three-dimensional-structure information: In a biological database, information regarding the three-dimensional relationships among elements in a molecular structure. [22]

Tiling: A technique used in three-dimensional surface segmentation wherein a surface is applied over manually or automatically segmented two-dimensional contours that have been stacked together, creating a continuous surface. [9]

Time-sharing mode: An interactive mode for communicating with a computer in which the operating system switches rapidly among all the jobs that require CPU services (see **batch mode**). [5]

Time trade-off: A common approach to utility assessment, comparing a better state of health lasting a shorter time, with a lesser state of health lasting a longer time. The time trade-off technique provides a convenient method for valuing outcomes that accounts for gains (or losses) in both length and quality of life. [3]

Tokenization: The process of breaking an unstructured sequence of characters into larger units called "token", e.g., words, numbers, dates, and punctuation. [8]

Token Ring: A type of local-area network, typically used by IBM systems (see also **Ethernet**). [5]

Topology: In networking, the overall connectivity of the nodes in a network. [5]

Touch screen: A display screen that allows users to select items by touching them on the screen. [5]

Track ball: An interactive device that uses a mounted ball, which, when rolled in its housing, manipulates a pointer on the computer screen. [5]

Transaction set: In data transfer, the full set of information exchanged between a sender and a receiver. [7]

Transcription: The conversion of dictated notes into ASCII text by a typist. [12]

Transducer: A device that produces electrical signals proportional in magnitude to the level of a measured parameter, such as blood pressure. [17]

Transformation-based learning: A method of machine learning in which structural transformations are acquired incrementally by attempting to convert a random or naive representation of a text into the target or correct representation. [8]

Transition matrix: A table of numbers giving the probability of moving from one state in a **Markov model** into another state or the state that is reached in a finite-state machine depending on the current character of the alphabet. [8]

Transition probabilities: The probabilities that a person will transit from one health state to another during a specified time period. [3]

Transmission Control Protocol/Internet Protocol (TCP/IP):   The standard protocols used for data transmission on the Internet and other common local- and wide-area networks. [5]

Treatment threshold probability: The probability of disease at which the expected values of withholding or giving treatment are equal. Above the threshold, treatment is recommended; below the threshold, treatment is not recommended and further testing may be warranted. [3]

Tree: In information retrieval, the hierarchically organized sets of index terms. [19]

Trigger event: In monitoring, events that cause a set of transactions to be generated. [7]

True-negative rate (TNR):   The probability of a negative result, given that the condition under consideration is false—e.g., the probability of a negative test result in a patient who does not have the disease under consideration (also called **specificity**). [3]

True-negative result (TN):   A negative result when the condition under consideration is false—e.g., a negative test result in a patient who does not have the disease under consideration. [3]

True-positive rate (TPR):   The probability of a positive result, given that the condition under consideration is true—e.g., the probability of a positive test result in a patient who has the disease under consideration (also called **sensitivity**). [3]

True-positive result (TP):   A positive result when the condition under consideration is true—e.g., a positive test result in a patient who has the disease under consideration. [3]

Turnaround document: A form that serves first as a summary form for presenting results and subsequently as a data collection form. [12]

Turnkey system: A computer system that is purchased from a vendor and that can be installed and operated with minimal modification. [6]

Tutoring system: A computer program designed to provide self-directed education to a student or trainee. [21]

Twisted-pair wires: The typical copper wiring used for routine telephone service but adaptable for newer communication technologies. [5]

Type checking: In computer programming, the act of checking that the types of values, such as integers, decimal numbers, and strings of characters, match throughout their use. [5]

Type I error: A false-positive error in an evaluation study such that the resource being studied is ineffective, but for some reason the study mistakenly shows that it is effective. [11]

Type II error: A false-negative error in an evaluation study such that the resource being studied is effective, but for some reason the study mistakenly fails to show that it is. [11]

Typology: A classification scheme (e.g., of evaluation methods). [11]

Ultrasonography: The use of pulses of high-frequency sound waves, rather that ionizing radiation, to produce images of body structures. [9,18]

Ultrasound (US):   A common energy source derived from high-frequency sound waves. [9,18]

Ultrasound imaging: The transmission of sound waves through the body, with analysis of the returning echoes to produce images. [9,18]

UMLS Semantic Network: A knowledge source in the **UMLS** that provides a consistent categorization of all concepts represented in the **Metathesaurus**. Each Metathesaurus concept is assigned at least one semantic type from the Semantic Network. [19]

Unicode: A representation for international character sets using 16 bits per character; ASCII is a small subset of Unicode. [5]

Unified Medical Language System (UMLS):   A terminology system, developed under the direction of the National Library of Medicine, to produce a common structure that ties together the various vocabularies that have been created for biomedical domains. [2,7,9,18,19]

Uniform Resource Locator (URL):   The address of an information resource on the World Wide Web. [5]

Uniform resource identifier (URI):   The combination of a URN and URL, intended to provide persistent access to digital objects. [19]

Uniform resource name (URN):   A name for a Web page, intended to be more persistent than a URL, which often changes over time as domains evolve or web sites are reorganized. [19]

Universal workstation: A computer of moderate size and cost that is used to access all computer resources connected to a network. [13]

Unit-dose dispensing: An approach to the distribution of drugs, whereby patients' drugs are packaged on a unit-of-dose basis to reduce wastage and to control drug use. [13]

Unobtrusive measures: Records or data for an evaluation that are accrued as part of a routine activity under study and therefore require no special intervention. [11]

Unsharp masking: A technique of image enhancement, in which a blurred image is subtracted from the original image to increase local contrast and to enhance the visibility of fine-detail (high-frequency) structures. [9]

Unstructured interview: An interview in an evaluation study in which there are no predefined questions to be asked. [11]

Usability: The characteristic of being convenient and practicable for use. Generally applied to whether a computer system is optimally usable by its intended audience. [4]

User interface: An application that allows users to enter data into a computer and that presents data to the user. [8]

User-interface layer: A conceptual level of a system architecture that insulates the programs designed to interact with users from the underlying data and the applications that process those data. [13]

Usual, customary, and reasonable fee: The typical fee used as the basis for billed charges and retrospective cost reimbursement. [23]

Utility: In decision making, a number that represents the value of a specific outcome to a decision maker (see, for example, **quality-adjusted life years**). [3,20]

Utilization review: In a hospital, inspection of patients' medical records to identify cases of inappropriate care, including excessive or insufficient use of resources. [13]

Validation: Verification of correctness. [6]

Validity check: In a database system or computer-based medical record system, a test (such as a range check or a pattern check) that is used to detect invalid data values. [12]

Variable: In evaluations, specific characteristics of subjects that either are measured purposefully by the investigator or are self-evident properties of the subjects that do not require measurement. [11]

Variable cost: A cost that changes with the volume of goods or services produced during a given period. [23]

Variable memory: See **random-access memory**. [5]

Vector-space model: A method of full-text indexing in which documents can be conceptualized as vectors of terms, with retrieval based on the cosine similarity of the angle between the query and document vectors. [19]

Vendor system: A host computer system owned by a third party that provides users with access to multiple databases or other services. [6]

Video display terminal (VDT):   An input–output device that is used for communication with a remote computer and that has a cathode-ray tube display for viewing output and a keyboard for entering data. [5]

View: In a database management system, a logical submodel of the contents and structure of a database used to support one or a subset of applications. [5,12]

View schemas: An application-specific description of a view that supports that program's activities with respect to some general database for which there are multiple views. [5]

Virtual addressing: A technique in memory management such that each address referenced by the CPU goes through an address mapping from the **virtual address** of the program to a physical address in main memory. [5]

Virtual memory: A scheme by which users can access information stored in auxiliary memory as though it were in main memory. Virtual memory addresses are automatically translated into actual addresses by the hardware. [5]

Virtual Private Network (VPN):   A secured communications channel, often used to secure access to resources within a company or organization by a user connecting from a remote site. VPNs typically operate over public networks using encryption to keep packet content from being disclosed. [5]

Virtual reality (VR):   A collection of interface methods that simulate reality more closely than does the standard display monitor, generally with a response to user maneuvers that heighten the sense of being connected to the simulation (see also **augmented reality**). [18,21]

Virus: A software program that is written for malicious purposes to spread from one machine to another and to do some kind of damage. Such programs are generally self-replicating, which has led to the comparison with biological viruses. [5]

Visible Human Project: A project of the National Library of Medicine in which detailed high-resolution images and other digital data were created from human cadavers (one male and one female) and made publicly available for research and education purposes. [19]

Visual-analog scale: A method for valuing health outcomes, wherein a person simply rates the quality of life with a health outcome on a scale from 0 to 100. [3]

Vital signs: A person's core temperature, pulse rate, respiratory rate, and arterial blood pressure. [17]

Viterbi algorithm: A procedure that computes the most likely sequence of states in a **Markov model,** given a sequence of symbols. [8]

Vocabulary: A dictionary containing the terminology of a subject field. [4, 7]

Volatile: A characteristic of a computer's memory, in that contents are changed when the next program runs and are not retained when power is turned off. [5]

Volume-based warping: A method for aligning the anatomical structures depicted in two image volumes as closely as possible by establishing a non-linear transformation (warp) that relates voxels in one volume to corresponding voxels in the other volume. Only voxel intensities are used to determine the warp. (see also **surface-based warping**). [9]

Volume performance standard (VPS): A system authorized by Congress for paying for Medicare physicians' services, intended to control volume. This approach may have instead motivated an increase in physician services as doctors sought to protect their real incomes in the face of controlled prices and a surplus of doctors (see **resource-based relative value scale**). [23]

Volume rendering: A method whereby a computer program projects a two-dimensional image directly from a three-dimensional **voxel** array by casting rays from the eye of the observer through the volume array to the image plane. [9]

von Neuman machine: A computer architecture that comprises a single processing unit, computer memory, and a memory bus. [5]

Voxel: A volume element, or small region of a three-dimensional digital image (see **pixel**). [9]

Waterfall model: A software development model in which development is seen as flowing steadily through the phases of requirements analysis, design, implementation, testing (validation), integration, and maintenance. [6]

Waveform template: A wave pattern that is stored in a computer and compared to collected waveforms, such as those acquired from patients. Used to identify and classify abnormal wave patterns. [17]

Wavelet compression: A method of lossy compression for grayscale and color images and video. Unlike methods such as JPEG and MPEG, which compress small blocks of 8×8 pixels, wavelet algorithms process the entire image, achieving compression ratios for grayscale images that can exceed 50:1. Nonuniform compression is possible, whereby different regions of an image can be compressed at different ratios. The methods are based on locally operative mathematical transforms into the frequency domain. [9, 18]

Web browser: A computer program used to access and display information resources on the World Wide Web. [5]

Web catalog: Web pages containing mainly links to other Web pages and sites. [19]

WebMedline: The first World Wide Web interface developed for searching the MEDLINE database. [19]

Weights: Values associated with the nodes of an artificial neural network; the weights propagate through the layers of the network to perform classification based on a set of inputs. [20]

White space: Spaces, punctuation, carriage returns, and other nonalphanumeric characters that appear in a text. [19]

Wide-area network (WAN):   A network that connects computers owned by independent institutions and distributed over long distances. [5,18]

Wildcard character: In search and retrieval applications, a method that allows unspecified single- or multiple-character expansion somewhere in a string that is being used as the basis for the search. [19]

Willingness to pay: An approach to valuing human life based on the values implied by the choices people make every day to change their probabilities of living or dying. For example, a person's implicit valuation for life could be calculated based on how much he is willing to pay for a car airbag that will reduce his chance of by death by a certain incremental amount. [3]

Word: In computer memory, a sequence of bits that can be accessed as a unit. [5]

Word size: The number of bits that define a word in a given computer. [5]

Working memory: In cognitive science, the portion of one's memory that is used to perform the tasks related to the current focus of attention. [4]

Workstation: A powerful desktop computer system designed to support a single user. Workstations provide specialized hardware and software to facilitate the problem-solving and information-processing tasks of professionals in their domains of expertise. [5]

World Intellectual Property Organization (WIPO):   An international organization, headquartered in Geneva and dedicated to promoting the use and protection of intellectual property. [19]

World Wide Web (WWW):   An application implemented on the Internet in which multimedia information resources are made accessible by any of a number of protocols, the most common of which is the **HyperText Transfer Protocol (HTTP)**. [5]

Worm: A self-replicating computer program, similar to a computer virus; a worm is self-contained and does not need to be part of another program to propagate itself. [5]

Write-it-once system: A type of paper-based billing system that uses carbon paper or photocopying to generate bills from patient-encounter information that has been transcribed onto ledger cards. [12]

Write once, read many (WORM):   A storage medium that is suitable for reuse but cannot be erased or rewritten. [5]

XML format: Content that is expressed using the **Extensible Markup Language (XML)**. [6]

X-ray: A type of **ionizing radiation** that has been harnessed to provide a technique of medical imaging, allowing the capture of views of structures within the body. [9]

X-ray crystallography: A technique in crystallography in which the pattern produced by the diffraction of X-rays through the closely spaced lattice of atoms in a crystal is recorded and then analyzed to reveal the nature of that lattice, generally leading to an understanding of the material and molecular structure of a substance. [22]

Name Index

Subject Index

Health Informatics Series
(formerly Computers in Health Care)

Public Health Informatics and Information Systems
P.W. O'Carroll, W.A. Yasnoff, M.E. Ward, L.H. Ripp, and E.L. Martin

Advancing Federal Sector Health Care
A Model for Technology Transfer
P. Ramsaroop, M.J. Ball, D. Beaulieu, and J.V. Douglas

Biomedical Informatics
Computer Applications in Health Care and Biomedicine, Third Edition
Edward H. Shortliffe and James J. Cimino

Filmless Radiology
E.L. Siegel and R.M. Kolodner

Cancer Informatics
Essential Technologies for Clinical Trials
J.S. Silva, M.J. Ball, C.G. Chute, J.V. Douglas, C.P. Langlotz, J.C. Niland, and W.L. Scherlis

Clinical Information Systems
A Component-Based Approach
R. Van de Velde and P. Degoulet

Knowledge Coupling
New Premises and New Tools for Medical Care and Education
L.L. Weed

Healthcare Information Management Systems
Cases, Strategies, and Solutions, Third Edition
M.J. Ball, C.A. Weaver, and J.M. Kiel

Organizational Aspects of Health Informatics, Second Edition
Managing Technological Change
N.M. Lorenzi and R.T. Riley

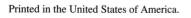
Printed in the United States of America.